Clinical Nuclear Medicine

Clinical Nuclear Medicine

THIRD EDITION

Edited by

M. N. Maisey

BSc MD FRCR FRCP
Division of Radiological Sciences
Guy's and St Thomas' Hospital
London, UK

K. E. Britton

MD MSc FRCR FRCP
Department of Nuclear Medicine
St Bartholomew's Hospital
London, UK

B. D. Collier

BA MA MD
Nuclear Medicine Department
Medical College of Wisconsin
Milwaukee, Wisconsin
USA

with the assistance of

Q. H. Siraj

MSc PhD

CHAPMAN & HALL MEDICAL
London · New York · Tokyo · Melbourne · Madras

Published by
Chapman & Hall, an imprint of Thomson Science, 2–6 Boundary Row, London SE1 8HN, UK

Thomson Science, 2–6 Boundary Row, London SE1 8HN, UK

Thomson Science, 115 Fifth Avenue, New York, NY 10003, USA

Thomson Science, Suite 750, 400 Market Street, Philadelphia, PA 19106, USA

Thomson Science, Pappelallee 3, 69469 Weinheim, Germany

First edition 1983
Second edition 1991
Third edition 1998

© 1983, 1991, 1998 Chapman & Hall

Thomson Science is division of International Thomson Publishing

Typeset in Palatino $9\frac{1}{2}/11$ by Best-set Typesetter Ltd., Hong Kong
Printed in Great Britain at the University Press, Cambridge

ISBN 0 412 75180 1

A catalogue record for this book is available from the British Library

Library of Congress Catalog Card Number: 97-76965

♾ Printed on acid-free text paper, manufactured in accordance with ANSI/NISO Z39.48-1992 (Permanence of Paper).

Contents

Contributors

Hussein M. Abdel-Dayem MD
Department of Radiology
New York Medical College and St Vincent's
    Hospital and Medical Center
New York, USA

Thérèse Benoit MD
Centre Hospitalier Universitaire de Liège
Service de Médicine Nucléaire
Liège, Belgium

A. Bertrand Brill MD PhD
Department of Radiology and Radiological
    Science
Vanderbilt University
Nashville, USA

Keith E. Britton MD MSc FRCR FRCP
Department of Nuclear Medicine
St Bartholomew's Hospital
London, UK

Julia W. Buchanan BS
Department of Radiology
The Johns Hopkins Medical Institutions
Baltimore, USA

John Buscombe MD MSc MRCP
Department of Nuclear Medicine
Royal Free Hospital
London, UK

V. U. Chengazi MB BS MSc PhD
Department of Nuclear Medicine
St Bartholomew's Hospital
London, UK

Elfy B. Chevretton BSc MS FRCS
Department of Oral Surgery
Guy's and St Thomas' Hospital
London, UK

Marco Chianelli, MD PhD
Servizio Medicina Nucleare
Istituto di Clinica Medica II
Università 'La Sapienza'
Roma, Italy

Marco Chinol PhD
Division of Nuclear Medicine
Istituto Europeo di Oncologia
Milano, Italy

S. E. M. Clarke MSc FRCP
Department of Nuclear Medicine
Guy's and St Thomas' Hospital
London, UK

A. J. Coakley MB ChB MSc FRCR FRCP
Department of Nuclear Medicine
Kent and Canterbury Hospital
Canterbury, UK

B. D. Collier BA MA MD
Nuclear Medicine Department
Medical College of Wisconsin
Milwaukee, USA

Durval C. Costa MD MSc PhD FRCR
Institute of Nuclear Medicine
UCL Medical School
Middlesex Hospital
London, UK

Peter Josef Ell MD MSc PD FRCR FRCP
Institute of Nuclear Medicine
Middlesex Hospital
London, UK

Ignac Fogelman BSc MD FRCP
Department of Nuclear Medicine
Guy's and St Thomas' Hospital
London, UK

David Gilday BEng, MD, FRCPC
Nuclear Medicine Division
The Hospital for Sick Children
Toronto, Canada

Marie Granowska MD MSc FRCR
Department of Nuclear Medicine
St Bartholomew's Hospital
London, UK

N. David Greyson MD FRCPC
University of Toronto
Department of Medical Imaging
St Michael's Hospital
Toronto, Canada

Milton D. Gross MD
Division of Nuclear Medicine
The Univerisity of Michigan
Ann Arbor, USA

L. Keith Harding BSc FRCR FRCP
Department of Physics and Nuclear Medicine
City Hospital NHS Trust
Birmingham, UK

David J. Hawkes PhD
Radiological Sciences
Guy's and St Thomas' Hospital
London, UK

**Stuart R. Hesslewood BPharm PhD
  MRPharmsS MCPP**
Radiopharmacy Department
City Hospital NHS Trust
Birmingham, UK

Andrew J. W. Hilson MA MSc FRCP
Department of Nuclear Medicine
Royal Free Hospital
London, UK

D. J. Hnatowich PhD
Department of Nuclear Medicine
University of Massachusetts Medical Center
Worcester, USA

C. A. Hoefnagel MD PhD
Department of Nuclear Medicine
Het Nederlands Kanker Instituut
Amsterdam, The Netherlands

Mario P. Iturralde MD DMC DM
Department of Nuclear Medicine
University of Pretoria
Pretoria, Republic of South Africa

Peter Jarritt BSc PhD
Institute of Nuclear Medicine
UCL Medical School
London, UK

David H. Keeling MA MB MSc FRCR FRCP
formerly at Department of Nuclear Medicine
Derriford Hospital
Plymouth, UK

Frederick Khafagi MB FRACP
St Andrew's War Memorial Hospital
Brisbane, Australia

Richard T. Kloos MD
Divisions of Endocrinology and Metabolism, and
  Nuclear Medicine
The University of Alabama at Birmingham
Birmingham, USA

Linda C. Knight PhD
Division of Nuclear Medicine
Department of Diagnostic Imaging and Sol
  Sherry Thrombosis Research Center
Temple University Hospital and School of
  Medicine
Philadelphia, USA

Colin R. Lazarus BPharm PhD MRPharmS
Department of Nuclear Medicine
Guy's and St Thomas' Hospital
London, UK

**Anne Lingford-Hughes MA PhD BM BCh
  MRCPsych**
Institute of Psychiatry
De Crespigny Park
London, UK

Homer A. Macapinlac MD
Nuclear Medicine Service
Department of Radiology
Memorial Sloan Kettering Cancer Center
New York, USA

B. J. McNeil, MD
Department of Radiology
Harvard Medical School
Cambridge
Massachusetts, USA

M. N. Maisey BSc MD FRCR FRCP
Division of Radiological Sciences
Guy's and St Thomas' Hospital
London, UK

Stephen J. Mather BPharm MSc MRPharmS PhD
Department of Nuclear Medicine
St Bartholomew's Hospital
London, UK

Alan H. Maurer MD
Departments of Diagnostic Imaging and Internal Medicine
Temple University Hospital and School of Medicine
Philadelphia, USA

P. J. Mountford BSc PhD CPhys FInstP FIPEMB
Division of Radiation Physics
North Staffordshire Hospital (Royal Infirmary)
Stoke-on-Trent, UK

M. J. O'Doherty MSc MD FRCP
Radiological Sciences
Guy's and St Thomas' Hospital
London, UK

Giovanni Paganelli MD
Division of Nuclear Medicine
Istituto Europeo di Oncologia
Milano, Italy

Adrian Parkin PhD FIPEMB
Medical Physics Department
St James' and Seacroft University Hospitals NHS Trust
Leeds, UK

Jim Patterson PhD
Department of Clinical Physics
Institute of Neurological Sciences
Southern General Hospital
Glasgow, UK

S. R. Payne MS FRCS FEBU
Department of Urological Surgery
Manchester Royal Infirmary
Manchester, UK

A. M. Peters MSc MD MRCP FRCR FRCPath
Department of Imaging
Imperial College School of Medicine
Hammersmith Hospital
London, UK

Lyn S. Pilowsky PhD MRCPsych
Institute of Psychiatry
De Crespigny Park
London, UK

Myron Pollycove MD
US Nuclear Regulatory Commission
Washington, DC, USA
Formerly at: Departments of Laboratory Medicine and Radiology
San Fransisco General Hospital
San Fransisco, USA

Pierre Rigo MD
Centre Hospitalier Universitaire de Liège
Service de Médicine Nucléaire
Liège, Belgium

Howard A. Ring MRCPsych MD
Academic Department of Psychological Medicine
St Bartholomew's and the Royal London School of Medicine
London, UK

Philip J. A. Robinson FRCR FRCP
Department of Clinical Radiology
St James' University Hospital
Leeds, UK

Henry D. Royal MD
Mallinckrodt Institute of Radiology
Washington University School of Medicine
St Louis, USA

Paul J. Ryan MSc MRCP
Nuclear Medicine Dept
Medway Hospital
Gillingham, UK

Brahm Shapiro MB ChB PhD
Department of Internal Medicine
The University of Michigan Medical Center and
   Ann Arbor Veterans Affairs Medical Center
Ann Arbor, USA

Alberto Signore MD
Servizio Medicina Nucleare
Istituto di Clinica Medica II
Università 'La Sapienza'
Roma, Italy

Edward B. Silberstein MD FACNP
Division of Nuclear Medicine
University of Cincinnati Medical Center
Cincinnati, USA

Qaisar H. Siraj MSc PhD
Nuclear Medicine Centre
A. F. Institute of Pathology
Rawalpindi, Pakistan

D. M. Swirsky MRCPath FRCP
Department of Haematology
Imperial College School of Medicine
Hammersmith Hospital
London, UK

H. J. Testa MD PhD FRCR FRCP
Department of Nuclear Medicine
Manchester Royal Infirmary
Manchester, UK

W. H. Thomson PhD
Department of Physics and Nuclear Medicine
City Hospital NHS Trust
Birmingham, UK

Sabah S. Tumeh MD FACR
Nuclear Medicine Division
Bon Secours DePaul Medical Center
Norfolk, USA

Henry N. Wagner Jr MD
Division of Radiation Health Science
The Johns Hopkins Medical Institution
Baltimore, USA

Richard L. Wahl MD
Division of Nuclear Medicine
University of Michigan Medical Center
Ann Arbor, USA

C. P. Wells MSc MIPEMB
Departments of Medical Physics
   and Nuclear Medicine
Kent and Canterbury Hospital
Canterbury, UK

David J. Wyper PhD
Department of Clinical Physics
Institute of Neurological Sciences
Southern General Hospital
Glasgow, UK

Preface to the first edition

Nuclear medicine is the bridge between a particular clinical problem and a relevant test using radionuclides. It began as a minor technical tool used in a few branches of medicine, notably endocrinology and nephrology. However, throughout the world it has now become established as a clinical discipline in its own right, with specific training programmes, special skills and a particular approach to patient management. Although the practising nuclear medicine physician must necessarily learn a great deal of basic science and technology, a sound medical training and a clinical approach to the subject remains of fundamental importance. It is for this reason that we have attempted in this book to approach the subject from a clinical standpoint, including where necessary relevant physiological material.

There exist many excellent texts which cover the basic science and technology of nuclear medicine. We have, therefore, severely limited our coverage of these aspects of the subject to matters which we felt to be essential, particularly those which have been less well covered in other texts – for example, the contents of Chapter 21 on Quantitation by Royal and McNeil. Similarly, we have included at the end of some chapters descriptions of particular techniques where we and the authors felt that it would be helpful. In order to emphasize the clinical approach of this book we have inverted the traditional sequence of material in chapters, presenting the clinical problems first in each instance. For similar reasons we have placed the chapters on Radiopharmaceuticals and Practical Instrumentation towards the end of the book.

Since medicine concerns the investigation, care and management of sick people who have specific problems, the virtues of a problem-orientated approach to the subject are becoming more widely recognized, particularly in the education of undergraduates. This approach has therefore been adopted in each chapter, making the overall structure of the book closer to that of a conventional textbook of medicine rather than a scientific treatise.

The contributors to this book come from both the United Kingdom and North America. As editors, in addition to requiring that authors should be expert in their field, we also wanted them to be particularly concerned about the day to day care of patients. We have endeavoured to emphasize the problem-orientated approach to clinical situations, whilst providing textual uniformity, without at the same time reducing the essentially individual contributions of each author.

We hope this textbook will be of value to a wide variety of medical professionals, including nuclear medicine clinicians in training, radiologists and clinicians from other specialities who use nuclear medicine in some form or other and require to know how it can help in solving their clinical problems. Finally, believing that medical students prefer the style of a textbook of medicine rather than that of a textbook of physics, we hope that the clinical priorities which have dictated the production of this book will encourage them to consult it.

M.N.M., K.E.B., London
D.L.G., Toronto

Preface to the third edition

Clinical nuclear medicine continues to develop with no sign of any diminishing impact. Since the first edition was published we have seen a progressive emphasis on providing functional information critical to good patient care. With tissue characterization techniques through receptor binding peptides, monoclonal antibodies and other agents, higher specificity is being added to sensitivity in oncology, endocrinology and infectious diseases. The cost-effectiveness of myocardial perfusion studies in ischaemic heart disease is now recognized. This edition reflects these growths and focuses with more emphasis on clinical applications of new tracers including positron emission tomography (PET), which is now widely accepted and becoming increasingly available. Therapeutic applications for radionuclides are expanding and effective and this ground is covered more extensively. As in previous editions we have also selected relevant topics which we believe to be of current importance rather than undertaking a comprehensive attempt to deal with all of basic science.

Our goal and that of our many new contributors remains the provision of a clinical text devoted to the role of radionuclide tracers for the best management of our patients. Nuclear medicine is now at the heart of mainstream medical practice, with an important role in every conventional clinical discipline, and the signs are that this will increase even more with a new emphasis on molecular medicine and the need to monitor disease states and therapeutic responses more critically.

M.N.M., K.E.B., London
B.D.C., Milwaukee

Clinical topics

CHAPTER 1

Radionuclide therapy

Bones and joints

E.B. Silberstein

INTRODUCTION

This chapter describes the use of beta- or electron-emitting radiopharmaceuticals for treating several painful musculoskeletal conditions. These radiopharmaceuticals emit negatively charged particles (beta particles or electrons) with a maximum range of approximately 1–11 mm (Tables 1.1 and 1.2), which can cause sub-lethal or lethal damage to cells by interacting with their DNA [1]. Radionuclide therapy, by eliminating the targeted cells responsible for tissue damage and the resultant pain, provides marked clinical benefit to the patient.

RADIONUCLIDE THERAPY OF SYNOVIAL DISEASE

ANATOMY AND PATHOPHYSIOLOGY

The normal synovial lining is largely composed of a one- to two-cell thick layer of type B synoviocytes, which are similar to fibroblasts. The normal synovial lining also contains about 10% of phagocytic type A synoviocytes that are similar to macrophages. The synovium transfers proteins and smaller molecules into and out of the joint spaces. The extracellular synovial matrix is primarily collagen and hyaluronate. The avascular cartilage beneath the synovium, provides a smooth articular surface and absorbs the energy load during weight-bearing.

Inflammatory joint disease affects at least 1% of the world's population. The inflammatory process, whatever its aetiology, leads to chemotactic recruitment of macrophages, lymphocytes and plasma cells, oedema of the synovial membrane and subsequent formation of synovial inflammatory granulation tissue called pannus, accompanied by an increased secretion of synovial fluid. In reactive arthropathy, the hyperplastic synovial lining may become hyperplastic and, depending on the severity and site of the involved joint, may become 1–7 mm thick [2]. Enzymes and other inflammatory mediators from the pannus progressively damage the cartilage; the pannus then invades, erodes and fragments the cartilage.

The damaging pannus can be surgically resected, but this invasive procedure, whether open or arthroscopically performed, is costly, requiring hospitalization and lengthy physical therapy. Since it is difficult to resect all the pathogenic synovium, recurrence is quite common in 3–5 years [3].

RADIATION SYNOVECTOMY

Nine radionuclides and 15 radiopharmaceuticals (four alone using yttrium-90), have been proposed or employed for ablation of the synovial lining (Table 1.1). In inflammatory arthropathies, where the type A synoviocyte predominates, particulate radiopharmaceuticals (radiolabelled colloids, macroaggregates and minerals) are phagocytosed by these macrophage-like cells, but it is not clear whether these are all distributed in the

Clinical Nuclear Medicine, 3rd edn. Edited by M.N. Maisey, K.E. Britton and B.D. Collier. Published in 1998 by Chapman & Hall, London. ISBN 0 412 75180 1

Table 1.1 Characteristics of radiopharmaceuticals employed for radiation synovectomy (listed in order of increasing beta-energy)

Radionuclide	Chemical form	Radiation	E_{max} in MeV (% abundance)	Physical half-life	Maximum soft-tissue penetration (mm)	Range of activity used (MBq)
Er-169	Citrate colloid	beta	0.34 (45%) 0.35 (55%)	9.4 days	0.9	9.25–37
Sm-153	Hydroxyapatite	beta, gamma	0.81 0.10 (28%)	1.95 days	2.5	148–518
Au-198	Gold colloid	beta, gamma	0.95 0.41 (96%)	2.7 days	3.9	18.5–370
Re-186	Sulphur colloid, hydroxyapatite	beta	1.07	3.7 days	4.5	74
Dy-165	Ferric hydroxide macroaggregate, hydroxide macroaggregate	beta, gamma	1.3 0.09 (4%)	140 minutes	5.7	9990–11 100
P-32	Chromic phosphate colloid	beta	1.7	14.0 days	7.9	11–222
Ho-166	Hydroxyapatite poly-L-lactate microspheres	beta, gamma	1.84 0.08 (4%)	27 hours	8.4	688
Re-188	Sulphur colloid	beta, gamma	2.2 0.155 (15%)	17 hours	11.0	No human data
Y-90	Silicate colloid, citrate colloid, calcium oxalate, ferric hydrate macroaggregate	beta	2.3	2.7 days	11.1	74–185

Table 1.2 Characteristics of radiopharmaceuticals employed for therapy of painful bone metastases (listed in order of increasing electron or beta-energy)

Radionuclide	Chemical form	Radiation	E_{max} in MeV (% abundance)	Physical half-life (days)	Maximum soft-tissue penetration (mm)	Usual range of activity administered (MBq)
Sn-117	DTPA chelate	electron, gamma	0.13, 0.15 0.161 (86%)	13.6	0.27	370–740
Sm-153	EDTMP chelate	beta, gamma	0.81 0.103 (28%)	1.95	2.5	330–1110
Re-186	HEDP chelate	beta, gamma	1.07 0.137 (9%)	3.7	4.5	1221–2516
Sr-89	Strontium chloride	beta, gamma	1.49 0.910 (0.01%)	50.5	7.0	111–148
P-32	Sodium orthophosphate	beta	1.7	14.0	7.9	148–888*

*Higher activities given in divided doses.

surface layer of cells or throughout the thickened pannus. Irradiation of the inflamed hypertrophied cell lining decreases fluid secretion causing a reduction in the intra-articular pressure. The destruction of the cells responsible for the secretion of destructive enzymes and cytokines causes a proportionate fall in their concentration [4].

Choice of radiopharmaceutical

The ideal radiopharmaceutical would have the following properties:

1. Absence of γ-ray emission.
2. β-particle energy sufficient to penetrate the thickened synovium but not sufficiently energetic to damage the underlying cartilage, bone or skin.
3. The radionuclide should be irreversibly bound to the particulate ligand.
4. The biological half-life of the radiopharmaceutical should approximate the physical half-life of the radionuclide.
5. No leakage should occur from the joint following injection.
6. The particles should be biodegradable to avoid causing a chronic inflammatory (foreign body) response.
7. Non-toxic and non-antigenic without any acute inflammatory properties.
8. Easily reproducible particle size.

Since samarium-153, gold-198, dysprosium-165, holmium-166 and rhenium-188, also emit γ-rays, depending on the activity employed, additional safety precautions may be required for these radionuclides. The β-particle ranges in Table 1.1 are adequate for applications in joints with thickened synovium even if phagocytosis occurs only at the synovial fluid–tissue interface. For joints of the fingers, with relatively thin diseased synovium, a low-energy radionuclide like erbium-169 is preferred [5,6].

Most of the radiopharmaceuticals listed in Table 1.1 are colloids in the sub-micron range. The smallest particles appear to have less tendency to remain in the joint space [5,7–13]. For example, there is 5–48% leakage of ^{198}Au-colloid (diameter in the 0.01 μm range) from the joint cavity to the draining regional lymph nodes, liver and spleen [8,9]. Most of these colloids are not biodegradable, i.e. there are no cellular enzyme systems to break them down. The reticuloendothelial system traps whatever leaks from the joint, and the type A synoviocyte retains much of what is instilled into the joints.

Hydroxyapatite, the major bone mineral, is biodegradable and has been labelled with ^{186}Re and ^{153}Sm with 95% efficiency. The cumulative leakage for ^{186}Re in a rabbit model was 3.05% but only 0.09% for ^{153}Sm. The latter was found to be distributed throughout the synovium. For this distribution, a relatively low-energy β-emitter such as ^{153}Sm should be effective, even in the largest joints [14]. ^{153}Sm-hydroxyapatite (particle diameter 5–45 μm), with activities of 4–14 mCi, has been injected into joints of patients with rheumatoid arthritis with 0–3% leakage seen as assessed by scintigraphy. Absence of leakage was reported in 54% (7/13) of the patients studied [15].

When leakage or drainage of these radiopharmaceuticals occurs, lymph nodes – being the closest tissue – receive the major radiation dose. The significant leakage from the joint space of gold-198 colloid to the draining groin nodes, can deliver nodal doses of 50 to 150 Gy [8]. Radiation doses to the nodes from yttrium-90 colloids have been estimated at 50–100 Gy and to the liver at 2.5–5 Gy [6]. Because of its short half-life, the lymph node doses from disprosium-165 are about 17 cGy [12].

Adverse effects

Injection of these radiopharmaceuticals into the joint space is frequently followed by an acute inflammatory reaction, which may be less severe if a radionuclide with lower activity (or higher specific activity) is employed, as has been suggested for ^{32}P-chromic phosphate, the longest-lived radionuclide employed for this purpose [10] (Table 1.1). Anticipation of this reaction has led 60% of European medical centres recently surveyed to co-inject a corticosteroid during radiation synovectomy [6].

Lymphocytes are highly radiosensitive, and radiation-induced lymphocyte chromosome aberrations have been used as biological dosimeters for decades [8]. Gold-198 colloid and yttrium-90 colloids have been associated with chromosome aberrations after intra-articular instillation in almost all cases examined [9]. Bed-rest seems to reduce leakage and the resultant number of lymphocyte chromosome aberrations significantly [18]. However, no increase in aberrations was found in seven patients treated with ^{32}P-chromic phosphate for haemophiliac synovitis [10].

In contrast to the systemic anti-rheumatic drugs, organ toxicity from this procedure is minimal. Radiation doses outside the joint have led to no sequelae (including lymphoproliferative disease) described in the medical literature.

Joint dosimetry

Variations in synovial thickness, joint dimensions, synovial fluid volume and degree of retention of radiopharmaceutical in the joint cavity, all make beta dosimetry problematic in this form of therapy [17]. Yttrium-90 colloid activity estimated to give an absorbed dose of 100 Gy to a 100 g synovium was described as efficacious in rheumatoid arthritis [13], and many investigators have subsequently used a 'calculated ^{90}Y dose equivalent' for determining the administered activity of other radionuclides [11], but these remain only crude dose estimates.

Technique

Arthrocentesis to instil these radiopharmaceuticals should be performed using a closed system with a three-way stopcock system, to permit a lidocaine flush after delivering the radiopharmaceutical [7]. The need for an intra-articular steroid to reduce acute radiopharmaceutical-induced inflammation is debatable [6]. A syringe shield is mandatory. The injected joint should be immobilized for at least several hours, and perhaps for 1–2 days, to reduce leakage.

Clinical results

The first use of radiolabelled colloids for treating arthritis was reported in 1952. This study and, 63 subsequent clinical reports, have been recently tabulated [7]. The measures of outcome reported by the many investigators have varied widely and have included pain reduction, improvement in range of motion, reduction in the size of effusion, changes in the degree of crepitus, or diminished knee circumference.

While little used in the United States, a recent survey documented 119 institutions in 23 European countries performing radiation synovectomy, as well as in Australia, Canada, South Africa and Mexico [6]. ^{90}Y was the most widely administered radiopharmaceutical. Of the diseases treated, rheumatoid arthritis comprised 71%, psoriatic arthritis 11%, osteoarthritis 7%; 'reactive' arthritis 5%, haemophiliac arthropathy 2%, anklylosing spondylitis 0.6%, pigmented villonodular synovitis 0.7%, crystal arthritis 0.3% juvenile chronic arthritis <0.1%, and 'other' 2%. The knee received almost 46% of all injections; fingers, 20%; wrist, 11%; ankle, 8%; shoulder, 6%; elbows, 6%; hip, 1%; 'other', about 3%. Repeat joint injections, or multiple joint injections in the same patient, were not uncommon [6].

Responses in very early rheumatoid arthritis (stage 1) have ranged from 53–100% with ^{90}Y and 68–90% with ^{165}Dy, but the definition of these re-

sponses has differed widely. Early rheumatoid arthritis always responds better than late disease [7]. There are no clinical studies allowing a direct comparison of different radiopharmaceuticals in rheumatoid arthritis. ^{90}Y silicate and ^{90}Y resin showed less leakage than ^{90}Y-ferric hydroxide and ^{90}Y-citrate, but no clinical correlates of these phenomena have been reported [13]. In a meta-analysis of yttrium-90 synovectomy, this radiopharmaceutical was superior to placebo but was not significantly different in efficacy from intra-articular corticosteroid [18].

Radiation synovectomy has also been successful in controlling the recurrent bleeding and improving range of motion in haemophiliac synovitis [19]. In contrast, radiation synovectomy does not have much efficacy in diminishing the symptoms of patients with degenerative osteoarthritis, presumably because the effect of this treatment is on synovium, which plays little role in producing the symptoms of osteoarthritis [7].

RADIOPHARMACEUTICAL THERAPY OF PAINFUL OSSEOUS METASTASES

The prevalence of pain in all patients with metastatic cancer has been estimated at 60–90%. In the United States, there are 125 000 cases of osseous metastases a year, two-thirds of those requiring an analgesic. Teletherapy is also quite efficacious for reducing or eliminating the pain of osseous metastases, and is the treatment of choice for single painful skeletal sites, impending pathological fractures, pain from cord compression due to epidural metastases, or pain from pressure on bone from soft-tissue metastases [20]. Teletherapy may be more difficult to employ in the presence of multiple painful metastases or in the thorax or abdomen where radiation-sensitive organs (e.g. lung and liver) limit the application of this treatment modality. Hemi-body radiation reduces pain in 70–80% of these patients, but has the problem of haematological and gastrointestinal adverse reactions [21].

RADIOPHARMACEUTICAL CHARACTERISTICS AND MECHANISM OF ACTION

An ideal radiopharmaceutical for treating the pain due to osseous metastases would have the following characteristics:

1. Selective localization and retention in the painful sites.
2. No radiation safety issues requiring hospitalization.
3. No organ toxicity.
4. A half-life of days to weeks.
5. Beta- or electron-emission of adequate energy to reach the tumour and other target cells from the site of bone localization.

The radiopharmaceuticals that have been employed for the treatment of pain from osteoblastic metastases are listed in Table 1.2. All of these localize in bone, either by substitution for a constituent (e.g. ^{32}P for stable phosphate and ^{89}Sr for calcium), by formation of hydroxides on bone (^{153}Sm and ^{117m}Sn) or by chemisorption to hydroxyapatite (^{153}Sm-EDTMP and ^{186}Re-HEDP). Reactive bone surrounding metastases retains ^{89}Sr and ^{186}Re far longer than the normal bone [22,23]. This phenomenon has not been examined for the other radionuclides listed in Table 1.2, but probably holds true for all of them.

The mechanism of pain relief cannot just be due to tumour shrinkage induced by radiation, since the pain may diminish, or even disappear, before the tumour has changed in size – as is frequently seen a few days after teletherapy has begun. A variety of local hormonal mechanisms for pain modulation may be affected by radiation.

The organ toxicity of these agents is solely myelosuppression, occurring between 3–8 weeks after administration; this is proportional in degree to the activity administered. The resultant pancytopenia is usually 30–70% of pre-treatment leucocyte and platelet counts, but concurrent disseminated intravascular coagulation, leading to severe thrombocytopenia, has been associated with at least two deaths [24]. All these radiopharmaceuticals have significant renal excretion, and renal dysfunction will therefore lead to an increase in bone and soft-tissue dose. Following injection, about 10% of patients will experience a self-limiting increase or 'flare' in pain within 10–14 days.

CLINICAL ISSUES

Beta- or electron-emitting radiopharmaceuticals are indicated for the treatment of bone pain due to metastases involving multiple skeletal sites with a documented osteoblastic response on bone scintigraphy. Marrow reserves must be adequate.

With spinal cord compression from vertebral tumour or pathological fracture – impending or actual – this form of therapy, if employed, must be used in conjunction with other forms of medical management directed at these complications [25]. When single vertebral lesions that have received a dose of 40–45 Gy become painful and cord compression is excluded, these agents are also indicated.

Recently, Silberstein and Taylor (1995) have published a *Procedure Guideline* for bone pain treatment [25]: patients should not have had recent myelosuppressive drugs or radiotherapy, and should possess adequate marrow reserves; active disseminated intravascular coagulation should be excluded; the radiopharmaceutical should be injected into an open and running intravenous line to avoid infiltration; and a plastic syringe shield (or equivalent) is recommended.

Some reduction in pain occurs in 60–80% of patients injected with any of the radiopharmaceuticals listed in Table 1.2 [23,26,30]. A small minority, perhaps 5–10%, receive complete relief. Unfortunately, we are unable to predict which patients will respond. Pain reduction occurs within a few days to 4 weeks after a single intravenous injection. Re-treatment is efficacious in 50–60% of patients after 12 weeks, and some patients have continued to respond to multiple injections. There is no evidence that any one of these radiopharmaceuticals is superior to the others in pain reduction, although ^{32}P may be more myelosuppressive than the others since it can be incorporated into the marrow DNA. There is no evidence of life prolongation with these radiopharmaceuticals [27]. However, compared with teletherapy alone, the combination treatment with strontium-89 and teletherapy has been shown to delay the time to pain recurrence and the onset of new painful sites [27].

REFERENCES

1. Phillips, T.L. (1991) Early and late effects of radiation on normal tissues, in *Radiation Injury to the Nervous System* (eds P.H. Gutin, S.D. Leibel and G.E. Sheline), Raven Press, Ltd., New York, pp. 37–55.
2. Hosain, F., Haddon, M.J., Hosain, H. *et al.* (1990) Radiopharmaceuticals for diagnosis and treatment of arthritis. *Nucl. Med. Biol.*, **17**(1), 151–5.
3. Gschwend, N. (1989) Synovectomy, in *Textbook of Rheumatology*, 3rd edn (eds W.N. Kelley, E.D. Harris, S. Ruddy and C.B. Sledge), W.B. Saunders, Philadelphia, pp. 1934–61.

4. Henderson, B. and Edwards, J.C.W. (1987) *The Synovial Lining: In Health and Disease*, Chapman & Hall, London.

5. Noble, J., Jones, A.G., Davis, M.A. *et al.* (1983) Leakage of radioactive particle systems from a synovial joint studied with a gamma camera: its application to radiation synovectomy. *J. Bone Joint Surg. (Am)*, **65**(3), 381–9.

6. Clunie, G. and Ell, P.J. (1995) A survey of radiation synovectomy in Europe, 1991–1993. *Eur. J. Nucl. Med.*, **22**(9), 970–6.

7. Deutsch, E., Brodack, J.W. and Deutsch, K.F. (1993) Radiation synovectomy revisited. *Eur. J. Nucl. Med.*, **20**(11), 1113–27.

8. Dolphin, G.W. (1973) Biological hazards of radiation. *Ann. Rheum. Dis.*, **32**(1), 23–8.

9. Stevenson, A.C., Bedford, J., Dolphin, G.W. *et al.* (1973) Cytogenetic and scanning study of patients receiving intra-articular injection of gold-198 and yttrium-90. *Ann. Rheum. Dis.*, **32**(1), 112–23.

10. Rivard, G.E., Girard, M., Lamarre, C. *et al.* (1985) Synoviorthesis with colloidal ^{32}P chromic phosphate for hemophilic arthropathy: clinical follow-up. *Arch. Phys. Med. Rehab.*, **66**, 753–6.

11. Zuckerman, J.D., Sledge, C.B., Shortkroff, S. *et al.* (1987) Treatment of rheumatoid arthritis using radiopharmaceuticals. *Nucl. Med. Biol.*, **14**(3), 211–18.

12. McLaren, A., Hetherington, E., Maddalene, D. *et al.* (1990) Dysprosium (^{165}Dy) hydroxide macroaggregates for radiation synovectomy – animal studies. *Eur. J. Nucl. Med.*, **16**(6), 627–32.

13. Gumpel, J.M., Beer, T.C., Crawley, J.C.W. *et al.* (1975) Yttrium-90 in persistent synovitis of the knee – a single centre comparison. The retention and extra articular spread of four ^{90}Y radiocolloids. *Br. J. Radiol.*, **48**(5), 377–81.

14. Chinal, M., Vallabhajosula, S., Goldsmith, S.J. *et al.* (1993) Chemistry and biological behavior of samarium-153 and rhenium-186-labeled hydroxyapatite particles: potential radiopharmaceuticals for radiation synovectomy. *J. Nucl. Med.*, **34**(9), 1536–42.

15. Clunie, G., Lui, D., Cullum, I. *et al.* (1995) Samarium-153 particulate hydroxyapatite radiation synovectomy: biodistribution data for chronic knee synovitis. *J. Nucl. Med.*, **36**(1), 51–7.

16. De la Chapelle, A., Oka, M., Rekonen, A. *et al.* (1972) Chromosome damage after intra-articular injection of radioactive yttrium. *Ann. Rheum. Dis.*, **31**(5), 500–12.

17. Johnson, L. and Yanch, V. (1991) Absorbed dose profile for radionuclides of frequent use in radiation synovectomy. *Arthritis Rheum.*, **34**, 1521–30.

18. Jones, G. (1993) Yttrium synovectomy: a meta-analysis of the literature. *Aust. N. Z. J. Med.*, **23**, 272–5.

19. Siegel, H.J., Luck, J.V., Siegel, M. *et al.* (1994) Hemarthrosis and synovitis associated with hemophilia: clinical use of P-32 chromic phosphate synoviorthesis for treatment. *Radiology*, **190**(1), 257–61.

20. Bates, T., Yarnold, J.R., Blitzer, P. *et al.* (1992) Bone metastasis consensus statement. *Int. J. Radiat. Oncol. Biol. Phys.*, **23**, 215–20.

21. Salazar, O.M., Rubin, P., Hendrickson, P.R. *et al.* (1986) Single dose half-body irradiation for palliation of multiple bone metastases from solid tumors. Final Radiation Therapy Oncology Group Report. *Cancer*, **58**, 29–36.

22. Blake, G.M., Zivanovic, M.A., McEwan, A.J. *et al.* (1986) Sr-89 therapy: strontium kinetics in disseminated carcinoma of the prostate. *Eur. J. Nucl. Med.*, **12**(5), 447–54.

23. Maxon, H.R., Schroder, L.E., Thomas, S.R. *et al.* (1992) Re-186 (Sn) HEDP for treatment of painful osseous metastases: initial clinical experience in 20 patients with hormone-resistant prostate cancer, *Radiology* **176**(1), 155–9.

24. Leong, C., McKenzie, M.R., Coupland, D.B. *et al.* (1994) Disseminated intravascular coagulation in 9 patients with metastatic prostate cancer: fatal outcome following strontium-89 therapy. *J. Nucl. Med.*, **35**(10), 1662–4.

25. Silberstein, E. and Taylor, A., Jr (1995) Procedure guideline for bone pain treatment: 1.0. *J. Nucl. Med.*, **37**(5), 881–4.

26. Silberstein, E.B. (1993) The treatment of painful osseous metastases with phosphorus-32-labeled phosphates. *Semin. Oncol.*, **20** (suppl. 2),10–21.

27. Porter, A.T., McEwan, A.J.M., Powe, J.E. *et al.* (1993) Results of a randomized phase III trial to evaluate the efficacy of strontium-89 adjuvant to local field external beam irradiation in the management of endocrine resistant metastatic prostate cancer. *Int. J. Radiat. Oncol. Biol. Phys*, **25**, 805–13.

28. Quilty, D.M., Kirk, D., Bolger, J.J. *et al.* (1994) A comparison of the palliative effects of strontium-89 and external beam radiotherapy in metastatic prostate cancer. *Radiother. Oncol.*, **31**, 33–40.

29. McEwan, A.J.B., Porter, A.T., Venner, P.M. *et al.* (1990) An evaluation of the safety and efficacy of treatment with strontium-89 in patients who have previously received wide field radiotherapy. *Antibody, Immunoconjugates and Radiopharmaceuticals*, **3**, 91–8.

30. Collins, C., Eary, J.F., Donaldson, G. *et al.* (1993) Samarium-153-EDTMP in bone metastases of hormone refractory prostate carcinoma: a Phase I/II Trial. *J. Nucl. Med.*, **34**(12), 1839–44.

Thyroid disease

S.E.M. Clarke

INTRODUCTION

Diseases of the thyroid constitute the most common form of endocrine disorders and, over the past 50 years, nuclear medicine has contributed significantly to the management of thyroid patients, both in terms of diagnosis and treatment [1]. Radionuclide therapy for both benign disease (thyrotoxicosis and goitre), and thyroid cancer, has served as a model for the development of other radionuclide therapies in the recent years.

The first reports of radionuclide therapy for thyrotoxicosis used iodine-130 and iodine-131 rapidly became the favoured radionuclide with β- and γ-ray emissions and a half-life suitable for therapy [2]. Although thyrotoxicosis was the initial indication for ^{131}I therapy, reports on treatment of differentiated thyroid cancer soon followed.

Surprisingly, given the length of time for which ^{131}I has been used, significant controversy persists as to which patients are suitable for treatment and what doses of radioiodine should be used.

In this chapter, the theory of radioiodine therapy will be explained, the clinical role explored and the practical aspects of treatment considered.

IODINE-131

The physical properties of ^{131}I are listed in Table 1.3. Iodine-131 has a physical half-life of 8.04 days, which is well suited to the biological half-life of iodine in patients with differentiated thyroid cancer. The medium energy beta-particle emission ($E_{max} = 0.61$ mev) with a path length of about 0.5 mm in tissue, ensures an intracellular radiation dose following the cellular internalization of ^{131}I. The gamma emissions of ^{131}I have both benefits and disadvantages. Gamma-ray emissions facilitate gamma-camera imaging, which enables tracer doses of ^{131}I to be used diagnostically and for dosimetry calculations, and also permits post-

therapy imaging to confirm uptake of the therapy dose in all known tumour sites.

The high-energy gamma emissions however, contribute to the unwanted whole-body radiation burden associated with radionuclide therapy and also to the radiation protection problems for the staff and the patients' relatives.

SYNTHESIS OF THYROID HORMONES

Thyroxine and triiodothyronine are synthesized in the thyroid follicular cells by the iodination of tyrosine (Figure 1.1). Iodine is taken up in the follicular cells by an active ATP-dependent transport mechanism through the stimulation of thyroid-stimulating hormone (TSH). The iodine pump increases in the presence of iodine deficiency. Peroxidase and hydrogen peroxidase enzymes oxidize the iodine, which is then linked to the tyrosine molecules in the tyrosine-rich thyroglobulin. The iodothyronines are produced, which couple to form triiodothyronine (T3) or tetra-iodothyronine (T4). The process of iodination is inhibited by the presence of excess iodine. The thyroglobulin is then hydrolysed, liberating T3 and T4, which are secreted into the circulation where they are bound to thyroid-binding globulin, thyroid-binding pre-albumin and albumin. This process of iodination is blocked by perchlorate and by the presence of excess iodine.

THE CONTROL OF THYROID HORMONE PRODUCTION

The production of TSH occurs in the anterior part of the pituitary. This production is in turn regulated by suppressants and stimulators. Thyroxine, T3, somatostatin and dobutamine all act as suppressors of TSH, and T4 is also believed to have a direct TSH-suppressing action.

The production of TSH is stimulated by thyrotropin-releasing hormone, which is found in various parts of the body including the hypothalamus. The release of TRH is inhibited by T4 and T3. TSH stimulates thyroid hormone production by stimulating cyclic AMP and by activating the incorporation of thyroglobulin in the thyroid follicular cells by a process of endocytosis.

Clinical Nuclear Medicine, 3rd edn. Edited by M.N. Maisey, K.E. Britton and B.D. Collier. Published in 1998 by Chapman & Hall, London. ISBN 0 412 75180 1

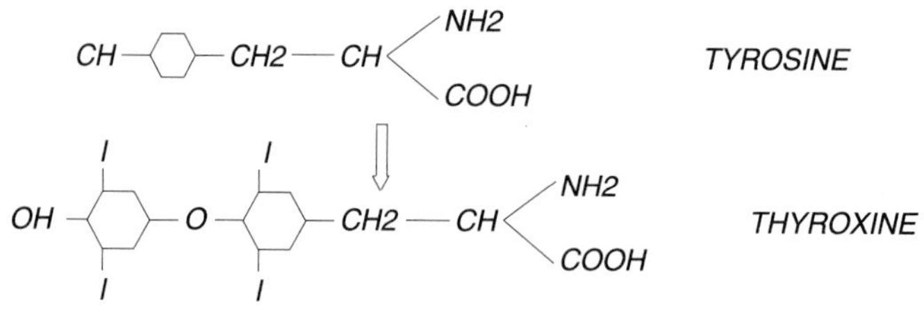

Figure 1.1   Synthesis of thyroxine by iodination of tyrosine molecule.

Table 1.3   Physical characteristics of iodine-131

Half-life	8.04 days
Principal gamma energies	80 keV
	284 keV
	364 keV
	637 keV
Beta E_{max}	0.61 MeV

PATHOLOGY OF THE THYROID GLAND

Like all endocrine organs, the thyroid gland may over- or under-produce hormones or be subject to malignant change. ^{131}I may be used to treat the various forms of thyroid hormone over-production, and also for the treatment of differentiated thyroid cancer.

THYROTOXICOSIS

The clinical symptoms of thyrotoxicosis are classically those of weight loss, heat intolerance, tremor and palpitations, increased bowel frequency and increased anxiety. The signs include tachycardia and tremor of the outstretched hands. There may be a bruit audible over the thyroid gland, and a systolic flow murmur may be audible over the precordium. In some patients – particularly those with severe disease or a prolonged period before diagnosis – evidence of proximal muscle wasting may be present.

There are two main pathological processes resulting in thyrotoxicosis. The first is a diffuse process affecting the whole gland; the second is a focal process affecting one or several areas of the gland. It is important to differentiate between these two main causes of thyrotoxicosis as the management of these pathologies differs.

Toxic diffuse goitre (Graves' disease)

Toxic diffuse goitre (Graves' disease) is an autoimmune process caused by the production of a stimulating antibody to the TSH receptor (Figure 1.2). The disease may be familial, although the pattern of inheritance is unclear. Various factors have been implicated in the development of Graves' disease and these include pregnancy and stress [3]. The autoimmune process not only affects the thyroid gland but may also affect the eyes in 50% of cases and, more rarely, can be associated with the development of pretibial myxoedema and thyroid acropathy. The causative antibody, variously known as thyroid-stimulating immunoglobulin or TSH-receptor antibody, may be assayed and can be demonstrated in 90% of patients with the clinical syndrome of Graves' disease. Although the level of antibody tends to correlate with the severity of clinical symptoms, this is not invariable. The link between TSH-receptor antibody and dysthyroid eye disease remains unclear. It would appear from various studies that the TSH-receptor antibody itself is not the causative factor in dysthyroid eye disease, and recent papers have implicated a 64 kDa protein present in the serum of patients with dysthyroid eye disease which reacts with pig eye muscle [4].

The management of toxic diffuse goitre (Graves' disease) in Europe is generally that of a prolonged course of anti-thyroid medication (carbimazole, methimazole or propylthiouracil). Data show that the continuance of treatment for 12–18 months results in an approximately 50% cure rate on discontinuing anti-thyroid medication [5]. Second-line treatment following failure of anti-thyroid medication, or in patients who are not responding to anti-thyroid treatment, is either ^{131}I or alternatively, surgery.

In the USA, there is a current trend to early ^{131}I treatment with little or no pre-treatment with anti-thyroid medication [6]. The value of pre-treatment with anti-thyroid medication however, is the potential cure rate in half the patients

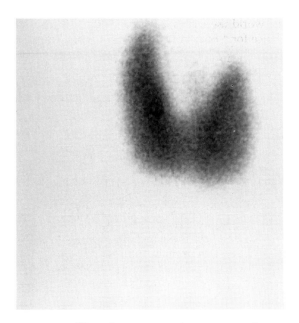

Figure 1.2 ^{99m}Tc thyroid scan of a patient with toxic diffuse goitre (Graves' disease) showing diffusely increased uptake and visualizing the pyramidal lobe.

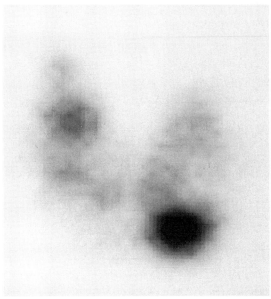

Figure 1.3 ^{99m}Tc thyroid scan of a patient with a multinodular goitre showing non-homogeneous uptake and developing autonomous nodules at left lower pole.

treated, and the rapid control of symptoms that cannot be achieved with ^{131}I, particularly in those patients who are markedly symptomatic [7].

Toxic nodular goitre (Plummer's disease)

In patients with multinodular goitres, there is an increased likelihood of the development of multiple focal areas of thyroid autonomy resulting in elevations of free T4 and free T3 levels. This form of Plummer's disease is particularly common in geographical areas where endemic goitre is prevalent. Germany, Austria and Switzerland are countries with a previous history of dietary iodine deficiency, and there is a higher prevalence of multinodular goitre in these countries compared with the UK [8] (Figure 1.3).

Patients may also develop a single nodule, which on isotope imaging is demonstrated to show increased uptake with suppression of the remainder of the gland. Uninodular toxic goitre is diagnosed using conventional biochemical tests and radionuclide imaging with technetium-99m (^{99m}Tc) or iodine-123 (^{123}I).

The presenting symptoms of uninodular or multinodular toxic goitre are similar to those of Graves' disease, but with the absence of eye signs, thyroid acropachy or pretibial myxoedema. This tends to be a disease of old people and, in the elderly, the clinical presentation may be non-classical with minimal signs and symptoms apart from tachycardia that may progress to atrial fibrillation.

DIAGNOSIS OF THYROTOXICOSIS

The diagnosis of thyrotoxicosis is made on the basis of history, clinical examination and investigations. The investigations include free T4, free T3 and ultra-sensitive TSH investigations. A ^{99m}Tc or an ^{123}I thyroid scan will differentiate toxic diffuse goitre from toxic nodular goitre. Thyroid-stimulating immunoglobulin measurement, if raised, will strongly support a diagnosis of toxic diffuse goitre (Graves' disease), as does the presence of dysthyroid eye disease.

RADIOIODINE THERAPY FOR THYROTOXICOSIS

SELECTION OF PATIENTS

Toxic diffuse goitre (Graves' disease)

As has already been stated, ^{131}I therapy usage is considered in patients who have completed a conventional 12- to 24-month course of anti-thyroid medication and whose thyroid function tests have again become elevated, or alternatively in patients who fail to respond to anti-thyroid medication. Patients who are poorly compliant in taking anti-thyroid medication should also be considered for radioiodine therapy.

As diffuse goitre (Graves' disease) frequently affects young and middle-aged women, the issue of using ^{131}I in women of childbearing years has been an issue of discussion. A recent survey of practice in Europe, Japan and the USA found that one-third of doctors in the USA believed ^{131}I to be an appropriate treatment for women of age 19. Only 4% of European doctors thought that ^{131}I was appropriate in such a case, although this does not reflect general European practice [9].

In the previous decades, such women were not selected for ^{131}I therapy because of the potential risk to the offspring. However, to date, no evidence has been presented to suggest damage to the offspring of patients treated with ^{131}I despite large patient population studies [10,11].

The use of ^{131}I in young patients remains controversial. In the USA, treatment of patients under the age of 18 with ^{131}I is now taking place routinely. In Europe, however, the concerns about radioiodine treatment in young patients with radiosensitive tissues has led to a general limitation of ^{131}I use to adults. However, it is important to recognize and consider the risks of thyroid surgery in children. It has been estimated that 16–35% of children treated with sub-total thyroidectomy experience acute complications with permanent complications occurring in up to 8% of children [12,13].

The marked variation in the use of ^{131}I throughout the world, both in terms of the patients who are selected for treatment and the protocols for treatment, is now recognized and surveys of practice undertaken in Europe, Japan, India and the USA confirm this variation [6,14–16].

The use of surgery as a second-line treatment, is less commonly used, although in certain parts of the world it remains the second-line treatment of choice for women of childbearing years. Kuma *et al.* [17] have shown clearly that there is an increased morbidity associated with surgery compared with ^{131}I therapy. There is also the risk of subsequent recurrence in the residual thyroid. Hypothyroidism is also a post-operative complication of surgery [17].

Toxic nodular goitre (Plummer's disease)

Patients with toxic nodular goitre are generally considered to be ideally suited for ^{131}I therapy. A short period of treatment using anti-thyroid medication is recommended in patients who are extremely symptomatic, and in the elderly. It is essential to ensure that the normal thyroid tissue is suppressed at the time of ^{131}I therapy, and this will require an adequate period of discontinuation of anti-thyroid medication before radioiodine treatment (Figure 1.4). In patients with mild to moderate elevations of thyroid hormone levels and who are relatively asymptomatic, direct treatment with radioiodine may be considered.

PRACTICAL ASPECTS OF THERAPY

Patients who have been selected for ^{131}I radioiodine treatment should have the implications of therapy explained clearly. It is generally considered good practice to render the patient euthyroid before treatment, as ^{131}I radioiodine administration will cause a transient elevation in free T4 and free T3 levels approximately 7 days following administration. In the symptomatically well-controlled patient this will have little effect, but in symptomatically toxic patients, this further elevation of thyroid hormone may trigger palpitations, atrial fibrillation and heart failure. This is a particular problem in the elderly. Symptomatic control may be achieved using beta blockade. Since carbimazole blocks the organification of iodine within the thyroid, carbimazole therapy should be discontinued at least 48 hours before therapy is undertaken to ensure adequate residence time of ^{131}I within the follicular cells.

The requirement to admit patients varies considerably across the world. In many countries in Europe, admission is required for doses of 185 MBq and above. In the USA, doses up to 1000 MBq may be given as an outpatient. Admission should be considered for the elderly with a risk of heart failure.

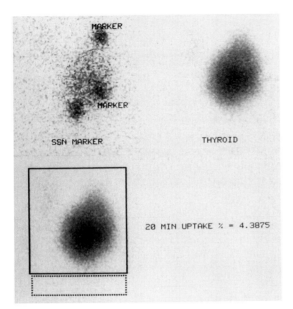

Figure 1.4 ^{99m}Tc thyroid scan showing an autonomously functioning thyroid nodule with complete suppression of the rest of the gland. The radiation dose to the suppressed areas of the gland will be extremely low compared with the dose to the toxic nodule. This explains why hypothyroidism is less common in radioiodine-treated Plummer's disease compared with Graves' disease.

Table 1.4 Precautions following radioiodine therapy

1. FOR 24 HOURS AFTER ^{131}I RADIOIODINE
   Drink plenty of fluids and empty bladder regularly
2. FOR 1 WEEK AFTER ^{131}I RADIOIODINE
   a) Carry this card with you at all times
   b) Avoid close contact with babies and small children (you will be advised in more detail about this
   c) Don't breastfeed your child
   d) Don't spend time with anyone who is pregnant
   e) Don't share a bed with your partner
   f) Don't go to the cinema or theatre or out to a restaurant
   g) Don't travel by public transport if your journey lasts longer than an hour
   h) Don't return to work unless permission is given by the doctor of physicist
   i) Keep your own cutlery and crockery separate from the rest of the family
3. FOR 4 MONTHS AFTER ^{131}I RADIOIODINE
   Don't become pregnant

Before therapy, patients should be asked to sign a consent form and should be informed of restrictions on working, contact with children and pregnancy before doing so [7,18]. The length of time for which restrictions should be observed varies by country, but time should be taken with the patient before treatment to ensure that appropriate restrictions are understood and will be adhered to.

Pregnancy and breast-feeding are absolute contraindications to radioiodine therapy, and it is recommended that a pregnancy test should be undertaken in women of childbearing years who are about to receive radioiodine therapy and in whom pregnancy may be an issue.

The restrictions on work and contact with small children will also depend on national dose limits, and these should be discussed with each patient individually [7,18]. Studies are now being undertaken following radioiodine therapy, and these data confirm that with adequate precautions, the dose to family members is minimal [19].

In patients in whom thyrotoxicosis is not well controlled before radioiodine therapy, it may be necessary to re-commence anti-thyroid medication for a short interval following treatment. All patients should be given written instructions about the precautions to be observed. In addition, the need to avoid pregnancy for 4 months following radioiodine treatment should be emphasized to female patients.

^{131}I may be administered in liquid form or as a capsule. The advantages of the capsule are those of radiation protection for staff administering the radioiodine; the disadvantages are those of expense and loss of flexibility in dose. Unusually, ^{131}I radioiodine may be given intravenously in patients in whom vomiting is a problem. ^{131}I should be administered in a designated area by trained staff in accordance with the national regulations.

Patients should be encouraged to drink large volumes of fluid for a 24-hour period following radioiodine therapy to lower the radiation dose to the bladder. Recommended precautions are included in Table 1.4.

DOSE CONSIDERATIONS

The determination of the dose of radioiodine to be administered in patients with thyrotoxicosis remains a topic of controversy. The controversy centres around whether it is possible to avoid hypothyroidism and successfully treat hyperthyroidism by using careful dosimetry calculations. Although much has been written on this subject, there appears to be no consensus as to the optimal protocol for deciding the dose. Current practice therefore ranges from the use of careful dose calculation to a fixed-dose protocol.

Dosimetry calculation

Various formulae have been generated which may be used to estimate the administered dose required to deliver an effective radiation dose to the gland to render the patient euthyroid and avoid unnecessary radiation being administered [20]. Most formulae require information on ^{131}I uptake and clearance of radioiodine by the gland, and the weight or volume of the gland. The percentage uptake and clearance of radioiodine may be estimated using tracer doses of radioiodine [21]. It is unclear, however, whether tracer doses may have the mild stunning effect on the thyroid follicular cells, thereby altering the uptake and clearance of subsequent therapy doses. In addition, variations in iodine intake in the diet may theoretically affect the reproducibility of radioiodine uptake and clearance.

The volume of the gland may be estimated using ultrasound measurements [22], but patients with Plummer's disease or in patients with Graves' disease in a multinodular goitre, the measured volume of the gland does not necessarily correspond to the functioning volume. It is therefore likely that ultrasound estimates of volumes are most accurate in patients with Graves' disease and least accurate in patients with Plummer's disease. ^{124}I-PET studies have been used by Flower *et al.* [23] to determine more accurately the functioning volume of the thyroid gland.

Results of studies published using these volume estimates to calculate administered dose, however, show that there continues to be an incidence of hypothyroidism and persisting hyperthyroidism in patients treated using these calculations. Other factors such as the duration of pretreatment with anti-thyroid medication and the issue of varying radiosensitivity may well explain why careful dosimetric measurements fail to predict reliably the dose that will render the patient euthyroid without subsequent hypothyroidism.

Low calculated dose protocols aim to deliver 80 Gy to the thyroid, whereas high calculated dose protocols aim to deliver 300 Gy. Willemsen *et al.* [24] have shown that the administered dose required to deliver a delivered dose of 300 Gy ranged from 240 to 3120 MBq.

Fixed-dose protocol

Fixed-dose protocols range from those that take count of the size of the gland, usually determined clinically by giving smaller doses to small glands on palpation and larger doses to clinically larger glands, and those protocols that attempt electively to ablate the thyroid gland.

As might be predicted, low-dose protocols result in a lower instance of hypothyroidism in the first year [23], but the long-term outcome shows a significant incidence of hypothyroidism at 15 years (35–40%) compared with 50–70% incidence using high-dose regimes [25–27].

The administered dose used in an attempt to ablate the thyroid gland varies world-wide, and is usually limited by the maximum permissible dose to be administered as an outpatient. In the USA, 1000 MBq may therefore be administered, whereas in the UK, 500 MBq is the standard upper limit for outpatient administration. Results in the UK published by Kendall-Taylor *et al.* [28] using a 500 MBq fixed-dose show that ablation was achieved in only 64% of patients with a small percentage of patients still remaining hyperthyroid following treatment.

The disadvantage of electively rendering a patient hypothyroid is that in effect, one pathology is exchanged for another. There is a need to ensure that patients who have been rendered hypothyroid remain on adequate replacement doses of thyroxine for life. The study by Kendall-Taylor *et al.* [28] demonstrated that 2% of patients who had been rendered hypothyroid and started on thyroxine were not taking treatment and a further 3% of patients had been recognized by their physicians to be non-compliant.

Hardisty *et al.* [26] explored the efficacy and cost-effectiveness of varying dose protocols, and concluded that both hypothyroidism and persisting hyperthyroidism were unavoidable whichever dose protocols were used. In addition, they noted that when both cost to the patients and the Health Service were considered, the use of high fixed-dose attempting to ablate the thyroid gland appeared more cost-effective [26].

SIDE EFFECTS AND COMPLICATIONS

The major complication of radioiodine therapy is hypothyroidism. This may occur in the early post-treatment period, particularly if higher administered doses are given. Alternatively, it may develop gradually in the years following treatment [26]. The later-onset hypothyroidism occurs at a rate of approximately 4% per year, and therefore it has been estimated that on follow-up after 25 years 100% of patients treated with radioiodine will be hypothyroid. It has been postulated that this long-term hypothyroidism relates in part to the natural outcome of Graves' disease [29]. The incidence of post-radioiodine hypothyroidism however, is markedly lower in patients treated for a solitary toxic nodule compared with those with Graves' disease [25,30]. This is undoubtedly due to the protection of the suppressed area of the gland at the time of treatment and emphasizes the need to ensure that patients have adequate time off anti-thyroid treatment before radioiodine therapy to ensure good suppression of the normal areas of the gland.

Careful follow-up of patients following radioiodine therapy is therefore mandatory, and should be coordinated by a trained thyroid practitioner. In the early post-therapy period, it is recommended that this follow-up is undertaken within a hospital environment. Subsequently, follow-up may be undertaken in conjunction with a community physician [7]. The management of these patients is greatly facilitated by computer-assisted follow-up programming.

Patients whose hypothyroidism develops rapidly following radioiodine treatment are frequently extremely symptomatic, whereas patients with delayed onset hypothyroidism may not present with classical hypothyroid symptoms. Weight gain and tiredness are key clinical symptoms in diagnosing post-therapy hypothyroidism.

Other side effects and complications of radioiodine therapy are remarkably few. Patients with large goitres may notice transient swelling of the goitre approximately 1 week following therapy and some discomfort may be associated with this swelling. As has been previously stated, there may be a transient rise in fT4 and fT3 levels 7–10 days following radioiodine treatment, and in patients who have been poorly controlled before radioiodine therapy there may be an exacerbation of palpitations and heart failure. Slight discomfort

of the salivary glands may be noted, but this is unusual with the doses used for thyrotoxicosis therapy. Iodine allergy is not a contraindication to radioiodine therapy.

In patients with large goitres in whom tracheal compression is present before therapy, a worsening of pressure symptoms in the immediate post-therapy period may be noticed. This complication is in fact rare. Patients with severe tracheal narrowing should be admitted for therapy with surgical cover. Surgery should be considered as an alternative to radioiodine therapy in this particular group.

Dysthyroid eye disease

There has been much discussion as to the effect of radioiodine therapy on dysthyroid eye disease. Reports in the literature yield conflicting information [31,32].

Catz and Tsao [31] have demonstrated that an improvement in ophthalmopathy can be obtained following ^{131}I radioiodine ablation of the thyroid, which they believe to be due to the destruction of the antigenic stimulus to antibody formation. Peqqequat et al. [33], using non-ablative doses, showed a varying response following therapy with some of the patients improving and a few patients deteriorating. Jones et al. [34] observed that while lid retraction improved following ^{131}I treatment in patients with Graves' ophthalmopathy, exophthalmos remained unchanged or deteriorated, and in 50% of the patients periorbital oedema was observed following treatment. It is therefore recommended that patients with severe dysthyroid eye disease should not be treated during an acute exacerbation. A course of high-dose steroids may be considered as a prelude to radioiodine therapy in this small percentage of patients. Tallstedt et al. [35] have studied the effects of thyroxine administered in the early post-radioiodine period, and they conclude that the early administration of thyroxine after radioiodine reduces the occurrence of Graves' ophthalmopathy.

RADIOIODINE THERAPY OF NON-TOXIC MULTINODULAR GOITRE

In recent years, the use of radioiodine in the treatment of non-toxic multinodular goitre has been

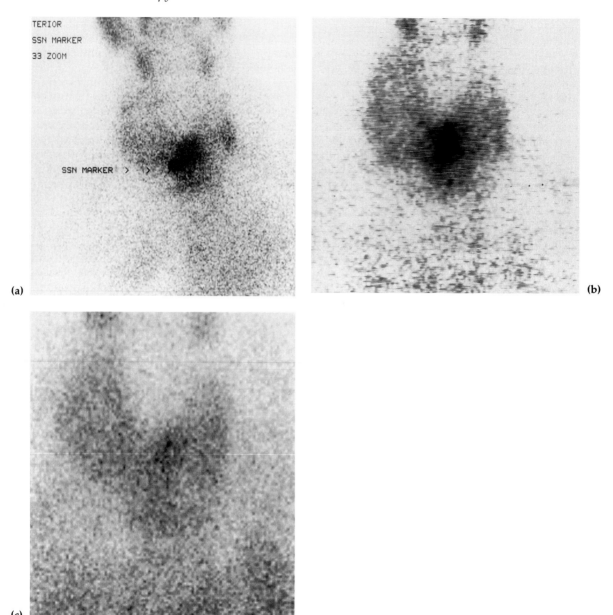

TERIOR
SSN MARKER
33 ZOOM

SSN MARKER >   >

(a)

(b)

(c)

Figure 1.5 ^{99m}Tc thyroid scan (a) showing a large multinodular goitre with retrosternal extension in a patient with pressure symptoms and stridor who was unsuitable for surgery. Following treatment with 400 MBq ^{131}I the pressure symptoms improved (b) and after a further 400 MBq (c) the goitre was notably smaller.

explored [36,37] (Figure 1.5). Radioiodine is particularly useful in elderly patients and those with medical contraindications to surgery. Goitre shrinkage is well documented, but multiple doses of radioiodine are frequently required. Varying dose regimes have been described on the basis of dosimetry calculation. High administered doses are required in view of the relatively low overall uptake compared with a toxic goitre. Although historically, patients with evidence of tracheal compression were not deemed suitable for radioiodine therapy, it is now apparent that the theoretical risk of increasing tracheal compression in the immediate post-treatment period does not in fact occur [37]. Nevertheless, in patients with significant stridor, admission is recommended.

Following radioiodine therapy, thyroid function tests should be performed at regular intervals. While hypothyroidism appears an uncommon complication, the development of hyperthyroidism with a picture suggestive of Graves' disease has been reported [38]. The mechanism for this is unclear, but it is presumed that the release of thyroid antigen may be the trigger for the development of autoimmune thyrotoxicosis. As these patients are frequently elderly and may have cardiovascular disease, careful follow-up is essential as hyperthyroidism may well exacerbate cardiac symptoms in this population.

RADIOIODINE THERAPY IN MALIGNANT THYROID DISEASE

Radioiodine therapy is used both as an adjunct to thyroid surgery in order to completely destroy the normal thyroid tissue and also to treat metastatic disease in patients with recurrent tumour.

PATHOLOGY OF THYROID CANCER

Malignancies of the thyroid may involve the thyroid follicular cells (papillary and follicular thyroid cancers), the parafollicular cells (medullary thyroid cancer) or be lymphoid in origin (primary lymphomas of the thyroid). Rarely, tumours such as breast cancer may metastasize to the thyroid.

Papillary thyroid cancer is the most common form of differentiated cancer, accounting for approximately 65% of all thyroid carcinomas. While some papillary tumours show a pure papillary form, many also exhibit follicular elements. Fine needle aspiration of a papillary thyroid cancer is usually diagnostic as the tumour cells demonstrate typical features of intranuclear grooving and 'orphan annie' nuclei. Papillary cancers may be found as unexpected asymptomatic lesions in patients undergoing thyroid surgery for benign disease. They are not infrequently multifocal, and spread into cervical lymph nodes is often discovered at the time of presentation. Distant metastases to lung and bone occur less frequently than with follicular tumours. Papillary cancers tend to develop in the third and fourth decades of life. While some pure papillary tumours do not retain the ability to take up iodine, those with follicular elements generally do so and ^{131}I may be used to treat local and distant metastatic spread.

Follicular thyroid cancers are diagnosed when capsular breakthrough of a follicular tumour is demonstrated. They cannot therefore be diagnosed by fine needle aspiration and lobectomy or total thyroidectomy is required in order to make the diagnosis.

Compared with papillary cancers, follicular thyroid cancers tend to occur in an older population,

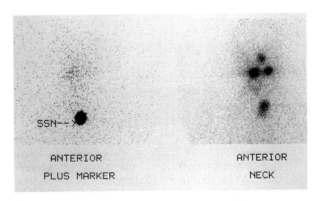

Figure 1.6 ^{131}I iodine scan of the head and neck in a patient following total thyroidectomy for papillary cancer showing residual thyroid tissue in the neck.

peaking in the fourth and fifth decades of life. Unlike papillary cancers, they metastasize more commonly to bone and lungs. Liver metastases are rare in both follicular and papillary cancers.

While the majority of follicular cancers take up ^{131}I radioiodine at the time of presentation, de-differentiation may occur, and these de-differentiated tumours being more aggressive frequently lose their ability to take up ^{131}I radioiodine. The Hurthle cell variant of follicular cancer is uncommon but is distinguished by the fact that only 10% of these tumours take up ^{131}I radioiodine. As medullary thyroid cancers and lymphomas do not take up ^{131}I radioiodine, its only role is in thyroid remnant ablation (see below).

THYROID ABLATION

The optimal management for patients having thyroid cancer diagnosed either by fine needle aspiration or at the time of surgery is total thyroidectomy. This may be achieved by a one-stage or a two-stage procedure. Despite careful surgery, however, it is extremely common to demonstrate small residues of normal thyroid tissue on post-operative imaging (Figure 1.6).

The data demonstrating an outcome advantage to complete ablation of normal thyroid tissue are unclear. While some series have demonstrated a reduction in relapse rate in patients treated with ^{131}I radioiodine post-surgery [39,40], others have failed to show any outcome benefit of radioiodine ablation [41,42]. Tubiana [43] has clearly demonstrated a benefit in outcome in patients with poor prognostic features. However, ablation of normal thyroid tissue undoubtedly aids follow-up in the following ways:

- Achieving a negative iodine tracer scan following complete ablation facilitates the interpretation of the subsequent radioiodine tracer scans and the appearance of iodine uptake in the neck subsequent to successful ablation can be reliably interpreted as recurrent tumour.
- As serum thyroglobulin levels play a key role in the follow-up of patients with differentiated thyroid cancer the achievement of undetectable thyroglobulin levels by total thyroid remnant ablation makes subsequent elevations of thyroglobulin levels interpretable as recurrent disease.

- As normal thyroid tissue will trap iodine more efficiently than will tumour cells, ^{131}I radioiodine therapy will be less immediately effective if recurrences occur as most of the treatment dose will be taken up by the remnant rather than the tumour recurrence.

ABLATION DOSES

One of the main problems of radioiodine thyroid ablation is the stunning effect of the tracer dose before administration of a therapy dose. There is now clear literature evidence confirming that even relatively low tracer doses of radioiodine will significantly reduce the uptake of a subsequent therapy dose [44,45]. It is therefore recommended that doses of 185 MBq or less are used in the tracer scan to minimize the stunning effect of the tracer dose. New techniques are currently being researched. Park *et al.* [46] are currently exploring the use of high doses of ^{123}I iodine with imaging up to 24 hours post-administration to determine the presence of remnant thyroid and to perform uptake measurements for dosimetry calculations. Further data are required to determine whether the substitution of ^{123}I will improve the efficacy of the subsequent therapy dose and reduce the number of ablation doses required, thereby reducing the requirement for admission with both cost savings and improvement in convenience to the patient.

The dose routinely used for ablation varies greatly world-wide. In the USA, 30 mCi (1000 MBq) is commonly used as this dose may be given as an outpatient. de Groot *et al.* [47] have shown that this leads to ablation in only 60% of cases, while Arad *et al.* [48] have reported on the use of fractionated doses using 30–50 mCi doses at weekly intervals. The success rate is disappointing, however, with only 25% of patients being ablated [48]. In Europe, larger ablation doses are generally used with 3.7 GBq being the standard dose [49] (Figure 1.7).

Post-therapy scans are recommended as, particularly with the higher doses, unsuspected metastatic tumour may also be detected (Figure 1.8).

Radioiodine may also be used to ablate remnant thyroid tissue in patients with medullary thyroid cancer while recognizing that these tumours themselves do not take up radioiodine. The rationale for this is the multicentricity of the tumours in patients with familial forms of the disease.

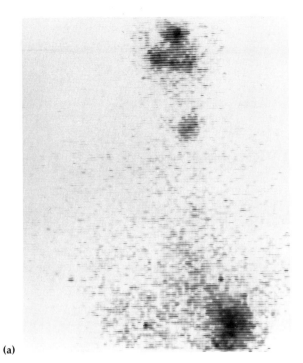
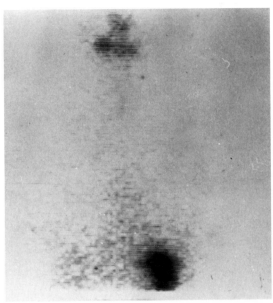

(a)   (b)

Figure 1.7 ^{131}I iodine scan in patient before (a) and after (b) successful ^{131}I iodine ablation with 3.7 GBq.

TREATMENT OF DIFFERENTIATED THYROID CANCER

Follicular cancers of the thyroid are usually well differentiated and demonstrate a capability of taking up iodine, although the uptake of iodine is significantly less than that of normal thyroid follicular cells. It has also been shown by Mazaferri *et al.* [40] that 50% of papillary carcinomas are also able to take up iodine and the presence of follicular elements on histology is an indicator of iodine uptake capabilities.

TSH levels must be high in order to ensure good uptake of ^{131}I radioiodine into recurrent sites of differentiated thyroid cancer. In patients with progressive disease, de-differentiation may occur and poorly differentiated tumour cells lose their ability to take up ^{131}I, although some may continue to secrete thyroglobulin into the circulation. Medullary thyroid cancers, anaplastic carcinomas of the thyroid and lymphomas of the thyroid do not take up ^{131}I which therefore has no role in therapy following ablation of remnant thyroid tissue.

After successful ablation of thyroid tissue with either surgery alone or a combination of surgery

and ^{131}I, the subsequent demonstration of focal areas of ^{131}I radioiodine uptake on whole-body imaging is strongly suggestive of recurrent thyroid tumour. The normal pattern of radioiodine by distribution however, must be taken into account when interpreting a whole-body scan. Activity is commonly seen in the salivary glands, nasopharynx, stomach, bowel and bladder (Figure 1.9). Care should also be taken to ensure that artefacts are not interpreted as focal areas of recurrent tumour. Since ^{131}I radioiodine is secreted in the saliva, contamination of pocket handkerchiefs is a not uncommon problem and may lead to a false-positive interpretation of a whole-body scan if care is not taken to ensure that no contamination object is imaged. Similarly, urine contamination of underclothes may cause artefacts in the region of the pelvis. ^{131}I radioiodine will successfully identify sites of both soft tissue and bone recurrence and may be the first indication of lung metastases.

Before undertaking an ^{131}I radioiodine tracer scan, the patient should be asked to discontinue thyroid replacement hormone. If the patient is taking thyroxine, a minimum of 4 weeks off treat-

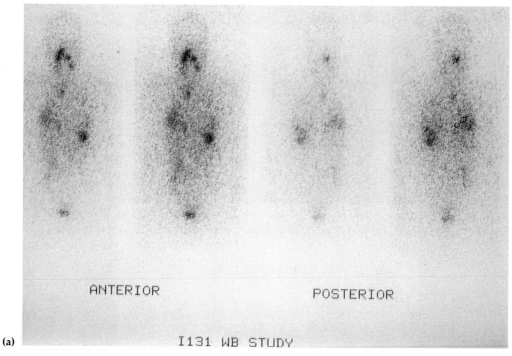

ANTERIOR   POSTERIOR

(a)   I131 WB STUDY

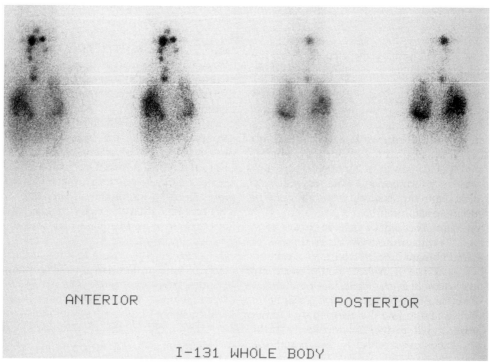

ANTERIOR   POSTERIOR

(b)   I-131 WHOLE BODY

Figure 1.8 ^{131}I iodine whole-body scans (a) before and (b) 1 week after a 5.5 GBq dose of ^{131}I iodine, showing metastases from a papillary cancer in the neck and lungs which appear more numerous and extensive on the post-therapy scan.

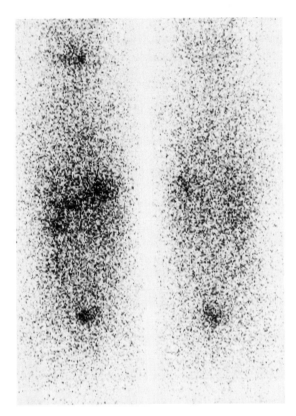

Figure 1.9 Normal whole-body ^{131}I iodine scan showing normal biodistribution in the salivary glands, saliva, stomach, bowel and bladder.

ment is required to ensure adequate TSH levels at the time of imaging. If the patient is taking T3, then a 2-week cessation of therapy is adequate. TSH levels must be measured at the time of undertaking ^{131}I imaging to ensure the patient's compliance with instructions and to confirm an adequate rise in TSH before a scan is interpreted as negative. Recent work at Sloane Kettering has suggested the use of re-combinant TSH in patients who have a poor TSH response or in those in whom the time delay necessitated in stopping thyroid hormone replacement is clinically unacceptable [50].

The use of low iodine diet in the period before tracer imaging will further enhance the avidity of thyroid tumour recurrence for ^{131}I radioiodine (Table 1.5).

The amount of ^{131}I radioiodine to be administered for the tracer scan again varies. The justification for a low tracer dose regime is the avoidance of possible stunning effects of the tracer dose on a subsequent therapy dose. There is little evidence in the literature however, to suggest that the stunning effects seen in the normal thyroid also occurs in thyroid tumour cells and as tumour cells are known to be less radio-sensitive than normal cells, it may be postulated that the stunning effect is less important when considering treatment of recurrence compared with ablation of thyroid remnants. The advantage of a high tracer dose (up to 400 MBq) is the higher sensitivity for detecting recurrent disease. The increase in sensitivity with dose is clearly evidenced by the fact that post-therapy scans not uncommonly show lesions that were not detected on a tracer scan [51].

Schlumberger [52] recommended a protocol which takes into account the lower sensitivity of the low dose tracer scan regime. It was proposed that patients with an elevated thyroglobulin level and a normal tracer scan should receive a therapy dose of ^{131}I radioiodine. Experience indicated that 50% of patients thus treated show uptake on the post-therapy scan [52].

A patient in whom a tracer scan is performed will be required to observe precautions as for a ^{131}I radioiodine dose for thyrotoxicosis if they are scanned as an outpatient. Again, extreme care must be taken to ensure that if the patient is a female, they are neither pregnant nor breast-feeding, as both conditions remain absolute contraindications to tracer scanning and subsequent therapy.

In those patients in whom the tracer scan confirms a focal area or areas of recurrence, therapy doses of ^{131}I may be administered. For this, the patient must be admitted into a designated room with en-suite bathroom facilities. Daily monitoring of the patient is required to ensure that the patient is not discharged until the radiation levels fall to those acceptable under national regulations

Table 1.5 Low iodine diet

Foods to avoid
1. Sea foods (e.g. shellfish, lobster, crab, prawns, scampi, etc.)
2. All other types of fish – fresh, frozen, canned, smoked or salted
3. All fish products (e.g. fish fingers, fish-cakes, fish-paste, etc.)
4. Vegetables: spinach – fresh or frozen, lettuce, watercress
5. Iodized salt in cooking

[53]. Visitors must be kept to a minimum, with visiting times being restricted to not more than 10 minutes per day.

As with thyrotoxicosis, there is a variation in practice concerning the use of dosimetry measurements obtained from the tracer scan in calculating the therapy dose. The pattern of practice varies between the use of a fixed dose ranging from 5 GBq to 7.4 GBq in some centres to an administered dose calculated from the uptake on the tracer scan. The advantage of the fixed-dose protocol is that it is simple and recognizes the problems associated with volume estimates of recurrent tumour and lack of reproducibility of results from a tracer study compared with the therapy. Again, it must be remembered that the reproducibility of uptake in the therapy dose compared with the tracer scan cannot be guaranteed in view of the potential stunning effect of the tracer scan dose. The dose to the tumour focus is dependent on the uptake of ^{131}I radioiodine within the tumour and its size, and small foci such as pulmonary metastases may receive doses of up to 30 000 rads.

Centres using dosimetric methods to estimate the dose for individual patients will variably base their dose on uptake and retention measurement obtained from the tracer scan or alternatively blood and urine collections and whole-body counting after tracer dose [54]. One approach utilizes so-called BEL dosimetry which calculates the dose to the blood from a tracer study. Doses are selected to give a maximum of 2 Gy to the blood, with no more than 4.4 GBq retained in the whole body at 48 hours [55,56]. Doses of up to 16.65 MBq (450 mCi) have been used with no permanent suppression of bone marrow observed. Benua *et al.* [55] however, have shown that average values of radiation delivered to the blood are significantly less than the predicted measurements after tracer doses. This observed fact obviously raises the whole question as to the value of estimating doses following dosimetry calculations. Kosal *et al.* [57] have shown that doses ranging from 400 to 29 000 rads may be delivered to the tumour using administered doses of 150–170 mCi. O'Connell *et al.* [58] have used PET in an attempt to more accurately define the volume of recurrent disease and have found that absorbed doses in excess of 100 Gy were found to eradicate cervical node metastases. Metastases that did not respond were calculated to have received less than 20 Gy [58].

After treatment, the patient should be reinstated on thyroid hormone replacement therapy. The whole process of rescanning and retreatment if required should not be repeated in under 6 months except in patients with rapidly progressive and life-threatening disease.

In patients with palpable recurrence localized to the neck, the use of surgery before radioiodine therapy should be considered to debulk the tumour and optimize the efficacy of radioiodine. The combination of surgery and radioiodine has a better outcome compared with the use of surgery alone [59].

The role of ^{131}I radioiodine in patients with Hurthle cell tumours is limited and McLeod *et al.* [60] reported that in their experience only 14% of Hurthle cell recurrent tumours take up radioiodine.

ACUTE SIDE EFFECTS FOLLOWING ^{131}I THERAPY FOR DIFFERENTIATED THYROID CANCER

As ^{131}I radioiodine is taken up and secreted by the salivary glands as well as by recurrent thyroid tumour sites, a significant radiation dose is received by the salivary glands. Becciolini *et al.* [61] have calculated the absorbed dose to the salivary glands based on external beam data to range between 0.24 and 2.29 Gy [61]. Patients are commonly aware of swelling and mild discomfort in the region of the salivary gland in the immediate post-therapy period and complain of alteration in taste with a metallic taste frequently noted. While these symptoms generally resolve after the first one or two treatments, subsequent treatments may result in a permanent reduction in salivary flow and a consequent dryness of the mouth and impaired sensation of taste. Attempts to reduce the radiation dose to the salivary glands have been made by suggesting patients chew gum or suck citrus sweets for 24 hours following therapy in order to increase salivary flow and thereby increase the rate of excretion of ^{131}I radioiodine from the salivary gland area. There is little data, however, to confirm the efficacy of this recommendation and indeed some have suggested that increasing salivary flow may increase radioiodine uptake into the salivary glands and therefore increase the overall dose received by the salivary glands.

Radiation doses to the bladder are minimized by ensuring a high urine output during the admission for therapy.

Some patients complain of nausea in the first 48 hours after therapy. This appears to be idiosyncratic. It is readily treated with conventional anti-emetics.

Transient episodes of marrow suppression have been observed in patients with widespread bone metastases. This appears to be a greater problem in patients of West African and West Indian background.

Transient impairment of testicular function has been demonstrated by Pacini *et al.* [62]. They concluded that approximately 25% of patients treated with ^{131}I suffered no alterations in FSH levels, whereas the remainder had transient rises in FSH levels. Patients treated repeatedly over a prolonged period had a reduced sperm count.

LONG-TERM COMPLICATIONS OF RADIOIODINE THERAPY FOR DIFFERENTIATED THYROID CANCER

Long-term side effects of ^{131}I therapy – apart from sialadenitis and xerostomia – are remarkably few. In patients with widespread lung metastases – particularly those with miliary metastases – caution must be taken in determining the dose to be administered in view of the risk of radiation fibrosis [63].

Leukaemia has been reported as a complication in patients receiving aggressive therapy with total administered doses exceeding 1 Ci with intervals of less than 6 months between treatments [55,63].

Cancer of the bladder is a theoretical long-term complication of ^{131}I radioiodine therapy given the radiation doses to the bladder in the early phases of treatment. Few reports of cases of cancer of the bladder have been made, although Edmonds and Smith [63] describe cases in patients who have received a cumulative dose of over 1 Ci. In patients with evidence of lymph node involvement at the time of initial surgery, external beam radiotherapy may be used in the post-operative period; this is recommended in those who have received over 1 Ci of administered radiation. Hall *et al.* [64], using the Swedish Cancer Registry, have followed a large cohort of patients with cancer of the thyroid treated with ^{131}I radioiodine, but have failed to show any long-term increase in incidence of solid tumours (including bladder tumours).

USE OF ADJUNCTIVE EXTERNAL BEAM RADIOTHERAPY

Patients who are found to have tumour spread to cervical lymph nodes at the time of primary surgery may be considered for external beam radiotherapy following surgery as an adjunct to ^{131}I radioiodine therapy. It is optimal to undertake ^{131}I radioiodine treatment before external beam therapy to avoid radiation damage to thyroid remnant and residual thyroid tumour cells which may reduce the efficacy of the radioiodine dose.

CONCLUSION

[131]I radioiodine remains the most frequently used form of radionuclide therapy with its clearly defined role in both benign and malignant disease. With 40 years of experience of use it has been shown to be safe and effective and the theoretical risks of tumour induction and chromosomal damage have not been demonstrated in practice.

Many of the lessons learned from the experience with ^{131}I radioiodine are now proving useful as new radionuclide therapies are developed and integrated into routine management.

REFERENCES

1. Williams, R.H., Tovery, B.T. and Jaffe, H. (1949) Radiotherapies. *Am. J. Med.*, **7**, 702–4.
2. Varma, V.M., Beierwaltes, W.H., Notal, M., Nishiyama, R. and Copp, J.E. (1970) Treatment of thyroid cancer. *JAMA*, **214**, 1437–42.
3. Safran, M., Paul, T.L., Roti, E. and Braverman, L.E. (1987) Environmental factors affecting autoimmune thyroid disease. *Endocrinol. Metab. Clin. North Am.*, **16**, 327–42.
4. Boucher, C.A., Bemard, B.F., Zhang, Z.G., Salvin, M., Rodien, P., Triller, H. and Wall, J.R. (1992) Nature and significance of orbital autoantigens and their autoantibodies in thyroid associated ophthalmopathy. *Autoimmunity*, **13**, 89–93.
5. Allanic, H., Fauchet, R. and Orgiazzi, A. (1990) Antithyroid drugs and Graves' disease: a prospective randomised evaluation of the efficacy of treatment duration. *J. Clin. Endocrinol. Metab.*, **70**, 675–9.
6. Klein, I., Becker, D.V. and Levey, G.S. (1994) Treatment of thyroid disease. *Ann. Intern. Med.*, **121**, 281–8.

7. Lazarus, J.H., Clarke, S.E.M., Franklyn, J.A. and Harding, L.K. (1995) *Guidelines – the use of radioiodine in the management of hyperthyroidism. The radioiodine audit subcommittee of the Royal College of Physicians Committee on Diabetes and Endocrinology and the Research Unit of the Royal College of Physicians.* Chameleon Press Ltd, London.

8. Subcommittee for the study of endemic goitre and iodine deficiency of the European Thyroid Association (1985) Goitre and iodine deficiency in Europe. *Lancet*, **i**, 1290.

9. Wartofsky, L., Glinoer, D., Solomon, B., Nagataki, S., Lagasse, R., Nagayama, Y. and Izumi, M. (1991) Differences and similarities in the diagnosis and treatment of Graves' disease in Europe, Japan and the United States. *Thyroid*, **1**, 129–35.

10. Hayek, A., Chapman, E.M. and Crawford, J.D. (1970) Long term results of treatment of thyrotoxicosis in children and adolescents with radioactive iodine. *N. Engl. J. Med.*, **283**, 949–53.

11. Sarkar, S.D., Beierwaltes, W.H., Gill, S.P. and Contey, B.J. (1976) Subsequent fertility and birth histories of children and adolescents treated with 131Iodine for thyroid cancer. *J. Nucl. Med.*, **17**, 460–4.

12. Bacon, G.E. and Laury, G.H. (1965) Experience with surgical treatment of thyrotoxicosis in children. *J. Pediatr.*, **67**, 1–5.

13. Ching, T., Warden, M.J. and Hefferman, R.A. (1977) Thyroid surgery in children and teenagers. *Arch. Otolaryngol.*, **103**, 544–6.

14. Schicha, H. and Scheidhauer, K. (1993) Radioiodine therapy in Europe – a survey. *Nuklearmedizin*, **32**, 321–4.

15. Kusakabe, K. and Maki, M. (1993) Radionuclide therapy of thyroid disease radioactive iodine therapy. *Japn. J. Nucl. Med.*, **30**, 813–19.

16. Mithal, A., Shah, A. and Kumar, S. (1993) The management of Graves' disease by Indian thyroidologists. *Nat. Med. J. India*, **6**, 163–6.

17. Kuma, K., Matsuzuka, F., Kobayashi, A., Hirai, K., Fukata, S., Tamai, H., Miyauci, A. and Sugawara, M. (1991) Natural course of Graves' disease after subtotal thyroidectomy and management of patients with postoperative thyroid dysfunction. *Am. J. Med. Sci.*, **302**, 8–12.

18. Singer, P.A., Cooper, D.S., Levy, E.G., Ladenson, P.W., Braverman, L.E., Daniels, G., Greenspan, F.S., McDougall, I.R. and Nikolai, T.F. (1995) Treatment guidelines for patients with hyperthyroidism and hypothyroidism. Standards of care committee. American Thyroid Association. *JAMA*, **273**, 808–12.

19. Thompson, W.H. and Harding, L.K. (1991) Radiation protection issues associated with nuclear medicine outpatients. *Nucl. Med. Commun.*, **16**, 879–92.

20. Shapiro, B. (1993) Optimization of radioiodine therapy: what have we learnt after 50 years. *J. Nucl. Med.*, **34**, 1638–41.

21. Bokisch, A., Jamitzy, T., Derwantz, R. and Biersack, H.J. (1994) Optimized dose planning of radioiodine therapy of benign thyroidal diseases. *J. Nucl. Med.*, **34**, 1632–8.

22. Tsuruta, M., Nagayama, Y., Izumi, M. and Nagataki, S. (1993) Long term follow-up studies on Iodine-131 treatment of hyperthyroid Graves' disease based on the measurement of thyroid volume by ultrasonography. *Ann. Intern. Med.*, **7**, 193–7.

23. Flower, M.A., al-Saadi, D., Harmer, C.L., McCready, V.R. and Ott, R.J. (1994) Dose response study on thyrotoxic patients undergoing positron emission tomography and radioiodine therapy. *Eur. J. Nucl. Med.*, **21**, 531–6.

24. Willemsen, U.F., Knesewitsch, P., Kreisig, T., Pickardt, C.R. and Kirsch, C.M. (1993) Functional results of radioiodine therapy with a 300 Gy absorbed dose in Graves' disease. *Eur. J. Nucl. Med.*, **20**, 1050–5.

25. Kinser, J.A., Roesler, H., Furrer, T., Grutter, D. and Zimmerman, H. (1989) Nonimmunogenic hyperthyroidism: incidence after radioiodine and surgical treatment. *J. Nucl. Med.*, **30**, 1960–5.

26. Hardisty, C.A., Jones, S.J., Hedley, A.J., Munro, D.S., Bewsher, P.D. and Weir, R.D. (1990) Clinical outcome and costs of care in radioiodine treatment of hyperthyroidism. *J. R. Coll. Physicians*, **24**, 36–42.

27. Johnson, J.K. (1993) Outcome of treating thyrotoxic patients with a standard dose of radioactive iodine. *Scottish Med. J.*, **38**, 142–4.

28. Kendall-Taylor, P., Keir, M. and Ross, W.M. (1984) Ablative radioiodine therapy for hyperthyroidism: long term follow up study. *Br. Med. J.*, **289**, 361–3.

29. Becker, D.R. (1982) Radioactive Iodine in the treatment of hyperthyroidism, in *Thyroid Disease* (ed. C. Beckers), Pergamon Press, Paris, pp. 145–8.

30. Ng Tang Fui, S.C. and Maisey, M.N. (1979) Standard dose of 131-Iodine therapy for hyperthyroidism caused by autonomously functioning thyroid nodules. *Clin. Endocrinol.*, **10**, 69–77.

31. Catz, B. and Tsao, J. (1965) Total 131-I thyroid remnant ablation for pretibial myxoedema. *Clin. Res.*, **13**, 130–2.

32. Hamilton, R., Mayberry, W., McConahey, W. and Hanson, K. (1967) Ophthalmopathy of Graves' disease: a comparison between patients treated surgically and patients treated with radioiodine. *Mayo Clin. Proc.*, **42**, 812–18.

33. Peququequat, E., Mayberry, W., McConahey, W. and Wyse, E. (1967) Large doses of radioiodine in Graves' disease: effect on ophthalmopathy and long acting thyroid stimulator. *Mayo Clin. Proc.*, **42**, 802–11.

34. Jones, D., Munro, D. and Wilson, G. (1969) Observations on the cause of exophthalmos after 131-Iodine therapy. *Proc. R. Soc. Med.*, **52**, 15–18.

35. Tallstedt, L., Lundell, G., Blomgren, H. and Bring, J. (1994) Does early administration of thyroxine reduce the development of Graves' ophthalmopathy after radioiodine treatment. *Eur. J. Nucl. Med.*, **130**, 494–7.

36. Wesche, M.F., Tie-v-Buul, M.M., Smits, N.J. and Wiersinga, W.M. (1995) Reduction in goiter size by 131I therapy in patients with non-toxic multinodular goitre. *Eur. J. Endocrinol.*, **132**, 86–7.

37. Huysmanns, D.A., Hermus, A.R., Corstens, F.H., Barentsz, J.O. and Kloppenborg, P.W. (1994) Large

compressive goiters treated with radioiodine. *Ann. Intern. Med.*, **121**, 757–62.

38. Nygaards, B., Hegedus, L., Gervil, M., Hjalgrim, H., Soe-Jensen, P. and Hansen, J.M. (1993) Radioiodine treatment of multinodular nontoxic goitre. *Br. Med. J.*, **307**, 828–32.

39. Beierwaltes, W.H. (1987) Carcinoma of the thyroid. Radionuclide diagnosis, therapy and follow-up. *Clin. Oncol.*, **5**, 23–7.

40. Mazzaferri, E.L. (1987) Papillary thyroid carcinoma: factors influencing prognosis and current therapy. *Semin. Oncol.*, **14**, 315–32.

41. Tubiana, M. (1985) Long term results and prognostic factors with differentiated thyroid carcinoma. *Cancer*, **55**, 794–804.

42. McConahey, W.M. (1986) Papillary thyroid cancer treated at the Mayo Clinic, 1946 through 1970: initial manifestations, pathologic findings, therapy and outcome. *Mayo Clin. Proc.*, **61**, 978–96.

43. Tubiana, M. (1982) Thyroid cancer, in *Thyroid Diseases* (ed. C. Beckers), Pergamon Press, Paris, pp. 182–227.

44. Jeevanram, R.K., Shah, D.H., Sharma, S.M. and Ganatra, R.D. (1986) Influence of initial large dose on subsequent uptake of therapeutic radioiodine in thyroid cancer patients. *Nucl. Med. Biol.*, **13**, 277–9.

45. Park, J.M. (1992) Stunned thyroid after high dose 131-I imaging. *Clin. Nucl. Med.*, **17**, 501–2.

46. Park, H.M., Perkins, O.W., Edmonson, J.W., Schnute, R.B. and Manatunga, A. (1994) Influence of diagnostic radioiodines on the uptake of ablative doses of iodine131. *Thyroid*, **4**, 49–54.

47. de Groot, L.J. and Reilly, M. (1982) Comparison of 30 and 50 mCi doses for 131-Iodine ablation. *Ann. Intern. Med.*, **96**, 51–2.

48. Arad, E., Flannery, K., Wilson, G. and O'Mara, R. (1990) Fractionated doses of radioiodine ablation of post surgical thyroid tissue remnants. *Clin. Nucl. Med.*, **16**, 676–7.

49. Kuni, C.C. and Klingensmith, W.C. (1980) Failure of low doses of ^{131}I to ablate residual thyroid tissue following surgery for thyroid cancer. *Radiology*, **137**, 773–4.

50. Braverman, L.E., Pratt, B.M., Ebner, S. and Longcope, C. (1992) Recombinant human thyrotropin stimulates thyroid function and radioactive iodine uptake in Rhesus monkeys. *J. Clin. Endocrinol. Metab.*, **74**, 1135–9.

51. Sherman, S.I., Tielens, E.T., Sostre, S., Wharam, M.D. Jr and Ladenson, P.W. (1994) Clinical utility of post-treatment scans in the management of patients with thyroid carcinoma. *J. Clin. Endocrinol. Metab.*, **78**, 629–34.

52. Schlumberger, M. (1988) Detection and treatment of lung metastases of differentiated thyroid cancer in patients with normal chest X-rays. *J. Nucl. Med.*, **29**, 1790–4.

53. Fruhling, J. (1994) Role of radioactive iodine in the treatment of differentiated thyroid cancer: physiopathological basis, results, considerations from the viewpoint of radioprotection. *Bull. Mem. Acad. R. Med. Belg.*, **149**, 192–206.

54. Maxon, H.R., Thomas, S.R. and Hertzberg, V.S. (1983) Relation between effective radiation dose and outcome of radioiodine therapy for thyroid cancer. *N. Engl. J. Med.*, **309**, 937–41.

55. Benua, R.S., Cieale, N.R. and Sonenberg, M. (1962) The relation of radioiodine dose to results and complications in the treatment of metastatic thyroid cancer. *Am. J. Roentgenol. Radiat. Ther. Nucl. Med.*, **87**, 171–82.

56. Leeper, R.D. and Shimaoka, K. (1980) Treatment of metastatic thyroid cancer. *Clin. Endocrinol. Metab.*, **9**, 383–404.

57. Kosal, K.F., Adler, S.F., Carey, J. and Beierwaltes, W. (1986) Iodine 131 treatment of thyroid cancer: absorbed dose calculated from post therapy scans. *J. Nucl. Med.*, **27**, 1207–11.

58. O'Connell, M.E., Flower, M.A., Hinton, P.J., Harmer, C.L. and McCready, V.R. (1993) Radiation dose assessment in radioiodine therapy. Dose–response relationships in differentiated thyroid cancer using quantitative scanning and PET. *Radiother. Oncol.*, **28**, 16–26.

59. Coburn, M., Teates, D. and Wanebo, H.J. (1994) Recurrent thyroid cancer. Role of surgery versus radioactive iodine *Ann. Surg.*, **219**, 587–93.

60. McCleod, M.K. and Thompson, W.T. (1990) Hurthle cell neoplasms of the thyroid. *Otolaryngol. Clin. North Am.*, **23**, 441–52.

61. Becciolini, A., Porciani, S., Lanini, A., Benucci, A., Castagnoli, A. and Pupi, A. (1994) Serum amylase and tissue polypeptide antigen as biochemical indicators of salivary gland injury during iodine–131 therapy. *Eur. J. Nucl. Med.*, **21**, 1121–5.

62. Pacini, F., Gasperi, M., Fugazzola, L., Cecearelli, C., Lippi, F., Centoni, R., Martino, E. and Pinehera, A. (1994) Testicular function in patients with differentiated thyroid carcinoma treated with radioiodine. *J. Nucl. Med.*, **35**, 1418–22.

63. Edmonds, C. and Smith, T. (1986) The long term hazards of treatment of thyroid cancer with radioiodine. *Br. J. Radiol.*, **59**, 45–51.

64. Hall, P., Holm, L.E. and Lundell, G.E. (1992) Cancer risks in thyroid cancer patients. *Br. J. Cancer*, **64**, 159–63.

Neuro-ectodermal tumours

C.A. Hoefnagel

INTRODUCTION

Since its first reported use in humans in 1981 [1], ^{131}I-meta-iodobenzylguanidine (MIBG) has been used with success for the scintigraphic diagnosis of a variety of neuroendocrine tumours [2]. Derived from the neural crest, many of these tumours maintain the characteristic features of these cells, such as an active uptake-1 mechanism at the cell membrane and neurosecretory storage granules in the cytoplasm, which are responsible for the specific uptake and retention of MIBG.

In comparison with antibodies and peptides that target cell membrane receptors, ^{131}I-MIBG – being a much smaller molecule – is concentrated intracellularly. The chemical structure of MIBG contains the benzyl group of bretylium and the guanidine group of guanethidine, and resembles products secreted by these tumours, such as catecholamines and serotonin.

In diagnostic scintigraphy, both ^{123}I-MIBG and ^{131}I-MIBG are sensitive and specific indicators of phaeochromocytoma, neuroblastoma and paraganglioma; this has led to the therapeutic use of ^{131}I-MIBG in these conditions. As the sensitivity for carcinoid and medullary thyroid carcinoma is lower, fewer of these patients can be treated. The basis for successful treatment is a high and selective tumour uptake with prolonged retention of MIBG. As a systemic treatment, ^{131}I-MIBG therapy will be directed at both the primary tumour and its distant metastases.

INDICATIONS AND PROCEDURAL ASPECTS

Any malignant neural crest tumour showing sufficient uptake and retention of ^{131}I-MIBG on a diagnostic tracer study is a candidate for ^{131}I-MIBG therapy. Apart from ^{131}I-MIBG concentration, the availability and feasibility of other treatment modalities and the patient's condition determines the indication. The principal indications for ^{131}I-MIBG therapy are malignant phaeochromocytoma, neuroblastoma (stages III and IV), malignant paraganglioma, medullary thyroid carcinoma, and symptomatic metastatic carcinoid tumours.

Contraindications to ^{131}I-MIBG therapy include pregnancy, breast-feeding, myelosuppression and renal failure. In addition, a relative contraindication is an unstable clinical condition of the patient, which does not allow isolation therapy.

Table 1.6 shows a checklist for preparation of patients for ^{131}I-MIBG therapy. Apart from assessing the various parameters regarding the extent of disease, the tumour response, and side effects, one must pay attention to the medication the patient is using, as many drugs are known or may be expected to interfere with the uptake and/or retention of ^{131}I-MIBG by the tumour [3]. Harvesting of bone marrow before ^{131}I-MIBG therapy may be considered, particularly in children with neuroblastoma and adults with extensive skeletal metastases. To protect the thyroid from uptake of free ^{131}I-iodide, 100–200 mg of potassium iodide (KI) is given orally daily.

An adequate infusion line must be in place, through which a fixed dose of 3.7–11.1 GBq of ^{131}I-MIBG with a high specific activity (up to 1.48 GBq/mg) is administered over a 1- to 4-hour period using a lead-shielded infusion pump [4]. An alternative approach is to administer a varying dose that has been assessed by a prior tracer study and aims for the maximal acceptable dose of 2 Gy to the bone marrow [5]. The treatment may be repeated at not less than 4-weekly intervals. To prevent acute effects from excess catecholamines in circulation, during or shortly after ^{131}I-MIBG infusion, administration of dibenzylene (α-blockade) and/or propranolol (β-blockade) may be indicated.

Patients may need to be isolated in compliance with local legislation, and encouraged to drink large volumes of fluid. Isolation may present practical difficulties when treating young children. Problems can be minimized by parents or other relatives becoming involved in their child's care, which, after proper instruction in issues of radiation protection, is both feasible and safe [6].

Before the administration of a therapeutic dose, quality control of ^{131}I-MIBG may be desirable by checking the radionuclide and radiochemical purity, as impurities will not contribute to tumour

Clinical Nuclear Medicine, 3rd edn. Edited by M.N. Maisey, K.E. Britton and B.D. Collier. Published in 1998 by Chapman & Hall, London. ISBN 0 412 75180 1

Table 1.6   Checklist for the preparation of a patient for therapy using ^{131}I-metaiodobenzylguanidine (MIBG)

- determination of the extent of disease (staging)
- identify volumetric and biochemical parameters (follow-up)
- blood counts, renal function, bone marrow condition (safety)
- stop any medication interfering with MIBG uptake/ retention
- if necessary, use propranolol and dibenzylene
- instruct patient in issues of radiation protection
- thyroid blockade: 100–200 mg KI orally daily for 2 weeks, starting 1 day before treatment
- install an adequate intravenous infusion line
- encourage the patient to drink large volumes of fluid
- for children: instruct parents involved in the patient care
- harvesting of bone marrow may be considered

targeting, and may add to the side effects of the treatment. High doses of ^{131}I-MIBG with a high specific activity are liable to autoradiolysis, which is dependent on the temperature, the volume, and stabilizing agents in the formulation [7].

CLINICAL APPLICATIONS

PHAEOCHROMOCYTOMA

Phaeochromocytoma is a tumour arising from chromaffin cells of the sympathoadrenal system. Approximately 85% are located in the adrenal medulla. Extra-adrenal primary tumours arising from the sympathetic paraganglia may be referred to as paragangliomas. Although only 10% of phaeochromocytomas are malignant, a higher percentage of malignancies may be found in tumours at extra-adrenal sites, or in those originating in childhood.

The clinical manifestations of phaeochromocytoma are highly variable and governed by the se-

cretion of catecholamines (dopamine, adrenaline and noradrenaline) by the tumour. The diagnosis may be suspected from clinical symptomatology, confirmed by biochemical measurements of increased levels of catecholamines and catecholamine metabolites in plasma and urine, and located by diagnostic imaging (CT, MRI and/or MIBG scintigraphy) [8].

Malignant phaeochromocytoma is a rare but ominous disease: the symptoms may be severe as a result of secretion of excess catecholamines, and the prognosis poor due to the occurrence of widespread metastases to lymph nodes, liver, lungs and bones.

Surgical resection is the treatment of choice. Inoperable or disseminated tumours may be treated symptomatically by α-methyltyrosine, interfering with the catecholamine synthesis, or by blocking the adrenergic effects with phenoxybenzamine (α-blockade) and propranolol (β-blockade), but none of these agents has any anti-tumour effect.

External beam radiotherapy has little value, other than local control of painful bone metastases, although objective remissions have been described. Combination chemotherapy is also of limited use and is associated with toxicity.

As more than 90% of phaeochromocytomas concentrate MIBG, therapeutic doses of ^{131}I-MIBG have been used to manage this condition since 1984 [9]. Although the main aim of this treatment is to attain objective tumour regression (Figure 1.10), other, more realistic goals are tumour arrest, reduction of the tumour function and palliation of symptoms such as hypertension, palpitations, sweating and bone pain.

In 1991, the results of ^{131}I-MIBG therapy in 117 patients treated in 14 centres world-wide were pooled [10]. A clinical response was defined as a >50% decrease in catecholamine excretion, a >50% reduction of the tumour volume, or significant

Table 1.7   Effect of ^{131}I-MIBG therapy on blood pressure and medication needs in a patient with malignant phaeochromocytoma (images shown in Figure 1.11)

Therapy	Blood pressure (mmHg)	Dibenzylene (α) (mg)	Propranolol (β) (mg)
MIBG nr 1	260/150	3 × 20	3 × 40
MIBG nr 2	95/65	3 × 20	2 × 40
MIBG nr 3	120/80	1 × 10	2 × 20
MIBG nr 4	140/95	1 × 10	None

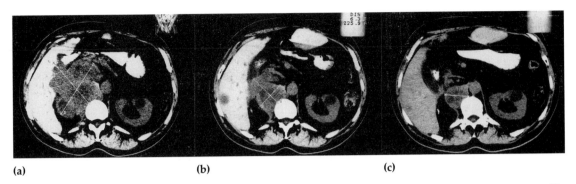

(a)   (b)   (c)

Figure 1.10 Objective partial remission of malignant phaeochromocytoma, metastatic to liver and lungs, by ^{131}I-MIBG therapy. Computed tomography showing the size of the abdominal tumour mass before (a), and after two (b) and four (c) consecutive treatments.

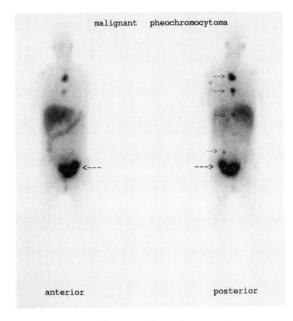

Figure 1.11 Malignant phaeochromocytoma metastatic to spinal and pelvic bones: ^{131}I-MIBG therapy, attaining only tumour arrest, leads to normalization of the blood pressure (Table 1.7), together with significant improvement of the patient's symptoms and condition.

scintigraphic improvement if lesions could not be measured. According to these criteria the overall response rate was 56%. Soft tissue metastases were found to respond better than skeletal metastases. In addition, subjective improvement of symptoms, decrease of blood pressure and pain relief were achieved in more than 60% of the patients (Figure 1.11; Table 1.7). For a widespread meta-

static disease, known to be either poorly or non-responsive to other treatment modalities, palliation and control of tumour function by ^{131}I-MIBG therapy may be clinically very beneficial. The therapy is non-invasive and minimal side effects have been observed.

PARAGANGLIOMA

Although there are only few reports in the literature which specifically describe ^{131}I-MIBG therapy of malignant paraganglioma, it is worthwhile to note that in most of these reports objective partial remission, pain relief and a dramatic improvement in the quality of life have been observed (Figure 1.12) [11].

NEUROBLASTOMA

Neuroblastoma is a malignant tumour of the sympathetic nervous system, occurring most frequently in children. Although most neuroblastomas arise from the adrenal gland and the abdominal sympathetic side-chain, the primary tumour may be located in the cervical or thoracic side-chain, or in the pelvis. Localized disease without distant metastases (TNM stages I and II) is treated by surgical excision and has a good prognosis; metastases to lymph nodes and other organs (TNM stages III–V) are correlated with a poor prognosis, and are treated by combination chemotherapy preceding surgery for the primary tumour. This is followed by post-operative chemotherapy, sometimes including high-dose chemotherapy (requiring autologous or allogeneic bone-marrow transplantation). Radiation therapy

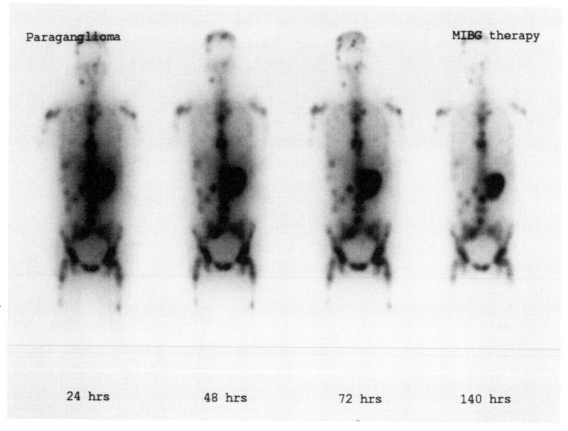

Paraganglioma   MIBG therapy

24 hrs   48 hrs   72 hrs   140 hrs

Figure 1.12   ^{131}I-MIBG therapy of malignant paraganglioma, metastatic to the liver and bone marrow, showing intense concentration and prolonged retention of ^{131}I-MIBG. The treatment led to a partial remission and significant improvement in the quality of life, despite myelotoxicity.

may be added [12]. This treatment regimen is characterized by a high initial response rate (up to 80% objective response), but most of the children relapse during or after treatment. This may be due to drug-resistance and/or unfavourable prognostic factors. Despite the combination of therapies, the 5-year survival rate remains only 10–20%. New approaches to the diagnosis and therapy of neuroblastoma include targeting of radionuclides via the immunological (monoclonal antibodies) and metabolic (MIBG) routes.

Pooled results of ^{131}I-MIBG therapy in a total of 273 neuroblastoma patients (predominantly children) reported by Troncone and Galli [10] indicate an overall objective response rate of 35%. Most of these patients had stage IV, progressive and intensely pre-treated disease, and ^{131}I-MIBG therapy

was instituted after other treatment modalities had failed. Nevertheless, in many children ^{131}I-MIBG therapy provided valuable palliation and improved the quality of life, and in contrast to combination chemotherapy had the advantage of being non-invasive.

In general, both the MIBG treatment and the isolation are well tolerated by children; haematological side effects may occur, predominantly as an isolated thrombocytopenia, which may be partly due to the radiation dose to the bone marrow, but may also be explained by selective uptake of ^{131}I-MIBG into the thrombocytes and megakaryocytes [13]. In patients with bone marrow involvement, MIBG therapy following chemotherapy should be utilized with care, as severe myelosuppression may occur [14].

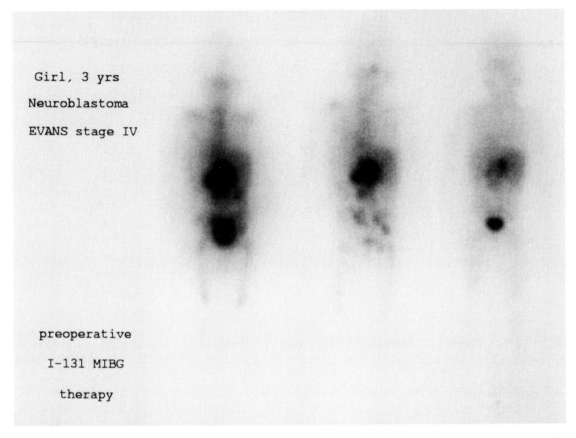

Girl, 3 yrs

Neuroblastoma

EVANS stage IV

preoperative

I-131 MIBG

therapy

Figure 1.13 ^{131}I-MIBG therapy at diagnosis in a 3-year-old girl with abdominal neuroblastoma metastatic to the bone marrow. Three consecutive treatments at 4-weekly intervals led to significant reduction of metastases and the tumour volume, enabling successful surgical resection.

Based on the observed response to ^{131}I-MIBG therapy in advanced neuroblastoma after conventional therapy and the non-invasiveness of this therapeutic modality, ^{131}I-MIBG is now integrated in the treatment protocol instead of pre-operative chemotherapy in children presenting with advanced disease/inoperable neuroblastoma. The objective is to reduce the tumour volume, enabling adequate surgical resection, and to avoid toxicity and the induction of early drug resistance. Chemotherapy is reserved for treating minimal residual disease post-operatively.

Initial results of pre-operative ^{131}I-MIBG therapy in 31 children demonstrated the feasibility and effectiveness of this approach: 19 of 27 evaluable patients (70%) had complete or >95% resection of the primary tumour or did not require surgery at all (Figure 1.13); only 11 patients developed isolated thrombocytopenia and moderate myelosuppression occurred in only two cases, despite the fact that the bone marrow was invaded in 16 patients [15]. As time progresses, survival statistics are emerging: the survival is 66% at 1 year, 53% at 2 years, 40% at 3 and 4 years, and 6/16 patients have survived more than 5 years.

MEDULLARY THYROID CARCINOMA

Medullary thyroid carcinoma (MTC) is a tumour of the C-cells, previously named parafollicular cells, which are derived from the neural crest. The incidence is 4–10% of all thyroid tumours, and in approximately 25% of the cases, the tumour occurs in a hereditary, familial form, in association with

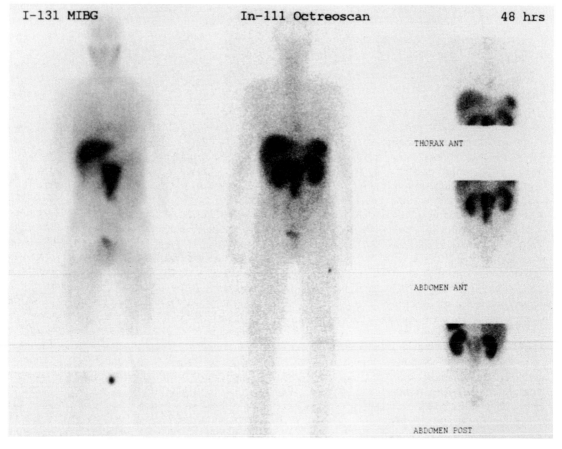

Figure 1.14   Comparative imaging using ^{131}I-MIBG (left) and ^{111}In-pentetreotide (right) of a carcinoid tumour in the upper median abdomen. Because of its more favourable biodistribution, ^{131}I-MIBG is preferred for radionuclide therapy.

other endocrine tumours (MEN type II syndrome) [16]. MTC produces calcitonin, the serum levels of which as well as those of carcinoembryonic antigen (CEA) serve as sensitive indicators of disease.

Unlike papillary and follicular thyroid carcinoma, MTC does not concentrate ^{131}I as iodide. Further, as only 30–35% of MTC concentrate ^{131}I-MIBG, diagnostic scintigraphy using ^{99m}Tc-pentavalent DMSA, ^{201}Tl-chloride and ^{111}In-pentetreotide are preferred for the locating of disease [2].

Radical surgical resection is the only curative treatment. For inoperable, recurrent and metastatic disease, local external beam radiotherapy may be helpful for disease in the neck and for painful bone metastases. The results of combination chemotherapy are disappointing. Octreotide can inhibit calcitonin secretion, giving symptomatic relief, but has no anti-tumour effect. In patients who show sufficient tumour uptake, radionuclide therapy using ^{131}I-labelled anti-CEA monoclonal antibody or MIBG may be palliative and might induce tumour regression.

A review of 22 reported cases of MTC treated with ^{131}I-MIBG reported an objective response rate of 38% and palliation in 50% of the patients [10]. Taking into account that only two patients showed complete remission, and partial remission was attained in one patient with an integrated treatment protocol involving surgery, ^{131}I ablation, radiotherapy and ^{131}I-MIBG therapy, the objective response appears to be limited, but it must be emphasized that in these patients with severely limited therapeutic options, the palliation of symptoms may be a worthwhile therapeutic goal.

CARCINOID

Carcinoid tumours arise from the enterochromaffin cells and account for 2% of gastrointestinal malignancies. Although the primary tumour may be located in the foregut, most carcinoids occur in the appendix, small intestine and rectum, and secrete a number of neuropeptides. Serotonin and its metabolite 5-hydroxy-indoleacetic acid (5-HIAA) are measured as tumour markers, and may give rise to the carcinoid syndrome of diarrhoea, flushing, bronchoconstriction and cardiac valvular abnormalities [17].

As ^{111}In-pentetreotide scintigraphy has a higher sensitivity (86%) than ^{131}I-MIBG (60–70%), it is preferred for diagnostic imaging, particularly when complemented by CT scanning [2]. Surgical resection is the best treatment for localized disease, and partial liver resection can be performed when liver metastases are confined to one lobe. Other palliative treatment modalities are hepatic artery embolization, octreotide therapy and α-interferon; results of external beam radiotherapy and combination chemotherapy are poor.

As more than 60% of carcinoids concentrate ^{131}I-MIBG, therapeutic doses may be administered for palliative treatment of symptomatic, metastatic disease (Figure 1.14). Cumulative results in 52 carcinoid patients showed an objective response rate of only 19%, but palliation was observed in 65% of all patients [10]. The palliative effect associated with a relative lack of objective response may be explained by observations that carcinoid liver metastases may present both as hot and cold lesions; ^{131}I-MIBG concentrates exclusively in the metabolically active metastases that are responsible for the patient's symptoms.

More recent results of ^{131}I-MIBG therapy at The Netherlands Cancer Institute in 30 patients with symptomatic, metastatic carcinoid showed no objective regression of tumours, but a symptomatic response with a mean duration of 8 months (range 2–24 months) in 60% of the cases, without significant side effects [18]. In carcinoid tumours not qualifying for ^{131}I-MIBG therapy because of insufficient tumour uptake, palliative treatment with high doses of unlabelled MIBG have reported to be beneficial in 60% of the cases (mean duration 4.5 months).

NEW DEVELOPMENTS

New applications of MIBG therapy include the use of other labels for MIBG such as ^{125}I-MIBG and [211]At-MABG. Because of their ultrashort pathway these radiopharmaceuticals may be of use in the treatment of minimal residual disease and bone marrow involvement, for which ^{131}I-MIBG is often myelotoxic [19,20].

The tumour targeting may be enhanced by administration of ^{131}I-MIBG by alternative routes, e.g. intra-arterially. By increasing the specific activity it is attempted to improve tumour uptake. A recent advance is the production of non-carrier-added MIBG [21]. However, from animal studies and experience with MIBG therapy in humans, it follows that the optimal specific activity may vary with the tumour type. Excess of unlabelled MIBG was found to decrease ^{125}I-MIBG uptake in PC12 phaeochromocytoma xenografts in nude mice, as well as in most normal tissues, but not to influence the uptake in SK-N-SH neuroblastoma [22], and in patients with carcinoid liver metastases increased ^{131}I-MIBG tumour/non-tumour ratios have been observed after treatment with unlabelled MIBG [18].

The therapeutic index may also be improved by a variety of pharmacological interventions aimed at increasing the uptake and retention of ^{131}I-MIBG, including induction of tumour cell differentiation (e.g. by retinoic acid or interferon), prolonging tumour retention time (e.g. by calcium-channel blockers) [23], and blockade of extra-tumoral specific uptake (e.g. by unlabelled MIBG or serotonin) or delaying its renal excretion.

By using the additive effects of other modalities, an attempt is made to enhance the anti-tumour effect, e.g. by combining ^{131}I-MIBG therapy with oxygen under hyperbaric conditions [24]. The response to ^{131}I-MIBG can be optimized by introducing it early on in an integrated protocol of tumour therapy with curative intent, as for neuroblastoma [15].

REFERENCES

1. Sisson, J.C., Frager, M.S., Valk, T.W. *et al.* (1981) Scintigraphic localization of pheochromocytoma. *N. Engl. J. Med.*, **305**, 12–17.

2. Hoefnagel, C.A. (1994) Metaiodobenzylguanidine and somatostatin in oncology: role in the management of neural crest tumours. *Eur. J. Nucl. Med.*, **21**, 561–81.

3. Khafagi, F.A., Shapiro, B., Fig, L.M. *et al.* (1989) Labetalol reduces iodine-131 MIBG uptake by pheochromocytoma and normal tissues. *J. Nucl. Med.*, **30**, 481–9.

4. Hoefnagel, C.A., Voûte, P.A., de Kraker, J. *et al.* (1987) Radionuclide diagnosis and therapy of neural crest tumors using Iodine-131 metaiodobenzylguanidine. *J. Nucl. Med.*, **28**, 308–14.

5. Lashford, L.S. Lewis, I.J., Fielding, S.L. *et al.* (1992) Phase I/II study of Iodine 131 metaiodobenzylguanidine in chemoresistant neuroblastoma: a United Kingdom Children's Cancer Study Group investigation. *J. Clin. Oncol.*, **10**, 1889–96.

6. Van der Steen, J., Maessen, H.J.M., Hoefnagel, C.A. *et al.* (1986) Radiation protection during treatment of children with ^{131}I-meta-iodobenzylguanidine. *Health Physics*, **50**, 515–22.

7. Wafelman, A.R., Suchi, R., Hoefnagel, C.A. *et al.* (1993) Radiochemical purity of ^{131}I-MIBG infusion fluids: a report from the clinical practice. *Eur. J. Nucl. Med.*, **20**, 614–16.

8. Bravo, E.L., Gifford, R.W. and Manger, W.M. (1993) Adrenal medullary tumors: pheochromocytoma, in *Endocrine Tumors* (eds L. Mazzaferri and N.A. Samaan), Blackwell, Oxford, pp. 426–47.

9. Sisson, J.C., Shapiro, B., Beierwaltes, W.H. *et al.* (1984) Radiopharmaceutical treatment of malignant pheochromocytoma. *J. Nucl. Med.*, **24**, 197–206.

10. Troncone, L. and Galli, G. (1991) Proceedings International Workshop on the role of [^{131}I]-metaiodobenzylguanidine in the treatment of neural crest tumors. *J. Nucl. Biol. Med.*, 35, 177–362.

11. Baulieu, J.-L., Guilloteau, D., Baulieu, F. *et al.* (1988) Therapeutic effectiveness of Iodine-131 MIBG metastases of a nonsecreting paraganglioma. *J. Nucl. Med.*, 29, 2008–13.

12. Voûte, P.A., de Kraker, J. and Hoefnagel, C.A. (1992) Tumours of the sympathetic nervous system. Neuroblastoma, ganglioneuroma and phaeochromocytoma, in *Cancer in children: Clinical management* (eds P.A. Voûte, A. Barrett and J. Lemerle), Springer, Berlin, pp. 226–43.

13. Rutgers, M., Tytgat, G.A.M., Verwijs-Janssen, M. *et al.* (1993) Uptake of the neuron-blocking agent meta-iodobenzylguanidine and serotonin by human platelets and neuroadrenergic tumour cells. *Int. J. Cancer*, **54**, 290–5.

14. Sisson, J.C., Hutchinson, R.J., Carey, J.E. *et al.* (1988) Toxicity from treatment of neuroblastoma with ^{131}I-meta-iodobenzylguanidine. *Eur. J. Nucl. Med.*, **14**, 337–40.

15. Hoefnagel, C.A., de Kraker, J., Valdés Olmos, R.A. *et al.* (1994) ^{131}I-MIBG as a first-line treatment in high-risk neuroblastoma patients. *Nucl. Med. Commun.*, **15**, 712–17.

16. Samaan, N.A., Ordóñez, N.G. and Hickey, R.C. (1993) Medullary thyroid carcinoma, in *Endocrine Tumors* (eds L. Mazzaferri and N.A. Samaan), Blackwell, Oxford, pp. 334–47.

17. Feldman, J.M. (1993) Carcinoid tumors, in *Endocrine Tumors* (eds L. Mazzaferri and N.A. Samaan), Blackwell, Oxford, pp. 700–22.

18. Taal, B.G., Hoefnagel, C.A., Valdés Olmos, R.A. *et al.* The palliative effect of metaiodobenzylguanidine (MIBG) in metastatic carcinoid tumors. *J. Clin. Oncol.*, **14**, 1829–38.

19. Sisson, J.C., Hutchinson, R.J., Shapiro, B. *et al.* (1990) Iodine-125-MIBG to treat neuroblastoma: preliminary report. *J. Nucl. Med.*, **31**, 1479–85.

20. Hoefnagel, C.A., Smets, L., Voûte, P.A. *et al.* (1991) Iodine-125-MIBG therapy for neuroblastoma. *J. Nucl. Med.*, **31**, 361–2.

21. Mairs, R.J., Russell, J., Cunningham, S. *et al.* (1995) Enhanced tumour uptake and in vitro radiotoxicity of no-carrier-added [^{131}I] metaiodobenzylguanidine: implications for the targeted radiotherapy of neuroblastoma. *Eur. J. Cancer*, **31A**, 576–81.

22. Rutgers, M., Buitenhuis, C.K.M. and Smets, L.A. Pre-dosing with MIBG to improve the relative neuroblastoma over normal tissue exposure of ^{131}I-MIBG in animal models. *Horm. Metab. Res.* (in press).

23. Blake, G.M., Lewington, V.J., Fleming, J.S. *et al.* (1988) Modification by nifedipine of ^{131}I metaiodobenzylguanidine kinetics in malignant phaeochromocytoma. *Eur. J. Nucl. Med.*, **14**, 345–8.

24. Voûte, P.A., van der Kleij, A.J., de Kraker, J. *et al.* (1995) Clinical experience with radiation enhancement by hyperbaric oxygen in children with recurrent neuroblastoma stage IV. *Eur. J. Cancer*, **31A**, 596–600.

FURTHER READING

Hoefnagel, C.A. (1989) *The Clinical Use of ^{131}I-meta-iodobenzylguanidine (MIBG) for the diagnosis and treatment of neural crest tumors.* Thesis, University of Amsterdam, ISBN 90-9003051-4.

Mazzaferri, L. and Samaan, N.A. (eds) (1993) *Endocrine Tumors*, Blackwell, Oxford.

Moertel, C.G. (1987) Karnofsky memorial lecture. An odyssey in the land of small tumors. *J. Clin. Oncol.*, **5**, 1502–22.

Troncone, L., Rufini, V., Montemaggi, P. *et al.* (1990) The diagnostic and therapeutic utility of radioiodinated metaiodobenzylguanidine (MIBG). 5 years experience. *Eur. J. Nucl. Med.*, **16**, 325–35.

Voûte, P.A., de Kraker, J. and Hoefnagel, C.A. (1992) Tumours of the sympathetic nervous system. Neuroblastoma, ganglioneuroma and phaeochromocytoma, in *Cancer in children: Clinical management* (eds P.A. Voûte, A. Barrett and J. Lemerle), Springer, Berlin, pp. 226–43.

Haematology

M. Pollycove

Phosphorus-32 has been used successfully to treat patients with polycythaemia vera (PV), since its introduction by John H. Lawrence in 1939 [1]. In more than 500 patients treated with ^{32}P, Lawrence, in 1955 [1] and Osgood, in 1965 [2] independently reported 13 years' mean survival after onset, with mean life spans of 70 years. Nevertheless, concern regarding induction of leukaemia by ^{32}P radiation was magnified by a review of the literature in 1965 [3]. The Polycythemia Vera Study Group (PVSG) was established in 1967 to determine the long-term complications and survival of patients in a prospective multicentric randomized clinical trial of phlebotomy, chlorambucil and ^{32}P therapy.

The initial protocol of the PVSG is shown in Figure 1.15 [4]. The median survival of chlorambucil-treated patients after entry into the study was 9 years. The incidence of acute leukaemia associated with chlorambucil therapy was 2.3 times greater than the comparable incidence in patients treated with ^{32}P [5]. Maximum PVSG follow-up of patients subsequently treated with hydroxyurea is 9 years, at which time the 8% incidence of acute leukaemia was approximately four times greater than the comparable incidence in patients treated with ^{32}P [5]. The median survival time of 11–12 years from PVSG clinical trial entry to death of patients treated with ^{32}P or with phlebotomy only, is comparable [4]. The incidence of acute leukaemia was approximately 1% in the phlebotomized patients and 8% in ^{32}P-treated patients. However, all patients receiving ^{32}P therapy experienced far fewer medical complications (thrombosis, fatigue, glossitis, cheilosis, etc.), fewer doctor visits, and a better quality of life than patients treated with phlebotomy [6]. Many haematologists regard phlebotomy as unacceptable for control of PV because of the 50% incidence of vascular accidents and the greater risk of early progression toward myelofibrosis with myeloid splenomegaly [7]. ^{32}P therapy remains the treatment of choice for patients with PV.

The importance of establishing or confirming a correct diagnosis of PV before initiating ^{32}P therapy cannot be overemphasized. An elevated haematocrit and red blood cell (RBC) count suggests the diagnosis of PV. However, these findings can occur with reduction of plasma volume by dehydration or chronic stress (pseudopolycythaemia), or with an increase in the RBC volume secondary to chronic hypoxia (secondary polycythaemia), or rarely due to erythropoietin-secreting tumours. However, none of these conditions is associated with several findings common in polycythaemia – i.e. splenomegaly, thrombocytosis, leucocytosis, increased leucocyte alkaline phosphatase, and increased serum B_{12} and serum B_{12} binders. These findings are included in the PVSG criteria for the diagnosis of PV shown in Table 1.8 [4]. An elevated RBC volume, unless masked by iron-deficiency anaemia, is essential for the diagnosis of PV. Also essential is the accurate measurement of RBC volume that requires the correct use of ^{51}Cr-labelled RBCs and correction for abnormal ratios of fat-to-lean tissue mass [8].

The aim of ^{32}P therapy is to maintain normal blood viscosity and coagulation by suppressing excessive haematopoiesis [9]. This can be accomplished by careful titration of haematocrit and platelets with judicious doses of ^{32}P so as to maintain the haematocrit at <50% and platelet count at $<450 \times 10^9/l$ – thereby avoiding the complications of thrombosis including cerebrovascular accident, myocardial infarction, peripheral arterial and venous occlusions, and pulmonary infarction. Status of the marrow, stage of the disease and symptoms related to enlargement of the spleen and liver must also be considered.

^{32}P therapy is initiated with intravenous administration of 2.3 mCi/m^2, approximately 4 mCi (1.5 $\times 10^8$ Bq) for a 70-kg person. One week later, the patient is phlebotomized to a haematocrit of ≤45%. This initial phlebotomy is best performed when radiation to the marrow suppresses the haematopoietic response to phlebotomy, thereby preventing additional excessive haematopoiesis and thrombocytosis. The same dose of ^{32}P is administered every 12 weeks until the haematocrit stabilizes at below 50% with platelet count at $<450 \times 10^9/l$. When response is suboptimal, the dose may be increased by 25%, but not to exceed 5 mCi. Infrequently, if stabilization is not achieved in 12–18

Clinical Nuclear Medicine, 3rd edn. Edited by M.N. Maisey, K.E. Britton and B.D. Collier. Published in 1998 by Chapman & Hall, London. ISBN 0 412 75180 1

Table 1.8   PVSG criteria for the diagnosis of polycythaemia vera [4]

A1. Increased RBC mass
    Male: ≥36 ml/kg
    Female: ≥32 ml/kg
	B1. Thrombocytosis
	    Platelet count >400 000/μl

A2. Normal arterial O_2 saturation (≥92%)	B2. Leucocytosis: >12 000/μl (no fever or infection)
A3. Splenomegaly	B3. Increased leucocyte alkaline phosphatase (>100 u/l)
	B4. Increased serum B_{12} binding capacity (>2200 pg/ml)

The diagnosis of PV is virtually certain in the presence of A1 + A2 + A3 or A1 + A2 + any two from category B.

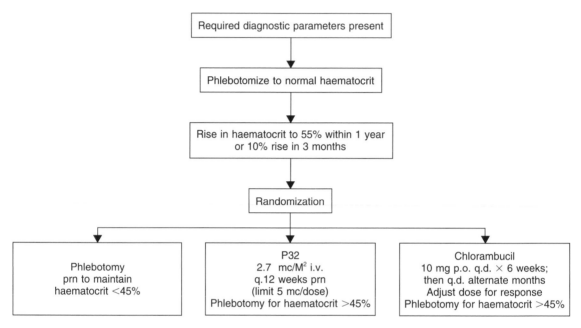

Figure 1.15   Schematic outline of Polycythemia Vera Study Group protocol Ol.

Table 1.9   PVSG criteria for the diagnosis of essential thrombocythaemia (Iland *et al.*, 1987)

1. Platelet count ≥1 000 000/μl
2. Megakaryocytic hyperplasia in the bone marrow
3. Absence of identifiable cause of thrombocytosis
4. Absence of the Philadelphia chromosome
5. Normal red cell mass (male <36 ml/kg, female <32 ml/kg), or haemoglobin <13 g/dl
6. Presence of stainable bone marrow iron, or no more than 1 g/dl increase in haemoglobin following 1 month of oral iron therapy
7. Absence of significant fibrosis (significant fibrosis defined as >1/3 cross-sectional area of bone marrow biopsy)
8. No more than two of the following:
   a. Mild fibrosis (defined as <1/3 area of bone marrow biopsy)
   b. Splenomegaly
   c. Leucoerythroblastic reaction

months, a further 25% increase in dose is indicated, but not to exceed a yearly dose of 15 mCi. An excessive dose may reduce platelets to <100 × 10^9/l, but haemorrhage is not a complication for it rarely occurs unless the platelet count is <25 × 10^9/l. The patient is then followed with complete blood count every 2–3 months and retreated at 6-monthly or longer intervals, adjusting the dose to maintain the blood cells at normal levels [9].

Essential thrombocythaemia is a related myeloproliferative disorder, characterized by persistent elevation of platelets ≥1000 × 10^9/l, normal red cell volume, and other findings shown in Table 1.9 [10]. ^{32}P therapy with 2.3–2.9 mCi/m^2 doses is given every 3 months as needed to control platelet levels below 450 × 10^9/l with no significant reactions [11].

REFERENCES

1. Lawrence, J.H. (1955) *Polycythemia: Physiology, Diagnosis, and Treatment Based on 303 Cases*, Grune and Stratton, New York.
2. Osgood, E.E. (1965) Polycythemia vera: age relationships and survival. *Blood*, **26**, 243–56.
3. Modan, B. and Lilienfeld, A.M. (1965) Polycythemia vera and leukemia: the role of radiation treatment. A study of 1222 patients. *Medicine*, **44**, 305–44.
4. Berk, P.D., Wasserman, L.R., Fruchtman, S.M. and Goldberg, J.D. (1995) Treatment of polycythemia vera: a summary of clinical trials conducted by the polycythemia vera study group, in *Polycythemia Vera and the Myeloproliferative Disorders* (eds L.R. Wasserman, P.D. Berk and N.I. Berlin), W.B. Saunders, Philadelphia, Chapter 15.
5. Landaw, S.A. (1995) Acute leukemia in polycythemia vera, in *Polycythemia Vera and the Myeloproliferative Disorders* (eds L.R. Wasserman, P.D. Berk and N.I. Berlin), W.B. Saunders, Philadelphia, Chapter 14.
6. Gardner, F.H. (1995) Early approaches in the treatment of polycythemia vera, in *Polycythemia Vera and the Myeloproliferative Disorders* (eds L.R. Wasserman, P.D. Berk and N.I. Berlin), W.B. Saunders, Philadelphia, Chapter 13.
7. Najean, Y., Dresch, C. and Rains, J.D. (1994) The very-long-term course of polycythemia: a complement to the previously published data of the Polycythemia Vera Study Group. *Br. J. Haematol.*, **86**, 233–5.
8. Pollycove, M. and Tono, M. (1996) Blood volume, in Diagnostic Nuclear Medicine (eds M.P. Sandler, R.E. Coleman, F.J.T.H. Wackers, J.A. Patton, A. Gottschalk and P.B. Hoffer), Williams and Wilkins, Baltimore, Chapter 42.
9. Hoffman, R. and Wasserman, L.R. (1979) Natural history and management of polycythemia vera. *Adv. Intern. Med.*, **24**, 255–85.
10. Iland, H.J., Laszlo, J., Case, D.C., Jr, Murphy, S., Reichert, T.A., Tso, C. and Wasserman, L.R. (1987) Differentiation between essential thrombocythemia and polycythemia vera with marked thrombocytosis. *Am. J. Hematol.*, **25**, 191–201.
11. Murphy, S., Rosenthal, D.S., Weinfeld, A. *et al.* (1982) Essential thrombocythemia response during first year of therapy with melphalan and radioactive phosphorus: a Polycythemia Vera Study Group report. *Cancer Treat. Rep.*, **66**, 1495–500.

Radioimmunological therapy

G. Paganelli, M. Chinol,
H.S. Stoldt, F. Aftab, J. Geraghty
and A.G. Siccardi

INTRODUCTION

Radioimmunotherapy (RIT) differs from conventional external beam radiation in that it is a form of systemically targeted therapy. Its anti-tumour effect is primarily due to the associated radioactivity of the radiolabelled antibody, which continuously emits exponentially decreasing low-dose-rate radiation. In some situations, the antibody itself may contribute to tumour cell killing. Important determinants of RIT are: the characteristics of the antibody (specificity, affinity, avidity, dose and immunoreactivity); the radionuclide label (emission properties and chemical stability of the radioimmunoconjugate); the targeted antigen (location, density, heterogeneity of expression, stability and modulation) and the nature of the targeted tumour (e.g. intrinsic radiosensitivity, proliferation rate, volume, tumour bed, etc.).

The range of radionuclides for radiolabelling antibodies is ever-increasing. Although the main mode of destroying tumour cells is generally by damaging the DNA, each radioisotope has a characteristic type and rate of decay that must be considered for its applicability for RIT. The chemistry involved in conjugating the antibody to the radioisotope is quite varied. Several radionuclides (e.g. ^{131}I and ^{125}I) can be directly conjugated to the antibody. Others involve binding of a chelator to the antibody followed by conjugation to the radioisotope; radiometals (e.g. ^{90}Y, ^{111}In and ^{186}Re) are coupled by this technique. The most important aspect of all the binding techniques is to avoid altering the antigen-binding region of the antibody in order to ensure optimal tumour concentration.

One of the main therapeutic advantages of radiolabelled monoclonal antibodies (MAb) is their potential to overcome the problem of tumour heterogeneity. Because the emitted radiation can penetrate up to several millimetres into the tissues, antigen-negative tumour cells that have no radiolabelled antibody localized on their surface may be killed by the so-called cross-fire effect.

SOLID TUMOUR CHARACTERISTICS

Solid tumours present a number of physical and biological characteristics that greatly influence the delivery and uptake of radiolabelled immunoreactive agents [1]. These characteristics include tumour size, tumour vascularity and capillary permeability, the lack of a well-established lymphatic drainage, and the type and amount of antigen expression.

Although tumours initially depend on existing vasculature, they soon develop new blood vessels that grow in an unpredictable manner. The result of this neovascularity is an uneven distribution of perfusion with regional tumour vascularity ranging from highly perfused regions to areas with negligible or absent vascularity. The delivery of blood-administered molecules to tumour cells is therefore non-uniform.

A second obstacle for tumour-targeting molecules is the abnormally high interstitial pressure found in all solid tumours [1,2]. The pressure of the interstitial matrix is greatest at the centre of a tumour where the blood supply is usually low or absent, and lowest at the periphery. Although low-molecular weight compounds leave the blood vessels preferentially by diffusion, the high-molecular weight monoclonal antibodies (molecular weight about 150kDa) extravasate by convection. These compounds move from a high-pressure area to a low-pressure area, but since tumours reveal a greatly increased interstitial pressure, molecules leave the circulation and travel through the interstitial matrix only very slowly. Although high-molecular weight antibodies also move by diffusion, they do this equally slowly. The permeability of the vascular epithelium to low-molecular weight compounds is greater, and, therefore, antibody fragments (one-third to one-half of the weight of the whole antibody) have the ability to diffuse more rapidly into the tumour due to poor lymphatic drainage from the tumours.

Clinical Nuclear Medicine, 3rd edn. Edited by M.N. Maisey, K.E. Britton and B.D. Collier. Published in 1998 by Chapman & Hall, London. ISBN 0 412 75180 1

Tumour-associated antigens (TAA) form some of the targets at which MAbs and other targeting vehicles can be aimed. The chemical nature of many of these target antigens has been characterized: examples include carcinoembryonic antigen (CEA), alpha-fetoprotein (AFP), human chorionic gonadotropin (hCG), tumour-associated glycoprotein (TAG-72) and prostatic acid phosphatase (PAP). Although antigens are present on/in tumour cells in relatively high concentrations, whole tumours often display intrinsic heterogeneity in antigen density. This characteristic also contributes to an uneven distribution of antibodies in the targeted tumours.

TAA are usually expressed by more than one type of carcinoma, but not all tumours of a given type will express a specific antigen. Antigen expression may also differ in the primary and in the metastatic lesion. Furthermore, antigen expression can be temporally modulated, i.e. antigens may be expressed at one time but may not be expressed at others [3].

MONOCLONAL ANTIBODIES

One of the first examples of an antibody response against a human tumour was described in 1951 in a patient with gastric cancer, who was inadvertently transfused with incompatible blood. The transfusion elicited an antibody response against the P1 blood group antigen. Although the patient was homozygous for the antigen, the tumour was found to express a P1-related antigen. The patient remained tumour-free for 25 years, possibly as a result of cytotoxic effects of anti-P1 antibody [4]. Because reactive antibodies were found more often in the sera of cancer patients, it was thought that patients whose cancer had undergone spontaneous or treatment-related regression harboured anti-cancer antibodies. Thus, a number of attempts were made to treat patients with different cancers types with blood, serum, or plasma thought to contain these anti-cancer antibodies. However, the results were rather disappointing.

ANTIBODY STRUCTURE

Antibody molecules are complex multi-chain proteins, which have been grouped into five distinct classes: IgG, IgM, IgA, IgD and IgE. These classes differ from each other in size, charge, amino acid composition and carbohydrate content. Each molecule is bifunctional, with one site binding to an antigen and the other to a host or complement. The antibody complex is composed of two identical heavy (H) and two identical light (L) chains forming a Y-shaped structure, stabilized by intra- and inter-chain disulphide bonds. The tips of the arms contain the antigen-binding variable regions and hence differ markedly from one antibody to the next. Each chain of an immunoglobulin molecule is divided into structural domains. The light chain has two domains, a variable (VL) and a constant domain (CL). The heavy chain folds to form VH, CH1, hinge, CH2, and CH3 domains (in an IgG molecule). The hinge region is the flexible portion of the Ig molecule. The antigen-binding sites are formed by six hypervariable loops: three from the VL domain (light chain) and three from the CH domain (heavy chain). The specificity and affinity of the antigen-binding sites are determined by these six hypervariable loops, termed the complementarity-determining regions or the CDRs [5].

Investigation of antibodies for clinical use began in the 1950s with the exploration of the concept of using polyclonal antibodies as carriers of isotopes to both malignant and normal tissues in the body [6]. This study demonstrated successful *in vivo* targeting of tumours in animals. Unfortunately, early clinical trials were marred by an inability to produce good radiolabelled sera against human tumours [7], and 25 years passed before any further developments were made in tumour targeting. The advent of the hybridoma technology described by Kohler and Milstein [8] for the production of MAbs, provided a major boost towards the use of antibody molecules as tools for tumour imaging and targeting. It was hoped that MAbs would bring new promise to cancer therapy and since then MAbs have been used extensively in cancer research, both as an aid to pathological diagnosis and in the detection of cancer by diagnostic imaging. The incorporation of radionuclides, toxins or chemotherapeutic agents with MAbs have yielded promising results in cancer therapy. MAbs also appear promising for developing assays that may be useful in screening for early cancer detection as well as in monitoring therapy for detecting microscopic recurrence (see Further reading: Britton and Granowska, 1988; DeLand, 1989).

PROBLEMS ASSOCIATED WITH MONOCLONAL ANTIBODIES

The murine origin of MAbs can give rise to several diagnostic and therapeutic problems in clinical practice. The relatively large size of an IgG antibody (150 kDa) can be a limiting factor in allowing adequate amounts of antibody to penetrate into tumours, thus leading to areas of suboptimal uptake [1]. A further clinical problem is the development of an immunological reaction against the antibody; repeated administrations of murine MAbs often leads to the generation of human anti-murine antibodies or HAMA [9]. This HAMA response leads to a rapid clearance of subsequent antibody administrations with immune-complex formation.

An attractive feature of RIT is the prospect that most normal tissues are spared from high radiation burden. Unfortunately, RIT has thus far failed to fulfil this expectation, mainly because only a very small amount of tagged MAb localises per gram of tumour (0.01%), while the remainder stays in the circulation conjugated to the radioisotope with toxic effects on tissues, especially the bone marrow [10]. As a consequence, the total radiation dose delivered to the tumour, is generally low, usually <2000 cGy and often <1200 cGy, especially with ^{131}I-labelled MAbs. Toxicity is principally thrombocytopenia, with nadirs appearing 4–6 weeks post-therapy; leucopenia also results

but is usually less severe. Among the leucocytes, the B-lymphocytes appear to be the most radio-sensitive [11]. The use of antibody fragments such as Fab or F(ab')$_2$ with a faster clearance than the whole antibodies, may counteract this problem, but it reduces the therapeutic efficacy of the radiolabelled fragments to tumour cells [12].

The generation of humanized and chimaeric antibodies, single-chain antibodies, antigen-binding peptides, and molecular recognition units (MRU) by utilizing recombinant DNA and gene transfection techniques can overcome these antibody and tumour-related problems [13,14]. Though trials establishing the role of these 'designer' molecules in animal models have shown promising results, their usefulness in the clinical setting yet remains to be established.

RADIOLABELLING OF MONOCLONAL ANTIBODIES

The labelling of MAbs can be achieved by attaching the radionuclide directly to the antibody or by coupling metallic radionuclides to chelators which are conjugated to the antibodies. The direct procedure is only applicable to a limited number of radionuclides, mainly iodine and technetium. The indirect method involving conjugation of chelating agents to MAbs allows labelling with practically all metallic radionuclides. The devel-

Table 1.10 Physical characteristics of potential therapeutic radionuclides

Radionuclides	Physical half-life	Decay mode (MeV)	Particle maximum range in soft tissue
[32]P	14.3 days	β (1.71)	8.7 mm
[67]Cu	2.58 days	β (0.54), γ (0.185)	1.8 mm
[89]Sr	50.5 days	β (1.49)	8.0 mm
[90]Y	2.67 days	β (2.28)	12.0 mm
[105]Rh	1.48 days	β (0.57), γ (0.320)	1.9 mm
[109]Pd	13.6 hours	β (1.0)	4.6 mm
[111]Ag	7.47 days	β (1.05), γ (0.34)	4.8 mm
[125]I	60.0 days	Auger, γ (0.027)	10 nm
[131]I	8.04 days	β (0.6), γ (0.364)	2.0 mm
[153]Sm	1.95 days	β (0.8), γ (0.103)	3.0 mm
[169]Er	9.5 days	β (0.34)	1.0 mm
[177]Lu	6.7 days	β (0.497), γ (0.208)	1.5 mm
[186]Re	3.77 days	β (1.08), γ (0.131)	5.0 mm
[188]Re	16.95 hours	β (2.13), γ (0.155)	11.0 mm
[198]Au	2.7 days	β (0.97), γ (0.411)	4.4 mm
[211]At	7.2 hours	α (6.8)	65 μm
[212]Bi	1.0 hours	α (7.8), γ (0.72)	70 μm

opment of bifunctional chelating agents (BCA) that form stable protein conjugates and tightly bind to metal ions, has made this a practical approach [15].

SELECTION OF RADIONUCLIDES

The choice of a particular radionuclide for a specific therapeutic application is governed by many key factors. The half-life of the isotope should be within a suitable range (varying from hours to several days) and match the kinetics of the protein, which may vary greatly if intact antibody or its fragments are used. The energy of the β- or α-particles should be also suitable and preferably should be accompanied by γ-ray photons for imaging (Table 1.10).

RADIOLABELLING TECHNIQUES

Direct methods of radioiodine labelling

Historically, antibodies have been radiolabelled with isotopes of iodine because of the widespread availability of ^{125}I and ^{131}I, and the ease of performing iodine attachment to the various amino acid residues of protein molecules. Iodine in the reduced form (iodide ion, I$^-$), which is the most stable for halogens in aqueous solution, does not react with protein molecules, but it can be oxidized to iodinium (I$^+$), allowing electrophilic substitution for hydrogen at the most electronegative sites of various amino acid residues. In the electrophilic reactions, the most reactive are the aromatic amino acids such as tyrosine or histidine, but under some conditions, phenylalanine and tryptophan can also be labelled. Many agents are available for oxidation of iodine, but chloramine-T, iodogen and lactoperoxidase are mainly employed for antibody labelling [16].

The *in vivo* use of any radioiodinated antibody requires pre-blocking of the thyroid gland with excess iodine to prevent radioiodine uptake following *in vivo* dehalogenation by enzymes.

Indirect methods of radioiodine labelling

Antibodies contain a large number of non-specific metal ion binding sites, but the *in vivo* metal ions tend to be transferred to other body proteins, mainly transferrin. Therefore, radiometals require to be attached tightly to MAbs via chelating groups that possess the right stereochemistry for binding radiometals and a reactive functional group for covalent linkage to amino acid residues on the antibody (BCA). The chelating agent is generally a polyaminocarboxylic acid, and the functional group may be a carboxylic mixed anhydride, a cyclic anhydride, a bromoacetyl group or isothiocyanate. The amino groups of lysine residues are used to anchor the chelating agents to the proteins [17].

The affinity of the antigen-binding region of the MAb for the antigen may be impaired by the conjugation of BCA with the lysine residues randomly dispersed in its light and heavy chains. Hence, the carbohydrate moieties of the Fc region and the sulphydryl group of the Fab' fragment, which are located away from the antigen-binding sites, have been proposed for the attachment of BCA.

Two widely used radionuclides for RIT, i.e. [186]Re and ^{90}Y, require a BCA for stable binding to MAbs; [186]Re may also be attached directly to an antibody [18,19]. Due to the difficulties of obtaining reduced rhenium and the consequent incorporation in a chelating system by ligand exchange, prelabelling techniques have been developed in which the chelating agent is initially labelled and then conjugated to the MAb [20].

Similarly, conjugates between macrocyclic chelators such as DTPA, that bind very tightly to ^{90}Y, prevent subsequent radiolabelling with MAbs, and require placement of a spacer group between the protein and the chelator to avoid steric hindrance. The more sophisticated chemistry behind this macrocyclic chelator, compared with an open-chain analogue, is justified with the remarkably high *in vivo* stability of the complex with consequent reduced bone accumulation of [90]Y [21].

Quality control of radiolabelled antibodies

In order to certify the pharmaceutical quality and to predict the *in vivo* behaviour, quality assurance tests need to be performed on the final preparation of the radiolabelled MAb, before administration. Many studies have shown that the presence of contaminating radiolabelled MAbs, which are either deactivated or are immunologically irrelevant, contributes to the augmented activity found in circulation and in normal tissues [22].

Radiochemical purity, defined as the percentage of total radioactivity bound to the MAb, is routinely determined for radiometallic MAbs by simple chromatographic techniques. More complex procedures such as high-performance liquid chromatography may provide valuable information about the final preparation such as the presence of cross-linked polymerized antibodies, and can also help in the separation of inactive antibodies, which have undergone structural modifications [23].

CLINICAL TRIALS

COLORECTAL CARCINOMA

Colorectal cancer (CRC) is one of the most common tumours affecting 1 in 20 in the United States. With the ever-increasing numbers of cases – just over 140 000 new cases are diagnosed in the United States each year – representing 15% of all cancers, this disease poses a major public health problem. Furthermore, the overall survival rate has remained approximately 45% (slightly better for colon cancer, slightly worse for rectal cancer) for decades.

Surgery has a lot to offer both in the diagnosis and treatment of colonic and rectal carcinoma and their polyp precursors. However, its role in the management of microscopic disseminated disease is limited. Both radiotherapy and chemotherapy have valuable objective response in the management of patients with disseminated disease, but at the expense of increasing morbidity and worsening the patient's quality of life. Furthermore, in the majority of patients that relapse despite the use of multiple and repeated chemotherapy regimens, the possibility of obtaining further control of the disease is very small and the future of the patient quite bleak. The administration of radiolabelled MAbs to target both the occult and the clinically detectable tumour deposits complements radiotherapy and chemotherapy. Because RIT incorporates the properties of localized radiation to the diseased tissues and the immunotoxic capability of the antibody, it potentially improves the prognosis.

Systemic RIT

In a phase I trial, 24 patients with TAG-72 antigen-expressing CRC were treated with increasing doses of ^{131}I-labelled CC49 MAb (20 mg), starting at 15 mCi/m^2 and escalating to 90 mCi/m^2 [24]. All patients had a poor response to conventional chemotherapy, had no prior radiotherapy and had not received murine MAb. None of the 24 patients developed any side-effects during radiolabelled MAb infusion; HAMA reaction was positive in all patients 4 weeks following the infusion. When the dose of the radiolabelled antibody was below 60 mCi/m^2, no haematological toxicity was noted; at a dose of 60 mCi/m^2, one patient developed grade II thrombocytopenia with its nadir 3 weeks after infusion; grade III and IV thrombocytopenia was observed with higher doses. There was also one case of grade IV lymphopenia at a dose of 90 mCi/m^2. As this was a phase I study, no major responses were noted; however, six patients were reported to have stable disease at 4 weeks following the infusion.

A phase II trial was conducted by Murray *et al.* [25] in 15 cases of CRC. All patients had prior chemotherapy. Patients were administered 75 mCi/m^2 ^{131}I-CC49 by the intravenous route. Non-haematological toxicity consisted of nausea, arthralgias, transient fever and chills, and transient blood pressure changes. At 4–5 weeks after treatment, reversible thrombocytopenia (grades III–IV) and reversible granulocytopenia (grades III–IV) were encountered in approximately 50% of the patients. HAMA reaction was positive in over 90% of the cases 6–8 weeks following MAb infusion. The half-life of ^{131}I after a single injection was 57.3 ± 13.4 hours (range 30.5–82.3 h). In addition, the calculated mean radiation dose to the bone marrow was 81.5 ± 18.4 rads (range 60.9–117 rads). A positive correlation ($r = 0.77$, $P < 0.001$) between the MAb half-life and the dose to the bone marrow, as well as a moderate correlation ($r = 0.59$, $P > 0.05$) between normalized radiation dose and decrease in platelet count was also seen. Despite adequate tumour localization with a sensitivity of 87%, no major tumour response was observed. Three patients had stable disease after 8 weeks and received a further injection of ^{131}I-CC49, but unfortunately, all of them had tumour progression 16 weeks after the second therapy.

Locoregional approach

The response of solid tumours to systemic RIT has been poor. Therefore, direct injection of MAbs into the peritoneal cavity has been proposed to increase the tumour-to-non-tumour ratio in intraperitoneal disease. Riva *et al.* [26] reported their experience in a clinical trial involving 31 patients with recurrent CRC using an anti-CEA FO23C5 MAb. All patients had surgical ablation of the tumour, and RIT was initiated as a third- or fourth-line therapy. The MAb was administered intraperitoneally, and repeated at 3- and 6-monthly intervals if the need arose. The ^{131}I dose on the average was 3641 MBq/ cycle and the antibody dose was 16.4 mg. The intraperitoneal route resulted in a satisfactory and long-lasting MAb tumour targeting; thus the radiation dose delivered to the neoplastic tissue was quite high, whereas the parenchyma of delicate tissues (liver, bone marrow, kidney and gut) was spared. The dosimetry values also validated the tumour-reducing effect of RIT. The objective response rates achieved were also quite striking: there were 10 complete tumour remissions lasting for a median of 23 months; partial remissions for a median of 8 months; and in eight cases, the disease process was stabilized (median duration 12 months); and the overall response rate was 41%. The most important factor in determining the response to treatment was the extent of the disease process (confined to the abdomen, less than three lesions and lesion diameter <2 cm). Histologically, RIT produced areas of necrosis and fibrosis in the involved lesions. The survival rate on an average was prolonged to 41 months. The intraperitoneal route of radiolabelled MAb delivery was well tolerated, even when the courses were repeated a number of times. A transient grade III reduction of platelets and WBCs was noted. To prevent the development of the HAMA, an immunosuppressive regimen consisting of cyclophosphamide and steroids was administered before each subsequent treatment.

Antibody fragments

In order to overcome the problem of inadequate penetration by the intact MAb, antibody fragments like F(ab')$_2$ with a molecular weight of 100 kDa have been tried in CRC. Ten patients with raised CEA levels were given ^{131}I-labelled anti-CEA intact IgG (A5B7), and nine patients received ^{131}I-labelled anti-CEA F(ab')$_2$ fragments of the same antibody. The mean percentage of the injected activity per kilogram in tumour at 4.25 hours was better with the antibody fragment (8.2%) than with intact antibody (4.4%). However, the tumour response rates were similar when comparing intact antibody versus antibody fragments [27]. In general, there is a lower toxicity associated with the F(ab')$_2$ compared with the whole antibody.

Chimaeric antibodies

With the recent developments in the field of genetic engineering, chimaeric antibodies have been tried, with the intent that they will excite a lower immunogenic response. Two clinical trials have been reported [28,29]. In both these series, two different chimaeric antibodies complexed to different radioactive isotopes have been utilized. Tumour was imaged in over 90% of cases with a lower toxicity to haematopoietic tissue. However, there was a higher uptake of antibody in the liver, together with the development of an anti-chimaeric antibody response. No major tumour responses were noted.

OVARIAN CARCINOMA

Ovarian carcinoma is a deadly disease, and is the fifth most common cancer-related mortality among women in the Western world. Only 35% of all women diagnosed with this disease survive for 5 years. The high death rate is attributable to an insidious onset, with most patients manifesting symptoms of the disease (e.g. epigastric pain and abdominal distension) at an advanced stage, when the tumour has spread outside the pelvis. Advances in cytoreductive surgery and post-operative chemotherapy have produced response rates of 60–85%, but with only a small improvement in the overall survival. However, approximately 50% of patients with an apparently complete response eventually relapse and the response rate with second-line chemotherapy in these patients is only 5–19%.

There have been several reports of radiolabelled MAbs being successfully tried for both diagnostic and therapeutic purposes. Especially in ovarian cancer, locoregional administration of MAb has been advocated to increase tumour-to-non-tumour ratio in intraperitoneal disease, and hence improve outcome. In a recent trial, 16 patients with advanced ovarian carcinoma underwent intraperitoneal RIT (mean dose of antibody 14 mg with 3700 GBq of iodine-131) [30]. All patients were given first-line chemotherapy and had minimal residual disease as diagnosed laparoscopically or following laparotomy. The results were quite encouraging with 31% of the patients showing a complete response, 38% showing no change, and the remaining 31% of the patients had disease progression. Of the five

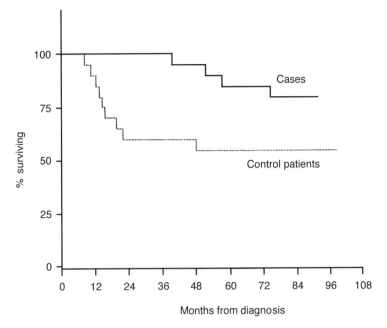

Figure 1.16   A Cox proportional hazards regression model predicting survival for recipients and non-recipients of adjuvant radioimmunotherapy. (Courtesy of Prof. A.A. Epenetos.)

patients who completely responded to RIT, only one was alive and disease-free at 34 months, while the other four relapsed after a mean disease-free interval of 10.5 months (range 3–16 months). One notable observation was the relapse site in two patients (inguinal and supraclavicular lymph node metastases). Only one patient developed a mild reversible bone-marrow toxicity. HAMA response was observed in 94% of the patients.

In a clinical trial, 25 patients with ovarian cancer (FIGO stages Ic to IV) received RIT in the form of ^{90}Y-HMFG1 in a stage I/II study (S. Nicholson *et al.*, unpublished data). All patients had optimal surgery followed by chemotherapy, and were classified through a second-look procedure as free of any macroscopic or microscopic disease. They were matched with control patients who also had adequate surgery and chemotherapy. Following ^{90}Y-based RIT, the 5-year-survival rate was in the region of 80% for treated cases as opposed to 55% for controls; the difference in survival is statistically significant ($P = 0.00335$) (Figure 1.16). The relative risk of death for the control group was 3.59 times greater than the RIT-treated cases.

Although most data concerning RIT describes its efficacy as a third- or fourth-line therapy, the data for its use as an adjuvant therapy has been described by Hird *et al.* [31]. This trial reports on 52 patients with grades I–IV ovarian carcinoma who received intraperitoneal ^{90}Y-labelled MAb following surgery and chemotherapy; 40% of these patients had no evidence of residual disease. Patients with bulky disease had a median survival of 11 months (range 2–31 months).

In summary, the data from these trials show that RIT – although still in its evolutionary phase – is a promising technique in killing residual malignant cells after debulking surgery and chemotherapy.

MALIGNANT ASTROCYTOMAS

Malignant glioma (or grade III–IV astrocytoma) accounts for about 75% of gliomas in adults. The patient, commonly stricken in the fifth decade of life, enters a cycle of repetitive hospitalizations and operations while experiencing the progressive complications associated with the relatively ineffective treatments of radiation and chemotherapy.

Some 80% of the patients die of tumour recurrence within 6–12 months. Therapeutic modalities are not highly effective. The average life expectancy of 17 weeks for untreated patients is improved by post-operative external beam radiation alone to 47 weeks, and by radiation combined with chemotherapy to 62 weeks [32].

Following intravenous injection, the extremely low amounts of radiolabelled MAbs that localize at the neoplastic target following their intravenous administration lead to the observation that the more promising results have been obtained by performing locoregional or intra-lesional RIT.

The injection of specific MAbs in a body cavity affected by neoplastic disease (e.g. peritoneum, skull, pleura, urinary bladder, etc.) has proven suitable for therapeutic purposes. In fact, the antibodies directly bind to their specific antigens for a sufficient length of time to achieve the degree of tumour irradiation necessary for the production of a therapeutic response.

Favourable clinical responses have been reported in patients with leptomeningeal neoplastic spread following intrathecal administration of ^{131}I-labelled MAbs [33].

A further step in the locoregional treatment of brain tumours is represented by the direct intra-tumoral administration of radiolabelled MAbs [34]. Since brain glioblastomas are confined within the skull, the intra-tumoral administration might theoretically achieve complete tumour sterilization and cure the patients.

RIT of malignant gliomas has been favoured by the observation that these tumours express high levels of tenascin, which is absent in normal brain tissue. Tenascin is uniformly distributed in viable neoplastic tissues and represents an excellent tumour target for anti-tenascin-specific antibodies. Two murine MAbs, BC-2 and BC-4, raised against two different epitopes on the tenascin molecule have been labelled with ^{131}I and used in patients with recurrent and bulky brain glioblastomas [35]. All patients had one or more operations and the majority were treated following tumour recurrence, and after completion of radiotherapy and chemotherapy regimens. Mean MAb doses of 1.93 mg labelled with an average of 551.3 MBq of ^{131}I were injected into the tumour or the site of disease through repeated administrations, until a cumulative tumour dose of >15 000 cGy was reached. When the therapeutic parameters obtained in this trial were compared with the values

observed in different series of patients either injected intraperitoneally or intravenously, the data suggested that the intra-tumoral route may be of particular interest in producing higher tumour doses and consequent lasting curative effects [36].

In a recent trial, the administered dose was increased to 3.0 mg of anti-tenascin MAbs labelled with 1100 MBq of [131]I [37]. The mean absorbed dose to the tumour was >25 000 cGy and produced an overall response rate of 34.7%.

These favourable parameters have produced encouraging clinical results in such highly aggressive and otherwise untreatable malignant gliomas, as partial or complete remission was observed in 36% of cases and the disease was stabilized in another 30% of patients, thus improving their duration of survival and their quality of life.

RIT OF DIVERSE TUMOURS

Breast cancer is yet another solid tumour where the clinical utility of RIT has been studied. In a phase I trial involving nine patients with stage IV breast cancer, ^{90}Y-labelled MAb was used in escalating doses [38]. Serial bone-marrow biopsies demonstrated a 1.7-fold ^{90}Y accumulation in the marrow at 48 hours compared with that at 24 hours. Because of the location of metastatic deposits, tumour response could be evaluated only in eight patients; four of these experienced partial response, one had a complete clinical response, and one patient experienced transient decrease in bone pain. The only toxicity was haematological with grade IV platelet toxicity requiring transfusion in four patients, and transient grade IV WBC toxicity in two patients that resolved in the next 3–9 days. Two additional clinical studies have reported encouraging results in the use of chimaeric antibodies in breast cancer RIT [39,40], but further investigations are clearly needed.

The clinical utility of radioimmunodetection utilizing MAbs to various melanoma-associated surface antigens has been documented by several investigators, but so far, there is little experience with RIT in metastatic melanoma.

NEW STRATEGIES: THE PRE-TARGETING APPROACH

Various groups have investigated the concept of tumour pretargeting based on the separate administration of MAbs and radiolabelled isotopes [41,42]. Their injection time can be delayed to a time when most of the primary MAb has been cleared from blood and normal tissues, and therefore, this strategy can achieve higher tumour-to-non-tumour ratios.

In pretargeting systems, MAbs first require their tagging to enable recognition by a second molecule. Four different types of tagged targeting vehicles for the use in pretargeting strategies have been described in the literature:

1. Biotin-conjugated or biotinylated antibodies.
2. Streptavidin-conjugated or streptavidinylated antibodies.
3. Bifunctional MAbs (Bs-MAbs).
4. Monoclonal antibody-oligonucleotide conjugates.

The biotinylation of MAbs is easily accomplished, and four to five biotin molecules can be incorporated per antibody molecule without loss of immunoreactivity; the use of a long spacer arm between the protein-binding site and biotin reduces steric hindrance of the subsequent avidin–biotin reaction [43].

The conjugation of streptavidin to MAb results in a molecular weight 40% greater than that of native MAb and therefore shows slower pharmacokinetics than MAb alone [44].

Bispecific antibodies with two different antigen-specific binding sites, one for the tumour-associated antigen and one for the radioactive effector compound, have been proposed [41]. Unpredictable pharmacokinetic properties due to the many chemical manipulations required in the production of coupled Fab' fragments [45], can partially be overcome by using Bs-MAbs produced by hybridomas [46].

The attachment of oligonucleotides to MAbs [47], typically binds three to five oligonucleotides per antibody molecule and, although it fully preserves their specificity, on the average it reduces the immunoreactivity by about 50% due to steric hindrance or charge interference. Being DNA-based conjugates, these targeting structures also need careful preservation and lose stability more rapidly than other MAb conjugates.

Once the tagged MAbs have targeted the preselected tumour antigens, a second conjugate that will recognize with high selectivity the tag on the first MAb is administered. Theoretically, this is best done at a time when the highest concentration of tagged MAbs are found on and in the tumour. The remaining tagged MAbs, which did not selectively bind to tumour antigens, must have been cleared from the normal tissues and blood, and must have been excreted. Also, the second molecule needs to be cleared rapidly from the normal tissues and blood after achieving its highest concentration on tumour-bound antibodies.

Most often, the second conjugates are radiolabelled avidin, streptavidin or biotin molecules, directed at the biotinylated or avidinylated MAbs. This pretargeting technique takes advantage of the avidin–biotin system that has been long and widely used for *in vitro* applications like immunocytochemistry, ELISA, and molecular biology. Due to the flexibility of this system, several protocols have been devised for its application in clinical trials [48]. Two major methods are presently used in clinical practice.

TWO-STEP APPROACH

This approach has been initially proposed based on the *in vitro* conjugation of streptavidin to the antibody, which is administered first and is followed by the injection of radiolabelled biotin 2–3 days later. A preliminary report on 10 patients with lung cancer showed decreased activity levels in all normal organs and blood. Clear images were obtained as little as 2 hours after the injection of ^{111}In-labelled biotin [49].

An alternative approach has also been used to target intraperitoneal tumours. When biotinylated MAbs are injected intraperitoneally, there is a rapid accumulation of antibodies in peritoneal tumour deposits, while most of the immunoglobulins that remain unbound leave the peritoneal cavity via the lymphatic system and eventually enter the blood pool. The first step of biotinylated MAbs is then followed 1–2 days later by the administration of radiolabelled streptavidin (Figure 1.17), thus exploiting at the best the specific binding of the biotinylated antibody onto the tumour [50].

THREE-STEP APPROACH

The locoregional approach described above is feasible when tumour is confined to the peritoneal cavity or in other locoregional approaches. In the presence of widespread disease, a systemic injection of the tracer is nonetheless required. A three-

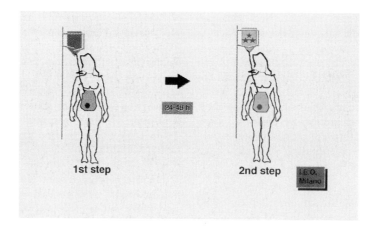

Figure 1.17   Two-step strategy. Biotinylated MAbs are injected (i.p.) and allowed to localize onto the target (1st step). Then 1–2 days later radioactive streptavidin is injected (i.p.) to target the tumour.

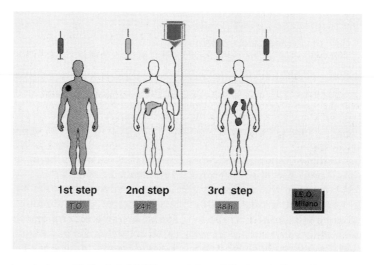

Figure 1.18   Three-step strategy. Biotinylated MAbs are injected (i.v.) and allowed to localize onto the target (1st step). One day later avidin and streptavidin are injected (i.v.) (2nd step). After 24 h, when unbound streptavidin and circulating avidin–MAb complexes have been cleared from circulation, radiolabelled biotin is injected (i.v.) (3rd step).

step approach has been designed for these cases, where conjugates need to be cleared not only from a well-defined body cavity, but from the entire blood pool (Figure 1.18).

Biotinylated MAbs are first injected (step 1) followed by injection of avidin/streptavidin 1 day later (step 2). The purpose of the second injection is twofold: (i) removal of excess circulating biotinylated antibodies in the form of cold com-plexes via avidin (fast clearance); and (ii) the tar-geting of tumour cells with streptavidin (slower clearance). Thereafter, radiolabelled biotin is in-jected (step 3), which binds selectively to strep-tavidin and thus to the tumour.

The three-step approach is designed to remove excess circulating biotinylated MAbs as cold com-plexes, which are taken up and metabolized by the liver. This is the major factor in background reduc-

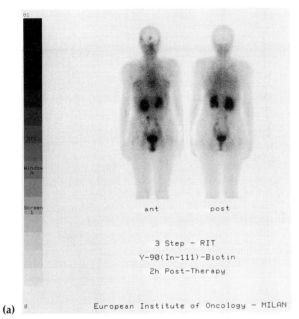

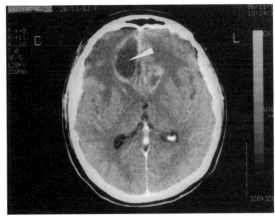

(a)

(b)

Figure 1.19 (a) Three-step RIT of a glioblastoma patient. The tumour was in progression after external radio-therapy and chemotherapy. Anterior and posterior whole body images, obtained 2 h after an i.v. injection of 3.7 GBq of ^{90}Y-DOTA–biotin spiked with 74 MBq of ^{111}In-DOTA–biotin, are shown. Note the rapid excretion of the radiotracer through the kidneys and the absence of activity in the liver and bone marrow. The tumour, located in the frontal hemisphere, is clearly visualized. (b) CT scan of the same patient 2 months after RIT. Compared with the pre-therapy CT scan, the tumour size is unchanged but the necrotic component is evident as a result of the ^{90}Y-radioimmunotherapy (see arrowhead). At present, 12 months after the treatment (18 months after diagnosis) the lesion size is slightly reduced and the patient is still in good condition with a Karnofski index of 90 (stable disease). This represents an excellent result in a patient with such a bleak prognosis.

tion and is obtained before label injection. More-over, the rapid blood clearance of the radio-labelled biotin allows imaging to be performed only 90–120 minutes after injection and with only very low background activity. In addition, another great advantage of this strategy is that of signal amplification, which may occur if avidin binds more than one, and up to four molecules of radio-active biotin per molecule of avidin.

CLINICAL APPLICATION OF AVIDIN–BIOTIN SYSTEM FOR THE THERAPY OF GLIOMAS

A therapy trial based on the three-step pretarget-ing was conducted in 19 patients with histological diagnosis of grade III–IV malignant glioma and immunohistochemical evidence of tenascin on tis-sue sections [51]. Doses of ^{90}Y from 1.48–2.96 GBq/ m^2 bound to 1–2 mg of biotin–DOTA were sys-

temically administered. The therapy was well tol-erated by all patients, and no acute or haemato-logical toxicity was observed. None of the patients developed HAMA and only one showed an anti-avidin immune response. All patients however, developed a moderate immune response to streptavidin.

While the dose delivered to the tumour was of 1520 ± 870 cGy, the absorbed dose was 270 ± 160 cGy to the kidneys, 150 ± 100 cGy to the liver, and 60 ± 30 cGy to the brain. All patients revealed the same activity profile in blood and this resulted in a mean absorbed dose of 80 ± 50 cGy to the bone marrow.

Of the 16 patients evaluated during a follow-up period of 2–12 months, one showed a complete response, four had a partial response, six cases were considered to have stable disease and five had progressive disease; in 58% of the patients refractory to other therapies there was an objective benefit. An example of high uptake in the tumour area (grade IV glioblastoma in the frontal hemisphere) 2 hours after therapy is shown in Figure 1.19(a); the CT scan of the same patient that was used to define the ROIs for the dosimetric calculations is shown in Figure 1.19(b).

In summary, the data showed that it was possible to administer high doses of ^{90}Y with low bone-marrow toxicity and that some cytotoxic effects to tumours were achieved. (For further reading, see Paganelli *et al.* (1995), Goodwin (1995) and Magnani *et al.* (1996).)

SUMMARY

The advent of the monoclonal antibody production raised the hope that RIT would have the great advantage of sparing most normal tissues while killing selectively malignant cells. Unfortunately, RIT has thus far gained limited acceptance mainly due to the low amount of radioactivity that can be targeted to the tumour and to the myelotoxicity which is typically the dose-limiting factor. Remarkable high therapeutic response rates have been obtained for tumours that are refractory to other therapies through the use of locoregional administration that allows the delivery of higher radiation doses to produce cytotoxic effects. New strategies based on pretargeting techniques have shown that higher doses of radioactivity can be administered systemically without associated bone marrow toxicity.

REFERENCES

1. Jain, R.K. (1994) Barriers to drug delivery in solid tumors. *Scientific American*, **7**, 42–9.
2. Jain, R.K. and Baxter, L.T. (1988) Mechanisms of heterogeneous distribution of monoclonal antibodies and other macromolecules in tumors: significance of elevated interstitial pressure. *Cancer Res.*, **48**, 7022–32.
3. Jain, R.K. (1987) Transport of molecules in the tumor interstitium: a review. *Cancer Res.*, **47**(12), 3039–51.
4. Levine, P., Bobbit O.B., Waller, R.K. *et al.* (1951) Isoimmunisation by a new blood factor in tumour cells. *Proc. Soc. Exp. Biol. Med.*, **77**, 403–11.
5. Roit, I.M., Brostoff, J. and Male, D.K. (1985) in *Immunology*, C.V. Mosby, Gower Medical Publishing, London, New York, pp. 5.1–5.10.
6. Pressman, D. and Korngold, L. (1953) *In vivo* localisation of anti-wagner osteogenic sarcoma antibodies. *Cancer*, **6**, 619–25.
7. Bale, W.F. and Spar, I.L. (1957) Studies directed towards the use of antibodies as carriers of radioactivity for therapy. *Adv. Biol. Med. Phys.*, **5**, 285–92.
8. Kohler, G. and Milstein, C. (1975) Continuous culture of fused cells secreting antibody of predefined specificity. *Nature*, **256**, 494–7.
9. Lange, M.K. and Martin, E.W. (1991) Monoclonal antibodies in imaging and therapy of colorectal cancer. *World J. Surg.*, **15**, 617–22.
10. Goldenberg, D.M. and Griffiths, G.L. (1992) Radioimmunotherapy of cancer: arming the missiles. *J. Nucl. Med.*, **33**, 1110–12.
11. Stein, R., Sharkey, R.M. and Goldenberg, D.M. (1991) Haematological effects of radioimmunotherapy in cancer patients. *Br. J. Haematol.*, **80**, 69–76.
12. Covell, D.G., Barbet, J., Holton, O.D. *et al.* (1986) Pharmacokinetics of monoclonal immunoglobulin G1 F(ab')$_2$, and Fab in mice. *Cancer Res.*, **46**, 3969–78.
13. Serafini, A.N. (1993) From monoclonal antibodies to peptides and molecular recognition units: an overview. *J. Nucl. Med.*, **34**, 533–6.
14. Milenic, D.E., Yokota, T., Filpula, D.R. *et al.* (1991) Construction, binding properties, metabolism and tumor penetration of a single-chain Fv derived from pancarcinoma monoclonal antibody CC49. *Cancer Res.*, **51**, 6363–71.
15. Eckelman, W.C. and Paik, C.H. (1989) Labeling antibodies with metals using bifunctional chelates, in *Antibodies in Radiodiagnosis and Therapy* (ed. M.R. Zalutsky), CRC Press, USA, pp. 103–28.
16. Eary, J.F., Krohn, K.A., Kishore, R. *et al.* (1989) Radiochemistry of halogenated antibodies, in *Antibodies in Radiodiagnosis and Therapy* (ed. M.R. Zalutsky), CRC Press, USA, pp. 83–102.
17. Meares, C.F. (1986) Chelating agents for the binding of metal ions to antibodies. *Nucl. Med. Biol.*, **13**(4), 311–18.
18. Washburn, L.C., Hwa Sun, T.T., Crook, J.E. *et al.* (1986) ^{90}Y-labeled monoclonal antibodies for cancer therapy. *Nucl. Med. Biol.*, **13**(4), 453–6.
19. Breitz, H.B., Weiden, P.L., Vanderheyden, J.L. *et al.* (1992) Clinical experience with rhenium-186-labelled monoclonal antibodies for radioimmunotherapy: results of phase I trials. *J. Nucl. Med.*, **33**, 1099–112.
20. van Gog, F.B., Visser, G.W.M., Klok, R. *et al.* (1996) Monoclonal antibodies labeled with rhenium-186 using the MAG3 chelate: relationship between the number of chelated groups and biodistribution characteristics. *J. Nucl. Med.*, **37**, 352–62.
21. Deshpande, S.V., DeNardo, S.J., Kukis, D.L. *et al.* (1990) Yttrium-90-labelled monoclonal antibody for therapy: labeling by a new macrocyclic bifunctional chelating agent. *J. Nucl. Med.*, **31**, 473–9.
22. Powe, J., Pak, K.Y., Paik, C.H. *et al.* (1984) Labeling monoclonal antibodies and F(ab')$_2$ fragments with ^{111}In using cyclic DTPA anhydride and their *in vivo* behavior in mice bearing human tumor xenografts. *Cancer Drug Delivery*, **1**, 125–34.
23. Hnatowich, D.J. (1990) Recent developments in the radiolabeling of antibodies with iodine, indium, and technetium. *Semin. Nucl. Med.*, **20**(1), 80–1.

24. Divgi, C.R., Scott, A.M., Dantis, L. *et al.* (1995) Phase I radioimmunotherapy trial with iodine-131-CC49 in metastatic colon carcinoma. *J. Nucl. Med.*, **36**, 586–92.

25. Murray, J.L., Macey, D.J., Kasi, L.P. *et al.* (1994) Phase II radioimmunotherapy trial with ^{131}I-CC49 in colorectal cancer. *Cancer* (Suppl.), **73**, 1057–66.

26. Riva, P., Tison, V., Arista, A. *et al.* (1993) Radioimmunotherapy of gastrointestinal cancer and glioblastomas. *Int. J. Biol. Markers*, **8**(3), 192–7.

27. Lane, D.M., Eagle, K.F., Begent, R.H.J. *et al.* (1994) Radioimmunotherapy of metastatic colorectal tumours with iodine-131-labelled antibody to carcinoembryonic antigen: phase I/II study with comparative biodistribution of intact and F(ab′)$_2$ antibodies. *Br. J. Cancer*, **70**, 521–5.

28. Wong, J.Y.C., Williams, L.E., Yamauchi, D.M. *et al.* (1995) Initial experience evaluating [90]Yttrium-radiolabelled anti-carcinoembryonic antigen chimeric T84.66 in a phase I trial. *Cancer Res.* (Suppl.), **55**, S5929–34.

29. Meredith, R.F., Khazaeli, M.B., Plott, W.E. *et al.* (1995) Initial clinical evaluation of iodine-125-labelled chimeric 17-1A for metastatic colon cancer. *J. Nucl. Med.*, **36**, 2229–33.

30. Crippa, F., Bolis, G., Seregni, E. *et al.* (1995) Single-dose intraperitoneal radioimmunotherapy with the murine monoclonal antibody I-131 Mov18: clinical results in patients with minimal residual disease of ovarian cancer. *Eur. J. Cancer*, **31A**, 686–90.

31. Hird, V., Maraveyas, A., Snook, D. *et al.* (1993) Adjuvant therapy of ovarian cancer with radioactive monoclonal antibody. *Br. J. Cancer*, **68**, 403–6.

32. Kornblith, P.L., Walker, M.D. and Cassard, J.R. (1985) Neoplasms of the central nervous system, in *Cancer: Principles and Practice of Oncology* (eds V.T.J. De Vita, S. Hellman and S.A. Rosenberg), Lippincott, Philadelphia, pp. 1437–510.

33. Moseley, R.P., Davies, A.G., Richardson, R.B. *et al.* (1990) Intrathecal administration of ^{131}I radiolabelled monoclonal antibodies as a treatment of neoplastic meningitis. *Br. J. Cancer*, **62**, 637–42.

34. Rowlinson-Busza, G., Bamias, A., Kraus, T. *et al.* (1991) Uptake and distribution of specific and control monoclonal antibodies in subcutaneous xenografts following intratumoral injection. *Cancer Res.*, **51**, 3251–9.

35. Zalutsky, M.R., Moseley, R.P., Coakam, H.B. *et al.* (1989) Pharmacokinetics and tumour localisation of I-131 labeled antitenascin monoclonal antibody 81C6 in patients with gliomas and other intracranial malignancies. *Cancer Res.*, **49**, 2807–10.

36. Riva, P., Arista, A., Sturiale, C. *et al.* (1992) Treatment of intracranial human glioblastoma by direct intratumoral administration of ^{131}I-labelled antitenascin monoclonal antibody BC-2. *Int. J. Cancer*, **51**, 7–13.

37. Riva, P., Arista, A., Sturiale, C. *et al.* (1994) Glioblastoma therapy by direct intralesional administration of I-131 radioiodine labelled antitenascin antibodies. *Cell Biophysics*, **24/25**, 37–43.

38. Schrier, D.M., Stemmer, S.M., Johnson, T. *et al.* (1995) Diethylenetriaminepentaacetic acid (DTPA)-BrE-3 and autologous hematopoietic stem cell support (AHSCS) for the treatment of advanced breast cancer: a phase I trial. *Cancer Res.*, **55** (Suppl.), S5921–4.

39. DeNardo, S.J., Mirik, G.R., Kroger, L.A. *et al.* (1994) The biologic window for chimeric L6 radioimmunotherapy. *Cancer*, **73** (Suppl.), 1023–32.

40. Richman, C.M., DeNardo, S.J., O'Grady, L.F. *et al.* (1995) Radioimmunotherapy for breast cancer using escalating fractionated doses of ^{131}I-labelled chimeric L6 antibody with peripheral blood progenitor cell transfusions. *Cancer Res.*, **55** (Suppl.), S5916–20.

41. Goodwin, D.A., Meares, C.F., McCall, M. *et al.* (1988) Pre-Targeted immunoscintigraphy of murine tumors with indium-111-labelled bifunctional haptens. *J. Nucl. Med.*, **29**, 226–34.

42. LeDoussal, J.M., Martin, M., Gautherot, E. *et al.* (1989) In vitro and in vivo targeting of radiolabelled monovalent and divalent haptens with dual specificity monoclonal antibody conjugates: enhanced divalent hapten affinity for cell-bound antibody conjugate. *J. Nucl. Med.*, **30**, 1358–66.

43. Paganelli, G., Malcovati, M. and Fazio, F. (1991) Monoclonal antibody pretargeting techniques for tumour localization: the avidin-biotin system. *Nucl. Med. Commun.*, **12**, 211—34.

44. Sung, C. and van Osdol, W.W. (1995) Pharmacokinetic comparison of direct antibody targeting with pretargeting protocols based on streptavidin-biotin binding. *J. Nucl. Med.*, **36**, 867–76.

45. LeDoussal, J.M., Barbet, J. and Delaage, M. (1992) Bispecific-antibody-mediated targeting of radiolabelled bivalent haptens: theoretical, experimental and clinical results. *Int. J. Cancer*, **7**, 58–62.

46. Suresh, M.R., Cuello, A.C. and Milstein, C. (1986) Bispecific monoclonal antibodies from hybrid hybridomas. *Methods Enzymol.*, **121**, 210–15.

47. Bos, E.S., Kuijpers, W.H.A., Meesters-Winters, M. *et al.* (1994) In vitro evaluation of DNA-DNA hybridization as a two-step approach in radioimmunotherapy of cancer. *Cancer Res.*, **54**, 3479–86.

48. Paganelli, G., Magnani, P., Zito, F. *et al.* (1991) Three-step monoclonal antibody tumor targeting in carcinoembryonic antigen-positive patients. *Cancer Res.*, **51**, 5960–6.

49. Kalofonos, H.P., Rusckowski, M., Siebecker, D.A. *et al.* (1990) Imaging of tumors in patients with indium-111-labelled biotin and streptavidin-conjugated antibodies: preliminary communication. *J. Nucl. Med.*, **31**, 1791–6.

50. Paganelli, G., Belloni, C., Magnani, P. *et al.* (1992) Two-step tumour targeting in ovarian cancer patients using biotinylated monoclonal antibodies and radioactive streptavidin. *Eur. J. Nucl. Med.*, **19**, 322–9.

51. Paganelli, G., Grana, C., Chinol, M. *et al.* (1996) Therapy trial in malignant glioma patients with Y-90-biotin in a 3-step pretargeting approach. *J. Nucl. Med.*, **37** (Suppl.), 169P.

FURTHER READING

Britton, K.E., Granowska, M. (1988) Experience with I-123 labelled antibodies, in *Radiolabelled Monoclonal Antibodies for Imaging and Therapy* (ed. S.C. Srivastava), Plenum, New York, pp. 177–92.

DeLand, F.H. (1989) A perspective of monoclonal antibodies: past, present, and future. *Semin. Nucl. Med.*, **19**(3), 158–65.

Goodwin, D.A. (1995) Tumor pretargeting: almost the bottom line. *J. Nucl. Med.*, **36**(5), 876–9.

Magnani, P., Paganelli, G., Modorati, G. *et al.* (1996) Quantitative comparison of direct antibody labeling and tumor pretargeting in uveal melanoma. *J. Nucl. Med.*, **37**, 967–1.

Paganelli, G., Magnani, P., Siccardi, A.G. *et al.* (1995) Clinical application of the avidin-biotin system for tumor targeting. in *Cancer Therapy with Radiolabeled Antibodies* (ed. D.M. Goldenberg), CRC Press, pp. 239–54.

Lymphoma

R.L. Wahl

INTRODUCTION

Lymphomas include Hodgkin lymphoma (HL) and non-Hodgkin lymphoma (NHL). Both types of lymphoma have multiple and complex methods of grading that are beyond the scope of this text but are reviewed elsewhere [1]. The diseases have a global presence, though prevalence of B- versus T-cell types of NHL vary geographically. In the United States, more than 80% of NHL are of B-cell origin, while the rest are of T-cell origin.

Nuclear medicine scanning plays an important role in the diagnosis and follow-up of treatment of lymphoma, especially ^{67}Ga scanning in Hodgkin lymphoma, and there is a growing role for FDG-PET in lymphoma imaging [2]. The frequency of NHL is increasing, with over 50 000 new cases diagnosed in the US in 1995, while HL was newly-diagnosed in about 8000 patients in the US during the same time [1]. While typically, lymphomas are initially responsive to chemotherapy and/or radiotherapy, up to one-third of patients with HL – and a much larger fraction of those with NHL – eventually have recurrent disease which ultimately is fatal [3]. Indeed, recent studies have suggested that only half of patients with advanced intermediate- or high-grade lymphoma can be expected to be cured by chemotherapy (with or without bone marrow transplantation). Low-grade NHL will often recur after initial successful treatment and become chemotherapy-resistant, ultimately leading to death [1,3,4]. The economic impact of the lymphomas is disproportionately large in relation to their frequency – and also when compared with some other forms of cancer – as lymphomas tend to affect younger patients than do many other common solid tumours. Thus, new and better methods are needed to treat lymphoma.

As recently as 1994, experts in nuclear medicine and oncology stated that 'in summary, we have not found a solid indication that radio-immunotherapy can at present make a significant contribution to the treatment of the cancer patient' [5]. However, another review, focused on lymphoma therapy, from the same time period by Grossbard et al. [3] felt 'the significant number of cure rates and partial responses seen with RIC (radioimmunoconjugate) therapy in these early studies of heavily pretreated patients portends an exciting future for this therapeutic modality'. As will be discussed in this chapter, multiple recent reports with several antibodies indicate that at least for lymphoma, this higher level of enthusiasm for radioimmunotherapy is justified.

The overall concept of radioimmunotherapy (RIT) of cancer is an old one. The first RIT of cancer was performed in a human patient in 1951 at the University of Michigan, where Beierwaltes et al. [6] successfully used ^{131}I polyclonal antibody to treat a patient with melanoma. The concept then and now, was to have a radiolabelled antibody with tumour specificity, which would selectively bind to the tumour, but less avidly bind to normal tissues *in vivo*. The selective *in vivo* targeting to tumours would result in tumour kill, but spare normal tissues. While the concept of specific targeting is appealing, and lymphoma was cured in animal models as early as 1974 by Ghose et al. using iodinated polyclonal anti-lymphoma antibodies, a much greater interest in RIT was aroused when monoclonal antibodies (MAbs) were developed, in 1975 [7,8]. Monoclonal antibodies and their isotypes are discussed elsewhere in this text and in several excellent reviews [3, 9]. The MAbs allowed for the uniform availability of pharmaceutical which was not possible with polyclonal antibodies. In most RIT studies to date, antibodies of murine origin have been used against a variety of tumour antigens. The results of RIT of solid tumours have been quite disappointing so far – mainly because too little radioantibody actually reaches the tumours and there is a high, non-specific localization in normal tissues. However, there has been a better success rate with RIT of lymphomas, and several radiolabelled MAb therapies of lymphoma are in advanced phase clinical trials. This chapter will review progress in this field and prospects for the future.

Clinical Nuclear Medicine, 3rd edn. Edited by M.N. Maisey, K.E. Britton and B.D. Collier. Published in 1998 by Chapman & Hall, London. ISBN 0 412 75180 1

TUMOUR ANTIGENS ON LYMPHOMA

The quest for 'tumour-specific antigens' has been a difficult one, and in solid tumours, none has yet been identified. In NHL, however, 'tumour-specific' antigens are present, and are the surface immunoglobulin present on the B-cells that have transformed into lymphoma. The antigen-combining site on this antibody present on the malignant B-cell surface is known as the antibody 'idiotype' and MAbs specifically reactive with the idiotype can be prepared. These 'anti-idiotypic' antibodies are, in some instances, totally specific for the lymphoma [3,9]. The disadvantage of the anti-idiotypic antibodies for RIT is that in many instances it is necessary to construct a patient-specific antibody to a patient-specific idiotype. This means that a unique radiopharmaceutical would need to be constructed for each individual patient. This would be prohibitively expensive for routine therapy and has been difficult to put into practice. While there are some idiotypes that are shared among different lymphomas (public idiotypes), these anti-idiotype approaches are probably not going to be as useful as had been hoped initially. Another disadvantage of idiotypic antigens is that these antibody molecules on the B-cell surface (which constitutes the idiotype) are commonly shed into the circulation. Thus, high levels of idiotype are often present in the circulation and can interfere with binding of intravenously administered radiolabelled antibody to idiotype on the B-cell and thus prevent the radioantibody from reaching a tumour [10].

More commonly used and targeted antigens in lymphoma have been the lymphocyte differentiation markers. Since there is a normal ontogeny of B- and T-cell development from marrow stem-cells to mature B- and T-cells, a variety of antigens are expressed at varying stages of development. These antigens are not tumour-specific, but are generally B- or T-cell-specific. They can be antigens that modulate or internalize, or antigens that are fixed onto the cell surface. The choice of antigen for RIT is extremely important. In general, it is better to attempt to use an antigen which is not expressed on stem-cells in the marrow but is expressed on the tumour. This reduces the likelihood of bone marrow ablation as a treatment-related complication. Antibodies need not be tumour-specific, rather they need to be on the tumour in high density, but not present on stem-cells. Several candidate antigens have been evaluated and will be discussed in the clinical results section.

There are also antigens which are not tumour-specific but which appear to be preferentially expressed in lymphomas. An example of this is the transferrin receptor which is over-expressed in lymphomas. Similarly, there is over-expression of ferritin, an intracellular protein, in lymphomas; this has been targeted by radiolabelled anti-ferritin antibodies. To date, the best therapeutic results with RIT have been seen with antigens which are cell line-specific, but not tumour-specific. Completely tumour-specific antigens are not necessary for RIT to be successful.

RADIOPHARMACEUTICALS

Several radioactive isotopes can and have been used for RIT. The most commonly used isotopes to date have been iodine-131 (^{131}I) and yttrium-90 (^{90}Y). ^{131}I is well known to practitioners in nuclear medicine and is both a γ- and β-ray emitter. While the γ-ray emission can result in considerable radiation to non-target tissues, it does allow for imaging. ^{90}Y has an energetic β-ray emission and no γ-ray emission. This lack of a γ-ray emission is something of a disadvantage if tracer imaging studies are to be used to determine how much radiopharmaceutical is to be administered for therapy.

Iodination of antibodies is reasonably straightforward and several methods are in use. Radiolabelling methods must be optimized for the specific antibody and label. Recently, radioiodine labels have been developed which are more stable than standard chloramine-T labelling. Labels that residualize within tumour are important for antigens which internalize, as internalized ^{131}I-MAb tends to be catabolized, dehalogenated and excreted, resulting in a low radiation dose to tumours [11].

^{90}Y, a radiometal, is attractive for RIT for several reasons: (i) its dose rate is higher than for ^{131}I; (ii) if ^{90}Y is internalized into a lymphoma cell by a modulating antigen, it will be retained in the cell; and (iii) there is no contaminating gamma radiation. By contrast, when ^{131}I-labelled antibody is internalized, in most instances (due to deiodination) it is not retained within the tumour cell. A disadvantage of ^{90}Y is that it can also be retained in normal tissues such as liver (where antibodies are normally catabolized), the kidneys and, most importantly, in the bone. Bone uptake of ^{90}Y has been a major problem with earlier chelating methods. If ^{90}Y detaches from the chelator molecule, it will bind avidly to bone and because of the long β-particle path length, will irradiate the adjacent bone marrow. This bone marrow irradiation can cause severe myelotoxicity. Major efforts have been focused at finding ^{90}Y chelating agents that bind stably to ^{90}Y so that it is not released as free ^{90}Y. Substantial progress has been made, but these agents have not been extensively evaluated in clinical studies. Results with ^{90}Y will be discussed in the clinical results section.

A variety of other radioactive isotopes have been used for lymphoma treatment. These include ^{67}Cu, which has been used to treat several patients. It has properties somewhat similar to those of ^{131}I, but without substantial γ-ray emission. Although ^{67}Cu is an interesting radiolabel and has produced a clinical response, it has limited availability at present [12]. Alpha-emitters have been evaluated in a preliminary form in animal models. Most are too short-lived to be useful in treatment of lymphoma, but they may be useful in the treatment of leukaemia or regional disease where very rapid antibody delivery to tumours will occur. They are beyond the scope of the current discussion other than to state that they are attractive, potentially because of their high dose-rate properties and high LET, but they have yet to be used clinically for the treatment of lymphoma [13].

In most RIT studies performed to date, radiolabelling has been performed at the clinical facility doing the treatment. This has limited the procedure and the therapy to academic institutions or centres with excellent radiopharmacy capabilities. Increasingly, as RIT becomes clinically available, these agents will be supplied as kits in which radiometal is added and injected into the patient, or in the form of totally synthesized radiopharmaceuticals. For instance, ^{131}I-labelled antibody may be supplied from a central radiolabelling facility, an approach which should make RIT techniques much more widely available.

RADIOIMMUNOTHERAPY OF LYMPHOMA: CLINICAL STUDIES

Clinical results of RIT in lymphoma can be divided into three segments: (i) results with Hodgkin lymphoma; (ii) results with non-Hodgkin lymphoma without bone-marrow transplantation; and (iii) results in non-Hodgkin lymphoma with bone-marrow transplantation.

HODGKIN LYMPHOMA

In 1985, when treating Hodgkin lymphoma (HL), Lenhard *et al.* [14] used ^{131}I-labelled polyclonal anti-ferritin antibodies for human therapy. They reported that some relief was achieved in over three-quarters of the patients with refractory HL, and objective tumour regressions occurred in 40% of patients. Herpst *et al.* [15] reported on the use of polyclonal ^{90}Y-labelled anti-ferritin in treatment of HL; 44 patients were entered and 39 treated. Several species of origin of polyclonal anti-ferritin antibodies were used. Doses ranged from 10 to 50 mCi of ^{90}Y-labelled antibody (2–5 mg), with up to five cycles of therapy being given. Some patients needed bone marrow transplant support, if they experienced toxicities. Larger ^{90}Y doses mainly caused haematopoietic toxicity. Among the 39 patients, there were 10 complete and 10 partial responses, two had stable disease, and 17 showed progression despite therapy [15]. There was substantial variability in pharmacokinetics, and about half the patients survived the therapy for more than 6 months. It was rare for complete response to be achieved after a single anti-ferritin treatment; however, these appear to occur more commonly after two to three treatments (9 of 10). The average tumour dose was 900 rad, indicating that only modest tumour targeting was achieved. This same ^{90}Y polyclonal anti-ferritin method of therapy was applied to patients with both radiolabelled antibody and high-dose chemotherapy followed by transplant in patients with poor-prognosis Hodgkin lymphoma [16]. Patients received the ^{90}Y-labelled anti-ferritin about 10–14 days before transplantation, followed by high-dose chemotherapy and bone marrow transplantation. Several patients died while undergoing the aggressive regimen, but several are alive more than 2 years after transplantation. This suggests that this method is active even in patients with chemotherapy-refractory tumour, and also that the combined approach with bone marrow transplantation carries with it substantial potential toxicity, including death. Nonetheless, these data clearly indicate that ^{90}Y polyclonal anti-ferritin is an active therapy of Hodgkin lymphoma.

NON-HODGKIN LYMPHOMA (NHL)

T-cell NHL

More clinical studies have been done in B-cell than T-cell lymphoma. However, cutaneous T-cell lymphoma was one of the first lymphomas studied with radioimmunotherapy using the ^{131}I-labelled T101 monoclonal antibody. Rosen *et al.* [19] reported on the use of ^{131}I-labelled T101 anti-CD5 monoclonal antibody in doses of about 100–250 mCi in five patients. Mixed responses and two partial responses were seen [19]. Essentially all of the patients developed human anti-murine antibodies (HAMA), although some could be retreated through the use of plasmapheresis to remove some of the HAMA from the serum. This high frequency of HAMA precluded continued studies with this reagent. Nonetheless, T101 did demonstrate the feasibility of treating T-cell lymphomas with ^{131}I-antibody and T-cell antibody. Patients with circulating antigen-positive cells with clinical leukaemia did not have the same level of response as was reported by Zimmer and colleagues in 1988 [18]. A small number of patients with acute T-cell leukaemia lymphoma were treated with 5–10 mCi of [90]Y -labelled anti-Tac antibody by Waldman *et al.* [19]; this reagent binds to the CD25 antigen. Myelosuppression was seen and modest anti-tumour response noted. These two studies indicate that treating T-cell lymphoma is feasible using radiolabelled MAbs, but that there are major obstacles with this approach.

B-cell NHL

The treatment of NHL with radiolabelled antibodies can be performed with two basic approaches. One involves millicurie doses of radiolabelled antibody which are relatively low and which do not sufficiently suppress the bone marrow so that bone marrow transplantation is necessary ('non-myeloablative'). The other approach is to give higher doses of radiolabelled antibody and support the patient with bone marrow transplantation ('myeloablative'). Clinical studies to date have been performed with lower doses of radiolabelled antibody given as a single dose or as multiple sequential injections. The results of these clinical trials will be reviewed briefly.

Several groups have investigated the treatment of NHL with non-myeloablative treatment, with most of the work having been done in B-cell lymphoma. As early as 1985, DeNardo *et al.* [12,20] treated a patient with ^{131}I-LYM-1 MAb and reported that the patient had a substantial clinical response and survived for 2 years after treatment. The authors recently summarized the results of 52 courses of RIT in patients with recurrent NHL with doses ranging from 10 to 100 mCi per cycle, in their 'low-dose fractionated phase I/II study' [12]. In this study, complete response was achieved in two patients and partial response in ten. Results suggested that in patients who received greater total millicurie doses (>180 mCi), the response rates were greater – at 94%. They also pointed out that unlabelled antibody was not effective in patients and thus the ^{131}I-LYM-1 was an essential component to the process [12, 20].

Using higher doses of radioactivity from 40–100 mCi/m^2 at 4-week intervals, Wilder and DeNardo and their colleagues observed seven complete responses and four partial responses. Since 21 patients were evaluated with a higher dose, a complete response rate of 33% and a partial response rate of 21% was identified. They observed, as have others, that tumour responses were rapid and complete with higher radioactivity doses administered. LYM-1 labelled with [67]Cu has also been used for RIT [12,20]. While experience with this agent has been limited, three patients have been reportedly treated, and one complete and one partial response noted. Per millicurie, [67]Cu delivers more radiation to the tumours than ^{131}I, but it is very limited in availability and requires special chelation chemistry to be effective in radioimmunotherapy. At present, it is unlikely that [67]Cu-labelled antibody will be widely applied to radioimmunotherapy.

Investigators at the University of Michigan evaluated the ^{131}I-labelled anti-CD37 monoclonal antibody (MB-1) in a dose escalation trial in patients with NHL [21]. In the trial, radiation dose was escalated based on estimated cGy to the whole body based on tracer studies using labelled antibody, as opposed to escalating dose based on millicuries or mCi/m^2. Of 12 patients studied, eight had intermediate- or high-grade lymphomas, seven of which were transformed, and four had low-grade lymphomas. All patients had been heavily pretreated with chemotherapy and one was status post bone marrow transplant. ^{131}I-MB-1 antibody was given at protein doses of 40 or 200 mg. Tumour targeting was modest, with only 39% of lesions detectable. Acute toxicity was minimal. Rapid declines in serum B-cells were seen, with delayed toxicity (mainly myelosuppression), especially thrombocytopenia. Two patients developed human anti-murine antibodies. The maximum tolerated dose was somewhat less than 50 cGy to the total body. Six patients had tumour responses post RIT. Four responses lasted longer than 1 month (2–6 months) and included a complete response, a partial response, a minor response, and a mixed response. Tumour dosimetry showed a mean 2.77 cGy/mCi reaching the tumour, versus 0.37 cGy/mCi for the whole body. Thus, selective tumour targeting of about seven- to eightfold was identified for the MB-1 antibody. Based on these data, ^{131}I-MB-1 at these protein and radiation doses, while having anti-tumour activity, was judged sub-optimal therapy.

Czuczman and colleagues from Memorial Sloan Kettering Cancer Center reported on the use of ^{131}I-labelled OK-B-7 monoclonal antibody (murine anti-CD21 monoclonal) [22]. These patients were treated in a phase I dose-escalation trial where dose-escalation was based on escalating millicurie doses. Therapy was performed with repeated 30–50 mCi (25 mg) of [131]I- OKB-7, administered several days apart to achieve total cumulative dose levels of between 90 and 200 mCi (range 90, 120, 160 and 200 mCi). Targeting to tumour was observed in eight of 18 patients; however, there was a high frequency of HAMA (occurring in 12 of 16 patients). As in the MB-1 study, significant non-haematological toxicity was rare and in this study was limited to asymptomatic hypothyroidism as evidenced by an increased TSH level. Bone marrow toxicity or myelosuppression was observed in one-third of patients. Out of the 18 patients, one partial response and 12 mixed responses were identified, with seemingly more frequent responses in patients given higher millicurie doses. The investigators observed that peripheral lymphadenopathy, large spleens and skin lesions responded most rapidly to treatment. A maximally tolerated cumulative dose of approximately 200 mCi was felt to be present for doses divided into 50 mCi aliquots. ^{131}I-OK-B7 had modest anti-tumour activity and was reasonably safe in the doses given, with the limitation to dosing being haematopoietic toxicity [22].

Investigators at the University of Michigan reported clinical results with ^{131}I-anti-CD20 IgGa murine MAb anti 'B-1' first in 1993 in nine patients [4], and in the follow-up article in 1996 on a total of 34 patients [23]. In this study, adults with B-cell NHL who were CD20-positive and who had failed at least one prior chemotherapy regimen were enrolled. Patients also had to have assessable and measurable disease by either physical examination or CT, and less than 25% of the marrow space involved by lymphoma cells. In addition, they had to have nearly normal organ function. The trial was conducted using sequential gamma-camera imaging and sequential conjugate counting assessments of radioactivity in the body by NaI probe. ^{131}I-anti-B1 is an ^{131}I-labelled mouse IgG2a MAb. Patients were first given tracer-labelled doses of ^{131}I-labelled anti-B1 15–20 mg (5 mCi) to assess radiolabelled antibody biodistribution and whole-body and organ dosimetry. Following the tracer dose, generally about 1 week later, a radioimmunotherapeutic dose of about the same protein mass, labelled with the quantity of ^{131}I that would deliver a specified radiation dose of the whole body as predicted by the tracer dose, was administered. Dose escalation was in groups of three to four patients, starting at a total-body dose of 25 cGy that was escalated to 85 cGy. To determine if radiolabelled antibody biodistribution could be optimized by changing the amount of unlabelled antibody predose, as had been shown in pre-clinical studies, some of the earlier patients in the study were given one or two additional tracer infusions on sequential weeks, each dose preceded by an infusion of either 135 mg of unlabelled anti-B1 or 685 mg of unlabelled anti-B1. The antibody dose resulting in the best tracer biodistribution was chosen for therapy. Later patients were given a single tracer dose immediately following an unlabelled antibody infusion of 685 mg.

As in the other trials with ^{131}I-labelled monoclonal antibodies to B-cell antigens, acute toxicity was modest and mainly immunological, and haematological toxicity was dose limiting. In this study, 75 cGy was established as the 'maximally tolerated' whole-body radiation dose (MTD) [4]. Of the 34 patients, 28 received radioimmunotherapy, with doses ranging from 34 to 161 mCi. Fourteen patients had a complete response and eight had a partial response. Thirteen patients with low-grade lymphoma responded, with 10 achieving complete response. Six of eight patients with transformed lymphoma responded. Thirteen of 19 patients whose disease was resistant to their last course of chemotherapy, and all patients whose disease had responded to chemotherapy

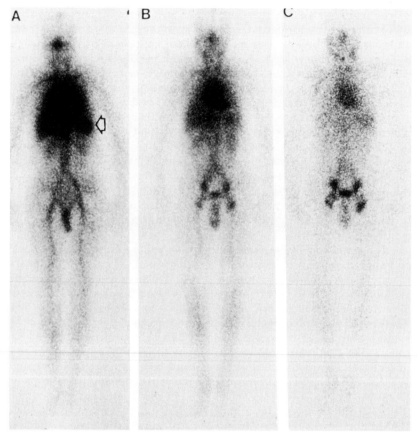

Figure 1.20   Sequential anterior whole body images following injection of 5 mg tracer dose of ^{131}I-anti-B1. Image A, soon after tracer injection, shows blood pool activity. Subsequent images show blood pool clearance and antibody accumulation in tumour sites, one to several days post injection (B, C).

immediately before radioimmunotherapy, showed a response. Median duration of complete remission was >15 months, with some of the remissions lasting in excess of 31 months. Patients with large tumour burdens and splenomegaly responded quite well to the treatment. None of the patients required infusion of bone marrow for haematopoietic support. In summary, ^{131}I-anti-B1 administered based on tracer study kinetics was capable of producing a high frequency of durable remissions with acceptable toxicity [4].

[131]I-anti-B1 is currently in phase III clinical investigation in the United States and Europe. An example of a radionuclide scan with ^{131}I-anti-B1 is shown in Figure 1.20, and Figure 1.21 shows an example of tumour response following ^{131}I-anti-B1 radioimmunotherapy.

Another phase I/II dose-escalation study with an anti-CD20 monoclonal antibody was performed by the group at Stanford University using anti-B1 and a different anti-CD20 MAb (Y2B8) [23]. In this case, murine ^{90}Y-labelled anti-CD20 was used as a therapeutic. Patients with relapsed low- to intermediate-grade NHL were treated. Biodistribution studies with [111]In- anti-CD20 MAb preceded the ^{90}Y therapy studies. A dose-escalation was performed with groups of three or four patients treated at doses of about 13, 20, 30, 40, and 50 mCi of ^{90}Y-anti-CD20. The major toxicity seen was haematological: leucopenia, granulocytopenia and thrombocytopenia were quite common. Grade 4 thrombocytopenia was seen in several patients receiving 30 mCi of ^{90}Y-MAb and at higher dose levels. Doses of 50 mCi ^{90}Y-MAb

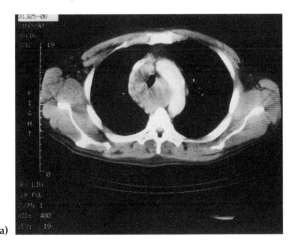
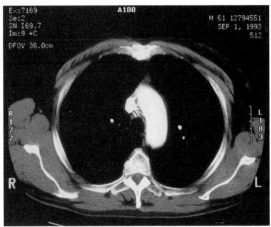

(a)
(b)

Figure 1.21 Pre-RIT CT scan (a) shows extensive mediastinal tumour burden, with tracheal narrowing. Scan (b) after non-myeloablative treatment with ^{131}I-anti-B1 shows complete response of NHL.

were generally quite toxic and required bone-marrow stem-cell support in several instances to achieve marrow reconstitution. In this study, at least three of the patients required transplantation to deal with radiation-induced toxicity. Despite the toxicity, the treatment showed considerable activity with the overall response rate following a single dose of ^{90}Y of 72%, with six complete responses and seven partial responses. Durations of responses range from 3 to more than 29 months after treatment. It should be noted that the first four patients on the study received anti-B1 MAb while the other 14 received the Y2B8 MAb, both anti-CD20.

Thus, with two different monoclonal antibodies and two different kinds of labels, anti-CD20 MAbs showed substantial therapeutic activity in the treatment of lymphoma. Furthermore, at lower doses of ^{131}I and ^{90}Y, the treatments were not myeloablative and thus presumably could be given at lower expense and less risk than the more aggressive myeloablative strategies.

Goldenberg [24] and subsequently Juweid and colleagues [25] reported on the use of LL2 labelled with ^{131}I as a treatment for lymphoma. LL2 is a murine IgG2a anti-CD22 MAb. Initially, Goldenberg reported on two partial responses and two mixed responses in five assessable patients with NHL [24]. Of interest is that one of the responses was seen with only 6.2 mCi of LL2. This trial was then expanded to treat 21 patients on an outpa-

tient basis using repeated injections of low doses of ^{131}I-LL2. The patients were treated with 15 to 343 mCi of +131I-LL2 for up to seven treatment cycles. Cumulative protein doses ranged from 1.1 mg IgG2a to 157 mg of F(ab')$_2$. Seventeen patients were assessable for treatment response and five showed anti-tumour activity [25]. One complete response was seen, two partial remissions and two minor responses. Responses were seen with both partial and complete responses noted for both F(ab')$_2$ and intact IgG treatment. When the dose was increased to 90 mCi/m^2 and bone-marrow transplantation support was provided, responses seemed more common [25]. As in other studies, anti-mouse antibodies were infrequent and only four patients developed HAMA. It is of note that the LL2 MAb is internalized and ^{131}I is not an optimal label for internalizing antibody. The authors state that they plan additional studies in patients with various forms of radioactive label such as ^{90}Y, which may be better suited to internalizing antibodies. Nonetheless, ^{131}I-LL2 does show activity in treatment of NHL and can achieve anti-tumour activity without bone marrow transplant support.

As discussed earlier, lymphomas have the unique attribute of bearing legitimate tumour-specific antigens on the cell surface, those being the surface immunoglobulin expressed by the malignant B-cells. Anti-idiotypic antibodies can be produced which are reactive with these antigenic determinants and targeted with radiolabelled antibody. Investigators at USCD evaluated the use ^{90}Y-labelled anti-idiotype antibody radioimmunotherapy in nine patients with relapsed B-cell lymphoma. Initial tracer targeting was with ^{111}In-labelled anti-idiotype antibody, this given after administration of between 1000 and 2320 mg of unlabelled MAb in an attempt to clear circulating idiotype from the circulation. One to four courses of treatment per patient were given, with the total dose of 10 to 54 mCi ^{90}Y-antibody per patient. Activity was seen against the lymphomas, with two of nine patients having a complete response, one a partial response, three stable disease and three progressive disease [10]. The time to tumour progression varied from 1 to 12 months. As with other radioimmunotherapies, toxicity was predominantly haematological with the need for transfusion support common. HAMA was not observed in these patients. The investigators felt the variable which best correlated with success or failure of treatment was the ability to clear the circulating idiotype from the blood with unlabelled anti-idiotypic antibody. When this clearance could not be achieved, successful tumour targeting was not likely and tumour therapy was unlikely to be successful. While logistically challenging and probably not practicable because of the difficulty in producing patient-specific radiopharmaceuticals, this study indicates that RIT of NHL is also possible using anti-idiotype antibodies labelled with ^{90}Y [10].

HIGH-DOSE RIT OF B-CELL NHL WITH TRANSPLANT SUPPORT

Press and colleagues at the University of Washington have used high doses of several ^{131}I-labelled murine MAbs reactive with CD20 (B1 and 1F5) and CD37 (MB-1) [11,26,27]. These investigators reported that they had evaluated 56 patients with lymphoma with labelled antibody infusions and 32 (57%) had been treated. Patients were treated based on having a 'favourable' biodistribution during the tracer study. This 'favourable biodistribution' meant that the tumour foci would receive more radiation dose than any other normal tissue. These investigators observed that patients with small spleens and low tumour burdens were more likely to have good targeting. They varied protein mass over several levels and found, depending on the kind of antibody used, different

protein masses were most appropriate. For the currently favoured antibody anti-B1, 2.5 mg/kg of antibody is used along with 10 mCi of ^{131}I for the tracer study. The therapy millicurie dose was dose-escalated. The dose-escalation study showed little toxicity up to organ doses of 2375 cGy (other than myelosuppression) but when the dose was increased to approximately 3100 cGy to the lungs, severe cardiopulmonary toxicity was seen. Thus, lower doses of radiation have been used subsequently and 2725 cGy is reported as the maximum tolerated organ dose. These investigators are currently investigating whether radioimmunotherapy can be combined with chemotherapy. Of 19 patients studied in phase I, 16 achieved complete response, two had partial response and one had a minor response. The mean response duration was in excess of 15 months and nine patients were reported in continuous complete remission at 14 months to >5 years after treatment without additional therapy. Ten patients entered into a phase II trial could not be evaluated as response was not yet complete, but had no evidence of progressive disease [28]. None of the patients has had a failure of bone-marrow grafting. Administered radiation activity has ranged from 345 to 785 mCi, delivering between 2700 and 9200 cGy to tumour sites. One patient who was treated with anti-idiotypic antibody achieved a complete response.

CONSIDERATIONS FOR THE NUCLEAR PHYSICIAN

The preceding clinical data indicate that multiple anti B-cell antibodies labelled with multiple radioisotopes show activity in the treatment of NHL and HL. While the optimal antibody/label combination is not yet fully resolved, very high response rates are being seen with ^{131}I-labelled antibodies.

The logistical considerations in ^{131}I-labelled antibody therapy differ depending on the country in which it is performed. Regulations on the amount of ^{131}I or therapeutic isotope in a patient who requires hospitalization vary significantly by country. In parts of Europe, as little as 2–5 mCi residual ^{131}I in the body may be sufficient to require the patient to be hospitalized. In contrast, new regulations in the United States, which will likely come into effect soon, potentially will allow for release of patients who have <100 mCi of ^{131}I in their body, if it can be shown that they are unlikely to expose the public to >500 mR of radiation following treatment. With appropriate behaviour and precautions, this can generally be achieved at the 100 mCi dose level. Thus, considerable differences exist in regulations which may mean varying ease in performance of RIT in different locales. In the light of the more liberal regulations proposed, it is easy to envisage giving relatively high doses of RIT to outpatient cases in the United States, with either ^{90}Y or ^{131}I as the label. In contrast, inpatient hospitalization will be likely necessary in other countries for several days to perhaps several weeks after treatment, depending on the radiolabel and millicurie dose. Despite these needs for hospitalization for radiation protection, RIT is still likely to be practical and cost-effective as it can be given as a single dose with a reasonably long duration response, in contrast to the repeated monthly doses given for chemotherapy.

Another practical consideration for the nuclear medicine physician administering the treatment, beyond radiation safety, is what activity level of the radiolabelled antibody should be given for treatment. Dosing in the trials performed to date have ranged from simple studies in which dose escalation has been based on escalating millicuries, to studies in which dose escalation has been made based on mCi/kg or mCi per m^2 of body surface area. More elaborate trials, in which patient tracer study kinetics have been used to plan patient dosing, are being carried out more frequently. These dosimetric studies are increasingly popular, as some of the anti-B-cell MAbs have substantial patient-to-patient variability in their clearance rates. For example, the anti-CD20 MAb anti-B1 can vary in clearance rate by a factor of at least two in patients with lymphoma. Thus, a patient who clears the radioantibody slowly would need a lower total millicurie dose than a patient who clears radioantibody rapidly, to achieve a similar radiation dose to the whole body. At present, strategies in which the tracer study is being used to plan the treatment millicurie dose are being used in some instances, while other studies are focusing on evaluating dose to organs or potentially in attempting to estimate radiation dose to the bone marrow.

Several recent reports have suggested that gamma scintigraphy of lymphoma patients which shows intense activity in the marrow may predict an increased likelihood of bone marrow toxicity [29,30]. It has been suggested in some algorithms that imaging of the bone marrow and quantitation of activity in the marrow may be important before determining the RIT dose. At present, the optimal method of dose planning in RIT is uncertain and marrow dosimetry is an evolving field of study. It is likely that if there is substantial variability in radioantibody clearance from patient to patient, that individualization of the patient therapy will be necessary based on the patient's pharmacokinetics. As an example, dosing based on 'whole-body dose' may be a reasonable and practicable means to allow some individualization of patient dosing without the necessity of repeated complex determinations of organ or bone-marrow dose [4]. Methods have been developed recently, which allow rapid calculation of patient therapy dose based on only a few data points if the tracer clearance is monoexponential [31]. This area of study is in rapid evolution, but it is likely that a reasonably simple method will have to be implemented, as complex dosimetric assessment pretreatment will be expensive and technically difficult. If complex dosimetry is needed to safely administer RIT, it will probably greatly slow the dissemination of the method. Another unresolved issue is whether tumour dosimetry is necessary to plan radioimmunotherapy – for example, if a tumour does not receive a specified radiation dose, will it be unlikely to respond? Clinical data in this area are still in evolution. With the ^{131}I-anti-CD20 MAb anti-B1, investigators at the University of Michigan have seen tumour responses at a variety of radiation doses, doses which are lower than those which might be expected to cause responses with standard external beam radiation [4]. This is concordant with the experience of multiple groups evaluating RIT. Because monoclonal antibodies have several activities beyond delivering radiation, it is probably not appropriate at present to deny patients therapy if tumour targeting is only modest. This is because intact monoclonal antibodies can fix complement, mediate ADCC, in some instances can potentially influence cell-surface receptors and can transduce signals. Furthermore, low-dose radiation may cause synchronicity or block the cell division cycle in a more radiosensitive portion, or induce apoptosis.

SUMMARY AND OUTLOOK

Just a few years ago, some experts in the field of RIT doubted if the technique would achieve any clinical success [5]. Although this concern remains valid for many solid tumours, it is clearly not the case for RIT of lymphoma, in which several different MAbs have demonstrated substantial therapeutic activity. It is possible that, before this text is revised, one or more MAbs will have made it into routine clinical practice in the United States and elsewhere. Thus, it is quite likely that radioimmunotherapy, which for many years was considered a dream, will finally become reality. It is likely that [131]I- or ^{90}Y-labelled MAbs, given at doses not requiring bone marrow transplant support, will be among the first agents available to nuclear medicine practitioners. It is probable that the practicality of these methods will depend on the local regulations for confining patients following radioactive therapy. Despite potential logistical difficulties, RIT of lymphoma is expected to become a more common part of the clinical armamentarium of nuclear medicine physicians in the next several years.

REFERENCES

1. Longo, D.L., Mauch, P., DeVita, V.T., Urba, W.J. *et al.* (1993) Lymphocytic Lymphomas (eds V.T. DeVita, S. Hellman and S.A. Rosenberg), *Can. Principles Practice of Oncology*, Lippincott, Philadelphia, PA, pp. 1859–927.
2. Shea, R. and Wahl, R.L. (1995) Oncology: Lymphoma, in *Principles of Nuclear Medicine*, 2nd edn (eds H.N. Wagner, Jr, Z. Szabo and J.W. Buchanan), Philadelphia, PA, pp. 1111–17.
3. Grossbard, M.L. and Nadler, L.M. (1993) Monoclonal antibody therapy for indolent lymphomas. *Semin. Oncol.*, **20**(5), 118–35.
4. Kaminski, M.S., Zasadny, K.R., Francis, I.R. *et al.* (1996) Iodine-[131]-Anti-B1 radioimmunotherapy for B-cell lymphoma. *J. Clin. Oncol.*, **14**(7), 1974–81.
5. Mello, A.M., Pauwels, E.K.J. and Cleton, F.J. (1994) Radioimmunotherapy: No news from the newcomer. *J. Can. Res. Clin. Oncol.*, **120**, 121–30.
6. Beierwaltes (personal communication).
7. Ghose, T. and Guclu, A. (1974) Cure of a mouse lymphoma with radio-iodinated antibody. *Eur. J. Cancer*, **10**(12), 787–92.
8. Kohler, G. and Milstein, C. (1975) Continuous cultures of fused cells secreting antibody of predefined specificity. *Nature*, **256**, 495–7.
9. Jurcic, J.G., Caron, P.C. and Scheinberg, D.A. (1995) Monoclonal antibody therapy of leukaemia and lymphoma. *Adv. Pharmacol.*, **33**, 287–314.
10. White, C.A., Halpern, S.E., Parker, B.A. *et al.* (1996) Radioimmunotherapy of relapsed B-cell lymphoma with yttrium-90 anti-idiotype monoclonal antibodies. *Blood*, **87**(9), 3640–9.
11. Press, O.W., Appelbaum, F.R., Eary, J.F. and Bernstein, I.D. (1995) Radiolabelled antibody therapy of lymphomas. *Important Adv. Oncol.*, 157–71.
12. Wilder, R.B., DeNardo, G.L. and DeNardo, S.J. (1996) Radioimmunotherapy: recent results and future directions. *J. Clin. Oncol.*, **14**(4), 1383–400.
13. Zalutsky, M.R. and Bigner, D.D. (1996) Radioimmunotherapy with x-particle emitting radioimmunoconjugates. *Acta Oncol.*, **35**(3), 373–9.
14. Lenhard, R.E., Order, S.E., Spunberg, J.J. *et al.* (1985) Isotopic immunoglobulin. A new systemic therapy for advanced Hodgkin's disease. *J. Clin. Oncol.*, **3**, 1296–300.
15. Herpst, J.M., Klein, J.L., Leichner, P.K., Quadri, S.M. and Vriesendorp, H.M. (1995) Survival of patients with resistant Hodgkin's disease after polyclonal yttrium-90 labeled antiferritin treatment. *J. Clin. Oncol.*, **13**(9), 2394–400.
16. Bierman, P.J., Vose, J.M., Leichner, P.K. *et al.* (1993) Yttrium-90 labeled antiferritin followed by high-dose chemotherapy and autologous bone marrow transplantation for poor-prognosis Hodgkin's disease. *J. Clin. Oncol.*, **11**(4), 698–703.
17. Rosen, S.T., Zimmer, A.M., Goldman-Leikin, R. *et al.* (1987) Radioimmunodetection and radioimmunotherapy of cutaneous T cell lymphomas using an ^{131}I-labeled monoclonal antibody: an Illinois Cancer Council Study. *J. Clin. Oncol.*, **5**(4), 562–73.
18. Kaplan, E.H., Goldman-Leikin, R.E., Radosevich, J.A. *et al.* (1989) *Cancer and Aging; Progress in Research and Treatment* (eds T.V. Zenser and R.M. Coe), Springer Publishing, New York, pp. 86–109.
19. Waldmann, T.A., White, J.D., Carrasquillo, J.A. *et al.* (1995) Radioimmunotherapy of interleukin-2R alpha-expressing adult T-cell leukaemia with Yttrium-90-labeled anti-Tac. *Blood*, **86**(11), 4063–75.
20. Lewis, J.P., DeNardo, G.L. and DeNardo, S.J. (1995) Radioimmunotherapy of Lymphoma: A UC Davis Experience. *Hybridoma*, **14**(2), 115–20.
21. Kaminski, M.S., Fig, L.M., Zasadny, K.R. *et al.* (1992) Imaging, dosimetry, and radioimmunotherapy with iodine-131-labeled anti-CD37 antibody in B-cell lymphoma. *J. Clin. Oncol.*, **10**(11), 1696–711.
22. Czuczman, M.S., Straus, D.J., Divgi, C.R. *et al.* (1993) Phase I dose-escalation trial of iodine-131-labeled monoclonal antibody OKB7 in patients with non-Hodgkin's lymphoma. *J. Clin. Oncol.*, **11**(10), 2021–9.
23. Knox, S.J., Goris, M.L., Trisler, K. *et al.* (1996) Yttrium-90 labeled anti-CD20 monoclonal antibody therapy of recurrent B-cell lymphoma. *Clin. Cancer Res.*, **2**, 457–70.
24. Goldenberg, D.M., Horowitz, J.A., Sharkey, R.M. *et al.* (1991) Targeting, dosimetry, and radioimmunotherapy of B-cell lymphomas with iodine-131-labeled LL2 monoclonal antibody. *J. Clin. Oncol.*, **9**(4), 548–64.
25. Juweid, M., Sharkey, R.M., Markowitz, A. *et al.* (1995) Treatment of non-Hodgkin's lymphoma with radiolabeled murine, chimeric, or humanized LL2, an anti-CD22 monoclonal antibody. *Cancer Res. Ctr*, **55**, 5899–907.

26. Press, O.W., Eary, J.F., Appelbaum, F.R. *et al.* (1993) Radiolabeled-antibody therapy of B-cell lymphoma with autologous bone marrow support. *N. Engl. J. Med.*, **329**(17), 1219–24

27. Press, O.W., Eary, J.F., Appelbaum, F.R. *et al.* (1995) Phase II trial of ^{131}I-B1 (anti-CD20) antibody therapy with autologous stem cell transplantation for relapsed B cell lymphomas. *Lancet*, **346**, 336–40.

28. Eary, J.F. and Press, O.W. (1996) High dose radioimmunotherapy in malignant lymphoma. *Rec. Res. Cancer Res.*, **141**, 177–82

29. Macey, D.J., DeNardo, S.J., DeNardo, G.L. *et al.* (1995) Estimation of radiation absorbed doses to the red marrow in radioimmunotherapy. *Clin. Nucl. Med.*, **20**(2), 117–25.

30. Juweid, M., Sharkey, R.M., Siegel, J.A. *et al.* (11995) Estimates of red marrow dose by sacral scintigraphy in radioimmunotherapy patients having non-Hodgkin's lymphoma and diffuse bone marrow uptake. *Cancer Res. (Suppl.)*, **55**, 5827–31.

31. Zasadny, K.R. and Wahl, R.L. (1996) A simplified method for determining therapeutic activity to administer for radioimmunotherapy. The Society of Nuclear Medicine 43rd Annual Meeting, Denver, CO, June 3–5, 1996. *J. Nucl. Med.*, **37**(5), 43P.

32. Macklis, R.M., Beresford, B.A., Palayoor, S. *et al.* (1993) Cell cycle alterations, apoptosis, and response to low-dose-rate radioimmunotherapy in lymphoma cells. *Radiat. Oncol.*, **27**, 643–50.

CHAPTER 2

Cancer imaging: principles and practice

S.E.M. Clarke and K.E. Britton

INTRODUCTION

Unlike the majority of imaging modalities used in the management of patients with suspected or proven malignancy, which rely on alterations in structure to visualize the tumour site, nuclear medicine imaging techniques utilize the ability to visualize alterations in metabolism. These alterations in metabolism may occur in the tissues surrounding the tumour site or may occur in the tumour itself. Radiopharmaceuticals used in tumour imaging may also be divided into those that are specifically taken up by tumours and those whose uptake is non-specific. These non-specific agents also localize in other pathological processes such as inflammation. In this chapter, the principles underlying the localization of radiopharmaceuticals used for tumour imaging will be discussed (Table 2.1) and the role of nuclear medicine in the management of cancer patients will be explored.

PRINCIPLES OF LOCALIZATION

UPTAKE IN TISSUE SURROUNDING A TUMOUR SITE

Tissue unaffected by the tumour

While the most obvious target site for tumour imaging is the tumour itself, the majority of radiopharmaceuticals used for tumour imaging in the past have localized in the normal tissues surrounding the tumour.

^{99m}Tc-labelled sulphur or tin colloid is taken up by the reticuloendothelial Kupffer cells of the liver. The uptake is uniform in normal liver tissue but the presence of hepatic metastases disturbs the normal liver architecture and there is no tracer uptake in the metastatic sites. The metastases therefore appear as photon-deficient or 'cold' areas in the liver.

This technique is obviously non-specific as any space-occupying lesion in the liver, such as a cyst, will yield an identical image appearance. ^{99m}Tc-labelled colloid liver imaging now plays little role in the detection of liver metastases as ultrasound scanning has proved to be a more cost-effective method. However, it is useful in monitoring the regression or progression of liver metastases since it is operator-independent and can provide a sequence of images that can be readily assessed by the clinician.

^{99m}Tc or ^{123}I thyroid imaging is an example of a radionuclide technique that may detect thyroid malignancy by the absence of tracer uptake in the tumour site(s) compared with that of normal thyroid tissue. Photon-deficient areas seen on a thyroid scan, particularly when solitary, raise the possibility of a thyroid malignancy as, in general, thyroid cancers fail to take up tracer. As with radionuclide liver imaging, these changes are non-specific as cysts and benign thyroid tumours will produce the same appearance. The combination of ultrasound scanning and radionuclide imaging greatly increases the diagnostic specificity, and combined imaging is an effective method of evaluating a palpable thyroid nodule.

Surrounding tissue affected by tumour

In the above examples, the tissue surrounding the tumour functions normally, but in the case of

Clinical Nuclear Medicine, 3rd edn. Edited by M.N. Maisey, K.E. Britton and B.D. Collier. Published in 1998 by Chapman & Hall, London. ISBN 0 412 75180 1

Table 2.1 The principles of radiopharmaceutical localisation

1. Uptake in tissue surrounding a tumour site
   a) Tissues unaffected by the tumour
   b) Tissues affected by tumour
2. Localization on tumour membranes
   a) Antigen/antibody reaction
   b) Receptor binding
3. Localization within tumour cells
   a) Tumour-specific metabolic tracers
   b) Non-specific tracers

^{99m}Tc-labelled methylene diphosphonate (^{99m}Tc-MDP) bone scan, the tissue surrounding the tumour site reacts with increased osteoblastic activity. An increase in tracer uptake is observed adjacent to the tumour. As diphosphonate uptake is proportional to osteoblastic activity, and since the changes in osteoblastic activity occur at an extremely early stage in the development of a bone metastasis, the radionuclide bone scan provides a sensitive tool for the detection of bone metastases. The technique is non-specific, and many benign conditions such as degenerative diseases and trauma will produce areas of increased uptake on a radionuclide bone scan. Single-photon emission computed tomography (SPECT) will increase the specificity of diagnosis, particularly in the spine as, for example, the exact localization of the area of increased uptake to the pedicle of a vertebra will increase the probability of the lesion being metastatic. X-rays of the suspicious area will also increase the diagnostic specificity for bone metastasis.

This uptake of diphosphonates by active osteoblasts has been utilized to develop a palliative therapy for pain due to bone metastases. Samarium-153-labelled ethylenediamine-tetramethylenephosphonate (^{153}Sm-EDTMP) and rhenium-186-labelled etidronate (^{186}Re-HEDP) (diphosphonates labelled with β-emitting radionuclides) are currently under evaluation as therapy agents. Strontium-89, which behaves like calcium, is taken up both into normal bone and sites of increased osteoblastic activity, but clears much more slowly from the abnormal sites. It has been shown to have a clear-cut role in palliating bone pain and in reducing the likelihood of developing new painful bone metastatic sites (see Chapter 1).

Angiogenesis is a phenomenon frequently observed in tumours and this increased vascularization may be demonstrated as increased blood pool if a dynamic study is performed or a radiolabelled red cell study undertaken. While this has little diagnostic utility, use may be made of tumour blood supply in therapy, particularly of liver metastases. ^{131}I-labelled lipiodol and ^{131}I-labelled ethiodol have been injected into the hepatic artery with successful reduction in the size of hepatic metastases. Blockage of the tumour capillary bed and delivery of a therapy radiation dose has also been achieved using ^{32}P- or ^{90}Y-labelled ceramic, resin or glass microspheres.

LOCALIZATION ON TUMOUR CELL MEMBRANES

Radiopharmaceutical localization may be achieved by binding to the tumour cell membrane. This may be achieved using an antigen–antibody reaction or by developing radiopharmaceuticals which bind to the receptors expressed on certain tumour cell membranes.

Monoclonal antibodies

Over the past decade, research has been undertaken to identify tumour-specific antigens expressed on the membranes of tumour cells. The identification of these antigens has allowed the development of monoclonal antibodies, which may be radiolabelled without losing their immunogenicity.

While initially, whole antibodies of the IgG type were labelled, fragments of IgG antibody are now also used; these exhibit more rapid blood and renal clearance than whole antibodies. These agents now have high specificity and sensitivity for tumour detection (Chapter 21). The liver uptake of the ^{111}In-labelled antibody also reduces the sensitivity of detection of liver metastases, but this is not a problem with ^{99m}Tc-labelled antibodies. Radiolabelled antibody fragments exhibit less non-specific uptake, but their rapid blood and renal clearance may lead to an overall lower target-to-background ratio in tumours with poor blood supply. They are effective in recurrent colorectal cancer [1].

A two-, or more, step targeting technique has been successfully developed using the biotin–avidin reaction. Unlabelled antibody is attached to either avidin or biotin and administered intravenously. After a suitable time interval, during which time the antibody has localized at tumour site(s), the radionuclide label attached to the recip-rocal biotin or avidin is injected and attaches to the antibody localized on the cell membrane. This technique reduces the amount of non-specific binding of antibody and increases target-to-background ratios (see Chapters 1 and 17).

Further measures to increase the specificity of monoclonal antibodies include the developments of chimeric antibodies, which have a murine vari-able region and a human constant region. The aim of these modified antibodies is to reduce non-specific uptake caused by the immunogenicity of the murine element of the antibody. Human anti-murine antibody (HAMA) develops in approxi-mately 50% of patients studied using more than 2 mg of monoclonal antibodies and these anti-bodies may affect the biodistribution of subse-quent doses of antibody, with the liver becoming the main site of uptake (Chapter 17).

Receptor binding

The presence of receptors on the cell membranes of certain tumour cells has led to the development of radiopharmaceuticals that bind to these mem-brane receptors. The most developed of these at present is the somatostatin analogue, octreotide, which binds to the somatostatin receptors on gastro- and neuroendocrine tumours and certain lymphomas. When labelled with ^{111}In, octreotide successfully images a large number of neuroendo-crine tumours including carcinoids, phaeo-chromocytomas, paragangliomas and melanomas [1a]. Small-cell lung cancers, certain central nervous system tumours and lymphomas are also imaged using ^{111}In-octreotide. The sensitivity of imaging most neuroendocrine tumours is of the order of 80% and non-specific uptake is minimal – apart from the liver and spleen, which reduces the sensitivity of imaging tumours in these areas. The specificity is also high (Chapter 17).

New receptor-binding peptides include ^{123}I-labelled vasoactive intestinal peptide (VIP), which binds well to gastrointestinal and pancreatic can-cers [1b], α-melanocyte-stimulating hormone for melanoma, ^{123}I-labelled insulin for hepatoma and radiolabelled neuropeptides for small-cell lung cancer.

Other receptor imaging systems are currently being explored. Radiolabelled forms of oestrogen and progestogen are being studied, but the pres-ence of oestrogen receptors on the cell-membranes of many body organs is likely to reduce the sensi-tivity of these agents.

LOCALIZATION WITHIN TUMOUR CELLS

Accessing the metabolic pathways of a tumour cell using radiolabeled analogues or substrates ena-bles the radiopharmaceutical to be incorporated into the tumour cell. If successful, the potential for using the radiopharmaceutical for therapy pur-poses is high since the radiation dose may be de-livered close to the target of the tumour cell nucleus. Unfortunately, the number of tumour cells that possess metabolic pathways that are am-enable to this method of approach is limited and at present is confined to ^{131}I for imaging differenti-ated thyroid tumours and ^{123}I-labelled metaiodo-benzylguanidine (^{123}I-MIBG) for imaging certain neuroendocrine tumours (Chapter 1). Ultimately, it is hoped that radiolabelled oligonucleotides will seek out and bind oncogenes that are the somatic mutational base of cancer (Chapter 17).

Less-specific techniques have also been devel-oped, which depend on accessing less tumour-specific pathways such as the pathway for glucose uptake. Although less specific, the enhanced tumour-cell uptake of tracers such as ^{18}F-DG com-pared with normal cells gives highly sensitive tumour imaging.

Tumour-specific agents

[131]**Iodine** Differentiated thyroid tumour cells of the follicular and papillary variety retain the abil-ity to trap and organify iodine. This accessible metabolic pathway, combined with the availabil-ity of a radioactive form of iodine, has been funda-mental to the development of radionuclide tumour imaging and therapy over the past 50 years. The radiopharmaceutical is specific to thy-roid cancer, although non-specific uptake in the salivary glands and excretion into the bowel and bladder may reduce the sensitivity of lesion detec-tion in the abdomen and pelvis. Therapy with ^{131}I is extremely successful in treating recurrent thy-roid cancer, and high tumour radiation doses may be achieved with sparing of surrounding normal tissues (Chapter 1).

[123/131]**I-MIBG** In 1982, the Ann Arbor group in Michigan developed a radiopharmaceutical for imaging the adrenal medulla, which is a guanethidine analogue that is taken up into the metabolic pathway of neuroendocrine cells. Over the past 15 years, the role of this radiopharmaceutical has been evaluated in both the diagnosis and therapy of certain neuroendocrine tumours, particularly phaeochromocytomas, neuroblastomas, carcinoid tumours, medullary thyroid tumours and paragangliomas. Unlike ^{111}In-octreotide, radiolabelled MIBG is not taken up into gastroendocrine pancreatic (GEP) tumours. The reason for this lack of uptake in certain neuroendocrine tumours is related to the absence of chromaffin granules [2].

Therapy with ^{131}I-MIBG has proved successful, particularly in neuroblastomas and carcinoid tumours (Chapter 1).

[99m]Tc(V)-DMSA An agent which has proved rather specific to one tumour type is [99m]Tc(V)-DMSA. The uptake of this radiopharmaceutical into sites of medullary thyroid cancer is well-documented but the mechanism of uptake and retention remains unknown (Chapter 10).

Non-specific agents

[67]Gallium citrate ^{67}Ga-labelled citrate has been used as a tumour imaging agent for many years. It is only relatively recently that an understanding of its mechanism of localization has been reached. It has been demonstrated that, as well as binding to leucocytes, ^{67}Ga also binds to transferrin in the blood, and the ^{67}Ga–transferrin complex binds to the transferrin receptors present on cell membranes, including the cell membranes of certain tumour cells. Once bound, the ^{67}Ga–transferrin complex is internalized into the cell by invagination of part of the cell membrane; the internalized ^{67}Ga is thought to bind to lactoferrin present in the cytoplasm.

[67]Ga is taken up into lymphoma cells as well as small-cell lung cancer cells. Uptake in many other tumour types has been described, but is less predictable. The sensitivity of tumour detection is reduced in the liver and abdomen due to non-specific uptake in the liver and excretion into the bowel.

While ^{67}Ga-labelled citrate plays a role as a tumour imaging agent, it lacks specificity as a result of uptake into sites of infection and inflammation. Although this may not be a problem when using gallium scans for the follow-up of patients with known lymphoma to monitor response to therapy and recurrence, it nevertheless limits the usefulness of ^{67}Ga in the diagnosis of lymphoma.

[201]Thallium As a potassium analogue, ^{201}Tl enters into the cells via the ATP-dependent sodium–potassium pump. Intracellularly, thallium is thought to localize in the mitochondria. [201]Tl uptake has been observed in a variety of tumour cells including bronchial carcinomas, lymphomas, thyroid tumours and a variety of bone and brain tumours. It is a non-specific agent however, and its main use is in the follow-up of patients with known malignancy, particularly for brain tumour recurrence and the responses of bone tumours to therapy.

[18]F-Fluorodeoxyglucose (^{18}F-FDG) This positron-emitting agent is proving to be a highly sensitive radiopharmaceutical for cancer imaging. It is taken up into cells in proportion to the activity of the glucose transporter protein and hexokinase II enzyme which relate to the degree of malignancy. Thus ^{18}F-FDG uptake is increased in relation to normal tissues and benign tumours. Because of the absence of a hydroxyl group in the 2-position, and following phosphorylation, it is unable to cross the cell membrane and remains trapped intracellularly. It is cost-effective in the staging and management of non-small cell lung cancer [2a] and is widely applied in staging and follow-up of many cancers. However, false positives may occur [2b].

Like ^{67}Ga-citrate, ^{18}F-FDG is a relatively non-specific tumour imaging agent since it is taken up by a wide variety of tumours including lymphomas. Uptake into benign tumours is generally less marked than into malignant tumours, and the 'standardized uptake value' (SUV) will usually differentiate malignant from benign lesions.

[11]C-Methionine It has been shown that cancer cells demonstrate increased transport and utilization of amino acids and this phenomenon has been the rationale for exploring the use of ^{11}C-methionine as a positron-emitting tumour imaging agent. Certain brain tumours, lymphomas and head and neck cancers may all be imaged with ^{11}C-methionine, and there is often a disparity between the uptake of ^{18}F-FDG and ^{11}C-methionine, particularly in low-grade brain tumours.

Other tumour agents   There are a number of other agents whose role in tumour imaging is currently being evaluated. These include ^{99m}Tc-MIBI and ^{99m}Tc-Tetrofosmin. These radiopharmaceuticals diffuse into tumour cells; their site of binding within the tumour cell is thought to be in the mitochondria. The main role for these agents at the present time is in imaging breast cancer. They are also taken up by lymphoma, myeloma and lung tumours. In the future the relationship between loss of uptake of the radiopharmaceutical and resistance to chemotherapy may prove extremely useful in the management of patients.

A number of compounds that are markers of hypoxia are now being developed. Since it is known that the centres of many tumours are relatively hypoxic (due to poor blood supply) and that these hypoxic areas are more radioresistant, the ability to define the hypoxic component of a tumour will be useful.

THE ROLE OF TUMOUR IMAGING AND THERAPY IN MANAGEMENT

Nuclear medicine now contributes significantly to clinical oncology. The current role of radionuclide techniques includes diagnosis, staging, follow-up and therapy of cancers.

DIAGNOSIS

Nuclear medicine studies contribute to diagnosis in a number of tumours. Using the simple technique of ^{99m}Tc-pertechnetate thyroid imaging combined with ultrasound, the possibility of thyroid malignancy is raised in patients shown to have thyroid nodules that are non-functioning on radionuclide imaging and solid on ultrasound imaging. Although only 10% of these lesions will prove to be malignant, they indicate that further investigation with fine needle aspiration is warranted.

Specific tumour imaging agents such as ^{123}I-MIBG and ^{111}In-octreotide contribute to the diagnosis of neuroendocrine tumours. The ^{123}I-MIBG study has a higher sensitivity than vanillylmandellic acid (VMA) levels in detecting a phaeochromocytoma due to the intermittent secretory nature of these tumours. Similarly, an ^{111}In-octreotide study may confirm a suspected diagnosis of a gastroendocrine pancreatic (GEP) tumour when other imaging techniques fail to localise a biochemically suspected primary tumour.

STAGING

The role of ^{99m}Tc-diphosphonate bone scans in staging patients with breast and prostate cancer is well-recognized, although in recent years its use in clinical stage I and II disease has diminished. The radionuclide bone scan remains the most effective means of imaging bone metastases with its combination of high sensitivity and whole-body information.

The role of ^{67}Ga in staging patients with lymphoma has also been well documented, although its ability to detect infra-diaphragmatic disease is inferior to its sensitivity above the diaphragm. The role of ^{18}F-FDG in staging a wide variety of tumours, particularly lymphomas, bronchial carcinomas and squamous carcinomas of the head and neck has been recognized.

FOLLOW-UP

At the present time, nuclear medicine tests play the greatest role in the follow-up of patients with proven malignancy. Since no test has a 100% sensitivity, it is helpful to study the patient before the initial intervention (e.g. surgery), to determine the uptake status of the primary tumour.

Radionuclide studies may be used to determine:

- the completeness of surgery or other primary intervention;
- the presence of recurrence;
- the response to second-line treatment;
- the appropriateness of certain therapies; and
- organ function following therapy.

Completeness of surgery

The completeness of surgery or other primary intervention is monitored successfully using radionuclide techniques in a number of clinical situations. Following thyroidectomy for thyroid malignancy, the radioiodine tracer scan will determine the presence of the thyroid remnant. Further surgery may be undertaken if the remnant is large, or therapy doses of ^{131}I used if the remnant is small.

^{99m}Tc(V)DMSA and ^{111}In-octreotide imaging is useful in detecting residual tumour post-operatively in patients with medullary thyroid cancer, although a good pre-operative assessment to determine the presence of involved nodes before surgery should facilitate a successful operation.

When radiotherapy or chemotherapy is the first-line treatment, radionuclide imaging may be used to determine the response of the primary tumour to therapy. [67]Ga has been shown in the past to be useful in assessing the presence of residual active tumour in patients treated with radiotherapy and or chemotherapy for lymphoma. CT and MRI are unable to determine whether a post-treatment residual mediastinal mass contains active tumour or not, and ^{67}Ga has been shown to be superior to these two anatomical techniques in this situation.

Recurrence

The presence of recurrence may be initially detected biochemically if an adequately specific biochemical marker exists. However, even a sensitive biochemical marker is unable to localize the recurrence or determine its suitability for further treatment.

A rising prostate-specific antigen (PSA) level in a patient with prostate cancer indicates recurrent disease, and a ^{99m}Tc-MDP bone scan or ^{111}In-labelled antibody against a prostate membrane-specific antigen (PMSA) will determine whether the recurrence is in the skeleton or in the soft-tissue [2c].

An ^{111}In-octreotide scan will show the site of recurrent neuroendocrine tumour in a patient whose biochemical markers become elevated and will also show whether the recurrence is in a site amenable to surgery. The presence of whole-body information will also accurately identify whether the recurrence is single and suitable for surgery or multiple requiring a more palliative approach.

^{18}F-FDG imaging is proving a sensitive method of detecting early local recurrence in patients with sarcoma and melanoma.

Tumour response

Tumour response to second-line treatment may be monitored using whole-body nuclear medicine imaging. ^{99m}Tc-MDP bone imaging remains the best method of monitoring the effects of chemotherapy in patients with breast cancer and bone metastases or in following patients undergoing

hormone manipulation with bone metastases in prostate cancer.

^{18}F-FDG imaging and other PET agents are now being assessed as a means of obtaining early information on the response of a tumour to second-line treatment such as chemotherapy since a reduction of uptake will precede the actual reduction in tumour mass (Chapter 3). Loss of uptake of radiolabelled monoclonal antibodies or receptor-binding peptides is also providing evidence of response.

Appropriateness of therapy

Evaluating the appropriateness of radionuclide therapy as an option in the treatment of malignancy may be determined using a tracer study. Unlike other second-line treatments such as chemotherapy, the tracer study can be used to select those patients for whom radionuclide therapy is likely to be helpful. This selection not only spares patients who show no uptake on the tracer study from unnecessary treatment, but also saves valuable resources.

The requirement for a positive ^{123}I-MIBG tracer study is a prerequisite of treatment with therapy doses of ^{131}I-MIBG in patients with neuroendocrine tumours. The tracer dose will confirm both the presence and degree of MIBG uptake and also enables dosimetry calculations to be performed as appropriate.

An ^{111}In-octreotide scan should be performed before undertaking therapy with somatostatin to confirm uptake, since the therapy is both expensive and has side effects, which may be avoided in scan-negative patients.

Organ function post-therapy

As many oncology therapies are toxic to normal tissues, the function of normal organs may require monitoring during certain therapies. Certain chemotherapy agents are nephrotoxic and monitoring of the glomerular filtration rate is required to guide the dose of chemotherapy that may be used. ^{51}Cr-EDTA is a well-established non-imaging technique for monitoring renal function in this situation.

Some chemotherapeutic agents such as adriamycin are cardiotoxic. Gated blood pool imaging is a reliable and reproducible technique for monitoring left ventricular ejection fraction in patients undergoing courses of chemotherapy.

THERAPY

As discussed in Chapter 1, the development of radionuclide therapy is one of the key areas of current nuclear medicine research and practice.

The successful use of ^{131}I for the treatment of patients with differentiated thyroid cancer has provided a model for the development of new agents such as ^{131}I-MIBG and the bone pain palliation agents.

Recent developments in radionuclide therapy include the use of ^{90}Y-octreotide in therapy and the successful ^{131}I monoclonal antibody B1 therapy for lymphoma (Chapter 1).

THE ROLE OF NUCLEAR MEDICINE IN MANAGEMENT

BREAST CANCER

Breast cancer provides a good example of the interaction between imaging techniques and clinical management of a common cancer and how present problems may be addressed in the future

(Table 2.2). There are over 24 000 new cases of breast cancer and over 15 000 deaths per annum in the UK. Breast cancer affects 1 in 14 women and 1 in 21 will die of the disease. The 5-year survival rate depends on staging: the rate is 98% for minimal disease and 85% for those with negative axillary nodes. However, in patients with axillary node involvement the 5-year survival drops to 55% and there is a 10% survival in those with distant metastases. While self-examination of the breast is recommended, it is unable to detect early disease. Mammography screening is the present conventional practice for detecting early breast cancer. However, its sensitivity varies from 55% to 94% and specificity from 88% to 99% [2d]. There are some situations where breast cancer is difficult to detect on mammography, particularly when there is a dense breast or a lot of fibroadenosis. In such cases, the ^{99m}Tc-sestamibi imaging technique introduced by Khalkali *et al.* [3] has proven beneficial [4,5]. The patient is imaged prone with a laterally placed gamma-camera over the dependent breast, at 10 minutes and 1 hour after the injection

Table 2.2 Clinical requirements for breast cancer

Detection of primary	Clinical examination Mammography Tc-99m MIBI Ultrasound, MRI
Distinction of benign from malignant	Fine needle aspiration or excision biopsy
Detection of axillary node involvement	Sentinal node probe detection RIS with Tc-99m SM3 Probability map or Tc-99m 170 H.82 or Tc-99m Mov 18 SPECT F-18 FDG-PET MRI
Detection of chest wall involvement	MRI
Extent of surgery	Perioperative probe for sentinel node
Detection of recurrences	Tc-99m MDP bone scan Radiological techniques RIS
Adjuvant therapy	Tamoxifen
Therapy of recurrence	Bone local: Radiotherapy Bone extensive: ^{89}Sr, ^{153}Sm or ^{186}Re, diphosphonates Soft tissue: chemotherapy

MIBI, Methoxyisobutylisonitrile; MRI, Magnetic Resonance Imaging; SPET, Single photon emission tomography; PET, Positron emission tomography; DG, Deoxyglucose; MDP, Methylene diphosphonate; RIS, Radioimmunoscintigraphy.

of 600 Mbq ^{99m}Tc-MIBI. Sensitivities over 90% are typical but inflammatory masses and fibroadenomata may also be positive, giving specificities of about 70%. It has recently been shown that the bone scanning agent ^{99m}Tc-MDP can also be used for this purpose when imaging is started at 10 minutes after injection [6].

Once the tumour has been identified using mammography and/or ultrasound, and if it is very small, a wire secured into the skin with its tip in the site of the tumour will allow the surgeon to perform excision biopsy; if the lump is larger, then fine needle aspiration is usually performed. Whereas previously, breast surgery was undertaken for any lump in the breast, surgical practice now considers that the best (i.e. most cost-effective) surgeon is the person with the highest malignant-to-benign ratio of breast masses excised. Thus, the distinction between the benign and malignant breast lumps has become even more important, and is usually made by fine needle aspiration or excision biopsy. Masses below 1 cm in diameter are difficult to detect using ^{99m}Tc-MIBI and here FDG-PET may be more sensitive [7].

The advent of segmental mastectomy as a valid surgical option, combined with the mammographic detection of early, small cancers of the breast, have led surgeons to question the need for axillary lymph node dissection in every patient.

Conventionally, axillary node dissection is performed in all patients with breast cancer to stage the disease and to guarantee local control in the axillae. It has a prognostic and therapeutic role, since the selection for chemotherapy is based on axillary node status. Surgery is the only currently reliable way of assessing nodal disease; unfortunately, to obtain this information, those women with node-negative disease have unnecessarily extensive surgery. Others argue that axillary lymph node dissection has only a prognostic aim. While it would be important to take away the axillary lymph nodes, which are macroscopically infiltrated by tumour, they consider that micrometastases do not affect the overall survival [8].

Axillary lymph node dissection is no longer performed for ductal carcinoma *in-situ* (DCIS) because of the extremely low rate of lymph node metastases. Routine node dissection for lesions larger than DCIS, but with extremely low likelihood of axillary node involvement, might also be abandoned [9]. If a pre-operative imaging technique were available to determine whether palpable or in particular, impalpable axillary lymph nodes were involved or not, the extent of surgery could be individually tailored.

Clinical assessment is unreliable, particularly in patients identified with early tumours as in a breast screening programme. ^{99m}Tc-MIBI is insufficiently accurate because axillary muscle uptake makes evaluation difficult. ^{18}F-FDG-PET studies show increased uptake in involved nodes and also in those with non-specific reaction to inflammation. A sensitivity of 72% and a specificity of 96% was found by Avril *et al.* [10]; nodes <2 cm were missed. The majority of the latter were with multiple node involvement however. Magnetic resonance imaging (MRI) is also being evaluated as a method for detecting lymph node involvement.

Radioimmunoscintigraphy (RIS) (Chapter 17) adds specificity to sensitivity in axillary node detection. It was first used for the breast by Epenetos *et al.* [11]. Radiolabelled anti-CEA has been used but the diffusion of the antigen into the axillary nodes means that visualization does not necessarily indicate the presence of cancer cells. McEwan *et al.* [12], using a ^{99m}Tc-labelled monoclonal antibody (17OH.82) against a synthetic glycoprotein antigen with planar and SPECT imaging, found a sensitivity of 90% and a positive predictive value of 95% for locoregional disease, mainly in patients with palpable nodes. Granowska *et al.* [13] and Biassoni *et al.* [14] used ^{99m}Tc-SM3 (stripped mucin) antibody against the mucin core protein, and were able to identify correctly the presence or absence of node involvement, the majority of nodes being clinically impalpable, and reported a sensitivity of 90% and a specificity of 84%. This was through serial planar imaging with statistical change detection analysis. The early 10-minute image of the axilla was compared with the later 18- to 22-hour image, on the basis that specific uptake increases with time whereas non-specific uptake decreases. Probability maps where significant change (with $P < 0.001$ coloured red, $P < 0.01$ coloured yellow, etc.) showed specific node involvement down to 0.35 g.

An alternative approach [15, 15a] is to use a pre-operative probe technique to identify the 'sentinel' node at operation after an injection of ^{99m}Tc-colloid, so that the surgeon can sample this node, which is then sent for frozen section; if positive, an axillary clearance follows. This approach requires that skipping of the first level nodes does not occur since the sentinel node is representative of the many lymphatic pathways from the breast to the axilla. But this approach is over 95% successful [16].

Breast metastases to bone may be identified by conventional bone imaging and palliation may be undertaken by β-emitting radionuclide therapy (Chapter 1). Bone-marrow imaging may show defects due to metastases not evident on bone imaging. Soft-tissue metastases may be detected by FDG-PET or by radioimmunoscintigraphy.

In conclusion, the combination of mammography, ^{99m}Tc-MIBI scintigraphy and biopsy identify the primary breast cancer; and FDG-PET or radioimmunoscintigraphy and/or MRI, and the sentinel node approach can determine axillary nodal involvement. If such a determination becomes reliable, then those that believe that axillary node status is only of prognostic value may be able to avoid axillary node surgery with its occasional unsightly and painful complications.

REFERENCES

1. Sirisrio, R., Podoloff, D.A., Patt, Y.Z. *et al.* (1996) Tc-99m-Immu4 imaging in recurrent colorectal cancer: efficacy and impact on surgical management. *Nucl. Med. Commun.*, **17**, 568–76.
1a. Krenning, E.P., Kwekkeboom, D.J., Bakker, W.H. *et al.* (1993) Somatostatin receptor scintigraphy with ^{111}In-DTPA-D-Phe and ^{123}I-Tyr^3-octreotide: the Rotterdam Experience with more than 1000 patients. *Eur. J. Nucl. Med.*, **20**, 716–31.
1b. Virgolini, I., Raderer, M., Kurtaran, A. *et al.* (1994) Vasoactive Intestinal Peptide receptor imaging for the localisation of intestinal adenocarcinomas and endocrine tumours. *N. Engl. J. Med.*, **331**, 1116–21.
2. Bomanji, J., Levison, D.A., Flatman, W.D. *et al.* (1987) Uptake of I-123 metaiodobenzylguanidine by pheochromocytomas, other paraganliomas and neuroblastomas: a histopathological comparison. *J. Nucl. Med.*, **23**, 973–8.
2a. Gambhir, S.S., Hoh, C.K., Phelps, M.E., Madar, I. and Maddahi, J. (1996) Decision tree sensitivity analysis for cost effectiveness of FDG-PET in the staging and management of non small cell lung carcinoma. *J. Nucl. Med.*, **37**, 1428–36.
2b. Strauss, L.G. (1996) Fluorine-18 deoxyglucose and false positive results: a major problem in the diagnostics of oncological patients. *Eur. J. Nucl. Med.*, **23**, 1409–15.
2c. Babaian, R.J., Sayer, J., Podoloff, D.A. *et al.* (1994) Radioimmunoscintigraphy of pelvic lymph nodes with ^{111}In-labelled monoclonal antibody CYT-356. *J. Urol.*, **152**, 1952–5.
2d. Elmore, J.G., Wells, C.K., Lee, C.H. *et al.* (1994) Variability in radiologists' interpretations of mammograms. *N. Engl. J. Med.*, **331**, 1493–9.
3. Khalkhali, I., Mena, I. and Diggles, L. (1994) A review of imaging techniques for the diagnosis of breast cancer: a new role of prone scintimammography using technetium-99m sestamibi. *Eur. J. Nucl. Med.*, **21**, 357–62.
4. Kao, C.K., Wang, S.J. and Liu, T.J. (1994) The use of technetium-99m methoxyisobutyl isonitrile breast scintigraphy to evaluate palpable breast masses. *Eur. J. Nucl. Med.*, **21**, 432–6.
5. Palmedo, H., Schomberg, A., Grunwald, F. *et al.* (1995) Mammoscintigraphy with Tc-99m MIBI in patients with suspicious breast nodules: a comparison of planar and SPECT imaging techniques. *Eur. J. Nucl. Med.*, **22**, 725.
6. Piccolo, S., Lastoria, S., Mainolfi, C. *et al.* (1995) Technetium-99m-Methylene diphosphonate scintimammography to image primary breast cancer. *J. Nucl. Med.*, **36**, 718–24.
7. Wahl, R.L., Cody, R.L., Hutchins, G.D. and Mudgett, E.E. (1991) Primary and metastatic breast carcinoma: initial clinical evaluation with PET with the radiolabelled glucose analogue 2-[F-18]-fluoro-2-deoxy-D-glucose. *Radiology*, **179**, 765–70.
8. Fischer, B., Redmond, C. and Fischer, E.R. (1985) Ten year results of randomized clinical trial comparing radical mastectomy and total mastectomy with or without radiation. *N. Engl. J. Med.*, **312**, 674–81.
9. Silverstein, M.J., Gierson, E.D., Waisman, J.R. *et al.* (1994) Axillary lymph node dissection for T1a breast carcinoma – Is it indicated ? *Cancer*, **73**, 664–7.
10. Avril, N., Janicke, F., Dose, J. *et al.* (1995) Evaluation of axillary lymph node involvement in breast cancer patients using F-18 FDG PET. *Eur. J. Nucl. Med.*, **22**, 733.
11. Epenetos, A.A., Britton, K.E., Mather, S. *et al.* (1982) Targetting of Iodine-123 labelled tumour-associated monoclonal antibodies to ovarian, breast and gastrointestinal tumours. *Lancet*, **ii**, 999–1005.
12. McEwan, A.H.B., Akran, U., Boniface, C. *et al.* (1994) Tc-99m MAb 170 H.82 in the evaluation of locoregional disease in patients with breast cancer. *Eur. J. Nucl. Med.*, **21**, S15.
13. Granowska, M., Biassoni, L., Carroll, M. *et al.* (1996) Breast cancer Tc-99m radioimmunoscintigraphy. *Acta Oncologica*, **35**, 319–21.
14. Biassoni, L., Granowska, M., Carroll, M.J. *et al.* (1997) Tc-99m labelled SM3 in the preoperative evaluation of axillary lymph nodes and primary breast cancer with change detection statistical processing as an aid to tumour detection. *Br. J. Cancer.* (in press).
15. Krag, D.N., Weaver, D.L., Alex, J.C. and Fairbank, J.T. (1993) Surgical resection and radiolocalisation of the sentinel lymph node in breast cancer using a gamma probe. *Surg. Oncol.*, **2**, 335–40.
15a. Paganelli, G., De Cicco, C., Cremonesi, M. *et al.* (1997) Gamma-probe guided resection of the sentinel node in breast cancer. *J. Nucl. Med.*, **38**, 97P.
16. Veronesi, U., Paganelli, G., Galimberti, V. *et al.* (1997) Sentinel node biopsy to avoid axillary dissection in breast cancer with clinically negative lymph nodes. *Lancet*, **349**, 1864–7.

CHAPTER 3

Clinical positron emission tomography

H.N. Wagner Jr, J.W. Buchanan and M.N. Maisey

INTRODUCTION

The clinical indications for positron emission tomography (PET) have increased dramatically in the past few years. Although PET continues to have a major role in patients with neurological, psychiatric and cardiovascular diseases, the area of most rapid growth has been oncology. ^{18}F-fluorodeoxyglucose (FDG) is the radiopharmaceutical most often used in patients with cancer, but a variety of peptides, amino acids, enzymes and proteins, which bind to specific recognition sites or receptors on cancer cells have been successfully labelled and are proving useful. Many studies now demonstrate that PET, and SPECT, reduce the overall cost of medical care, because they increase the certainty of diagnosis and clinical stage of disease, and therefore eliminate the expense of unnecessary or unproductive testing or treatment. These studies are also very useful in planning and monitoring treatment.

Nuclear medicine is now best thought of as molecular nuclear medicine. Exciting studies are underway, which will define the extended role of radiopharmaceuticals in genetics, pharmacology, molecular biology and physiology. Chemical changes can almost always be detected before there are clinical signs of disease and, when these are measured, a more specific characterization of the disease is possible. For example, if a metastatic breast tumour contains oestrogen receptors, it can be treated with the oestrogen receptor-antagonist tamoxifen. Both the planning of treatment and the response to treatment can be based on regional biochemistry.

Positron emission tomography makes it possible to measure the rate of chemical reactions within the human body thereby allowing *in vivo* identification of a disease at the molecular as well as the cellular level. PET imaging is revolutionizing medicine by making it possible for the first time to measure *in vivo* chemistry, expressing the results in absolute units of metres, kilograms and seconds (the MKS system), rather than in relative terms such as the percentage of the administered dose of radioiodine accumulated by the thyroid, or the amount of thallium-201 in one part of the myocardium compared with another. PET is bringing about a new way of looking at disease by making it possible to define disease in terms of regional chemistry. By measuring regional chemistry in normal persons to provide standards, the diseases can be defined as deviations from the norm by statistical analysis. It is often possible to use the patient as his or her own control – by comparing the metabolic or chemical activity in an area of the body with its normal contralateral counterpart.

Although the use of radioactive tracers to measure regional chemistry was first introduced for the study of the thyroid gland with radioactive iodine almost 50 years ago, only recently has the concept been applied widely to the study of other organs such as the brain and heart. In theory, when we

Clinical Nuclear Medicine, 3rd edn. Edited by M.N. Maisey, K.E. Britton and B.D. Collier. Published in 1998 by Chapman & Hall, London. ISBN 0 412 75180 1

can measure the rate of a chemical process in an organ or part of an organ, there is the possibility of at least two diseases, one in which the rate of the chemical process is abnormally slow, and another in which the process is abnormally fast.

PET imaging provides information about *in vivo* regional chemistry with a sensitivity and specificity comparable with that obtained by radio-immunoassay in studies of body fluids. Other imaging modalities, such as computed tomography (CT) and magnetic resonance imaging (MRI), provide predominantly anatomical information. By measuring regional chemistry, PET can at times detect abnormalities before anatomical changes have occurred, for example in epilepsy [1,2], Huntington's disease [3,4] or cerebrovascular disease [5].

PET helps us to understand the 'chemical language' of the body. The studies fall into three categories: regional blood flow, substrate metabolism, and information transfer. In the latter category, PET makes it possible to identify 'recognition' sites involved in the energy supply to the cell or in regulatory processes, for example, via neurotransmitters and neuroreceptors. Since most drugs act by blocking or stimulating these recognition sites, PET imaging can be used to monitor the effects of drugs on receptors, and it shows promise in improving the treatment of depression, Parkinson's disease, epilepsy, tardive dyskinesia, Alzheimer's disease, and substance abuse. The use of simple probe detector systems makes it possible to monitor the response of a given patient to drug treatment [6]. Such measurements can increase the effectiveness and decrease the incidence of untoward side effects.

NUCLEAR ONCOLOGY

Positron emission tomography scanning can help in the care of patients with cancer by providing information useful in the planning and monitoring of treatment. PET can be used to measure the rate of utilization of important biochemical substrates such as sugars and amino acids that supply energy to tumours, and in pharmacokinetic and pharmacodynamic studies of cancer chemotherapeutic agents. It can also be used to assess the effectiveness of surgery, radiation and chemotherapy. PET can document the extent of tumours, and their progression or regression with different forms of treatment, at a time when modi-

fications can be made in the treatment plan. Until now, treatment has been based primarily on histopathological examination of biopsies; biochemical characterization may be an even better way to classify tumours.

Almost all types of cancer have been studied with PET, for example, melanoma, head and neck (Figure 3.1), renal, thyroid, bone, soft-tissue, pancreatic and ovarian cancers. FDG is used most often, but other agents that target specific cellular receptors or functions are being developed at a rapid rate. New PET instrumentation makes it possible to image the whole body in a relative short period of time, and PET is playing a major role not only in diagnosis but in staging, treatment planning and monitoring of patients with cancer.

LUNG CANCER

Lung cancer is the most common type of cancer world-wide and is usually fatal. Early diagnosis and treatment may increase survival time. When a solitary pulmonary nodule is seen on a chest radiograph, it must be determined whether it is benign or malignant and, if cancer is found, the stage of the disease must be established. Often the differentiation cannot be made with CT or MRI, and it is necessary to obtain tissue for histological examination. This involves an invasive procedure such as bronchoscopy, percutaneous biopsy or open-lung biopsy, and it may be necessary for the patient to undergo this more than once during the course of therapy. FDG-PET can usually answer the question about the pathology of a solitary nodule and spare the patient the more invasive and expensive procedures. Figure 3.2 shows the use of FDG-PET to establish the metastatic spread of lung cancer.

Patz *et al.* [7] initially studied 51 patients with solitary pulmonary nodules, and reported the sensitivity of FDG-PET for the detection of carcinoma at 100% and the specificity at 89%. In a more recent multicentre trial, the sensitivity was similar and the specificity a little lower, which was attributed to the fact that FDG is also taken up by active infective or inflammatory lesions [8]. In patients with nodules that show FDG uptake, the biopsy can be directed to this area. A logical paradigm to follow in patients at a low risk for cancer or those with a high risk of operative complications, would be to combine FDG-PET data with

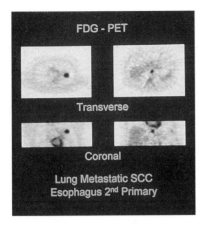

Figure 3.1 A patient with a history of head and neck cancer had a left lung opacity on a chest CT scan. The PET study shows a lung metastasis and a focus of centrally located activity at the level of the diaphragm (right). The CT was normal at this site. Oesophagoscopy and biopsy revealed squamous cell carcinoma of the oesophagus and needle biopsy of the lung confirmed metastatic squamous cell cancer. (Courtesy of Peter E. Valk, MD, Northern California P.E.T. Center, Sacramento, CA.)

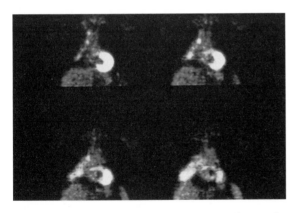

Figure 3.2 A FDG study in a patient with a right lower-lobe lung cancer shows that the disease has metastasized to the right hilar and right mediastinal areas. The four coronal sections are going anterior to posterior through the lung. (Courtesy of R. Edward Coleman, MD, Duke University.)

the clinical and other available information, and closely follow the patient at 3-monthly intervals so as to avoid an immediate invasive test. If the suspicious lesion does not accumulate FDG, then the patient can be considered not to have cancer. Many thoracotomies could be avoided in patients who have solitary nodules which do not accumulate FDG.

BRAIN TUMOURS

One of the first uses of PET imaging was in brain tumours. Measurements of the rate of ^{18}F-FDG uptake in lesions in the brain seen by CT or MRI after therapy for brain tumours are made in order to discriminate between tumour recurrence and radiation necrosis (Figure 3.3) [9,10]. Subsequently, another substrate, ^{11}C-methionine, was used to delineate the boundaries of brain tumours, providing information of value in directing stereotactic biopsy, planning the approach and extent of brain surgery, and permitting differentiation of the metabolizing brain tumour from simple disruption of the blood–brain barrier [11,12]. ^{11}C-Thymidine has been used to measure nucleotide metabolism and utilization in DNA synthesis, which reflects cell proliferation [13].

In some tumours, such as pituitary adenomas, PET can detect the presence of receptors in the tumour. Using the dopamine receptor binding agent ^{11}C-N-methylspiperone, it has been possible to classify pituitary adenomas according to whether they possess dopamine receptors [14,15] (Plate 1). If the tumours contain such receptors, they can be treated chemically rather than surgically, i.e. by administering the dopamine receptor agonist, bromocriptine.

BREAST CANCER

Breast cancer is an example of the use of PET to assess the presence of receptors in tumours. ^{18}F-labelled oestradiol accumulation as determined by PET makes it possible to tailor the treatment of a specific patient on the basis of the number of oestrogen and progesterone receptors. A tumour containing oestrogen receptors is more likely to be treated successfully with oestrogen receptor-blocking drugs, such as tamoxifen, than cancers that do not contain oestrogen receptors. The presence of progesterone receptors as well as oestrogen receptors is the best prognostic sign. Radioactive tracers that bind to oestrogen receptors make it possible to assess the status of the primary breast cancer and regional metastatic deposits [16]. ^{18}F-FDG and ^{18}F-oestradiol have been used to

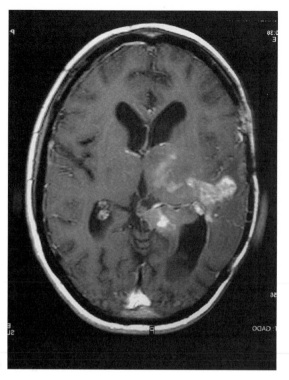

(a)

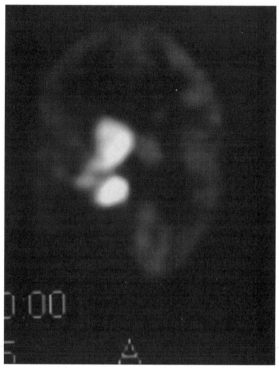

(b)

Figure 3.3 A 40-year-old woman with an oligodendroglioma which had been treated returned with recurrent symptoms. The contrast MRI study (a) shows diffuse areas of contrast enhancement in the right hemisphere which could be either recurrent tumour or necrosis. The FDG-PET (b) study shows marked hypermetabolism in the right hemisphere documenting recurrent tumour. The abnormality was biopsied and proved to be anaplastic oligodendroglioma. (Courtesy of R. Edward Coleman, MD, Duke University.)

assess the response of breast tumours to tamoxifen therapy [17]. Tamoxifen has been labelled with fluorine-18 and used to image the receptors on breast tumours [18]. This makes it possible to predict which patients will respond to tamoxifen therapy [19].

Increased metabolic activity is seen in both primary and metastatic breast cancer, and FDG-PET is particularly useful in patients with dense breasts when mammography may not provide a definitive diagnosis. FDG-PET is also useful in staging disease in the axillary nodes. ^{11}C-Tyrosine was shown to be a better PET radiotracer than FDG because of its lower accumulation in fibrocystic disease [20].

These are examples of the new biochemical approach to the characterization of disease, an approach directly related to prognosis and therapy. Histopathology alone need no longer be the only criterion for diagnosis, prognosis and therapy.

COLORECTAL CANCER

Colorectal cancer is a common form of malignancy, which if discovered very early, is often curable. The prognosis for patients who have recurrent disease is not very good, but improves if the new or metastatic lesions are surgically removed. With CT, it is often difficult to distinguish between a new lesion and a scar (Figure 3.4). FDG-PET has been used effectively in patients with recurrent colorectal cancer [21]. Valk *et al.* [22] found that the surgical management was changed in 30/88 (34%) of the patients studied. The PET study demonstrated unresectable disease in 17 patients and located unknown sites of potentially resectable tumour in seven patients. Exploratory

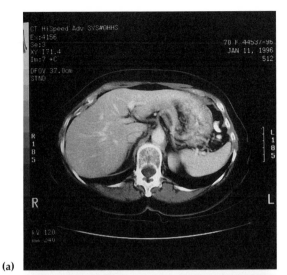

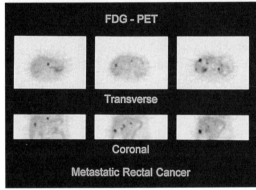

(a)

(b)

Figure 3.4 A patient with a history of colon cancer was found to have an elevated carcinoembryonic antigen (CEA) level. A CT scan (a) was normal. This corresponds to the middle transverse FDG-PET study (b) of the liver which shows multiple metastases which were confirmed by biopsy. (Courtesy of Peter E. Valk, MD, Northern California P.E.T. Center, Sacramento, CA.)

laparotomy was avoided in four patients and the surgical approach was changed in two. PET has also been useful in staging colorectal cancer by demonstrating metastatic spread to the liver, lymph nodes and pelvis. Another study, which compared FDG-PET and CT in 62 patients, reported that the sensitivity in detecting liver metastases was 97% with 13% false-positives [23].

NEUROLOGICAL DISEASES

DEMENTIA

Dementias fall broadly into two categories: those treated successfully by specific medical means, and those in whom the only treatment consists of supportive care. Some 30% of demented elderly patients suffer from impairment of brain blood flow from blocked blood vessels. Another 20% of dementias are caused by diseases for which there are specific treatments, one of the most common being drug intoxication. Older people often take many medicines, which can either singly or in combination cause dementia. Depression is also common in the elderly and can be associated with increased forgetfulness and confusion. If diagnosed correctly, depression is often treated successfully. Hyper- or hypothyroidism and vitamin B_{12} deficiency are other causes of dementia, which if recognized, can be treated. Subdural haematomas can lead to dementia and may be the result of unrecognized or minor trauma.

The diagnosis of Alzheimer's disease is usually made by exclusion of the other causes. Because the disease is so progressive, it is important to make the diagnosis in the early stages, which can be made with a 90% accuracy on the basis of clinical and psychological testing in about 50% of the patients who first come to medical attention because of memory loss. Usually, the diagnosis is not made before thousands of dollars have been spent on diagnostic tests.

Alzheimer's disease accounts for about 50% of demented patients. The disease is characterized by abnormally accelerated neuronal death, especially pronounced in the hippocampus, parietal, temporal and, to a lesser degree, frontal lobes. As a result of the neuronal degeneration, there is a secondary loss of blood flow, oxygen utilization and glucose metabolism in the involved regions. The most characteristic pattern seen on PET scans in patients with Alzheimer's disease is bilateral hypometabolism and decreased blood flow in the parietal and temporal regions [24]. The magnitude and the extent of the hypometabolism seem to correlate with the severity of the cognitive symptoms. It has recently been shown that the posterior cingulate cortex is the brain region that shows the earliest sign of reduced FDG metabolism in patients who subsequently develop symptoms which fulfil the NINCDS/ADRDA criteria for probable Alzheimer's disease [25].

With the discovery of abnormal genes in patients with Alzheimer's disease and the prospect of drugs to control or slow the degenerative changes, it is important to make the diagnosis as early as possible. When members of families at-risk for Alzheimer's disease were studied with genetic testing and FDG-PET, it was found that those with the abnormal gene had significantly reduced parietal metabolism and their left-to-right parietal asymmetry was higher than the family members who did not express the genetic abnormality [26]. The combination of genetic testing and PET will increase the certainty of the diagnosis and provide a way to follow the effectiveness of treatment.

STROKE

Stroke is another condition in which PET can aid in the care of the patient. The metabolic abnormalities seen on PET are frequently more extensive than the corresponding CT findings in stroke patients [5,27]. The pattern of metabolic abnormalities in PET correlate with the clinical syndrome and with the degree of eventual recovery.

PET imaging provides a powerful method for quantitative, non-invasive measurement of the physiological and biochemical consequences of cerebral ischaemia. In addition to being an important prognostic test, PET imaging can lead to more effective treatment of an individual patient, as well as providing a better understanding of the pathogenesis of the disease. PET tracers used for quantitatively measuring regional cerebral blood flow include ^{15}O, $^{11}CO_2$, $C^{18}F_4$ and $^{13}NH_3$.

EPILEPSY

Epilepsy is one of the most common diseases of the brain. Many patients have partial epilepsy, i.e. seizures that begin in a focus, often in the temporal lobe, and then spread over large areas of the cortex. For most patients with partial epilepsy, diagnosis and classification depends on the use of surface electroencephalography (EEG), which records the summation of electrical activity associated with neuronal activity. For the approximately 20% of patients whose seizures are uncontrolled by medication, surgical therapy becomes a possibility if the site of origin of the seizure can be determined. Anatomical imaging techniques such

as CT or MRI reveal lesions in only a minority of patients, so that certainty of diagnosis may require intra-operative electrocorticography and chronic direct recordings from stereotactically implanted depth electrodes. The results are often conflicting, and the procedure is invasive and accompanied by certain risks. PET imaging can provide independent confirmatory information about the site of the epileptogenic lesion.

During focal seizures, brain metabolism and blood flow are increased at the site of onset of the epileptic activity, which spreads as the seizure activity is propagated. Between the seizures (interictal state), both metabolism and blood flow are reduced at the site(s) where seizures begin. PET was first applied in epilepsy in 1980 [28]. It was found that PET imaging could localize the focal changes in cerebral metabolism and perfusion and provide unique diagnostic information, which would be valuable in the management of patients with epilepsy. A variety of examinations have proved to be useful: glucose utilization (FDG), oxygen utilization ($^{15}O_2$), and cerebral perfusion ($^{13}NH_3$ and $H_2^{15}O$).

PET scans performed during partial seizures have shown marked increases in local brain metabolism and perfusion at the site of seizure onset, but because of propagated neuronal activity, the ictal scans are less useful in predicting epileptic origin than those made during the interictal state – PET scans made during non-focal seizures showed a generalized increase in brain metabolism and perfusion [1,28]. In patients with petit mal seizures, there is a diffuse increase of metabolism at the time of the seizure.

Interictal PET scans are better in delineating the offending focus from which the seizure originates, rather than measuring the increased regional blood flow or metabolic activity during the seizures themselves. The results of interictal PET scans in patients with partial epilepsy have been compared with the results of CT and EEG in multiple reports. Approximately 70% of the patients with partial complex epilepsy demonstrate zones of hypometabolism or decreased cerebral blood flow at the site of origin of the seizure. At times, focal abnormalities may be identified with PET even if EEG data do not reveal a clear-cut focus. In such cases, PET is particularly useful in localizing the site. In most cases however, EEG will verify the site as being the source of the seizures. Furthermore, there has been an excellent correlation between the site of hypometabolism as determined by PET and the presence of a pathological abnormality in the surgical specimen, even in cases where lesions have not been detectable by MRI or CT.

Other neurological and psychiatric diseases and conditions in which PET studies have contributed both to patient care and a better understanding of the disease process include Parkinson's disease and other movement disorders, head trauma, chronic pain, AIDS dementia, alcoholism, cocaine abuse, schizophrenia and depression.

CARDIOVASCULAR DISEASES

While many PET studies of the heart, such as measurements of regional glucose metabolism, involve the use of cyclotron-produced radionuclides, measurements of regional myocardial blood flow can be measured with a tracer available from a generator. Rubidium-82 has a 76-second half-life and is obtained from the parent radionuclide strontium-82, which has a 25-day half-life [29]. For studies of myocardial blood flow, rubidium-82 is administered in ionic form as it is eluted from the generator [30]. Other PET tracers used to measure myocardial blood flow include $^{13}NH_3$, $H_2^{15}O$ and ^{62}Cu-PTSM. Copper-62 is available from a generator whereas nitrogen-13 and oxygen-15 are cyclotron-produced. An advantage of PET is that it is possible to obtain quantitative measurements of myocardial blood flow expressed in ml/min/100 g of tissue. Attenuation correction with PET is more accurate than with SPECT which results in better quantification.

^{18}F-Deoxyglucose, ^{11}C-acetate and ^{11}C-palmitate are used with PET to assess substrate metabolism by the heart. Several radiopharmaceuticals have been used to study the autonomic innervation of the heart including ^{11}C-hydroxyephedrine, an analogue of norepinephrine (noradrenaline) that is used for visualizing sympathetic nerve terminals, and ^{11}C-CGPP-12177 that binds to post-synaptic receptor sites [31,32].

Coronary artery disease is often present in persons with no symptoms, although chest pain may be the presenting complaint. The first sign of heart disease in many persons is sudden death. Approximately 60% of patients who have coronary artery disease die suddenly from heart attack or develop a myocardial infarction without prior symptoms [33–35]. The accuracy of exercise thallium-201 imaging for detecting coronary artery disease is approximately 80–90% in symptomatic patients – but is much lower in asymptomatic individuals. Rest-exercise ventricular function studies with technetium-99m tracers have a sensitivity similar to that of thallium-201 imaging [36]. Gould and colleagues [37] have advocated the use of PET imaging with rubidium-82 as a means of screening high-risk patients to detect asymptomatic coronary artery disease. PET scanning has also been used to differentiate damaged from necrotic myocardium in patients with myocardial infarction. This presence of damaged myocardium is an important consideration in selecting patients for revascularization procedures.

The accuracy of myocardial perfusion imaging with PET in the diagnosis of coronary artery disease has been documented [37,38]. The patients are examined during supine bicycle exercise [38] or after intravenous administration of dipyridamole [39].

Gould *et al.* [37] have reported that the sensitivity of PET for diagnosing coronary artery disease is >95% with a similar specificity, even in asymptomatic individuals. PET perfusion studies are more accurate than the non-invasive studies presently being used in the evaluation of patients with suspected coronary artery disease.

Myocardial viability is determined with ^{18}F-deoxyglucose [40]. It is possible to identify areas that are ischaemic but contain viable myocardium. Although in the fasting state, 95% of the energy requirements of the myocardium are normally supplied by fatty acids, ischaemic myocardium shifts from fatty acid to glucose metabolism. ^{18}F-FDG accumulation in ischaemic myocardium is greater than in normally perfused myocardium. In contrast, necrotic myocardium does not accumulate ^{18}F-FDG. Before coronary artery bypass graft surgery, viable myocardium can be characterized as regions of decreased blood flow and maintained FDG accumulation; such regions often have decreased contractility. Myocardial scarring is characterized by both decreased regional blood flow and FDG accumulation. In a UCLA study, regional wall-motion improved after bypass grafting in 85% of the segments identified as viable by their metabolism of glucose. On the other hand, 96% of segments identified as scar did not show an improvement in regional wall motion. In another study of patients with previous infarction, PET studies identified viable myocardium in many segments with fixed defects on thallium imaging. In patients with acute infarction, areas of matching decreases in flow and FDG did not recover contractile function. In approximately 50% of segments with FDG accumulation but decreased flow, regional function improved 6 weeks later.

THE FUTURE

The development of regional pharmacies to distribute PET radiopharmaceuticals to hospitals and clinics that are unable to obtain and support a cyclotron will extend the benefits of PET to more patients. We have seen this happen as many radiopharmaceuticals first developed for PET subsequently have been successfully labelled with ^{99m}Tc, ^{123}I or ^{111}In and translated into SPECT studies. The new SPECT camera systems, which are capable of imaging positron-emitting isotopes, will also extend the use of PET, particularly FDG. As more and more 'outcome' studies are published, it will become increasingly convincing that PET is no longer just a research tool limited to large academic centres. In many clinical situations, patients' problems cannot be answered completely with anatomical imaging studies, laboratory data and physical examination, or a combination of these. PET is expensive to install and maintain, but the results it produces reduce the overall cost to the healthcare system by avoiding unnecessary and unfruitful diagnostic tests, operative procedures and prolonged hospitalizations. When the proper question is asked about a particular patient, it is often possible to tailor a PET study, which will answer the question with a molecular or biochemical understanding of the problem. We are moving into an era when it will be possible to treat each patient based on his or her specific regional molecular diagnosis, rather than relying on statistical norms.

REFERENCES

1. Engel, J. Jr, Lubens, P., Kuhl, D.E. and Phelps, M.E. (1985) Local cerebral metabolic rate for glucose during petit mal absences. *Ann. Neurol.*, **17**, 121–8.
2. Frost, J.J. and Mayberg, H.S. (1995) Epilepsy, in *Principles of Nuclear Medicine, Second Edition* (eds H.N. Wagner, Jr, Z. Szabo and J.W. Buchanan), W.B. Saunders Co., Philadelphia, pp. 564–73.
3. Kuhl, D.E., Phelps, M.E., Markham, C.E. *et al.* (1982) Cerebral metabolism and atrophy in Huntington's disease determined by FDG and computed tomographic scan. *Ann. Neurol.*, **12**, 425–34.
4. Kuwert, T., Lange, H.W., Langen, K.J., Herzog, H., Aulich, A. and Feinendegen, L.E. (1990) Cortical and subcortical glucose consumption measured by PET in patients with Huntington's disease. *Brain*, **113**, 1405–23.
5. Heiss, W.-D. and Podreka, I. (1995) Cerebrovascular disease, in *Principles of Nuclear Medicine, Second Edition* (eds H.N. Wagner, Jr, Z. Szabo and J.W. Buchanan), W.B. Saunders Co., Philadelphia, pp. 564–73.
6. Lee, M.C., Wagner, H.N., Tanada, S., Frost, J.J., Bice, A.N. and Dannals, R.F. (1988) Duration of occupancy of opiate receptors by naltrexone. *J. Nucl. Med.*, **29**, 1207–11.
7. Patz, E.J., Lowe, V.J., Hoffman, J.M., Paine, S.S., Burrowes, P., Coleman, R.E. and Goodman, P.C. (1993) Focal pulmonary abnormalities: evaluation with F-18 fluorodeoxyglucose PET scanning. *Radiology*, **188**, 487–90.
8. Lowe, V.J., DeLong, D.M., Hoffman, J.M. and Coleman, R.E. (1995) Optimum scanning protocol for FDG-PET evaluation of pulmonary malignancy. *J. Nucl. Med.*, **36**, 883–7.
9. Patronas, N.J., Di Chiro, G., Brooks, R.A. *et al.* (1982) Work in progress. ^{18}F-fluorodeoxyglucose and PET in the evaluation of radiation necrosis of the brain. *Radiology*, **144**, 885–9.
10. Glantz, M.J., Hoffman, J.M., Coleman, R.E. *et al.* (1991) Identification of early recurrence of primary central nervous system tumors by [^{18}F]fluorodeoxyglucose positron emission tomography. *Ann. Neurol.*, **29**, 347–55.
11. Kameyama, M., Shirane, R., Itoh, J. *et al.* (1990) The accumulation of ^{11}C-methionine in cerebral glioma patients studied with PET. *Acta Neurochir.*, **104**, 8–12.
12. Ogawa, T., Kanno, I., Shishido, F. *et al.* (1991) Clinical value or PET with ^{18}F-fluorodeoxyglucose and L-methyl-^{11}C-methionine for diagnosis of recurrent brain tumor and radiation injury. *Acta Radiol.*, **32**, 197–202.
13. Conti, P.S. (1995) Brain and Spinal Cord, In *Principles of Nuclear Medicine, Second Edition* (eds H.N. Wagner Jr, Z. Szabo and J.W. Buchanan), W.B. Saunders Co., Philadelphia, pp. 1041–54.
14. Muhr, C., Bergstrom, M., Lundberg, P.O. *et al.* (1986) Dopamine receptors in pituitary adenomas: PET visualization. *J. Comput. Assist. Tomogr.*, **10**, 175–80.
15. Wagner, H.N. Jr and Conti, P.A. (1991) Advances in medical imaging for cancer diagnosis and treatment. *Cancer*, **67**, 1121–8.
16. McGuire, A.H., Dehdashti, F., Siegel, B.A., Lyss, A.P., Brodack, J.W., Mathias, C.J., Mintun, M.A., Katzenellenbogen, J.A. and Welch, M.J. (1991) Positron tomographic assessment of 16-(^{18}F)fluoro-17-estradiol uptake in metastatic breast carcinoma. *J. Nucl. Med.*, **32**, 1526–31.
17. Flanagan, F.L., Dehdashti, F., Mortimer, J.E., Siegel, B.A., Jonson, S. and Welch, M.J. (1996) PET assessment of response to tamoxifen therapy in patients

with metastatic breast cancer. *J. Nucl. Med.,* **37**(Suppl.), 99P.

18. Young, H., Carnochan, P., Trivedi, M., Potter, G.A., Eccles, S.A., Haynes, B.P., Jarman, M. and Ott, R.J. (1995) Pharmacokinetics and biodistribution of radiolabelled idoxifene: prospects for the use of PET in the evaluation of a novel antioestrogen for cancer therapy. *Nucl. Med. Biol.,* **22**(4), 405–11.

19. Inoue, T., Yang, D.J., Oriuchi, N., Wallace, S., Buzdar, A., Tansey, W., Kim, E.E., Cherif, A., Kuang, L.-R. and Podoloff, D.A. (1996) Positron emission tomography with F-18 fluorotamoxifen in patients with breast cancer. *J. Nucl. Med.,* **37**(Suppl.), 86P.

20. Kole, A.C., Nieweg, O.E., Pruim, J., Hoekstra, H.J., Plukker, J.Th.M., Paans, A.M.J., Koops, S.H. and Vaalburg, W. (1996) L-1-[^{11}C]-Tyrosine, a better PET tracer for breast cancer: visualization and quantification of metabolism. *J. Nucl. Med.,* **37**(Suppl.), 86P.

21. Strauss, L.G. and Conti, P.S. (1991) The applications of PET in clinical oncology. *J. Nucl. Med.,* **32**, 623–48.

22. Valk, P.E., Abella-Columna, E., Tesar, R.D., Pounds, T.R., Haseman, M.K. and Myers, R.W. (1996) Diagnostic accuracy and cost-effectiveness of whole-body PET-FDG imaging in recurrent colorectal cancer. *J. Nucl. Med.,* **37**(Suppl.), 132P.

23. Hustinx, R., Paulus, P., Daenen, F., Jerusalem, G., Jacquet, N. and Rigo, P. (1996) PET imaging of liver metastases: a retrospective study. *J. Nucl. Med.,* **37**(Suppl.), 250P.

24. Kuhl, D.E., Metter, E.J., Riege, W.H. *et al.* (1983) Local cerebral glucose utilization in elderly patients with depression, multiple infarct dementia and Alzheimer's disease. *J. Cereb. Blood Flow Metab.,* **3**(Suppl. 1), S494–5.

25. Minoshima, S., Giordani, B.L., Berent, S., Frey, K.A., Foster, N.L. and Kuhl, D.E. (1996) The posterior cingulate cortex: the earliest metabolic reduction in Alzheimer's disease as revealed by PET. *J. Nucl. Med.,* **37**(Suppl.), 163P.

26. Small, G.W., Saxena, G.W., Mazziotta, J.C. *et al.* (1996) Strategies using PET for early detection of Alzheimer's disease. *J. Nucl. Med.,* **37**(Suppl.), 79P.

27. Kushner, M., Reivich, M., Fieschi, C., Silver, F., Chawluk, J., Rosen, M., Greenberg, J., Burke, A. and Alavi, A. (1987) Metabolic and clinical correlates of acute ischemic infarction. *Neurology,* **37**, 1103–10.

28. Kuhl, D.E., Engel, J., Jr, Phelps, M.E. and Selin, C. (1980) Epileptic patterns of local cerebral metabolism and perfusion in humans determined by emission computed tomography of ^{18}FDG and ^{13}NH$_3$. *Ann. Neurol.,* **8**, 348–60.

29. Yano, Y., Budinger, T.F., Chiang, G., O'Brien, H.A. and Grant, P.M. (1979) Evaluation and application

of alumina-based Rb-82 generators charged with high levels of Sr-82/85. *J. Nucl. Med.,* **20**, 961–6.

30. Yano, Y., Cahoon, J.L. and Budinger, T.F. (1981) A precision flow-controlled Rb-82 generator for bolus or constant-infusion studies of the heart and brain. *J. Nucl. Med.,* **22**, 1006–10.

31. Syrota, A., Merlet, P. and Delforge, J. (1995) Cardiac neurotransmission, in *Principles of Nuclear Medicine, Second Edition* (eds H.N. Wagner, Jr, Z. Szabo and J.W. Buchanan), W.B. Saunders Co., Philadelphia, pp. 759–73.

32. Schwaiger, M. and Ziegler, S. (1996) Cardiac application of positron emission tomography, in *Diagnostic Nuclear Medicine, Third Edition* (eds M.P. Sandler, R.E. Coleman, F.J.Th. Wackers, J.A. Patton, A. Gottschalk and P.B. Hoffer), Williams and Wilkins, Baltimore, pp. 517–42.

33. Lown, B. (1979) Sudden cardiac death: the major challenge confronting contemporary cardiology. *Am. J. Cardiol.,* **43**, 313–28.

34. Reunanen, A., Aromaa, A., Pyorala, X., Punsar, S., Maatela, J. and Knekt, P. (1983) The Social Insurance Institution's coronary heart disease study: baseline data and 5-year mortality experience. *Acta Med. Scand.,* **Suppl. 673**, 67–81.

35. Kannel, W.B. and Abbott, R.D. (1984) Incidence and prognosis of unrecognized myocardial infarction. An update on the Framingham Study. *N. Engl. J. Med.,* **311**, 1114–7.

36. Jones, R.H., McEwan, P., Newam, G.E. *et al.* (1981) Accuracy of diagnosis of coronary artery disease by measurement of left ventricular function during rest and exercise. *Circulation,* **64**, 586–601.

37. Gould, K.L., Goldstein, R.A., Mullani, N.A. *et al.* (1986) Noninvasive assessment of coronary stenoses by myocardial perfusion imaging during pharmacologic coronary vasodilation. VIII. Clinical feasibility of positron cardiac imaging without a cyclotron using generator-produced rubidium-82. *J. Am. Coll. Cardiol.,* **7**, 775–89.

38. Tamaki, N., Yonekura, Y., Senda, M. *et al.* (1985) Myocardial positron computed tomography with ^{13}N-ammonia at rest and during exercise. *Eur. J. Nucl. Med.,* **1**(1), 246–51.

39. Gould, K.L. (1978) Noninvasive assessment of coronary stenosis by myocardial perfusion imaging during pharmacological coronary vasodilation. I. *Am. J. Cardiol.,* **41**, 267–8.

40. Schwaiger, M., Brunken, R., Grover-McKay, M., Krivokapich, J., Child, J., Tillisch, J.H., Phelps, M.E. and Schelbert, H.R. (1986) Regional myocardial metabolism in patients with acute myocardial infarction assessed by positron emission tomography. *J. Am. Coll. Cardiol.,* **8**, 800–8.

CHAPTER 4

Paediatric issues

D.L. Gilday

SPECIAL CONSIDERATIONS IN CHILDREN

The practice of nuclear medicine is quite different for children. In addition, consideration must be given to patient motion, fear and parental involvement. The diseases of childhood are very different from those of adulthood and often have a very fast time course. Therefore, there is a need for automating nuclear medicine techniques for paediatric patients.

CHILD INTERACTION

As children are easily frightened by the unknown, especially in a hospital where they may have had previous phlebotomies and tests, it should be the goal of the nuclear medicine department to provide a quiet and friendly environment. The staff should behave in a calm and relaxed manner, with a kind, confident and sympathetic approach towards the child. The nuclear medicine technique(s) used should be tailored to the child. The study should be designed to minimize the length of time the child must lie still. Thus, long dynamic studies are modified to sequential static images, allowing the child to move between images such as in the gastric emptying and transit studies.

All children old enough to comprehend (usually about the age of three), should have the procedure explained to them in simple words, appropriate to their level of understanding. It is also important to gain the parent's cooperation as their attitude can positively or negatively influence their child. The positive aspects of the study should be empha-sized and the negative aspects minimized. It is crucial never to mislead the child about what is about to happen. A child's trust in the staff may be difficult to obtain, and once obtained it can be easily jeopardized.

Maintaining close physical contact with the patient and talking to them while the study is being performed, distracts their attention from the procedure itself, and often gains greater cooperation. The most valuable distracter is a television set, a video recorder and a good video movie (The *Lion King* is very good for all ages). Soothers, stickers, and awards for being injected all help to make it easier to get a first-class result.

Parents usually accompany the child during the test unless the procedure requires a sterile field. It has been our experience that with well-trained staff and cooperative parental involvement, it is rare to have problems with a study. An occasional child with a disciplinary problem is likely to be less cooperative in the presence of parent(s). In such cases, it is helpful if the parent stays in the waiting room.

In a younger patient, careful restraint is frequently necessary but should be used in moderation. The goal is to prevent motion and also an accidental fall from an imaging stretcher or couch. Babies can be restrained by the use of sandbags alongside the body and across the knees and arms. Wrapping the baby in a 'papoose'-like manner with blankets is often the best approach. This provides adequate restraint without causing discomfort. Older uncooperative children are best immobilized with restrainers strapped around the stretcher top using Velcro straps.

Clinical Nuclear Medicine, 3rd edn. Edited by M.N. Maisey, K.E. Britton and B.D. Collier. Published in 1998 by Chapman & Hall, London. ISBN 0 412 75180 1

SEDATION

If moderate restraint is not successful then sedation is required for a technically satisfactory study. This is especially true for lengthy procedures such as SPECT or whole-body imaging. Sedation is recommended in overly anxious patients who refuse to cooperate, very young or hyperactive patients who are unable to remain still, and retarded patients who lack the mental capacity to follow simple instructions.

Sedation may take several forms. In the correct setting sedation with intravenous Nembutal (pentobarbital sodium) is very effective. Using a dose of 5 mg/kg up to a maximum of 100 mg, we administer half the volume rapidly, wait 60 seconds and then administer one-quarter of the dose. This usually puts the child to sleep in about 2–3 minutes. If not, then the remaining one-quarter dose is given. The child remains asleep for about 45–60 minutes. The advantage of this technique is that the child falls asleep very quickly, it is more reliable than the intramuscularly injected Nembutal, and the child recovers faster. With all sedatives, the child's cardiac and respiratory status must be closely monitored. We currently use an automated pulse oximeter.

Nembutal is contraindicated in neonates less than 2 months of age. This group lacks adequate levels of the liver enzymes, which are required to metabolize Nembutal before it acts *in vivo*. In place of Nembutal, we use an elixir of Phenergan (promethazine) and chloral hydrate, 30–45 minutes before scanning. The effect is less pronounced than with Nembutal, but it is usually adequate and the patient arouses readily.

Valium and Nembutal suppositories have all been found to be inadequate; none produces the deep sleep required to perform nuclear medicine procedures on the patient.

INJECTION TECHNIQUES

Injection of radiopharmaceuticals in small children presents several minor problems, all of which are easily surmounted by modifying the techniques used in adults. Very small children will be completely covered by the head of a large field-of-view camera. This increases the child's anxiety and makes injection difficult. This can often be solved by placing the child supine on the stretcher top with the camera positioned underneath.

Lucite stretcher tops or gantries prevent excessive attenuation of photons. In smaller children, for head, feet or hand imaging, holding the child directly on the camera collimator can act as an extension of the stretcher.

Finding a suitable vein for intravenous injections is rarely a problem. Although the antecubital fossa frequently has the largest vein, the elbows are less easily immobilized than the hands or feet, and the latter are often preferable injection sites. Scalp veins are also easily accessible, but are used as a last resort as a small area of hair must be shaved to find them. Jugular injections are mandatory for left-to-right shunt evaluations. With procedures requiring repeated blood sampling (e.g. glomerular filtration rate determination), the insertion of an angiocath is the best approach.

Our injection apparatus consists of a 10-ml syringe of saline connected with extension tubing to a three-way stop-cock which is connected to the syringe containing the radiopharmaceutical. The outflow channel is then attached to the previously established intravenous line or a scalp vein needle is used to obtain intravenous access. This system allows the dose syringe to be completely isolated from the saline. Once the needle is properly positioned – confirmed by injecting some saline into the vein – the radiopharmaceutical is pushed into the extension tube and then the input channel is changed to the saline syringe, the contents of which force the bolus into the vein. Any remaining saline is used to flush the dose syringe to ensure that all of the dose gets into the patient (especially important with small volume doses).

RADIOPHARMACEUTICAL DOSAGE

The amount of radioactivity can be readily calculated by referring to a chart (Figure 4.1). The patient's dose is determined by weight and the percentage of the standard adult dose is determined according to the patient's body surface area. This is possible because the chart estimates body surface area from the child's weight. This dose calculation permits distribution of tracer per unit area of organ rather than per kg of body weight.

It is very important to establish the minimum dose for each radiopharmaceutical. To get an adequate study, especially a dynamic one, there have to be enough photons detected per unit time to

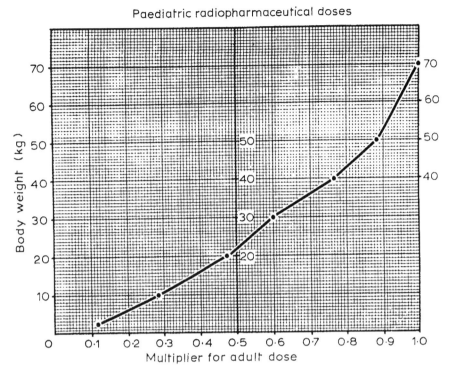

Figure 4.1 Radiopharmaceutical dosage schedule based on a body surface area using weight to determine the percentage of adult dose to administer.

adequately assess the patient's problem. It is better to ensure a slightly higher delivered radiation dose than to have an uninterpretable study. This is especially true in children where one wants the imaging time to be as short as possible so as to avoid motion. The risk from the higher radiation dose is negligible, especially if it is outweighed by the clinical benefit derived from the procedure.

IMAGE EVALUATION

It is very important to view all images on the imaging workstation so as to take optimal advantage of the windowing capability. In musculoskeletal imaging, it is very important to see the physes (growth zones) clearly, and this is best achieved with the aid of a computer workstation. At the same time, spiral and bucket-handle fractures may require lowering the upper window limit. Reviewing a voiding cystogram dynamically may help in detecting a hint of reflux that may not be apparent on the hard copy.

MUSCULOSKELETAL PROBLEMS

The two major indications for bone scintigraphy in non-malignant diseases are the investigation of bone pain and fever/infection. Plain film examination should be carried out first. Frequently, computed tomography (CT) is also done to detect a lesion. Our standard technique is to acquire blood pool images and static or SPECT images of the areas of clinical interest. We use the highest resolution system available, since in small children and infants it is important to obtain top-quality images. We often use magnification with converging or pin-hole collimation.

OSTEOMYELITIS

The ability to diagnose osteomyelitis clinically is variable. The child may present with joint pain, joint tenderness, limited range of motion, soft-tissue swelling, erythema, fever and bacteraemia. Differentiation of osteomyelitis from cellulitis or

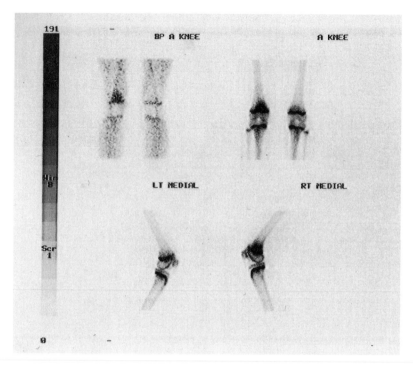

Figure 4.2   Acute osteomyelitis. There is increased tracer in the lateral epiphysis of the right femur, which is seen to be hyperaemic. This is typical in location and appearance of acute osteomyelitis. Note the loss of demarcation of the physis and the metaphysis.

septic arthritis may be clinically difficult, and unfortunately, the radiological examination is often normal. Occasionally, soft-tissue swelling is present. Only rarely are the frank bone changes of osteomyelitis seen, due to the fact that most parents of children with these symptoms seek immediate medical advice, and generally a treatment of intravenous antibiotic is promptly started. Using combined blood pool and bone scintigraphy, we have found it possible to differentiate osteomyelitis from cellulitis very early in the course of the child's illness [1]. Bone scintigraphy is especially valuable in assessing areas such as the pelvis and spine, which are difficult to evaluate radiologically.

A typical bone scan appearance of osteomyelitis is a well-defined focus of increased radioactivity within the bone that is associated with an identical area of hyperaemia on the blood pool images (Figure 4.2). This is most often located in the metaphysis of a long bone (although occasionally other bones may be involved), especially if a puncture wound has occurred. This appearance is specific for osteomyelitis, and is readily differentiated from the patterns of cellulitis and septic arthritis. Occasionally, there is generalized hyperaemia of a limb, which tends to mask the typical appearance.

In a child with acute osteomyelitis, the hyperaemia involving the metaphysis of the long bone is usually seen between 24 and 36 hours after the onset of symptoms. Bone images may be positive as early as 24 hours, but usually become positive between 36 and 72 hours. If the findings are not typical of osteomyelitis then gallium imaging is the simplest solution for determining whether there is an infection (Figure 4.3). Although radiological abnormalities, such as indistinct fat-lines and soft-tissue swelling, permit the presumptive radiological diagnosis of osteomyelitis, it usually requires 8 days to demonstrate demineralization, whereas the bone changes are usually evident on bone scintigraphy by 3 days. We are confident that if a child has clinical symptoms suggesting osteomyelitis and a normal or a suggestive plain X-ray examination, then bone imaging is the ex-

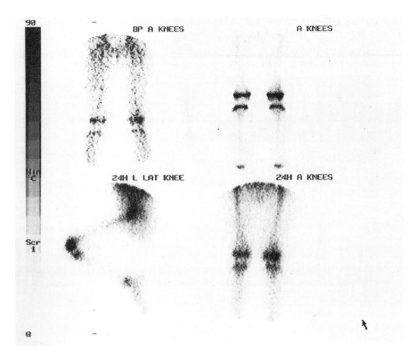

Figure 4.3 Acute osteomyelitis. There is increased tracer medially in the proximal metaphysis of the right femur, which is seen to be hyperaemic. Because of this unusual location for acute osteomyelitis, a gallium scan was performed. This confirms the diagnosis of acute osteomyelitis as the gallium to normal bone ratio is higher than that of the bone scan.

amination of choice for establishing the diagnosis [1–3].

In the spine, the blood pool images are less valuable due to the underlying abdominal and thoracic organs. However, with the addition of bone SPECT, osteomyelitis or discitis involving the spine is readily detected.

CELLULITIS

Cellulitis has a distinctive appearance which is a diffuse increase in radioactivity involving both the soft tissues and the bone. This is more readily apparent on the blood pool than on the bone images. The appearance is due to a diffuse soft-tissue hyperaemia. This is readily distinguished from the appearance described above for osteomyelitis.

SEPTIC ARTHRITIS

Septic arthritis has a similar appearance, but the hyperaemia involves both sides of the joint (Figure 4.4). Subchondral bone on either side of the af-

fected joint has markedly increased metabolism. An important point regarding the method of diagnosis and treatment of septic arthritis of the hip is to do a needle aspiration of the hip. There is no role for imaging of any type in the diagnosis of septic arthritis of the hip. Although ultrasound has been used to demonstrate increased fluid in the hip joint, it is imperative not to delay the aspiration. The aspiration decreases the intracapsular pressure, and this minimizes the possibility of necrosis of the femoral head. After the aspiration, the patient can have a bone scintigram to determine whether or not concomitant osteomyelitis is present.

LEGG–PERTHES' DISEASE

Avascular necrosis of the femoral head (e.g. Legg–Perthes' disease) is usually detected radiologically. In those patients where the radiographs are normal or show mild capsular distention, the use of magnetic resonance imaging (MRI) has become the main means of evaluating the hip. Bone scintigraphy can be used either as an adjunct to determine degree of viability, or to detect avascular necrosis in the presence of an inconclusive MRI. Bone scintigraphy, especially when using pinhole magnification, remains an excellent test for detecting avascular necrosis of the femoral head (Figure 4.5).

SICKLE CELL DISEASE

The child with sickle cell disease frequently presents with an acute onset of bone pain, and may occasionally have fever. The main dilemma is to determine whether the child has had a sickle cell crisis with marrow ischaemia or has osteomyelitis. Our current approach is to use ^{99m}Tc sulphur colloid to image the marrow and then follow with a bone scan using ^{99m}Tc-MDP. If the marrow scan shows ischaemia and the bone scan is normal or cold, the study is terminated and the diagnosis of sickle cell crisis is made/presumed (Figure 4.6). However, if the bone scan is hot, then it is important to carry on and do a gallium study. This is especially true if the marrow does not show a cold defect at the site of the hypermetabolic bone scan lesion. If the bone scan is abnormal and the gallium scan normal, then most likely the diagnosis is post-ischaemic healing. The diagnosis is consistent with osteomyelitis if both the bone and gallium scans are abnormal in the appropriate pattern, i.e. usually involving a metaphysis.

SPONDYLOLYSIS

In many cases of spondylolysis, the pars interarticularis defect may not be 'easily' identified on the spinal radiographs. SPECT bone imaging has the ready advantage of being able to detect not only the reparative attempts of the defect but also allows visualization of the increased bone stress at the articular facets. By locating the site of increased bone metabolism, SPECT can help differentiate between a bilateral pars defect and bone stress. The lesion of spondylolysis abnormalities will be more posterior (Figure 4.7).

CHILD ABUSE

Our sociomedical legal system has developed an enlightened sensitivity to child abuse. The estimated incidence of reported child abuse has increased from 30/1000 in 1985 to 45/1000 in 1992. The incidence of skeletal injury in these children is approximately 20%, and is more common among

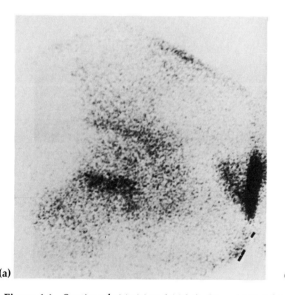
(a)

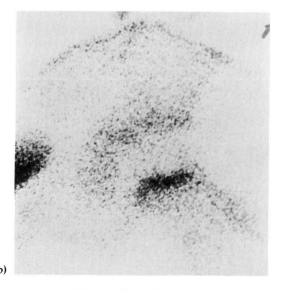
(b)

Figure 4.4 Septic arthritis (a) and (c) left, (b) and (d) right posterior views, (e) pelvic X-ray. Initially, the left femoral capital epiphysis showed reduced tracer accumulation (b) and after surgical relief of the increased intracapsular pressure there was increased tracer metabolism in the femoral head (d) indicating a return of blood flow.

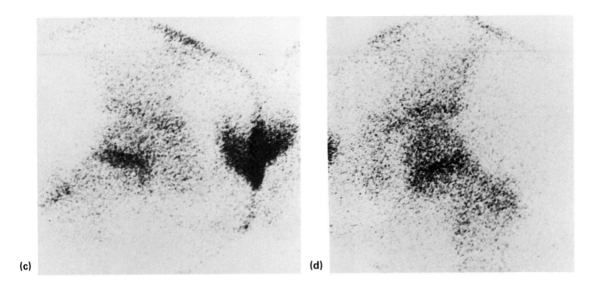

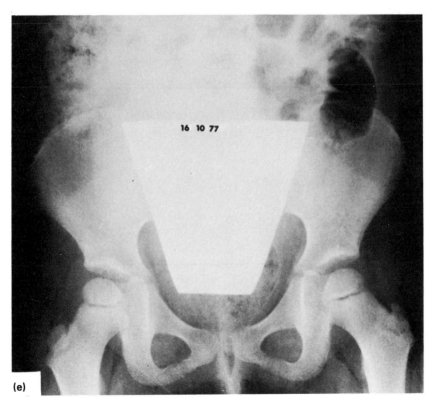

16 10 77

Fig. 4.4 *Continued.*

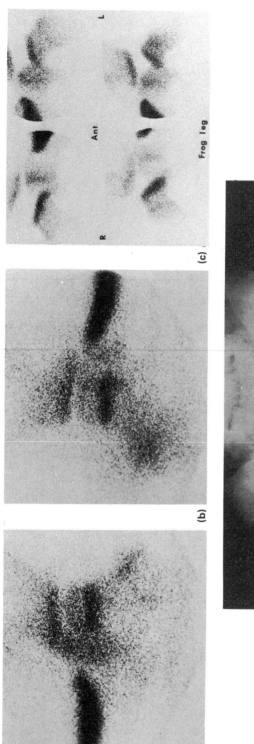

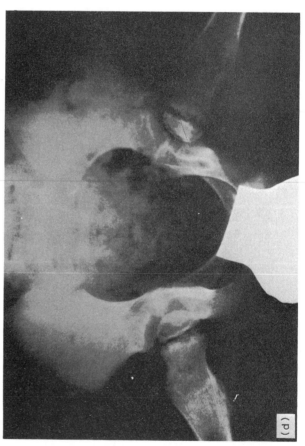

Figure 4.5 Legg–Perthes disease. (a,b) Normal magnification view of the femoral heads. (c) Bilateral avascular femoral capital epiphyses. (d) The radiograph demonstrates typical Legg–Perthes involvement on the left.

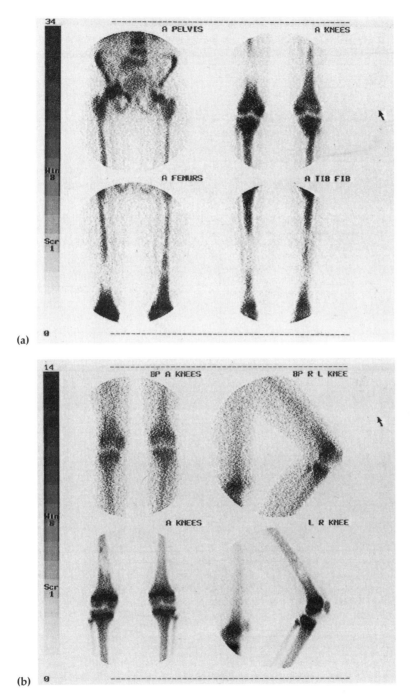

Figure 4.6 Sickle cell crisis (a) bone marrow scan, (b) bone scan. Multiple sites of decreased marrow activity in the diaphysis of each distal femur, both tibiae and the left femoral capital epiphysis. Note that in the MDP bone scan the same areas are either photopenic or normal, indicating a sickle cell crisis rather than osteomyelitis.

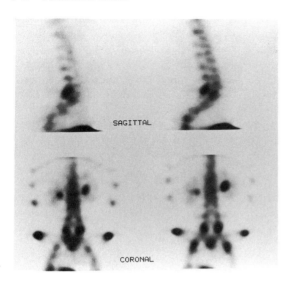

Figure 4.7 Spondylolysis. An excellent example of attempted repair of the pars interarticularis defects seen bilaterally on the SPECT bone scan.

those under 1 year of age. The fractures are usually multiple, involving the long bones, skull, vertebrae, ribs, and facial bones, and usually show different stages of healing. In most paediatric hospitals, the approach is to radiograph the clinically affected body parts. If the suspicion of child abuse arises, then a total-body radiographic examination is undertaken, and a total-body bone scan is next performed to locate any unsuspected bony injuries. Metaphyseal–epiphyseal injury is common. Careful positioning and correct window and level settings are important to avoid the pitfall of 'blooming' in the image, which may obscure a mild abnormality. Accurate interpretation will depend on assessment of the intensity and shape of abnormality. Prime sites of investigation are the ribs, costovertebral junctions, spine, and diaphyses of long bones (Figure 4.8). If the bone scan is normal at 3 days or more after injury, then there is a very low probability of bony injury. Disadvantages of the bone scan include an inability to determine the type, extent, and age of each injury; poor

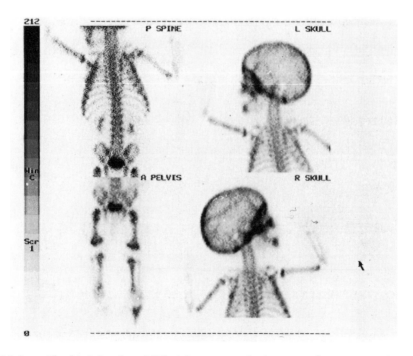

Figure 4.8 Child abuse. The third, fourth and fifth right costovertebral junctions have increased activity, indicating healing trauma. Both femora, both tibiae and both humeri show increased activity in the diaphyses, typical of subperiosteal new bone formation as a result of trauma. Note the linear increase in activity in the right parietal bone due to a skull fracture (not normally as well seen as in this case).

bone accumulation of the ^{99m}Tc-MDP in cases of severe malnutrition; it is also not possible to differentiate systemic and metabolic disorders associated with trauma from trauma alone. If one (or more) area is found to be abnormal, then high-resolution multiple-view radiographs are obtained to confirm the diagnosis and also to help date the injury. With greater recognition of this problem, more studies are being undertaken. Skull radiography is performed suited for detecting trauma to the calvarium, as the scan is very poor in detection of fractures of the flat bones of the skull.

MALIGNANT TUMOURS

Although it is important to detect primary and secondary malignancies, the real goal is to first assess the potential response to therapy as a failure is extremely disappointing. If one is aware of the potential of poor chemotherapeutic response then it would alter the management protocol.

OSTEOGENIC SARCOMA

Osteogenic sarcomas usually occur in the metaphyses of long bones, common sites being the distal femur or the proximal tibia. The common age range is from 10 to 17 years. Occasionally, several sites may be involved at the time of presentation. The plain film is always abnormal, but the appearance can mimic other diseases such as chronic osteomyelitis. An untreated osteogenic sarcoma has a typical bone scan appearance. It demonstrates an uneven intensely increased distribution of tracer in the metaphysis. The blood pool image shows an increased blood volume within the tumour. The flow study however, shows markedly increased blood flow when compared with what would be expected from the blood pool image. This is due to the presence of arteriovenous connections with direct arteriovenous shunting (Figure 4.9). Recently there have been attempts to determine the potential response to chemotherapy by measuring the washout of ^{99m}Tc-MIBI during the 3 hours after injection. The theory is that if the tracer is washed out, the P1 glycoprotein content will be high and thus the sarcoma will not respond (Figure 4.10). In addition, the primary site will initially metabolize thallium/sestamibi, which has the same appearance as the lesion seen on the bone scan. After chemotherapy, there is often a marked reduction in thallium/sestamibi activity,

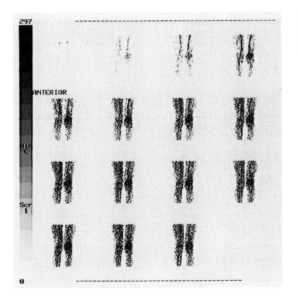
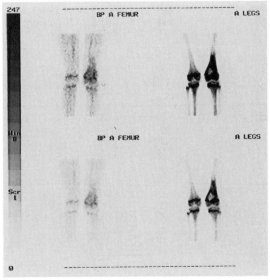

Figure 4.9 Osteogenic sarcoma. The radionuclide angiogram (left) demonstrates arteriovenous shunting typical of osteogenic sarcoma. The blood pool image (left side of right image) does not capture the shunting, but does reflect the bone repair in response to the tumour.

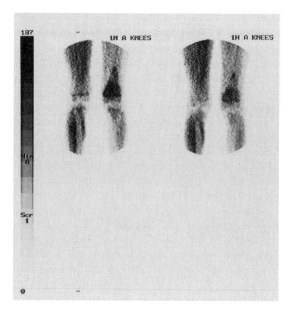

Figure 4.10   Osteogenic sarcoma. The sestamibi activity in the 1-minute image (left) is quite intense. Although there is some decrease by 1 hour (right), there is still considerable activity present. This patient responded well to chemotherapy.

whereas the ^{99m}Tc-MDP scan may show little change. This indicates that there has been a histological response to chemotherapy. However, the bone itself is still attempting to heal and thus there will be very little change on the bone scan. Nadel [4] has shown a good correlation between the histological response and the reduction in thallium/ sestamibi activity after chemotherapy in eleven children.

EWING'S SARCOMA

There are several differences between Ewing's sarcoma and osteogenic sarcoma. The site is usually not metaphyseal, but rather diaphyseal or in the flat bones (Figure 4.11) and there is no arteriovenous shunting. However, the thallium/sestamibi uptake is comparable with that seen in osteogenic sarcoma. On the bone scan, the lesion may be obscured by the bladder or intestinal activity in the pelvis.

LYMPHOMA

Gallium-67 scanning has replaced bone scanning in the evaluation of children with lymphomas.

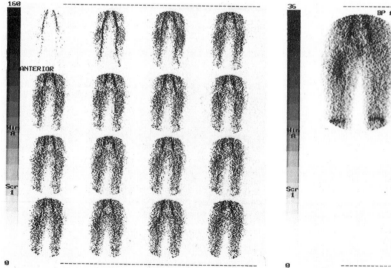

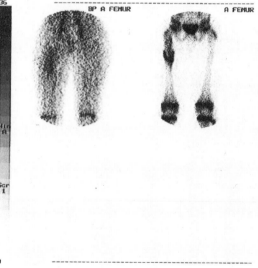

Figure 4.11   Ewing's sarcoma. the radionuclide angiogram (left) demonstrates a lack of arteriovenous shunting typical of Ewing's sarcoma. The bone scan demonstrates increased activity at the tumour site (right) and it is also hyperaemic in the blood pool images (middle). This is typical of Ewing's sarcoma, as there is little arteriovenous shunting.

^{99m}Tc-MDP scan has no place in the evaluation of childhood lymphoma, unless it is being used to evaluate an orthopaedic problem [5]. In children, the Hodgkin and non-Hodgkin lymphomas and the Burkitt's lymphoma are all quite gallium-avid. The presenting site as well as metastases are both readily identified. The post-laxative 72-hour scan usually shows any involvement of abdominal nodes. SPECT can be added to better depict lesions in the abdomen when colonic activity is present.

LANGERHANS CELL HISTIOCYTOSIS

Langerhans cell histiocytosis (formerly called histiocytosis X) presents in many variations, from a solitary mass or painful bone lesion to a very aggressive disseminated disease, that is usually fatal. Approximately 50% of the children present with bone lesions only. The preferred method of investigation is radiographic skeletal survey. However, the radiographic study can miss 20–30% of bone lesions that can be seen on the ^{99m}Tc-MDP whole-body scan [6]. Since the MDP scan also misses a number of lesions that can be seen on the radiographs, the two techniques in combination give the best yield.

The bone scan typically demonstrates a focal rim of increased activity with a photopenic centre at the lytic site. However, there can be false-negative scans with rapidly destructive lesions (Figure 4.12). Therefore, we perform both bone scans and radiographs in all children suspected of having histiocytosis X. It is important to correlate all modalities and, if the face is involved, CT may be especially helpful.

NEUROBLASTOMA

Neuroblastoma is a common childhood tumour that frequently metastasizes to bone. Bone scans are more sensitive than radiographic skeletal surveys. Between 30–70% of the lesions seen on bone scans are normal on X-ray. Therefore, a radionuclide skeletal survey should be the primary investigation. The bony involvement is usually seen as multiple foci of increased activity in metaphyses, which are usually asymmetric, and may involve the skull, vertebrae, ribs, pelvis, and the long bones [7]. Frequently, symmetric metaphyseal involvement is seen, especially around

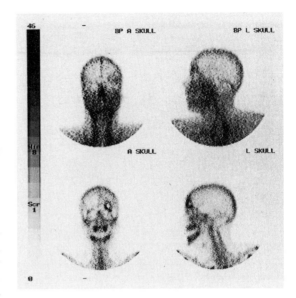

Figure 4.12 Langerhans cell histiocytosis. There is a photopenic lesion just above the left orbit, which has a reactive component at the orbit. The eosinophilic granuloma is mildly hyperaemic.

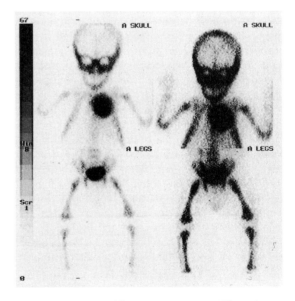

Figure 4.13 Neuroblastoma metastases. The primary tumour has accumulated the tracer, which is typical of most thoracic neuroblastomas. The metaphyses of the femora and tibiae show the typical metastases. The demarcation between the physis and metaphysis is lost.

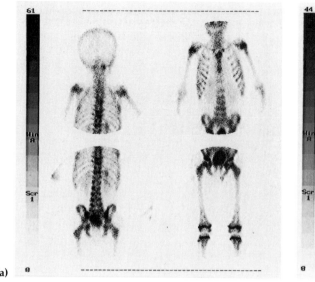
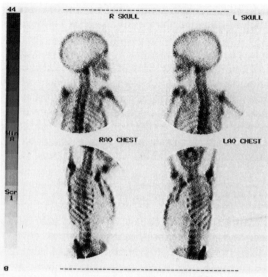

(a)   (b)

Figure 4.14   Neuroblastoma metastases. This case demonstrates mixed 'cold' and 'hot' metastases of neuroblastoma. Cold photopenic lesions are present in the spine (a) and ribs (b). Hypermetabolic lesions are present in the ribs (b) and metaphyses of long bones (a).

the knees involving both femora and tibiae (Figure 4.13). The physis is normally slightly elliptical in infants under 18 months of age, and is plate-like in older children. The metaphyseal border is always well-demarcated. When the uptake in the physis is wedge-shaped or globular, or if there is blurring of the metaphyseal border, metastasis should be suspected, even if the involvement is symmetric. Occasionally, if the tumour is very destructive, the metaphysis may be photon deficient (Figure 4.14).

The primary tumour accumulates ^{99m}Tc-MDP in 50–70% of cases (Figure 4.13). The mechanism of uptake is unknown, but may be related to dystrophic calcification in the tumour. When the primary tumour is intra-abdominal, renal abnormalities such as non-function, obstruction, or inferior and/or lateral displacement are commonly seen. In any child suspected of having neuroblastoma or abdominal tumour blood pool and sequential renal scans should be performed during the first 15 minutes after ^{99m}Tc-MDP injection.

^{131}I-metaiodobenzylguanidine (^{131}I-MIBG) was first described in 1983 and was rapidly and enthusiastically adopted for both the investigation and therapy of neuroblastoma [8]. Before this, the ^{99m}Tc-MDP bone scan was the only way to determine skeletal involvement by neuroblastoma in children. The problem with ^{99m}Tc-MDP bone scanning was that the studies required great care to avoid false-negative interpretations, even though the skeletal lesions have a significant lesion-to-background activity level. It was because of this – and the generally poor ability to detect soft-tissue or marrow neuroblastoma lesions – that ^{123}I- or ^{131}I-MIBG was so quickly adopted. However, Gordon *et al.* [9] bring a strong concern forward about the use of MIBG scanning as the sole test for the detection of skeletal neuroblastoma lesions. They found that ^{131}I-MIBG revealed more extensive skeletal disease than ^{99m}Tc-MDP, but all had abnormal bone scans. On the other hand, five patients had normal ^{123}I-MIBG with abnormal ^{99m}Tc-MDP studies of the skeleton.

In view of the inability of ^{123}I- or ^{131}I-MIBG scanning to detect all of the neuroblastoma bony lesions, all children with a diagnosis of neuroblastoma must have both the MIBG and MDP scanning in order to stage and monitor their neuroblastoma involvement.

GASTROINTESTINAL SYSTEM

LIVER DISEASE

With the widespread use of ultrasound, CT and MRI, there is little call for sulphur colloid liver/spleen imaging in paediatrics. The most common indication for imaging the spleen is in children with congenital heart disease, where the presence of a spleen can help define the prognosis. Situs inversus, polysplenia and asplenia can be of importance in determining the type of congenital heart disease. In children with haematological disorders, the presence of an accessory spleen can be of vital importance in explaining red cell destruction after a splenectomy. Imaging with heat-damaged red cells is the best way to detect an accessory spleen.

BILIARY DISEASE

One of the more difficult but rewarding investigations in paediatrics is the evaluation of neonatal jaundice. The problem of differentiating neonatal hepatitis from biliary atresia is extremely difficult to achieve with 100% reliability [10]. In neonates with biliary atresia, there is good extraction of the tracers in the first 60 minutes (extraction fraction usually in excess of 85%) but none is excreted into the duodenum. At 24 hours, no radiotracer is seen in the bowel (Figure 4.15). However, with neonatal hepatitis, there is reduced hepatic extraction fraction and delayed clearance with some radiotracer appearing in the bowel within 24 hours [11]. We have found that although no neonate with biliary atresia will excrete the radiotracer; a similar result is seen in a significant number of babies with neonatal hepatitis. Therefore, although the presence of tracer in the bowel eliminates the possibility of biliary atresia (Figure 4.16), the converse is not true as other conditions such as neonatal hepatitis, bile duct paucity syndrome and total parenteral nutrition can be a cause of non-excretion of the radiotracer into the bowel. A most important aspect of this study is to premedicate the patient for 5 days with phenobarbital (2.5 mg/kg, twice daily for 5 days) before injecting the biliary radiopharmaceutical [12].

Another important role for biliary imaging in paediatrics is the evaluation of a choledocal cyst. While this is usually detected as a cystic structure on ultrasound, the radionuclide evaluation aims to determine the physiological nature of the cyst. It is important that the cyst be seen to communicate with the hepatic duct system and to fill. In the post-operative period, the study demonstrates the easy flow of the radiopharmaceutical through the biliary tract.

ASPIRATION

The role of gastro-oesophageal reflux as the cause of symptoms and more specifically lung disease is well-defined. However, it is difficult to determine whether or not the reflux is the cause of the repeated pulmonary infections. In the past, the use of ^{99m}Tc-sulphur colloid in a formula or milk to monitor reflux and aspiration in children has been used to see if refluxed gastric contents are aspirated. We have been much more successful using the salivogram as suggested by Heyman *et al.* [13]. This study is performed by instilling a drop of radiotracer (any ^{99m}Tc-labelled radiopharmaceutical will suffice) into the mouth and letting the child swallow their radioactive saliva. This is carried out three times. Dynamic imaging is done of the thorax and upper abdomen. After the three salivograms, a long-exposure image (2–3 minutes) of the thorax is acquired to detect any aspiration. This procedure is very physiological as it mimics the normal state of the pharyngeal motility (Figure 4.17). In children with cerebral palsy or other neurological disorder that affects pharyngeal mechanics the study can show the presence of aspiration. It is an easy test to do and to interpret.

GASTRIC TRANSIT

The rate of gastric emptying is very important in many paediatric gastroenterological problems and can be readily assessed. The percent retention at 30, 60 and 120 minutes is calculated. There are no good normal-value studies, due to the fact that it is unethical to do control studies in children. However, some data have become available which indicate the normal range. A group of effectively normal children aged under 24 months were found to have <50% retention at 120 minutes (M.J. Gelfand, personal communication). In older children some data are available which suggest that retention at 60 minutes should be <50%. In dumping syndromes one is looking for faster than normal emptying. This has not been defined, but in our experience there should be at least 30% retention at 1 hour. In children with severe feeding

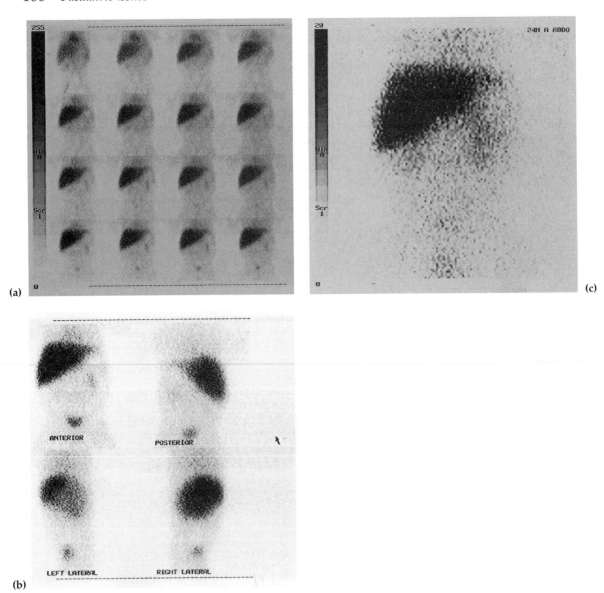

Figure 4.15   Biliary atresia. The liver extracts the tracer reasonably well (a) but there is no evidence of excretion after 4 hours (b) and 24 hours (c). This is typical of biliary atresia.

problems this test can be used to assess the efficacy of the formula being used to minimize emesis [14].

PERTECHNETATE ABDOMINAL IMAGING

The aetiology of rectal bleeding in infants and children is often obscure. In a 10-year period from 1952 to 1962, 801 patients were admitted to The Hospital for Sick Children with a history of rectal bleeding, i.e. approximately 80 per year. Of 61 patients in whom all examinations were negative and who underwent laparotomy, 31 had negative findings and a Meckel's diverticulum was present in 24, of whom 20 had gastric mucosa [15]. Meckel's diverticulum is a common congenital

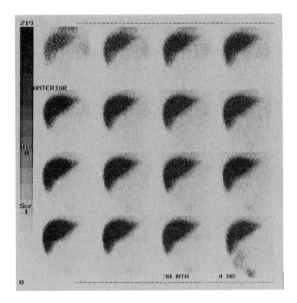

Figure 4.16 Neonatal hepatitis. Although the extraction is better than would be expected there is excretion by 4 hours.

anomaly (0.3–3% in mature individuals); however, a relatively small percentage (average 20%) of these patients have ectopic gastric mucosa within their Meckel's diverticulum.

The initial descriptions by Duszynski and colleagues [16] describe successful detection of Meckel's diverticulum with a rectilinear scanner. However, the test was not specific in their hands (as intussusceptions and polyps were also positive) and it took 2 hours from the time of injection to complete the study. Rosenthal, who performed this study using a gamma-camera, had an accuracy rate of 5/8 but still did not have a specific investigation [17]. He carried out such gamma-camera studies by imaging at 15, 30, 45 and 60 minutes after injection. In a multi-institutional paper [18], the results had greater than 80% accuracy in children who had a laparotomy.

There is a rapid increase in radioactivity in the stomach as the pertechnetate is secreted by the gastric mucosa. Renal and bladder activity are present as 20% of the injected pertechnetate is ex-

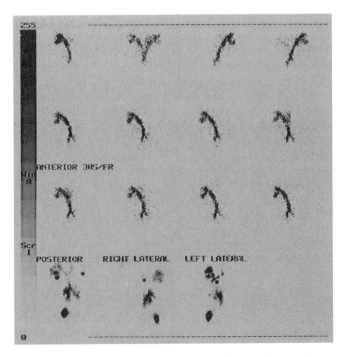

Figure 4.17 Salivogram aspiration. After the tracer was placed in the mouth it can be seen in the trachea (motion in frames 2–4). The tracer moves into each proximal bronchus. The posterior and lateral views are used to help localization with markers on the shoulders.

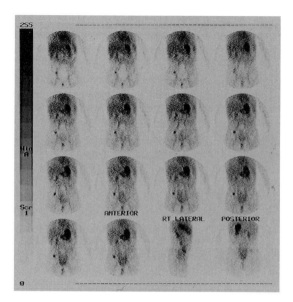

Figure 4.18 Meckel's diverticulum containing ectopic gastric mucosa. The images from 1 to 14 minutes show pertechnetate accumulating in the ectopic gastric mucosa, parallelling that of the stomach. Posterior and right lateral images are seen at 20 minutes to better differentiate the ectopic mucosa from other normal structures (renal pelves).

creted by the kidneys. The early sequential views permit monitoring of the rate of accumulation of pertechnetate in the stomach during the first 15 minutes. The posterior views at 15 and 30 minutes demonstrate the location of the renal pelves. Other than these normal structures, there should not be any focus of activity throughout the abdomen in the area of the small bowel, although ureters and the iliac vessels are sometimes seen.

In the child with a Meckel's diverticulum, the time sequence of radioactive concentration within the ectopic gastric mucosa parallels that in the normal gastric mucosa of the stomach (Figure 4.18). This important feature helps to differentiate ectopic gastric mucosa from inflammatory causes that tend to accumulate the radioactivity at a slower rate; it also can help to differentiate an extrarenal pelvis from a Meckel's diverticulum.

Problems occur in interpreting this study. The early appearance of the radiopharmaceutical in the ureters may simulate a focal lesion posteriorly at the pelvic brim due to a slight hold-up at this location while the child is supine. This fades with time and usually disappears during the prone and lateral views and, in the subsequent anterior views, there should not be much activity within the ureter. Occasionally, a Meckel's diverticulum may overlie an existing structure that contains radioactivity such as the ureter. Then the diagnosis of Meckel's diverticulum is difficult unless the bowel moves during the study. If not, a repeat study may show the focal accumulation to have moved. In some patients there is rapid movement of the tracer into the duodenum, which causes confusion; however, the lateral and posterior views help demonstrate the location of such increased activity. To minimize the excretion of the pertechnetate into the lumen of the stomach or out of the ectopic gastric mucosa we suggest premedication 1 hour before the study with ranitidine 5 mg/kg to a maximum of 50 mg infused in 20 ml of saline over 20 minutes. Any other lesion which contains ectopic gastric mucosa can produce the correct time sequence but may assume a different shape, such as duplication of the small bowel. Inflammatory bowel disease (e.g. gastroenteritis or regional enteritis) produces abnormal scans but the distribution of activity is diffuse or the time sequence is different.

Our results would suggest that the pertechnetate abdominal scan can detect ectopic gastric mucosa with an accuracy of at least 95%. This is a significant improvement over previously published reports, and is attributable to sequential early imaging, multiple views at 15 and 30 minutes and the use of ranitidine (or cimetidine).

GENITOURINARY PROBLEMS

TECHNIQUE CONSIDERATIONS

In children of all ages, various radionuclide renal studies are widely used to evaluate kidneys depending on the problem being investigated. In conjunction with ultrasound, the radionuclide renal tests have almost completely replaced the intravenous urogram. When interpreted with the ultrasound study, the two usually give a complete picture of the state of the kidneys. In neonates with compromised renal function, the study is the most accurate method for determining the function of each or both kidneys [19].

Serial assessment of renal function is important to paediatric nephrology/urology, particularly in children with hydronephrosis, vesicoureteral reflux, after acute pyelonephritis and those who may require evaluation post-operatively. The decision of whether to do a nephrectomy or a reconstructive procedure may be a difficult one, especially in the child whose contralateral kidney is already jeopardized. One of the factors influencing this decision is the degree of function of the affected kidney. In our centre we have found that renal scanning with technetium-99m diethylene-triamine penta-acetic acid (^{99m}Tc-DTPA), which has >95% excretion by glomerular filtration, provides a simple and relatively non-invasive method for assessing the relative function on each side and for measuring the glomerular filtration rate (GFR). In children with severe hydronephrosis, ^{99m}Tc-dimercaptosuccinic acid (^{99m}Tc-DMSA) can be substituted to better assess relative renal function. A separate filtration rate for each kidney may be calculated from these two measurements and used to assess the patient pre-operatively and to follow post-operative changes.

Dynamic images of the kidneys are taken every minute for 15 minutes after the injection of a renal radiopharmaceutical which is usually ^{99m}Tc-DTPA. Additional images are taken as necessary. In children under the age of 1 month, we substitute ^{99m}Tc- MAG3, as it has more rapid clearance of the kidneys and is thus better visualized in children who have compromised renal function. In children with hypertension or who have had a renal transplantation, we will record the radionuclide angiogram for the first minute after intravenous bolus injection of the radiopharmaceutical. Differential renal function is determined by placing regions-of-interest over each kidney and subtracting a local background. The reference image is the composite from 0 to 2 minutes. The net amount of each kidney is summed together to obtain the total and a ratio is deduced. This provides a measure of the functioning renal mass of one kidney relative to the other. Correction factors for kidney depth have been used in other centres, but we have not found these to be necessary. Although ^{99m}Tc-DTPA is essentially a glomerular filtration agent and theoretically may not reflect tubular function, we have found that in almost all cases this provides a simple and useful index. In a series of 13 cases in which the differential renal function measured by radionuclide techniques was compared with split creatinine clearances, the correlation coefficient was 0.96 [20]. If one kidney has markedly decreased or delayed function and is not well visualized between 1 and 3 minutes, the differential renal analysis cannot be performed between the two kidneys. It is also difficult to assess kidneys that are extremely hydronephrotic with thinned parenchyma containing less radioactivity than background due to large amounts of non-radioactive urine in the calyces and renal pelvis. In these cases, the differential renal analysis may have less validity as it is difficult to define accurately the functioning parenchyma and avoid the areas not containing radioactivity. If the information is vital, the study is repeated with ^{99m}Tc- DMSA and the relative renal mass measured at 2–3 hours. The differential renal function analysis is a relative measure only and an apparent decrease on one side may be due to improvement on the other side. Although the images obtained from the renal scan usually indicate the side that has changed, accurate diagnosis may be difficult unless a GFR is performed at the same time.

One advantage of using ^{99m}Tc-DTPA is that the GFR may be measured at the same time by taking two plasma samples, one at 90 minutes and one at least 30 minutes later and then plotting the plasma disappearance curve. The results have a good correlation when compared with 24-hour urinary creatinine clearances (correlation coefficient of 0.91). By multiplying the percentage obtained from the differential renal functional analysis by the GFR, individual filtration rates for each kidney may be determined [21]. A variety of pure imaging techniques have been used to evaluate GFR without taking a blood sample. In paediatric patients these uptake GFR measurements have not correlated with the two-sample method as well as in the case of adults.

The use of ^{99m}Tc-DTPA renal imaging is helpful in assessing renal function in patients with vesicoureteral reflux, pelviureteric junction obstruction, ureterovesical junction obstruction, posterior urethral valves and prune belly syndrome. It is particularly useful in the neonate and young infant in whom a drastic improvement in renal function may be seen following surgery and as much as a 20 percentile increment (for example from 10–30%) in the renal differential obtained. Radionuclide measurement has become an integral part of urological assessment in paediatrics.

PELVI-URETERIC OBSTRUCTION

The child with pelvi-ureteric obstruction is usu-ally evaluated pre- and post-operatively for the degree of relative renal function, absolute renal function and rate of egress of the radioactive urine from the kidneys. Interestingly, in young children with antenatal hydronephrosis, many have in-creased renal mass on the side of the hydroneph-rosis. This has been confirmed in ^{99m}Tc-DMSA studies carried out subsequent to the original Lasix (frusemide) washout study. In cases where an obstructive component to urine flow is sus-pected, a Lasix stress test is begun between 10 and 30 minutes after the injection of ^{99m}Tc-DTPA. Intra-venous Lasix (1.0 mg/kg; maximum 20 mg) is given and images recorded for 20 minutes. The clearance rate is calculated using the computer. This permits a quantitative method of determin-ing the effect of surgery and/or post-operative complications on the renal drainage system. Nor-mal $t_{1/2}$ values are <8–10 minutes. This value may be higher (up to 20 minutes) in grossly dilated pelves or after surgery. In cases where the $t_{1/2}$ is >10 minutes, then a retention at 20 minutes is cal-culated from:

$$\frac{\text{zero} - \text{time value of kidney radioactivity} - 20-\text{minute value}}{\text{zero} - \text{time value of kidney radioactivity}} \times 100$$

If the patient has a $t_{1/2}$ of 20 minutes, then the retention value at 20 minutes should be 50%; thus, the two converge at this point. The Lasix washout study appears to reflect the state of urinary flow better than the Whitaker test in the post-operative period (Figure 4.19) [22].

In children who have had repair of a pelvi-ureteric junction obstruction or have had reimplantation of the ureters as an anti-reflux sur-gical procedure, there will be a significant delay of about 6 months before there is a change in the relative renal function. When evaluated after that time, they usually drain normally. Several important points have to be made regarding as-sessing Lasix washout curves. First, in those per-formed on normal kidneys that have already emptied their pelves, the $t_{1/2}$ would be invalid. When there is poor renal function, the kidneys cannot be evaluated as there may be poor, if any, response to the Lasix stimulation. In large hydronephrotic kidneys (of >70 ml capacity), there will be a significant delay in emptying,

even though there may be no mechanical obstruction.

RENAL TRANSPLANT ASSESSMENT

In children with a renal transplant, the renal scan is used during the first 2 weeks to evaluate the effectiveness of the transplant surgery. As the art of renal transplantation has improved signifi-cantly, the need for an immediate renal evaluation is less important. We now generally do one study in the first 48–72 hours if the urine output is nor-mal and blood pressure and creatinine are as ex-pected. The first GFR estimate is made at 2 weeks after transplantation, and then on a regular basis until the child has only yearly re-evaluations. The most important observations are the GFR estimate and whether or not there is any evidence of renal infarct.

URINARY TRACT INFECTION

In children with upper urinary tract infection, radionuclide techniques are the primary investi-gative modalities. The direct radionuclide cysto-gram is the most sensitive method for detecting reflux, which is often a prelude to an upper uri-nary tract infection. Radionuclide cystography is a well-tried technique that has proven to be very successful [23]. Recently, computer-analysed an-terograde voiding cystography has been tried and appears to be almost as accurate as the retrograde version. This could be preferred as it is more physiological. However, due to reflux and other problems, the generally preferred method is still the catheter voiding cystogram (Figure 4.20). The detection rate of reflux is at least as good or better than that of the voiding cystourethrogram, signifi-cantly less than that of the radiological study [24]. In addition, the monitoring of the bladder and ureters is constant throughout both filling and emptying phases – something not feasible using fluoroscopy.

If the patient has an upper urinary tract infec-tion, then the child must be evaluated to deter-mine whether or not acute pyelonephritis is present [25]. If the child is sick enough to be admit-ted to hospital, then a DMSA-SPECT study should be performed to determine whether or not pyelonephritis is present. Ultrasound should also be performed to see if there is dilatation of the renal pelvis. Finally, a cystogram should be taken

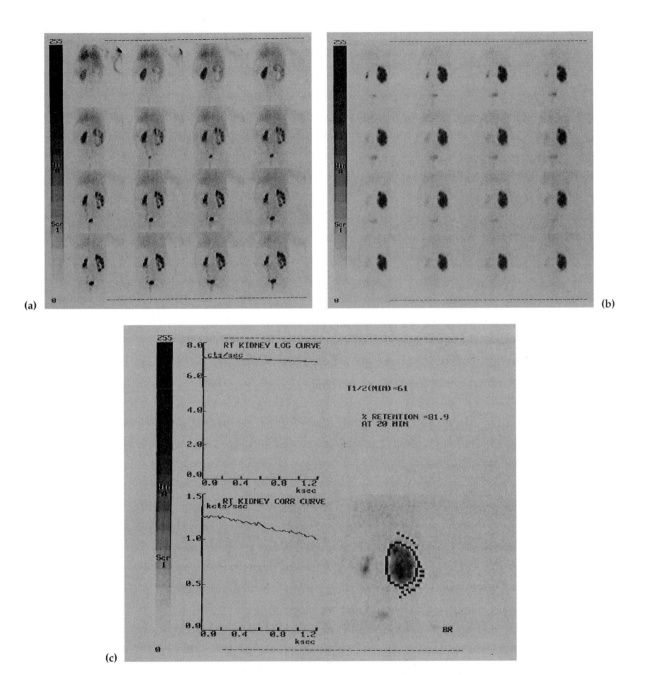

Figure 4.19 Pelviureteric obstruction. The left kidney is normal. The right kidney shows marked caliectasis, but retains good function (a). After administration of Lasix, there was no emptying of the renal pelvis (b). The $t_{\frac{1}{2}}$ was 61 minutes (normal <20 min) and the 20-minutes retention was 81.9% (normal <50%) (c).

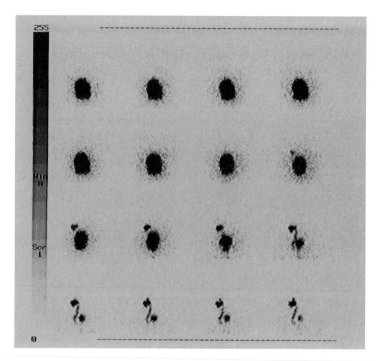

Figure 4.20 Vesicoureteric reflux. After instilling 150 ml of radioactive saline, reflux occurred up the left ureter and filled the pelvis, which is dilated. The reflux persisted after voiding.

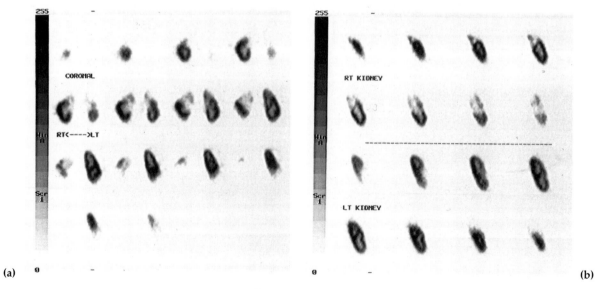

(a)   (b)

Figure 4.21 Acute pyelonephritis. SPECT with ^{99m}Tc-DMSA (a) coronal and (b) sagittal sections. The right kidney shows a marked reduction of tracer in the upper pole without loss of volume. This is typical of pyelonephritis.

to see whether reflux is present. If the child has an upper urinary tract infection without being sick enough to be admitted to hospital, the first study should be a cystogram, followed, if there is reflux, by ultrasound and DMSA studies. Similarly, if there are repeated urinary tract infections at the time of presentation, this patient should be investigated in a similar manner.

Acute pyelonephritis appears as a non-segmental single or multifocal reduction in cortical accumulation of the ^{99m}Tc-DMSA (Figure 4.21). In the acute phase, it is sometimes difficult to do SPECT imaging. Although it is better in defining the location of the lesions, it has only a marginal increase in sensitivity. Planar with oblique images is a satisfactory substitute. Subsequent ^{99m}Tc-DMSA scans to monitor the progress of acute pyelonephritis should probably be done using SPECT imaging. Certainly in our hands and others, it has been shown that SPECT may not increase the sensitivity in diagnosing disease, but is useful in diagnosing the size and multiplicity of lesions [26].

A major concern after an episode of acute pyelonephritis is the development of scars. In this case, SPECT imaging appears to be the method of choice [26]. Not only is it easier to define whether scars are present or not, but location and definition are also enhanced. In addition, it is much easier to differentiate between splenic impression of the upper pole of the left kidney and a true scar (Figure 4.22). Cortical mantle thickness is also much more readily defined.

KIDNEY TRAUMA

Traumatic lesions of the kidney can also be easily defined by DMSA-SPECT imaging. Although ultrasound, CT and intravenous pyelograms (IVPs) are the common methods for evaluating trauma, sometimes the degree of functional impairment is important to know. In some institutions, SPECT imaging may be more easily and less expensively obtained. Sensitivity of DMSA-SPECT imaging for renal trauma is extremely high and compares favourably with CT but is superior to ultrasound and IVP. In fact, combined SPECT liver and spleen imaging as well as renal imaging is extremely sensitive for the overall detection of trauma of both organs. Usually, the abnormality is that of a band or section of the kidney which has depressed renal

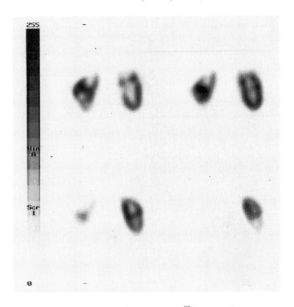

Figure 4.22 Pyelonephritic scars. ^{99m}Tc-DMSA images. The upper pole of each kidney demonstrates a cortical defect with loss of volume. The right kidney has a second defect in the lower pole. These are typical of scars.

function. Sometimes, the abnormality may be iatrogenic after interventional angiography.

RENAL ARTERY STENOSIS

Subsegmental or segmental renal artery stenosis is difficult to detect by the traditional nuclear medical techniques, even by ^{99m}Tc-DTPA imaging with captopril. In this case, we see a subsegmental or segmental reduction in ^{99m}Tc-DMSA accumulation within the kidney. This is much more easily seen with SPECT than planar imaging.

CEREBROSPINAL FLUID PROBLEMS

The cerebrospinal fluid (CSF) is produced primarily in the choroid plexus of the ventricles, but is also produced throughout the subarachnoid space. The predominant flow is normally directed from the ventricles out into the foramina in the fourth ventricle, and from there out into the subarachnoid cisterns, and around the brainstem, then up through the tentorial hiatus between and over the hemispheres. Although water and ions are secreted and absorbed throughout the system,

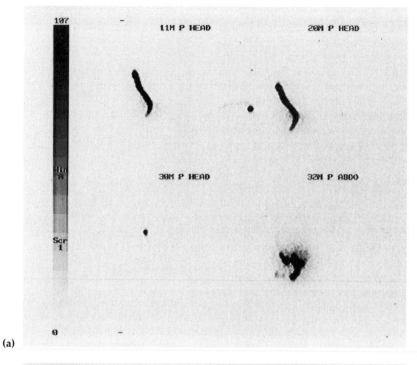

(a)

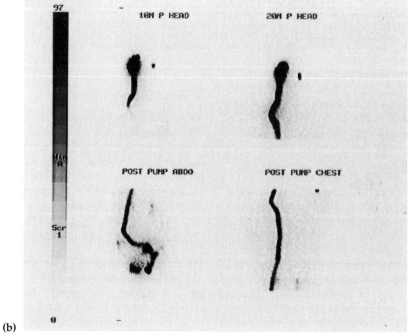

(b)

Figure 4.23 Patent right and blocked left ventriculoperitoneal shunt. The right ventriculoperitoneal shunt shows rapid tracer movement down the distal limb and after compression of the reservoir empties into the peritoneal cavity (a). The left one does not empty, even after compression of the reservoir, but the distal limb fills, indicating it is obstructed distally (b). The activity in the peritoneal cavity is from the prior right ventriculoperitoneal shunt examination.

albumin and chelates do not readily diffuse across the subarachnoid membrane. The CSF protein is mainly reabsorbed parasagittally at the arachnoid villae projecting into the venous sinuses and by the epidural veins in the vertebral column.

With the widespread use of MRI of the brain, the role of CSF imaging is less vital to the diagnosis of extraventricular hydrocephalus. Now, the main uses are the evaluation of shunt patency and the presence and location of leaks.

EVALUATION OF CSF DIVERSIONARY SHUNTS

The clinical evaluation of CSF diversionary shunt function is often difficult. Usually, the problem of whether or not the overall shunt function is adequate is apparent from a change in symptomatology. However, shunt function is usually evaluated clinically by observing the compression of the reservoir and its subsequent refilling. If the reservoir is difficult to compress, the obstruction is usually considered to be distal, whereas if the reservoir compresses easily but fills slowly, it is considered to be proximal.

Once the needle is introduced into the reservoir, 37 MBq of freshly prepared ^{99m}Tc- DTPA, in 0.1 ml, is introduced into the reservoir and an image taken. One-minute images of the reservoir and the distal limb are then acquired. The images are repeated at 5, 10, 15 and 20 minutes. At this point, the patient is allowed to sit or walk so that the increased hydrostatic pressure in the ventricles will drive the CSF through the system to its destination. Usually, this will occur in all patients with a functioning shunt. If there is no flow of the tracer through the shunt apparatus, then the reservoir is compressed five to ten times in patients with ventriculoperitoneal shunt, and the head and torso images repeated to confirm the lack of flow. If the tracer readily enters the abdomen but does not disperse throughout the peritoneal cavity, the patient is rotated and moved about so as to try and disperse the tracer. This manoeuvre will help to differentiate between a loculation and normal pooling. The reservoir images are used to determine the qualitative clearance rate. The distal limb images are used to delineate the movement of the tracer out of the shunt tubing and its movement around the abdomen (ventriculoperitoneal shunts) or the presence of kidneys (ventriculoatrial shunts). The images are compared to determine the clearance of the tracer from the reservoir during the supine phase of the study and the effect of hydrostatic pressure on the system is evaluated after the upright images.

In a review, we studied 67 ventriculoatrial and 164 ventriculoperitoneal shunts. Of these, 105 studies were normal and none had subsequent documentation of shunt malfunction. Of the 103 blocked shunts, 98 had the site correctly predicted. A variety of clinical and surgical results were found for the 23 poorly functioning shunts (Figure 4.23).

These results indicate that, in general, the radionuclide assessment of shunt function is quite satisfactory. However, in some of the cases when there was a discrepancy between the radionuclide results and the clinical or surgical findings, it indicated that the shunt study only evaluates the function at the time of the study. This was exemplified in one child whose shunt was obstructed by scan, but at surgery, the reservoir externalized, and there was no sign of malfunction. However, when the surgeon had reconnected the reservoir to the distal tube, it suddenly appeared to be blocked, and indeed was. This type of intermittent obstruction can occur when the distal catheter imbeds itself into the peritoneum or the bowel. Our overall evaluation of the distal tubing is much better than that of the ventricular tube assessment as the latter requires an indirect means for determining its state of function.

PAEDIATRIC CARDIOLOGY

Nuclear cardiology procedures are as important in the diagnosis and management of many cardiac abnormalities in infants and children as they are in adults. The functional and structural information obtained from echocardiography – in conjunction with nuclear cardiology where needed – has replaced the need for diagnostic cardiac catheterization in most cases.

Echocardiography and functional information, nuclear cardiology is used for specific functional information, e.g. ejection fraction, myocardial perfusion.

RADIONUCLIDE ANGIOCARDIOGRAPHY

For diagnosis, radionuclide angiocardiography allows separation of the cardiac chambers in time as well as in space so that individual chambers, particularly when in an unusual location, can be identified and the direction of blood flow through the chamber determined. However, the small size of the cardiac chambers and the more rapid transit of activity through the central circulation in children limits the anatomical resolution that is possible. The indications in congenital heart disease, are as follows:

1. The asymptomatic patient with a murmur suggestive of congenital heart disease such as a ventricular septal defect.
2. Repetitive evaluation when a diagnosis has already been established to define changes.
3. Determination of patency of temporary surgical shunts.

The first-pass technique involves the injection of tracer as an intravenous bolus, preferably via a jugular vein. The sequential passage of the bolus is followed through the heart with a gamma-camera using a high-sensitivity collimator. The nuclear angiogram is performed by injecting a small bolus <0.5 ml of ^{99m}Tc–pertechnetate into an external jugular vein via a 19- or 21-gauge scalp vein needle. The needle is attached to a three-way stopcock and extension tube. The radioactivity is injected into the extension tube by the stopcock once the needle is properly placed in the vein. The dose is then flushed into the vein with 10 ml of saline, such that a short, sharp bolus results. This is important, as erroneous results are usually produced if prolongation or fragmentation of the bolus occurs. The bolus may also be delayed when there is obstruction to the venous return to the heart, elevated pulmonary venous pressures or obstructive valvular disease. Currently, we record the transit of the bolus at 10 frames per second. Acquisition zoom is used in imaging very small children, especially neonates.

SHUNT QUANTIFICATION

Left-to-right shunts

Left-to-right shunt estimation is the most common indication for radionuclide angiocardiography. Computer quantification was first described by Maltz and Treves in 1973 [27]. A time–activity histogram is generated from the passage of the radioactive bolus through the lungs. By applying a least-squares fit to a gamma variate function of this pulmonary flow, the latter can be accurately estimated. By subtracting the fitted curve from the raw data, a pulmonary recirculation curve is obtained. The ratio of the area under the first transit curve to the area under the recirculation curve is the pulmonary/systemic flow ratio (Q_P/Q_S).

This analysis is comparable with the dye dilution technique and is more readily performed. A good correlation was obtained ($r = 0.82$, $P < 0.001$) in a group of 86 patients. The main difficulty with this technique is to determine whether or not the gamma variate fit to the raw data is satisfactory, but a computerized curve-fit–analysis routine will improve the quality of the fit. Experience is most valuable in obtaining correct and consistent results. The fit of the recirculation curve is critical in small shunts, especially as the shape of the fitted curve can change due to the shape of the bolus. Factors such as poor bolus injection, superior vena cava obstruction, a large heart in a small chest (which causes difficulty in placing a region of interest over the lung alone), single ventricle or large ventricular septal defect (VSD) (chamber mixing) will all make the study uninterpretable.

Right-to-left shunts

^{99m}Tc- labelled macroaggregates (MAA) embolize in the pulmonary circulation and normally do not appear in the systemic circulation following intravenous injection. If there is a right-to-left shunt, the MAA appear in the systemic circulation and may be quantitated by whole-body imaging. The shunt can be measured using the following:

$$\% \text{ Right-to-left shunt} = \frac{(\text{Total-body counts} - \text{Total lung count}) \times 100}{\text{Total-body count}}$$

Imaging of the body should not be delayed after injection of MAA, as rapid loss of ^{99m}Tc occurs from the particles, possibly due to fragmentation, and a consequent overestimate of shunt size will occur. Since there is the possibility of particles entering the systemic circulation, the number of particles should be restricted to about 50 000.

EQUILIBRIUM BLOOD POOL IMAGING

Besides wall motion, quantification of ventricular function – that is ejection fraction (EF), stroke volume, systolic and diastolic volumes – and atrial kick contribution to the EF can be readily obtained. These are important parameters in determining the extent or severity of the disease and are a rapid, non-invasive method of following the patient's clinical course. Differentiation of time–activity curves also allows the maximum rate of construction and expansion to be determined.

This technique is used primarily to evaluate children with heart failure as a prelude to transplantation, children undergoing chemotherapy with cardiotoxic drugs, and children with compromised ventricular function such as those associated with tricuspid atresia.

MYOCARDIAL PERFUSION IMAGING

Myocardial perfusion imaging is now well established in children. The imaging technique is the same as that used for adults and uses ^{99m}Tc-sestamibi. For a same-day protocol, the rest phase is performed preferably early in the morning, followed by the stress phase in the afternoon.

The common indicators are children with familial hypercholesterolaemia [28], anomalous left coronary artery, vasculitis (Kawasaki's disease), systemic lupus erythematosus, the total anomalous great vessels switch procedure and atrophic cardiomyopathies. Evaluation of the extent and progression of ischaemia can be determined accurately by ^{99m}Tc-sestamibi imaging.

Although the presence of an anomalous left coronary artery is uncommon, it is important to make this diagnosis in the child presenting with cardiac symptoms. Similarly, after coronary artery surgery the vessel flow may be compromised and all such patients should be evaluated 6 months after surgery. The extent of myocardial ischaemia and infarction can readily be obtained from careful interpretation of the sestamibi tomogram. Some prognostic information can be derived by observing the amount of left ventricular myocardium rendered ischaemic by the anomalous origin of the left coronary artery. In some patients with extensive collateral circulation between the right and left coronary systems, the degree of ischaemia may be small. Repeat studies can follow the progression of ischaemia and help to determine timing of surgical intervention. Pre- and post-operative perfusion studies help evaluate the results of surgical correction.

In children with familial hypercholesterolaemia, there is a need to detect early the presence of coronary vessel narrowing. These children respond very well to aggressive management. Perfusion SPECT imaging of the myocardium has proved to be the best detection mechanism for early narrowing of coronary artery vessels in this population. Patients in our hypercholesterolaemia clinic are evaluated annually with stress myocardial perfusion imaging. The lesions that we see are often reversible, although occasionally they may be fixed. After aggressive therapy, there has been a very good improvement in the perfusion to the affected portion of the myocardium. Indeed, a number of defects including several fixed defects have completely reversed.

Children undergoing the 'switch' procedure for complete correction of total anomalous great vessels frequently have to be evaluated post-operatively as there is a significant morbidity associated with this procedure [29]. In some children the ischaemic areas will improve and can be demonstrated in follow-up studies.

REFERENCES

1. Gilday, D., Paula, D.J. and Patterson, J. (1975) Diagnosis of osteomyelitis in children by combined blood pool and bone imaging. *Radiology*, **117**, 331.
2. Hamdan, J., Asha, M. *et al.* (1987) Technetium bone scintigraphy in the diagnosis of osteomyelitis in childhood; review by radionuclide bone scan. *Pediatr. Infect. Dis.*, **6**, 529–32.
3. Kim, E.E., Podoloff, D.A., Lowry, P.A. and Harle, T.S. (1989) Radionuclide imaging in the evaluation of osteomyelitis and septic arthritis. *Crit. Rev. Diagn. Imaging*, **29**(3), 257–305.
4. Nadel, H. (1993) Thallium-201 for oncological imaging in children. *Semin. Nucl. Med.*, **23**, 243–54.
5. Mouratidis, B., Ash, J. *et al.* (1994) Comparison of bone and 67-Gallium scintigraphy in the initial diagnosis of bone involvement in children with malignant lymphoma. *Nucl. Med. Commun.*, **15**, 144–7.
6. Schaub, T., Ash, J. *et al.* (1987) Radionuclide imaging in Histiocytosis-X. *Pediatr. Radiol.*, **17**, 397–404.
7. Howman-Giles, R., Gilday, D. *et al.* (1979) Radionuclide skeletal survey in neuroblastoma. *Radiology*, **131**, 497–502.
8. Jacobs, A.D.M., Desprechins, B., Otten, J., Ferster, A., Jonckheer, M.H., Mertens, J., Ham, H.R. and Piepsz, A. (1990) Consolidating the role of ^{123}I-MIBG-scintigraphy in childhood neuroblastoma: five years of clinical experience. *Pediatr. Radiol.*, **20**(3), 157–9.
9. Gordon, I., Peters, A. *et al.* (1990) Tc-99m bone scans are more sensitive than I-123 mIBG scans for bone imaging in neuroblastoma. *J. Nucl. Med.*, **31**, 129–43.
10. Majd, M., Reba, R.C. and Altman, R.P. (1981) Hepatobiliary scintigraphy with 99m-Tc-PIPIDA in the evaluation of neonatal jaundice. *Pediatrics*, **67**, 140–5.

11. Howman-Giles, A., Moase, R. *et al.* (1993) Hepatobiliary scintigraphy in a pediatric population: determination of hepatic extraction fraction by deconvolution analysis. *J. Nucl. Med.*, **34**, 214–21.
12. Majd, M., Reba, R.C. and Altman, R.P. (1981) Effect of phenobarbital on 99Tc-IDA scintigraphy in the evaluation of neonatal jaundice. *Semin. Nucl. Med.*, **11**, 194–204.
13. Heyman, S. and Respondek, M. (1989) TI-detection of pulmonary aspiration in children by radionuclide salivagram. *J. Nucl. Med.*, **30**, 697–9.
14. Fried, M., Khoshoo, V. *et al.* (1992) Decrease in gastric emptying time and episodes of regurgitation in children with spastic quadriplegia fed a whey-based formula. *J. Pediatr.*, **120**, 569–72.
15. Shandling, B. (1965) Laparatomy for rectal bleeding. *Pediatrics*, **35**, 787.
16. Duszynski, D.O., Jewett, T.E. and Allen, J.E. (1970) The visualization of Meckel's diverticulum with 99m Tc-pertechnetate. *Surgery*, **68**, 567–70.
17. Rosenthal, L., Henry, J.N., Murphy, D.A. and Freeman, L.M. (1972) Radiopertechnetate imaging of the Meckel's diverticulum. *Radiology*, **105**, 371–3.
18. Conway, J. (1976) The sensitivity, specificity and accuracy of radionuclide imaging of Meckel's diverticulum. *J. Nucl. Med.*, **17**, 553.
19. Martin, D.J., Gilday, D.L. and Reilly, B.J. (1975) Evaluation of the urinary tract in the neonatal period. *Radiol. Clin. N. Am.*, **13**, 359.
20. Pieretti, R., Gilday, D. and Jeffs, R. (1974) Differential kidney scanning in pediatric urology. *Urology*, **4**, 665.
21. Ash, J. and D. Gilday (1980) Renal nuclear imaging and analysis in pediatrics. *Urol. Clin. N. Am.*, **7**, 201.
22. Krueger, R., Ash, J.M., Silver, M. *et al.* (1980) Primary hydronephrosis: assessment of the diuretic renogram, pelvic perfusion pressure, post operative findings and renal and ureteral histology. *Urol. Clin. N. Am.*, **7**, 231.
23. Conway, J. (1976) Effectiveness of direct and indirect radionuclide cystography in detecting vesicoureteral reflux. *J. Nucl. Med.*, **17**, 81.
24. Pollet, J.E., Sharp, F. and Smith, F.W. (1979) Radionuclide imaging for vesicorenal reflux using intravenous 99m Tc-DTPA. *Pediatr. Radiol.*, **8**, 165–7.
25. Jantausch, B., Wiedermann, B. *et al.* (1992) *Escherichia coli* virulence factors and 99mTc-dimercaptosuccinic acid renal scan in children with febrile urinary tract infection. *Pediatr. Infect. Dis. J.*, **11**, 343–9.
26. Mouratidis, B., Ash, J. and Gilday, D.L. (1993) Comparison of planar and SPECT 99Tcm-DMSA scintigraphy for the detection of renal cortical defects in children. *Nucl. Med. Commun.*, **14**(2), 82–6.
27. Maltz, D. and Treves, S. (1973) Quantitative radionuclide angiography: determination of $Q_p:Q_s$ in children. *Circulation*, **47**, 1049–56.
28. Mouratidis, B., Vaughan-Neil, E. *et al.* (1992) The detection of silent coronary artery disease in adolescents with familial hypercholesterolaemia utilizing SPECT 201-thallium scanning. *J. Cardiol.*, **70**, 1109–12.
29. Vogel, M., Smallhorn, J. *et al.* (1991) Assessment of myocardial perfusion in patients after the arterial switch operation. *J. Nucl. Med.*, **32**, 237–41.

SECTION TWO

Clinical systems

CHAPTER 5

Infection and immunology

HIV disease and other immunosuppressed patients

M. J. O'Doherty

INTRODUCTION

The use of imaging in the immunosuppressed patient provides a new variety of causes for abnormalities of common scans. An awareness of the cause(s) is the prime need, and therefore, it is essential to be informed of the immune competence of an individual when reporting scans and to have a high level of suspicion.

Immunosuppression, as a result of T- or B-cell dysfunction, may be associated with a variety of illnesses. These may be a direct result of the disease, the therapy given for the disease, or the result of inadequate therapy. The problems in the immunosuppressed individual may be considered in relation to: the underlying disease, e.g. leukaemia, lymphoma, human immunodeficiency virus or congenital immune deficiency; the chemotherapy or drug treatment used; the organ transplanted (heart, lung, liver, kidney, bone marrow) and the possibility of rejection.

With the increasing use of cytotoxic drugs for treating a variety of diseases, the nuclear physician has a battery of tests available for monitoring iatrogenic disease: the use of bone scans may be the first pointer to avascular necrosis associated with steroid therapy; renal dysfunction associated with a number of cytotoxic agents used in oncology can be monitored with ^{51}Cr-EDTA, and this should also be used to monitor the effects of cyclosporin therapy of non-malignant diseases (e.g. dermatological diseases, fibrosing lung disease, etc.); and the use of gated blood pool scans to follow the effect of cardiotoxic agents.

A difficulty in patients with underlying malignant diseases is that the occurrence of a fever may be associated with a recurrence of the malignancy or an occurrence of infection. The type(s) of infection will to some extent depend on the underlying cause of immunosuppression; thus HIV infection is often associated with different infective processes compared with iatrogenic or malignant cause.

In a patient with fever (pyrexia) of unknown origin (PUO or FUO), the clinician may wish to know whether focal infection, a diffuse inflammatory/infective process affecting one or more organs, or recurrent underlying disease is the cause of the pyrexia.

There are a variety of nuclear medicine tests available to seek infection or tumour; some of these have been discussed in other chapters. This section will deal with the application of radionuclide investigations to the HIV-infected individual and to various transplant groups. The possible investigations currently available are shown in Table 5.1, and this list is gradually expanding.

The pulmonary system is the most commonly affected system in the immunocompromised host, and is associated with high mortality. There are differences in the incidence of disease processes

Clinical Nuclear Medicine, 3rd edn. Edited by M.N. Maisey, K.E. Britton and B.D. Collier. Published in 1998 by Chapman & Hall, London. ISBN 0 412 75180 1

Table 5.1 Inflammation and infection scanning in the immunosuppressed

Gallium-67
White cell imaging
   ^{99m}Tc-HMPAO or ^{111}In-oxine/tropolonate
   Autologous
   Donor
Polyclonal immunoglobulins
HIgG
Antigranulocyte antibody
Anti-E Selectin
Other inflammatory peptides
^{99m}Tc Infecton
Specific antibodies against bacterial/protozoal antigens
^{99m}Tc DTPA permeability study
^{18}F-FDG imaging

affecting individuals that are dependent on the cause of the immunosuppression. The causes of fever in the acutely immunosuppressed patient will often be treated with empirical use of antibiotics, since the conditions causing the fever or deterioration are likely to be due to bacterial sepsis. However, in the chronically immunosuppressed, there may also be differences – for instance, transplant patients on chemotherapy have a higher incidence of cytomegalovirus (CMV) pneumonia compared with HIV-infected patients [1]. The HIV-infected patients have a higher incidence of *Pneumocystis carinii* pneumonia, bacterial pneumonias (e.g. *Streptococcus* pneumonia) and mycobacterial infections. Infections with various fungal diseases may occur in either group. The chest radiograph seldom allows a confident specific diagnosis, and a number of studies have shown that high-resolution CT (HRCT) can be helpful in the management of patients with pulmonary complications (see review by Worthy *et al.*, 1995).

HIV-POSITIVE PATIENTS

PULMONARY SYSTEM

Pneumocystis carinii pneumonia (PCP) is still the most common chest infection in HIV-positive patients, although there is an increasing problem with bacterial infections including *Streptococcus* pneumonia, *Haemophilus influenzae, Pseudomonas* infections and mycobacterial infection. Some 10–15% of patients with PCP have a normal or atypical chest X-ray (CXR). A further diagnostic difficulty with the so-called 'typical PCP CXR' is the differentiation of PCP from other causes of an abnormal CXR – such as mycobacterial infections, Kaposi's sarcoma (KS), lymphocytic interstitial pneumonitis, or non-specific interstitial pneumonitis. HRCT can be of help, although in one study, two observers made a confident diagnosis in only 48% of the cases, most of whom had PCP or KS.

A number of nuclear medicine investigations have been used to evaluate the cause(s) of breathlessness and fever; these are discussed below.

Gallium-67 citrate

Scans are usually performed at 24, 48 and occasionally 72 hours after injecting 74–185 MBq of ^{67}Ga. Patients with PCP normally show diffuse distribution throughout both lung fields, such that a negative cardiac silhouette is seen [2,3]; this diffuse uptake has been documented with CMV. The uptake can be graded, and should be equal to, or higher than, that in the liver, to enable a confident diagnosis of diffuse lung disease, but the uptake is highly variable in PCP (Figure 5.1), and occasionally it is lower (above soft tissue activity, but less than the liver uptake).

The sensitivity and specificity of ^{67}Ga are 80–90% and 50–74% respectively [4], rising to 100% in those patients with a normal CXR [5]. Early scanning at 4 hours has been used, and the ratio between lung and liver uptake recorded to distinguish between a normal and an abnormal scan, although limitations with this approach would be expected in patients with liver disease. Atypical uptake confined to the upper lobes can be seen with PCP. One advantage of ^{67}Ga is that uptake throughout the body can be observed, and thus lung uptake with associated parotid uptake is suggestive of interstitial pneumonitis or sarcoidosis. Diffuse or patchy lung uptake with high lymph node uptake may be due to atypical mycobacterial infection, but may equally be due to lymphoma associated with an opportunistic lung infection. In patients with a lung infiltrate on the CXR, a gallium scan may show either lobar or multiple lobar focal defects, due to infection or tumour (Figure 5.2). If this uptake is associated with bone involvement, then atypical fungal infection or lymphoma should be considered in the differential diagnosis. In the presence of an abnormal CXR, the scan may be useful if it is entirely normal, since this would be consistent with KS; if

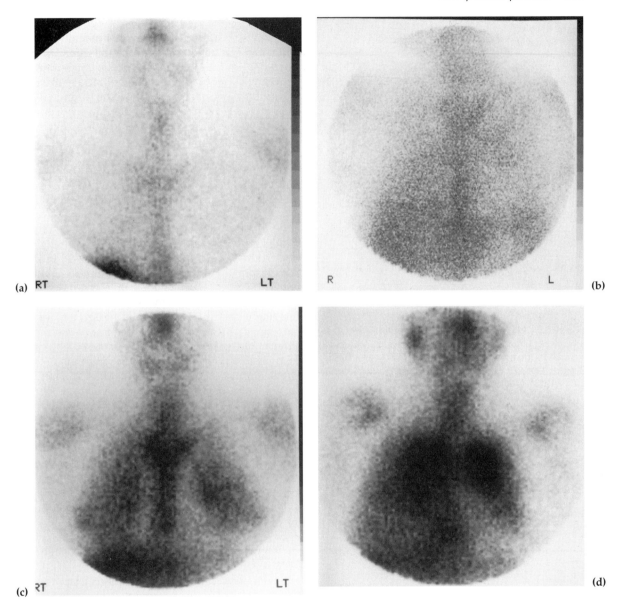

(a) RT   LT

(b) R   L

(c) RT   LT

(d)

Figure 5.1 Gallium-67 scan appearances in patients with *Pneumocystis carinii* pneumonia. The scan shows (a) normal uptake, (b) low-grade uptake in the lung, (c) uptake greater then bone marrow but less than the liver, and (d) uptake higher than the hepatic uptake. (Figure reproduced from O'Doherty, M.J. and Nunan, T.O. (1993) Nuclear medicine and AIDS. *Nucl. Med. Commun.*, **14**, 830–48, with permission.)

the scan is abnormal then superadded infection should be considered.

Gallium undoubtedly has a role in the investigation of a persistent PUO in this patient group when there are no specific localizing features or in patients with a wasting syndrome to exclude focal pathology.

Thallium-201 has been used in a small number of patients to localize KS. Following injection of approximately 90 MBq of ^{201}Tl, images acquired

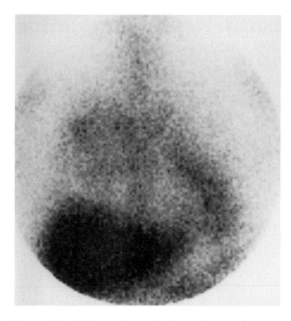

Figure 5.2 Gallium-67 uptake in a patient with pneumococcal pneumonia. The scan shows increased uptake present in the upper right lung and the lower left lung. (Figure reproduced from O'Doherty, M.J. and Nunan, T.O. (1993) Nuclear medicine and AIDS. *Nucl. Med. Commun.*, **14**, 830–48, with permission.)

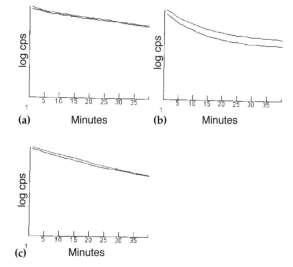

Figure 5.3 Lung ^{99m}Tc DTPA transfer curves in (a) a patient who had no evidence of lung disease; (b) when the patient developed *Pneumocystis carinii* pneumonia; and (c) after therapy.

immediately after the injection and up to 3 hours later showed uptake in the skin lesions, lymph nodes and the lung (lung uptake was confirmed as due to KS in one-third of the patients). It is not known whether thallium is taken up in persistent generalized lymphadenopathy, which may present a source of confusion. Fluorodeoxyglucose (FDG) and methionine PET studies have also not shown conclusive uptake.

Antibody studies

The advantage of using antibodies available in the kit form over leucocyte imaging is a shorter preparation time and reduced blood handling. Currently, these products use indium-111 as the radionuclide, and therefore there is potentially a time delay before the study can be performed. Localization of ^{111}In-polyclonal antibodies (^{111}In-HIgG) has been demonstrated in lungs infected with PCP in both animal and human studies. Imaging with ^{111}In-HIgG and ^{99m}Tc-HIgG has been performed, with the former having superior sensitivity and specificity than the latter. This was thought to be due to the later imaging with ^{111}In-HIgG. Diffuse uptake was seen with PCP and focal uptake with bacterial infections. Poor uptake of antigranulocyte antibody in HIV patients with infection has been demonstrated [6].

Imaging of PCP has been performed in HIV-positive patients using ^{99m}Tc-labelled Fab' fragment raised in mice against *Pneumocystis carinii*. In this selected population, the 24-hour images had a sensitivity of 86% and a specificity of 87%. The technique raises the interesting possibility of its use in the detection of extrapulmonary disease.

Lung ^{99m}Tc-DTPA transfer

The method is described in the section on pulmonary imaging. The use of the technique in HIV-positive patients has been described and reviewed recently [7]. The half-time of DTPA transfer in HIV-positive patients is described normally by a single exponential curve with mean half-times of 20 min for smokers and 60 minutes for non-smokers (k values 2.5%/min and 0.8%/min); approximately 10% of smokers may have a multiexponential curve. In our studies, the appearance of a biphasic curve and a rapid first component [half-time of <4 min (12.5%/min)] is the hallmark of alveolitis (Figure 5.3). In patients with HIV infection, PCP is still the most likely cause of alveolitis

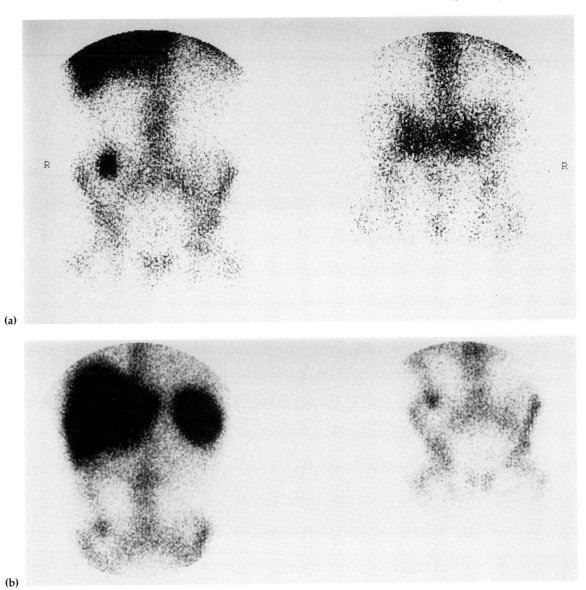

(a)

(b)

Figure 5.4 An indium-111 donor leucocyte scan in a patient with HIV infection and a pyrexia. (a) The 4-h images demonstrate accumulation of leucocytes in the right iliac fossa. (b) The 24-h images demonstrate communication of the abscess with tracking of the leucocytes around the large bowel.

– hence the biphasic pattern – although this pattern may also be seen in patients with CMV infection, lymphocytic interstitial pneumonitis and non-specific interstitial pneumonitis. In this patient population, the test has a high sensitivity and specificity for PCP, but there are false-negative results [8]. The false-negative results usually show an abnormally fast transfer rate, but not with a typical biphasic pattern, and therefore further investigation (e.g. sputum examination or bronchoscopy) is suggested rather than initiation of treatment for PCP. In other bacterial infections, the transfer times are not biphasic (except for *Legionella pneumophila*) [9]. Rosso *et al.* [10] have demonstrated by using only the first 7 minutes of the time–activity curve that the clearance rate for PCP is higher than for other pulmonary conditions. The biggest area of overlap was in patients who had a cytotoxic lymphocyte alveolitis. The most interesting comparison from this study was with ^{67}Ga scintigraphy, which was shown to have lower sensitivity than ^{99m}Tc DTPA (72% versus 92%) for infectious pulmonary complications. This was even more marked for patients who had a normal CXR and normal blood gases. A normal CXR with normal DTPA clearance virtually excluded pulmonary infection/inflammation that needed therapy.

ABDOMINAL DISEASE

Abdominal disease is common in association with HIV infection, and may include opportunistic infections or any of the causes of intra-abdominal pathology in non-HIV-infected individuals. Inflammation/infection can be detected with ^{67}Ga and by using either autologous or donor leucocytes labelled with technetium-99m (^{99m}Tc-

Human immunoglobulin, ^{99m}Tc-HIg) or indium-111 (^{111}In-HIg) [11]. The investigation of choice will be dependent on the clinical problem suspected. If infection is suspected to be within the bowel or in the soft tissues, leucocyte scanning is a more appropriate investigation. However, a ^{67}Ga scan would be more effective where the disease process is likely to involve the lymph nodes. Donor leucocytes are safe and either ^{111}In-oxine or ^{99m}Tc-exametazamine can be used as the label [12]) (Figures 5.4 and 5.5). Alternatively, ^{111}In-polyclonal antibodies or ^{99m}Tc-HIgG may be used to image inflammation in the bowel or sites of infection [13].

Non-specific accumulation of ^{67}Ga in the bowel limits its use in inflammatory bowel disease. However, it has been suggested that the isotope may have a particular use in HIV-positive patients. Large bowel uptake on a scan has to be regarded with caution, since varying degrees of uptake are seen without any evidence of pathogens in the bowel. Occult malignancies of the stomach, particularly lymphoma, have been revealed by gastric uptake of ^{67}Ga in patients with AIDS, but also

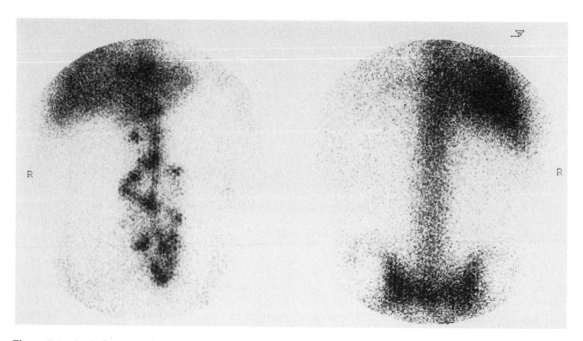

Figure 5.5 An indium-111 donor leucocyte scan in a patient with HIV infection who developed a pyrexia 10 days post-splenectomy. The scan appearances show the absent spleen and the diffuse uptake in the abdominal wound infected with *Staphylococcus aureus*.

'innocent' uptake has been shown in one patient with AIDS.

Other potential problems that may occur in the gastrointestinal tract of HIV-positive patients include gastrointestinal haemorrhage, tumour involvement of the bowel with lymphoma or KS and unusual infections resulting in sclerosing cholangitis (cryptosporidiosis, CMV). The use of iminodiacetic acid agents to examine the biliary tree may be more sensitive than ultrasound in demonstrating strictures and promoting the need for further investigation and therapy.

Gallium scans should be part of the investigation of weight loss in patients with wasting syndrome, since the test is easy to perform and will exclude the presence of abnormal lymph nodes, soft tissue tumours and focal infections as a cause of wasting.

^{18}FDG-PET studies have demonstrated the ability to show abnormal lymph nodes and soft tissue tumours as well as bone tumours. The technique provides a method of examining the abdomen with little bowel interference. A difficulty appears to be variable uptake in persistent generalized lymphadenopathy. There is a high uptake in pulmonary infections (e.g. mycobacterial and streptococcal pneumonia).

NEUROLOGICAL DISEASE

Neurological complications may occur in up to 30% of AIDS patients. The nervous system may be directly affected by the HIV infection, which may result in acute HIV meningoencephalitis (acute seroconversion illness), vacuolar myelopathy, or the AIDS dementia complex. Non-viral causes of a diffuse encephalitis such as *Cryptococcus neoformans* and *Toxoplasma gondii*, may also result in focal lesions throughout the brain. The prevalence of these infections varies throughout the world. Primary cerebral lymphoma is a relatively common tumour in patients with HIV and commonly occurs as multifocal lesions with a poor response to therapy.

Cerebral perfusion anomalies associated with HIV disease have been demonstrated using ^{123}I-IMP (isopropyl-*p*-iodoamphetamine hydroacetate) and ^{99m}Tc-exametazamine; although both radiotracers reflect blood flow, Pohl *et al.* [14] have shown that there are differences between the two agents, with the latter showing larger defects on the scan. Both agents have demonstrated

abnormalities in blood flow corresponding to focal signs or symptoms in patients, whereas in contrast, the abnormalities on CT or MRI are less marked or absent. Abnormalities have been found in early HIV infection with no demonstrable cognitive dysfunction. In HIV-1 AIDS dementia complex, the scan shows hypoperfusion in the frontal and parietal lobes, which is often bilateral, and there may be a relative increase in activity in the basal ganglia. Advanced dementia is associated with more extensive blood flow disturbances and frequently there is cerebellar involvement.

FDG-PET scans have also been demonstrated to be abnormal in patients with AIDS dementia complex. Brunetti *et al.* [15] have demonstrated an improvement in ^{18}FDG distribution with the introduction of zidovudine (antiviral therapy) to a small number of patients.

One of the difficult areas to be assessed is the presence of space-occupying lesions, and their differentiation into lymphoma, progressive multifocal leucoencephalopathy and cerebral toxoplasmosis. MRI is more sensitive than CT for demonstrating the presence of space-occupying lesions. The presence of progressive multifocal leucoencephalopathy is also clearly delineated with MRI, with greater sensitivity than CT; lesions may be found with increased signal intensity without mass effect on dual-echo MRI in the periventricular and subcortical white matter of the parieto-occipital or frontal lobes, but also abnormalities can be found elsewhere including the posterior fossa, corpus callosum and basal ganglia. An FDG-PET study suggested that a low ^{18}FDG uptake in the region of a focal space-occupying defect seen on CT or MRI is suggestive of opportunistic infection, whereas high uptake is in keeping with cerebral lymphoma [16]. Similar results may be possible with thallium-201, since high uptake in brain tumours has been found on both early and delayed imaging, which is different from studies obtained from patients with cerebral oedema and infection. This needs further study before acceptance into clinical practice and the possible additional information with ^{11}C-methionine needs evaluation.

A further role for perfusion and metabolic imaging will be to assess the effect of various therapies. There is a potential role for metabolic scanning in focal abnormalities for distinguishing between tumours and opportunistic infections, to enable appropriate treatment and/or further investigation.

MUSCULOSKELETAL SYSTEM

Standard imaging methods can be used to investigate the variety of conditions normally common to the patient's age group. In younger patients, the presence of non-Hodgkin's lymphoma may provide a variety of scan appearances such as abnormal bone or marrow scans.

Recently, the condition of bacillary angiomatosis has been described in HIV-positive patients. These patients have angiomatous skin lesions that are similar to KS, but a Rickettsia-like organism, similar to that causing cat scratch disease, can be found in the lesion, and unlike KS, there may be bone involvement at distant sites. Baron *et al.* [17] showed that approximately 35% of patients with bacillary angiomatosis may have multiple bone involvement that may be asymptomatic, but would serve to distinguish between the skin pathology from KS and other causes of multiple bone uptake with skin lesions such as due to atypical mycobacterial infection (Figure 5.6). The bone and skin lesions can be treated with erythromycin, with subsequent bone scans returning to normal.

Abnormal soft tissue uptake seen in the bone scans of young patients may be expected to be found in drug-induced myositis (e.g. zidovudine-induced myositis), KS, or other causes of poly-

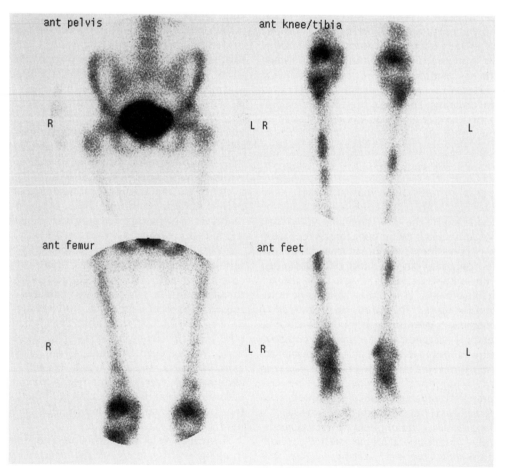

Figure 5.6 An HIV-infected patient with a pyrexia and skin lesions. The bone scan demonstrates multiple areas of increased uptake within the tibia and femora. A diagnosis of *Mycobacterium kansasii* infection was made.

myositis. Gallium is avidly accumulated in myositis but should not be associated with KS, and if the above appearance is seen on a bone scan, it may be used to distinguish between KS and polymyositis. Accumulation in bones and joints may be due to inflammatory disease associated with Reiter's syndrome, or other reactive joint conditions, or arthropathies secondary to haemophilia. In these reactive arthropathies, ^{67}Ga and ^{111}In-leucocyte scanning can be positive, and therefore, may not distinguish these from infected joints. The symmetry of the uptake may be the only pointer.

OTHER SYSTEMS

There is also a role for other radionuclide tests, although the specific abnormalities found are likely to be due to diseases that also afflict non-HIV-positive patients. HIV infection can affect the myocardium directly and result in myocarditis. Both CMV and toxoplasma can also cause similar inflammatory problems. Therefore, the presence of myocardial uptake on a gallium scan would be consistent with any inflammatory aetiology. Renal tract investigations may show increased uptake of gallium in HIV nephritis, as well as in other causes of nephritis (infectious or drug-induced) or tumour involvement.

OTHER IMMUNOSUPPRESSED CONDITIONS

Scanning in patients with transplants is highly specialized and dependent on the transplant. Thus, liver and renal transplants may utilize techniques to examine perfusion, and in the case of liver transplantation the iminodiacetic acids to look for biliary leaks. The issues are often related to the drugs used to immunosuppress the patients or rejection. With heart and lung transplantation, early reports suggest that quantitative ventilation/perfusion scans could detect early rejection with non-homogeneity developing in the perfusion scan. ^{99m}Tc-DTPA clearance has been used with the finding of a very rapid clearance in those patients who are developing rejection; the data suggest that this is a simple method of monitoring patients and is more sensitive than FEV_1 measurements. However, other pathology such as CMV and PCP, would give similar clearance changes.

HRCT has been used in patients who have non-AIDS immunosuppression. The role is to direct interventional procedures. Janzen *et al.* [18] demonstrated that bronchoalveolar lavage or transbronchial biopsy were most likely to yield diagnostic information if the HRCT was abnormal in the central one-third of the lung.

REFERENCES

1. Murray, J.F., Garay, S.M., Hopewell, P.C., Mills, J., Snider, G.L. and Stover, D.E. (1987) Pulmonary complications of the acquired immunodeficiency syndrome: an update. *Annu. Rev. Respir. Dis.*, **135**, 504–9.
2. Bitran, J., Beckerman, C., Weinstein, R., Bennet, C., Ryo, U. and Pinsky, S. (1987) Patterns of gallium-67 scintigraphy in patients with acquired immunodeficiency syndrome and the AIDS related complex. *J. Nucl. Med.*, **28**, 1103–6.
3. Kramer, E.L., Sanger, J.J., Garay, S.M. *et al.* (1987) Gallium-67 scans of the chest in patients with acquired immunodeficiency syndrome. *J. Nucl. Med.*, **28**, 1107–14.
4. Tumeh, S.S., Belville, J.S., Pugatch, R. and McNeil, B. (1992) Ga-67 scintigraphy and computed tomography in the diagnosis of pneumocystis carinii pneumonia in patients with AIDS. A prospective comparison. *Clin. Nucl. Med..*, **17**, 387–94.
5. Tuazon, C.V., Delaney, M.D., Simon, G.L. *et al.* (1985) Utility of gallium-67 scintigraphy and bronchial washings in the diagnosis and treatment of *Pneumocystis carinii* pneumonia in patients with the acquired immunodeficiency syndrome. *Annu. Rev. Respir. Dis.*, **132**, 1087–92.
6. Prvulovich, E.M., Miller, R.F., Costa, D.C. *et al.* (1995) Immunoscintigraphy with a ^{99m}Tc-labelled anti-granulocyte monoclonal antibody in patients with human immunodeficiency virus infection and AIDS. *Nucl. Med. Commun.*, **16**, 838–45.
7. O'Doherty, M.J. (1995) ^{99m}Tc DTPA transfer/permeability in patients with HIV disease. *Q. J. Nucl. Med.*, **39**, 231–42.
8. Leach, R., Davidson, C., O'Doherty, M.J., Nayagam, M., Tang, A. and Bateman, N. (1991) Noninvasive management of fever and breathlessness in HIV positive patients. *Eur. J. Respir. Med.*, **4**, 19–25.
9. O'Doherty, M.J., Page, C.J., Bradbeer, C.S. *et al.* (1989) The place of lung 99mTc DTPA aerosol transfer in the investigation of lung infections in HIV positive patients. *Resp. Med.*, **83**, 395–401.
10. Rosso, J., Guillon, J.M., Parrot, A. *et al.* (1992) Technetium-99m-DTPA aerosol and gallium-67 scanning in pulmonary complications of human immunodeficiency virus infection. *J. Nucl. Med.*, **33**, 81–7.
11. Fineman, D.S., Palestro, C.J., Kim, C.K. *et al.* (1989) Detection of abnormalities in febrile AIDS patients with In-111-labelled leucocyte and Ga-67 scintigraphy. *Radiology*, **170**, 677–80.
12. O'Doherty, M. J., Revell, P., Page, C.J., Lee, S., Mountford, P. J. and Nunan, T.O. (1990) Donor leu-

cocyte imaging in patients with AIDS. A pre-liminary communication. *Eur. J. Nucl. Med.*, **17**, 327–33.

13. Miller, R.F. (1990) Nuclear medicine and AIDS. *Eur. J. Nucl. Med.*, **16**, 103–18.

14. Pohl, P., Riccabona, G., Hilty, E. *et al.* (1992) Double tracer SPECT in patients with AIDS encephalopathy: a comparison of 123I-IMP with ^{99m}Tc-HMPAO. *Nucl. Med. Commun.*, **13**, 586–92.

15. Brunetti, A., Berg, G., Di Chiro, G. *et al.* (1989) Reversal of brain metabolite abnormalities following treatment of AIDS dementia complex with 3′ azido-2′-3′-dideoxythymidine (AZT, zidovudine): a PET FDG study. *J. Nucl. Med.*, **30**, 581–90.

16. Hoffmann, J.M., Waskin, H.A., Schifter, T. *et al.* (1993) FDG-PET in differentiating lymphoma from nonmalignant central nervous system lesions in patients with AIDS. *J. Nucl. Med.*, **34**, 567–75.

17. Baron, A.L., Steinbach, L.S., Leboit, P.E., Mills, C.M., Gee, J.H. and Berger, T.G. (1990) Osteolytic lesions of bacillary angiomatosis in HIV infection: radio-logic differentiation from AIDS-related Kaposi sarcoma. *Radiology*, **177**, 77–81.

18. Janzen, D.L., Adler, B.D., Padley, S.P.G. *et al.* (1993) Diagnostic success of bronchoscopic biopsy in immunocompromised patients with acute pulmonary disease: predictive value of disease distribution as shown on CT. *Am. J. Roentgenol.*, **160**, 21–4.

FURTHER READING

O'Doherty, M.J. and Nunan, T.O. (1993) Nuclear medicine and AIDS. *Nucl. Med. Commun.*, **14**, 830–48.

O'Doherty, M.J. and Miller, R.F. (1996) *Nuclear Imaging of the Lung in AIDS. AIDS and Respiratory Medicine* (eds A. Zunila, M. Johnson and R.F. Miller), Chapman & Hall, London.

Worthy, S., Young Kang, E. and Muller, N.L. (1995) Acute lung disease in the immunocompromised host: differential diagnosis at High Resolution CT. *Semin. Ultrasound, CT and MRI*, **16**, 353–60.

Infection

J. Buscombe

INTRODUCTION

Infection remains a major source of morbidity and mortality in the modern world. Although many cases of infection may be treated in the community by oral antibiotics, this has led to the emergence of new strains of pathological organisms which are resistant to multiple antibiotics. An example is the methicillin-resistant *Staphylococcus aureus* (MRSA), which is now almost endemic in UK hospitals, and has also appeared in most other developed nations. While this bacterium by itself does not kill the host, it leads primarily to the breakdown of surgical wounds, debilitating the patient, and then secondarily, to an often fatal infection.

It was assumed that antibiotics would be the cure for all infections. However, if the dosage is inadequate to eradicate infection, re-activation can occur. This is particularly true for mycobacterial disease. Re-activated infection, having been previously exposed to antibiotics, has an increased possibility of being resistant to anti-bacterial drugs, and can transmit this resistance to other microorganisms using subcellular DNA packages called plasmids. Imaging for early diagnosis and to confirm the eradication of infection will become increasingly more important in providing optimal patient management.

The advent of multi-resistant strains of pathological organisms has coincided with technological developments in modern medicine, and modern medical life-support measures can keep patients with severe systemic disease and/or severe trauma alive. These patients may have attenuation of the classical signs of infection – fever, pain, loss of function, tissue swelling and rubor. A patient with multi-organ failure may only exhibit a rise in body temperature and possibly no obvious localizing signs. Patients who are being given drugs that modify the immune system, as part of cancer therapy, to reduce the effect of autoimmune disease, or to prevent rejection of a do-nated organ, may be as susceptible to infection as those with human immunodeficiency virus (HIV). These patients may exhibit a poor inflammatory response, with limited or absent symptoms and signs may enable a life-saving diagnosis to be made. In such patients, rapid and accurate diagnostic imaging may be extremely beneficial.

The inherent advantage of nuclear medicine over structural imaging modalities is that it is unaffected by changes in anatomy, which can occur after surgery or when there is scarring as a result of a previous infection. With radionuclide techniques, multiple sites of infection can be imaged without any extra radiation burden to the patient. Scintigraphic imaging can be used to monitor the effect of therapy on a site of known infection where anatomical imaging is not useful. One such example is *Pneumocystis carinii* pneumonia, where it is not unknown for the chest radiograph to be negative in the active infection stage, but become positive after successful treatment. However, the importance of a close relationship between anatomical and functional imaging is stressed because these studies are complementary, and not competitive. For example, ultrasound and CT can be used to localize precisely an area of abnormal uptake seen on a nuclear medicine study performed to localize infection. Likewise, the nature of an unexplained abnormality on an anatomical imaging method may be elucidated by the correct application of a specific nuclear medicine test such as a labelled leucocyte study.

It is important, however, that patients are not subjected to multiple tests using ionizing radiation without good reason, and a knowledge of the radiation exposure from the different radionuclide tests used for imaging infection is essential for the judicious use of these investigations (Table 5.2).

NON-SPECIFIC METHODS

BONE SCINTIGRAPHY

One of the most common scintigraphic tests used for the identification and localization of infection is dynamic bone scintigraphy. This normally includes a dynamic first phase covering the first 30–

Clinical Nuclear Medicine, 3rd edn. Edited by M.N. Maisey, K.E. Britton and B.D. Collier. Published in 1998 by Chapman & Hall, London. ISBN 0 412 75180 1

Table 5.2 Effective dose equivalent (EDE) to patients from different techniques used to image infection

Radiopharmaceutical	Administered activity (MBq)	EDE (mSv)
^{67}Ga citrate	150	18
^{In}111-labelled leucocytes	20	12
^{99m}Tc-HMPAO leucocytes	200	3
Chest X-ray CT (estimate)	–	4

60 seconds post-injection of a bone-seeking agent such as ^{99m}Tc-MDP. During this time the arterial supply and capillary flow and early venous phases can be seen. Asymmetrically increased arterial flow is suggestive of increased vascular supply to that area; this is non-specific but can occur at sites of infection and inflammation. A second 'blood pool' phase is used to determine capillary dilatation at a site of infection/inflammation, which results from local vasodilatation secondary to histamine and other mediators of inflammation. The capillaries become 'leaky' to small molecules, and therefore some of the activity may be extravascular rather than intravascular. A third phase is related to increased diphosphonate uptake at sites of bone infection and inflammation. If the third phase is normal, soft tissue infection is more likely than infection in the bone. Increased activity at a site in all three phases is suggestive, but not proof, of bone infection. While these techniques have high sensitivities (>90%), the specificity can be as low as 33% [1].

However, in some clinical situations, a positive three-phase bone scan is sufficient to confirm the clinical diagnosis: in children with discitis and in patients with a vertebral body abscess a positive bone scan result should then lead to urgent intervention, normally including a CT-guided biopsy, and possibly surgical drainage. Performing another more specific nuclear medicine test may delay urgently needed treatment with disastrous consequences. Bone scintigraphy is not useful in determining the resolution of bone infection as a study may be positive 12 or more months after infection has cleared. More specific infection studies are indicated.

HEPATOBILIARY SCINTIGRAPHY

Hepatobiliary scintigraphy with ^{99m}Tc-labelled iminodiacetic acids (^{99m}Tc-IDAs) is useful in the diagnosis of gallbladder infection. In acute cholecystitis, non-visualization of the gallbladder by 60 minutes is more sensitive and specific than ultrasound. The sensitivity of the test can be enhanced by giving morphine during the study.

Chronic infection of the biliary ducts can result in poor clearance of ^{99m}Tc-IDAs from the hepatic ducts, at the sphincter of Oddi, and the appearance of beading if there are biliary strictures. These tests are rarely used in diagnosis but may be an unsuspected finding in a patient being investigated for food-related right upper abdominal pain.

RADIOCOLLOID SCANNING

While CT and ultrasound have replaced colloid scanning for the identification of space-occupying lesion(s) in the liver, ^{99m}Tc-sulphur colloid scintigraphy may still have a place in the identification of liver abscesses in countries with limited health resources. The study is cheaper than CT and less operator-dependent than ultrasound. The sensitivity and localization of lesion(s) can be improved by the application of single-photon emission computed tomography (SPECT).

STATIC RENAL IMAGING

^{99m}Tc-dimercaptosuccinic acid (^{99m}Tc-DMSA) studies are widely used as a screening test for acute pyelonephritis. Early changes are characteristically seen as an area of reduced uptake, with an indistinct edge. The outer contour of this area can be concave, or if there is sufficient local swelling, convex. The whole kidney may be involved, giving a universally reduced uptake.

The scan should be performed as part of the initial assessment of patients before antibiotics have been given. Comparison with a follow-up DMSA study after 6 weeks will help determine the extent of any subsequent scarring (Figure 5.7).

CEREBRAL INFECTION

The use of non-specific blood–brain barrier scintigraphy using ^{99m}Tc-pertechnetate, ^{99m}Tc-DTPA or ^{99m}Tc-glucoheptanate is now universally reserved for those cases where there is a high index of suspicion for a cerebral abscess and limited or no access to CT or MRI. However, because of the non-

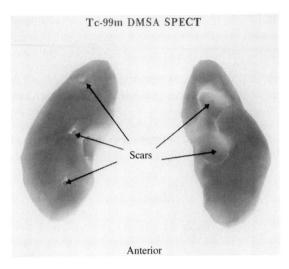

Tc-99m DMSA SPECT

Scars

Anterior

Figure 5.7 Anterior view of a volume-rendered three-dimensional SPECT image of two scarred kidneys imaged with ^{99m}Tc-DMSA.

specificity of this method, the results must be treated with caution.

SPECIFIC METHODS

GALLIUM-67 SCINTIGRAPHY

It is now 25 years since gallium-67 citrate (^{67}Ga) was first used in the identification of infection. Originally developed as a tumour imaging agent, 'non-specific' uptake was noted at sites of infection. This was first exploited in 1973 and ^{67}Ga quickly became a popular test for identifying infection. The 3.26-day half-life was an advantage, and because of this the material could be kept in stock and used as required. Unfortunately, the long half-life and pharmacokinetics of the tracer results in a significant radiation dose to the patient. Four characteristic γ-rays are emitted with peak energies of 394, 300, 190 and 90 KeV. The 394 KeV has a low yield (about 5%) and though it cannot contribute to imaging, it does contribute to scatter seen in the image. This is true with the medium-energy collimators supplied by some manufacturers, which will collimate the 300 KeV γ-ray, but the 394 KeV γ-ray will penetrate the septa and produce a poor image. Therefore, with some gamma-cameras a high-energy collimator is required, but this reduces sensitivity.

As ^{67}Ga is essentially an iron analogue, it quickly binds to the plasma protein transferrin after injection, so there is a significant blood pool activity until about 24 hours post-injection. During this time, most of the excretion of the tracer is urinary; after 24 hours, elimination is via the bowel, either in the terminal ileum or proximal colon. If the patient suffers from iron overload, very little bowel excretion occurs, blood pool activity remains high, and urinary excretion continues (Figure 5.8).

The consequence of these routes of excretion is that uptake seen in the kidneys and bladder over the first 24 hours, and in the gut after 24 hours, can be physiological. It is therefore normal practice to perform the earliest imaging at 48 hours post-injection for the abdomen and pelvis, though in the chest, head and limbs, earlier images can be obtained if the blood pool activity has reduced sufficiently. Any uptake in the large bowel should be followed by sequential imaging; if activity at a particular site within the large bowel increases

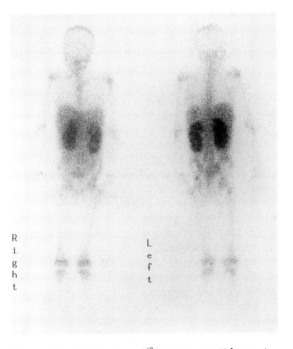

Right

Left

Figure 5.8 Distribution of ^{67}Ga citrate, at 48 hours, in a child with iron overload. Note the high renal uptake and marked bone uptake; long bone epihyses are seen. Note the absence of gut activity.

Table 5.3 Physiological uptake of ^{67}Ga into organs and tissues

Liver
Spleen
Bone marrow
Bone
Colon
Lacrimal glands
Salivary glands
Nasal mucosa
External genitalia
Breasts (especially lactation)
Gastric mucosa
Bone epiphysis

Table 5.4 Non-infection pathological distribution of ^{67}Ga citrate

Pathological uptake	Cause
Pulmonary, hilar	Idiopathic, lymphoma Sarcoid
Pulmonary, diffuse	Sarcoid, chemotherapy Radiotherapy
Breast	Combined oral contraceptive, cancer
Salivary glands	Sarcoid, Sjögren's, radiotherapy
Renal	Nephritis, anaemia, iron overload
Lymph nodes	Sarcoid, lymphoma, cancer
Wounds	Wound healing
Bones/joints	Fractures, gout, arthritis, sarcoid

with time, then infection is more likely. However, this rule does not apply to severely constipated patients and those with paralytic ileus.

Other sites of physiological activity of ^{67}Ga include the red bone marrow, the liver, and to a lesser extent the spleen. There is some excretion of the tracer into the lacrimal and salivary glands as well as the nasal mucosa. In women, breast uptake is seen in the luteal phase of the menstrual cycle, and is associated with pregnancy and lactation, but this is not invariable. ^{67}Ga can be excreted in the milk, and therefore precautions on interruption of feeding as recommended nationally should be used in nursing mothers.

Uptake of ^{67}Ga can also occur in a wide range of tissues (Table 5.3) and non-infected pathologies (Table 5.4). The patient's medical history may be required to ensure correct interpretation of a ^{67}Ga study. Despite these difficulties, ^{67}Ga has a wide range of clinical uses and is probably an under-utilized technique. In most countries, a ^{67}Ga scan is

still cheaper than a CT scan and is able to pick up a wide range of infections. It is also useful in localizing bacterial and protozoal infections. With care, good images are attainable, and excellent quality SPECT images of any part of the body should be available at 48 hours post-injection. In looking for small abscesses or lymph node involvement, for example in tuberculosis, SPECT is recommended as it is possible to see para-aortic and hilar lymph nodes more clearly.

INDIUM-111-LABELLED LEUCOCYTES

Thakur and his colleagues [2] were the first to successfully separate mixed leucocytes and label them in saline with a lipophilic amine indium-111 oxine. Since then, an additional method has been described using ^{111}In tropolonate in plasma. In both cases, a mixed population of leucocytes is labelled, though granulocytes predominate. Upon re-injection of the ^{111}In-labelled leucocytes there is early retention of activity within the lungs. However, if the cells are not severely damaged in the labelling procedure lung uptake should be negligible by 3–4 hours.

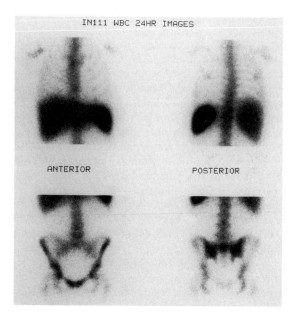

Figure 5.9 Normal distribution of ^{111}In-labelled leucocytes at 24 hours, with activity limited to the spleen, liver and bone marrow.

While it is possible to perform some *in vitro* studies of the viability of the labelled leucocytes, a simple test is to ensure that all lung activity has cleared by 4 hours post-injection. If diffuse lung activity remains at this time, and the patient does not have a known or suspected diffuse lung infection, then the viability of the cells and the interpretation of any subsequent images must be questioned. At 4 hours, there is normal distribution of the labelled leucocytes in the reticuloendothelial system, particularly in the spleen. Liver uptake is more than that seen on ^{67}Ga citrate scan. No activity should be seen, either in the bowel or urinary system, 24 hours after injection of the ^{111}In-labelled leucocytes. Radiolabelling does lead to premature death of these cells, and imaging beyond their mean survival of 24 hours is not recommended. The photon flux and physical characteristics of the γ-rays emitted from the ^{111}In is better for gamma-camera imaging than ^{67}Ga, except in the feet and the hands, where counts may be low, good quality images should be available at 24 hours post-injection (Figure 5.9).

The lack of physiological bowel or urinary activity makes this an ideal agent in patients with suspected intra-abdominal infection, as all activity outside the reticuloendothelial system can be considered pathological.

TECHNETIUM-99m-LABELLED LEUCOCYTES

The physical characteristics of ^{99m}Tc are near ideal for the modern gamma-cameras. The dosimetry of the isotope is good allowing a reasonable activity to be given for obtaining high-quality scans. Imaging time can be extended to 24 hours – the expected life span of a labelled leucocyte.

The earliest techniques by Hanna *et al.* [3] used a ^{99m}Tc-labelled colloid, which was used to label leucocytes isolated in colloid or in whole blood as a semi *in vitro* method. Experience of this method outside Australia is limited, though there is some evidence that while it works well, non-specific colonic activity is seen in the whole blood-labelling technique, presumably as a result of significant levels of free colloid. Recently, this approach has been re-introduced, and may become commercially available.

The most common method of labelling leucocytes with ^{99m}Tc is by using a preparation of leucocytes in plasma and incubating with the lipophilic amine, hexamethylpropyleneamineox-

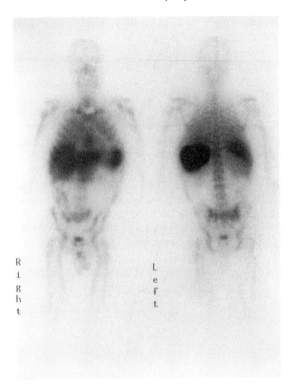

Figure 5.10 Anterior and posterior whole-body images performed 2.5 hours post-injection in a patient where the leucocytes labelled with ^{99m}Tc-HMPAO have been damaged. Note the persistent lung activity and colonic activity in the absence of gut pathology.

ime (HMPAO-exametzine) [4]. There is labelling of both granulocytes and lymphocytes and good labelling efficiencies of 50–60% can be obtained such that imaging can be performed up to 24 hours post-injection. However, biliary excretion has been noted by 3 hours post-injection, and therefore in the abdomen a 30- to 60-minute and 3- to 4-hour imaging protocol is recommended. There is no doubt that if the red blood cells are damaged, either during venepuncture or in the labelling process, there is significant ^{99m}Tc-HMPAO outside the leucocytes, and the biliary and gut activity is increased. The cells must be carefully handled, and if the plasma shows that significant haemolysis has taken place at some point before the labelling procedure, a fresh blood sample must be taken (Figure 5.10). Outside of the abdomen imaging can continue for up to 24 hours post-injection, and this is recommended in suspected bone and joint infections.

The single exception to this rule is the suspected Crohn's abscess, where a 24-hour image of the abdomen to show increasing activity adjacent to but separate from the colon is diagnostic.

As some radiolabelled product is excreted in the urine, the patient should void before each set of images. In common with all labelled leucocyte preparations, damaged cells will accumulate in the lungs, though some lung activity in the 30–60 minute image is expected, this should subsequently clear on the delayed images. Despite these apparent drawbacks, the versatility of this leucocyte-labelling method with ^{99m}Tc – and the fact that in most cases imaging is usually completed within 3 hours – means that many nuclear medicine departments find little use for other infection-specific imaging methods.

COLLOIDS

Colloids of nanometre size are preferentially phagocytosed by macrophages. Therefore, by injecting radiolabelled nanocolloids, it should be possible to achieve *in vivo* macrophage labelling for imaging sites of infection. Good-quality images of peripheral bone and joint infections have been reported, using ^{99m}Tc nanocolloids particularly in chronic osteomyelitis. However, there is still significant bone marrow and liver uptake, which together with the non-specific bowel activity, limits its use in soft tissue abdominal infection. The sensitivity of this method appears lower than labelled leucocytes and the specificity is about 50% for infection.

RADIOLABELLED IMMUNOGLOBULINS

A further approach to the problem of imaging infection without the need for cell labelling, is to use radiolabelled immunoglobulins. Using purified and pasteurized pooled human immunoglobulin, it is possible to attach ^{111}In via a DTPA linker and ^{99m}Tc via an iminothioline linker.

^{111}In-labelled human immunoglobulin (^{111}In-HIg) has the advantage of imaging beyond 24 hours. It appears to have a high sensitivity and specificity in a wide range of infections including those caused by viral, bacterial and protozoal agents [5]. As the HIg is basically non-

immunogenic, blood pool activity remains high, and late imaging at 24 and 48 hours post-injection produces the best results. The mechanism of action appears to be related to increased capillary permeability at the site of infection combined with the transfer of the ^{111}In radiolabel to local proteins. ^{111}In-labelled pooled IgM has also been used, but does not appear to offer any advantage over the IgG product. As ^{111}In is expensive, is not available in many countries, and has poor imaging characteristics, further work has been done using ^{99m}Tc HIg. This agent is commercially available in most of Europe, and appears to localize well at sites of soft tissue or bone infection in the periphery. The best images are seen 4–6 hours post-injection, as there is washout of the ^{99m}Tc-HIg after this time. High blood pool levels and normal colonic excretion significantly reduce its effectiveness within the chest, abdomen or pelvis.

IMMUNOSCINTIGRAPHY

Immunoscintigraphy of infection depends on raising a monoclonal antibody, normally murine, against an antigen found on the cell surface of granulocytes. Such an antigen, a 9 kDa glycoprotein, has been used to raise a series of monoclonal antibodies. Initially, labelling was with ^{123}I, but most experience is with the ^{99m}Tc-labelled products. There is a good body of evidence that ^{99m}Tc anti-granulocyte antibodies (^{99m}Tc-AGAB) have a high sensitivity and specificity for a wide range of soft tissue and bone infections [6]. As no cell labelling is required, imaging can be completed within 3–4 hours of injection of the antibody. However, there are significant problems in the production of the antibodies and there is also a risk of inducing human anti-mouse antibodies within the patient. This will reduce the effectiveness of future immunoscintigraphy in that patient and there is a slight risk of anaphylaxis. A further problem is that these antibodies have a preferred targeting of the pre-myleocytic cells in the marrow. This may lead to rapid marrow uptake of the ^{99m}Tc-AGAB, leaving little circulating antibody to image any infection.

While general applications remain limited, immunoscintigraphy offers a degree of specificity that is not available with other methods. There has been some work showing encouraging results with ^{99m}Tc anti-T-lymphocyte antibody in the diagnosis of active tuberculosis. A specific antibody has been raised against *Pneumocystis carinii* and, though this has only been used in a small group of patients, its sensitivity is high but specificity unproven [7].

LABELLED ANTIBIOTICS

Pathophysiologically, there is little difference between non-infective inflammation and infection. Both processes result in capillary dilatation, increased capillary permeability, the release of inflammatory mediators (mostly proteins) and the migration of inflammatory cells (both granulocytes and lymphocytes), the only difference being the presence or absence of a pathological microorganism.

Most of the methods described either use the passage of radiolabelled inflammatory cells to the site of infection or label proteins (e.g. human IgG) that are found at the site of inflammation. Hence, it is not unexpected to find that such methods will not discriminate between infection and inflammation.

A novel approach has been to label the antibiotic ciprofloxacin with ^{99m}Tc. This product, named 'Infecton' has been compared with labelled leucocyte imaging in 56 patients with a wide range of bone and soft tissue infections [8]. The sensitivity of ^{99m}Tc Infecton was 84% for infection compared with 81% for labelled leucocytes, and specificity was particularly high at 96% compared with that of labelled leucocytes (71%). Bone marrow activity of ^{99m}Tc Infecton is low, and if these early results are confirmed the test may be useful in infections of the axial skeleton and around joint prostheses. However, whether it can be used in non-bacterial infections remains unclear.

NEW AGENTS

There are many mediators of infection that can be labelled and used for imaging. Some are toxic and can cause significant side effects if administered to a patient, an example being interleukin-1 and the interferons. Interleukin-2 (Il-2) is less toxic and attaches readily to T-lymphocytes. With Il-2 it is possible to image tuberculosis, but the agent is not specific for any granulomatous disease and many auto-immune conditions.

Peptides that either recognize an antigen present on the surface of activated granulocytes or other mediators of the inflammatory response may be used. These agents, labelled with ^{99m}Tc, have had a limited success but few if any will be commercially available over the next decade. They are potentially as specific as antibodies, but have the advantage of being non-allergenic.

A newer research approach has been to use liposomes to deliver a radioactive tag to granulocytes *in vivo*. Liver clearance of liposomes is high but can be reduced by manipulating the surface of the liposome to appear like water to the hepatocyte – the so-called 'stealth-liposomes'. However, work on this idea has not yet progressed beyond the preclinical stage.

CLINICAL APPLICATIONS OF INFECTION IMAGING METHODS

OSTEOMYELITIS

Bone infection can be identified by dynamic bone scintigraphy. However, the specificity of this method is low, since similar findings may be found in tumours or secondary to trauma. More specific imaging with either ^{67}Ga citrate or labelled leucocytes should be undertaken if the identification of infection is required, either for initial diagnosis or after antibiotic therapy. There appears to

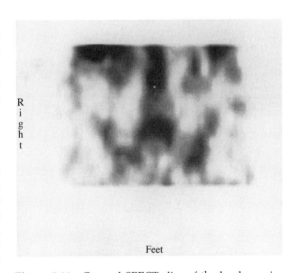

Right

Feet

Figure 5.11 Coronal SPECT slice of the lumbar spine obtained with ^{67}Ga 48 hours post-injection, showing intense uptake in the 5th lumbar vertebra which has an enterococcal abscess.

be little to suggest that any particular test is ideal in the diagnosis of osteomyelitis. Theoretically, it is thought that agents such as ^{67}Ga citrate and ^{99m}Tc HIg, which do not rely on the transit of leucocytes, may be of more use in chronic infection. There is little evidence to support this hypothesis except in the spine, though 24-hour imaging of suspected infection with ^{111}In or ^{99m}Tc labelled leucocytes is recommended.

A preparation of radiolabelled pure granulocytes may be of some advantage in the patients with chronic osteomyelitis, but this technique is not widely used.

There are however, two situations in which labelled leucocyte scintigraphy is not recommended. The first is a suspected tuberculous bone abscess and the second a spinal abscess. In both cases, ^{67}Ga citrate imaging should be performed (Figure 5.11). Labelled leucocyte imaging is particularly useless in the vertebral abscess where the infected vertebrae will appear 'cold' as there is no normal bone marrow uptake of the leucocytes,

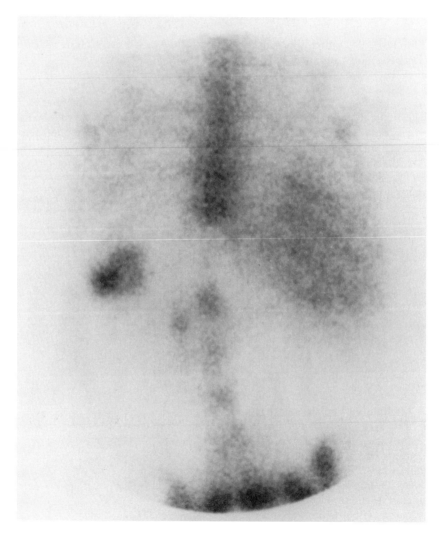

Figure 5.12   3.5-hour image with ^{99m}Tc-HMPAO-labelled leucocytes, showing no uptake in the site of a vertebral abscess involving the first two lumbar vertebrae.

but transit of labelled leucocytes into the abscess is so restricted that no active accumulation occurs (Figure 5.12). Unfortunately, the appearance of a 'cold' vertebral body in such a study is non-specific and has been reported in metastases and myeloma.

These techniques offer both high sensitivity and specificity for bone infection and in combination with the dynamic bone scintigraphy should prove diagnostic in most patients.

SUSPECTED INFECTED PROSTHETIC JOINTS

The incidence of joint prosthesis infection has fallen over the recent years; about 1% of hip and 4% of knee prostheses may become infected. The standard practice is to first perform a dynamic bone scintigram. If this is negative then the probability of infection is low. However, in some patients with uncemented hip prosthesis, loosening and infection may occur without changes on the bone scintigrams. Therefore, specific studies for infection should be considered in all patients with a positive dynamic bone scintigram and those with uncemented hip prosthesis and other signs that they may have infection such as persistent pain, history of wound infection, raised blood leucocyte count or raised erythrocyte sedimentation rate (ESR) and C-reactive protein (CRP).

There may be some advantage in using techniques which do not rely on labelled leucocytes in patients with hip prosthesis. This is particularly true of uncemented femoral components where native bone marrow is not removed but pushed

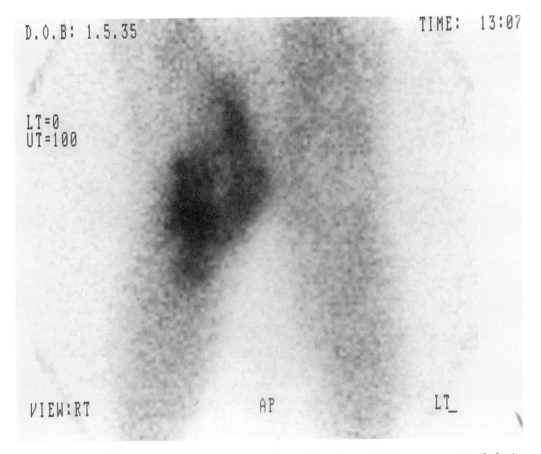

D.O.B: 1.5.35   TIME: 13:07

LT=0
UT=100

VIEW:RT   AP   LT_

Figure 5.13 Uptake of ^{67}Ga around an infected knee prosthesis. Note that activity is seen around both the femoral and tibial components, but none is seen in the synovium.

down the femoral shaft by the prosthesis. They can form into islands of marrow which have the appearance of focal infection when using labelled leucocyte or anti-granulocyte antibody scans. In both these cases higher sensitivities have been recorded for both ^{111}In and ^{99m}Tc human immunoglobulins [9].

An alternative is to perform a ^{99m}Tc nanocolloid scan in addition to the labelled leucocyte scan to map bone marrow. If the pattern of uptake in and around the hip is concordant then an infection in unlikely.

There is a significant difference in imaging the prosthetic hip and knee. The knee joint is often replaced secondarily to rheumatoid infection and post-operative synovial inflammation is not uncommon. The symptoms and signs are similar to infection and, as none of the techniques commonly described is able to distinguish infection and inflammation, synovial uptake of ^{67}Ga, labelled leucocytes and human immunoglobulin is not uncommonly seen. The pattern of uptake around the synovium but not the joint replacement should help to differentiate between the two (Figure 5.13).

In comparison with dynamic bone scintigraphy the specificity of ^{67}Ga, labelled leucocytes or other techniques is much higher but without loss of sensitivity. The failure of other imaging techniques such as ultrasound, CT and MRI in this area has meant that these are the only techniques which can be recommended in patients with a suspected infected joint prosthesis. [99m]Tc Infecton is showing promising results.

CHEST INFECTION

Pulmonary infections in the non-immuno-compromised patients are normally bacterial and most of these will be identified by increasing accumulation of ^{67}Ga, labelled leucocytes or ^{111}In HIg over time. Diagnostic imaging with labelled leucocytes can be performed 4 and 24 hours post-injection, with ^{67}Ga citrate and ^{111}In HIg 24 hours post-injection. [99m]Tc HIg is not indicated in the chest infections: both diffuse and focal accumulation of these agents have been recorded and lobar pneumonia produces characteristic pictures of a single lobar or segmental uptake.

Tuberculosis will be best imaged by ^{67}Ga citrate: focal and diffuse intrapulmonary uptake will be seen often with associated hilar lymph node up-

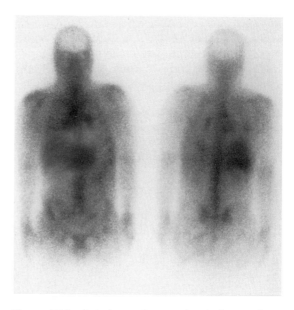

Figure 5.14 Anterior and posterior 48-hour whole-body images in a patient with a 6-month history of fever and weight loss. There is abnormal uptake in the liver, hilar and mediastinal lymph nodes. Biopsy demonstrated infection with *Mycobacterium tuberculosis*; however, changes are non-specific and can be seen in sarcoid.

take (Figure 5.14). While there is evidence that, at least in the immunocompromised, nuclear medicine techniques are more sensitive than planar radiology [10], it is unlikely that suspected pulmonary infection will be a major indication for such studies but pulmonary infection may be found in patients imaged for other reasons, e.g. post-operative fever (Figure 5.15).

ABDOMINAL AND PELVIC INFECTION

The abdomen may contain significant focal infection, without localizing signs, particularly in the elderly. The first investigation normally performed if intra-abdominal or intra-pelvic infection is suspected is ultrasound. However, the method is operator-dependent and large tracts of the abdomen may not be correctly imaged. Abdominal CT is of particular use around the liver and pelvis or in the fat patient. Except in the latest generation of spiral CT machines, non-contiguous slices are performed 1–2 cm apart. Hence, a small abscess may be missed between slices.

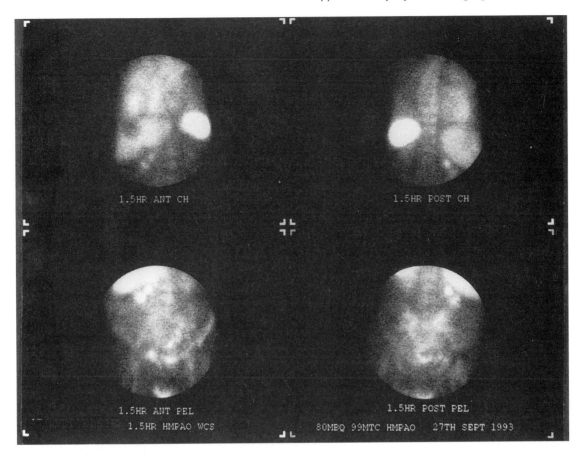

Figure 5.15 1.5-hour ^{99m}Tc-HMPAO-labelled leucocyte scan in an elderly female patient showing uptake in the left iliac fossa due to diverticular abscess, under the liver secondary to metastatic abscesses, and in the lungs due to bronchopneumonia. This study illustrates that multiple sites of infection can be identified using nuclear medicine techniques (the 'cold' area in the liver was a simple cyst).

Therefore, as soon as ultrasound and CT have failed to find evidence of infection the patient should be promptly imaged with labelled leucocytes. ^{67}Ga citrate is not appropriate as the physiological uptake in the terminal ileum and colon from 24 hours post-infection makes interpretation of colonic and pericolonic infection difficult.

The value of labelled leucocytes will be greatly enhanced in these often severely ill patients if the service can deliver an answer on the day of request. This has been done using the 1- and 3-hour imaging protocol with ^{99m}Tc-HMPAO leucocytes [11]. Similar results have also been obtained within 4 hours post-injection with ^{99m}Tc anti-granulocyte antibodies.

Comparisons with other imaging techniques are limited, however. In an extensive study comparing ^{111}In and ^{99m}Tc-HMPAO-labelled leucocytes with ultrasound in patients with suspected intra-abdominal infection, there was no difference in the results obtained using the two different types of labelled leucocytes [12]. The sensitivity of the labelled leucocyte studies was 76% compared with 71% for ultrasound, though the authors noted that liver infections were missed by the former technique. The liver, as part of the reticuloendothelial system, has a physiological accumulation of labelled leucocytes which can mask any labelled leucocytes in a liver infection. If an area of the liver has absent or reduced activity in the 1-hour image but normal activity in the 4-hour

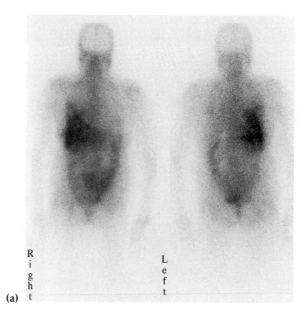

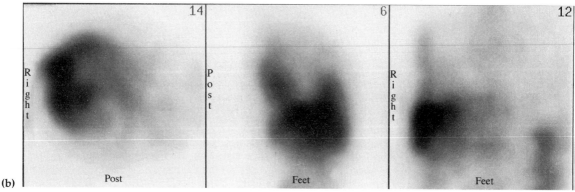

Figure 5.16 (a) Anterior and posterior 48-hour whole-body ^{67}Ga images suggest infection near the liver and possibly right chest. (b) A SPECT study with transaxial, sagittal and coronal slices demonstrate that the abscess lies mainly around the upper outer part of the liver and under the diaphragm in the sub-phrenic space.

image, then liver abscess must be considered. An additional liver colloid subtraction image can be performed which will not only localize intrahepatic infections but also allow visualization of subphrenic infections. SPECT may also be of use in identifying liver or subphrenic abscess (Figure 5.16).

There is some dissociation of the ^{99m}Tc from the HMPAO-labelled leucocytes seen at 1 hour postinjection and resulting in physiological kidney and bladder activity. Therefore, ^{111}In-labelled leucocytes may be preferable if an infection of the renal tract or lower pelvis is suspected.

PYREXIA OF UNKNOWN ORIGIN

Very few patients fit into the Petersdorf description of a patient with at least 2 weeks' fever, the cause of which is unknown 1 week after hospital investigations are initiated. This leisurely approach to diagnosis is not acceptable to modern health economics. However, there is a group of patients who present with persistent undiagnosed fever. Only 50% will be found to have fever, 25% will have another medical cause such as lymphoma and in 25% no cause will be found. It is not surprising that nuclear medicine techniques in common with other techniques often fail to provide the answer to the patient's fever.

If the fever is chronic (greater than 2 weeks' duration) infection is less common and ^{67}Ga imaging may be more appropriate than labelled leucocytes. However, less specific localization in non-infected pathology such as lymphoma may lead to a diagnostic CT or ultrasound-directed biopsy.

The single biggest advantage of nuclear medicine in cases of unknown fever is that head-to-foot imaging can be performed easily. A negative ^{67}Ga study makes the presence of significant infection unlikely.

In conclusion, imaging infection with nuclear medicine techniques is an under-used approach but one that is useful in a wide variety of clinically important infections. It is complementary to anatomical imaging and can be used to guide both ultrasound- and CT-directed biopsy. The ability to image the whole body makes it ideal in many patients without localizing symptoms or signs. Although a variety of agents is available, each individual patient and their clinical problem will direct the clinician to the study most likely to contribute to localizing that patient's infection.

REFERENCES

1. Schaweker, D.S. (1992) The scintigraphic diagnosis of osteomyelitis. *Am. J. Roentgenol.*, **158**, 9–18.
2. Thakur, M.L., Lavender, P., Arnot, R.N. *et al.* (1977) ^{111}In-labeled autologous leucocytes in man. *J. Nucl. Med.*, **18**, 1012–19.
3. Hanna, R., Lomas, F. and Teverdel, A. (1984) Radiochemistry and biostability of autologous leucocytes labelled with ^{99m}Tc-stannous colloidin whole blood. *Eur. J. Nucl. Med.*, **9**, 216–19.
4. Roddie, M.E., Peters, A.M., Danpure, H.J. *et al.* (1988) Imaging inflammation with ^{99m}Tc hexamethyl-propyleneamine oxime (HMPAO) labelled leucocytes. *Radiology*, **166**, 767–72.
5. Oyen, W.J.G., Claessens, R.A.M.J., van der Meer, J.W.M. *et al.* (1992) Indium-111 labeled human nonspecific immunoglobulin G: a new radiopharmaceutical for imaging infectious and inflammatory foci. *Clin. Infect. Dis.*, **14**, 1110–18.
6. Scuik, A., Bandau, W., Vollet, W. *et al.* (1991) Comparison of technetium-99m polyclonal human immunoglobulin and technetium-99m monoclonal antibodies for imaging chronic osteomyelitis; first clinical results. *Eur. J. Nucl. Med.*, **18**, 401–7.
7. Goldenberg, D.M., Sharkey, R.M., Udem, S. *et al.* (1994) Immunoscintigraphy of *Pneumocystis carinii* pneumonia in AIDS patients. *J. Nucl. Med.*, **34**, 1028–34.
8. Vinjamuri, S., Hall, A.V., Solanki, K.K. *et al.* (1996) Comparison of ^{99m}Tc infection imaging with radiolabelled white cell imaging in the evaluation of bacterial infection *Lancet*, **347**, 233–5.
9. Oyen, W.J.G., Claessens, R.A.M.J., van Horn, J.R., van der Meer, J.W.M. and Corstens, F.H.M. (1991) Scintigraphic detection of bone and joint infections with indium-111 labeled nonspecific human IgG. *J. Nucl. Med.*, **31**, 403–12.
10. Buscombe, J.R., Oyen, W.J.G., Corstens, F.H.M., Ell, P.J. and Miller, R.F.A. (1995) Comparison of ^{111}In-HIg scintigraphy and chest radiology in the identification of pulmonary infection in patients with HIV infection. *Nucl. Med. Commun.*, **16**, 327–35.
11. Mountford, P.J., Kettle, A.G., O'Doherty, M.J. *et al.* (1990) Comparison of ^{99m}Tc HMPAO leucocytes with ^{111}In-oxine leucocytes for localising intra-abdominal sepsis. *J. Nucl. Med.*, **31**, 311–15.
12. Weldon, M.J., Joseph, A.E., French, A., Saverymuttu, S.H. and Maxwell, J.D. (1995) Comparison of technetium-99m hexamethylpropylene-amineoxime labelled leucocytes and indium-111 oxine labelled granulocyte scanning and ultrasound in the diagnosis of intra-abdominal abscess. *Gut*, **37**, 551–64.

FURTHER READING

Becker, W., Goldenburg, D.M. and Wolf, F. (1994) The use of monoclonal and antibody fragments in the imaging of infectious lesions. *Semin. Nucl. Med.*, **12**, 142–53.
Buscombe, J.R. (1995) Radiolabelled immunoglobulins. *Nucl. Med. Commun.*, **16**, 990–1001.
Datz, F.L. (1994) Indium-111-labeled leucocytes for the detection of infection: current status. *Semin. Nucl. Med.*, **12**, 92–109.
Palestro, C.J. (1994) The current role of gallium imaging in infection. *Semin. Nucl. Med.*, **12**, 128–41.
Peters, A.M. (1994) The utility of (^{99m}Tc) HMPAO leucocytes for imaging infection. *Semin. Nucl. Med.*, **12**, 110–27.

Autoimmune diseases

A. Signore and M. Chianelli

INTRODUCTION

Autoimmune diseases can be defined as diseases resulting from an immune aggression of a self-tissue and leading to its complete destruction. The hallmark of autoimmune diseases is the presence of circulating antibodies and activated lymphocytes, which react against self-antigens. Measurement of specific autoantibody titre is currently used for diagnostic purposes and for therapy follow-up as this indicates the presence of the ongoing autoimmune process, although the relationship between the antibody titre and the severity and/or the extent of disease is still unclear.

RELEVANT PATHOPHYSIOLOGY

Almost all body tissues have been described as possible targets for an autoimmune reaction, the pathogenesis of which is still incompletely understood. Among the factors involved in the genesis of autoimmunity, either a loss of thymic tolerance or a failure of peripheral anergy against self-antigens, and in some cases, a cross-reaction with bacterial, viral and retroviral antigens, has been described. There is an undoubted genetic predisposition for autoimmune diseases, since they are associated with MHC- and non-MHC-related genes.

Several classifications of autoimmune diseases have been proposed, based on the clinical and pathogenetic findings; in particular, they can be classified as either systemic or organ-specific diseases, depending on whether the response is primarily against widespread or tissue-specific antigens. An important clinical characteristic of autoimmune diseases, that reflects the common genetic predisposition, is the associated high frequency of polyglandular autoimmune syndromes (Table 5.5).

It is important to emphasize that these diseases are characterized by a long asymptomatic prodromal period, during which lymphocytes (activated T-helper and cytotoxic), plasma cells and macrophages infiltrate the target tissue [1–4]; autoantibodies can also be detected in the patient's serum, and have a predictive value [5]. Infiltrating mononuclear cells release several cytokines (e.g. IL-1, IL-2, IL-4, IL-10, IL-12, IFN-γ, etc.) *in situ*, and their complex network seems to be important in the clinical evolution of the disease. Thus, therapeutic approaches that interfere with cytokine production have proved successful in altering the natural history of the disease. When there is an acute inflammation or superimposed infection, polymorphonuclear cells can also migrate into the target tissue – this often occurs in autoimmune diseases of the gut (e.g. Crohn's disease and ulcerative colitis).

The clinical diagnosis of an organ-specific autoimmune disease is commonly made when symptoms of target tissue hypofunction appear. Thyroid Graves' disease is an exception, since the presence of anti-TSHr antibodies stimulate the thyroid function, and therefore, an early diagnosis of hyperthyroidism can be made and therapy started before the thyroid is destroyed by infiltrating lymphocytes.

Immunologically, autoimmune diseases are quite heterogeneous. As shown in Table 5.6, in some cases there is a prevalence of humoral immunity (i.e. production of autoantibodies), and in others, cellular immunity predominates (i.e. a decrease in circulating T-suppressor cells, an increase in activated T-cells and mononuclear cell infiltration of the target tissue). However, the same disease in different subjects may appear with a different involvement of the two compartments.

Thus, in most organ-specific autoimmune diseases, the detection of lymphocytes infiltrating the target tissue represents an important additional marker, together with the measurement of circulating autoantibody titre, for early diagnosis, early treatment and therapy follow-up. For histological examination, tissue specimens can be obtained from thyroid, gut, joints, skin and kidney, but for other tissues (e.g. parathyroid, adrenals, pancreas, gonads, pituitary gland, brain, etc.), biopsies can be difficult to obtain. Therefore the opportunity to image infiltrating lymphocytes in these tissues is an important goal for nuclear medicine.

Clinical Nuclear Medicine, 3rd edn. Edited by M.N. Maisey, K.E. Britton and B.D. Collier. Published in 1998 by Chapman & Hall, London. ISBN 0 412 75180 1

Table 5.5 Autoimmune polyglandular syndromes

	Type 1	Type 2	Type 3
Diagnostic features	Onset in childhood Non HLA associated Siblings affected Mucocutaneous candidiasis	Onset in adulthood HLA B8, DR3 associated Multiple generations affected No mucocutaneous candidiasis	
Frequency of autoimmune disease association	Hypoparathyroidism (82%) Adrenal insufficiency (75%) Mucocutaneous candidiasis (67%) Alopecia (30%) Malabsorption (23%) Primary hypogonadism (15%) Pernicious anaemia (14%) Active chronic hepatitis (12%) Chronic thyroiditis (11%) Vitiligo (9%) Type 1 diabetes mellitus (3%)	Adrenal insufficiency (100%) Primary hypothyroidism (75%) Graves' hyperthyroidism (70%) Type 1 diabetes mellitus (52%) Primary hypogonadism (34%) Vitiligo (5%) Pernicious anaemia (<1%) Coeliac disease (?) Myasthenia gravis (?)	Autoimmune thyroiditis (100%) Type 1 diabetes mellitus (?) Pernicious anaemia (?) Vitiligo (?) Alopecia (?) Autoimmune gastritis (?)

Table 5.6 The spectrum of autolmmune diseases

← *Cellular Immunity Involvement*
Multiple sclerosis
    Crohn's disease
        Dermatomyositis
            Scleroderma
                Ulcerative colitis
                    Sjogren's syndrome
                        Primary hypogonadism
                            Primary myxoedema
                                Hashimoto's thyroiditis
                                  Addison's disease
                                    Type 1 diabetes mellitus
                                    Active chronic hepatitis
                                    Primary biliary cirrhosis
                                      Coeliac disease
                                        Graves' thyroiditis
                                          Rheumatoid arthritis
                                            Atrophic gastritis
                                              Pernicious anaemia
                                                Myasthenia gravis
                                                  Systemic lupus erythematosus
                                                  Humoral Immunity Involvement →

RADIOPHARMACEUTICALS FOR THE STUDY OF AUTOIMMUNE DISEASES

As mentioned above, most organ-specific autoimmune diseases are characterized by a chronic infiltration of the target tissue by mononuclear cells, with little or no haemodynamic changes, and poor symptoms of inflammation. Tissue mononuclear cell infiltration precedes and persists until target cells are destroyed and symptoms of hypofunction appear. Thus, functional imaging of the tissue is generally not useful for early diagnosis. It may just support the clinical diagnosis (i.e. thyroid iodine uptake in Hashimoto's thyroiditis) or be used in some cases for therapy follow-up (i.e. liver colloid scintigraphy in chronic hepatitis). By contrast, it has a relevant diagnostic and therapeutic importance: the possibility to detect and quantify the tissue mononuclear cell infiltration (i.e. what causes the autoimmune disease). Low-molecular weight radiolabelled receptor ligands should be used – they can pass through the intact capillary endothelium and bind specifically to infiltrating cells. Radiolabelled granulocytes cannot be used for the detection of tissues infiltrated by mononuclear cells. However, in some auto-immune diseases such as Crohn's disease and rheumatoid arthritis, typical signs of acute inflammation coexist with chronic lymphocytic infiltration. In these cases, radiolabelled granulocytes or mixed leukocytes can be used. Other techniques can also be employed such as the use of macromolecules like nanocolloids and non-specific human immunoglobulin, that accumulates at sites of acute inflammation as a result of non-specific extravasation. A brief description of the most relevant radiopharmaceuticals for the study of autoimmune diseases will follow.

RADIOLABELLED AUTOLOGOUS LYMPHOCYTES

Several studies have reported the use of ^{111}In-labelled lymphocytes in normal subjects and in patients with malignancies. Good results were obtained in patients with haematological tumours and organ-specific autoimmune diseases [6–8]. However, their use was discontinued when *in vitro* studies reported that lymphocytes were highly sensitive to radiation damage [9,10].

RADIOLABELLED MIXED LEUCOCYTES

Inflammatory foci can be detected by radiolabelled leucocytes. Following intravenous injection into patients, they migrate specifically into inflamed tissues by adhering to the activated endothelium and following a gradient of chemotactic factors [11]. Leucocytes can be labelled with ^{111}In-oxine or ^{111}In-tropolonate, and more recently, the use of ^{99m}Tc-hexamethylpropyleneamineoxime (^{99m}Tc-HMPAO) has been introduced [12]. ^{99m}Tc-HMPAO-labelled leucocytes are preferred, particularly in paediatric patients, and when better resolution is needed, for example, in the diagnosis of small bowel involvement in patients with Crohn's disease.

TECHNETIUM-LABELLED NANOCOLLOIDS

[99m]Tc-labelled nanocolloids are small particles, 30 nm in diameter, produced from albumin, that are taken up by the reticuloendothelial system

(RES) cells; they are rapidly cleared from the circulation following uptake by the liver, spleen and bone marrow. They leak into inflamed tissues non-specifically as a result of increased vascular permeability, and accumulate at the site of inflammation following phagocytosis by macrophages [13].

The uptake of ^{99m}Tc-nanocolloids in inflamed lesions is relatively small compared with that of other radiopharmaceuticals [14], but as a result of their rapid blood clearance, a good target-to-background ratio is obtained at early time points and the scan is usually completed in an hour. They are especially used for the study of inflammatory processes of the musculoskeletal system.

NON-SPECIFIC HUMAN IMMUNOGLOBULINS

The use of radiolabelled non-specific human immunoglobulins (HIg) has been recently introduced for detecting sites of inflammation/infection [15]. They produce no allergic reactions or any side effects, and are commercially available and provided in a ready-to-use kit form. Although their mechanism(s) of action has not yet been completely clarified, their accumulation seems to be mainly non-specific as a result of leakage into the inflamed site. They are available labelled with ^{99m}Tc or [111]In. The mechanism of accumulation is the same for both radiopharmaceuticals. The biodistribution of the two tracers is similar. Both accumulate in the liver and have slow kinetics. Diagnostic images are usually acquired at late time points (6–24 hours). However, compared with ^{99m}Tc-HIg, the use of ^{111}In-labelled HIg results in a higher concentration in inflamed tissue, due to accumulation of free ^{111}In resulting from the local metabolism of ^{111}In-HIg.

The major indication for the use of radiolabelled HIg is the study of inflamed/infected joints and/or bone, where they give excellent results [16]. They can successfully be used in many diseases, such as rheumatoid arthritis, with a diagnostic accuracy comparable with that of radiolabelled white blood cells.

ANTIBODIES AGAINST GRANULOCYTE OR LYMPHOCYTE ANTIGENS

Radiolabelled antibodies recognizing lymphocyte antigens such as CD3 or CD4, have been used for the study of autoimmune diseases [17,18]. BW250/183 is a monoclonal antibody recognizing the non-specific cross-reacting antigen 95 (NCA-95) that is expressed on human granulocytes, promyelocytes and myelocytes. It was commercially available and provided as a ready-to-use kit for [99mTc] labelling. Localization of inflammatory processes is thought to be mediated by migration of circulating radiolabelled granulocytes and by non-specific extravasation of the free antibody into the inflamed focus. Following binding to bone marrow (55%), liver (10%), spleen (6%) and peripheral organs, the antibody is rapidly cleared from the circulation and low values of circulating radioactivity are obtained [19].

Radiolabelled antibodies have a long plasma half-life and give a high background radioactivity that decreases slowly with time. A long interval (6–24 hours) is usually required between the administration of the labelled MAb and the acquisition of images in order to have a good target-to-background ratio. They are of heterologous origin and may induce production of human anti-murine antibodies (HAMA) with the possible development of allergic reactions, anti-idiotypic antibody and altered pharmacokinetics.

RADIOLABELLED SOMATOSTATIN ANALOGUES

Radiolabelled somatostatin analogues have extensively been used for the detection of neuroendocrine tumours [20]. Somatostatin receptors (SSRs) have also been observed on human lymphoid tissue, although the identification of the receptor-bearing cells is still unclear [21]. Hyperexpression of the SSRs has been reported in intestinal samples from patients with active ulcerative colitis and Crohn's disease; SSRs were localized in intramural veins, and were not detected in non-inflamed control intestine [22]. SSRs have also been identified *in vitro* in patients with active rheumatoid arthritis [23] and *in vivo* in the thyroid of patients with Graves' thyroiditis [24].

RADIOLABELLED INTERLEUKIN-2

A new radiopharmaceutical for the detection of lymphocytic infiltration is radiolabelled interleukin-2 (IL-2), a low-molecular weight (15.5 kDa) cytokine that binds to a specific receptor expressed by activated lymphocytes [25]. Radio-

labelled IL-2 has a rapid plasma clearance and diagnostic images can be acquired an hour after the injection with a good target-to-background ratio. With the doses used for diagnostic imaging (<50 μg), no side effects have been reported [26]. Radiolabelled IL-2 has recently been used with promising results in clinical trials for the study of autoimmune diseases such as Crohn's disease, coeliac disease, type 1 diabetes mellitus and autoimmune thyroiditis [27].

CLINICAL APPLICATIONS

We will describe the use of nuclear medicine techniques in a few autoimmune diseases in which the role of these techniques for diagnostic and follow-up purposes is clearly established.

RHEUMATOID ARTHRITIS

Rheumatoid arthritis is a chronic autoimmune disease characterized by severe short- and long-term complications of the joints. Chronic mononuclear cell infiltration of the synovial membrane and subsequent erosion of cartilage and bone lead to joint ankylosis. The typical haemodynamic changes of acute inflammation and the persistence of the chronic infiltrate are both present.

Specific and non-specific signs of inflammation are normally used for the clinical diagnosis and follow-up of the disease. Systemic treatment with anti-inflammatory drugs (steroidal and non-steroidal), is commonly employed for relief of symptoms and to delay disease progression. Treatment is usually life-long and is accompanied by several side effects; local therapy is also used and has the advantage of higher local concentrations and fewer side effects. It would be very useful for the prevention of disease progression to diagnose affected joints before they become clinically evident and local therapies could be applied before complications develop. Rheumatoid arthritis has been extensively studied by nuclear medicine techniques and all radiopharmaceuticals tested showed accumulation in the inflamed joints [28].

In a comparative study, [99mTc]-HIg, [99mTc]-nanocolloid and [99mTc]-HMPAO-labelled leucocytes, showed a similar diagnostic accuracy [29] (Figure 5.17). The use of a [99mTc]-labelled MAb (OKT3) has been recently described in patients with rheumatoid arthritis [18]; in this study, the

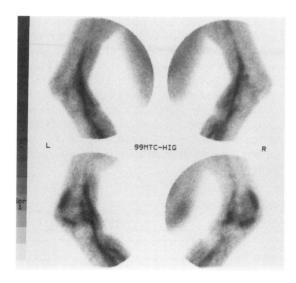

99MTC-HIG

Figure 5.17 γ-Camera images of the left (L) and right (R) knees in a normal subject (upper panels) and in a patient affected by rheumatoid arthritis (lower panels) after administration of ^{99m}Tc-HIg. In the patient's knees, HIg accumulates in the synovial fluid, whereas in the normal subject circulating radioactivity is detectable only in major blood vessels.

accumulation of the radiolabelled MAb correlated with the intensity of the inflammation, and also detected active joints that were clinically asymptomatic. The use of this antibody was however, associated with side effects due to the release of cytokines following binding of the MAb to the CD3 molecule.

Anti-CD4 radiolabelled antibodies have also been used in patients with rheumatoid arthritis. In a comparative study using the anti-CD4 and ^{99m}Tc-labelled polyclonal human immunoglobulins, both preparations showed similar accumulation in the inflamed joints. However, the anti-CD4 antibody showed a higher target-to-background ratio owing to the faster clearance of background radioactivity as a result of greater binding to the liver and the spleen [17].

CROHN'S DISEASE

Crohn's disease is characterized by a chronic mononuclear cell infiltration of the intestinal wall and hypertrophy of local lymphoid tissues [30]. Immune erosion of the intestinal wall may lead to severe complications of the affected bowel such as stenosis and ulceration, that may require surgical

resection. In over 70% of patients, relapse of the disease is noted within 1 year after the intervention. In the early relapse phase, the symptoms are infrequent and non-specific, and conventional X-ray examinations are negative. Since effective therapies are available, early diagnosis of the relapse might allow prompt initiation of therapy to prevent the onset of complications and the need for further surgical resection [31].

Good results are obtained in Crohn's disease by radiolabelled autologous leucocytes for preoperative evaluation of disease extent and for early diagnosis of relapse [32] (Plate 2). If ^{111}In-labelled leucocytes are used, the severity of the inflammatory process can also be quantified by measuring the percentage of radioactivity excreted in the stools as a result of the migration of radiolabelled leucocytes into the intestinal lumen. In normal subjects, this is less than 2% in the 4 days after the scan. Affected bowel is usually detected 3 hours after the injection.

The BW250/183 monoclonal antibody has given good results in the study of chronic inflammatory bowel disease. Accumulation increased over 24 hours after the injection, but there was no excretion of the radiolabel into the intestinal lumen and quantitative studies could not be performed. In a recent study, ^{123}I-labelled IL-2 was successfully used in patients with Crohn's disease for the detection of bowel infiltrating lymphocytes [27]. Nanocolloids cannot be reliably used for the study of gastrointestinal inflammation, probably owing to the slow and low uptake and also due to the physiological intestinal excretion of the tracer [33].

AUTOIMMUNE THYROID DISEASES

Autoimmune thyroid diseases, including Graves' disease, primary myxoedema and Hashimoto's thyroiditis, appear related in certain aspects of their pathogenesis and clinical course. Evidence of humoral immunity is provided in all of these disorders by the presence of antibodies against thyroid peroxidase (formerly known as microsomal antigen) and often against thyroglobulin. Titres tend to be highest in Hashimoto's disease and lowest in primary hypothyroidism at the time it is diagnosed. More specific to Graves' disease are circulating autoantibodies that are capable of binding to the thyroid-stimulating hormone receptor (TSHr) on the surface of thyroid cells, and stimulate cell growth and hormone production. However, these factors are also sometimes found in the serum of patients with Hashimoto's disease.

Graves' disease, primary myxoedema and Hashimoto's thyroiditis all share evidence of cell-mediated immunity against thyroid antigens, and are characterized by a varying degree of infiltration by lymphocytes and plasma cells. The infiltrating cells collect in aggregates, forming lymphoid follicles with germinal centres [34,35].

Exophthalmos is a frequent manifestation of Graves' disease that may lead to severe complications. It is caused by muscle hypertrophy and lymphocytic infiltration of the retro-orbital space, that may eventually turn into fibrosis. Exophthalmos is usually treated with corticosteroids and/or cyclosporin, or by local X-ray therapy. It would be extremely important to be able to diagnose the state of activity of the disease and to differentiate between active infiltration and fibrosis, because of the difference in their treatment.

Current diagnosis of thyroid autoimmunity is based on the detection of autoantibodies (anti-TSHr, anti-TPO and anti-TG), and clinical signs and symptoms. However, the relationship between autoantibodies and disease activity is still unclear, and it is generally believed that the activity of the autoimmune process is determined by the intensity of intra-thyroidal lymphocytic infiltration. *In vivo* measurement of thyroid cellular infiltration, particularly in patients with undetectable serum thyroid autoantibodies, would be ideal for evaluating the disease activity, determining the need for therapy and for monitoring the efficacy of treatment.

Accumulation of ^{111}In-labelled lymphocytes has been shown in the thyroid glands of patients with Hashimoto's thyroiditis (Plate 3) and primary myxoedema, but not in patients with Graves' disease [8].

The use of ^{111}In-octreotide has also been investigated in patients with Graves' disease, and a positive correlation between disease activity and accumulation of the agent in the thyroid and retro-orbital space of patients with exophthalmos has been reported [24,36]. However, these findings have not been confirmed by other investigators [37,38]. Further studies are required to help elucidate the potential value of this compound in Graves' disease.

In a recent study in patients with Hashimoto's thyroiditis, it was possible to highlight the presence of activated lymphocytes by gamma-camera imaging using ^{99m}Tc-labelled IL-2 (Plate 4). No correlation was detected between the degree of thyroid accumulation of ^{99m}Tc-IL-2 and the autoantibody titre [26]. This interesting finding suggests that the humoral immunity and cell-mediated immunity are not directly related, and that both should be evaluated for the assessment of disease activity.

COELIAC DISEASE

Coeliac disease is characterized by a mononuclear cell infiltration of intestinal mucosa, mainly localized in the duodenum and jejunum [30]. Diagnosis of the disease is based on the detection of anti-gliadin and anti-endomysium antibodies, and the more important histological finding of lymphocytic infiltration and atrophy of the mucosa. Biopsy can be performed, only down to the first loop of the jejunum; with more distal involvement, biopsy is likely to produce false-negative results.

The opportunity of detecting the presence of lymphocytic infiltration by external imaging could be used as an alternative to biopsy, and has the advantages of being non-invasive and of delineating the full extent of the disease. In this respect, attempts made by using radiolabelled IL-2 scintigraphy have been encouraging [27]. This technique may help to evaluate correctly the extent and severity of the disease, together with the possibility to follow-up the efficacy of diet (Plate 5). An important application of this technique can be the screening for coeliac disease in at-risk subjects and the siblings of patients discordant for jejunal biopsy and autoantibodies.

TYPE 1 DIABETES MELLITUS

Type 1 (insulin-dependent) diabetes mellitus (IDDM), is a disease characterized by an auto-immune destruction of insulin-secreting β-cells, mediated by mononuclear cells. Chronic lymphocytic infiltration of β-cells is observed in two animal models of IDDM – the bio-breeding (BB) rat and the non-obese diabetic (NOD) mouse, long before the onset of hyperglycaemia, and persists until the clinical onset [39]. In humans, lymphocytic infiltration of the endocrine pancreas is observed in patients soon after the diagnosis of diabetes [40], and a preclinical period of infiltration is thought to be present long before the clinical onset of the disease [41].

Indirect signs of the ongoing autoimmune process include the appearance in the peripheral blood of islet cell antibodies (ICA), insulin autoantibodies (IAA) and other circulating markers [42,43]. Their relation with the underlying autoimmune process however, is unknown, and a significant number of subjects with autoantibodies do not develop clinical diabetes [44].

An ability to detect lymphocytic infiltration before the clinical onset of the disease could be used for the selection of patients for preventive therapeutic trials and for monitoring the efficacy of therapy regimens.

There have been attempts to detect pancreatic lymphocytic infiltration in the past by using autologous radiolabelled lymphocytes. Kaldany, *et al.* [7] attempted to image the infiltrated pancreas in a few newly diagnosed patients but without convincing and conclusive results. Gallina *et al.* [45] showed that ^{111}In-labelled lymphocytes did not image the infiltrated pancreas in BB rats. This might be explained by the pathophysiology of the immune process that leads to β-cell destruction. It is a slowly progressive phenomenon that is thought to be operative for years before the clinical diagnosis; moreover, infiltrating cells are supposed to be generated by *in situ* clonal expansion and not through migration from the peripheral blood. A recent study on pancreas sections obtained from newly diagnosed diabetic patients showed a typical finding of cell-mediated immunity: among infiltrating cells, over 80% were lymphocytes, the majority of which were CD8-positive; moreover, there was no accumulation of IgG or C3 in the infiltrated islets of Langerhans, and within a panel of adhesion molecules studied, only ICAM-1 was moderately hyperexpressed on very few endothelial cells [46]. The lack of haemodynamic changes and of endothelial activation support the *in situ* clonal expansion hypothesis, and provides an explanation for the failure of autologous lymphocytes to migrate and to image the infiltrated pancreas in this pathological condition.

A preliminary study with radiolabelled IL-2 in high-risk subjects showed that this technique may be useful for early diagnosis of pancreatic infiltration and possibly for monitoring the efficacy of preventive treatments [47].

Finally, a significant accumulation of radiolabelled HIg has been shown in the pancreas of approximately 50% of newly diagnosed type 1 diabetic patients [48], probably as a consequence of the presence of immune complexes or secondary to increased vascular permeability. This may help identify patients who may benefit from adjuvant immunotherapy at the time of diagnosis, with an aim to induce clinical remission.

REFERENCES

1. Wall, J.R., Baur, R., Schleusener, H. and Bandy-Dafoe, P. (1983) Peripheral blood and intrathyroidal mononuclear cell populations in patients with autoimmune thyroid disorders enumerated using monoclonal antibodies. *J. Clin. Endocrinol. Metab.*, **56**, 164–8.
2. Selby, W.S., Janossy, G., Bosil, M. and Jewell, D.P. (1984) Intestinal lymphocyte subpopulations in inflammatory bowel disease: an analysis by immunohistological and cell isolation techniques. *Gut*, **25**, 32–40.
3. Foulis, A.K., Liddle, C.N., Farquharson, M.A., Richmond, J.A. and Weir, R.S. (1986) The histopathology of the pancreas in type 1 (insulin-dependent) diabetes mellitus: a 25-year review of deaths in patients under 20 years of age in the United Kingdom. *Diabetologia*, **29**, 267–74.
4. Pallone, F., Fais, S., Squarcia, O., Biancone, L., Pozzilli, P. and Boirivant, M. (1987) Activation of peripheral and intestinal lamina propria lymphocytes in Crohn's disease. In vivo state of activation and in vitro response to stimulation as defined by the expression of early activation antigens. *Gut*, **28**, 745–9.
5. Giananni, R., Pugliese, A., Bonner-Weir, S., Shiffrin, A.J., Soeldner, J.S., Erlich, H., Awdeh, Z., Alper, C.A., Jackson, R.A. and Eisenbarth, G.S. (1992) Prognostically significant heterogeneity of cytoplasmic islet cell antibodies in relatives of patients with type I diabetes. *Diabetes*, **41**, 347–53.
6. Lavender, J.P., Goldman, J.M., Arnot, R.N. and Thakur, M.L. (1977) Kinetics of indium-111-labelled lymphocytes in normal subjects and in patients with Hodgkin's disease. *Br. Med. J.*, **2**, 797–9.
7. Kaldany, A., Hill, T., Wentworth, S., Brink, S.J., D'Elia, J.A., Clouse, M. and Soeldner, J.S. (1982) Trapping of peripheral blood lymphocytes in the pancreas of patients with acute-onset insulin-dependent diabetes mellitus. *Diabetes*, **31**, 463–6.
8. Pozzilli, P., Pozzilli, C., Pantano, P., Negri, M., Andreani, D. and Cudworth, A.G. (1983) Tracking of indium-111-oxine-labelled lymphocytes in autoimmune thyroid disease. *Clin. Endocrinol. (Oxford)*, **19**, 111–16.

9. Ten Berge, R.J.M., Natarajan, A.T., Hardeman, M.R., van Royen, E.A. and Schellekens, P. (1983) Labelling with Indium-111 has detrimental effects on human lymphocytes: concise communication. *J. Nucl. Med.*, **24**, 615–20.

10. Signore, A., Beales, P., Sensi, M., Zuccarini, O. and Pozzilli, P. (1983) Labelling of lymphocytes with Indium-111-oxine: effect on cell surface phenotype and antibody-dependent cellular cytotoxicity. *Immunol. Lett.*, **6**,151–4.

11. Zakhireh, B., Thakur, M.L., Malech, H.L., Cohen, M.S., Gottschalk, A. and Root, R.K. (1979) Indium-111-labeled polymorphonuclear leukocytes: viability, random migration, chemotaxis, bactericidal capacity and ultrastructure. *J. Nucl. Med.*, **20**, 741–7.

12. Peters, A.M. (1994) The utility of ^{99m}Tc-HMPAO-leukocytes for imaging infection. *Semin. Nucl. Med.*, **24**, 110–27.

13. De Schrijver, M., Streule, K., Senekowitsch, R. and Fridrich, R. (1987) Scintigraphy of inflammation with nanometer-sized colloidal tracers. *Nucl. Med. Commun.*, **8**, 895–908.

14. McAfee, J.G., Gagne, G., Subramanian, G. and Schneider, R.F. (1991) The localisation of indium-111-leucocytes, gallium-67, polyclonal IgG and other radioactive agents in acute focal inflammatory lesions. *J. Nucl. Med.*, **32**, 2126–31.

15. Fischmann, A.J., Rubin, R.H., Khaw, B.A., Callhan, R.J., Wilkinson, R., Keech, F., Nedelman, M., Dragotakes, S., Kramer, P.B. and LaMuraglia, G.M. (1988) Detection of acute inflammation with ^{111}In-labelled nonspecific polyclonal IgG. *Semin. Nucl. Med.*, **18**, 335–44.

16. Oyen, W.J.G., van Horn, J.R., Claessens, R.A.M.J., Sloof, T.J.J.H., van der Meer, W.M.J. and Corstens, F.H.M. (1992) Diagnosis of bone, joint and joint prosthesis infections with indium-111-labelled human immunoglobulin G scintigraphy. *Radiology*, **182**, 195–9.

17. Kinne, R.W., Becker, W., Schwab, J., Horneff, G., Schwarz, A., Kalden, J.R., Emmrich, F., Burmester, G.R. and Wolf, F. (1993) Comparison of ^{99m}Tc-labelled specific murine anti-CD4 monoclonal antibodies and nonspecific human immunoglobulins for imaging inflamed joints in rheumatoid arthritis. *Nucl. Med. Commun.*, **14**, 667–75.

18. Marcus, C., Thakur, M.L., Huynh, T.V., Louie, J.S., Leibling, M., Minami, C. and Diggles, L. (1994) Imaging rheumatic joint disease with anti-T lymphocyte antibody OKT-3. *Nucl. Med. Commun.*, **15**, 824–30.

19. Becker, W., Goldenberg, G.M. and Wolf, F. (1994) The use of monoclonal antibodies and antibodies fragments in the imaging of infectious lesions. *Semin. Nucl. Med.*, **24**, 1–13.

20. Krenning, E.P., Kwekkeboom, D.J., Pauwels, S., Kvols, L.K. and Reubi, J.C. (1995) Somatostatin receptor scintigraphy. *Nucl. Med. Annual*, 1–50.

21. Reubi, J.C., Waser, B., Horisberger, U., Krenning, E., Lamberts, S.W.J., Gebbers, J.O., Gersbach, P. and Laissue, J.A. (1993) In vitro autoradiographic and in vivo scintigraphic localisation of somatostatin receptors in human lymphatic tissue. *Blood*, **82**, 2143–51.

22. Reubi, J.C., Mazzucchelli, L. and Laissue, J. (1994) Intestinal vessels express a high density of somatostatin receptor in human inflammatory bowel disease. *Gastroenterology*, **106**, 951–9.

23. Van Hagen, P.M., Markusse, H.M., Lamberts, S.W.J., Kwekkeboom, D.J., Reubi, J.C. and Krenning, E.S.P. (1994) Somatostatin receptor imaging: the presence of somatostatin receptor in rheumatoid arthritis. *Arthritis Rheum.*, **37**, 1521–7.

24. Postema, P.T.E., Wijnggaarde, R., Vandenbosch, W.A., Koij, P.P.M., Oei, H.Y., Hennemann, G., Lamberts, S.W.J. and Krenning, E.P. (1995). Follow-up in (In-111-DTPA-D-Phe-1)octreotide scintigraphy in thyroidal and orbital Graves' disease (abstract). *J. Nucl. Med.*, **36** (Suppl.), 203P.

25. Signore, A., Parman, A., Pozzilli, P., Andreani D. and Beverley, P.C.L. (1987) Detection of activated lymphocytes in endocrine pancreas of BB/W rats by injection of 123-iodine-labelled interleukin-2: an early sign of Type 1 diabetes. *Lancet*, **2**, 536–40.

26. Chianelli, M., Signore, A., Biassoni, L., Sobnak, R., Procaccini, E., Ronga, G., Plowman, N., Grossman, A., Britton, K.E. and Mather, S.J. (1995) In vivo targetting of activated lymphocytes by ^{99m}Tc-labelled IL2. Biodistribution in normal subjects and studies in patients (abstract). *J. Nucl. Med.*, **36** (Suppl.), 228P.

27. Signore, A., Picarelli, A., Chianelli, M., Biancone, L., Annovazzi, A., Tiberti, C., Anastasi, E., Multari, G., Negri, M., Pallone, F. and Pozzilli, P. (1996) 123I-Interleukin-2 scintigraphy: a new approach to assess disease activity in autoimmunity. *J. Pediatr. Endocrinol. Metab.*, **9**(Suppl.1), 139–44.

28. De Bois, M.H.W., Pauwels, E.K.J. and Breedveld, F.C. (1995) New agents for scintigraphy in rheumatoid arthritis. *Eur. J. Nucl. Med.*, **22**, 1339–46.

29. Liberatore, M., Clemente, M., Iurilli, A.P., Zorzin, L., Masini, M., Di Rocco, E. and Centi Colella, A. (1992) Scintigraphic evaluation of disease activity in rheumatoid arthritis: a comparison of technetium-99m human non-specific immunoglobulins, leucocytes and albumin nanocolloids. *Eur. J. Nucl. Med.*, **19**, 853–7.

30. Podolsky, D.K. (1991) Inflammatory bowel disease (I). *N. Engl. J. Med.*, **325**, 928–38.

31. Podolsky, D.K. (1991) Inflammatory bowel disease (II). *N. Engl. J. Med.*, **325**, 1008–18.

32. Saverymuttu, S.H., Peters, A.M., Crofton, M.E., Rees, H., Lavender, J.P., Hodgson, H.J. and Chadwick, V.S. (1985) ^{111}Indium autologous granulocytes in the detection of inflammatory bowel disease. *Gut*, **26**, 955–60.

33. Wheeler, J.G., Slack, N.F., Duncan, A., Palmer, H. and Harvey, R.F. (1990). Tc-99m-nanocolloids in inflammatory bowel disease. *Nucl. Med. Commun.*, **11**, 127–33.

34. Weetman, A.P. and McGregor, A.M. (1984) Autoimmune thyroid disease: developments in our understanding. *Endocr. Rev.*, **5**, 309–15.

35. DeGroot, L.J. and Quintans, J. (1989) The causes of autoimmune thyroid disease. *Endocr. Rev.*, **10**, 537–57.

36. Diaz, M., Bokisch, A., Kahaly, G. and Hahn, K. (1993) Preliminary results of somatostatin receptor scintigraphy in endocrine ophthalmology. *Eur. J. Nucl. Med.*, **20**, 844 (abstract).

37. Eberhardt, J.U., Oberwöhrmann, S., Clausen, M., Schulte, H., Epe, B. and Henze, E. (1993) Accumulation of ^{111}In-Octreotide in the orbital and thyroid regions of patients with Graves' disease and with exophthalmos. *Eur. J. Nucl. Med.*, **20**, 844 (abstract).

38. Bohuslavizki, K.H., Oberwörhmann, S., Brenner, W., Eberhardt, J.U., Mönig, H., Clasen, M., Sippel, C., Wolf, H., Epe, B. and Henze, E. (1995) ^{111}In-octreotide imaging in patients with long-standing Graves' ophthalmopathy. *Nucl. Med. Commun.*, **16**, 912–16.

39. Makino, S., Kunimoto, K., Muraoka, Y., Katagiri, K. and Tochino, Y. (1980) Breeding of a non-obese, diabetic strain of mice. *Exp. Anim.*, **29**, 1.

40. Bottazzo, G.F., Dean, B.M., McNally, J.M., MacKay, E.H., Swift, P.G.F. and Gamble, D.R. (1985) In situ characterization of autoimmune phenomena and expression of HLA molecules in the pancreas in diabetic insulitis. *N. Engl. J. Med.*, **313**, 353–60.

41. Eisenbarth, G.S. (1986) Type I diabetes: a chronic autoimmune disease. *N. Engl. J. Med.*, **314**, 1360–7.

42. Lendrup, R., Walker, G., Cudworth, A.G., Theophanides, C., Pyke, D.A., Bloom, A. and Gamble, D.R. (1976) Islet-cell antibodies in diabetes mellitus. *Lancet*, **ii**, 1273–6.

43. Dean, B.M., Becker, F., McNally, J.M., Tarn, A.C., Schwartz, G. and Bottazzo, G.F. (1986) Insulin autoantibodies in the pre-diabetic period: correlation with islet cell antibodies and development of diabetes. *Diabetologia*, **29**, 339–42.

44. McCulloch, D.K., Claff, L.J., Kahn, S.E. *et al.* (1990) Subclinical beta-cell dysfunction is not always progressive among first-degree relatives of Type I diabetes: five years' follow-up of the Seattle study. *Diabetes*, **39**, 549–56.

45. Gallina, D.L., Pelletier, D., Doherty, P., Koevary, S.B., Williams, L.M., Like, A.A., Chick, W.L. and Rossini, A.A. (1985) [111]Indium-labelled lymphocytes do not image or label the pancreas of BB/W rats. *Diabetologia*, **28**, 143–7.

46. Somoza, N., Vargas, F., Roura-Mir, C. *et al.* (1994) Pancreas in recent onset insulin-dependent diabetes mellitus changes in HLA, adhesion molecules and autoantigens, restricted T cell receptor Vb usage, and cytokine profile. *J. Immunol.*, **153**, 1360–77.

47. Signore, A., Chianelli, M., Picarelli, A., Ferretti, E., Multari, G. and Pozzilli, P. (1995) In vivo detection of pancreatic T-lymphocytes: a new tool for IDDM prediction? *Autoimmunity*, **21** (Suppl.), P64.

48. Signore, A., Barone, R., Procaccini, E., Annovazzi, A., Chianelli, M., Scopinaro, F., Ronga, G., Multari, G., Looman, W.J.M. and Pozzilli, P. (1996) In vivo measurement of immunoglobulin accumulation in the pancreas of recent onset type 1 diabetic patients. *Clin. Exp. Rheumatol.*, **14** (Suppl.15), S41–5.

FURTHER READING

Chianelli, M., Mather, S.J., Martin-Comin, J. and Signore, A. (1997) Radiopharmaceuticals for the study of inflammatory processes: a review. *Nucl. Med. Commun.*, **18**, 437–55.

Higgins, C.B. and Auffermann, W. (1994) *Endocrine Imaging*, Thieme Medical Publishers, Inc., New York.

Roitt, I. (1994) *Essential Immunology*, 8th edn, Blackwell Scientific Publications, London.

CHAPTER 6

Cardiovascular

Myocardial ischaemia

P. Rigo and T. Benoit

INTRODUCTION

The first application of a tracer technique in humans was the measurement of cardiovascular physiological function, when Blumgart, in 1927, used the timing of a tracer injected into a peripheral vein to measure circulation times in health and disease [1]. Subsequently, this was developed by Veal, Prinzmetal and others, as a method of measuring cardiac output and pulmonary transit times. This has evolved into a wide variety of highly sophisticated functional imaging and measurement techniques, which continues to contribute to our understanding of cardiac physiology and the management of patients with cardiac diseases.

Nuclear medicine techniques rely on the tracer principle to provide information on the cardiovascular system without interfering with its function. Despite their considerable sophistication, the resolution of the imaging equipment remains rather gross (around 1 cm for single-photon emission and 0.5 cm for positron emission tomography). The selectivity of the tracers provides functional rather than morphological information at the capillary, cellular or even molecular level [2]. For instance, perfusion can be assessed either as the retention of labelled microspheres at the capillary level, normalized for the input function, or as the cellular

uptake of compounds with a high extraction, trapped into the cell as a result of passive diffusion, active transport, membrane potential, metabolism or combination thereof. As another example, the use of ligands and specially receptor antagonists offers for the first time the possibility to study ligand–receptor activity *in vivo*. In most situations, the nuclear medicine techniques provide functional information that complements the anatomical information available through radiological techniques, or quantitative measurements that are more difficult or impossible to obtain using echography or other techniques.

The principal nuclear cardiology studies are concerned with the assessment of regional perfusion, the measurement of global and regional ventricular function and circulatory dynamics, the identification of myocardial necrosis, the measurement of myocardial metabolism and the evaluation of the integrity of myocardial neurohumoral control. Nuclear medicine techniques are also available to assess the pulmonary and systemic circulations.

Coronary artery disease (CAD) is the most important cardiac pathology in the adult population of the Western world, which leads to abnormal myocardial perfusion and myocardial ischaemia that may result in angina, impaired myocardial function, myocardial infarction and/or sudden death. Coronary angiography is routinely used to demonstrate the morphological abnormalities of the coronary artery system, and describe them in terms of the most severe narrowing in the three major coronary arteries. This approach ignores

Clinical Nuclear Medicine, 3rd edn. Edited by M.N. Maisey, K.E. Britton and B.D. Collier. Published in 1998 by Chapman & Hall, London. ISBN 0 412 75180 1

however, the length of lesions, their presence in series and the diffuseness of arterial involvement. Comparative studies of angiography and physiological measurements of coronary flow have shown that the angiographic estimates of severity correlate poorly with true obstruction, except when the stenosis is very severe (>90%) or very slight (<10%) [3]. Nuclear medicine provides techniques able to demonstrate the functional consequences of coronary artery stenoses that are most importantly abnormalities of regional and global myocardial perfusion and function. This will be the primary focus of this chapter.

ANATOMY AND PATHOPHYSIOLOGY

A knowledge of the anatomy and physiology of the coronary circulation as well as of the haemodynamic effects of coronary stenosis is required to fully understand and interpret cardiac imaging studies.

ANATOMY

Coronary arteries

The coronary vascular supply is through three main vessels: the left anterior descending and the circumflex (major branches of the left main coronary artery), and the right coronary artery. These give off numerous branches (of variable physiological importance), the diagonal and marginal branches being the largest. The left coronary artery predominates in humans, but there is considerable inter-individual variation in the contribution of the right coronary artery. Three types of distribution are described depending on the origin of the posterior descending branches: most often (in 84%) this branch originates from the right coronary artery (right predominant distribution); in 12% of the cases, it originates from the left circumflex (left distribution); and in about 4% of the population, there are two posterior descending branches (balanced distribution).

These anatomical variations complicate the relationship between individual arteries and their myocardial territories of supply. It is usual to assign the anterior wall and septum to the left anterior descending, the lateral wall to the circumflex, and the inferior wall to the posterior descending branch, or more precisely if the type of coronary distribution is known. The apex can be supplied by any of the three main arteries.

Coronary collaterals

Coronary arteries do not behave as terminal arteries as collateral channels are potentially present. Underdeveloped in normal individuals, they become critically important in patients with progressively developing significant coronary artery lesions. However, coronary collaterals also appear as a marker of the severity of coronary lesions. Patients with collaterals therefore frequently have more symptoms and signs of ischaemia than patients without collaterals, and the effectiveness of collaterals to protect the myocardium has been the subject of debate. Data in patients with complete occlusion but no infarct attest to the potential effectiveness of collateral protection. Thallium-201 has also been used in selected patients with multiple vessel disease to demonstrate relative collateral protection [4]. Overall, patients with severe coronary artery disease and collaterals are more likely to develop scintigraphic abnormalities at exercise, and specially under vasodilator stress, than patients without collaterals.

CORONARY BLOOD FLOW REGULATION

Oxygen demand and flow coupling

Myocardial oxygen requirements are high, even at rest (6–8 ml/min/100 g), and increase with cardiac work. Volume of work can be increased without a proportional increase in oxygen consumption, but there can be up to five-fold increase with changes in pressure, contractility and heart rate.

The most potent factor regulating coronary flow is the tight coupling between flow and myocardial oxygen demand that appears to adapt on a beat-by-beat basis to oxygen consumption. Indeed, changes in oxygen extraction are limited by the high basal oxygen extraction in the coronary circulation.

Numerous other factors intervene to regulate the coronary circulation. Among them, it is important to consider the left ventricular compression forces, the diastolic time (as coronary flow occurs mainly in diastole), capillary recruitment, perfusion pressure, neural regulation (parasympathetic and sympathetic innervation and humoral effects), endothelium-derived vasoactive substances, as well as changes induced by metabolic demands or drugs.

Coronary autoregulation

The various individual factors regulating myocardial blood flow result in an integrated mechanism known as coronary autoregulation. Due to this phenomenon, coronary artery resistance adjusts to balance changes in perfusion over a wide range of pressures (from 50 to 150 mmHg) and maintain a relatively constant coronary flow.

Reactive hyperaemia

Changes in coronary resistance are also responsible for the development of reactive hyperaemia. This phenomenon mediates an immediate rise in coronary blood flow, upon release of a temporary occlusion, even of brief duration. This rise is out of proportion to the oxygen debt incurred during occlusion and sufficient to repay this debt three to five times. Release of the endothelium-derived relaxant factor and other mediators, and contribution of ATP-sensitive potassium channels, appear responsible for reactive hyperaemia, but no single factor or mechanism regulates coronary flow, in all or even in specific circumstances.

Coronary flow reserve

The interaction between coronary perfusion pressure and coronary artery resistance is also illustrated by variations in coronary flow reserve. Coronary flow at rest remains normal during progressive coronary artery narrowing as a result of changes in distal resistance until the arterial lumen is severely reduced to stenosis reflecting advanced disease (±90%). However, the capacity to increase flow to high levels, in response to exercise or pharmacological stimulation, becomes impaired with mild coronary artery stenosis. Coronary flow reserve in normal and stenotic coronary arteries was first described by Gould *et al.* in 1974 [5] (Figure 6.1). It is defined as the ratio of maximum flow under stress or pharmacological vasodilatation to resting flow. Coronary flow reserve begins to decrease in the presence of a 40–50% diameter stenosis, provided a stimulus increasing normal flow to 4–5 times the baseline value is used. It is abolished for 90% stenoses when resting flow begins to drop.

Variations in distal coronary resistance at rest explain maintenance of normal resting flow in the presence of proximal stenosis, as the perfusion pressure responsible for flow is the total pressure across the proximal and distal vascular bed, including the site of stenosis. As long as the resistance at the level of the stenosis is smaller than the distal bed resistance, it has little effect on flow.

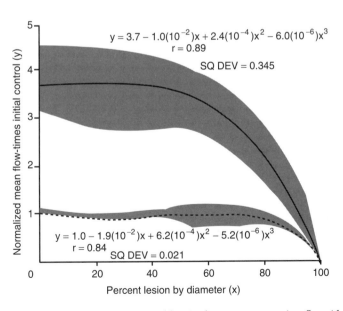

Figure 6.1   Effect of the progressive reduction in vessel luminal patency on resting flow (dashed line) and hyperaemic response (solid line) in experimental animals. (Reproduced with permission from Gould *et al.* [5].)

When the stenosis becomes more severe however, the distal bed becomes fully dilated and loses its ability to autoregulate, leading to fall in resting coronary flow with further stenosis. This reasoning outlined here for single coronary artery lesions is also valid for stenoses in series.

Changes in cardiac work-load conditions such as changes in aortic pressure and heart rate, can alter resting or maximum coronary flow. Absolute coronary flow reserve, defined as the maximum flow divided by the resting flow (measured by flowmeter), is therefore not load-independent. Relative maximal flow reserve, defined as maximum flow in the stenotic artery normalized to normal maximum flow in the absence of stenosis, is however, load-independent.

Imaging relative flow reserve

Nuclear medicine myocardial perfusion studies are based on the concept of relative coronary flow reserve [5]. Flow reserve in myocardial territories supplied by stenotic arteries is compared with flow reserve in regions with intact arteries and flow (Figure 6.2). Even in patients with severe multiple vessel disease, an area usually persists with normal or near-normal perfusion that can serve as reference. However, in patients with severe balanced lesions, underestimation of disease severity is possible, but this has not proven a frequent problem in clinical practice.

The relative distribution of flow and perfusion tracers reflects the effects of stenosis independent of other physiological parameters (i.e. pressure, work-load, hypertrophy, vasomotor tone, etc.), and provides unique information complementary to morphological data and even to absolute flow data. Alteration of regional coronary flow reserve is the first parameter to be compromised when there is a stenotic lesion of a coronary artery. A 40–50% stenosis will decrease the measured coronary reserve and can be detected by perfusion imaging using techniques, whether exercise or vasodilator or inotropic drug, that induce marked increase in coronary blood flow and unmask focally diminished flow reserve without necessarily producing ischaemia or regional dysfunction. Myocardial ischaemia, when present, can further affect the loading conditions, and results in decreased regional coronary flow, further enhancing the discrepancy between regions with abnormal and normal flow reserve [6].

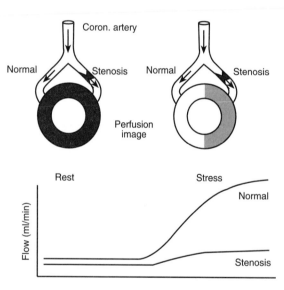

Figure 6.2 Schematic representation of the principle of rest/stress myocardial perfusion imaging. Resting flow and flow reserve in myocardial territories supplied by a stenotic artery (right) is compared with flow reserve in regions with intact arteries and flow (left). At rest, blood flow is normal and homogeneous. At stress, flow increases more in the normal vessel than in the stenosed vessel and resulting flow and tracer distribution is heterogeneous. [Reproduced with permission from Wackers, F.J.Th., *J. Nucl. Med.*, **35**, 729 (1994).]

Available methods to increase coronary blood flow

Dynamic exercise is most frequently used to increase coronary blood flow, and results in a large increase in cardiac output and decrease in systemic vascular resistance. The sympathetic drive induces vasoconstriction of capacitance veins, and combines with the pumping effect of muscular contraction and decreased systemic resistance to increase venous return and ventricular volume. Stroke volume increases as a result of both the Frank–Starling effect and increased contractility. Blood pressure also increases together with the stroke volume and heart rate. Myocardial wall tension and myocardial oxygen demand therefore also rise. The increased myocardial oxygen demand associated with dynamic exercise is the potential cause of myocardial ischaemia. The ability of exercise to achieve maximal flow is limited and depends on patients' activity, and on symptoms such as dyspnoea, fatigue, claudication, arthritis or chest pain.

It is also possible to increase coronary blood flow using drugs such as dipyridamole, adenosine and dobutamine. Dipyridamole is capable of increasing coronary blood flow five-fold. Its mechanism of action has not been fully elucidated, but probably involves an increase in local adenosine levels. Combined with exercise, it is capable of increasing coronary blood flow even further. Adenosine is produced naturally by myocardial cells in response to hypoxia or increased oxygen demand. It is a potent vasodilator, acting on specific adenosine receptors. This produces a rise in intracellular cAMP level, which in turn leads to vascular smooth muscle relaxation. Dobutamine has predominantly β_1 agonist activity. It produces a dose-related increase in myocardial oxygen demand and increases coronary blood flow approximately two-fold.

RELATIONSHIP BETWEEN FLOW, METABOLISM AND FUNCTION

Myocardial ischaemia

Myocardial ischaemia occurs whenever the balance between the oxygen demand and myocardial blood flow delivery is altered. The condition can therefore result either from a transient reduction in coronary blood flow or from an increased myocardial oxygen demand without appropriate increase in blood flow.

Transient or permanent reduction in coronary blood flow occurs as a result of vasoconstriction, platelet aggregation, coronary thrombosis or other causes. The mechanisms involved in clinical spontaneous ischaemic syndromes are believed to be vasoconstriction in variant angina, platelet aggregation in unstable angina and coronary thrombosis in acute myocardial infarction. Alterations in coronary blood flow, among other factors, are also involved in chronic stable angina. Indeed, chronic angina results primarily from an increase in myocardial oxygen demand unmatched by a concomitant increase in flow because of a fixed coronary lesion limiting the regional flow reserve. Symptoms of myocardial ischaemia are usually quite predictable due to the fixed nature of the atherosclerotic lesion. They are, however, modulated by baseline myocardial oxygen consumption and by variations in the previously described factors affecting coronary blood flow.

Variation in myocardial oxygen consumption results from voluntary or involuntary changes in cardiac activity. Oxygen demand mainly depends on the pressure developed by the contractile ventricles as well as the frequency of this pressure generation. A smaller demand is related to myocardial contractility, while the mechanical work itself is undemanding. The integrated area below the ventricular pressure curve over time (tension–time index) is linearly related to oxygen consumption. It is clinically approximated by the product of rate and pressure. Changes in heart rate and/or blood pressure are therefore usually associated with clinical symptoms of ischaemia.

Ischaemic cascade

As seen earlier, the cascade of abnormalities resulting from coronary artery lesions and leading to myocardial ischaemia begins with impaired flow reserve (Figure 6.3). A relative decrease in blood flow is then successively associated with metabolic, functional (first diastolic then systolic) and electrocardiographic abnormalities. The symptoms of angina pectoris are a rather late sign and may be missing. Decreased delivery of oxygen results in cessation of aerobic metabolism, increased anaerobic utilization of glucose with lactic acid production, and acidosis and energy depletion. Reduction in myocardial blood flow promptly results in a decrease in regional ventricular function (Figure 6.4), apparently related to an inability to cycle calcium normally to the myofilament, and associated with a depletion in high-energy phosphates. Prolonged ischaemic episodes can lead to progressive cellular necrosis involving, in order of priority, the vulnerable subendocardial layers of the myocardium and progressing toward

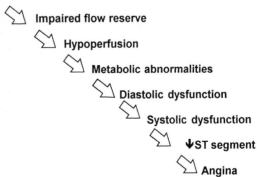

Figure 6.3 Cascade of abnormalities resulting from coronary lesion and progressing to clinical angina.

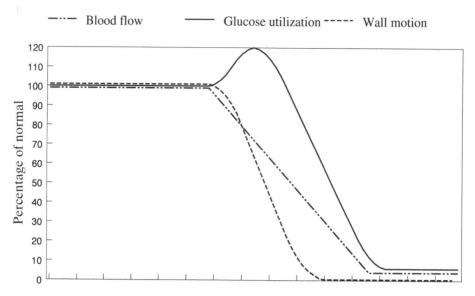

Figure 6.4 Schematic diagram illustrating the relationship between blood flow, myocardial wall motion and glucose utilization with ischaemia of progressive severity. Glucose utilization may first be enhanced in mild to moderate ischaemia (especially in relation to blood flow); however, it decreases in severe ischaemia and necrosis.

the epicardium. Ischaemic alterations are usually completely reversible if flow is restored within 15–20 minutes, but clinical and experimental situations have been described where dysfunction persists in the absence of progression to myocardial infarction. As some of these patients may benefit from revascularization procedures, the need for diagnostic assessment of these conditions has become important in patients with CAD and depressed left ventricular function.

Myocardial stunning

The term myocardial stunning has been coined by Braunwald and Rutherford [7] based on initial experimental evidence by Heyndrickx *et al.* [8]. It is a form of myocardial injury that results in prolonged impairment of contractile function following blood flow restoration to previously ischaemic myocardium. This regional dysfunction resolves spontaneously over the course of several hours or days without requiring revascularization.

Both ischaemic and reperfusion injuries appear to play a role in stunning, but the exact pathophysiological mechanism remains unclear. Altered calcium kinetics and free radical injury are likely to be involved. An important feature of

stunned myocardium is its maintained reactivity to inotropic stimulation such as adrenergic stimulation (a feature used in dobutamine echocardiography) or to the addition of extracellular calcium.

Initially described in experimental animals, stunning has now been shown to have reasonably frequent clinical occurrence. It is mainly observed in patients submitted to reperfusion therapy for impending myocardial infarction, but can also be encountered after balloon angioplasty and in patients with unstable angina or variant angina.

Myocardial hibernation

In contrast to myocardial stunning where myocardial injury occurs despite or because of reperfusion, the regional left ventricular dysfunction in myocardial hibernation reflects an adaptive new state where myocardial energy requirements adjust to the available blood flow, substrates and oxygen supply.

The pathophysiological mechanisms responsible for myocardial hibernation are not clearly elucidated as there are no experimental models of chronic hibernation. However, short-term models of hibernation exist, and these are mainly based on repetitive episodes of ischaemia leading to functional impairment and matched blood flow changes without persisting metabolic evidence for ischaemia. Inotropic reserve in these models, elicited by catecholamine stimulation, can only be maintained temporarily and disappears with time. Similarly, it has been proposed that myocardial hibernation in humans might be the consequence of multiple ischaemic episodes and represent repetitive episodes of stunning (Figure 6.5). Several groups have used regional myocardial blood flow measurements in patients with CAD and chronic regional left ventricular dysfunction thought to represent hibernation as arguments for this hypothesis [9]. Indeed, they have measured blood flow, within or close to normal range in these cases – results suggestive of a pathophysiological mechanism closer to stunning. These observations require critical reassessment of current hypotheses but several potential problems have to be kept in mind. Some of the perfusion measurements have been performed with water ($H_2^{15}O$) and this PET technique yields measurement of flow to the perfusable tissue rather than to the effective tissue mass and the

perfusable tissue fraction also needs to be taken into account. Further, use of this technique requires the evaluation of large areas defined by regions-of-interest which may dilute results in the most affected regions. It is also possible that hibernation and stunning might coexist in the same patient. Hibernating regions at rest might develop ischaemia during exercise (due to change in left ventricular end diastolic pressure or in perfusion pressure) and post-ischaemic stunning might be superimposed on the basal hibernating state.

The potential heterogeneity of hibernating myocardium is also attested by results of myocardial biopsy samples taken from patients with chronic ischaemic heart disease and contractile dysfunction [10]. In general, in these samples, high-energy phosphate concentrations are not reduced reflecting lack of ongoing ischaemia, but accumulation of glycogen and ultrastructural de-differentiation with loss of sarcomere are heterogeneous and mixed with varying degrees of fibrosis. It is unlikely that de-differentiated myocardium could respond to inotropic stimulation such as with dobutamine.

The clinical importance of stunning and hibernation comes from the potential functional im-

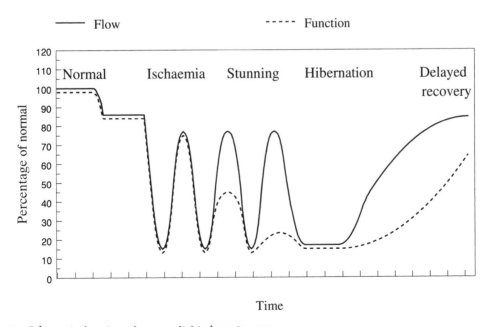

Figure 6.5   Schematic drawing of myocardial ischaemic patterns.

provement implicit in the definition of these abnormalities. Numerous patients suffer from chronic CAD and severe left ventricular dysfunction unresponsive to medical treatment. Bypass surgery is either considered too hazardous because of poor function or is not considered because of lack of angina pectoris. A substantial number of patients with severe CAD or ischaemic cardiomyopathy could benefit from revascularization surgery if they could be positively identified. As we will see later, imaging agents reflecting myocardial blood flow, cation influx or metabolic activity have potential to provide information regarding reversibility of dysfunction. FDG–PET evaluation of glucose metabolism appears as the best method and possibly the only one to reliably differentiate hibernating myocardium from partial necrosis.

EVALUATION OF MYOCARDIAL PERFUSION

PERFUSION TRACERS

The ideal radiopharmaceutical to evaluate regional myocardial perfusion should be taken up by the myocardium in direct linear proportion to flow over a wide range of blood flow values and not be affected by changes in cellular metabolism. It should have a high extraction from the blood on its first passage through the heart, and extraction should not vary with flow. It should remain stable in the myocardium for the period of acquisition, but subsequently rapid elimination should allow repeated studies under different conditions. It should not be toxic, have a high photon flux of gamma rays of optimal energy for detection with a standard gamma-camera (140 keV), have a low radiation burden to the patient, be easy to prepare and in the end be cheap. Unfortunately, none of the available compounds fulfil all these requisites.

Thallium-201

Thallium is the most commonly used radionuclide for myocardial perfusion studies. Because of the large experience with its use – and despite some limitations – it is the standard against which other tracers must be judged. Thallium has a physical half-life of 73 hours. It emits gamma photons (135 and 167 keV with low abundance) but the main emission are the mercury X-rays (69–80 keV; 88% abundance).

Thallium is administered intravenously at a usual dose of 80–120 MBq. Blood clearance of thallium is rapid and it has a high first-pass myocardial extraction (up to 80%). Active transport using the sodium–potassium ATPase-dependent exchange mechanism is responsible for approximately 60% of thallium transfer. The remainder probably enters passively along the electropotential gradient. The extraction efficiency is reduced by acidosis and hypoxaemia, but these effects may not be significant until close to cell death [11]. After its initial distribution, thallium does not remain fixed in the myocardium but is progressively released, and its net extraction diminishes over time (±50% after 5 min). Persistence of thallium in the myocardium over time reflects a dynamic process of continuous uptake and release. This phenomenon can explain the progressive redistribution of thallium after injection at stress or during ischaemia, with gradual normalization of the images reflecting normalization of the haemodynamic conditions. Redistribution requires persistence of an adequate amount of thallium in the circulation from the release by other organs or from reinjection. Reinjection has been recommended because of the reported lack of redistribution to ischaemic non-infarcted tissue, which is attributed to insufficient levels of circulating thallium. Redistribution in hibernating myocardium is more difficult to understand as flow remains abnormal. It could reflect progressive equilibration among regions with different exchange kinetics, or result from alternating episodes of flow improvement following periods of severe flow reduction (repeated stunning hypothesis). Distribution of thallium within the myocardium is not entirely proportional to blood flow, as at high flow rates, extraction becomes rate-limiting. In animal experiments, this proportionality to flow is maintained in non-viable tissues for some time after a prolonged occlusion (3 hours). It is therefore recommended to delay studies aimed at assessing reperfusion to avoid underestimation of infarct size with thallium.

Technetium-labelled agents

The need to develop technetium-labelled myocardial perfusion tracers has arisen from the recognition of the limitations of thallium for this indication including: (i) inadequate physical properties with a long half-life, poor imaging characteristics and high dosimetry; (ii) limitations imposed by thallium redistribution on the realization of acute studies (e.g. during unstable angina or at the acute stage of myocardial infarction) where the need to image immediately after tracer injection and before intervention frequently interferes with the performance of the study; (iii) limitations imposed on diagnosis of reversible perfusion deficits by the lack of complete thallium redistribution; and (iv) the inability of thallium to provide simultaneous evaluation of perfusion and function.

Several technetium-labelled tracers are now available for clinical use. They belong to two main pharmacological classes, lipophilic cations and neutral compounds. The myocardial uptake of lipophilic cations was first noted by Deutsch *et al.* [12] and is a feature common to a wide variety of technetium-99m complex types, including the isonitriles (e.g. sestamibi) and the phosphine complexes (e.g. tetrofosmin and furifosmin).

Sestamibi The blood clearance of sestamibi is very rapid with a $t_{1/2}$ of a few minutes, both at rest and exercise. Its uptake mechanism has been well worked out. Sestamibi diffuses passively through the capillary membrane. Its permeability surface product is lower than that of thallium, resulting in a lower instantaneous extraction than thallium. Sestamibi accumulation in the cell is governed by the transmembrane potential and the Nernst equation, and it accumulates in mitochondria, where its concentration can reach 140 times that of the blood. It remains trapped in living cells, with little secondary release and its net extraction at 5–10 minutes is high (almost equivalent to thallium) (Figure 6.6). Significant redistribution does not occur within 3–4 hours, mainly because the blood activity decreases very rapidly with elimination through the liver and kidneys. The 24-hour urinary excretion is 27% and the 48-hour faecal excretion is 37%. Sestamibi does not appear to be metabolized [13].

Tetrofosmin Several technetium diphosphine complexes have been investigated for myocardial imaging. The DMPE complex had significant heart uptake, but imaging was impaired by high liver uptake and poor blood and liver clearance in humans, in striking opposition to animal data. Functionalized diphosphine complexes like tetrofosmin have had more success. This compound is rapidly cleared from the blood. Its distribution

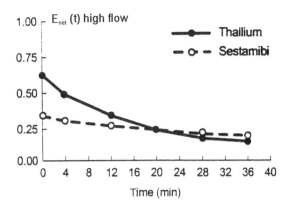

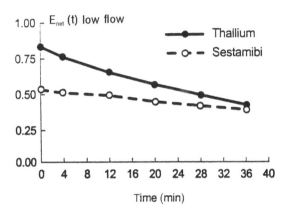

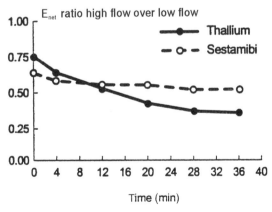

Figure 6.6 Net extraction (E_{net}) of thallium and sestamibi over time at high and low flow. The ratio of E_{net} at high over low flow is potentially indicative of the value to separate regions with normal and abnormal coronary reserve. As is seen from the plot, that ratio decreases with time for thallium while it is more stable for sestamibi. Crossover occurs after 10 minutes. [Data from Marshall *et al.*, *Circulation*, **82**, 998–1007 (1990); reproduced by permission of the American Heart Association.]

into the myocardium is proportional to blood flow, but it also accumulates in other organs (liver, spleen, kidneys and skeletal muscles). There is little redistribution in the myocardium over 3 hours. The mechanism of uptake is probably related to diffusion along an electropotential gradient and similar to that of sestamibi. The excretion is through the hepatobiliary and urinary routes [14].

Furifosmin Another cationic phosphine ligand, Q12, also provides favourable characteristics for myocardial imaging. Its blood clearance is slower than that of the other technetium-labelled compounds, but its liver and gallbladder clearance is faster. The uptake of Q12 in the myocardium follows microsphere determined blood flow linearly up to 2 ml/g/min. Myocardial uptake is 2.3% of the injected dose with no evidence of redistribution. The elimination is both hepatobiliary and renal [15].

Neutral compounds Neutral compounds for myocardial imaging remain unavailable in Europe. Some experience has been accumulated with teboroxime, a lipophilic compound which diffuses quickly into the cell membrane, most likely due to passive transport. The cardiac uptake of teboroxime is high (>3% of the injected dose), the first-pass extraction is >70%, and the myocardial clearance ($t_{1/2}$) is 5–15 minutes. Rapid back-diffusion of the tracer reduces the net extraction however. Imaging must be started immediately, and completed within 5 minutes to compensate for this rapid clearance. Differential washout might provide the equivalent of redistribution.

^{99m}Tc-NOET is a new neutral imaging agent. It has a high first-pass extraction, but slow blood washout (15 and 90 minutes activity of 37% and 18% respectively). Redistribution is observed in models of coronary ligature followed by reperfusion, making this tracer potentially different from the other technetium-labelled agents.

PET perfusion tracers

A number of tracers are available to study myocardial perfusion using PET [16]. ^{11}C-labelled microspheres constitute the reference agent, but require injection in the left atrium or ventricle. Accurate measurement of regional myocardial blood flow can be obtained using this tracer and the reference sample technique.

^{15}O-labelled water, administered either as $C^{15}O_2$ inhalation (owing to rapid transformation in the lungs by carbonic anhydrase) or as $H_2^{15}O$ infusion, has a high extraction and volume of distribution, but requires a PET system capable of fast dynamic acquisitions. Tracer kinetic modelling provides accurate determination of regional myocardial blood flow corrected for spillover of blood activity, partial-volume effect and the incomplete volume of distribution of water. Images of regional myocardial blood flow however, cannot be obtained directly, but require subtraction of the early blood pool phase.

Cationic tracers, such as $^{13}NH_3^+$, ^{82}Rb or ^{38}K, are alternative agents for the assessment of myocardial blood flow. Ammonia is trapped in the cell by incorporation into glutamine while the other cations enter via active transport. Kinetic modelling can be used to calculate myocardial uptake (clearance) of the tracer (FxE) and thereby myocardial blood flow (provided the relation between F and E and between FxE and E is known). As compared with results obtained with similar SPECT cationic tracers, determination of absolute myocardial blood flow yields a significant advance in the pathophysiological analysis of disease processes but clinical accuracy is not markedly enhanced by visual or normalized assessment of the PET images.

PERFUSION IMAGING

Imaging schedules

Various imaging schedules have been proposed depending on tracer selection and clinical objectives. A stress–redistribution protocol is possible with thallium, but the available technetium-labelled tracers do not redistribute and require single-day or separate-day rest–stress or stress–rest protocols. The objective of perfusion imaging is to provide a simple and fast procedure to detect, localize and measure perfusion defects, and to define their reversibility. Most centres prefer a single-day protocol, while some laboratories still adopt separate-day protocols for inpatients or patients without transportation problems; flexibility is the rule.

Diagnostic thallium studies should be started with exercise, as the tissue distribution changes with time and the half-life and retention of the tracer in the myocardium is long. Thallium should be injected at peak exercise; imaging should begin as soon as possible and be completed by 30 minutes to avoid redistribution. Indeed, as thallium continuously moves in and out of the cell, there is slow equilibration between the intracellular thallium content and the lower intravascular concentration. The pattern of distribution changes reflects the changing conditions: therefore images acquired shortly after injection reflect myocardial perfusion during stress while those acquired several hours later tend to reflect the distribution of viable myocardium.

Comparison of stress and redistribution images leads to description of fixed or reversible abnormalities corresponding to infarcted or reversibly ischaemic myocardium (Plate 6). This classification is however simplistic, since redistribution is frequently incomplete and the redistribution images underestimate the presence of reversible ischaemia. Reinjection of thallium, 1–4 hours after exercise or on a separate day, leads to improvement in up to one-third of fixed defects, and a separate day protocol is therefore recommended for detection of viable myocardium.

When technetium-labelled tracers are used, diagnostic studies are also probably best started with exercise, as no resting control is needed when the exercise study remains negative. In patients with known disease however, the resting study should be performed first, to avoid superimposing exercise-induced defects on the resting data, resulting in a potential underestimation of the degree of reversibility. Imaging delay after injection should be kept as small as possible for patients' convenience. Such delay depends on lung and liver tracer kinetics; a flexible delay – as available with current tracers – allows the study of patients with unstable conditions as well as facilitating logistic problems (e.g. distance between stress laboratory and imaging suite, camera availability, etc.).

Preparation for exercise and choice of stress type

It is generally recommended that cardioactive drugs be discontinued before diagnostic work-up. However, for functional evaluation of patients with known disease, and in patients with unstable conditions, therapy withdrawal may not be indicated. It should be kept in mind that in these conditions, scintigraphy may underestimate the extent of potential ischaemic changes, although it remains more sensitive than the stress ECG

for that purpose. Before the test, the patients should avoid drinks or drugs containing caffeine or theophylline derivatives. This allows dipyridamole or adenosine to be used as a substitute to exercise in patients with limited exercise capability.

The injection is given close to the end of a maximum symptom-limited exercise. The patient should continue to exercise for 1–2 minutes after injection, to allow tracer uptake by the myocardium before regression of the pathological changes associated with exercise. This is particularly important with the current technetium-labelled tracers, which have a lower peak extraction fraction and therefore require more circulation time for complete extraction. It may be necessary to reduce the work-load slightly to allow the patient to continue exercise for 60–90 seconds after injection, rather than stopping exercise too early. Reasons for stopping including maximal exercise, angina or other clinical symptoms such as arrhythmias, shortness of breath or hypotension should be documented.

Dipyridamole is injected intravenously at a dose of 0.56 mg/kg over 4 minutes. A higher dose (up to 0.80 mg/kg) is sometimes recommended. An interesting option is to combine dipyridamole with exercise at a low, moderate or even maximal level as it increases the sensitivity of the test, decreases the side effects of the drug and maintains the flow gradient after exercise is stopped. The tracer injection should be given at a minimum of 2 minutes after the end of the dipyridamole infusion, but can be delayed further when using a combined dipyridamole–exercise protocol [17].

Adenosine has similar effects to dipyridamole, but its action and side effects are easier to control as its plasma half-life is less than 10 seconds. It is infused for 6 minutes at a dose rate of 140 µg/kg/min with injection of the perfusion tracer at 4 minutes. Like dipyridamole, it should not be given to patients with spastic airways disease.

Dobutamine, a β-agonist with a plasma half-life of less than 2 minutes, provides an alternative approach to increase myocardial oxygen demand and coronary flow by increasing heart rate, blood pressure and contractility. It is infused in stages starting at 5 µg/kg/min and increasing to a maximum of 40 µg/kg/min. Intravenous atropine is frequently given to reach the target heart rate but it should preferably be given at the onset of the test. Arbutamine is a similar β-agonist agent with a slightly different haemodynamic profile (more prominent effect on heart rate). β-agonists are considered safe in patients with coronary artery disease, but more ventricular arrhythmias occur with their use than with vasodilators or exercise. They are also safe in patients with spastic pulmonary disease. However, the positive inotropic and chronotropic effects of β-agonists make them unsuitable in patients with contraindication to dynamic exercise, in particular, aortic stenosis and unstable angina. Their action is antagonized by β-blockers, and these should logically be discontinued 48 hours before the study, although some studies have shown perfusion abnormalities, even in patients on β-blockers.

Planar imaging

Planar imaging is the classical technique. It has a proven efficacy for disease detection with approximate sensitivity and specificity figures of 80% and 90%, respectively. It is however, less effective than tomography in defining individual vessel lesions and disease extent. Planar imaging is well-suited for thallium. Although image quality is probably better using technetium-labelled tracers, lesion contrast may be diminished by shine-through of normal regions. Planar imaging is performed in three or four projections: anterior, left anterior oblique 45°, 70° left anterior oblique and/or left lateral. The latter views should be performed with the patient lying on his/her right side. Each view should be acquired over 5 minutes to collect sufficient data for statistical analysis.

Planar images are difficult to read and require experienced observers. Available data suggest improved reproducibility and accuracy of reading when a standardized acquisition and display format is used and when quantification is performed comparing a patient's data with a normal database. Reproducibility of reading is higher for technetium agents than for thallium [18].

SPECT acquisition

Single-photon emission computed tomography (SPECT) acquisition is usually performed over 180° (from left posterior oblique to right anterior oblique). A minimum of 30 projections should be acquired; 30–40 seconds per projection are considered adequate. The total time varies between 10 and 30 minutes, depending on the type of camera used (one to three heads). A matrix size of 64×64 and a field-of-view of 40 cm are adequate, given the resolution of current cameras (with preferably a high-resolution collimator) and the influence of cardiac motion.

Image reconstruction is performed from the set of two-dimensional (2D) projections to obtain a three-dimensional (3D) representation of the data. Tomographic reconstruction is usually performed with the back-projection technique. Appropriate choice of filter determines the final resolution and contrast of the image. Butterworth filters (order 5 or 6, cut-off frequency .25 cycles/pixel) are frequently applied. Iterative reconstruction results in better representation of the original data with less artefacts (no activity outside the object and no negative values), but is more time consuming. Attenuation correction using transmission data is now becoming available, and will probably become standard in the future, but problems (mainly related to scatter correction) remain to be solved.

At present, SPECT imaging appears to be superior to planar imaging, particularly when using technetium-labelled tracers. It provides better visualization of the three-dimensional distribution of the tracer, and has been shown to be more effective than planar imaging in defining the extent of disease. Background subtraction is not necessary, and in fact is not recommended. Standardized reorientation has been defined [19], but the use of oblique radial long-axis slices gives more advantages including control of reorientation, easier registration and quantification (Plate 7).

Image quantitation

Visual analysis forms the basis of image interpretation and is necessary to evaluate the potential impact of confounding factors such as attenuation and gastrointestinal artefacts. It should be supplemented in all cases by quantitative analysis to provide objective and reproducible decision criteria.

Increased thallium uptake in the lungs is related to the extent and severity of CAD, the degree of left ventricular functional impairment and the increase in pulmonary capillary pressure during exercise. It is an important predictor of future cardiac events in coronary patients. Lung uptake can be assessed subjectively but should preferably be quantitated as the lung-to-myocardial ratio. Quantification of planar images is usually performed using horizontal or circumferential profiles. However, planar quantification is complicated by the variable effect of background and the lack of an adequate program to correct for it. Reorientation is usually not performed and this also complicates the analysis of horizontal profiles.

Quantification of SPECT images may be obtained using short-axis and long-axis circumferential profiles. More comprehensive quantification is provided by polar map display (Plate 8). These can be constructed using either a set of short-axis slices or a set of oblique radial long-axis slices. The latter analyses the activity distribution over the entire ventricle, whereas use of short-axis slices often leads to truncation at the apex and at the base. Polar maps can provide quantitative evaluation of myocardial tracer uptake percentage of the reference zone, usually the zone with highest counts (when the reference zone is not in its usual position, a value different from 100% may be chosen to match the normal database) [20].

Polar maps are also useful to evaluate the extent and severity of perfusion defects (Plate 9), provided that the distortions resulting from the polar projections are accounted for. Abnormal areas are quantified in reference to a normal population database, specific for the tracer and protocol used. Pixel-by-pixel lower limit of normal thresholds are calculated using the distribution of normal values. Several groups have used 2.5 standard deviations below the mean as this threshold, though others use varying thresholds optimized using receiver operating characteristic (ROC) curves in the different areas of the polar map. It is not surprising that these thresholds can be empirically rather than statistically defined, as normalized data do not necessarily conform to a normal distribution. Separate databases for men and women are recommended.

The advantage of the polar map is that all areas of the myocardium are represented in a single image, but this image is less familiar to cardiologists. Also, 2D representation of 3D data leads to size distortion. When stress and rest or redistribution polar plots are compared, the projection of both studies must be identical, and this may be difficult to obtain in pathology.

Recently, a new programme has been introduced to quantify tomographic perfusion studies using radial slices and a polar map. The advantages of this program rely on an optimized scheme for reorientation (see Plate 7). Only the long axis must be defined to sample the heart from apex to base, without truncation or the need to set apical or basal limits. As sampling is performed over 360°, the activity is analysed automatically in the region of the valve plane, where no muscular wall is present. Background activity is determined and used as baseline to quantify the severity of the perfusion defects. It is not used, however, to increase image contrast or to manipulate images before threshold determination or quantification. Finally, radial slices are the optimal reorientation method for gated studies [21].

Three-dimensional representation of the heart is also possible using for instance 'bullet' models that can be viewed from varying angles on the computer screen. These models are optimal to superimpose anatomical or other information on the myocardial walls (for instance the coronary arteries) but are more difficult to use in prints.

Gating of myocardial perfusion images

Gated acquisitions have usually not been found useful with thallium, but their use should become more widespread with technetium-labelled agents in the planar or tomographic mode. Gating provides better evaluation of frozen diastolic images without the blurring effect of wall motion. In addition, there is no variation in partial-volume effects due to wall thickening.

Gating also allows simultaneous evaluation of perfusion and function through analysis of wall motion or wall thickening [22]. For instance, abnormalities of wall motion in the presence of restored or maintained perfusion tracer uptake in the setting of fibrinolysis post-myocardial infarction are typical of stunned, recoverable myocardium. Wall motion and wall thickening can be appreciated visually or with the use of parametric imaging. Changing counts resulting from changes in resolution related count recovery or partial-volume effects can probably be used to appreciate wall thickening.

CARDIAC BLOOD POOL IMAGING

BLOOD POOL AGENTS

The study of global or regional myocardial function utilizes radiotracers that remain in the vascular compartment for the period of the study. Most technetium-labelled compounds transit rapidly through the lungs without trapping and fulfil these requirements during first pass, but ^{99m}Tc-pertechnetate or ^{99m}Tc-DTPA are usually preferred for the sake of simplicity or because DTPA is rapidly cleared from the blood allowing repeated injections. Rarely ^{81}Rb/^{81m}Kr maybe used to study the right ventricular function.

Labelled red cells are the preferred agents to label the blood pool. They can be used both for first-pass and equilibrium studies. Labelling involves preconditioning of the red cells with stannous chloride with subsequent addition of technetium. Technetium reduced within the cell by the stannous ion remains trapped. Labelling can be performed using *in vivo* (injection of stannous chloride followed 20–30 minutes later by technetium), *in vitro* (addition of ^{99m}Tc to a preconditioned red cells suspension in vitro followed by incubation and wash) or *in vivo–in vitro* techniques (combination of both methods). Using these techniques, more than 95% of the ^{99m}Tc is bound to red cells (after 10–15 minutes in the case of *in vivo* labelling) and high contrast is achieved between cardiac blood pool and surrounding tissue. The effective half-life in the blood is 6 hours, and adequate to perform serial or intervention ventricular function studies.

The opportunity exists to use technetium-labelled perfusion tracers to study perfusion and function simultaneously. Global function measurements of the right and left ventricles can indeed be performed during first-pass despite some initial lung uptake and concurrent myocardial uptake. As seen earlier, evaluation of regional and global left ventricular function can alternatively be obtained through planar or tomographic gating of the ventricular tracer distribution.

RADIONUCLIDE VENTRICULOGRAPHY

Radionuclide ventriculography consists of synchronized imaging of the intracardiac blood pools following the administration of a technetium-labelled blood pool agent.

First-pass image acquisition

First-pass acquisition follows the transit of the tracer through the right heart chambers, the lungs, the left heart chambers and the aorta. The spatiotemporal separation of these chambers allows the use of an anterior or right anterior oblique projection that best identifies the atria and the ventricles. Tracer concentration in the ventricles is high but variable and background activity minimal. Study of the time–activity curves of the different structures allows determination of the cardiac output and transit times, as well as the detection of an early recirculation caused by a left-to-right shunt. Data corresponding to the right and/or left ventricular transit can also be reframed at a high temporal resolution to provide images of an average cardiac cycle and be further processed like an equilibrium study. Alternatively, the time–activity curve can be used directly to calculate the global ejection fraction, but regional wall motion cannot be assessed in this manner.

Equilibrium image acquisition

Acquisition at equilibrium provides images with better statistics and with higher spatial and temporal resolution. Images are synchronized using the ECG R-wave as a reference to provide an average cardiac cycle series (Figure 6.7). The computer acquires a number of images (16 to 64) within each R-R interval, depending on the required time resolution, and sorts the images according to their position within the cardiac cycle. This sorting is done either directly or retrospectively (from a buffer) after acquisition in list mode. In patients with arrhythmia this makes it possible to select the cardiac cycles to be studied and reject others. However, we prefer to use a large acquisition window to obtain average cycle information and to correct the end-of-cycle images for undersampling. This can be done with precision by correcting for difference in the time each image has been exposed.

The left anterior oblique view (35 to 45° LAO with 5–10° craniocaudal obliquity, the 'best septal view') is the only view that adequately separates all cardiac chambers and is therefore used for quantitative analysis of left ventricular function. Other projections are however necessary to analyse regional wall motion: the anterior or 20° RAO projection to explore the anterior wall, the right ventricular free wall and frequently part of the inferior wall, and the left lateral projection for the posterolateral wall.

Tomographic imaging of the cardiac blood pool is now possible, using for instance 64 projections around 360° and acquiring up to 16 images at each projection. The long data acquisition and process-

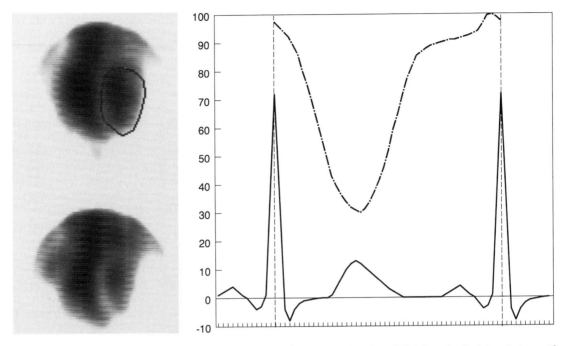

Figure 6.7   Synchronized diastolic and systolic images of the cardiac blood pool (LAO projection) in relation with the ECG reference (R wave trigger) and the resulting left ventricular (LV) time-activity curve.

ing times have limited the applications of this technique. It should however gain more acceptance in the near future due to the increasing computer memory and power, and the potential of tomography to obtain realigned long-axis view and to better avoid cavity superimpositions [23].

Equilibrium-gated radionuclide ventriculography can also be performed during exercise or coupled to pharmacological stress or unloading. Stress techniques (e.g. exercise, pacing, dobutamine or isuprel, cold pressor test), aim to detect the occurrence of regional ischaemic dysfunction or the global consequences of alterations in cardiac haemodynamics secondary to ischaemia or changes in the loading conditions. Unloading techniques such as the use of nitrates look for improved global or regional function as evidence for preserved myocardial function and viability.

Image processing and scintigraphic parameters

Image processing involves several steps to normalize uneven sampling as a consequence of arrhythmias, to smooth the data both spatially and temporally, and to create parametric images such as phase and amplitude Fourier images.

ROI determination over the ventricles and background can be made automatic or rely on contours evident on the parametric images. Standardization of the ROI selection is necessary to guarantee reproducibility as it influences the results. The background region, in particular, must be chosen with care as it has been shown that background subtraction performs as a normalization factor rather than determining the true background level. It should be chosen differently whether a single diastolic ROI or multiple systolic and diastolic ROIs are chosen. As the tracer is uniformly distributed in the blood at equilibrium and its concentration remains constant, the activity on the images is proportional to the underlying blood volume. Therefore, the time–activity curves constructed over the left and right ventricles are proportional to their time–volume curves, after background subtraction and calibration. These curves are therefore used to calculate the main parameters of cardiac function.

Global function The left ventricular ejection fraction assesses the left ventricular pump function but remains influenced by the loading conditions. Only a ratio of activity is necessary to determine the ejection fraction:

$$EF = \frac{\text{diastolic counts} - \text{systolic counts}}{\text{diastolic counts} - \text{background counts}}$$

Radionuclide angiography is the only technique that allows ejection fraction determination without geometric assumption, avoiding the errors resulting from the inadequacy of the geometric model in patients with wall motion abnormalities. It is therefore superior to echocardiography and X-ray ventriculography, particularly for abnormal ventricles. The measurements are reproducible to within 5 percentage points both at rest and during dynamic exercise.

Other functional parameters can be extracted from the time–activity curve including the ejection velocity, the filling velocities (maximum and mean) and their timing. Normalization of these indices to either end-diastolic counts or stroke counts is usually performed. These indices can also be calculated regionally.

Determination of ventricular volumes The measurement of absolute ventricular volumes has proven more difficult than the measurement of relative ventricular volume. It requires the determination of a conversion factor (activity per area to activity per ml) as well as correction for attenuation and background. While the blood activity can easily be determined by blood sampling, the other factors are not easy to evaluate accurately. Tomography can however, define a geometrical sample within the left ventricle. If the actual count in this sample can be determined free of attenuation and superimposition, and if the total left ventricular counts are known then the total left ventricular volume can be extrapolated. However, this technique has not yet found widespread application.

It should be pointed out that despite some inaccuracy, volume determination remains useful to follow a patient acutely or even chronically as long as the same methodology is used.

Regional function Regional analysis is performed either by dividing the cavity in a number of segments (8 to 12 sectors in a radial symmetry around the geometric centre of gravity) and calculating for each segment the time–activity curves and the derived parameters. This approach can recognize wall motion abnormalities as well as compensatory hyperkinesia.

The other approach is based on the calculation of parametric images reflecting cardiac function on a pixel-by-pixel basis. Although simple parametric images such as the stroke volume images or the ejection fraction images have been used, the most popular and most effective parametric images are the Fourier amplitude and phase images. Indeed, the cardiac cycle as any periodic phenomenon can be represented as a sum of sinusoids of increasing frequency and decreasing amplitude. The first harmonic contains already a large part of the information of the time–activity curve, with higher harmonics adding fine structure such as diastasis and atrial contraction. The first harmonic allows pixel-by-pixel calculation of the amplitude (i.e. that is the maximal variation of the sinusoid), and of its phase (i.e. that is the delay between the time reference and the minimum value). Colour-coded images representative of the amplitude and phase of regional volume variations depict hypokinetic and dyskinetic areas as regions with reduced amplitude and delayed phase. Ischaemic myocardium has both a reduced and delayed or even paradoxical wall motion, and the combined amplitude and phase images are more accurate for detecting abnormal function than methods that look only at the extent of contraction [24].

IMAGING OF MYOCARDIAL NECROSIS

INFARCT-AVID AGENTS

Several tracers have been developed to identify irreversibly damaged myocardium. After a first attempt using tetracycline derivatives, experience has been gained using bone-seeking agents, and in particular pyrophosphate. Subsequently, antibodies to cardiac myosin have been proven to be more specific. Recently, the use of glucaric acid has been proposed but little experience is available with this tracer.

^{99m}Tc-Pyrophosphate

In patients with myocardial infarction, pyrophosphate accumulation is maximum 2–4 days after the acute event, sooner if the infarct-related vessel is patent. Pyrophosphate accumulation parallels myofibrillar degeneration, a pathological event characterized by mitochondrial calcium deposition and suggestive of necrosis with reperfusion. Pyrophosphate binds to calcium phosphate crystalline structures within the mitochondria, but a diffuse cellular deposition is probably associated. Concentration is maximal in areas of moderate reduction in myocardial blood flow, but decreases in regions with severe reduction of flow. In contrast, the accumulation of antimyosin antibodies is greatest in regions of lowest myocardial blood flow.

Antimyosin antibodies

Myosin is one of the myofibrillar proteins and represents a large target within the myocardium (40–50 mg/g). It is not exposed to circulating antibodies as long as the sarcolemmal membrane remains normal. Myocyte necrosis and cell membrane disruption allow antimyosin antibodies to attach to the exposed myosin filaments. Myocardial uptake is highly specific for myocyte necrosis, though this is encountered not only in acute myocardial infarction but also in patients with myocarditis or anthracycline toxicity as well as in cardiac allograft rejection. Antibodies can be labelled with indium or technetium. With indium, imaging is preferably performed 24–48 hours after injection, a time when optimal images are available. In the days following infarction, cardiac myosin disappears gradually and the uptake progressively fades. No uptake should be seen at the site of an old infarction, but positive images may reflect ongoing necrosis.

HOT-SPOT IMAGING

Imaging of myocardial necrosis with pyrophosphate or antimyosin antibodies has long been done using planar technique. Currently however, tomography is the technique of choice and allows better separation of the myocardial and extramyocardial tracer uptake (especially the bones in the case of pyrophosphate). Dual-tracer imaging with thallium or another blood flow agent has also been recommended to provide better delineation of the necrotic area in relation to the remaining myocardium. The timing of these studies depends on the clinical indications and on the tracer used and is discussed elsewhere.

IMAGING MYOCARDIAL METABOLISM

TRACERS OF MYOCARDIAL METABOLISM

The myocardium has high energy demand devoted primarily to mechanical work, while 20% is used for maintenance of cellular integrity. It derives most of its energy from fatty acid consumption but choice of substrate depends on availability. Carbohydrate loading increases glucose utilization as insulin rises and free fatty acid levels decrease. During exercise, lactate is an important alternate source of energy. Ischaemia impairs free fatty acid utilization and alters the balance of substrate metabolism. The glycolytic flux is increased until accumulation of metabolites such as lactate inhibits glycolysis.

^{18}F-FDG

Both natural substrates and analogues have been used to study myocardial substrate utilization. Kinetic modelling of ^{11}C-glucose has however proven complex, and most experience has been acquired using ^{18}F-FDG. ^{18}F-FDG competes with glucose for transmembranous transport and is phosphorylated by hexokinase. However, it is not a substrate for phosphoisomerase and it accumulates in the cell.

Exogenous glucose utilization can be derived from ^{18}F-FDG uptake through knowledge of the blood glucose level and input function, if an appropriate correction for the difference in affinity between FDG and glucose is applied (lumped constant).

Single-pass ^{18}F-FDG extraction is low, but largely variable, and yields cumulative uptake of 1–6% of the injected dose. These large variations in uptake reflect the metabolic, physiological and pathological conditions under study. The primary clinical application of FDG in the heart is to identify jeopardized but viable myocardium using the FDG/flow mismatch pattern [25].

Fatty acids

Cardiac fatty acid metabolism has primarily been studied using ^{11}C-palmitate. This compound represents 25–30% of the circulating fatty acids in the blood and it circulates bound to albumin. It has a high extraction and, therefore, its initial distribution is proportional to blood flow. Its clearance from the myocardium is bi-exponential and reflects β-oxidation then incorporation into the lipid pool. However, the clinical application of this tracer has been hampered by modelling complexities and by the recognition of back-diffusion of unmetabolized tracer contaminating the early clearance phase and data interpretation in pathological conditions. Little experience is available with the use of [18]F- or ^{11}C-labelled fatty acid analogues such as the β-methylheptadecanoic acid, but their metabolic characteristics differ from normal substrates. ^{123}I-labelled fatty acids also differ from normal substrates because of the size of the heteroatom. Their initial kinetics are nevertheless similar to ^{11}C-palmitate and their clearance has been shown to be influenced by metabolic or haemodynamic interventions known to modify substrate utilization. The use of iodinated fatty acid is complicated by rapid dehalogenation and the build-up of iodine background activity. Use of iodophenyl derivatives in part circumvents that difficulty but further modifies the metabolic behaviour of these tracers.

Recently, the use of β-methyl iodophenylpentadecanoic acid, an analogue with prolonged myocardial retention, has been shown useful to study myocardial viability in comparison with a blood flow tracer as flow/metabolism mismatch (partially preserved flow with depressed fatty acid uptake) [26].

[11]C-Acetate

[11]C-Acetate has been proposed as a more direct alternative to study myocardial oxidative metabolism. It is highly extracted and metabolized only by the TCA cycle. Clearance of acetate correlates with myocardial oxygen consumption (MVO$_2$) and is only minimally influenced by myocardial substrate availability. Acetate kinetics corrected for ^{11}C metabolite contamination allows non-invasive quantitative assessment of myocardial oxygen consumption.

POSITRON EMISSION TOMOGRAPHY

Positron emission tomography (PET) is an imaging technique that displays the 3D distribution of β+ emitters within an object. Positrons travel a very short mean distance within matter. After absorption of their kinetic energy they undergo an annihilation reaction with an electron and emit two 511-keV γ-rays in almost opposite directions (180°). These γ-rays are detected in coincidence (by opposing detectors within a very short time-window) by the PET camera, which can

therefore localize the origin of the annihilation somewhere along that coincidence line without requiring collimation. Coincidence detection also allows accurate determination of tissue attenuation. Indeed, as the total distance travelled by the two photons is independent of the position of origin of the annihilation reaction, whether within or outside the body, tissue attenuation can be measured by comparing, line-by-line, the count rate of a ring or rotating rod source, with and without interposition of the object. Recent developments have allowed the performance of transmission studies during or after the emission acquisition, i.e. in the presence of the emission tracer. This will do much to expedite data acquisition and to simplify positron tomography in clinical circumstances.

These physical principles confer many essential advantages to PET over SPECT, including the potential for true quantitative measurement of radioactivity within the object in μCi per ml as a function of time, higher sensitivity resulting from the electronic collimation and 3D acquisition algorithms, as well as improved spatial resolution. The principal benefit of PET is related to the nature of the principal positron-emitters available for medical studies. The cyclotron-produced positron-emitters include oxygen-15, nitrogen-13 and carbon-11 with physical half-lives of 2, 10 and 20 minutes respectively. These elements constitute the components of organic substances. Tracers with longer half-lives including [18]F ($t_{1/2}$ 110 min) and [76]Br ($t_{1/2}$ 16 hours), are also frequently used, incorporated as tracers in ligands or analogue substrates. Rubidium-82 and potassium-38 are additional compounds used as cations to study regional myocardial blood flow.

OTHER IMAGING AGENTS

Radiopharmaceuticals have been developed with a high affinity for the pre-synaptic uptake nerve terminal transport mechanism of the sympathetic system. These noradrenaline analogues are subject to the uptake-1 mechanism and undergo vesicular storage. ^{11}C-metahydroxyephedrine and ^{123}I-MIBG are the principal tracers used. Their retention is altered by pharmacological intervention (desipramine or reserpine), by sympathetic denervation or injury (e.g. ischaemic injury) as well as by heart failure.

Other tracers have been developed to study the

post-synaptic receptors (e.g. ^{11}C-CGP 12177). Indium-labelled platelets, monoclonal antibodies against platelets and peptides specific for the GP IIb/IIIa activated platelet receptor are being developed to visualize venous and arterial thrombi as well as pulmonary emboli.

Low-density lipoproteins (LDL) labelled with indium, iodine or technetium, are cleared by the liver as a function of the density of its receptors. LDL accumulate in atherosclerotic plaques, particularly in lipid-rich lesions, but imaging is difficult due to persisting blood pool activity and low target-to-background ratio.

CLINICAL APPLICATIONS

DETECTION OF MYOCARDIAL ISCHAEMIA AND DIAGNOSIS OF CAD

Clinical manifestations of CAD

Despite recent improvement, CAD remains the major cause of premature death and disability in Western countries, and constitutes a very significant economic burden. The risk factors for CAD have been identified and include family history, age, sex, blood lipid disorders, smoking, hypertension and obesity. Correction of risk factors at the clinical as well as at the preclinical stages of the affection can improve the prognosis.

Initial manifestations of CAD consist of sudden death, myocardial infarction and angina. Sudden death occurring within 1 hour of onset of symptoms is most often the result of CAD. Its principal mechanism appears to be ischaemia-induced ventricular tachycardia or fibrillation. Coronary thrombosis plays an essential role in the development of an acute myocardial infarction. It is indeed present in most patients studied by angiography early on. Coronary thrombosis is apparently triggered by plaque rupture. Unstable plaques with a larger lipid core are more vulnerable to rupture than many plaques corresponding to more severe stenoses organized by thicker fibrous caps. Both types of plaques frequently coexist in the same patient. Early diagnosis is therefore mandatory to decrease mortality and avoid permanent sequelae. Diagnosis relies on subjective or objective signs of myocardial ischaemia and infarction or on morphological evidence of coronary stenosis (angiography).

Symptoms and signs of myocardial ischaemia

Symptoms Patients' symptoms are most important. Chest pain is classified as typical or atypical angina or non-cardiac pain. Typical angina has a pressure-like character, is localized in the midsternal region, is induced by stress and has typical irradiation; it is relieved by rest and nitrates. Atypical pain lacks key elements, while non-cardiac pain lacks most elements, and is most frequently suggestive of a visceral or parietal origin.

Physical examination In patients with chronic CAD, physical examination is frequently non-contributory, although it can provide evidence of left ventricular dysfunction in severe or advanced cases. Risk factors and the clinical presentation are frequently combined to evaluate the pre-test likelihood for CAD in symptomatic patients.

Electrocardiography The resting ECG can provide clues to the presence of CAD. Pathological Q waves or absent R waves can suggest the presence of a previous, eventually silent myocardial infarction. ST-T wave changes at rest are most often non-specific unless transient and recorded during ischaemic symptoms. The exercise ECG is more useful as exercise is one of the most common ways to increase myocardial oxygen demand and induce ischaemia. Exercise can elicit typical chest pain or demonstrate reduced exercise tolerance or ECG changes 'typical' for CAD. However, exercise ECG gives many false-negative and false-positive results and its sensitivity and specificity are not perfect. Indeed, ECG changes as well as angina are late occurrences in the ischaemic cascade. False-positive results are more frequent in women.

Imaging The increased efficacy of combining diagnostic information from independent tests performed simultaneously or in succession has been demonstrated (Bayesian approach). Myocardial perfusion imaging can provide information on the presence, site, extent and reversibility of stress-induced perfusion abnormalities.

Radionuclide ventriculography during stress evaluates the effect of ischaemia on global and regional function [27]. Ischaemia induces wall motion abnormalities, leading to global function alterations. A drop in ejection fraction of at least 5% from baseline is required, given the variability of repeated baseline measurements (±5%). This contrasts with the expected increase in ejection fraction normally observed during exercise (±5–10%). Also, the left ventricular end-systolic volume increases followed by the end-diastolic volume (changes in left ventricle volume are however affected by the patient's position during exercise as the basal end-diastolic volume is larger in the supine than in the upright posture and less subject to variations). Ejection fraction changes are affected by loading conditions and have proven less specific than perfusion abnormalities to detect coronary lesions. Alterations in ejection fraction are also frequently observed in patients with non-coronary heart disease such as hypertension, cardiomyopathies, myocarditis and valvular heart disease. Ejection fraction changes are probably also less sensitive in patients with mild lesions as they require occurrence of ischaemia in contrast to relative flow reserve abnormalities. Regional wall-motion abnormalities should be more specific than global function changes as they are less affected by variations in loading conditions. The limited number of available projections as well as the limited time for analysis during ischaemia, limit the potential usefulness of regional wall-motion abnormalities. In particular, tomographic imaging cannot be performed during exercise. Similar considerations are also true regarding the comparison of myocardial perfusion imaging and stress or dobutamine echocardiography. The requisite for ischaemia makes it less sensitive in cases of mild single-vessel disease, while patient's motion and breathing, limited sampling and limited timing curtail the quality of stress echocardiography. Residual myocardial ischaemia within or around a zone of myocardial infarction is also better depicted by exercise myocardial perfusion imaging than by exercise echocardiography as the latter method has difficulty judging the degree and the extent of wall motion abnormalities in and around an infarct zone.

Myocardial imaging to diagnose CAD

Myocardial imaging is most frequently performed in symptomatic patients with low to intermediate probability for CAD, i.e. men with atypical chest pain together with some risk factors, or women with more typical chest pain. It is also useful in patients with non-diagnostic ECGs (hypertension, pacemaker-related or conduction disturbances, drug-induced ST-T changes, etc.) as well as in patients unable to exercise properly. Pharmacological stress (dipyridamole, adenosine or dobutamine) is frequently proposed as an alternative to exercise in combination with myocardial imaging in these patients (Table 6.1). As the patient's exercise tolerance may be difficult to predict and considering the pathophysiological basis of myocardial perfusion imaging, the most effective approach is probably systematically to propose a combination test associating dipyridamole or adenosine with exercise. This approach maximizes coronary blood flow and combines the benefits of the relative perfusion reserve mechanism with the information and advantages of exercise (for instance on image quality through reduction of splanchnic blood flow). This combined stress is safe and well tolerated and even diminishes the side effects usually associated with dipyridamole or adenosine. The effectiveness of myocardial perfusion scintigraphy in detecting perfusion abnormalities associated with CAD has been the subject of many studies. Most have assessed the sensitivity and specificity of the technique using coronary angiography as the standard. The wisdom of this approach can be debated but no substitute reference is currently widely available. Pooled reviews of such studies reveal sensitivity and specificity of 80% and 92% respectively, significantly better than those of exercise ECG (sensitivity 64%, specificity 82%) (Table 6.2) [28].

The value of myocardial imaging to screen asymptomatic patients with low disease probability has not been established. Indeed, in these groups of patients, any test without perfect specificity will produce more false-positive results than true-positive results and overall diagnostic accuracy will be low.

A special situation is that of vascular patients with claudication, abdominal aortic aneurysm or carotid lesions in whom one wishes to ascertain the risk of vascular surgery. These patients have medium to high prevalence of coronary artery disease, though the information required is not really diagnostic but rather prognostic. In this group, systematic performance of myocardial imaging appears inefficient as patient's stratification can also be done using clinical risk factors. Selective performance of myocardial imaging in clinically higher-risk patients allows further stratification into a low-risk group and a very high-risk group in which surgery must be postponed until after a full cardiac work-up and treatment or even cancelled [29].

Table 6.1 Stressors for myocardial perfusion

End-point	Exercise Ischaemia	Dipyrimadole Flow disparity	Adenosine Flow disparity	Dobuutamine Ischaemia
Convenience logistics	More demanding	Easy	Easy	Longer protocol
Experience	Largest	Large	Large	Moderate
Side effects	Determined by ischaemia	Nausea, flush	AV-block, nausea, flush	Arrhythmias

From Sochor *et al.* [54], by permission of Kluwer Academic Publishers.

Table 6.2 Sensitivity and specificity of pharmacological stress ^{201}Tl scintigraphy for detection of coronary artery disease

Authors	No. of patients with CAD	Without CAD	Sensitivity (%)	Specificity (%)
Dipyridamole				
Albro	51	11	67	91
Leppo	40	20	93	80
Schmoliner	60	–	95	–
Francisco	51	35	90	96
Timmis	20	–	85	–
Narita	35	15	69	100
Machencourt	58	10	90	90
Okada	23	7	91	100
Sochor	149	45	92	81
Ruddy	53	27	85	93
Taillefer	19	6	79	86
Adenosine				
Verani	73	16	83	94
Coyne	47	53	83	75
Iskandrian	132	16	92	88
Nguyen	53	7	92	100
Total	864	268	85.7	90.3

CAD, coronary artery disease.
From Sochor *et al.* [54], by permission of Kluwer Academic Publishers.

Myocardial infarction can sometimes remain silent, specially in diabetic patients. These patients will usually be identified on the occasion of a routine ECG. Confirmation of the presence of necrosis by exercise myocardial imaging is very useful in these patients as the test is also able to evaluate the extent of the disease.

Myocardial imaging to evaluate the extent of disease

Patients with a high probability for CAD (i.e. a typical history as well as positive risk factors) do not usually require imaging for diagnosis. However, it is frequently performed to evaluate the location and extent of the disease and to aid in the planning of therapy. Assessment of disease extent is necessary for a complete evaluation of the patients with ischaemic heart disease, even with overt clinical signs or known disease including known previous myocardial infarction. Extent of disease and its functional repercussion are indeed the principal factors determining prognosis and influencing therapy selection [30].

Several parameters are included under the term 'disease extent'. One is the severity of stenosis varying from a minimal plaque to a complete coronary occlusion with or without collaterals. Another is the site of a lesion and its relation to the distal perfusion bed (area at-risk). Yet another is the number of lesions, whether in series or in parallel, affecting one or several vessels, taking also into consideration the special significance of the left main stem and of the proximal left anterior descending artery (LAD), given their large territories and their potential immediate significance.

Extent of disease also concerns functional consequences of lesions, transient or fixed dysfunction, as well as the haemodynamic consequences of complications such as mitral regurgitation, septal rupture or left ventricular aneurysm.

Choice of techniques to assess extent of disease

Imaging of regional myocardial function and perfusion are the techniques that can best define the extent of disease. Other non-invasive techniques lack sensitivity and specificity for the detection of multiple vessel disease or proximal disease or even left mainstem lesions.

The localizing value of the exercise ECG is notoriously poor, although functional impairment and reduced exercise tolerance increase the probability of multiple vessels or proximal lesions. Concomitant haemodynamic changes (blood pressure drop or increased left ventricle filling pressure) improve the value of information provided but lack sensitivity.

SPECT has considerably improved, over planar acquisition, the ability of perfusion imaging to define the extent of disease [31]. Compared with projections, SPECT diminishes overlaps between vascular territories and provides more segments to identify different vascular lesions. The relationship between specific lesions and segments is also closer with SPECT. Even though the advantages of SPECT to define the extent of disease are clear-cut, this does not imply that it will detect all lesions. Due to the relative nature of perfusion imaging, regions with milder disease might appear normal, especially in patients with triple-vessel disease where such regions could possibly be taken as the reference. Furthermore, the exercise tolerance of patients with multiple-vessel disease is primarily affected by the most severe lesion. In rare cases, patients with balanced stenoses might have balanced perfusion abnormalities complicating

evaluation. However, evidence of some perfusion heterogeneity as well as of ventricular dilatation enables recognition of most of these patients [32].

The sensitivity to detect multiple-vessel disease using perfusion imaging is influenced by the presence of a previous myocardial infarction. Detection of a second lesion is generally enhanced when the first lesion corresponds to infarction rather than to another ischaemic area. However, the presence of a large infarct may complicate visualization of further ischaemia. Quantification has proven very important for assessing patients with prior infarct and suspected additional ischaemia. The ability of bull's-eye programmes to summarize the perfusion images in one comprehensive view, rather than to compare images of uncertain alignment, is the major contributing factor together with the assessment of size and severity of the defect. In our experience, the value of quantification to confirm evidence for residual ischaemia in patients with previous infarction is considerable.

Patients with left main disease, multiple-vessel disease and also probably severe proximal disease (at least in the LAD), especially when associated with mild or moderate ventricular dysfunction, are at increased risk for myocardial infarction or death, and should be revascularized. Defining the extent of disease by perfusion imaging thus appears a highly effective strategy. Complementary information on global and regional function – whether acquired by gating of perfusion images, radionuclide ventriculography or echocardiography – is also important in view of the increased risk and potential intervention benefits in patients with left ventricle dysfunction. Selection of patients for angiography can be done quite effectively and results in a high proportion of patients treated by revascularization making optimal use of generally limited resources. Systematic performance of angiography in all patients with CAD to confirm diagnosis and define disease extent has been advocated but does not seem warranted. It is more costly, carries more risk to the patient and in fact provides less prognostic information than is available using stress myocardial imaging as it shows the anatomy of the lesions rather than their functional significances. Experience has shown a tendency to intervene on anatomical lesions regardless of symptoms, natural history data or functional significance when angiography is performed first. Given current knowledge on a lesion's functional significance and site of subsequent obstruction in patients with documented CAD, no lesion should be dilated without adequate proof that it is responsible for ischaemia or malperfusion.

Assessment of the functional significance of coronary lesions

Demonstration of a lesion of borderline angiographic significance frequently leaves the cardiologist in doubt as to whether that lesion is responsible for the patient's symptoms, and whether to dilate it. Qualitative angiographic criteria have rather poor reproducibility and accuracy and in many cases cannot be used for decision making. Techniques are needed to assess the significance of lesions depicted by angiography, and SPECT myocardial perfusion imaging is frequently used to find out if a lesion can be demonstrated to produce perfusion abnormalities and/or objective signs of myocardial ischaemia.

The potential of myocardial imaging to assess the significance of a given lesion however, varies with the extent of coronary artery disease. In patients with single-vessel disease, perfusion imaging has a high sensitivity (90%) for detecting significant (>70% luminal narrowing) lesions. It has been shown that the detection sensitivity drops with the angiographic severity of the lesions, but this finding might simply reflect the increasing frequency of patients in whom the angiographic abnormality is in fact not functionally significant.

Patients with multiple-vessel lesions present a more difficult evaluation problem [33]. These patients may develop angina and stop exercising when ischaemia occurs in the territory of the most significant lesion. The detection sensitivity for the second and the third lesion is therefore less than optimal. Tomographic studies have indicated a sensitivity value of around 70% in these situations, and this should be kept in mind when requesting such a study.

The situation is somewhat different when the patient has prior myocardial infarction in the territory of the first coronary artery obstruction and the significance of a second lesion is sought. The detection sensitivity for a left anterior descending abnormality after a small inferior infarct is almost as high as that for a first lesion. The detection

sensitivity for a right coronary artery or a left circumflex lesion after a first large anterior myocardial infarction is somewhat lower but much improved by tomography.

A similar situation is encountered in patients with multiple-vessel disease and symptomatic angina pectoris who are not candidates for bypass surgery because of refusal or contraindications for surgery. In these patients, rather than attempt complete revascularization by angioplasty, it is possible to use perfusion imaging to identify the lesion responsible for initial manifestations of ischaemia and symptoms, the so-called 'culprit lesion', and to attempt – in priority – dilatation of this lesion without unduly prolonging the procedure. Subsequent scintigraphic evaluation is then required to evaluate the functional result in the region of the dilated artery, to detect the presence of residual ischaemia elsewhere and the need for secondary procedures [34].

Effectiveness of collateral supply

Regions distal to coronary occlusion may remain completely or partially viable due to collateral supply. Collaterals are however difficult to visualize angiographically. Myocardial imaging can be used to assess their functional effectiveness. A normal perfusion pattern in a collateral-dependent region is infrequent at stress but indicative of optimal collateral supply. An exercise-induced perfusion defect is more frequently observed, indicative of an adequate collateral supply at rest but of the inability of the collateral bed to meet the increased demand of exercise. Finally, an abnormal perfusion pattern at rest indicates partial or total necrosis (depending on defect severity) and the inadequacy of the collateral supply.

ACUTE ISCHAEMIC SYNDROMES

Emergency room

Patients with acute chest pain of unusual characteristics (e.g. pain *de novo*, severe or prolonged pain) are usually admitted to the emergency room for further diagnosis and treatment. However, not all patients have myocardial infarction, unstable angina or even coronary artery disease. The history may be atypical, laboratory tests may be inconclusive or uninterpretable and it may be difficult to reach a clinical diagnosis without further testing. Patient care and economic constraints require strategies to confirm or rule out acute is-chaemia as the cause of symptoms as simply and as early as possible. Nuclear medicine evaluation of perfusion and function have been considered for this purpose as ischaemia is characterized by perfusion and functional abnormalities. Perfusion tracers have usually been selected for this purpose because they are considered more specific for coronary artery disease. Initial studies were per-formed with thallium in patients presenting to the emergency room [35]. Patients in this study could be separated in two groups. The first group in-cluded patients with perfusion abnormalities who had CAD corresponding to either acute ischaemia or acute myocardial infarction or scar. The evolu-tion and/or repeated scanning was necessary for differential diagnosis but all patients were at high-risk, warranting hospitalization to the coronary care unit. The second group comprised of patients without perfusion abnormalities and therefore without ischaemia or infarction. Some had no CAD, others had CAD but no current ischaemia, while in some patients of this group, the ischaemia had already resolved and it was considered that they could be managed more conservatively, and were therefore either admitted to an ordinary ward or discharged and referred to the outpatient clinic.

Unstable angina

Angina is considered unstable if 'crescendo' (abruptly increasing in frequency and/or sever-ity), if '*de novo*', especially when progressive, and if occurring at rest without provocation. The basis for instability is the complicated or ulcerated plaque leading to platelet deposition and a vicious cycle of increased vasomotor tone, thrombus for-mation and embolization. These conditions lead to recurrent prolonged cardiac pain at rest and re-quire careful attention as these patients have a high risk for myocardial infarction and death without adequate treatment.

The diagnosis of unstable angina pectoris is pri-marily clinical supported by the 12-lead ECG demonstrating suggestive evidence for ischaemia in the absence of myocardial infarction signs. However, confirmation of the site and extent of ischaemia is frequently needed as part of the patient's management. Nuclear medicine in this indication offers the ability of the technetium-labelled perfusion tracers to freeze the perfusion distribution and obtain 'ischaemic fingerprint'

even if imaging is performed at a time when therapy has been successful and ischaemia has al-ready cleared.

In comparative studies, sestamibi SPECT imaging at rest had a higher sensitivity and better accuracy for ischaemic changes than the ECG obtained during, as well as between, episodes of pain (sensitivity 96% and specificity 79% for sestamibi versus 35% and 68% for ECG) [36]. Repeated imaging, first during pain and then in normal resting conditions, further improved specificity. Based on current experience, myocar-dial imaging is useful to rule out ischaemia in some uncertain cases, to identify the culprit vessel and the involved territory, and to aid in the selection of patients for coronary angiography.

Myocardial infarction

Appropriate use of nuclear medicine techniques depends on an active nuclear cardiology service with adequate equipment, preferably SPECT and portable cameras and the ability to acquire images in the emergency room and coronary care unit.

Infarct detection In some patients, the diagnosis of an acute myocardial infarction may be difficult when the combination of history, ECG and en-zymes remains inconclusive. Patients admitted late after the onset of chest pain, those with a pacemaker or a conduction disorder, those with peri-operative infarction, and those with possible right ventricular extension most frequently pose diagnostic problems. Nuclear medicine tech-niques may be helpful in these patients.

Technetium-pyrophosphate can identify acute myocardial infarction with a high sensitivity (at least 85%) when given 1–4 days after the event. Bone and skeletal muscle activities as well as per-sistent blood pool activity are the cause of some difficulties partially overcome nowadays by tomo-graphic acquisition. Uptake in areas of old infarct or of aneurysm as well as uptake in cases of unsta-ble angina reduce specificity (unstable angina up-take might however reflect limited but true cellular injury).

[111]In-labelled monoclonal antibodies against hu-man myosin, used as Fab' fragments, have high specificity for uptake by irreversibly injured myocytes. They also have high sensitivity for the diagnosis of acute infarction. A report from a

multicentre study indicates a 98% sensitivity in Q-wave infarct, 84% in non Q-wave infarct [37]. Specificity is 93% if one excludes patients with unstable angina in whom frequent focal uptake again suggests occurrence of some myocardial damage. The value of infarct-avid imaging is also related to its prognostic information as large infarct and ongoing uptake are considered pejorative signs.

Perfusion tracers, thallium as well as technetium-labelled agents, have diagnostic value in acute infarction. For instance, in some infarct locations, especially those caused by lesions of the circumflex artery, the ECG changes can be minimal or even absent. Patients with posterior or posterolateral infarct are frequently misdiagnosed as having non-transmural infarct while the myocardial perfusion scans show large defects typical of transmural infarctions. Clinical evidence of previous infarction may disappear with time. Retrospective diagnosis may be difficult in some patients where the ECG normalizes or becomes non-specific, due to changes related to conduction disturbances or pacemaker. It is important to demonstrate the presence of coronary disease as this diagnosis has important therapeutic and prognostic implications and is essential for the patient's management.

The use of perfusion tracers in acute myocardial infarction has however concentrated on the evaluation of infarct size as well as on the assessment of the risk area and myocardial salvage.

Use in patients submitted to fibrinolysis
Patients admitted with an evolving acute myocardial infarction are considered for fibrinolytic therapy. Knowledge of the size of the area at risk is important to determine the need for aggressive therapy and to separate patients into groups likely or unlikely to benefit from fibrinolysis, as the latter should not be subjected to the therapeutic risk. Clinical factors such as the time delay after onset of chest pain and early ECG signs are of help and commonly used, but myocardial imaging with a non-redistributing tracer can be of further help. It is indeed possible, for instance with sestamibi, to inject the tracer acutely when its distribution represents the status of perfusion before intervention and to obtain later images (after stabilization of the patient) of the initial area at risk without delaying essential treatment. Assessment of individual treatment effects can then be judged from com-

parative images obtained after a second post-therapy injection, hours or days later and this is the only readily available method able to directly assess myocardial salvage in individual patients [38] (Plate 10).

Several studies have been reported in patients undergoing thrombolytic therapy. Large variations in areas at risk are noted and the size of the perfusion defect cannot be predicted from the clinical presentation, the location of infarction neither the site of occlusion, proximal or distal. Indeed, many factors including collateral flow, vascular tone, humoral and neuronal stimuli play a role in determining occurrence of ischaemia or necrosis. Patients with an open artery, most often resulting from fibrinolytic therapy, have smaller defects on the second study as compared with the initial study. The full extent of improvement in perfusion is however observed fairly late after therapy (6–14 days) or even later [39,40]. It is thus possible to determine early on the amount of myocardium at risk in the setting of acute myocardial infarction. A significant correlation is found between the left ventricular ejection fraction and the final defect size, suggesting that sestamibi uptake reflects viable myocardium.

While it is often not possible to obtain a pre-fibrinolysis study, imaging early after therapy remains of value. A small perfusion defect confirms fibrinolysis efficacy unless the area at risk was initially limited. A large perfusion defect indicates unsuccessful reperfusion or lack of benefit and this information can be used to decide on the need for emergency angiography, depending on the patient's status and history.

Another study has also shown the value of later images to demonstrate then confirm potential perfusion improvement later after infarction [40]. This latter improvement probably represents delayed recovery from hibernating myocardium. The ability to predict this improvement is advantageous for prognosis and the patient's management.

Complications of acute myocardial infarction
Complications of infarction during the acute phase include heart failure and cardiogenic shock, associated right ventricular infarction, rhythm disturbances, aneurysmal transformation, valvular leakage (principally mitral) resulting from ischaemic papillary muscle dysfunction or rupture, as well as rupture of the free wall or of the septum.

Radionuclide angiography is an accurate technique to evaluate cardiac function and to detect areas of dysfunction in the left as well as in the right ventricle and is therefore useful to sort out the various dysfunctions leading to failure or shock. In particular, its role in the assessment of right ventricular myocardial infarction, to recognize the formation and operability of an aneurysm, to measure the regurgitant fraction and estimate the size of a left to right shunt in case of an intraventricular septal rupture has been demonstrated.

Information on regional myocardial function can also be derived using wall-motion data. However, following successful reopening of an occluded vessel, salvaged myocardium can remain akinetic and is therefore difficult to differentiate from necrotic muscle. Special studies are necessary in these cases to assess myocardium viability.

Left ventricular thrombi are another complication detectable by echocardiography or alternatively by radionuclide angiography or labelled platelets techniques. The latter can be used to assess the 'thrombogenic activity' of the thrombus.

MANAGEMENT OF PATIENTS AFTER ACUTE MYOCARDIAL INFARCTION

Patients surviving an acute myocardial infarction remain at increased risk of cardiovascular complications and their management is determined by the need to identify patients in whom further events such as reinfarction or death will occur in order to prevent those events. Approximately 5–7% of patients with an acute myocardial infarction die during the year following their hospital discharge (the hospital mortality rate has decreased during the past decade, but long-term survival improves more slowly).

Most reinfarctions and deaths, of which about 20% are sudden, occur within the first 6 months after the acute event. The extent of myocardial damage, the degree of global pump dysfunction, the extent and severity of residual myocardial ischaemia and the propensity to electrical instability are the major determinants of prognosis.

Extent of myocardial damage

The extent of myocardial damage is related to the location of the infarct (anterior versus inferior) as well as to the type of infarct (Q-wave versus non Q-wave). The extent of damage cannot however, be inferred from simple ECG or enzymatic criteria due to confounding factors, for instance the contribution of right ventricular myocardial infarction to enzyme release. Perfusion imaging is probably the best current technique to measure infarct size, provided that both defect extent and defect severity are taken into account. Infarct size on the other hand closely correlates with indices of global left ventricular function such as the left ventricular ejection fraction, provided that the measurement is made late after the myocardial infarction. Indeed, early on, the ejection fraction is also influenced by transient dysfunction (stunning or hibernation), by sympathetic stimulation with compensatory hyperkinesia of non-infarcted territories and by the unadjusted effects of mechanical complications. The Mayo Clinic Group has proposed to use a perfusion-derived infarct size index to predict the late left ventricular function level and recognize patients with stunning or hibernation or sympathetic stimulation [39].

Most of the prognostic information is present in the ejection fraction measured at rest as opposed to perfusion imaging where the extent of stress-induced ischaemia carries the information. It is therefore likely that radionuclide ventriculography and perfusion imaging provide complementary prognostic information, hence the efforts to combine them, for instance using gated perfusion imaging.

Radionuclide ventriculography can also be used to document the efficacy of therapy such as angiotensin-converting enzyme inhibitors on ventricular size and function. Echocardiography is more commonly used perhaps because of its availability but the nuclear technique is superior both in quantitative accuracy and in reproducibility.

Residual myocardial ischaemia

The development of angina early in the course of myocardial infarction is believed to imply a poor outcome. Demonstration of provoked myocardial ischaemia has also been shown to have prognostic significance. The prognostic role of exercise ECG to select patients with residual ischaemia remains debated. The value of ST segment depression initially described in selected patients is now considered insignificant based on large patient numbers. The better sensitivity and accuracy of cardiac imaging techniques is useful to improve prognostic accuracy. Several variables determined from perfusion imaging are powerful prognostic indicators. Extensive perfusion defects, reversible ischaemia – in particular at a distance from myocardial infarction – and increased lung uptake of thallium indicate a poor prognosis. Prediction value is superior to exercise ECG and to coronary angiography. Perfusion imaging defines both a group at lower risk (patients with fixed perfusion defects limited to one coronary artery bed) and a group at higher risk (combination of large defect, ischaemia with multivessel extension and signs of left ventricular dysfunction). For instance, in a study of 140 asymptomatic patients followed for a mean of 15 months after acute myocardial infarction, exercise ECG, thallium imaging and coronary angiography all predicted the seven deaths reasonably accurately. Thallium imaging was much better however for the prediction of nonfatal reinfarction, identifying 95% of the 43 patients compared with 53% and 61% respectively for ECG and angiography [41].

The best moment to perform prognostic investigations after myocardial infarction has been the subject of debate. The trend toward early discharge has pushed these investigations forward to a time when a maximal exercise test is impossible. However, the use of dipyridamole or adenosine allows safe optimal testing as early as 3–5 days after the event.

ASSESSMENT OF CORONARY ANGIOPLASTY AND CORONARY ARTERY BYPASS GRAFT SURGERY

Percutaneous transluminal coronary angioplasty (PTCA)

PTCA is an attractive technique that carries less risk of morbidity at a lower cost as compared with coronary artery bypass graft surgery (CABG). Unfortunately, restenosis occurs in many patients (30–40%), predominantly during the first 6 months after the intervention. Only stenosis responsible for documented myocardial ischaemia should be dilated and therefore the question of whether to dilate a mild stenosis is or should be frequently asked and these patients referred for exercise myocardial imaging.

Another potential question concerns the need for intervention on several vessels. In these patients, the localizing value of perfusion imaging is the key for interpretation. For instance, in

patients after myocardial infarction, assessment of both the presence of residual ischaemia in the infarct-related vessel and of ischaemia at a distance is necessary. Also, in patients with multiple vessel stenoses of varying severity or in high-risk patients with complex lesions, identification of the culprit vessel (lesion responsible for most severe ischaemia) allows a decision to be made on the dilatation's priorities and to reduce risks.

Inadequate results after PTCA may be caused by inadequate dilatation of the treated artery, by complications of the procedure (i.e. dissection or thrombosis), by residual stenosis elsewhere, or by restenosis. However, shortly after PTCA transient perfusion imaging abnormalities may reflect an altered perfusion reserve in the dilated territory resulting from arterial disruption or increased vasomotor tone but are not predictive of the long-term results. It may therefore be necessary to delay routine exercise myocardial imaging for 2–3 months after PTCA at a time when these transient problems have resolved and the incidence of restenosis increases. Residual myocardial ischaemia reflecting incomplete revascularization will also be evident at that time. Scintigraphy is superior to clinical and ECG signs of residual ischaemia as it has higher sensitivity and better localizes the area of ischaemia in relation to the known anatomy.

Clinical signs of restenosis are not very reliable, nor is the ECG very sensitive or specific for detecting restenosis. Myocardial imaging on the contrary is highly accurate to 'predict' restenosis early or to detect it at 6 months when most protocols have performed re-angiography [42]. Currently however, the need to detect asymptomatic restenosis is questioned as these stenoses are primarily made of fibrotic tissue and are thought to be unlikely to progress to occlusion. If this hypothesis is confirmed, the need for systematic evaluation of patients post-PTCA will be reduced.

Coronary artery bypass graft surgery

CABG has, over the past 20 years, profoundly altered the fate of patients with CAD. First performed for symptomatic relief, it also can provide functional improvement at rest and mainly after exercise and can improve prognosis. Patients with severe disease, either left main or multiple-vessel disease, and altered left ventricular function are the principal beneficiaries in terms of life expectancy. The principal role of nuclear medicine techniques is to help in the differential diagnosis of suboptimal results, perioperative complications, persistence of anginal pain, lack of functional improvement or functional alterations.

Diagnosis of perioperative infarction can be difficult as a result of ECG and enzyme changes subsequent to the intervention. Necrosis-specific tracers can recognize such an infarct early on. Perfusion imaging can also document a new or larger perfusion defect if a previous normal scan can be assumed or if a preoperative scan is available for comparison. Incomplete revascularization can result from an incomplete procedure or from an early graft obstruction. Obstruction of an initially patent graft can lead to recurrent ischaemia or to myocardial necrosis, especially if disease in the native coronary artery has progressed. Rest and stress perfusion scans can document ischaemia and necrosis but should be interpreted with the information of the preoperative angiographic results and of the surgical procedure. Progression of disease in the non-grafted arteries will usually be the cause of later events.

Pre- and post-operative reference scans are most helpful to interpret later images and assess the need for reinterventions. Valuable information about the patient's prognosis post-bypass is also provided by the nuclear medicine investigations. Indeed, variables of myocardial perfusion and ventricular function continue to be predominant in patients after surgery.

DETECTION OF JEOPARDIZED BUT VIABLE MYOCARDIUM

Definition

Perfusion and metabolic tracers play an increasing role in the assessment of reversibly asynergic myocardium such as occurring in stunning and hibernation. These conditions have been described earlier. The term 'viable' refers *sensu stricto* to myocardium which is alive and does not imply any particular state of function, perfusion or metabolism. Normal myocardium is obviously alive as are some myocytes within an area of partial necrosis or myocardium salvaged by thrombolysis even if jeopardized by a residual stenosis. Unfortunately, the term 'viable' is sometimes used interchangeably with jeopardized or with hibernation, leading to much confusion.

Population under concern

The patient population primarily concerned by 'viability' studies is not as large as originally thought. Only patients with left ventricular dysfunction or signs of heart failure and ischaemic cardiomyopathy require demonstration of viable myocardium to support the indication of coronary reperfusion rather than transplantation or medical therapy. In patients whose primary symptom is angina, the choice of therapy is primarily based on the need for revascularization. Accurate simple evaluation of myocardial viability would however be useful to assess the need and priority for bypass to achieve complete beneficial revascularization.

Tools

Several methods are available to detect and identify jeopardized myocardium or reversible chronic dysfunctioning myocardium. First, evaluation of regional function helps to categorize patients' segments with normal motion or mild to moderate hypokinesia as having persisting viability. Severe hypokinesia, akinesia or dyskinesia can be further stratified by inotropic stimulation or unloading. Improvement in regional function is considered evidence for viability. Improvement following low-dose dobutamine probably corresponds to stunning. Larger doses of dobutamine may also elicit some functional improvement in patients with subendocardial myocardial infarction or partial thickness infarction by stimulating the subepicardium, but revascularization does not lead to functional improvement in these patients [43].

Flow is compromised in ischaemic or jeopardized myocardium. Progressive alterations of flow corresponds to progressive loss of viability and diminished potential for recovery. Quantitative flow measurements, as can be done by PET, are therefore one of the best parameters to indicate potential for functional recovery.

Single-photon tracers however do not measure flow but estimate tracer uptake affected by partial volume and resolution effects, attenuation and other factors. Tracers indicative of membrane integrity such as cations (^{82}Rb, ^{38}K or ^{201}Tl) remain in viable cells but their release from necrotic cells is accelerated. The rate of rubidium and potassium release has been proposed to indicate non-viable myocardium [44].

Use of thallium The ability of thallium to redistribute is also useful. As the ultimate thallium distribution is determined by viability, any area with uptake superior to background levels must contain some viable myocardium. Significant uptake (>50%) as compared with normal suggests probable functional recovery after revascularization [45] (Figure 6.8). Sufficient time must be allowed for redistribution however, as its rate is related to resting perfusion. Four hours redistribution may be insufficient and thallium reinjection or preferably resting injection with delayed imaging is the preferred strategy. Different degrees of redistribution after reinjection, rest injection or rest plus redistribution might suggest more profound alterations such as hibernation and myocyte dedifferentiation (Table 6.3).

Use of technetium-labelled tracers The use of technetium-labelled perfusion agents also provides information on jeopardized myocardium. The uptake of a tracer such as sestamibi is primarily reflecting relative perfusion although its mitochondrial concentration and retention require

membrane integrity and cell viability. Lack of sestamibi concentration therefore clearly reflects low perfusion and necrosis and no falsely positive uptake is encountered like with thallium. Conversely significant uptake reflects both reasonable perfusion and viability and leads toward viable tissue and potential functional recovery [46] (Figure 6.8).

Intermediate uptake is however, more difficult to categorize as the absence of redistribution does not provide a qualitative parameter on which to base prediction. Rather, careful quantitative analysis of tracer uptake at rest and comparison of stress–rest data is necessary. Analysis of defect severity on a continuous scale (from 0 to 100% severity, normal uptake to background level) rather than use of a discrete threshold has been shown to predict variable probabilities of recovery (Figure 6.9). Evidence for residual ischaemia from the stress–rest comparison is also evidence for retained viability and potential for functional recovery.

Due to physical tracer differences, quantitative estimates of perfusion defects obtained by thal-

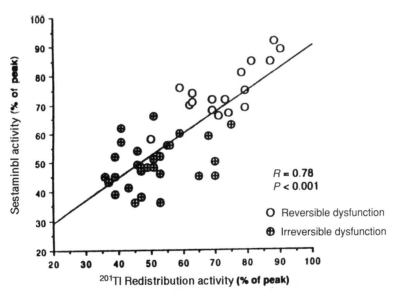

Figure 6.8 Comparison of the preoperative regional thallium and sestamibi activity is related to recovery (open circles) and lack of recovery (crossed circles) of regional function after revascularization. Both tracers provide discrimination of these two groups with some overlap. (Reproduced from Udelson *et al.* [46], by permission of the American Heart Association.)

Table 6.3   Single-photon tracers for myocardial viability assessment

Scintigraphic pattern	Interpretation
Reversibility of defects	
• Stress-induced defect	→ ischaemic, hence viable myocardium
• Rest defect with redistribution	→ severely ischaemic but still viable myocardium
Severity of resting defects	
• Mild to moderate (<60% hypoperfusion severity)	→ viable myocardium
• Intermediate (60%≥ ≤80% hypoperfusion severity)	→ undetermined, to be explored by PET
• Severe (>80% hypoperfusion severity)	→ scarred myocardium

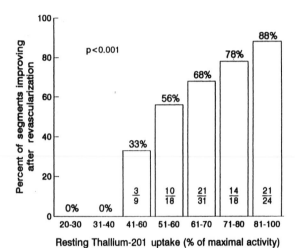

Figure 6.9   The need to assess defect severity on a continuous scale is illustrated by this graph. Progressively increasing cut-off for 'viability' progressively increases the percentage of segments improving after revascularization. [Reproduced from Perrone-Filardi *et al.*, *Circulation*, **91**, 2556–65 (1995), by permission of the American Heart Association.]

lium and sestamibi are different. This invalidates much of the literature reports which have compared thallium and sestamibi using identical arbitrary thresholds optimized for thallium. Furthermore, many of these reports have not used an adequate standard such as recovery of function to compare the merits of both tracers, but have naively assumed that the tracer showing more viable segments was the more accurate. It has now been shown that thallium uptake and redistribution are sensitive but not specific parameters to predict functional recovery and that false-positive predictions are frequent [47].

Use of metabolic tracers: ^{18}F-FDG   Finally, evaluation of myocardial metabolic shifts in conjunction with regional perfusion appears as the best method to evaluate retained viability and potential for recovery [48]. Irreversible scar has minimal if any metabolic use of any substrates whether fatty acids, glucose, acetate, ketone bodies, amino acids or oxygen. Ischaemic or jeopardized myocardium undergoes metabolic impairment in a progressive manner. Aerobic metabolism of fatty acids, acetate and ketone bodies is affected first as oxygen supply diminishes. Glucose utilization persists later as it can be used both in aerobic and in anaerobic pathways. Glucose or ^{18}F-FDG uptake is therefore increased in relation to flow in patients with myocardial ischaemia or hibernating myocardium.

PET perfusion/metabolism protocols for viability have been primarily performed in the postprandial state as glucose utilization is dependent on substrates availability. In these conditions, both normal myocardium and ischaemic or hibernating myocardium would demonstrate FDG uptake. Interpretation of the perfusion and metabolic images is usually performed on data normalized on the basis of the flow distribution: the region with maximum flow serves as the 100% uptake reference for both FDG and flow data. Interpretation is based on the ratio between the uptake of the perfusion tracer and FDG, but also on the relative value of normalized perfusion and FDG uptakes (Table 6.4). FDG uptake below 50% of reference is indeed rarely associated with recovery of function even if the FDG to flow ratio is increased. Quantitative evaluation of flow and glucose metabolism have also been used but the large variability in normal parameters makes their use less discriminant.

Table 6.4 Flow metabolism and functional alterations in various ischaemic syndromes at rest

	Blood flow	Function	FDG uptake	Low dose Dobutamine effect	Interpretation
1	Normal	Normal	Normal	↑	Normal
2	Normal	Depressed	Normal	↑	Stunning
3	Mildly decreased	Depressed	Normal	↑	Stunning
4	Mildly decreased	Depressed	Low Normal	→	Admixture: normal/scar
5	Moderately decreased	Akinetic	Normal or ↑	?	Repetitive stunning
6	Abnormal	Akinetic	Normal or ↑	→	Hibernating
7	Abnormal	Akinetic	Decreased	→	Admixture: hibernating/scar
8	Abnormal	Akinetic	Abolished	→↓	Scar
9	(Abnormal)	Normal	(Abnormal)	?	Dissociation*

*Temporal (transient ischaemia), spatial (malregistration) or artifacts.

Two different patterns of FDG/flow mismatch have been demonstrated (Plate 11). In the first pattern, the mismatch involves the entire myocardial segment with abnormal perfusion and normal or near-normal FDG uptake. This demonstrates that the myocardium is viable but underperfused and that it is metabolically embarrassed having switched from normal aerobic fatty acids metabolism to glucose metabolism. This is the pattern most frequently seen in hibernating myocardium. In the other, the mismatch involves only the periphery of an infarct and is most frequently seen in reperfused myocardial infarction with partial salvage but ongoing ischaemia at the periphery of the infarct.

Also, two different patterns of perfusion/metabolism matching have been described. In one, profound perfusion and FDG defects correspond to transmural infarction. In the other, both perfusion tracer and FDG uptakes are abnormal and similar but uptake is partially preserved. This pattern corresponds to partial myocardial infarction and to non-transmural or subendocardial infarction, although PET does not really allow identification of the various layers of the myocardium. This pattern therefore represents a mixture of viable and non-viable tissue within the infarcted area. Little or no improvement should be expected after reperfusion of segments with a match pattern, while improvement is mainly observed in patients with complete mismatch pattern and hibernating myocardium. This improvement can however, be considerably delayed.

Recent data have demonstrated that use of the concept of perfusion/metabolism mismatch does not require availability of a PET scanner but can be explored using conventional cameras equipped with a 511-keV collimator. If this is confirmed by additional studies, FDG could become more widely available for clinical practice.

Use of metabolic tracers: fatty acids Alternatively, another approach uses iodine-labelled fatty acids to document the anaerobic myocardial metabolic shift and does not require use of a PET camera. The proposed technique uses a fatty acid analogue, β-methyl iodophenyl penta-decanoic acid (BMIPP), as a marker of fatty acids uptake and utilization. This tracer is used in conjunction with a perfusion tracer, for instance sestamibi. If the myocardium remains viable, the metabolic deficit and hence the lack of uptake and utilization of BMIPP are out of proportion to the blood flow decrease and this results in a flow/metabolism mismatch: relatively preserved flow, abolished fatty acid utilization. Validity of this concept has been reported in patients post-myocardial infarction and fibrinolysis where this pattern has been shown to be indicative of delayed functional recovery [49].

^{11}C-Acetate has also been used to assess viability. This tracer is a direct substrate of the tricarboxylic acid cycle and indicates myocardial oxygen consumption. Quantitative estimates of acetate utilization have been proposed to identify residual oxidative metabolism and viability [50].

Perfusable tissue index Another positron emission tomographic technique used to identify viable and potentially hibernating myocardium is calculation of the water-perfusable tissue index from kinetic analysis of water ($H_2{}^{15}O$) as a perfusion tracer. This index is a measure of the proportion of tissue into which water perfuses rapidly and hence the proportion of viable myocytes as opposed to fibrotic tissue. Areas with reduced function but without significant reduction of this index may recover function after revascularization.

As can be seen, numerous techniques and approaches are available to study jeopardized but viable myocardium. Given the relatively limited target population, a consensus approach is needed. Standard perfusion imaging can be used to stratify most patients into viable or scar groups. Intermediate patients require further testing. In those, use of FDG appears as the most straightforward technique provided that it can be made more widely available.

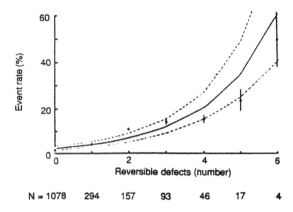

Figure 6.10 Cardiac event rate in relation to the number of segments with redistribution on exercise thallium-201 image. The event rate increased exponentially with the extent of ischaemia. (Reproduced from Ladenheim *et al.* [51], by permission from the American College of Cardiology.)

PROGNOSIS OF PATIENTS WITH CAD

The evaluation of prognosis in patients with CAD may well be the most important contribution of nuclear techniques. Numerous reports have indeed documented their particular prognostic value at various stages of the disease.

In patients with known disease, prognosis is related not only to the presence of CAD but also to its extent and severity and to the consequences of the disease on cardiac function. The extent of ventricular dysfunction, global and regional, is an important prognostic factor in symptomatic patients. The role of nuclear cardiology procedures is therefore to recognize patients at high risk in whom consideration should be given of more invasive procedures as well as patients with low or very low risk in whom no further testing but only regular follow-up is indicated.

Patients with stable CAD

The powerful prognostic role of an abnormal perfusion scan has been largely demonstrated using thallium and planar imaging, but is now confirmed with technetium-labelled tracers and SPECT. The increased risk is directly related to the extent of ischaemic myocardium (Figure 6.10). A 1-year follow-up of 1689 patients with CAD but without prior infarction has showed that the extent and severity of the reversible thallium defects were independent predictors of cardiac events [51]. The event rate at 1 year varied between 0.4%

in patients with normal perfusion to 78% in patients with both severe and extensive perfusion defects. The same group demonstrated the incremental prognostic power of thallium imaging over history and exercise ECG. Similar results obtained with SPECT were reported more recently [52]. Several studies have also demonstrated the prognostic value of non-exercise (dipyridamole or pacing) myocardial perfusion imaging.

Equally important is the ability to identify those patients at low risk, and who are unlikely to benefit from additional costly procedures. Patients with a normal radionuclide perfusion study have a very low cardiac event rate, usually lower than 1% per year, a figure approaching that of the age-matched normal population. This is observed even for long-term follow-up (10 years) and also in patients with proven coronary artery disease. The good prognosis of patients with normal exercise nuclear scans (adequately performed and correctly interpreted), even with angiographically significant disease, is important to underline because it highlights the essential difference between angiography and perfusion scintigraphy. Angiography provides a crude visual estimate of anatomical severity. It has large intra- and interobserver variability and a poor association with post-mortem anatomy. Perfusion scintigraphy provides an estimate of the functional severity of the lesions at the capillary level. Discordance does not necessarily reflect 'another false-negative scintigraphic result', but rather the lack of functional significance of an anatomical lesion. Although false-negatives do occur, the prognostic data should comfort both the nuclear medicine physician and the cardiologist on the significance of the scintigraphic results.

Risk stratification after myocardial infarction

The value of stress myocardial perfusion imaging to define the extent of the infarct and the presence of residual ischaemia has been previously described in the section on post-infarction management. Also, intravenous dipyridamole can be substituted for exercise as the cardiac stressor but the presence of reversible defect then becomes the principal prognostic finding while the others, extent of disease and mainly lung uptake, lose their

importance. The principal rationale for pharmacological testing is to allow early stratification (2–4 days after the event).

The prognostic significance of metabolic/perfusion mismatch has been reported in patients with severe coronary disease and left ventricular dysfunction [53]. Two studies have reported the high risk associated with mismatch in non-reperfused patients. The prognosis of patients with mismatch undergoing revascularization is considerably improved. By contrast, patients without mismatch have 'low' event rate, irrespective of therapy (Figure 6.11).

The prognostic value of myocardial perfusion imaging has also been established in patients studied before vascular surgery (mainly in patients with positive clinical risk factors) and in patients with unstable angina.

While most previous reports were performed

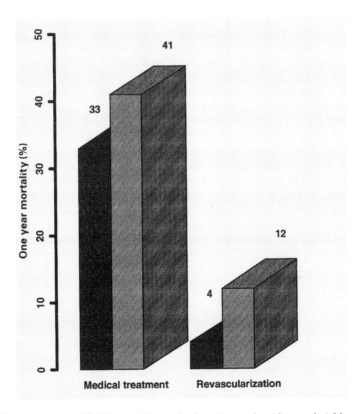

Figure 6.11 Mortality in patients with left ventricular dysfunction and evidence of viable myocardium as determined by PET and FDG/blood flow mismatch. Patients treated medically had higher 1-year mortality than patients undergoing revascularization. [Dark panels: data from Eitzman *et al.*, *J. Am. Coll. Cardiol.* (1992); light panels: data from DiCarli *et al.*, *Am. J. Cardiol.* (1994).]

using thallium, sufficient data are now available to support the contention that similar results can be obtained using technetium-labelled perfusion tracers.

REFERENCES

1. Blumgart, H.L. and Weiss, S. (1927) Studies on the velocity of blood flow: VII. The pulmonary circulation time in normal resting individuals. *J. Clin. Invest.*, **4**, 399–425.
2. Wagner, H.N., Jr (1995) Nuclear Medicine: What it is, what it does, in *Principles of Nuclear Medicine* (eds H.N. Wagner, Z. Szabo and B.S. Buchanan), W.B. Saunders Company, Philadelphia, 1995, pp. 1–8.
3. Marcus, M.C., Skorton, D.J., Johnson, M.R. *et al.* (1988)Visual estimates of percent diameter stenosis: 'a battered gold standard'. *J. Am. Coll. Cardiol.*, **11**, 882–6.
4. Rigo, P., Becker, L.C., Griffith, L.S.C., Alderson, P.O., Bailey, I.K., Pitt, B., Burow, R.D. and Wagner, H.N., Jr (1979) Influence of coronary collateral vessels on the results of thallium-201 myocardial stress imaging. *Am. J. Cardiol.*, **44**, 452–8.
5. Gould, K., Lipscomb, K. and Hamilton, G. (1974) Physiologic basis for assessing critical coronary stenosis. Instantaneous flow response and regional distribution during coronary hyperemia as measures of coronary flow reserve. *Am. J. Cardiol.*, **33**, 87–94.
6. Maseri, A., L'Abbate, A., Pesola, A. *et al.* (1977) Regional myocardial perfusion in patients with atherosclerotic coronary artery disease at rest and during angina pectoris induced by tachycardia. *Circulation*, **55**, 423–33.
7. Braunwald, E. and Rutherford, J.D. (1986) Reversible ischemic left ventricular dysfunction: Evidence for the 'hibernating myocardium'. *J. Am. Coll. Cardiol.*, **8**, 1467–70.
8. Heyndrickx, G., Millard, R., McRitchie, R. *et al.* (1975) Regional myocardial function and electrophysiologic alterations after brief coronary occlusion in conscious dog. *J. Clin. Invest.*, **56**, 978–85.
9. Marinho, N.V.S., Keogh, B.E., Costa, D.C. *et al.* (1996) Pathophysiology of chronic left ventricular dysfunction. New insight from the measurement of absolute myocardique blood flow and glucose utilization. *Circulation*, **93**, 737–44.
10. Maes,. A., Flameng, W., Nuyts, J. *et al.* (1994) Histological alterations in chronically hypoperfused myocardium: correlation with PET finding. *Circulation*, **90**, 735–45.
11. Zimmermann, R., Mall, G., Rauch, B. *et al.* (1995) Residual 201-Tl activity in irreversible defects as a marker of myocardial viability – clinicopathological study. *Circulation*, **91**, 1016–21.
12. Deutsch, E., Glavan, K.A., Sodd, V.J., Nishiyama, H., Ferguson, D.L. and Lukes, S.J. (1981) Cationic Tc-99m complexes as potential myocardial imaging agents. *J. Nucl. Med.*, **22**, 897–907.
13. Jones, A.G., Davidson, A., Abrams, M.J. *et al.* (1984) Biological studies of a new class of technetium complexes: the hexakis (alkylisonitrile) technetium (I) cations. *Int. J. Nucl. Med. Biol.*, **11**, 225–34.
14. Zaret, B.L., Rigo, P., Wackers, F.J.T., Hendel, R.C., Braat, S., Iskandrian, A.S., Sridhara, S., Jain, D., Itti, R., Serafini, A.N., Goris, M.L., Lahiri, A. and the Tetrofosmin International Trial Study Group (1995) Myocardial perfusion imaging with technetium-99m tetrofosmin: comparison to thallium-201 imaging and coronary angiography in a phase III multicenter trial. *Circulation*, **91**, 313–19.
15. Gerson, M.C., Millard, R.W., Roszell, N.J. *et al.* (1994) Kinetics properties of 99mTc-Q12 in canine myocardium. *Circulation*, **89**, 1291–300.
16. Schwaiger, M. and Muzik, O. (1991) Assessment of myocardial perfusion by positron emission tomography. *Am. J. Cardiol.*, **67**, 35–43.
17. Iskandrian, A.S., Verani, M.S. and Heo, J. (1994) Pharmacological stress testing: mechanism of action, hemodynamic responses and results in detection of coronary artery disease. *J. Nucl. Cardiol.*, **1**, 94–111.
18. Wackers, F.J., Bodenheimer, M., Fleiss, J.M. *et al.* and the multicenter study on silent myocardial ischemia (MSSMI) Thallium-201 investigators. (1993) Factors affecting uniformity of interpretation of planar Thallium-201 imaging in a multicenter trial. *J. Am. Coll. Cardiol.*, **21**, 1064–74.
19. From the Committee on advanced cardiac imaging and technology, Council on clinical cardiology, American Heart Association; Cardiovascular Imaging Committee, American College of Cardiology; and Board of directors, Cardiovascular Council, Society of Nuclear Medicine. (1992) Standardization of cardiac tomographic imaging. *Circulation*, **86**, 338–9.
20. Garcia, E.V., Cooke, C.D., Van Train, K.F. *et al.* (1990) Technical aspects of myocardial SPECT imaging with technetium-99m sestamibi. *Am. J. Cardiol.*, **66**, 23E–31E.
21. Benoit, T., Vivegnis, D., Foulon, J. and Rigo, P. (1996) Quantitative evaluation of myocardial SPECT imaging: application to the measurement of perfusion defect size and severity. *Eur. J. Nucl. Med.*, **23**, 1603–12.
22. Chua, T., Kiat, H., Germano, G. *et al.* (1994) Gated technetium-99m sestamibi for simultaneous assessment of stress myocardial perfusion, post-exercise regional ventricular function and myocardial viability: correlation with echocardiography and rest thallium-201 scintigraphy. *J. Am. Coll. Cardiol.*, **23**, 1107–14.
23. Corbett, J.R., Jansen, D.E., Lewis, S.E. *et al.* (1985) Tomographic gated blood pool radionuclide ventriculography: analysis of wall motion and left ventricular volumes in patients with coronary artery disease. *J. Am. Coll. Cardiol.*, **6**, 349–58.
24. Neumann, D.R., Go, R.T., Myers, B.A. *et al.* (1993) Parametric phase display for biventricular function from gated cardiac blood pool single-photon emission tomography. *Eur. J. Nucl. Med.*, **20**, 1108–11.

25. Schelbert, H. (1991) Positron emission tomography for the assessment of myocardial viability. *Circulation*, **84**, I122–31.

26. Knapp, F.F., Ambrose, K.R. and Goodman, M.M. (1986) New radioiodinated methyl-branched fatty acids for cardiac studies. *Eur. J. Nucl. Med.*, **12**, S39–44.

27. Borer, J.S., Bacharach, S.L., Green, M.V. *et al.* (1977) Real-time radionuclide cineangiography in the non invasive evaluation of global and regional left ventricular function at rest and during exercise in patients with coronary artery disease. *N. Engl. J. Med.*, **296**, 839–44.

28. Rozanski, A. and Berman, D.S. (1987) The efficacy of cardiovascular nuclear medicine exercise studies. *Semin. Nucl. Med.*, **17**, 104–20.

29. Van Damme, H., Piérard, L., Gillain, D. *et al.* (1997) Cardiac risk assessment before vascular surgery: a prospective study comparing clinical evaluation, dobutamine stress echocardiography, and dobutamine Tc-99m Sestamibi tomoscintigraphy. *J. Cardiovasc. Surg.*, **5**, 54–64.

30. CASS Principal Investigators and Associates. (1983) Coronary Artery Surgery Study (CASS): a randomized trial of coronary artery bypass surgery. *Circulation*, **68**, 939–50.

31. Fintel, D.J., Links, J.M., Brinker, J.A. *et al.* (1989) Improved diagnostic performance of exercise thallium-201 single photon emission tomography over planar imaging in the diagnosis of coronary artery disease: a receiver operating characteristic analysis. *J. Am. Coll. Cardiol.*, **13**, 600–12.

32. Weiss, A.T., Berman, D.S., Lew, A.S. *et al.* (1987) Transient ischaemic dilatation of the left ventricle and stress thallium-201 scintigraphy: a marker of severe and extensive coronary artery disease. *J. Am. Coll. Cardiol.*, **9**, 752–9.

33. Rigo, P., Bailey, I.K., Griffith, L.S.C. *et al.* (1980) Value and limitations of segmental analysis of stress thallium myocardial imaging for localization of coronary artery disease. *Circulation*, **61**, 973–81.

34. Breisblatt, W.M., Barnes, J.V., Weiland, D. and Spaccavento, J. (1988) Incomplete revascularization in multivessel percutaneous transluminal coronary angioplasty: the role for stress thallium-201 imaging. *J. Am. Coll. Cardiol.*, **11**, 1183–90.

35. Wackers, F.J.Th. (1980) Thallium-201 myocardial scintigraphy in acute myocardial infarction and ischemia. *Semin. Nucl. Med.*, **10**, 127–45.

36. Gregoire, T. and Theroux, P. (1990) Detection and assessment of unstable angina using myocardial perfusion imaging: comparison between technetium-99m sestamibi Spect and 12-lead electrocardiogram. *Am. J. Cardiol.*, **66**, 42A–46E.

37. Johnson, L.L., Seldin, D.W., Becler, L.C. *et al.* (1989) Antimyosin imaging in acute transmural myocardial infarctions: results of a multicenter clinical trial. *J. Am. Coll. Cardiol.*, **13**, 27–35.

38. Gibson, W.S., Christian, T.F., Pellikka, P.A. *et al.* (1992) Serial tomographic imaging with Technetium-99m-Sestamibi for the assessment of infarct-related arterial patency following reperfusion therapy. *J. Nucl. Med.*, **33**, 2080–5.

39. Christian, T.F., Behrenbeck, T., Pellikka, P.A. *et al.* (1990) Mismatch of left ventricular function and infarct size demonstrated by Technetium-99m isonitrile imaging after reperfusion therapy for acute myocardial infarction: identification of myocardial stunning and hyperkinesia. *J. Am. Coll. Cardiol.*, **16**, 1632–8.

40. Galli, M., Marcassa, C., Bammo, R. *et al.* (1994) Spontaneous delayed recovery of perfusion and contraction after the first five weeks after anterior infarction: evidence for the presence of hibernating myocardium in the infarcted area. *Circulation*, **90**, 2386–92.

41. Gibson, R.S., Watson, D.D., Craddock, G.B. *et al.* (1983) Prediction of cardiac events after uncomplicated myocardial infarction: a prospective study comparing predischarge exercise thallium-201 scintigraphy and coronary arteriography. *Circulation*, **68**, 321–36.

42. Wijns, W., Serruys, P.W., Simoons, M.L. *et al.* (1985) Predictive value of early maximal exercise test and thallium scintigraphy after successful percutaneous transluminal coronary angioplasty. *Br. Heart J.*, **53**, 194–200.

43. Afridi, I., Kleinman, N.S., Kaizer, A.E. and Zaghbi, W.A. (1995) Dobutamine echocardiography in myocardial hibernation: optimal dose and accuracy in predicting recovery of ventricular function after coronary angioplasty. *Circulation*, **91**, 663–70.

44. Gould, K.L., Yoshida, K., Hess, M.J. *et al.* (1991) Myocardial metabolism of fluorodeoxyglucose compared to cell membrane integrity for the potassium analogue rubidium-82 for assessing infarct size in man by PET. *J. Nucl. Med.*, **32**, 1–9.

45. Ragosta, M., Beller, G.A., Watson, D.W. *et al.* (1993) Quantitative planar rest-redistribution 201-Tl imaging in detecting of myocardial viability and prediction of improvement in left ventricular function after coronary bypass surgery in patients with severely depressed left ventricular function. *Circulation*, **83**, 1630–41.

46. Udelson, J., Coleman, P., Matherall, J. *et al.* (1994) Predicting recovery of severe ventricular dysfunction: comparison of resting scintigraphy with thallium-201 and Tc-99m sestamibi. *Circulation*, **89**, 2552–61.

47. Arnese, M., Cornel, J., Salustri, A. *et al.* (1995) Prediction of improvement of regional left ventricular function after surgical revascularization: a comparison of low dose dobutamine echocardiography with thallium-201 single photon emission computed tomography. *Circulation*, **91**, 2748–52.

48. Maddahi, J., Schelbert, A., Brunken, R. *et al.* (1994) Role of thallium-201 and PET imaging in evaluation of myocardial viability and management of patients with coronary artery disease and left ventricular dysfunction. *J. Nucl. Med.*, **35**, 707–15.

49. Franken, P.R., Dendale, P., De Geeter, F. *et al.* (1996) Prediction of functional outcome after myocardial infarction using BMIPP and sestamibi scintigraphy. *J. Nucl. Med.*, **37**, 718–22.

50. Gropler, R.J., Geltman, E.M., Sampath Kumaran, K. *et al.* (1992) Functional recovery after coronary

revascularization for chronic coronary artery disease is dependent on maintenance of oxidative metabolism. *J. Am. Coll. Cardiol.*, **20**, 569–77.

51. Ladenheim, M.L., Pollock, B.H., Rozanski, A. *et al.* (1996) Extent and severity of myocardial hypoperfusion as predictors of prognosis in patients with suspected coronary artery disease. *J. Am. Coll. Cardiol.*, **7**, 464–71.

52. Machecourt, J., Longere, P., Fagret, D. *et al.* (1994) Prognostic value of thallium-201 single-photon emission computed tomographic myocardial perfusion imaging according to extent of myocardial defect. *J. Am. Coll. Cardiol.*, **23**, 1096–106.

53. Di Carli, M., Davidson, M., Little, R. *et al.* (1994) Value of metabolic imaging with positron emission tomography for evaluating prognosis in patients with coronary artery disease and left ventricular function. *Am. J. Cardiol.*, **73**, 527–33.

54. Sochor, H., Bourguignon, M., Braat, S.H. *et al.* (1996) Pharmacological stress testing with ^{99m}Tc sestamibi. *Dialogues in Nuclear Cardiology*, **3**, 1–31. Kluwer, Dordrecht.

Other cardiac applications

P. Rigo

INTRODUCTION

The ability of tracer techniques to assess non-invasively the various cardiac functional parameters has led to their widespread use in many patients with non-coronary heart diseases. Many applications rely on techniques to assess circulatory flow patterns and cardiac pump function, and benefit from the quantitation and reproducibility characteristics of the tracer procedures.

PATHOPHYSIOLOGY

The primary aims of the circulation comprise the delivery of oxygen and energy substrates to various parts of the body, the transport of numerous substances including hormones, and the washout of metabolic by-products.

With each beat, the cardiac pump carries blood into the lungs and the systemic circulation. The heart is a muscular bag functionally divided into two parts. The right heart receives desaturated venous blood through the venae cavae (superior and inferior) into the right atrium, and the right ventricle (RV) and pumps it via the pulmonary artery into the pulmonary circulation where it is oxygenated. The pulmonary circulation is a low-resistance system and consequently the pressure in the right heart remains low. The left heart receives the oxygenated blood via the pulmonary veins into the left atrium and the left ventricle (LV), which is pumped to the systemic circulation through the aorta. The pressure in the left heart is considerably higher than in the right heart in order to overcome the peripheral vascular resistance of the systemic vascular bed.

The morphology of the heart is adapted to these pressure differences: the left ventricle is much thicker than the right ventricle and has a concentric shape, while the right ventricle attaches to the septum-like bellows. The right ventricular contraction therefore results in part from the left ventricular contraction, and there is ventricular interdependence. The four cardiac chambers are contained by the pericardium, a rather stiff membrane; therefore changes (mainly acute) in the volume of one cavity influence the others and increases this interdependence.

The cardiac cycle alternates between diastole and systole. A sequence of electrical events triggers mechanical events and produces pressure and flow. In early diastole, the atria and ventricles are relaxed. The atrioventricular valves are open and blood flows from the atria to the ventricles. The aortic and pulmonary valves are closed to prevent backflow from the great vessels. Most of the ventricular filling occurs passively during the early diastole, while the atrial contraction, in response to atrial activation, later contributes the last 10–20% of filling and serves mainly to prepare closure of the atrioventricular valves. The rise in pressure resulting from ventricular contraction in response to electrical depolarization first causes a complete closure of the atrioventricular valves and then opens the aortic and pulmonary valves to allow ejection of the stroke volume. The ventricular ejection fraction (EF) is the fraction of the end-diastolic ventricular volume ejected during systole. The sinoatrial node is the normal pacemaker, whose fastest inherent rhythm supersedes other sites with automaticity. The impulse is conducted by a specialized conduction system (Purkinje system) through the myocardium. The atrioventricular node is responsible for the delay necessary for optimal atrioventricular synchronization. Rapid conduction along the bundle of His and the Purkinje system allows efficient and almost simultaneous stimulation of ventricular walls in an orderly manner.

The cardiac pump function is regulated beat-by-beat by the preload, the afterload and the inotropic level. The preload determines the initial length of the muscle fibres before contraction, and depends upon venous return and the atrial contraction together with the residual volume. The afterload results from the stresses imposed on the ventricle during systolic shortening including peripheral resistance, aortic impedance, blood mass and viscosity. The inotropic level determines the contractile force and is dependent on the neurohumoral regulation of the heart as well as its frequency. Cardiac frequency is also by itself one of the most important means of adjusting cardiac

Clinical Nuclear Medicine, 3rd edn. Edited by M.N. Maisey, K.E. Britton and B.D. Collier. Published in 1998 by Chapman & Hall, London. ISBN 0 412 75180 1

function to the circulatory demands. Others factors include increased stroke volume, through increased EF and/or end-diastolic volume. Peripheral circulatory adjustments such as blood flow redistribution to working regions or increased oxygen extraction are also effective. Long-term adjustment includes ventricular dilatation and hypertrophy.

Pathology determines: (i) volume and/or flow overload (with increased preload) in valvular regurgitant lesions, intracardiac shunts, transposition and arteriovenous fistulas (pulmonary or systemic); (ii) pressure overload (with increased afterload), for instance in aortic stenosis or hypertension; and (iii) alterations in the mass or contractile properties of the cardiac muscle. Other lesions affect the transmission of cardiac impulses or the coordination of contraction. The various forms of cardiovascular adaptation can maintain satisfactory compensation despite progressive alteration in cardiac function and reserve. Heart failure primarily results from progressive mismatch between imposed afterload and preload reserve [1]. Altered ventricular reserve makes patients more sensitive to afterload, and the pump function deteriorates when the afterload is increased. This effect becomes most prominent when the preload reserve is exhausted and when the contractile state can no longer be increased.

TECHNIQUES

The radiopharmaceuticals and techniques used to assess ventricular function have been described in the previous chapter. The count–volume proportionality of gated blood pool scans allows assessment of cardiac volume as well as global and regional ventricular function. It is also possible to calculate cardiac output either as the stroke volume times heart rate or using first pass as the product of equilibrium activity and blood volume divided by the integral of the extrapolated cardiac time–activity curve [2].

Several techniques have been devised to assess valvular regurgitation [3–7]. The standard approach compares the total ventricular stroke volume to the reference pulmonary or systemic stroke volume measured by a variety of techniques (most often the cardiac output divided by heart rate). In patients with single ventricular regurgitation (aortic and/or mitral for the LV;

tricuspid and/or pulmonary for the RV), the contralateral ventricle can be used to calculate the reference stroke volume, and this particular feature has led to the development of the stroke volume ratio [4,5] (Plate 12). This approach assumes equal detection efficiency of both ventricular stroke counts in the left anterior oblique (LAO) projection or during first pass – an assumption that is not entirely satisfactory, particularly in patients with LV failure. Several adaptations have therefore been proposed to correct for this problem. In particular, the Fourier phase and amplitude images are quite useful for tracing the outline of proper regions-of-interest over the left and right ventricles [8], but it is not advisable to compute either the stroke counts or the stroke ratio using the amplitude image as this may introduce errors in regions with asynergy [9]. Factor analysis of first pass-data is an attractive technique, but has been seldom used [7]. SPECT radionuclide angiography, also under-utilized, has the potential to improve ventricular sampling and the accuracy of the stroke volume ratio [10].

All of the proposed methods have sources of inaccuracies, and in my opinion, methods that require absolute quantification of ventricular volumes are more prone to these errors than the others. However, these methods are useful in conjunction with other measurements for the overall functional assessment of patients with valvular heart diseases.

CLINICAL APPLICATIONS

VALVULAR AND CONGENITAL HEART DISEASES

Intracardiac shunts and valvular regurgitation impose abnormal flow patterns and ventricular volume overload conditions, which can be readily appreciated using radionuclide angiography and perfusion imaging (Table 6.5). Advances in the radionuclide angiographic measurement of ventricular volumes (diastolic, systolic, forward ejection, regurgitant, right or left, etc.) have made it a practical technique for the detection, quantitation and functional assessment of valvular regurgitation and shunts. Pressure overload and associated ventricular hypertrophy can be recognized both on radionuclide angiography (as a widening of the right and left ventricular separation) and on myo-

Table 6.5 Haemodynamic repercussions in various cardiac disorders

	Volume overload	Dilatation	Hypertrophy
Compensated aortic stenosis		LA	LV++
Decompensated aortic stenosis		LV,LA	LV
Aortic regurgitation	LV	LV	LV
Mitral stenosis		LA	RV
Mitral regurgitation	LV	LA,LV	(RV)
Tricuspid regurgitation	RV	RV,RA	(RV)
Pulmonary regurgitation	RV	RV	RV
Atrial septal defect (+ anomalous venous return)	RV	RV,(RA)	
Patent ductus	LV	LV	
Ventricular septal defect	LV(RV)	LV(RV)	RV

cardial perfusion imaging, specially tomographic (increased wall thickening frequently associated with reduced cavity dimensions). Assessing the severity of hypertrophy is however difficult, as the image depends on camera resolution, tracer energy, type of filtering, partial-volume effect, etc. Radioactive tracer studies help quantify the effect of valve disease on chamber size and function, assess the prognosis, facilitate therapeutic decision and monitor the effects of therapy [11].

Aortic stenosis

Aortic stenosis primarily affects the left ventricle and produces progressive hypertrophy. The left ventricle becomes elongated while the aortic root widens due to post-stenotic dilatation. The EF is not initially affected but the ejection phase is prolonged and ejection velocity decreases. The diastolic part of the LV volume curve may also be affected. Left atrial dilatation may reflect increased LV filling pressure, but the right side of the heart usually remains normal unless decompensation occurs. Left ventricular hypertrophy has been shown to regress after aortic valve replacement with concomitant improvement in cardiac function. In the presence of aortic stenosis, perfusion defects suggestive of regional myocardial ischaemia may be observed using myocardial perfusion imaging in the absence of angiographically significant coronary artery lesions [12].

Aortic regurgitation

Aortic regurgitation induces LV dilatation, primarily diastolic. Initially, the ventricle appears elon-

gated but with progressive disease the regurgitant fraction increases and the cavity tends to become more globular. Exercise capacity can long be maintained as the regurgitant fraction decreases with exercise. Left ventricular dysfunction can be difficult to recognize initially. The ejection fraction response to exercise must be interpreted with caution as the EF can decrease in the absence of LV dysfunction as a result of changes in the loading conditions and decreases in regurgitation. Measurement of the exercise end-systolic volume (ESV) or of the end-systolic (ES) pressure-volume slope appears to be the most reliable indicator of LV dysfunction [13]. Also, the regurgitant volume over EDV index, easily calculated using radionuclide angiography as EF × RF, indicates the extent of the potential surgical benefit [14]. According to Bonow and Epstein [15], 50% of the patients with pre-operative LV dysfunction do not do well after valve replacement, if surgery is delayed until the onset of severe symptoms or of moderate to severe LV dysfunction. Postoperative improvement in left ventricular systolic function is related to early reduction in left ventricular dilatation after surgery.

Mitral stenosis

Left atrial dilatation consecutive to mitral stenosis is easily identified on gated blood pool scan. Also, the diastolic filling phase of the LV volume curve is characteristically modified: slow monotonous filling with loss of atrial contribution even when the patient remains in sinus rhythm. The LV dimensions are normal or small, as the left ventricle may be underfilled. Left ventricular EF usually remains normal but can be moderately diminished as a result of rheumatic myopathy, underfilling or of the rigidity of the LV walls adjacent to the mitral valve. Secondary pulmonary hypertension leads to RV hypertrophy recognizable on perfusion imaging, or to right ventricular dilatation with concomitant tricuspid regurgitation in the later stages.

Mitral regurgitation

Left atrial and left ventricular dilatation coincide in mitral regurgitation. The left ventricle appears globular and can overlap the left atrium in the LAO projection, making the left atrial enlargement more difficult to recognize, unless the patient and camera are properly positioned with some craniocaudal obliquity. Chronic mitral regurgitation can be tolerated for a fairly long period of time. Because of the low-impedance ejection resulting from regurgitation, the EF long remains normal and is not a good sign of LV dysfunction. ESV determination at rest, and particularly during exercise, is a better indicator of disease progression. Development of pulmonary hypertension is more common in cases of concomitant mitral stenosis and leads to RV hypertrophy followed by RV dysfunction – another important sign of functional deterioration. The clinical and scintigraphic pattern of acute mitral regurgitation is different as the left atrium has no time to dilate and pulmonary venous congestion develops more rapidly.

Most patients with mitral valve prolapse have normal LV function and only minimal or mild regurgitation. Diminished LV functional reserve observed in a small subgroup of patients has suggested the presence of a cardiomyopathic process [16]. Progression of the disease with ruptured chordae tendineae or secondary to endocarditis can lead to significant mitral regurgitation that may require surgical correction.

Tricuspid regurgitation

Tricuspid regurgitation usually develops as a consequence of RV dilatation, but the tricuspid valve can also be affected by rheumatic disease, right ventricular myocardial infarction, endocarditis, etc.). Tricuspid regurgitation leads to right atrial dilatation as well as hepatic and venous congestion. Reflux of activity into the jugular or hepatic vein can sometimes be observed during first-pass studies, while systolic liver pulsations can be appreciated on the equilibrium amplitude images. Right ventricular volume overload can also be appreciated using the stroke volume ratio approach (RV stroke volume/LV stroke volume) provided that the LV stroke volume is not affected (as with pure mitral stenosis or after successful mitral valve replacement) [17]. Right ventricular hypertrophy can be appreciated on the perfusion scan, but its development varies according to the aetiology of tricuspid regurgitation.

Left-to-right shunts

Left-to-right shunts produce pulmonary recirculation, that can best be appreciated during first-pass acquisition using pulmonary region-of-interest. The pulmonary time–activity curve represents the transit of the total injected activity in the pulmonary bed followed by the transit of the shunted fraction in the same pulmonary bed. The counting efficiency is maintained throughout, and all that is required for quantification is homogeneous bolus distribution and an accurate curve stripping technique to separate the shunt recirculation from the first transit and subsequent systemic recirculation. Several activity and area ratios have been proposed but the gamma variate fitting technique of Maltz and Treves has yielded the best results [18]. This technique accurately measures left-to-right shunts and is probably better than oximetry, particularly in cases of anomalous pulmonary venous return and of shunts at the atrial level when an accurate mixed venous sample cannot be obtained.

Equilibrium gated acquisitions are also useful for assessing the site and magnitude of the ventricular volume overload and its repercussions on cardiac function. Shunts at the atrial level overload the right ventricle with the result that the RV stroke volume exceeds the LV stroke volume. Left-to-right shunts associated with a patent ductus arteriosus overload the left ventricle, and the LV stroke volume exceeds the RV stroke volume. Shunts at the ventricular level (ventricular septal defects) are more complex but systolic left-to-right shunting usually predominates and overloads the left ventricle. In simple situations, the stroke volume ratio (expressed as RVSV/LVSV or LVSV/RVSV depending on which ventricle is overloaded), corrected for results in normal subjects, can be used to estimate the Q_P/Q_S [19]. RV hypertrophy is common in patients with congenital abnormalities and can be visualized using perfusion imaging.

HYPERTROPHIC CARDIOMYOPATHY AND CARDIAC HYPERTROPHY

Severe hypertrophic cardiomyopathy can result from severe hypertension, which can be idiopathic but is more frequently seen in patients with chronic renal failure. It primarily affects the LV diastolic function, and the LV volume curve reveals delayed LV filling and the absence of diastasis. It is difficult to separate patients with severe concentric hypertrophy from those with idiopathic hypertrophic cardiomyopathy or obstructive cardiomyopathy using radionuclide imaging. However, asymmetric hypertrophy of the high septum may at times be evident on the blood pool images as well as on the perfusion scans.

PET imaging in hypertrophic cardiomyopathy has revealed regional disparities in perfusion and metabolism. Myocardial perfusion is mildly depressed in the interventricular septum. The uptake of ^{11}C-palmitate is also reduced but its kinetics appears rather homogeneous. In contrast, ^{18}F-FDG accumulation in the septum is markedly reduced in comparison with the posterolateral wall [20].

In patients with a milder form of hypertrophy such as seen in patients with systemic hypertension, the LV systolic dysfunction does not usually develop until late in the course of the disease. Diastolic dysfunction however, appears much earlier, but can improve with regression of hypertrophy as a result of antihypertensive therapy.

DILATED CARDIOMYOPATHY AND MYOCARDITIS

Severe ventricular dysfunction has many causes since it can result from the end-stage evolution of most cardiac diseases. Cardiomyopathy may either be primarily myocardial in origin or secondary to myocardial damage caused by alcohol, drugs, viral infection, metabolic defects, etc. The utilization of metabolic substrate (mainly fatty acids) appears heterogeneous in many patients with cardiomyopathy, although no specific pattern can be described. In some patients, glucose loading increases rather than decreases fatty

acid utilization rate, supporting the hypothesis of an impairment of substrate utilization in these patients.

Duchenne muscular dystrophy is a generalized muscular disorder that also affects the heart. In this disorder, myocardial abnormalities predominantly involve the posterobasal and posterolateral segments of the left ventricle where fibrotic degeneration is often observed on pathological examination. PET studies have confirmed reduced blood flow in these areas, which have also been observed on thallium scans. A concomitant increase in FDG uptake in these regions has also been reported, but the significance of these findings remains hypothetical [21].

While the pattern of regional abnormalities is not specific for the aetiology of cardiomyopathies, it can be used to distinguish patients with true cardiomyopathies from patients with ischaemia-induced severe LV dysfunction. In the latter group, the RV function is often spared. Furthermore, in necrosis and ischaemia, the metabolic abnormalities are more localized and frequently affect large segments of the myocardium, which is in contrast to the more heterogeneous pattern seen in cardiomyopathy.

Patients with myocarditis must be distinguished from patients with cardiomyopathy, as this distinction has important prognostic and therapeutic implications. Myocarditis or inflammation of the cardiac muscle, most often affects the young and is usually of viral origin. It can be associated with pericarditis. The infectious agent may be a cardiotropic virus (Coxsackie or echo virus) or a virus that primarily affects other organs (e.g. influenza virus, adenovirus, cytomegalovirus, HIV, etc.). Definitive diagnosis of myocarditis should be based on a demonstration by endomyocardial biopsy of histopathological evidence of lymphocytic infiltration associated with myocyte necrosis, but technical difficulties and sampling errors limit the clinical role of biopsy. Antimyosin immunoscintigraphy, although nonspecific, provides a sensitive means of detecting myocardial necrosis associated with myocarditis. Patients with biopsy-positive myocarditis have positive antimyosin scans [22]. Also, a negative scan is highly predictive of a normal biopsy. However, a number of patients with positive scans have negative biopsy results, and it is difficult to ascertain whether this represents false-positive antimyosin scans or reflects limitations of the biopsy. In this patient group with altered LV function, patients with abnormal antimyosin scans have better clinical outcome regardless of the biopsy result [22]. Indeed, an increase in the LVEF occurs in more than 50% of patients with a positive antimyosin scan, but this is infrequently seen in patients with negative scans. This improvement probably reflects the spontaneous functional improvement frequent in active myocarditis and the diagnostic value of the antimyosin scan irrespective of biopsy results.

Myocyte necrosis associated with myocarditis, displays a different antimyosin uptake pattern than that seen with myocardial infarction. The most frequent pattern associated with acute myocardial infarction is localized uptake in the territory supplied by the artery involved. However, myocarditis has a more diffuse and heterogeneous uptake pattern, and this feature can be helpful in distinguishing patients with myocarditis and chest pain but without coronary artery disease [23].

Myocyte necrosis and degeneration (with or without inflammatory infiltration) is also a feature of the cardiac pathology of several systemic diseases including systemic lupus erythematosus, polymyositis, phaeochromocytoma and rheumatic carditis. Positive antimyosin scans have been reported in these diseases.

Amyloidosis, a rare disease, primarily affecting elderly patients, causes a restrictive form of cardiomyopathy. Recently, myocardial amyloid involvement has been detected using ^{99m}Tc-aprotinin [24].

MONITORING DRUG TOXICITY

Indium antimyosin antibodies have also been used to document cardiac toxicity in patients on antineoplastic chemotherapy using cardiotoxic agents like anthracycline. However, an increased accumulation of this tracer was seen in the majority of patients who received $500\,mg/m^2$ of adriamycin (doxorubicin) despite a normal EF during rest and exercise, and therefore the technique is not useful for monitoring the development of drug intolerance.

On the other hand, the assessment of cardiac function by means of serial gated blood pool scans has proven useful for monitoring the cardiotoxic effect of antineoplastic chemotherapy, and allows pre-clinical detection of cardiac damage. As first reported by Lefrak *et al.* [25], heart failure developed in relatively few patients receiving a cumulative dose of less than $550\,mg/m^2$ while the incidence of congestive heart failure as well as morbidity was more in patients receiving higher doses. The cumulative doxorubicin dose is now limited to $550\,mg/m^2$ but some patients are unusually sensitive while others can benefit from higher doses. Radionuclide evaluation of left ventricular function has proven the best method for identifying any untoward effects in sensitive patients. Patients in whom LV function pro-

Table 6.6 Guidelines for monitoring doxorubicin cardiotoxicity by serial radionuclide angiocardiography

Baseline evaluation:
Baseline radionuclide angiocardiography (RNA) at rest to estimate LVEF prior to the commencement of doxorubicin therapy or before $100\,mg/m^2$ of doxorubicin has been given.

Subsequent evaluations:
Subsequent studies are performed 3 weeks after the indicated last dose of doxorubicin and before the consideration of next dose at the following intervals:
I. Patient with normal baseline LVEF (50%).
   A. Second study after $250–300\,mg/m^2$.
   B. Repeat study after $400\,mg/m^2$ in patients with known heart disease, hypertension, radiation exposure, abnormal ECG, or cyclophosphamide therapy; or after $450\,mg/m^2$ in the absence of above risk factors.
   C. Obtain sequential studies thereafter before each dose.
     Discontinue doxorubicin therapy one functional criteria for cardiotoxicity develop, i.e., absolute decrease in LVEF 10% (EF Units) to a level <50% (EF Units).
II. Patients with abnormal baseline LVEF (<50%)
   A. *With baseline LVEF <30%, doxorubicin should not be started.*
   B. With baseline LVEF >30% and <50%, perform study before each dose.
     Discontinue doxorubicin with absolute decrease in LVEF 30%.

gressively deteriorates during therapy are at a high risk for developing congestive heart failure. However, if therapy is stopped, the ventricular function usually stabilizes.

Schwartz *et al.* [26] have devised a monitoring protocol (Table 6.6) that allowed them to produce a four-fold reduction in clinical congestive heart failure in more than 1500 patients receiving doxorubicin over a 7-year period. In patients with initially normal LV function, the EF should be measured after a cumulative dose of $400\,mg/m^2$ and before each subsequent dose. Discontinuation of therapy should be considered whenever the EF falls below the normal value or, depending on its initial value, decreases by 10 points or drops below 30 points.

Evaluation of exercise EF or of diastolic function parameters might provide a more sensitive evidence of myocardial damage but would be less specific and might unduly deprive some cancer patients of an effective antineoplastic drug.

COR PULMONALE

Patients with progressive long-standing pulmonary arterial hypertension and RV pressure overload, first develop RV hypertrophy, and then ventricular dysfunction and dilatation with a reduced EF characteristic of cor pulmonale [27]. Measurement of RVEF is therefore useful to confirm suspected cor pulmonale, evaluate therapeutic response and assess prognosis. Patients with RV failure are at a high risk of developing secondary problems such as ventilatory deterioration caused, for example, by pulmonary infection(s), and have a decreased survival.

Acute right ventricular dysfunction results from an acute rise in pulmonary resistance as may for instance occur with pulmonary embolism. In these cases, RV failure may be accompanied by alterations in the LV filling pattern resulting from decreased inflow or from ventricular interference.

Detection of patients with LV dysfunction superimposed on respiratory disorders is also clinically difficult and can be an important contribution of blood pool imaging in patients with dyspnoea.

CARDIAC TUMOURS

Intracavitary cardiac tumours such as myxomas produce filling defects on the first pass or equilib-

rium blood pool images. They should be differentiated from intracardiac thrombi. The pathological context and the location of the filling defect can be of some help but positive identification of active thrombi using labelled platelets is more reliable. Pericardial and myocardial tumours can interfere with the cardiac function through inflow or outflow obstruction as well as through myocardial replacement. Although these consequences can be depicted, it is not easy specifically to ascertain their origin.

PERICARDIAL EFFUSIONS

Large pericardial effusions also interfere with cardiac function. They surround the myocardium and can be seen on blood pool images as a halo of decreased activity separating the cardiac blood pool from the activity in the lungs and the liver. The sensitivity and specificity of the 'halo' sign is not high, specially where the effusion is less than 100 ml in volume.

ROLE OF NUCLEAR MEDICINE IN PATIENTS WITH VENTRICULAR ARRHYTHMIAS

Radionuclide angiography can be used to visualize the ventricular activation sequence, and therefore to study the site of origin and sequence of ventricular activation in patients with conduction abnormalities, pre-excitations or ventricular tachycardia. These techniques have occasionally been found useful in patients evaluated before surgical or catheter interruption of an accessory pathway or destruction of the site of origin of a tachycardia. Arrhythmogenic right ventricular dysplasia can cause fatal ventricular arrhythmia in otherwise asymptomatic young patients. The dysplastic tissue can be recognized during surgery and autopsy, and can be visualized by contrast angiography or MRI. The complex anatomy of the right ventricle however, makes the interpretation of angiographic images difficult, and the reproducibility of the scan diagnosis is suboptimal. It is easier to detect global and regional RV wall motion abnormalities using gated blood pool studies specially with the use of Fourier phase and amplitude images (Plate 13). However, acquisition of high-count-rate images (in multiple projections) as well as adequate temporal sampling is mandatory. Use of three harmonic Fourier analysis has been recommended [28]. A localized decreased amplitude and phase delay during sinus rhythm and in the absence of right bundle branch block is observed. It translates into a phase dispersion with an enlarged phase standard deviation and primarily affects the infundibulum, the apex or the basal portion of the inferior wall and the free right ventricular wall [29]. During ventricular tachycardia, activation originates between the normal and abnormal areas defined during sinus rhythm. At least three views (anterior, LAO and left lateral) are needed and the septum must be visualized. Tomography can also be helpful if statistics are maintained.

Blood pool studies are also useful for assessing the impact of atrial contribution in atrioventricular pacing and to help differentiate LV failure from respiratory insufficiency in patients with dyspnoea and atrial fibrillation.

Alterations in the cardiac autonomic innervation are believed to play a role in the genesis of cardiac arrhythmias. In particular, an imbalance of the cardiac sympathetic innervation with a predominance of the activity of the left sympathetic nerves has been reported in patients with long QT syndromes and left stellectomy has been shown to improve survival in some of these patients. The possibility of using ^{123}I-MIBG to image the heterogeneity of sympathetic innervation in patients with long QT syndromes has been reported but results need to be confirmed. Heterogeneous focal denervation is also thought to be implicated in the arrhythmias of diabetics with cardiac neuropathy, and in patients after myocardial infarction or after cardiac surgery, and could be imaged using ^{123}I-MIBG or ^{11}C-hydroxyephedrine.

CONTRIBUTION OF RADIONUCLIDE IMAGING TO THE EVALUATION OF PATIENTS WITH HEART FAILURE

Radionuclide imaging can contribute significantly to the functional and aetiological evaluation of patients with cardiac insufficiency. Indeed, this diagnosis is heralded by deterioration of cardiac function, first at stress and, secondarily, also at rest. Cardiac dilatation is accompanied by global or regional dysfunction so that the end-systolic volume is primarily involved.

Tachycardia at rest is a part of the compensating mechanism and a reliable sign of dysfunction. The EF is diminished in proportion to the severity of the disease and is one of the best indicators that is

especially useful for prognostic purposes. Alteration in cardiac output is a later manifestation of the problem. The severity of heart failure is influenced by the pattern of myocardial damage and by the presence of complications, specially the occurrence of regurgitation. Mitral regurgitation can well be a cause of failure, but can also be a consequence of cardiac and mitral annulus dilatation. In the context of CAD, focal dysfunction such as that occurring in patients with an isolated LV aneurysm carries a better prognosis than diffuse hypokinesia. Similarly, it has been recognized that patients with biventricular involvement have a more severe prognosis than patients with isolated alteration of LV function.

Determination of the underlying aetiology of heart failure is important in patient management. Patients with coronary artery disease (CAD) develop heart failure, most frequently as a result of extensive myocardial damage (necrosis) or superimposed complications (aneurysm, mitral valve dysfunction, ventricular septal rupture, etc.). However, ventricular dysfunction can also result from stunned myocardium (post-reperfusion) or from chronic hibernating myocardium. The incidence of jeopardized but viable myocardial tissue in patients with reperfused myocardial infarction is high.

In patients without CAD, results of metabolic imaging can demonstrate heterogeneous tracer uptake with diminished perfusion and metabolism (after correction for heart rate and blood pressure) consistent with LV dysfunction. These studies appear more important for analysing the pathophysiology of cardiomyopathies than as a guide to clinical management. More important clinically is exclusion of active myocarditis and mapping of neuronal sympathetic activity. Patients with active myocarditis can be identified using indium-labelled antimyosin monoclonal antibodies. Left ventricular functional improvement is more frequent in the post-therapeutic follow-up of patients with antimyosin uptake than in patients without demonstrated uptake. Merlet *et al.* [30] have indicated the role of MIBG imaging as a prognostic indicator in patients with severe LV dysfunction and congestive cardiomyopathy. Lack of MIBG uptake reflects either a diminution of myocardial neuronal noradrenaline storage capacity or diminished reuptake capacity. It is associated with increased circulating catecholamines and β-receptor down-regulation. It separates a group of patients with increased risk of cardiac death. These important data require confirmation using PET quantitative techniques.

Myocardial uptake of ^{111}In-labelled antimyosin antibodies is also used to detect suspected rejection of human transplanted hearts. Diffuse or focal tracer uptake reflects myocyte necrosis associated with inflammatory infiltration [31]. However, low-grade rejection can persist up to one year after transplantation, and antimyosin scanning should be restricted to the surveillance of patients after the lapse of one year after surgery. In this group, antimyosin can significantly reduce the number of required biopsies.

REFERENCES

1. Ross, J. (1976) Afterload mismatch and preload reserve: a conceptual framework for the analysis of ventricular function. *Prog. Cardiovasc. Dis.*, **18**, 255.
2. Van Dyke, D., Anger, H.O., Sullivan, R.W. *et al.* (1972) Cardiac evaluation from radioisotope dynamics. *J. Nucl. Med.*, **13**, 585–92.
3. Sandler, H., Dodge, H.T., Hay, R.E. and Rackley, C.E. (1963) Quantification of valvular insufficiency in man by angiocardiography. *Am. Heart J.*, **65**, 501–13.
4. Rigo, P., Alderson, P.O., Robertson, R.M. *et al.* (1979) Measurement of aortic and mitral regurgitation by gated blood pool scans. *Circulation*, **60**, 306–12.
5. Janowitz, W.R. and Fester, A. (1982) Quantitation of left ventricular regurgitant fraction by first pass radionuclide angiocardiography. *Am. J. Cardiol.*, **49**, 85–92.
6. Klepzig, H., Standke, R., Nickelsen, Th. *et al.* (1984) Volumetric evaluation of aortic regurgitation by combined first-pass/equilibrium radionuclide ventriculography. *Eur. Heart. J.*, **5**, 317–25.
7. Philippe, L., Mena, I., Sarcourt, J. and French, W.J. (1988) Evaluation of valvular regurgitation by factor analysis of first pass angiography. *J. Nucl. Med.*, **29**, 159–67.
8. Makler, P.T., McCarthy, D.M., Velchik, M.G. *et al.* (1983) Fourier amplitude radio: a new way to assess valvular regurgitation. *J. Nucl. Med.*, **24**, 204–7.
9. Adam, W.E., Tarkowska, A., Bitter, F. *et al.* (1979) Equilibrium (gated) radionuclide ventriculography. *Cardiovasc. Radiol.*, **2**, 161–73.
10. Ohtake, T., Nishikawa, J., Machida, K. *et al.* (1987) Evaluation of regurgitant fraction of the left ventricle by gated cardiac blood-pool scanning using SPECT. *J. Nucl. Med.*, **28**, 19–24.
11. Boucher, C.A., Okada, R.D. and Pohost, G.M. (1980) Current status of radionuclide imaging in valvular heart disease. *Am. J. Cardiol.*, **46**, 1153–63.
12. Bailey, G.Y., Come, P.C., Kelly, D.T. and Burow, R.D. (1977) Thallium myocardial perfusion imaging in aortic valve stenosis. *Am. J. Cardiol.*, **40**, 889–99.
13. Dehmer, G.J., Firth, B.G., Hillis, L.D. *et al.* (1981) Alterations in left ventricular volumes and ejection fraction at rest and during exercise in patients with aortic regurgitation. *Am. J. Cardiol.*, **48**, 17–6.
14. Levine, H.J. and Gaasch, W.H. (1983) Ratio of regurgitant volume to end diastolic volume: a major determinant of ventricular response to surgical correction of chronic volume overload. *Am. J. Cardiol.*, **52**, 406.
15. Bonow, R.O. and Epstein, S.E. (1987) Is preoperative left ventricular function predictive of survival and functional results after aortic valve replacement for chronic aortic regurgitation? *J. Am. Coll. Cardiol.*, **10**, 713–16.
16. Gottdiener, J.S., Borer, J.S., Bacharach, S.L. *et al.* (1981) Left ventricular function in mitral valve prolapse: assessment with radionuclide cineangiography. *Am. J. Cardiol.*, **47**, 7-13.
17. Chevigne, M. and Rigo, P. (1982) Quantification of isolated tricuspid regurgitation by gated cardiac blood pool scan. *Eur. J. Nucl. Med.*, **7**, 39–40.
18. Maltz, D.L. and Treves, S. (1973) Quantitative radionuclide angiocardiography. Determination of Qp:Qs in children. *Circulation*, **47**, 1049–56.
19. Rigo, P. and Chevigné, M. (1982) Measurement of left to right shunts by gated radionuclide angiography. Concise communication. *J. Nucl. Med.*, **23**, 1975–9.
20. Grover-McKay, M., Schwaiger, M., Krivokapich, J. *et al.* (1989) Regional myocardial blood flow and metabolism at rest in mildly symptomatic patients with hypertrophic cardiomyopathy. *J. Am. Coll. Cardiol.*, **13**, 317–24.
21. Perloff, J.K., Henze, E. and Schelbert, H.R. (1984) Alterations in regional myocardial metabolism, perfusion, and wall motion in Duchenne muscular dystrophy studied by radionuclide imaging. *Circulation*, **69**, 33–42.
22. Dec, G.W., Palacios, I.F., Fallon, J.T. *et al.* (1990) Antimyosin antibody cardiac imaging: its role in the diagnosis of myocarditis. *J. Am. Coll. Cardiol.*, **167**, 97–104.
23. Narula, J., Khaw, B.A., Dec, G.W. *et al.* (1993) Recognition of myocarditis masquerading as myocardial infarction. *N. Engl. J. Med.*, **328**, 100–4.
24. Aprile, C., Marinone, M.G., Saponaro, R. *et al.* (1996) Detection of myocardial amyloid involvement with Tc-99m aprotinin. *J. Nucl. Med.*, **37**, 185P.
25. Lefrak, E.A., Pitha, J., Rosenheim, S. and Gottlieb, J.A. (1973) A clinicopathologic analysis of adriamycin cardiotoxicity. *Cancer*, **32**, 302–14.
26. Schwartz, R.G., McKenzie, W.B., Alexander, J. *et al.* (1997) Congestive heart failure and left ventricular dysfunction complicating doxorubicin therapy. Seven-year experience using serial radionuclide angiocardiography. *Am. J. Med.*, **82**, 1109–18.
27. Berger, H.J., Matthay, R.A., Lohe, J. *et al.* (1978) Assessment of cardiac performance with quantitative radionuclide angiocardiography: right ventricular ejection fraction with reference to findings in chronic obstructive pulmonary disease. *Am. J. Cardiol.*, **41**, 897–905.

28. Valette, H., Bourguignon, M.H., Merlet, P. *et al.* (1990) Improved detection of anterior left ventricular aneurysm with multiharmonic Fourier analysis. *J. Nucl. Med.*, **31**, 1303–6.
29. Le Guludec, F., Bourguignon, M.H., Sebag, C. *et al.* (1987) Phase mapping of radionuclide gated biventriculograms in patients with sustained ventricular tachycardia or Wolff Parkinson White syndrome. *Int. J. Cardiac Imaging*, **2**, 117–26.
30. Merlet, P., Valette, H., Dubois Randé, J.L. *et al.* (1992) Prognostic value of cardiac MIBG imaging in patients with congestive heart failure. *J. Nucl. Med.*, **33**, 471–7.
31. Frist, W., Yasuda, T., Segall, G. *et al.* (1987) Noninvasive detection of human cardiac transplant rejection with 111-indium antimyosin Fab imaging. *Circulation*, **67**, V81–5.

Peripheral vascular disease

P. J. A. Robinson and A. Parkin

INTRODUCTION

Occlusive disease of the peripheral arteries is a common cause of morbidity which is likely to increase further in an ageing population. The major underlying pathology is arterial atheroma, the effect of which can be modified and accelerated in patients with systemic hypertension or diabetes. The techniques described below are also applicable in patients with the less common varieties of peripheral arterial disease, including Raynaud's syndrome, vibration white finger, Buerger's disease, inflammatory vasculitides (e.g. Takayasu's disease) and the various vascular entrapment syndromes.

Therapeutic manoeuvres include measures directed at the underlying cause (e.g. stopping smoking, better control of diabetes or hypertension, steroid therapy for inflammatory vasculitides), but in the majority of patients interventions are aimed at improving or redistributing blood flow to the affected limbs.

The measurement of limb blood flow or tissue perfusion is valuable in the diagnosis of peripheral arterial disease, in the measurement of severity of functional disturbance, in monitoring the progress of disease, and in measuring the effectiveness of treatment. Nuclear medicine techniques can also be useful in confirming the patency of grafts, demonstrating aortic aneurysms or occlusions and detecting wound or graft infections after surgery.

DIAGNOSIS AND TREATMENT OF PERIPHERAL ARTERIAL DISEASE

DIAGNOSIS

Patients with large-vessel atheroma or arterial entrapment present with pain in the leg or arm caused by muscle ischaemia precipitated by exercise. Those with more advanced atheroma or with primary small-vessel disease may suffer from pain at rest and ischaemic changes in the skin leading eventually to tissue death and peripheral gangrene. Exercise-induced leg pain may also result from ischaemia of nerve roots (cauda equina syndrome) [1] and other skeletal or neurogenic causes [2]. Most patients with peripheral arterial disease will have abnormal pulses on clinical examination, but in a minority the peripheral pulses are normal. Non-invasive investigation of patients suspected of having occlusive peripheral vascular disease (PVD) includes exercise testing, plethysmography, Doppler ultrasound studies and flow measurement by nuclear medicine techniques.

Exercise testing using a treadmill provides appropriate physiological stress for estimating the severity of blood flow impairment but has the disadvantage that the end points are determined by the patient and are not objective. A significant proportion of patients (43% in one study [3]) cannot complete a standard exercise test owing to concurrent cardiac, respiratory, neurological or musculoskeletal disease [3–5].

Venous occlusion plethysmography is a well-tried physiological technique, but has poor reproducibility and has not been validated in patients with severe disease, primarily because of the poor signal-to-noise ratio at low flow rates [6]. The ankle-to-brachial pressure index (ABPI) is the ratio between the pressures required to occlude the arterial pulses at the wrist and ankle. ABPI measurement is a useful screening test for the detection of aortoiliac and femoropopliteal disease. The technique cannot be applied in patients who have no pulses at the ankle or in those with heavily calcified peripheral arteries. The method, although simple, has limited precision and reproducibility [7] and it also assumes normality of the radial pulse which may be inappropriate in patients with widespread vascular disease. Some patients with reduced hyperaemic flow have normal ABPI [3].

Estimation of arterial flow by direct Doppler measurement over the femoral artery has also been fairly widely used. This approach is quick and elegant but is handicapped by its operator dependence. The reproducibility of flow measurements is not as good as with the radionuclide technique described below [5], the method assumes a relationship between flow and velocity which is

Clinical Nuclear Medicine, 3rd edn. Edited by M.N. Maisey, K.E. Britton and B.D. Collier. Published in 1998 by Chapman & Hall, London. ISBN 0 412 75180 1

unreliable in the presence of turbulence and, most importantly, it takes no account of collateral flow which is often significant in patients with aorto-iliac disease [8].

TREATMENT

Drug treatment of chronic occlusive arterial disease is of only limited value and although increasing emphasis has been placed recently on the use of graded exercise as a valuable therapeutic manoeuvre, the mainstay of treatment is the anatomic improvement of peripheral blood flow. This may be by surgery on the occlusive lesions (embolectomy, thrombectomy, endarterectomy, profundoplasty), by bypass procedures using autologous vein grafts or prostheses, or by endovascular approaches using percutaneous balloon angioplasty, insertion of stents and reopening of occlusions with various laser and atherectomy devices. Since all of these methods of treatment require detailed demonstration of arterial anatomy, X-ray angiography is an essential prelude to intervention. However, angiography has two major disadvantages – firstly, it is invasive and so inappropriate for screening and follow-up examinations, and secondly it gives only indirect and imprecise indications of the severity of blood flow impairment, particularly in patients with primary small-vessel disease. In addition, like the ultrasound techniques, angiography investigates the patient at rest, so the vasodilatation and redistribution of blood flow which occur during exercise are not visualized.

RADIONUCLIDE IMAGING AND CLEARANCE TECHNIQUES

FIRST-PASS ANGIOGRAPHY

Rapid non-invasive imaging of large arteries or grafts can be obtained by dynamic acquisition following the intravenous bolus injection of ^{99m}Tc-pertechnetate or ^{99m}Tc-labelled red blood cells. The technique can be used to detect the presence and patency of major peripheral arteries, bypass grafts, aneurysms or pseudoaneurysms [9–11]. Although qualitative, the technique is simple to perform and can be offered as an alternative to Doppler examination, or as a second-line test in patients with inadequate or unexpected Doppler results.

MICROSPHERE ANGIOGRAPHY

Peripheral perfusion has been studied by injection of ^{99m}Tc-labelled microspheres into the femoral arteries or abdominal aorta [12]. The technique has the major disadvantage of requiring intra-arterial catheterization, and it is also dependent on mixing of the injected tracer with arterial blood, which is a dubious assumption particularly in the presence of turbulent flow.

XENON CLEARANCE

The inert gases are freely diffusible within tissues so the rate of disappearance of ^{133}Xe from a site of injection may be regarded as a good indicator of tissue perfusion. This technique has been applied to leg muscle [13] and to subcutaneous adipose tissue in the foot [14]. Its results describe blood flow in only a small area of tissue, may be influenced by skin contamination and retention of tracer in fat. Probably for these reasons this test has not been widely adopted in clinical practice.

PERFUSION IMAGING WITH THALLIUM-201

When injected intravenously during exercise, ^{201}Tl is distributed in proportion to blood flow to the myocardium and skeletal muscle. Obtaining images of the thighs and calves shortly after administration of 80 MBq of ^{201}Tl during maximal exercise allows qualitative assessment of perfusion to the major muscle groups of the leg. In patients with truly unilateral disease, assessment of severity and extent can be made by comparing the two sides, but most patients with occlusive PVD have bilateral disease, even if their symptoms are limited to one limb. It may help to compare calf versus thigh uptake within each leg, and also to compare the immediate post-exercise images with 'redistribution' images obtained 4 hours later. If whole-body images are obtained, the calf and thigh uptake can be expressed as a proportion of whole body activity so a degree of quantitation can be achieved [15].

PERFUSION IMAGING WITH METHOXYISOBUTYL NITRILE

^{99m}Tc-MIBI improves on ^{201}Tl because it can be labelled on site in the nuclear medicine department, and it also provides much better counting statistics relative to the absorbed dose to the patient. Its handling at cellular level is different from ^{201}Tl in that there is no redistribution, so if rest and exercise studies are both required, then two separate procedures must be performed. In practice, resting studies are unlikely to be helpful since some patients with severe PVD have normal resting flows [16]. The technique requires intravenous injection of 400–550 MBq of ^{99m}Tc-MIBI during maximal exercise, with imaging of both legs and, preferably, whole-body activity measurement [17]. Assessments using comparison of left versus right, thigh versus calf, and rest versus stress images have been suggested. Using the ratio of local muscle uptake to whole-body activity, a good separation between groups of patients with PVD and control subjects has been found [17], but correlation with angiographic findings has been disappointing [18]. This technique looks promising but requires validation with reproducibility studies and more extensive clinical application in order to assess its role.

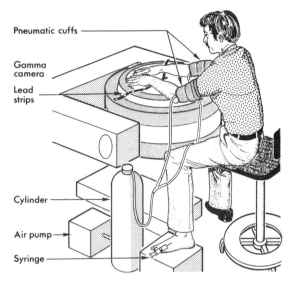

Figure 6.12 Diagrammatic representation of the method for measurement of limb blood flow during reactive hyperaemia. (Reproduced with permission from Parkin *et al.* [23].)

GRAFT INFECTION

Post-operative infection around vascular grafts can be difficult to detect by ultrasound or computed tomography particularly in the presence of haematoma or serous effusions. Scintigraphy with ^{99m}Tc-HMPAO-leucocytes is often helpful [19] although imaging using ^{111}In-leucocytes is probably more reliable [20].

MEASUREMENT OF LIMB BLOOD FLOW (LBF)

The object of this technique is to measure the maximum blood flow which the cardiovascular system can deliver to the affected limbs, using an inexpensive and readily available blood pool label. By dividing the measured flow by the limb volume, a result is obtained in terms of absolute flow per unit volume of tissue (ml/min/100 ml of tissue). The technique, as described by Parkin *et al.* [21], requires the following steps:

1. The circulation to the affected limbs (both legs or both arms) is isolated by placing sphygmomanometer cuffs around the limbs at knee or elbow level and inflating the cuffs very rapidly using a large volume gas reservoir, up to a pressure of 300 mmHg (Figure 6.12). This pressure is sufficient to occlude both arterial inflow and venous outflow and effectively isolates the limbs from the rest of the circulation.

2. ^{99m}Tc-labelled human serum albumin (HSA) or red blood cells (400 MBq) is then given intravenously into one of the uninvolved limbs. A period of 3 minutes has been shown to be long enough to allow thorough mixing of the labelled material within the blood compartment and also to produce a near-maximal reactive hyperaemia in the occluded limbs; occluding the peripheral circulation for longer becomes progressively more uncomfortable for the patients and offers only a very marginal increase in the reactive hyperaemia achieved.

3. Immediately before releasing the cuffs, a venous blood sample is obtained from the uninvolved limb contralateral to the site of tracer injection.

4. After 3 minutes of occlusion, the cuffs are abruptly released with the affected limbs in position over a large field-of-view gamma-camera. Image data is acquired at 1 frame per second for 100 seconds and time–activity

curves created from regions of interest around each limb (Plate 14). The curves show three distinct phases: (i) a linear inflow phase during which radiolabelled blood is flowing into the limb while unlabelled blood is flowing out; (ii) a mixing phase when labelled inflow continues while the outflow consists of a mixture of labelled and unlabelled blood; and (iii) an equilibrium phase resulting from complete mixing of the unlabelled blood from the isolated limbs with the rest of the circulation. The gradient of the linear inflow phase (G counts/s/s) represents the rate of arrival of arterial blood during reactive hyperaemia and is derived by a least squares regression algorithm.

5. The activity in the venous blood sample is measured on the gamma-camera to determine the concentration (C) of tracer in blood (counts/s/ml). Blood flow to the limbs can then be calculated: flow $F = G/C \times 60$ ml/min.

6. The volume of the limbs is then measured by water displacement, allowing final results to be expressed in terms of ml/min/100 ml of tissue. Where appropriate, separate regions-of-interest and volume measurements can be made for the foot and calf, or for the hand and forearm. In order to correct for underestimation due to absorption of radioactivity within the limb itself, the measured flow is multiplied by a correction factor of 1.3 (legs) or 1.1 (arms), derived from calibration of scintigraphic measurements with measured activity contained in perspex models of the leg and arm [21,22].

The reproducibility of the method, tested in a population of normal controls and patients with various degrees of PVD, is high, with the correlation coefficient between paired observations being >0.98 for legs and 0.96 for arms [23]. The approach has a number of advantages over other non-invasive tests for diagnosing and measuring the severity of occlusive arterial disease.

- The method is reproducible and relies on objective measurement criteria.
- The technique uses inexpensive consumables and requires no special apparatus apart from the cuff inflation device which is of a fairly simple mechanical construction.
- The technique does not require collaboration from the patient to undertake exercise.
- The reactive hyperaemia provides a reproducible level of ischaemic stress.

- Unlike the treadmill test which may be limited by symptoms in a single limb, the maximum flow to both limbs is assessed.
- The method is equally applicable to arms or legs and, if required, separate measurements can be made for ankle, foot, hand and forearm.
- The measurement includes inflow from collateral vessels as well as the main axial arteries.
- An absolute measurement is obtained and with volume calibration the flow can easily be compared with that in other patients; measurements can be tested against expected ranges for normals, patients with claudication, patients with rest pain, etc.
- The method is applicable for repeated measurements, e.g. pre- and post-surgery or angioplasty.

The hazards and limitations of the technique are few. The estimated effective dose equivalent from the use of 400 MBq of ^{99m}Tc-HSA or RBC is about 2.4 mSv [4].

Adverse reactions to HSA are described, but in over 5000 procedures carried out at St James's Hospital, no significant complications occurred. The technique measures global limb blood flow rather than muscle perfusion, but in the presence of reactive hyperaemia the relative contribution of skin flow is small. The use of limb volume measurement to calibrate flow does mean that muscle perfusion will tend to be underestimated in patients with oedema, but this occurs in only a small minority of patients. It may be thought that the period of arterial occlusion which is inherent in the method is undesirable in patients who have recently undergone graft surgery. Studies in the immediate post-operative period are avoided, but follow-up measurements on patients are carried out from 3 weeks after surgery onwards with no adverse consequences, even when the graft passes through the area of occlusion.

CORRELATION BETWEEN LBF AND ARTERIOGRAPHY

In occlusive PVD, symptoms are the result of impaired function (blood flow), whereas treatment involves changing the anatomy by angioplasty or surgery. The correlation between anatomic disturbance, as shown by angiography, and functional disturbance as determined by LBF measurement presents some difficulties. The major limitation is that the arteriogram is a qualitative display of structure, with hardly any functional component. In patients with disease at a single level, the degree of arterial stenosis has some (limited) validity as a predictor of flow impairment. However, most patients have multifocal disease so it is difficult to attribute significance to stenoses at different levels and to predict the result of correction of one or more segments of disease. LBF measurement does not provide the whole answer to this, but it helps by stratifying the patients in terms of functional impairment, and measures the severity of disease in the asymptomatic leg of patients with unilateral presentation. Using an arbitrary scoring system, an estimate of disease severity can be made from a peripheral arteriogram. Comparing this with LBF measurements in a large cohort of patients with intermittent claudication shows good correlation in the group as a whole, although there is a substantial scatter among paired measurements in individual patients [4]. Interestingly, in patients presenting with ischaemic pain at rest, the correlation is poorer. The disparity between the arterial anatomy and tissue perfusion is much more apparent in patients with rest pain, suggesting that there is a major component of small vessel disease in these cases. This pattern is also found in patients with inflammatory vasculitides, Raynaud's disease and vibration white finger [4,24].

APPLICATIONS OF LBF MEASUREMENT

CLAUDICATION

Normal values for LBF in the arms and legs are shown in Table 6.7. In patients with intermittent claudication, maximal hyperaemic flow is substantially reduced, typically to about 3–5 ml/min/ 100 ml of tissue. It is noteworthy that in patients with unilateral claudication, LBF in the contralateral (non-symptomatic) limb is also substantially reduced, typically about 5–7 ml/min/100 ml tissue [4]. As expected, in patients with asymmetric disease, the blood flow to the more severely symptomatic leg is less than that to the contralateral leg. In some patients however, the degree of disparity is small compared with the clinical discrepancy between peripheral pulses and the anatomic differences between the two sides shown at angiography. In such cases, successful surgery or angioplasty on the apparently worse leg may lead to little clinical benefit since the patient may then be limited by symptoms on the opposite side. One of the major advantages of LBF measurement compared with treadmill testing is that the information provided about flow in the non-symptomatic limb may indicate a requirement for bilateral rather than unilateral intervention.

In patients presenting with a history suggestive of intermittent claudication but with unexpected or conflicting clinical findings and Doppler indices, LBF measurement is also useful. In those with significant arterial disease confirmed on subsequent arteriography, blood flow is always reduced, while in patients with underlying neurological or orthopaedic problems, the flow is often normal [25]. LBF measurement can be used to select which patients need invasive investigation, and can also indicate the contribution of vascular disease to symptoms in patients with multiple causes of limb pain.

ISCHAEMIC REST PAIN

Assessment of flow in patients presenting with rest pain or ischaemic skin changes is particularly

Table 6.7   Typical hyperaemic limb blood flow values

Subject limbs	LBF in ml/min/100 ml tissue	Reference
Legs of normal controls	10–22	[4]
Claudicants, symptomatic legs	2–8	[3]
Claudicants, asymptomatic legs	4–12	[3]
Rest pain patients, symptomatic legs	0.5–4	[4]
Rest pain patients, asymptomatic legs	2–8	[4]
Arms of normal controls	20–45	[22]
Arms with brachial artery occlusion	3–8	[23]
Hands of normal controls	22–50	[22]
Hands in occupational Raynaud's (VBF)	6–25	[24]

difficult. The patients are usually unable to perform a treadmill test, Doppler studies are handicapped by the absence of peripheral pulses, and methods depending upon plethysmography or radionuclide clearance are limited by poor signal-to-noise ratio at very low flow rates. The LBF technique described above has the advantage that the inflow signal is virtually noise free since the baseline is zero, and the linear inflow phase is substantially prolonged in patients with severe disease so that a fairly precise and reproducible gradient measurement can be made. Flow measurements in patients with ischaemic rest pain are typically in the range of 0.5–2 ml/min/100 ml tissue.

With more aggressive reconstructive surgery, the incidence of amputation has declined, but one of the residual problems in patients facing this radical surgery is the determination of a level through which amputation should be performed with expectation of healing. Studies in a fairly small population of patients have indicated a tendency for successful healing of a below-knee amputation to occur when the calf blood flow is greater than about 2 ml/min/100 ml and a potential requirement for above-knee amputation when the calf blood flow is less than this, but these figures should be regarded only as rough guidelines, not as absolute indicators.

ARM ISCHAEMIA

Hyperaemic blood flow to the forearm is sharply reduced in patients with brachial artery occlusion following cut-down for cardiac catheterization, but shows only a minor decrease in patients retaining peripheral pulses after the procedure [23]. 'Vibration white finger' (VBF) is a variety of Raynaud's disease precipitated by occupational exposure to vibratory tools, and is now regarded as an industrial disorder. The majority of patients tested have diminished hyperaemic flow to the hands (Plate 15), suggesting a mechanism of structural damage in addition to vasospasm [24].

EFFECTS OF THERAPY

Measurement of LBF before and after angioplasty or surgical bypass shows results which correlate well with clinical outcomes (Figure 6.13 and Plate 16). Patients with a good clinical outcome after intervention typically have flow improvement in the range of 70–100%, whereas those in which the

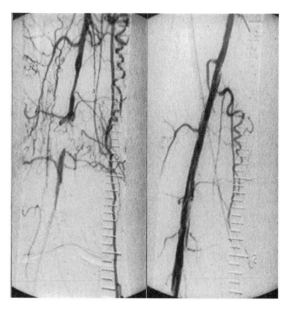

Figure 6.13   Same patient as Plate 16. Subtraction angiogram showing femoral artery occlusion (left) and successful recanalization by angioplasty (right).

clinical outcome is poor have little or no change in LBF [4,5,26,27]. Conversely, patients showing a significant increase in LBF after angioplasty almost invariably report an improvement in symptoms. A third possible outcome – seen in a minority of patients – is that in spite of improvement in blood flow to the treated limb, walking is limited by other factors, either pain in the contralateral side or angina. Interestingly, LBF measurements carried out before and after profundoplasty in a small group of patients showed no change, even when symptoms were improved, suggesting that this particular surgical procedure may not influence flow in the calf although flow to the thigh muscles may be increased. The natural history of occlusive PVD shows a tendency to continual decline in hyperaemic blood flow in patients who are untreated, and in those who are treated unsuccessfully. One interesting finding is that in patients with unilateral disease which is treated successfully, the rate of deterioration of the opposite limb may be reduced [27].

REFERENCES

1. Blau, J.N. and Logue, V. (1961) Intermittent claudication of the cauda equina. *Lancet*, **i**, 1081–6.

2. Evans, J.G. (1964) Neurogenic intermittent claudication. *Br. Med. J.*, **2**, 985–7.
3. Wilkinson, D., Vowden, P., Parkin, A. *et al.* (1987) A reliable and readily available method of measuring limb blood flow in intermittent claudication. *Br. J. Surg.*, **74**, 516–19.
4. Parkin, A., Robinson, P.J., Martinez, D. *et al.* (1991) Radionuclide limb blood flow in peripheral vascular disease: a review of 1100 measurements. *Nucl. Med. Commun.*, **12**, 835–51.
5. Gehani, A.A., Thorley, P., Sheard, K. *et al.* (1992) Value of a radionuclide limb blood flow technique in the assessment of percutaneous balloon and dynamic angioplasty. *Eur. J. Nucl. Med.*, **19**, 6–13.
6. Figar, S. (1959) Some basic deficiencies of the plethysmographic method and possibilities of avoiding them. *Angiology*, **10**, 120–5.
7. Baker, J.D. and DeEtte Dix, P.A.C. (1980) Variability of Doppler ankle pressures with arterial occlusive disease. An evaluation of ankle index and brachial:ankle pressure gradient. *Surgery*, **89**, 134–7.
8. John, H.T. and Warren, R. (1961) The stimulus to collateral circulation. *Surgery*, **49**, 14–25.
9. Grime, J.S., Critchley, M., Whitehouse, G.H. *et al.* (1986) A method of radionuclide angiography and comparison with contrast aortography in the assessment of aorto-iliac disease. *Nucl. Med. Commun.*, **7**, 45–52.
10. Hayek, M.E., Ludwig, M.A., Fischer, K. *et al.* (1988) The use of scintiangiography with technetium 99m in the diagnosis of traumatic pseudoaneurysm. *J. Vasc. Surg.*, **7**, 409–13.
11. Oshima, M., Ijima, H., Kohda, Y., *et al.* (1984) Peripheral arterial disease diagnosed with high-count-rate radionuclide arteriography. *Radiology*, **152**, 161–6.
12. Rhodes, B.A., Greyson, N.D., Seigel, M.E. *et al.* (1973) The distribution of radioactive microspheres after intra-arterial injection in the legs of patients with peripheral vascular disease. *Am. J. Roentgenol.*, **118**, 820–5.
13. Lassen, N.A., Lindbjerg, I.F. and Dahn, I. (1965) Validity of the Xe 133 method for measurement of muscle blood flow evaluated by simultaneous venous occlusion plethysmography. *Circ. Res.*, **16**, 287–93.
14. Jelnes, R., Bulow, J. and Tonnesen, K.H. (1987) Subcutaneous adipose tissue blood flow in the forefoot during 24 hours. Labelling pattern and reproducibility. *Scand. J. Clin. Lab. Invest.*, **47**, 223–7.
15. Segall, G.M., Lang E.V., Lennon, S.E. *et al.* (1992) Functional imaging of peripheral vascular disease: a comparison between exercise whole-body thallium perfusion imaging and contrast arteriography. *J. Nucl. Med.*, **33**, 1797–800.
16. Williams, C.A. and Lind, A.R. (1979) Measurement of forearm blood flow by venous occlusion plethysmography. Influence on hand blood flow during sustained and intermittent isometric exercise. *Eur. J. Appl. Physiol.*, **42**, 141–9.
17. Miles, K.A., Barber, R.W., Wraight, E.P. *et al.* (1992) Leg muscle scintigraphy with ^{99m}Tc-MIBI in the assessment of peripheral vascular (arterial) disease. *Nucl. Med. Commun.*, **13**, 593–603.
18. Bajnok, L., Kozlovszky, B., Varga, J. *et al.* (1994) Technetium-99m sestamibi scintigraphy for the assessment of lower extremity ischaemia in peripheral arterial disease. *Eur. J. Nucl. Med.*, **21**, 1326–32.
19. Krznaric, E., Nevelsteen, A., Van Hoe, L., *et al.* (1994) Diagnostic value of 99mTc-d,l-HMPAO-labelled leukocyte scintigraphy in the detection of vascular graft infections. *Nucl. Med. Commun.*, **15**, 953–60.
20. Brunner, M.C., Mitchell, R.S., Baldwin, J.C. *et al.* (1989) Prosthetic graft infection: limitations of indium white blood cell scanning. *J. Vasc. Surg.*, **3**, 42–8.
21. Parkin, A., Robinson, P.J., Wiggins, P.A. *et al.* (1986) The measurement of limb blood flow using technetium-labelled red blood cells. *Br. J. Radiol.*, **59**, 493–7.
22. Parkin, A., Wilkinson, D., Smye, S.W. *et al.* (1989) The clinical application of forearm and hand blood flow measurements using a gamma-camera. *Surgery*, **106**, 26–32.
23. Parkin, A., Smye, S.W., Bishop, N. *et al.* (1989) Forearm blood flow measurements using technetium-99m human serum albumin following brachial arteriotomy. *J. Nucl. Med.*, **30**, 45–50.
24. Greenstein, D., Parkin, A., Maughan, J. *et al.* (1994) Perfusion defects in vibration white finger: a clinical assessment using isotope limb blood flow. *Cardiovasc. Surg.*, **2**, 354–8.
25. Parkin, A., Maughan, J., Robinson, P.J. *et al.* (1994) Radionuclide limb blood flow measurements to resolve diagnostic problems in vascular surgery. *Nucl. Med. Commun.*, **15**,148–51.
26. Thorley, P.J., Sheard, K.L., Sivananthan, U.M. *et al.* (1994) Limb blood flow measurement in technically successful balloon angioplasty. *Br. J. Radiol.*, **67**, 764–9.
27. Thorley, P.J., Sheard, K.L. and Rees, M.R. (1993) Does peripheral angioplasty compromise limb blood flow? *Br. J. Radiol.*, **66**, 506–9.

Venous thrombosis

L. C. Knight and A. H. Maurer

INTRODUCTION

Deep venous thrombosis (DVT), or the formation of thrombi in the deep veins of the extremities, is a common disorder. There is a strong association with certain clinical risk factors, as listed in Table 6.8.

The development of DVT in an extremity is usually asymptomatic; however, symptoms when present are usually due to the effects of obstruction and/or accompanying inflammation. The non-specificity of clinical signs (e.g. pain, swelling and tenderness in an extremity) for DVT is well recognized. About 70% of patients with clinical signs and symptoms of DVT have no evidence of DVT by objective testing and are found to have another cause of the symptoms such as: cellulitis, muscle tear, tendon rupture, haematoma or rupture of a popliteal cyst [1].

Pulmonary embolism (PE) is the most important complication of venous thrombosis, and can be fatal. Other complications include chronic pain, swelling and skin ulceration due to post-phlebitic syndrome, discomfort in lower limb(s) due to acute DVT, and the potential side effects of treatment.

Early institution of anticoagulant therapy is important in preventing complications. Because of its potentially significant side effects it is not desirable to begin anticoagulant treatment unless the diagnosis of thrombosis has been confirmed. A simple objective test to diagnose accurately the presence of DVT is very important to define the patients who need therapy.

ANATOMY AND PATHOPHYSIOLOGY

LOCATION OF PERIPHERAL THROMBI

Thrombi may technically form in any blood vessel. Venous thrombi usually occur in the deep veins of the lower limbs and can involve the deep veins of the calf, the deep veins above the knee (popliteal veins), and the more proximal (femoral, deep femoral or iliac) veins. The veins of the leg are shown in Figure 6.14. Venous thrombosis of the lower limb may also involve the superficial veins, which often occurs in varicosities. Thrombosis in the superficial veins is usually benign and self-limiting, unless it accompanies DVT.

Most lower-extremity thrombi start in the calf. If left untreated, many of these propagate into the more proximal deep veins. Isolated proximal vein thrombosis is uncommon in general surgical or medical patients. In patients after hip surgery or hip fracture, however, 40–45% of thrombi are in proximal veins, and many of these are without associated calf vein thrombi.

AETIOLOGY AND PATHOGENESIS

Venous thrombosis occurs when there is a shift in the normal balance between thrombotic factors and protective mechanisms. Normally, a low level of blood coagulation is occurring continuously, but this fails to develop into DVT because of protective mechanisms. An excess of coagulation stimulation or a breakdown in protective mechanisms can shift the balance. Vascular damage during hip surgery can lead to exposure of blood to sub-endothelium, which supports platelet adhesion and aggregation, accumulation of leucocytes, and activation of the coagulation pathway. Activation of endothelial cells by cytokines released as a result of non-local tissue injury or inflammation can stimulate endothelial cells to release tissue factor and plasminogen activator inhibitor-1 (PAI-1), and can reduce the amount of exposed thrombomodulin (a thrombin suppressor). Tissue thromboplastin can be released as a result of vascular wall damage, endothelial cell activation, or by activated leucocytes migrating to an area of vascular damage. Some malignant cells contain a protease which can activate coagulation factor X. Thus, many of the known clinical risk factors for thrombosis are related to initiation of coagulation: major surgery or trauma, malignancy and myocardial infarction (Table 6.8).

Venous stasis plays a critical role in coagulation by permitting the interaction among coagulation proteins as they sequentially activate the other

Clinical Nuclear Medicine, 3rd edn. Edited by M.N. Maisey, K.E. Britton and B.D. Collier. Published in 1998 by Chapman & Hall, London. ISBN 0 412 75180 1

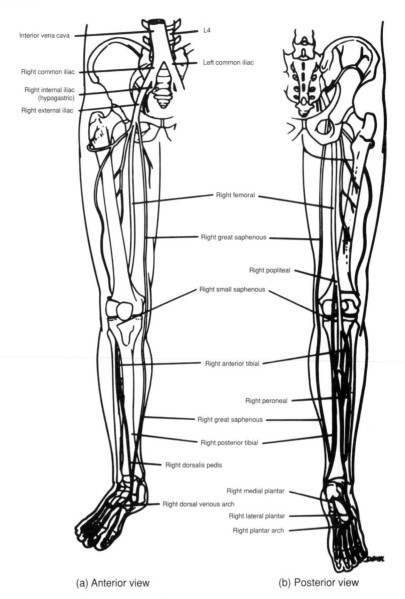

Interior vena cava
L4
Right common iliac
Left common iliac
Right internal iliac (hypogastric)
Right external iliac
Right femoral
Right great saphenous
Right popliteal
Right small saphenous
Right anterior tibial
Right peroneal
Right great saphenous
Right posterior tibial
Right dorsalis pedis
Right medial plantar
Right dorsal venous arch
Right lateral plantar
Right plantar arch

(a) Anterior view

(b) Posterior view

Figure 6.14 Principal veins of the pelvis and right lower extremity. (Reprinted from *Principles of Human Anatomy*, 6th edn (ed. G.J. Tortora), HarperCollins, New York, 1992, with permission.)

proteins which ultimately convert fibrinogen to fibrin. Normally, these proteins are swept away and diluted by the flowing blood before they can interact to the extent necessary to induce thrombosis. Even though natural inhibitors to activated clotting factors may be produced by the vessel wall, stasis may impede their access to the clotting factors. Platelets play a role in venous thrombosis in that they act as a surface upon which clotting factors can assemble and accelerate the coagulation cascade. Stasis may explain the association between thrombotic risk and clinical conditions

Table 6.8 Clinical risk factors for development of deep venous thrombosis (DVT)

Specific risk factors	Incidence of DVT (%)
Surgery	
hip (or hip fracture)	49–75*
knee	50
abdominothoracic	14–33
urologic	22–51
hysterectomy	7–27
Cancer	33–60
Myocardial infarction	34–40
Post-partum period	0.3–2.0 per month
Stroke	30
Paralysis	12
General risk factors	
Increasing age	
Previous DVT (3- to 5-fold increase)	
Immobilization >1 week	
Oral contraceptive use	
Chemotherapy	

* Associated with a 10–13% incidence of fatal pulmonary embolism.

such as paralysis or prolonged bed rest. Venous dilatation may be associated with advanced age (especially if varicose veins are present, or if the patient is bedridden). This may contribute to local stasis, explaining these clinical risk factors. The contribution of stasis also explains why DVT usually occurs in the legs, regardless of where trauma occurs. Zones of stasis are most commonly found in the legs, in valve cusp pockets in either the calf or the thigh, or in large venous sinuses in the calf.

Decreased protective mechanisms may contribute further to the formation of DVT. For example, decreased fibrinolytic activity has been reported to be present in patients in the early post-operative period and in women taking oral contraceptives. Fibrinolytic activity has been found to be lower in leg veins than arm veins, and this gradient is more pronounced in the elderly.

COMPOSITION OF THROMBI

All thrombi are composed of fibrin, platelets and other trapped blood elements. The relative proportions of these components are based on flow conditions at the location of the thrombus. Venous thrombi often form in areas of stasis or sluggish flow, and consist mainly of fibrin with many trapped red cells and plasma proteins, alternating with layers of aggregated platelets ('red' thrombi). Arterial thrombi often form in areas of rapid flow, and are composed mainly of platelet aggregates held together with thin fibrin strands ('white' thrombi). As long as the balance is in favour of thrombosis rather than lysis, additional thrombus elements may continue to deposit on the lesion, because its surface of exposed fibrin and activated platelets is thrombogenic. As a thrombus enlarges, the flow dynamics in the blood vessel may change and alter the composition of the newer parts of the lesion. Thus, a single lesion may have one 'red' composition end where there is in an environment of static flow, while the other end of the thrombus may be 'white' because there is locally rapid flow. Changes in composition also occur as thrombi resolve. If this occurs, it is the result of invasion by leucocytes, which cause platelets to be lysed and replaced by fibrin. Fibrinolytic enzymes from leucocytes and endothelial cells then slowly digest the fibrin, and endothelial cells spread over the surface of the thrombus. Because endothelial cells are not as thrombogenic as exposed platelets and fibrin, this deters further thrombus deposition.

Often, thrombi do not spontaneously resolve. They may continue to propagate, completely occluding the blood vessel. A portion of the thrombus may also break away (embolize) and cause an obstruction of a pulmonary artery in the lungs (pulmonary embolus).

THERAPY

Venous thrombosis can be prevented by reducing the coagulability of blood by the use of anticoagulants (heparin or warfarin sodium), as well as reducing venous stasis by mobilization of patients and use of compression stockings or mechanical devices which increase blood flow in the legs. Existing thrombi can be encouraged to resolve by removing the thrombotic stimulus and shifting the balance towards clot lysis. Complete lysis of small calf thrombi is more likely than of large proximal thrombi, even with heparin therapy. The goals of treatment of existing thrombi are to prevent extension and occlusion, and prevent embolization. Anticoagulants are usually effective in preventing acute extension of thrombus, but it is more difficult to prevent a recurrence. Once a thrombus has formed and resolved, vessel scarring predisposes a patient to recurrence of DVT.

Thrombolytic drugs such as streptokinase, urokinase and tissue plasminogen activator have also been used, particularly when rapid lysis of a massive pulmonary embolism is desired. Use of thrombolytic agents is less common in treatment of DVT. The incidence of bleeding has been shown to be more than twice as high among patients treated with thrombolytics than among those treated with heparin. Theoretically, thrombolytic drugs might reduce the incidence of post-thrombotic syndrome and DVT recurrence, because they induce more complete clot lysis than heparin. This has, however, not been conclusively demonstrated in the limited clinical trials reported.

Other treatments for DVT include vena caval interruption with a Greenfield filter or some other device to capture emboli. This option is usually used when anticoagulant therapy is contraindicated because of the risk of haemorrhage. Surgical embolectomy is used rarely when urgent removal of a massive saddle embolus is needed to restore blood pressure. Venous thrombectomy in the lower extremities often provides immediate relief from venous obstruction, but re-thrombosis almost always occurs. In

the lower limbs, the surgical approach is usually reserved for treatment of cases where extensive venous obstruction jeopardizes the viability of the limb, although even here anticoagulation may be preferable.

VALUE OF PRE-TREATMENT DIAGNOSTIC TESTS IN DVT

Thrombi confined to the calf may resolve on their own and even if they embolize, the emboli are small and usually not fatal. However, untreated calf vein thrombi are at risk for propagating into the proximal veins. Thrombi extending into the proximal veins can give rise to pulmonary embolism which can produce clinical symptoms or, ultimately, death. If thrombi resolve on their own, the slow process involves organization and recanalization, and may predispose patients to post-phlebitic syndrome when venous valves are damaged. After one episode of DVT, patients are predisposed to recurrence.

Therefore, it is clear that patients with venous thrombosis should be given early and adequate therapy to dissolve thrombi. It is not acceptable to administer therapeutic levels of anticoagulation in the absence of known thrombosis, because of the risks of anticoagulation. The morbidity from anticoagulant therapy is higher than the morbidity of performing contrast venography, which is considered the most invasive of the objective tests for DVT. The main side effect of anticoagulation is bleeding. In addition, there is a risk of skin necrosis from oral warfarin, particularly in patients with Protein C or Protein S deficiency. The use of thrombolytic drugs is associated with the potential for severe, even life-threatening bleeding.

RADIONUCLIDE DIAGNOSIS OF DVT

The available radionuclide tests for diagnosing DVT can be grouped into two categories: (i) indirect methods using non-specific radiotracers, which basically delineate anatomy; and (ii) direct tests using thrombus-specific radiotracers that bind to molecular sites on venous thrombi with exposed fibrin or platelets allowing visualization of actively forming thrombi. The indirect tests have the advantage of being readily available, but the information gained is more limited than with thrombus-specific agents. In general, thrombus-specific radiopharmaceuticals are preferable to the non-specific ones, but many are currently of limited availability.

RADIONUCLIDE VENOGRAPHY

Principle of the test

In this technique, a particulate radiotracer with short lifetime in the blood circulation is used, usually ^{99m}Tc-macroaggregated albumin (^{99m}Tc-MAA). The radiotracer is injected simultaneously into the dorsal pedal veins of both feet, and flushed in with saline. Tourniquets are placed around both ankles, and sometimes at both knees, before injection to direct the tracer into the deep veins. Static (10-s) views of the calves, thighs and pelvis are acquired, the tourniquets are then removed and the static views repeated. After mild exercise (flexing each foot against the resistance of the technician's hand), another set of static images may be taken to look for areas of retained radiotracer (hot spots). These may result from either pooling in the venous valves or non-specific binding to acute mural thrombi. Finally, images of the lungs are taken as in a lung perfusion study. This study therefore can be done as an alternative to antecubital injection of ^{99m}Tc-MAA in a routine lung perfusion study. Examples of clinical images are shown in Figures 6.15 and 6.16.

The basics of interpretation

A normal study should show uninterrupted passage of radiotracer through the deep veins of the legs to the inferior vena cava. The criterion for the presence of DVT is an abnormal pattern such as collaterals, filling defects in the deep system and residual hot spots. The use of hot spots as a criterion for positivity is controversial, however. Occlusive thrombi do not always trap particles [2], and non-thrombus-related trapping frequently occurs [3]. With this technique, it is not possible to distinguish between chronic and acute thrombi [4]. There are other possible difficulties. Injecting simultaneously into both feet is not always technically feasible, especially in oedematous limbs [5]. Care must be taken in deciding whether deep veins are filled, as filling of the saphenous vein instead of the femoral vein may not be recognized. Similarly, the presence of normal variants such as duplicated veins may be a source of misinterpretation. Varicose veins can lead to an appearance of prominent collaterals in the absence of thrombi.

Lymphoedema and cellulitis can cause non-specific retention and abnormal flow patterns [6]. Finally, the technique is inaccurate below the knee because of inadequate filling of the numerous calf veins with the small volume of radiotracer [7].

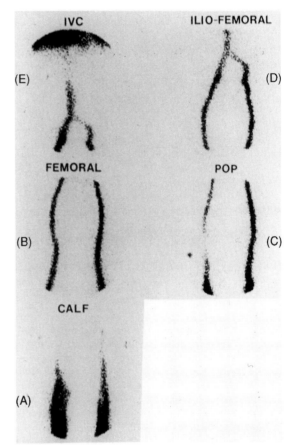

Figure 6.15 Normal ascending radionuclide venogram. With tourniquets applied tightly at the ankles and just below the knees, blood flow is directed preferentially towards the deep venous structures. Images are then acquired sequentially centred first over the calves, then the knees, thighs, and pelvis as the bolus is observed on the persistence scope to ascend the leg. The initial image of the calves (A) shows normal filling of the anterior and posterior tibial veins. The sequential images (B-E) then show normal, symmetrical venous flow through the popliteal, femoral, and iliac veins with ultimate visualization of activity in the inferior vena cava and lungs. (Images provided courtesy of Dr Robert Henkin, Loyola University.)

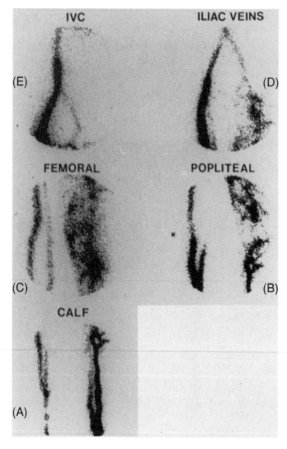

IVC
ILIAC VEINS
(E)
(D)
FEMORAL
POPLITEAL
(C)
(B)
CALF
(A)

Figure 6.16 Abnormal ascending radionuclide venogram showing deep venous thrombosis (DVT) in the left femoral vein (on the right in these anterior images). The study was performed as described in Figure 6.15. The initial image of the calves (A) shows dilatation on the left but no obstruction to flow in the tibial veins. The popliteal veins also appear patent (B). Images centred over the thighs show evidence of soft tissue swelling on the left with extensive collaterals and occlusion (non-visualization) of the left femoral vein (C-E). (Courtesy of Dr Robert Henkin, Loyola University.)

EQUILIBRIUM BLOOD POOL VENOGRAPHY

Principle of the test

An alternative technique for radionuclide venography uses ^{99m}Tc-labelled autologous red blood cells to provide a map of venous blood pool after the labelled red cells have equilibrated throughout the blood. This is usually done by injecting *in vitro*- or *in vivo*-labelled cells into an antecubital or other suitable vein. If desired, the labelled cells may be administered via the pedal veins for an ascending venogram as described above, following which equilibrium imaging is performed. Static views of 1000 K-count each are acquired for clear delineation of the blood vessels. The vascular pattern seen is of the venous system, as the arteries contain a smaller volume of blood and are usually not visualized. Examples of clinical images are shown in Figures 6.17 and 6.18.

The basics of interpretation

The criteria for the presence of DVT are as follows:

1. The absence of a vein that is normally visualized. This indicates total or near-total occlusion of vessel and is the most reliable sign.
2. Failure to visualize a segment of a vein, or an abrupt interruption of a venous channel.
3. In conjunction with 1 or 2, a significant increase in background activity in the symptomatic limb. This is indicative of small superficial collaterals that develop to compensate for severe obstruction of the deep system.

Because this method does not require pedal injections or tourniquets, it is technically less demanding and more comfortable for the patient compared with the ascending venogram. Reported sensitivities range from 77–100%, specificities 71–94%. The most accurate results are for the thigh [8]. Small lesions, floating thrombi, or lesions in small calf veins are not reliably identified.

Potential pitfalls

If there are extensive collaterals, it may be difficult to identify a small obstruction in the deep venous system. Administration of the labelled cells via an ascending venogram performed with tourniquets may be helpful in this case, to provide an initial view of only the deep system without the visual interference of surface vessels. If the patient is imaged in a standing position, involuntary muscle contractions may compress veins, especially in the calf. For this reason, imaging should be performed with the patient relaxed and recumbent on an imaging table. This technique requires meticulous attention to detail for a technically good study. Good red cell labelling is essential. Because of the wide variation in normal vascular patterns, significant

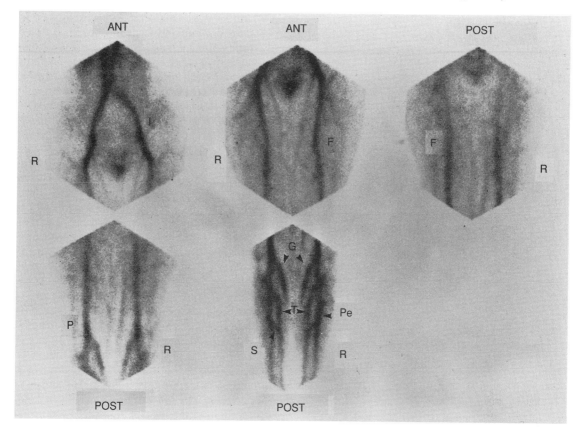

Figure 6.17 Normal equilibrium blood pool venous imaging. After radiolabelling of the patient's red cells, high-resolution images of the lower extremities can be obtained which detail primarily the venous system due to preferential pooling of blood within the veins. I, iliac vein; F, superficial femoral vein; P, popliteal vein; Pe, paired peroneal veins; T, paired posterior tibial veins; G, medial gastrocnemius or sural veins; S, soleal vein. (Reproduced with permission from Lisbona, R. (1986) Radionuclide blood-pool imaging in the diagnosis of deep-vein thrombosis of the leg, in *Nuclear Medicine Annual 1986* (eds L.M. Freeman and H.S. Weissman), Raven Press, New York, pp. 161–93.)

experience of the interpreter in recognizing normal variants and sites of extrinsic compression is very important.

GENERAL COMMENTS

Many different techniques have been reported and there is little standardization. Strict interpretation criteria must be followed to maintain reasonable sensitivity and specificity. Neither ascending venography nor equilibrium blood pool imaging is helpful in distinguishing intraluminal obstruction from extravascular compression [5].

^{125}I-FIBRINOGEN UPTAKE TEST (FUT)

Principle of the test

Fibrinogen normally circulates in the blood as an inactive precursor for fibrin. The technique is most useful for screening asymptomatic high-risk patients. It requires an active thrombotic process, and is less suitable for evaluating symptomatic patients for existing DVT. When the coagulation cascade has been activated, thrombin is formed which catalyses conversion of fibrinogen to fibrin. Fibrin spontaneously polymerises into a clot. If there is an active thrombotic process, radiolabelled fibrinogen is likewise converted into

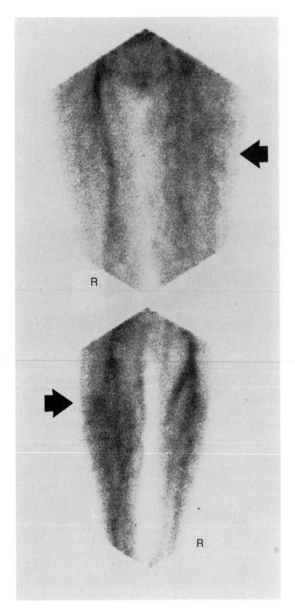

Figure 6.18 Example of abnormal equilibrium blood pool venous imaging showing left femoral and calf DVT. These images show marked soft tissue swelling on the left with extensive collaterals in the calf and thigh (arrows). There is absence of visualization of the left femoral vein indicating occlusive clot. (Reproduced with permission from Lisbona, R. (1986) Radionuclide blood-pool imaging in the diagnosis of deep-vein thrombosis of the leg, in *Nuclear Medicine Annual 1986* (eds L.M. Freeman and H.S. Weissman), Raven Press, New York, pp. 161–93.)

fibrin and is deposited in a forming thrombus. After sufficient deposition has occurred, coupled with sufficient background clearance, the thrombus-bound radiolabel may be detected over the background. Because the low-energy gamma emissions of ^{125}I are readily attenuated by overlying tissue, it does not provide images. Counts are obtained using a hand-held probe, and are recorded at marked points from ankle to mid-thigh. The test is best used in asymptomatic high-risk patients for surveillance. In post-operative patients, the tracer is injected within 1 day after surgery. Counts are collected at bedside daily for 1 week to look for acute thrombus formation. It may be necessary to perform a second injection of labelled fibrinogen if circulating counts become too low before the surveillance period is completed.

The basics of interpretation

The criteria for evidence of thrombus formation have been established as the following: increased counts (20% higher) compared with contralateral side, compared with the same point on the previous day, or compared with points on same leg at adjacent positions more proximal or distal.

The method is useful only from ankle to mid-thigh, because excessive attenuation in the upper thigh and proximity to the bladder (with excreted ^{125}I iodide) make detection of proximal DVT inaccurate.

The radiopharmaceutical is no longer available in many parts of world, presumably because of concern about viral contamination of human blood plasma used as the starting material for isolation of fibrinogen.

Recent studies determining the accuracy of ^{125}I FUT compared with contrast venography reveal that the test is neither as sensitive nor as specific for acutely forming DVT as was originally thought [9]. When evaluated by anatomic region, both sensitivity and specificity for calf vein thrombi are low (59% and 79%) and sensitivity for thrombi in the thigh is very low (18%) [10].

Future prospects

Other fibrin-directed radiopharmaceuticals are currently under development. The potential radiopharmaceuticals are intended to bind to fibrin already deposited on the surface of a thrombus and permit rapid imaging of existing DVT. The agents being evaluated include labelled fibrinogen, fibrin fragments, anti-fibrin mono-clonal antibodies, and tissue plasminogen activator.

INDIUM-111-OXINE-LABELLED AUTOLOGOUS PLATELETS

Principle of the test

Platelets are isolated from patient's blood, labelled with ^{111}In-oxine (commercially available as a label for leucocytes) and resuspended in the patient's own citrated plasma, then re-injected [11,12]. The isolation and labelling process requires about 2 hours. The labelled platelets join the unlabelled platelets in the patient's blood circulation to deposit in actively forming thrombi. After adequate deposition has occurred and blood background has disappeared sufficiently, gamma-camera images are acquired which may show areas of increased uptake corresponding to acute thrombi. Examples of clinical images are shown in Figures 6.19 and 6.20. Imaging is usually performed at 4 hours and repeated at 18–24 hours. The time delay required depends upon how acute the thrombi are, because this affects the rate at which platelets are depositing. Because of the long circulating half-life of ^{111}In-labelled platelets, further imaging at 48 and even 72 hours can be performed. Anterior views should be used for the thighs and pelvis; however, posterior views should be acquired for the calves and popliteal region.

Notes

As with the fibrinogen uptake test, there is usually a time delay before adequate deposition in thrombus occurs, coupled with sufficient decrease in background, for detection of uptake at the site of thrombus. Thus, ^{111}In-oxine platelets are well suited to surveillance testing. In some cases in which acute thrombus formation is ongoing, labelled platelets may provide images within 1–4 hours post-injection. For such cases, autologous platelets have been labelled with ^{99m}Tc-exametazime (HMPAO) [13].

Because there is currently no approved method for *in vivo* platelet labelling, *in vitro* labelling of platelets is the only option at present. This *in vitro* labelling requires special expertise in handling blood to avoid viral transmission to workers, and to avoid contamination of the patient's platelets with bacteria. Special equipment is required, such as a sterile laminar-flow cabinet and an adjustable-

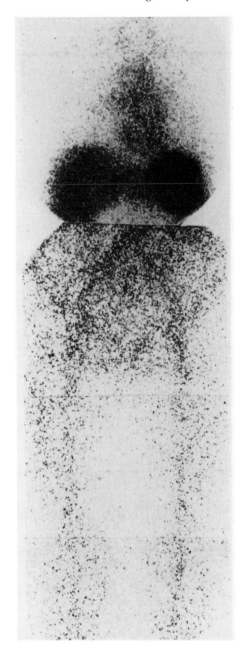

Figure 6.19 Normal ^{111}In-oxine platelet study. Composite anterior image 24 hours after injection of labelled platelets. There is normal sequestration of labelled platelets in the liver and spleen, with normal blood pool. No focal areas of increased accumulation are seen. (Reproduced from Clarke-Pearson *et al.* (1985) *Surgery*, **98**, 98–104, with permission.)

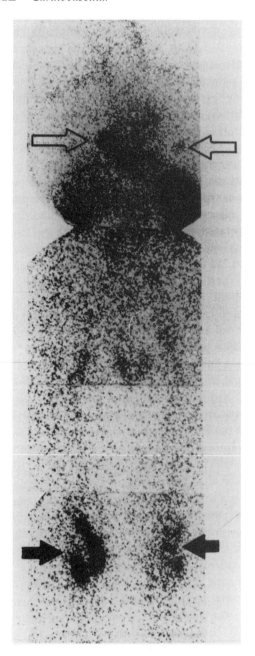

Figure 6.20 Abnormal ^{111}In-oxine platelet study in a postoperative patient. Composite anterior image shows bilateral calf and popliteal venous thrombosis (solid arrows) and bilateral pulmonary emboli (open arrows). The thrombi and emboli were confirmed by venography and pulmonary arteriography. (Reproduced from Clarke-Pearson *et al.* (1985) *Surgery*, **98**, 98–104, with permission.)

speed centrifuge. Special training for labelling personnel is advisable to minimize inadvertent platelet activation through improper handling. The labelling may be performed in-house with ^{111}In-oxine (approved for labelling white blood cells), or commercial labelling may be available by an outside service.

The basics of interpretation

Criteria for a positive study are focal areas of increased activity corresponding to a vascular structure, as demonstrated in Figure 6.20. Increased uptake confined to the inguinal area has been found to be non-specific for thrombi, and probably represents pooling of blood [14]. An asymmetric pattern in the 4-hour image is non-specific because of extensive blood pool at this time. Imaging should be repeated at 24 hours.

Labelled platelets have been found to work best for imaging fresh thrombi [15]. Older thrombi and pulmonary emboli do not reliably accumulate fresh platelets. The effect of ongoing heparin or warfarin therapy is controversial. Some reports indicate that anticoagulants may interfere with platelet uptake even in fresh thrombi; however, others believe that positive platelet images may be obtained although at a later time than if anticoagulants were not administered. Some investigators have shown that temporary suspension of anticoagulant therapy may permit thrombus images to be obtained with labelled platelets [14]. The safety and utility of temporarily withholding anticoagulants for platelet imaging needs to be evaluated.

Future prospects

Other platelet-directed radiopharmaceuticals are currently under development. The potential radiopharmaceuticals are intended to bind to activated platelets already deposited on the surface of a thrombus and permit rapid imaging of existing DVT. The agents under evaluation include monoclonal antibodies and peptides which recognize receptors on the surface of platelets. Most are directed at the glycoprotein IIb/IIIa receptor.

CLINICAL APPLICATIONS

The approach to diagnosis will vary depending on the clinical setting. For DVT there are four major clinical settings.

1. A suspected first episode in a symptomatic patient. Non-scintigraphic tests such as compression ultrasonography and impedance plethysmography are usually used with confidence in this setting, in which thrombi are usually large and proximal.
2. A suspected recurrence in a symptomatic patient. In this setting, venographic findings may be inconclusive because of obliteration and recanalization which disrupt the familiar pattern of venous opacification. Impedance plethysmography may be falsely positive because of a persistent obstruction to venous outflow, or falsely negative because of the development of large collateral channels in response to the prior episodes of DVT [16]. Compression ultrasound depends extensively on lack of compressibility of veins to make a diagnosis of thrombus. In recurrent DVT, however, patent but scarred veins may be incompressible. Labelled platelets should be useful in diagnosing an acute recurrence.
3. The screening of a high-risk asymptomatic patient. In post-surgical patients, the majority of thrombi at 10 days post-surgery are non-occlusive, particularly above the knee [17]. This limits the ability of the flow-dependent tests to identify them. Surveillance testing with ^{111}In-labelled platelets or ^{125}I-fibrinogen would be useful in this setting.
4. Improved scintigraphic detection of pulmonary emboli. Since pulmonary emboli arise from thrombi in the deep veins, using thrombus-imaging radiopharmaceuticals to diagnose the presence of DVT could improve the specificity of an observed perfusion defect in V/Q studies. This could be done by performing an ascending venogram using ^{99m}Tc-MAA before perfusion imaging using the same dose. Alternatively, a thrombus-specific radiopharmaceutical such as labelled platelets could be used to image the extremities, as a complement to a traditional V/Q scan. In the future, new radiopharmaceuticals may permit direct visualization of pulmonary emboli in addition to deep venous thrombi.

REFERENCES

1. Zorba, J., Schier, D. and Posmituck, G. (1986) Clinical value of blood pool radionuclide venography. *Am. J. Roentgenol.*, **146**, 1051–5.
2. Rosenthall, L. and Greyson, N.D. (1970) Observations on the use of 99mTc albumin macroaggregates for detection of thrombophlebitis. *Radiology*, **94**, 413–16.
3. Webber, M.M., Bennett, L.R., Cragin, M. and Webb, R.J. (1969) Thrombophlebitis – demonstration by scintiscanning. *Radiology*, **92**, 620–3.
4. Holden, R.W., Klatte, E.C., Park, H.M. *et al.* (1981) Efficacy of noninvasive modalities for diagnosis of thrombophlebitis. *Radiology*, **141**, 63–6.
5. Oster, Z.H., Atkins, H.L. and Trivedi, M. (1987) Radionuclide venography vs Tc-99m-RBC equilibrium angiography: a comparative paired study. *Eur. J. Nucl. Med.*, **13**, 174–82.
6. Gomes, A.S., Webber, M.M. and Buffkin, D. (1982) Contrast venography vs. radionuclide venography: A study of discrepancies and their possible significance. *Radiology*, **142**, 719–28.
7. Vittadini, A., Franchi, R. and Barbieri, L.L. (1980) Isotope phlebography in the study of lower extremity venous thrombosis. *Eur. J. Nucl. Med.*, **5**, 135–43.
8. Lisbona, R. (1986) Radionuclide blood-pool imaging in the diagnosis of deep-vein thrombosis of the leg, in *Nuclear Medicine Annual 1986* (eds L.M. Freeman and H.S. Weissman), Raven Press, New York, pp. 161–93.
9. Lensing, A.W.A. and Hirsh, J. (1993) ^{125}I-fibrinogen leg scanning: reassessment of its role for the diagnosis of venous thrombosis in post-operative patients. *Thromb. Haemost.*, **69**, 2–7.
10. Sautter, R.D., Larson, D.E., Bhattacharyya, S.K. *et al.* (1979) The limited utility of fibrinogen I-125 leg scanning. *Arch. Intern. Med.*, **139**, 148–53.
11. Thakur, M.L., Welch, M.J., Joist, J.H. and Coleman, R.E. (1976) Indium-111-labeled platelets: studies on preparation and evaluation of in vitro and in vivo functions. *Thromb. Res.*, **9**, 345–57.
12. Thakur, M.L., Walsh, L., Malech, H.L. and Gottschalk, A. (1981) Indium-111-labeled human platelets: improved method, efficacy, and evaluation. *J. Nucl. Med.*, **22**, 381–5.
13. Becker, W., Börner, W. and Borst, U. (1988) ^{99m}Tc hexamethylpropyleneamineoxime (HMPAO) as a platelet label: evaluation of labelling parameters and first in vivo results. *Nucl. Med. Commun.*, **9**, 831–42.
14. Seabold, J.E., Conrad, G.R., Kimball, D.A., Ponto, J.A. and Bricker, J.A. (1988) Pitfalls in establishing the diagnosis of deep venous thrombophlebitis by indium-111 platelet scintigraphy. *J. Nucl. Med.*, **29**, 1169–80.
15. Moser, K.M., Spragg, R.G., Bender, F., Kanopka, R., Hartman, M.T. and Fedullo, P. (1980) Study of factors that may condition scintigraphic detection of venous thrombi and pulmonary emboli with indium-111-labeled platelets. *J. Nucl. Med.*, **21**, 1051–8.
16. Hull, R.D., Carter, C.J., Jay, R.M. *et al.* (1983) The diagnosis of acute, recurrent, deep-vein thrombosis: a diagnostic challenge. *Circulation*, **67**, 901–6.
17. Ascani, A., Radicchia, S., Parise, P., Nenci, G.G. and Agnelli, G. (1996) Distribution and occlusiveness of

thrombi in patients with surveillance detected deep vein thrombosis after hip surgery. *Thromb. Haemost.*, **75**, 239–41.

FURTHER READING

Colman, R.W., Hirsh, J., Marder, V.J. and Salzman E.W. (eds), *Haemostasis and Thrombosis. Basic Principles and Clinical Practice*, 3rd edn. J.B. Lippincott, Philadelphia, 1994.

Comerota, A.J., Knight, L.C. and Maurer, A.H. (1988) The diagnosis of acute deep venous thrombosis: noninvasive and radioisotopic techniques. *Ann. Vasc. Surg.*, **4**, 406–24.

Knight, L.C. (1990) Radiopharmaceuticals for thrombus detection. *Semin. Nucl. Med.*, **20**(1), 52–67.

Knight, L.C. (1993) Scintigraphic methods for detecting vascular thrombus. *J. Nucl. Med.*, **34**, 554–61.

Lisbona, R. (1986) Radionuclide blood-pool imaging in the diagnosis of deep-vein thrombosis of the leg, in *Nuclear Medicine Annual 1986* (eds L.M. Freeman and H.S. Weissman), Raven Press, New York, pp. 161–93.

Rodrigues, M. and Sinzinger, H. (1994) Platelet labeling. Methodology and clinical applications. *Thromb. Res.*, **76**(5), 399–432.

CHAPTER 7

Pulmonary and thoracic

Pulmonary embolism

H. D. Royal

INTRODUCTION

Much has been written about pulmonary embolism in the medical and surgical literature. Despite this interest in pulmonary embolism, the scientific basis for our beliefs about the condition is quite weak. In this section, mostly conventional ideas about pulmonary embolism will be discussed; however, readers are encouraged to develop a healthy scepticism about what we think we know about pulmonary embolism.

RELEVANT ANATOMY AND PHYSIOLOGY

Most pulmonary emboli are clots which originate in the venous system. When these clots break loose from their site of origin – usually veins in the lower extremities – they return to the right atrium and right ventricle through the major venous vessels. The emboli usually will continue unimpeded out from the pulmonary artery until they occlude a vessel that is similar in size to the clot.

The main pulmonary artery divides progressively until there are approximately 300 million pre-capillary arterioles that are 20–30 μm in size. These arterioles further divide into pulmonary capillaries that are 5–8 μm in size. Red blood cells (8 μm in diameter) are deformed before they can squeeze through these tiny vessels. The divisions of the pulmonary artery are conveniently called generations. The first division of the main pulmonary artery (left and right pulmonary arteries) are second-generation vessels, the lobar arteries are third-generation vessels and the segmental arteries are fourth-generation vessels. The smallest vessels that can be examined for pulmonary emboli by arteriography are subsegmental vessels (fifth generation) [1].

The segmental arteries are 4–5 mm in size and they provide blood flow to a segment of the lung which is tens of centimetres in size. The high sensitivity of perfusion imaging for the detection of pulmonary emboli is due to the fact that a small (4–5 mm) embolus acutely causes a much larger (tens of centimetres) perfusion defect. Emboli usually are dissolved by the body's own endogenous thrombolytic processes. Dissolution can occur rapidly (24–48 hours), especially in young patients without pre-existing heart or lung disease. If pulmonary arteriography is to be performed after ventilation–perfusion imaging, it should not be delayed for longer than 24 hours if the sensitivity of pulmonary arteriography is to be maximized.

The morbidity and mortality of pulmonary embolism is caused by an acute elevation of pulmonary vascular resistance and subsequent right heart failure. Healthy lungs have a large vascular reserve. For example, during exercise the cardiac output and pulmonary blood flow can increase several fold without an increase in the pulmonary artery pressure. Even unhealthy lungs have a large vascular reserve. Most smokers who have a

Clinical Nuclear Medicine, 3rd edn. Edited by M.N. Maisey, K.E. Britton and B.D. Collier. Published in 1998 by Chapman & Hall, London. ISBN 0 412 75180 1

pneumonectomy for lung cancer have no or only a small increase in the resting pulmonary artery pressure. These observations would suggest that a large percentage of the pulmonary vascular bed would have to be occluded by emboli in order to have a significant effect on pulmonary artery pressures.

The physiological principle that is exploited by pulmonary perfusion imaging is that intravenously injected microemboli will be trapped in the arterioles of the lung in proportion to regional pulmonary blood flow. Severe pulmonary hypertension and a large anatomic right-to-left shunt are relative contraindications to perfusion imaging. In patients with pulmonary hypertension, the particles occlude a larger fraction of the cross-sectional area of the pulmonary vascular bed and may increase an already severely elevated pulmonary artery pressure. Despite this concern, there is no alternative safer method to evaluate pulmonary perfusion in these patients. In patients with right-to-left shunts, some of the injected particles will be diverted into the systemic circulation and will embolize pre-capillary arterioles throughout the body. Fortunately, this has not been associated with any documented untoward sequelae, but the theoretical risk remains of concern. When a patient with either pulmonary hypertension or a right-to-left shunt is studied with ^{99m}Tc-MAA, the number of particles injected can be reduced to 100 000 to make the examination as safe as possible.

The hypoxia associated with pulmonary emboli can not be explained by simple occlusion of pulmonary vessels. Occlusion of vessels will increase the dead space of the lung but another mechanism must be invoked to explain the hypoxia. The hypoxia is likely caused by the release of vasoactive substance that causes intrapulmonary shunting of blood.

CLINICAL SETTING

Pulmonary embolism may present with myriad findings, most of which are non-specific [2,3]. Moreover, pulmonary embolism is often asymptomatic. Hence, it is difficult to provide rigid guidelines regarding the indications for ventilation–perfusion scintigraphy in suspected pulmonary embolism. The most common presenting symptoms and signs in patients with pulmonary embolism are dyspnoea and tachypnoea.

Strong risk factors for pulmonary embolism include recent surgery, trauma (especially to the lower extremities), prolonged bed rest, hypercoagulable states, venous disease, and pre-existing cardiopulmonary disease.

Since emboli can resolve within several days, especially in young patients who have no underlying cardiopulmonary disease, ventilation–perfusion scintigraphy should be obtained within 24 hours of the acute event that initiated the clinical suspicion for pulmonary embolism. Additionally, there is a tendency with increasing delay for ventilation–perfusion studies to give equivocal results more frequently both because of thrombolysis and partial resolution of perfusion defects and because of the development of matching radiographic abnormalities. However, in patients with pulmonary oedema or with acute bronchospasm, a more definitive ventilation–perfusion study may be obtainable if it is performed after initial treatment of these conditions.

In patients with abnormal chest radiographs, ventilation–perfusion scintigraphy is predictably less helpful overall than in patients with normal radiographs [4]. This is because most radiographically apparent infiltrates or pleural effusions cause perfusion defects, and thus it is generally difficult to exclude pulmonary embolism with high confidence in most such patients (i.e. perfusion defects due to pulmonary embolism complicated by pulmonary infarction cannot be distinguished from perfusion defects due to pneumonia or other causes of an infiltrate).

Despite the problems of interpretation caused by chest radiograph abnormalities, ventilation–perfusion scintigraphy is still indicated [5,6]. In patients with focal radiographic abnormalities, a diagnosis of pulmonary embolism can be still be made if radiographically normal areas of the lungs exhibit ventilation–perfusion abnormalities characteristic of pulmonary embolism. This is likely in patients with pulmonary embolism, since emboli are usually multiple and they are distributed in the lung according to pulmonary blood flow. Since blood flow is generally best to radiographically normal areas of the lung, such regions have a higher chance of encountering pulmonary emboli.

Ventilation–perfusion imaging is often requested in patients with congestive heart failure.

The patients are short of breath and it is usually clear that they have congestive heart failure. The clinical concern is determining why the patient acutely went into heart failure. What tipped the balance? If there is no clearly identifiable cause for the patient's acute decompensation, then to consider the possibility of a pulmonary embolus in these chronically ill patients is reasonable. Two questions emerge. The first is 'When is ventilation–perfusion imaging most likely to be diagnostic in these patients, who most likely have diffuse infiltrates on their chest radiograph?' The second is 'What findings on ventilation–perfusion imaging are likely in patients with congestive heart failure?'

Several factors must be considered in order to decide when ventilation–perfusion imaging is best performed in patients with congestive heart failure. On the one hand, aggressive treatment of the congestive heart failure will usually greatly improve the chest radiograph abnormalities over a period of 24–48 hours. Improvement in these radiographic and clinical abnormalities will often make the results of ventilation–perfusion imaging more definitive. On the other hand, a delay in the diagnosis of pulmonary embolism is undesirable. This tension is usually resolved in the following way. If the patient has an identifiable cause for his/her decompensation, is treated aggressively for congestive heart failure and responds well to treatment, there is little need to look for alternative causes for the patient's decompensation. If the patient has no readily identifiable cause for his/her decompensation or does not respond well to treatment, ventilation–perfusion imaging is indicated and may be performed acutely.

In patients with a diffusely abnormal chest X-ray, the diagnosis of pulmonary embolism can still be made using ventilation–perfusion imaging. Pulmonary emboli cause focal and randomly distributed perfusion defects that follow the segmental anatomy of the lung, whereas a diffuse pulmonary process such as congestive heart failure tends to cause ill-defined large perfusion defects that do not follow the segmental anatomy of the lung and heterogeneity of perfusion. Even when the results of ventilation–perfusion scintigraphy are non-diagnostic (i.e. indeterminate or intermediate probability), the information obtained is useful to guide subsequent pulmonary angiography.

TECHNICAL FACTORS

VENTILATION IMAGING

Ventilation imaging is performed along with perfusion imaging to improve the specificity of this diagnostic procedure. Perfusion defects generally are present in regions of obstructive airways disease (because the regional alveolar hypoxia leads to reflex arteriolar vasoconstriction in the same area). The use of ventilation imaging permits detection of localized ventilatory abnormalities and allows perfusion defects to be classified as matched or mismatched with respect to abnormal ventilation; it is well established that mismatched perfusion defects are much more likely to be due to pulmonary emboli than are matched defects.

Four types of ventilation studies can be performed using either ^{133}Xe, ^{99m}Tc-labelled aerosol, ^{99m}Tc-labelled gas or ^{81m}Kr. ^{133}Xe is a radioactive, inert gas that is most commonly used for ventilation studies. Successful ^{133}Xe ventilation imaging requires a moderate degree of patient cooperation. The ventilation study consists of three distinct phases: (i) first breath; (ii) equilibrium; and (iii) washout (Figure 7.1).

During the first breath phase, the patient is instructed to take a deep breath (from end-expiratory to end-inspiratory capacity) and to hold this breath for about 20 seconds, if possible. At the start of this deep inspiration, ^{133}Xe gas can be introduced as a bolus injection into the tubing through which the patient inhales. Alternatively, the xenon could be injected into the reservoir of a closed spirometer before the first breath phase (Figure 7.2). The advantage of injecting the xenon into the tubing is that nearly all of the xenon will be in the patient's lungs during the first breath phase; therefore, the number of counts in a 20-second image of the lungs will be several times greater than if the xenon was injected into the reservoir of the spirometer. The disadvantage of injecting a bolus of xenon into the tubing is that the xenon will not be uniformly mixed in the inspired air. Inadequate mixing can create artefacts in the image because the early portions of each breath preferentially ventilate the lower portions of the lung (in a upright patient). If the xenon is injected after inspiration has begun, the lower lung may artefactually appear to be hypoventilated. Fortunately, this problem is rarely seen when careful attention is paid to injecting the xenon at the beginning of inspiration. During this

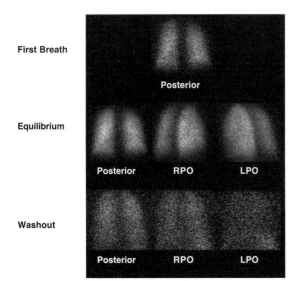

First Breath

Posterior

Equilibrium

Posterior　　RPO　　LPO

Washout

Posterior　　RPO　　LPO

Figure 7.1 Normal ^{133}Xe ventilation. The ^{133}Xe ventilation study consists of three distinct phases: (i) First breath; (ii) equilibrium; and (iii) washout. During the equilibrium and washout phases, posterior oblique images can be obtained in cooperative patients who are able to sit on a swivel stool. Near-complete washout of activity occurs rapidly (3–5 min) in this patient with normal ventilation.

first breath, the radioactive gas is distributed within the lungs roughly in proportion to regional alveolar ventilation; areas of the lung that are poorly ventilated contain less of the radioactive gas.

During the next phase of the study the patient rebreathes the radioactive gas from a closed spirometer system for several minutes. During this time, most of the aerated portions of the lungs will achieve a uniform (equilibrium) concentration of ^{133}Xe. The equilibrium images, therefore, reflect the regional distribution of aerated lung volume, but they generally provide no information about the rate of ventilation since all but the most poorly ventilated zones of lung (e.g. bullae) will achieve equilibrium (Figure 7.3).

During the washout phase, the patient breathes room air, resulting in clearance of the radioactive gas from the lungs. The non-radioactive room air rapidly dilutes the radioactive gas in well-ventilated lung zones. However, there is delayed clearance of ^{133}Xe from areas of the lung that are poorly ventilated; therefore, these appear as areas of increased activity on the washout images. Since

it generally is much easier in scintigraphic studies to see zones of relatively increased activity rather than areas of decreased activity, the washout images are more sensitive for detecting regional obstructive airways disease than are either the first breath or rebreathing images. The exception to this generalization is when the poorly ventilated areas of the lung do not reach equilibrium. If little xenon enters the poorly ventilated areas then no delay in the washout of activity from these areas may be appreciated.

Because of downscatter from the 140 keV photon of ^{99m}Tc into the 81 keV energy window for ^{133}Xe, it is more difficult to perform xenon imaging after the injection of ^{99m}Tc-MAA than before injection. Downscatter from the ^{99m}Tc becomes most important during the critical washout phase of the xenon study when there is little xenon remaining in the lungs (Figure 7.4). If the xenon ventilation study is to be performed after the ^{99m}Tc-MAA injection, the downscatter problem can be partly mitigated by taking three actions. First, patients can be injected with less ^{99m}Tc-MAA (e.g. 80 MBq rather than 160 MBq) and can inhale more ^{133}Xe (e.g. 700 MBq rather than 350 MBq). Second, an image of the downscatter of ^{99m}Tc into the ^{133}Xe energy window can be obtained before the patient inhales the xenon. Third, the xenon can be injected into the tubing connected to the face mask rather than into the reservoir of the spirometer in order to maximize the count rate during the first breath phase of the ventilation study.

Despite the problem of downscatter, performing xenon ventilation studies after the perfusion study has two advantages. First, the ventilation study can be performed in the view which best demonstrates the perfusion defect. Second, the ventilation study can be performed only in patients who have defects on their perfusion study. Ventilation imaging with ^{127}Xe [primary photon energies 172 (25%), 203 (68%), 375 (17%) keV] would also eliminate problems due to downscatter; however, ^{127}Xe is not widely available.

A second type of ventilation scintigraphy, ^{99m}Tc-labelled aerosol imaging, can be performed. The aerosol is most commonly labelled using ^{99m}Tc-DTPA. Aerosol imaging is particularly useful in patients who must undergo bedside studies. For radiation safety reasons, ^{133}Xe ventilation imaging cannot be performed routinely in patients who must stay in the intensive care unit. Xenon ventilation studies require a cumbersome system to trap

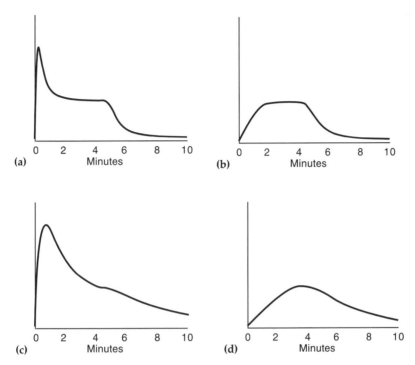

Figure 7.2 ^{133}Xe activity versus time curve. The curve shape depends on how the xenon is administered and on the patient's ventilatory function. For schematic curves (a) and (c), the xenon was introduced as a bolus injection into the tubing through which the patient inhales, resulting in a high initial xenon activity in the lungs. When the xenon is injected into the reservoir bag of the spirometer (curves (b) and (d)), the initial activity of xenon in the lungs is much less. Curves A and B depict the prompt equilibrium and washout that would be expected in patients with normal ventilation. Curves C and D never reach equilibrium and show slow washout consistent with obstructive airways disease.

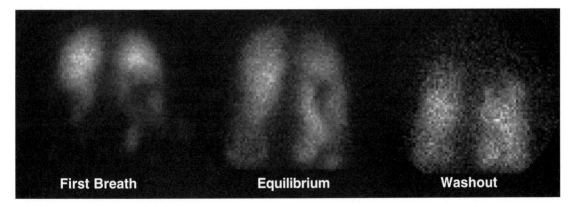

Figure 7.3 Abnormal ventilation due to α_1-antitrypsin deficiency. During the first breath there is near-normal ventilation of both lung apices. At equilibrium, the xenon activity is more uniformly distributed throughout the lung. Marked retention of activity (trapping) is seen in the lower two-thirds of both lungs during washout. In α_1-antitrypsin deficiency, ventilation is best preserved in the lung apices. In patients with obstructive airways disease who do not have α_1-antitrypsin deficiency, ventilation is best preserved in the lung bases. (See also Figure 7.7.)

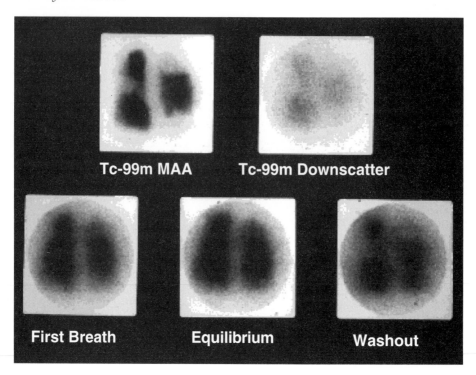

Tc-99m MAA   Tc-99m Downscatter

First Breath   Equilibrium   Washout

Figure 7.4 [99mTc] downscatter. When [99mTc]-MAA perfusion scintigraphy is performed before [133Xe] ventilation scintigraphy, some of the scattered 140 keV photons from [99mTc] will be detected in the [133Xe] energy window. In order to minimize the potential for confusion, it is helpful to obtain an image of the [99mTc] downscatter before beginning the [133Xe] ventilation study. In this patient with pulmonary embolism, the non-uniform activity seen on the washout image is due to [99mTc] downscatter and not to ventilatory abnormalities.

the exhaled gas and a specialized ventilation system to exhaust any of radioactive gas that is not trapped. However, the short half-life of [99mTc] (6 hours) and the ability to trap exhaled aerosol easily make it possible to perform aerosol imaging at the bedside without significant radiation hazard.

[99mTc]-DTPA aerosol is generated by a jet nebulizer and consists of droplets that are approximately 0.8 μm in diameter [7]. Under normal physiological conditions, inhaled aerosol droplets are uniformly deposited in bronchioles and alveoli. Airway obstruction causes turbulent airflow with resultant impaction of aerosol droplets in larger bronchi and reduced peripheral deposition of the tracer. Hence, the presence of regional airways disease generally can be inferred from the aerosol images.

Tachypnoea alone causes turbulent airflow (and increased central airway deposition of aerosol), and can make interpretation of aerosol images more difficult. Unfortunately, the sick patients in whom bedside studies are required often are tachypnoeic. Tracheal intubation and increased airway secretions also increase central deposition of aerosol. Despite these problems, aerosol imaging improves the specificity of portable studies for the diagnosis of pulmonary embolism, by comparison with perfusion imaging alone, and also allows recognition of so-called 'reverse ventilation–perfusion mismatch' – decreased ventilation with better maintained or normal perfusion (failure of hypoxic vasoconstriction) (Figure 7.5). Patients with this finding, which is seen in a small fraction of bedside ventilation–perfusion studies, are generally hypoxaemic because of the concomitant functional intrapulmonary right-to-left shunting.

An advantage of aerosol imaging over [133Xe] imaging is that aerosol, once deposited in the alveoli, remains there for some time (Table 7.1) [8]. It is possible, therefore, to obtain multiple ventila-

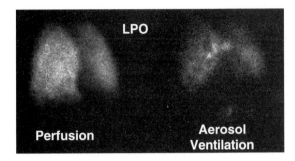

Figure 7.5 Reverse ventilation perfusion mismatch. In this patient, there is decreased ventilation to the left lower lobe but perfusion is well-preserved. Reverse ventilation–perfusion mismatches are due to the loss of the normally potent vasoconstriction that occurs in response to alveolar hypoxia.

Table 7.1 Lung clearance times*

^{99m}Tc-Imaging agent	Normal (n = 22)	Smokers (n = 14)	Abnormals (n = 14)
^{99m}Tc-DTPA aerosol	52.5 ± 29.5	28.3 ± 15.6	4.8 ± 5.7
^{99m}Tc-pertechnegas	10.1 ± 2.4	7.0 ± 1.1	2.5 ± 0.7

*Values are in minutes (mean ± SD).
Data are from Monaghan *et al.* [8].

tion images with aerosols for comparison with the perfusion study. Only one or a limited number of views can be obtained with ^{133}Xe.

An important technical concern about the use of ^{99m}Tc aerosol studies is that the same radionuclide is being used to map ventilation and perfusion. Activity from the first study (perfusion or ventilation) will be indistinguishable from activity from the second study. The simplest way to minimize this problem is to ensure that the activity used for the second study results in a count rate that is at least four to five times greater than the count rate of the first study.

Generally, it is best to perform the ^{99m}Tc aerosol study first, since it is much easier to administer larger amounts of ^{99m}Tc-MAA than it is to administer a large amount of ^{99m}Tc aerosol. Typically, rebreathing ^{99m}Tc aerosol for 5 minutes results in the deposition of <2mCi of activity within the lungs. The actual amount of activity within the lungs of each patient can be determined with reasonable certainty by comparing the observed

count rate with the count rate obtained after a known amount of ^{99m}Tc-MAA is injected intravenously. Generally, an 8mCi injection of ^{99m}Tc should increase the count rate following ^{99m}Tc aerosol ventilation imaging by a factor of 5. It is important to document the change in count rate, since the expected change will not occur if a significant portion of the ^{99m}Tc-MAA is extravasated. Achieving the desired ratio of count rates will be much more difficult if the ^{99m}Tc aerosol study is performed after the ^{99m}Tc perfusion study. In this case computer subtraction of images may be necessary. This process imposes the added burden that the patient can not move between the time when the most suspicious perfusion image is obtained and the ventilation image is obtained.

Failure to achieve the necessary ratio of count rates can result in major errors. If the perfusion study is obtained first, perfusion defects may erroneously appear to be matched by ventilatory abnormalities. If the ventilation study is obtained first, perfusion defects due to pulmonary embolism may not be appreciated because ventilation in the region of the perfusion abnormality is normal.

Technegas and pertechnegas have not received approval for routine use in the United States but this agent is widely used in Australia and in Europe [9–11]. The technetium-labelled gas is produced using a generator system that uses a graphite crucible filled with 0.1ml of pertechnetate. After drying, this crucible is rapidly heated to ~2500°C to produce the technetium-labelled gas. This dry gas consists of carbon particles. Technegas is produced when the gas is made in an atmosphere of 100% argon. Pertechnegas is produced when the gas is made in an atmosphere of 95% argon and 5% oxygen. Technegas is cleared very slowly, if at all from the lungs. Pertechnegas is soluble and is absorbed rapidly from the lungs with a $t_{1/2}$ of ~10 minutes in patients with no underlying lung pathology (Table 7.1). More rapid absorption is seen in patients with pulmonary pathology, including smokers. Using either agent, it is possible to obtain multiple, high-quality ventilation views.

When compared with ^{99m}Tc aerosols, ^{99m}Tc-labelled gases have the following advantages. First, there is less central airways deposition of the tracer. Second, the patient needs to take only a few breaths of the gas to obtain a satisfactory count rate compared with several minutes of breathing with aerosols. The major potential problem with ^{99m}Tc gases is the same problem that was discussed in detail for ^{99m}Tc aerosols. That is, the same radionuclide is used for both ventilation and perfusion; thus, it is essential to document that the count rate of the second study is four to five times greater than that of the first study. As with aerosols, it is generally best to perform the ^{99m}Tc gas ventilation study before the ^{99m}Tc-MAA perfusion study. The more rapid clearance of ^{99m}Tc-pertechnegas from the lung compared with ^{99m}Tc aerosols is also an advantage, since the problems caused by the residual administered ventilation agent diminish more rapidly with time.

Krypton-81m can also be used for ventilation imaging. Unlike imaging with xenon, krypton images are obtained while the patient rebreathes krypton. Because of its short half-life (13 seconds), krypton decays before it reaches portions of the lung that are poorly ventilated. Therefore, poorly ventilated areas of the lung have decreased activity when compared with well-ventilated areas. Since ventilation images are obtained while the patient continuously rebreathes krypton, images can be obtained in multiple views. In addition, ventilation images can be obtained either immediately before or immediately after each perfusion image. The relatively high photon energy of krypton (190 keV) allows for the acquisition of high-quality ventilation images after ^{99m}Tc-MAA has been injected. High-quality ^{99m}Tc perfusion images can also be obtained after a krypton ventilation image because the krypton in the lungs disappears rapidly (due to its short physical half-life) when the krypton is eliminated from the inspired air. This ability to acquire alternately the ventilation and perfusion images minimizes any differences in the views that are obtained. The relatively high photon energy of krypton necessitates the use of a medium-energy collimator; therefore, image resolution is degraded when compared with ^{99m}Tc images acquired with a low-energy collimator.

The major disadvantages of krypton are that it is expensive and not widely available; moreover, its short half-life mandates that a generator must be used. Unfortunately, krypton's parent, rubidium-81, is less than ideal, having a relatively short half-life (4.6 hours). Thus, a new krypton generator needs to be ordered for every day of use. Several (8–10) patients need to be studied with each generator in order for the costs to be similar to that for other ventilation agents. Another problem is that

^{81m}Rb emits many high-energy photons that require considerable shielding, thus making the generator system heavy and awkward.

Several paired comparison studies have shown that the type of ventilation imaging performed does not significantly influence the accuracy of interpretation of ventilation–perfusion studies in patients with suspected pulmonary embolism. When quantitative information about ventilation is desired, ventilation imaging with xenon or krypton is recommended. Because of deposition of activity in the central airways, quantitation with aerosols or with ^{99m}Tc-labelled gases may be inaccurate. Typical acquisition parameters for each type of ventilation study are listed in Table 7.2.

PERFUSION SCINTIGRAPHY

Regional pulmonary perfusion is evaluated by imaging the distribution of ^{99m}Tc-macro-aggregated albumin (MAA). This radiopharmaceutical consists of particles of denatured albumin, most of which are 20–40 μm in size (range 10–90 μm). When injected intravenously, these particles are uniformly mixed with blood before they are trapped in the pre-capillary arterioles of the lungs. Thus, they distribute in the lungs in proportion to regional pulmonary blood flow. In patients with relatively normal lungs, only about 0.03 to 0.3% of the 300 million pre-capillary arterioles will be temporarily occluded by the 100 000 to 1 000 000 albumin particles that are injected. The particles are 'biodegradable', and are cleared from the lungs with a half-time of several hours (chiefly by breaking into smaller particles which are then phagocytosed by the cells of the reticuloendothelial system).

INTERPRETATION OF VENTILATION–PERFUSION STUDIES

The interpretation of ventilation–perfusion studies in patients with suspected pulmonary embolism is based on the theoretical premise that uncomplicated pulmonary embolism typically impairs perfusion but not ventilation (a ventilation–perfusion mismatch) (Figure 7.6), whereas airway disease typically reduces both ventilation and perfusion (a ventilation–perfusion match). This simple concept, however, has not proved entirely reliable in practice. Hence, more complicated criteria have been developed based on correlations of

Table 7.2 Acquisition parameters for ventilation–perfusion studies

Radiopharmaceutical	Administered activity	View	Acquisition time or counts	Matrix size	Pixel depth
Ventilation					
Xenon-133 gas (one view usually posterior)	370–740 MBq	Wash in	20 s 1 frame	64 × 64 or 128 × 128	8 bits
		Equilibrium	3–5 min 1 frame per 20 s		
		Washout	3–6 min 1 frame per 20 s		
^{99m}Tc-labelled aerosol	35–75 MBq	4–6 views	100–300 K	128 × 128	16 bits
^{81m}Kr	Not applicable	4–6 views	100–300 K	128 × 128	16 bits
Pertechnegas Technegas	35–75 MBq	4–6 views	100–300 K	128 × 128	16 bits
Perfusion					
^{99m}Tc MAA	75–300 MBq	4–6 views	300–1000 K	128 × 128 or 256 × 256	16 bits

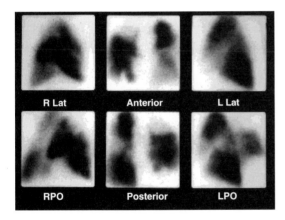

Figure 7.6 Perfusion defects due to pulmonary embolism. Perfusion defects that follow the segmental anatomy of the lung and have nearly absent perfusion are most characteristic of pulmonary embolism. The segmental anatomy of the lung is very well demonstrated on this perfusion study. In particular, note the absence of the four basal segments of the right lower lobe on the RPO view and the absence of the superior segment of the left lower lobe on the LPO view.

radiographic and scintigraphic findings. Because of the importance of the chest radiograph in these schemes, patients should have a recent chest radiograph (standard examination, if possible). The definition of recent depends on the clinical circumstances. Certainly a chest radiograph should be obtained after the patient's most recent acute event. For example, if a patient had the acute onset of shortness of breath 1 hour ago and the most recent chest radiograph is 2 hours old, the chest radiograph should be repeated, even if the ventilation–perfusion study was normal. The rationale behind this recommendation is that a normal ventilation–perfusion study can not reliably exclude other important causes for acute pulmonary symptoms such as a small pneumothorax. On the other hand, if the patient has no clearly defined acute event (e.g. unexplained worsening chronic dyspnoea on exertion or onset of atrial fibrillation 3–4 days ago), a 2- to 3-day-old chest radiograph that is concordant with the scintigraphic findings may be sufficient.

The multiple sets of criteria have been proposed for the interpretation of ventilation–perfusion studies (Table 7.3) [12,13]. All of these criteria are useful summaries of some of the factors to consider when interpreting ventilation–perfusion studies. Perfusion defects are characterized by their size (in reference to the expected size of the pulmonary segments) as: small, <25% of a segment; moderate, 25–75% of a segment; and large, >75% of a segment. By following these criteria, a physician can arrive at a reasonable first approximation of the interpretation of the study. This first approximation should then be modified based on logic and other factors not adequately considered by these simplistic sets of interpretation crite-

Table 7.3 V/Q criteria for categorizing probability of pulmonary embolism [13]

Probability of pulmonary embolism	Sullivan (based on McNeil)	Biello	PIOPED	Revised PIOPED
Normal	No Q defects	No Q defects	No Q defects. Q outlines exactly the shape of the lungs on CXR	Same as PIOPED
Very low			≤3 small Q defects with normal CXR	
Low	Multiple V/Q matches. Single subsegmental V/Q mismatch	Small V/Q mismatches. V/Q matches without corresponding CXR changes. Q defect << CXR density	Non-segmental Q defect. 1 mod V/Q mismatch, with normal CXR. Q defect << CXR density. Large or mod V/Q matches, involving ≤4 segments in 1 lung and ≤3 segments in 1 lung region with normal CXR or findings << Q defects. >3 small Q defects with normal CXR	Non-segmental Q defect. Any Q defect << CXR abnormality. V/Q matches provided that there are clear CXR and some areas of normal perfusion in the lungs*. Any number of small Q defects with a normal CXR
Intermediate	Q defect with matched density on CXR. Mixed V/Q mismatches and matches. Single segment, lobe or lung V/Q mismatch. Multiple subsegmental V/Q mismatches	Severe diffuse OPD with Q defects. Single medium or large V/Q mismatch. Q defect same size as CXR change	Anything not falling into normal, very low, low, or high probability categories. Borderline high or borderline low. Difficult to categorize as low or high	1 mod to 2 large V/Q mismatches or the arithmetic equivalent in moderate or large and moderate defects†. Single V/Q match and normal CXR. Difficult to categorize as low or high, or not described as low or high
High	Multiple segmental or larger V/Q mismatches	≥2 medium or large V/Q mismatches. Q defect >> CXR density	≥2 large V/Q mismatches, with normal CXR or findings << Q defects. ≥2 mod V/Q mismatches and 1 large V/Q mismatch without CXR findings. ≥4 mod V/Q mismatches without CXR findings	≥2 large V/Q mismatches or the arithmetic equivalent in moderate or large and moderate defects†

*Very extensive defects can be categorized as low probability. Single V/Q matches are borderline for low probability and thus should be categorized as intermediate in most circumstances by most readers, although individual readers may correctly interpret individual scans with this pattern as showing low probability.
†Two large V/Q mismatches are borderline for high probability. Individual readers may correctly interpret individual scans with this pattern as showing high probability for PE. In general, it is recommended that more than this degree of mismatch be present for inclusion in the high probability category.
V, ventilation; Q, perfusion; CXR, chest radiograph; OPD, obstructive pulmonary disease; <<, substantially smaller than; >>, substantially larger than; non-segmental Q defect, very small effusion, cardiomegaly, enlarged aorta, hila or mediastinum, elevated diaphragm. Biello criteria: small =<25% of a segment; medium = 25–90% of a segment; large = >90% of a segment. PIOPED criteria: small = <25% of a segment; moderate = 25–75% of a segment; large = >75% of a segment.

ria. Additional factors that may influence the interpretation of ventilation–perfusion studies are listed in Table 7.4.

Published sets of interpretation criteria have several major shortcomings [14]. The most basic shortcoming is that these criteria have irrevocably confused the concepts of: (i) the results of the test; and (ii) the post-test probability of pulmonary embolism. According to Bayes' theorem, the post-test probability of pulmonary embolism cannot be calculated without combining the results of the ventilation–perfusion study with the pre-test probability of pulmonary embolism. The words most commonly recommended to express the results of ventilation–perfusion imaging ('Low/Intermediate/High Probability for Pulmonary Embolism') are frequently misinterpreted as the post-test probability [15,16]. This sloppy thinking can greatly affect practical decisions that physicians make about individual patient management. For example, respected authors make sweeping recommendations about patient management based solely on the results of ventilation–perfusion imaging without accounting for the patient's pre-test probability of disease. Such recommendations are nonsense, since (according to Bayes' theorem) the post-test probability of pulmonary embolism can easily be greater in a patient with a 'low' ventilation–perfusion study result and a high pre-test probability than it is in a patient with an 'intermediate' study result and a low pre-test probability. Reporting the results of ventilation–perfusion imaging as likelihood ratios rather than probabilities would help to eliminate this confusion [17].

An illogical discontinuity of published interpretation criteria is the interpretation of three small-sized ventilation–perfusion mismatches versus three moderate-sized mismatches. The recommended interpretation of the former is 'low probability for pulmonary embolism' and the latter

Table 7.4 Additional factors affecting the interpretation of ventilation–perfusion studies

- The presence of the 'stripe sign' (a non-pleural-based and presumably non-embolic perfusion defect)
- The chronicity of radiographic or scintigraphic findings
- Alternative diagnosis is more tenable
- Perfusion defects ill-defined
- Perfusion defects not randomly distributed according to anticipated relative pulmonary blood flow

is 'high probability for pulmonary embolism'. Unfortunately, reliably distinguishing between a small size perfusion defect and a moderate size perfusion defect is difficult. One observer may think that the perfusion defect is 24% of a segment (small defect) and another observer may consider it is 26% of a segment (moderate defect). There is no rational justification for such a large change in interpretation due to such a small change in the perceived size of the perfusion defects.

With most sets of published interpretation criteria, four categories of interpretation ('normal', 'low', 'intermediate' and 'high') are possible; however, in practice, 'low', 'intermediate' and 'high' are used much more frequently then is the 'normal' category. The dividing line between 'normal' and 'low' is difficult to define unambiguously; therefore, many medical centres reserve the use of 'normal' for unequivocally normal studies. Effectively, a three-category interpretation scheme is used. This represents an only minimal improvement over a binary (positive, negative) interpretation scheme. A much more realistic interpretation scheme would be one that allowed for a continuous spectrum of test results expressed as likelihood ratios. The average likelihood ratio for low (~0.1), intermediate (~1.0) and high results (~10) could be used as reference points on this continuous spectrum. Interpreters could estimate the likelihood ratio for a particular test result based on whether they perceived the result to be close to the average test result or greater than or less than the average test result. The estimated likelihood ratio could than be combined with the estimated pre-test probability in order to determine an estimate of the post-test probability.

Current interpretation schemes do not account for the severity of pulmonary embolus. No overt distinction is made between an interpretation of 'intermediate probability' of a single embolus or 'intermediate probability' of massive pulmonary embolism yet patient management must be based on a balance between the risks of anticoagulation, the risk of recurrent pulmonary embolism and the risk of pulmonary arteriography.

The clinical significance of small emboli has been the subject of increasing debate [18]. Another pressing problem is how the presence of pleural effusions, common in patients with congestive heart failure, should be incorporated into the interpretation. Some nuclear medicine experts believe that the results of ventilation–perfusion imaging must be placed in the intermediate category when a pleural effusion of any size is present [19]. Others believe that the results of ventilation–perfusion imaging can still be placed in the low category if the perfusion defect caused by the pleural effusion is small and there are not moderate to large defects in the radiographically more normal areas of the lung. This problem is unresolved.

The ventilation and perfusion abnormalities caused by chronic obstructive pulmonary disease (COPD) are very different than the abnormalities expected with pulmonary emboli (Figures 7.3 and 7.7). COPD usually causes large, ill-defined perfusion abnormalities that do not follow the segmental anatomy of the lung. Ventilation is also abnormal in these areas of abnormal perfusion. In the past, many experts believed it was not possible

confidently to exclude pulmonary embolism in patients with diffuse COPD. The results of the PIOPED study (see Gottschalk *et al.*, 1993a,b) have suggested that the presence of diffuse COPD may not be as great a problem as it was once thought to be.

Substances other than thrombi can cause pulmonary emboli. These substances include air, fat, tumour and amniotic fluid emboli, as well as particulates injected by drug addicts. Massive air emboli can mimic thromboemboli on pulmonary ventilation–perfusion studies. A possible distinguishing feature is that perfusion defects caused by air embolization may resolve more quickly than thrombotic emboli. Other microemboli such as fat, amniotic fluid or tumour usually cause a distinctive appearance on pulmonary perfusion imaging. Since the emboli are small, they are

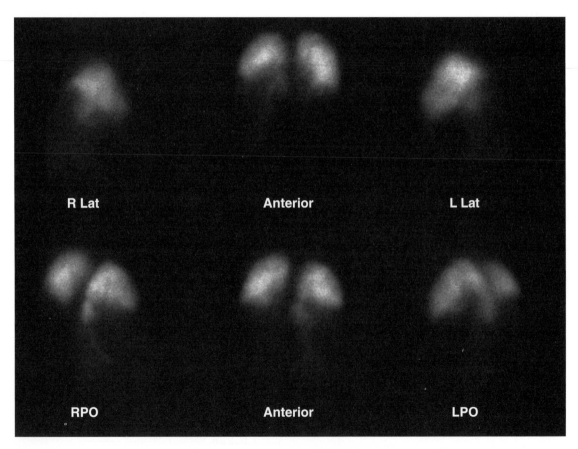

Figure 7.7 Abnormal perfusion due to α_1-antitrypsin deficiency. This perfusion study is from the same patient as the abnormal ventilation study in Figure 7.3. The ventilation and perfusion abnormalities are matched.

trapped in the distal vessels and especially affect perfusion to the surface of the pulmonary segments. Because of this, the pulmonary segments are prominent. This appearance has been referred to as segmentalization of the lung or the 'mulberry' pattern.

UTILITY ANALYSIS

Utility analysis is useful to better understand how the results of ventilation–perfusion imaging should be used to make decisions about patient management. With utility analysis, the best possible patient outcome has the highest possible utility. The highest possible utility is often arbitrarily set to a value of 100 and less desirable patient outcomes are given values between 0 and 100, where 0 is assigned to the worst possible outcome, death.

Assigning intermediate utilities to intermediate outcomes requires expert judgement that takes into consideration patient values. Despite the difficulties involved in assigning exact values for intermediate utilities, it is relatively easy to order common outcomes according to their approximate values. For example, for a patient being evaluated for pulmonary embolism who does not have pulmonary embolism (Table 7.5), the outcome with the highest utility is that the patient is not subjected to the morbidity associated with pulmonary arteriography and that the patient is not treated with anticoagulants. The next best outcome is that the patient would be subjected to a pulmonary arteriogram to prove that they did not have pulmonary embolism. The worst outcome would be that the patient would be subjected unnecessarily to the morbidity of anticoagulation.

Three outcomes are also possible in patients with pulmonary embolism. The best possible outcome would be to receive anticoagulation. The

utility of this outcome must be less than the utility of not having pulmonary embolism and being subjected unnecessarily to the morbidity of anticoagulation (the worst outcome above) since the patient will be subjected to the morbidity of treated pulmonary embolism in addition to the morbidity of anticoagulation. The next best outcome would be to treat for pulmonary embolism only after having had a diagnostic pulmonary arteriogram. The patient suffers the morbidity of anticoagulation, treated pulmonary embolism and pulmonary arteriography. The worst outcome is for a patient with pulmonary embolism to receive no treatment.

Once the value of these six utilities has been estimated, it can be shown mathematically that the expected utility (Figure 7.8(a)) for any prevalence of pulmonary embolism is equal to the lines connecting the utilities for zero prevalence (no pulmonary embolism) and 100% prevalence (pulmonary embolism). The oft-cited recommendation that pulmonary arteriography be obtained in patients with an intermediate probability result on ventilation–perfusion imaging studies is based on the fact that (according to Figure 7.8(a)) the highest expected utility is gained by performing pulmonary arteriography in patients with post-test probabilities for pulmonary embolism between 20% and 80%. However, the reality is that only a small proportion of patients who have intermediate probability results on ventilation–perfusion imaging studies are referred for pulmonary arteriography. How can we explain the discordance between what is done clinically and what is predicted by the utility analysis that has been presented? Are patients being denied optimal diagnosis and treatment?

So far, the utility analysis has ignored two important factors. First, there is the confusion between the results of ventilation–perfusion imaging

Table 7.5 Expected utilities

Patients without pulmonary embolism		*Patients with pulmonary embolism*	
Outcome	*Expected utility*	*Outcome*	*Expected utility*
No treatment	100	Anticoagulation	70
Pulmonary arteriography and no anticoagulation	95	Pulmonary arteriography and anticoagulation	65
Anticoagulation	80	No treatment	50

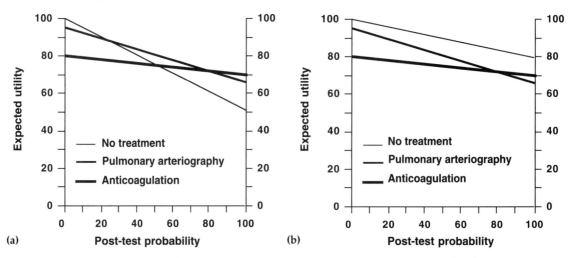

Figure 7.8 Expected utility. (a) The values for the expected utilities from Table 7.5 for the three main patient management options have been plotted on the left *y*-axis for patients with no pulmonary embolism and on the right *y*-axis for patients with pulmonary embolism. It can be shown mathematically that the expected utility for any prevalence of pulmonary embolism is equal to the lines connecting the utilities for zero prevalence (no pulmonary embolism) and 100% prevalence (pulmonary embolism). With these conventional expected utilities, pulmonary arteriography has the highest expected utility when the post-test probability is >20% and <80%. (b) If the morbidity of untreated pulmonary embolism is less than the morbidity of treated pulmonary embolism (due to the significant morbidity of anticoagulation) then the expected utility is greatest with no treatment for any prevalence of pulmonary embolism. Although the morbidity of untreated pulmonary embolism is conventionally regarded as high, there are very few data concerning the natural history of untreated pulmonary embolism. Some have suggested that not all small pulmonary emboli have to be treated [18]. One of the most valuable, but as yet rarely appreciated, roles of ventilation–perfusion imaging is in risk stratification.

and post-test probability. The *x*-axis in Figure 7.8 refers to the post-test probability, not to the results of ventilation–perfusion imaging. The likelihood ratio of the average intermediate result is close to 1.0. Mathematically, this means that the average intermediate ventilation–perfusion imaging result does not change the pre-test probability of pulmonary embolism. If the pre-test probability was low, the post-test probability would also be low. Likewise, the post-test probability will be high when the pre-test probability is high.

A second, equally important factor is that the utilities used in the utility analysis are based on average values and traditional views regarding the morbidity of untreated pulmonary embolism, the morbidity of anticoagulation, and the improvement of morbidity for treated pulmonary embolism. Under some circumstances, it is possible that the morbidity of untreated pulmonary embolism may be small [20]. For example, if a patient has no evidence for deep venous thrombosis of the lower extremities by non-invasive test-

ing, was not at high risk for pelvic vein thrombosis, was rapidly recovering from an acute illness, and had only a few perfusion abnormalities that resulted in the intermediate likelihood ratio results of the ventilation–perfusion imaging study, then the morbidity of untreated may be lower then the morbidity from anticoagulation. Under these circumstances [utility of untreated pulmonary embolus is 80, not 50] (Figure 7.8(b)), no treatment or pulmonary arteriography would be indicated.

One of the unheralded but important roles of ventilation–perfusion imaging may be in risk stratification. The natural history of untreated pulmonary embolism has not been studied. The only prospective randomized controlled study of anticoagulation in the treatment of pulmonary embolism was published in 1960 [21]. The diagnosis of pulmonary embolism was based on the clinical findings and the control patients were treated with prolonged bed rest (presumably to prevent embolization of a deep venous thrombus). No ventilation–perfusion imaging studies or pulmonary arteriograms were performed. The study was halted after excess mortality and morbidity in the untreated patients reached statistical significance. Presumably, these patients with clinically diagnosed pulmonary embolism had extensive pulmonary emboli and they are not representative of the much larger number of patients in whom the clinical diagnosis of pulmonary embolism can not be made without sophisticated diagnostic testing. However, since this study, treatment of arteriographically demonstrable pulmonary embolism has been generally regarded as essential.

The combination of non-invasive testing of the lower extremities and ventilation–perfusion imaging may be a powerful predictor of prognosis. Lower-extremity testing provides a measure of the potential for additional emboli, whereas ventilation–perfusion imaging depicts the balance between current pulmonary clot burden and the body's endogenous thrombolytic mechanisms. Support for the prognostic value of ventilation–perfusion imaging comes from several papers that report good outcomes in patients who had low probability results who were not treated for pulmonary embolism.

Comparing the results of ventilation–perfusion scintigraphy with those of pulmonary angiography addresses the wrong question. This analysis simply compares the results of Test 1 (ventilation–perfusion scintigraphy) with Test 2 (pulmonary angiography). The important clinical question is, 'Which patients with venous thromboembolism benefit from anticoagulation?' Although posing this question may seem heretical to some, no study has been performed to show that patients with 'small' emboli and no evidence for deep venous thrombosis (negative serial impedance plethysmograms or Doppler studies) benefit from anticoagulation. Studies performed at this and other medical centres have shown that patients with low-probability ventilation–perfusion studies who are not treated with anticoagulants nor have underlying cardiac and pulmonary disease have a very low incidence of subsequent events due to suspected or documented thromboembolism [22–24].

REFERENCES

1. Osler, R.F., Zuckerman, D.A., Gutierrez, F.R. and Brink, J.A. (1996) Anatomic distribution of pulmonary emboli at pulmonary angiography: implications for cross-sectional imaging. *Radiology*, **199**, 31–5.
2. Stein, P.D., Terrin, M.L., Hales, C.A. *et al.* (1991) Clinical, laboratory, roentgenographic, and electrocardiographic findings in patients with acute pulmonary embolism and no pre-existing cardiac or pulmonary disease. *Chest*, **100**(3), 604–6.
3. Fennerty, A.G., Shetty, H.G., Paton, D., Roberts, G., Routledge, P.A. and Campbell, I.A. (1990) Clinical presentation and investigation of patients proceeding to isotope lung scanning for suspected pulmonary embolism. *Postgrad. Med. J.*, **66**(774), 285–9.
4. Worsley, D.F., Alavi, A., Aronchick, J.M., Chen, J.T., Greenspan, R.H. and Ravin, C.E. (1993) Chest radiographic findings in patients with acute pulmonary embolism: observations from the PIOPED study. *Radiology*, **189**(1), 133–6.
5. Worsley, D.F., Alavi, A., Palevsky, H.I. and Kundel, H.L. (1996) Comparison of diagnostic performance with ventilation–perfusion lung imaging in different patient populations. *Radiology*, **199**(2), 481–3.
6. Stein, P.D., Coleman, R.E., Gottschalk, A., Saltzman, H.A., Terrin, M.L. and Weg, J.G. (1991) Diagnostic utility of ventilation/perfusion lung scans in acute pulmonary embolism is not diminished by pre-existing cardiac or pulmonary disease. *Chest*, **100**(3), 604–6.
7. Kohn, H., Mostbeck, A., Bachmayr, S. *et al.* (1993) 99m-Tc-DTPA aerosol for same-day post-perfusion ventilation imaging: results of a multicentre study. *Eur. J. Nucl. Med.*, **20**, 4–9.
8. Monaghan, P., Provan, I., Murray, C. *et al.* (1991) An improved radionuclide technique for the detection of altered permeability. *J. Nucl. Med.*, **32**, 1945–9.
9. Mackey, D.W.J., Jackson, P., Baker, R.J. *et al.* (1997) Physical properties and use of pertechnegas as a ventilation agent. *J. Nucl. Med.*, **38**, 163–7.
10. James, J.M., Herman, K.J., Lloyd, J.J. *et al.* (1991) Evaluation of 99m-Tc Technegas ventilation scintigraphy in the diagnosis of pulmonary embolism. *Br. J. Radiol.*, **64**(764), 711–19.
11. Cook, G. and Clarke, S.E.M. (1992) An evaluation of technegas as a ventilation agent compared with krypton-81m in the scintigraphic diagnosis of pulmonary embolism. *Eur. J. Nucl. Med.*, **19**, 770–4.
12. Sostman, H.D., Coleman, R.E., DeLong, D.M., Newman, G.E. and Paine, S. (1994) Evaluation of revised criteria for ventilation–perfusion scintigraphy in patients with suspected pulmonary embolism. *Radiology*, **193**(1), 103–7.
13. Kwok, C.G., Skibo, L.K. and Segall, G.M. (1996) Low probability lung scan in a patient at high risk for pulmonary embolism. *J. Nucl. Med.*, **37**, 165–70.
14. Gray, H.W. (1993) Reporting of lung scans: the future beckons. [editorial]. *Nucl. Med. Commun.*, **14**, 1–3.
15. Gray, H.W., Mckillop, J.H. and Bessent, R.G. (1993) Lung scan reports: interpretation by clinicians. *Nucl. Med. Commun.*, **14**, 989–94.
16. Gray, H.W., Mckillop, J.H. and Bessent, R.G. (1993) Lung scan reporting language: what does it mean? *Nucl. Med. Commun.*, **14**, 1084–7.

17. Jaeschke, R., Guyatt, G.H. and Sackett, D.L. (1994) Users' guides to the medical literature. III. How to use an article about a diagnostic test. B. What are the results and will they help me in caring for my patients? The Evidence-Based Medicine Working Group. *JAMA*, **271**(9), 703–7.

18. Kelley, M.A., Carson, J.L., Palevsky, H.I. and Schwartz, J.S. (1991) Diagnosing pulmonary embolism: new facts and strategies. *Ann. Intern. Med.*, **114**(4), 300–6.

19. Goldberg, S.N., Richardson, D.D., Palmer, E.L. and Scott, J.A. (1996) Pleural effusion and ventilation/perfusion scan interpretation for acute pulmonary embolus. *J. Nucl. Med.*, **37**(8), 1310–13.

20. Stein, P.D., Henry, J.W. and Relyea, B. (1995) Untreated patients with pulmonary embolism. Outcome, clinical, and laboratory assessment. *Chest*, **107**(4), 931–5.

21. Barritt, D.W. and Jordan, S.C. (1960) Anticoagulant drugs in the treatment of pulmonary embolism. A controlled trial. *Lancet*, **i**, 1309–12.

22. Bellomo, R., Low, R., Pianko, S. *et al.* (1994) The 1-month outcome of patients with a low probability technegas ventilation/perfusion lung scan. *Nucl. Med. Commun.*, **15**, 505–10.

23. Lee, M.E., Biello, D.R., Kumar, B. and Siegel, B.A. (1985) 'Low-probability' ventilation perfusion scintigrams: clinical outcomes in 99 patients. *Radiology*, **156**, 497–500.

24. Kahn, D., Bushnell, D.L., Dean, R. and Perlman, S.B. (1989) Clinical outcome of patients with a 'low probability' of pulmonary embolism on ventilation–perfusion lung scan. *Arch. Intern. Med.*, **149**(2), 377–9.

FURTHER READING

Carson, J.L., Kelley, M.A., Duff, A. *et al.* (1992) The clinical course of pulmonary embolism. *N. Engl. J. Med.*, **326**, 1240–5.

Freitas, J.E., Sarosi, M.G., Nagle, C.C., Yeomans, M.E., Freitas, A.E. and Juni, J.E. (1995) Modified PIOPED criteria used in clinical practice. *J. Nucl. Med.*, **36**(9), 1573–8.

Gottschalk, A., Juni, J.E., Sostman, H.D. *et al.* (1993a) Ventilation-perfusion scintigraphy in the PIOPED study. Part I. Data collection and tabulation. *J. Nucl. Med.*, **34**(7), 1109–18.

Gottschalk, A., Sostman, H.D., Coleman, R.E. *et al.* (1993b) Ventilation-perfusion scintigraphy in the PIOPED study. Part II. Evaluation of the scintigraphic criteria and interpretations. *J. Nucl. Med.*, **34**(7), 1119–26.

Gottschalk, A., Stein, P.D., Henry, J.W. and Relyea, B. (1996) Can pulmonary angiography be limited to the most suspicious side if the contralateral side appears normal on the ventilation/perfusion lung scan? Data from PIOPED. Prospective Investigation of Pulmonary Embolism Diagnosis. *Chest*, **110**(2), 392–4.

Gottschalk, A., Stein, P.D. and Henry, J.W. (1996) Patient stratification by cardiopulmonary status in the diagnosis of pulmonary embolism. *J. Nucl. Med.*, **37**(4), 570–2.

Henry, J.W., Stein, P.D., Gottschalk, A. and Raskob, G.E. (1996) Pulmonary embolism among patients with a nearly normal ventilation/perfusion lung scan. *Chest*, **110**(2), 395–8.

Lung cancer

H. D. Royal

Conventional ventilation–perfusion imaging occasionally is useful in the evaluation of patients with lung tumours. In addition, other single photon emitting radiopharmaceuticals have been recently introduced to better determine the extent of disease at the time of diagnosis and at various times during subsequent follow-up. Oncological applications of FDG-PET imaging are increasing in number. Data supporting the cost-effectiveness of FDG-PET imaging in differentiating benign from malignant pulmonary neoplasms and in determining the extent of disease at the time of initial diagnosis are accumulating.

ROLE OF CONVENTIONAL VENTILATION–PERFUSION IMAGING

Occasionally, when ventilation–perfusion imaging is performed in a patient suspected of pulmonary embolism, a dominant ventilation–perfusion match is found suggesting an endobronchial obstruction as the potential cause for the patient's pulmonary symptoms (Figure 7.9). Recognition of this distinctive appearance is important because the diagnostic approach and treatment of a patient with an endobronchial obstruction is very different than the diagnostic approach and treatment of a patient with pulmonary embolism. Endobronchial obstruction may be caused by a mucus plug or by a malignant lung tumour. In these patients, bronchoscopy or chest computed tomography is often a more appropriate next step than is pulmonary arteriography. In addition, treatment to improve the clearance of secretions from the airway are more appropriate than anticoagulants if the cause of the patient's hypoxia is due to mucous plugging of the airways. Rarely a hilar cancer or lymph node will obstruct a pulmonary artery and leave the airway intact. This possibility should be considered, in addition to the diagnosis of pulmonary embolism, whenever there is a large dominant ventilation–perfusion mismatch.

PRE-TREATMENT EVALUATION OF PULMONARY FUNCTION

Quantitative ventilation–perfusion imaging is occasionally ordered in patients with known lung tumours before surgery and, less frequently, before radiation therapy in order to predict their post-treatment pulmonary function. The predicted post-treatment function is calculated by multiplying the pre-treatment FEV_1 times the percentage of lung function that is expected to remain post-treatment. For example, if the pre-operative FEV_1 were 1500 ml/min and if the right lung received 55% of total pulmonary blood flow, the predicted post-operative pulmonary function following a left pneumonectomy would be 825 ml/min (0.55×1500).

Not all lung cancer patients need to have quantitative pre-treatment pulmonary imaging. The patients with borderline pre-treatment pulmonary function ($FEV_1 < 1.5$–2.0 l/min) will benefit most from a quantitative evaluation. As a rule of thumb, patients whose predicted post-treatment FEV_1 exceeds 700 ml/min are less likely to be respirator-dependent following therapy.

QUANTITATIVE VENTILATION–PERFUSION IMAGING

Quantitative pulmonary perfusion imaging is readily performed in most nuclear medicine facilities. The special requirement is that the study must be acquired digitally. Typically, the size of the acquisition matrix will be 128×128 8-bit pixels or 256×256 8-bit pixels. Once the study is acquired, regions-of-interest are drawn over both lungs (some facilities also draw background regions of interest). The percent of the injected activity in each lung is determined by dividing the (background-corrected) counts in each lung by the (background-corrected) counts in both lungs. This fraction is multiplied by 100 to express the results as a percentage (Figure 7.10).

Ideally, the counts from both an anterior and a posterior view are used. On the anterior view, the contribution of the left lung tends to be underestimated due to attenuation of some of the left lung counts by the heart. On the posterior view, the

Clinical Nuclear Medicine, 3rd edn. Edited by M.N. Maisey, K.E. Britton and B.D. Collier. Published in 1998 by Chapman & Hall, London. ISBN 0 412 75180 1

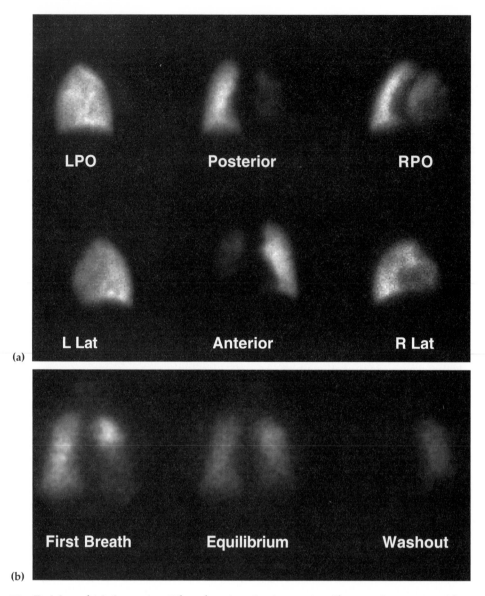

LPO   Posterior   RPO

L Lat   Anterior   R Lat

(a)

First Breath   Equilibrium   Washout

(b)

Figure 7.9   Endobronchial obstruction. When there is a dominant area of hypoperfusion (a) and hypoventilation (b) involving an entire lobe or lung, an endobronchial obstruction due to benign or malignant causes should be considered.

contribution of the left lung tends to be overestimated because the loss of lung due to displacement by the heart is not fully appreciated. Some advocates maintain that it is important to take the geometric mean (square root of anterior counts × posterior counts) of the counts; however, results obtained by using the arithmetic mean are very similar. Significant errors in the estimates of re-gional perfusion may occur following a ^{99m}Tc aerosol study.

Some proponents recommend dividing each lung region into thirds (upper, middle, lower) and calculating the percentage of blood flow to each third of the lung. The rationale for this recommendation is to estimate the effects of a partial pneumonectomy. Unfortunately, the lobar

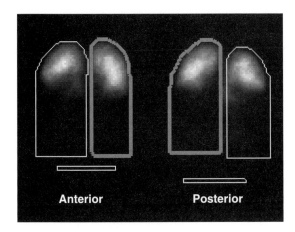

Figure 7.10 Quantitative pulmonary perfusion

	Right	Left
Anterior	49%	51%
Posterior	48%	52%
Geometric mean	49%	51%

To calculate relative pulmonary perfusion, regions-of-interest are drawn around each lung. In this example, background regions-of-interest were also drawn. This patient has α_1-antitrypsin deficiency (also see Figures 7.3 and 7.7).

anatomy of the lung is not consistent with these three arbitrary regions of interest.

Quantification of relative pulmonary ventilation is done less often, is more complex and less reliable. Several radiopharmaceuticals are available for pulmonary ventilation studies; however, some are less suitable for quantitative studies. Aerosol ventilation agents are the least satisfactory. Patients in whom quantitative pulmonary scintigraphy is indicated are likely to have underlying lung disease which will cause deposition of the aerosol in the central airways. Therefore, the counts in lung regions-of-interest will not be related simply to relative ventilation. Use of aerosols for quantifying relative pulmonary ventilation is therefore not recommended.

The simplest ventilation agent to use to quantifying relative pulmonary ventilation is ^{81m}Kr. Because of its short half-life (13 seconds), an equilibrium image of a patient rebreathing ^{81m}Kr approximates regional rates of ventilation. ^{81m}Kr decays before it is able to reach the poorly ventilated areas of the lung. Regional ventilation can be estimated by using the same approach, as was described earlier for estimating regional pulmo-

nary perfusion. The disadvantage of using ^{81m}Kr is that its short half-life requires the use of a generator system. The mother radionuclide is rubidium-81, the half-life of which is only 4.7 hours; therefore, a new generator system must be acquired daily. The requirement to purchase a new generator daily makes the use of ^{81m}Kr inconvenient and expensive.

^{133}Xe has been used most widely for measurement of regional pulmonary ventilation, though its use introduces some new problems as ventilation imaging with this agent is a dynamic process. Measurements of regional rates of ventilation are best done using the 'height over area' method, though unfortunately, this approach requires special analysis software that is not widely available. An alternative, less accurate but more practical approach is to modify slightly the routine xenon ventilation study to consist of an initial 40-second period of tidal breathing instead of an initial breath-holding image taken at end-inspiratory capacity. The quantitative analysis of the 40-second initial tidal breathing images would be similar to the analysis that was described above for measuring regional pulmonary perfusion.

TUMOUR IMAGING

Several fundamentally different approaches to lung tumour imaging have been or are being explored. These include the use of ^{67}Ga, or more recently ^{201}Tl, to detect and determine the stage of lung tumours. ^{67}Ga has been used to determine the response to treatment in patients with lymphoma. In particular, it has been used in patients who presented initially with bulky mediastinal disease to distinguish between residual scar tissue and persistent disease [1]. Care must be taken to not mistake thymic rebound with recurrent mediastinal disease, especially in children and young adults.

Several monoclonal antibodies against lung tumours are being developed for diagnosis and therapy, though as yet, the role of these needs to be defined [2]. Since radionuclide techniques are conducive to whole-body examinations, these antibodies will hopefully result in the earlier detection of metastatic disease. Ultimately, treatment with monoclonal antibodies may be possible.

Somatostatin receptors are present in many lung cancers, especially small-cell carcinomas. Between 50 and 75% of small-cell lung cancer (SCLC) tumours have specific high-affinity binding sites for somatostatin. In one study, 88% of primary tumours but only 66% of metastatic deposits were seen in patients with small-cell carcinomas [3]. Metastatic disease in and adjacent to the liver, spleen and kidneys was most difficult to detect due to the fact that the radiopharmaceutical normally accumulates in these organs.

Imaging lung cancers with [57]Co-bleomycin has been used in Europe and Israel to predict response to treatment [4] as well as in the staging and diagnosis of lung cancers. Although a negative study does not exclude mediastinal/hilar involvement, a positive study almost certainly indicates such involvement; hence, mediastinoscopy can be avoided in most patients in whom a bleomycin study indicates mediastinal/hilar involvement. These promising results must be replicated by

others and be shown to be cost-effective before bleomycin imaging is accepted as a clinical test.

The final approach to imaging lung tumours is to study their glucose metabolism [5,6] (Figure 7.11). Three distinct patient populations have been studied. The first is patients with a solitary pulmonary nodule. The clinical question in this population is whether the nodule is benign or malignant. If the results of FDG-PET imaging were definitive in some patients, unnecessary biopsies could be avoided. The second population is patients with biopsy-proven cancer who are being staged to see if they are candidates for curative lung resection. More accurate staging would help to avoid fruitless surgery. The third population is patients with treated lung cancers where the question is whether a persistent residual mass represents scarring or recurrent disease. The oncological ap-

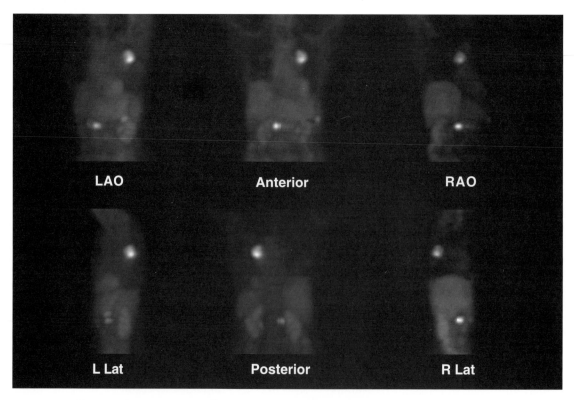

Figure 7.11   ^{18}F-FDG-PET study. These ^{18}F-FDG-PET images were obtained from a 70-year-old woman with a solitary pulmonary nodule that was thought to be due to a primary lung tumour. Focal uptake in the pancreas indicated that the lung tumour was not resectable and that the primary was pancreatic cancer. Prior work-up including CT was negative except for the lung mass. In this patient, futile lung surgery was avoided because of the results of the PET study.

plications for PET hold great promise for the future.

REFERENCES

1. Weiner, M., Leventhal, B., Cantor, A. *et al.* (11991) Gallium-67 scans as an adjunct to computed tomography scans for the assessment of residual mediastinal mass in pediatric patients with Hodgkin's disease. A pediatric oncology group study. *Cancer*, **68**, 2478–80.
2. Breitz, H.B., Sullivan, K. and Nelp, W.B. (1993) Imaging lung cancer with radiolabeled antibodies. *Semin. Nucl. Med.*, **23**, 127–32.
3. Kirsch, C.M., von Pawel, J., Grau, I. and Tatsch, K. (1994) Indium-11 pentreotide in the diagnostic work-up of patients with bronchogenic carcinoma. *Eur. J. Nucl. Med.*, **21**, 1318–25.
4. Even-Sapir, E., Bettman, L., Iosilevsky, G. *et al.* (1994) SPECT quantitation of cobalt-57-bleomycin to predict treatment response and outcome of patients with lung cancer. *J. Nucl. Med.*, **35**, 1129–33.
5. Gambhir, S.S., Hoh, C.K., Phelps, M.E., Maddar, I. and Maddahi, J. (1996) Decision tree sensitivity analysis for cost-effectiveness of FDG-PET in the staging of non-small-cell lung carcinoma. *J. Nucl. Med.*, **37**, 1228–36.
6. Lewis, P., Griffin, S., Marsden, P. *et al.* (1994) Whole-body ^{18}F-fluorodeoxyglucose positron emission tomography in preoperative evaluation of lung cancer. *Lancet*, **344**, 1265–6.

Other pulmonary applications

M. J. O'Doherty

INTRODUCTION

Airway diseases are a major cause of morbidity and mortality in the UK, accounting for a large number of visits of patients to the primary care physicians. The variety of diseases include pulmonary inflammation and infection, as well as lung cancer, the most common cancer in men. The lung presents a huge exposed surface to the air allowing the entrance of a variety of particulate matter onto the epithelial surfaces. These particulate substances encompass a range of pathogens (e.g. bacteria, viruses, fungi, etc.) as well as particulate matter, which may promote an antigenic response (e.g. pollens, house dust, mite, etc.), particles that are potentially carcinogenic as in cigarette smoke, or fibres such as asbestos producing other responses in the pleura.

The huge exposed surface is of course important for gas exchange, but is also potentially available for the absorption of drugs across the epithelial-endothelial interface. The delivery of drugs to the lung to treat respiratory disease has been established using a variety of particle generators. The lung represents a body organ that may be studied with a variety of radionuclide techniques; areas of possible interest are outlined in Table 7.6. The major use of pulmonary nuclear medicine is in the investigation of ventilation/perfusion inequality, particularly with reference to pulmonary emboli. However, there are a variety of other areas requiring the use of radionuclide techniques to explore pulmonary pathophysiology.

INFLAMMATION AND INFECTION

The initiation of an inflammatory response is linked to changes in the vascular supply to the affected part of the lung. Such changes include hyperaemia and increased vascular permeability, leading to swelling of local tissues due to interstitial oedema. Damage to the endothelium and epithelial surface of the lung leads to leakage of fluid, proteins and cells into the airspaces. The primary response may be to damage the epithelium, resulting in cell death and damage to the vascular endothelium. These inflammatory responses may be excessive, leading to alveolar flooding or consolidation, and affecting the aeration of the distal bronchioles and alveoli due to constriction of smooth muscle in the airways, and also by collapse and mucus plugging of airways. Airway diseases will affect the air supply to these regions, and the concomitant vasoconstriction will compromise the blood supply. Conversely, inflammation within the vascular supply due to arteritis may affect ventilation to a lesser extent. These abnormalities can be detected using conventional ventilation/perfusion imaging.

Severe widespread damage to the lung resulting in the syndrome of adult respiratory distress can be caused by a variety of disease processes. This condition results in the need to ventilate the patient, with few other therapeutic options available at the current time. A greater understanding of the physiology, and a marker for its severity – other than blood gases – would be potentially helpful in the assessment of new treatments. A number of nuclear medicine techniques, including lung epithelial transfer/permeability and endothelial permeability measurements, have been used to assess damage.

Inflammation and infection in the lung are most commonly assessed using gallium-67 imaging, but other agents including somatostatin, J001, labelled antibodies and labelled leucocytes, are also used. ^{67}Ga has been used in the assessment of granulomatous disease for many years; its role has been extended by the advent of HIV infection and by its application in a variety of other diseases that affect the thorax, and this will be discussed.

Finally, the use of aerosols in the lung, both as therapeutic and investigative agents, deserves a mention. A variety of devices have been used to deliver aerosols to patients' lungs, for pulmonary scanning and for medication in the form of bronchodilators, steroids, antibiotics, surfactants, etc. The use of radiolabels provides a rapid means of assessing the pulmonary delivery of drugs and allows comparison of patient response to the amount of drug delivered [1].

Clinical Nuclear Medicine, 3rd edn. Edited by M.N. Maisey, K.E. Britton and B.D. Collier. Published in 1998 by Chapman & Hall, London. ISBN 0 412 75180 1

Table 7.6   Radionuclides and imaging the lung

Single photon imaging	Positron emission imaging
Mucociliary clearance	Regional vascular volume
Aerosol deposition of drugs	Regional lung density
Lung permeability/transfer	Regional metabolism
Ventilation/perfusion imaging – pulmonary emboli	Receptor imaging
Preoperative lung cancer assessment	Ventilation/perfusion imaging
Congenital vascular/ventilation anomalies	Vascular/endothelial permeability
Vascular/endothelial permeability	Inflammation and infection
Inflammation and infection	Tumour imaging
Tumour imaging	

LUNG PERMEABILITY MEASUREMENTS

An assessment of the integrity of the alveolar capillary interface has been performed using molecules delivered to the alveolar airspace to examine the epithelial integrity, and to the capillary bed to examine the endothelial permeability. Radiopharmaceuticals of various shapes, sizes and charge, have been used for the assessment of permeability, ^{99m}Tc-DTPA (diethylenetriaminepentaacetic acid) being the most common. The procedure for measuring ^{99m}Tc-DTPA transfer is simple, and the measure indicates the integrity of the alveolar–capillary interface [2]. The alveolar–capillary interface represents a large surface exposed to air, through which gas exchange occurs, but this barrier also allows soluble compounds to cross. The rate at which these molecules can cross the barrier is dependent on several factors, including membrane pore radii size, membrane charge, presence or absence of surfactant, the molecular gradient, etc. The transfer of molecules of different size and charge is used for elucidating disease processes.

Measurements made with the radionuclide techniques are not direct estimates of permeability, since this would require a knowledge of the rate of flux of a molecule along a known concentration gradient across a known surface area. Therefore, all that these methods measure is the flux of the radionuclide, that is at best, an indirect measure of permeability.

Initial studies by Taplin and colleagues [3] showed that ^{99m}Tc-pertechnetate clearance from the lung was very rapid, both in normal and abnormal subjects, whereas the higher molecular weight ^{99m}Tc-DTPA cleared more slowly; this has subsequently been confirmed by using molecules of even greater size. Other alterations to clearance have been found by changing the lipophilicity and the charge of the compound by using charged or neutral dextrans and using exametazamine, antipyrine, etc. Alterations in permeability have been found in a variety of conditions including smoking [4], collagen diseases, and fibrosing alveolitis. Permeability may also be altered by the use of various drugs (both chemotherapeutic and recreational), and by administration of carbon monoxide and histamine. There are a variety of physiological factors that affect permeability, including exercise and the lung region (upper regions are more permeable than lower). The permeability measures are normally associated with a monoexponential clearance; however, biexponential clearance has been observed with respiratory distress syndrome and with alveolitis associated with *Pneumocystis carinii* pneumonia. Barrowcliffe and Jones [5] demonstrated fast clearance values with multi-exponential clearance in several patients; this phenomenon has been observed by other groups in severe lung injury [5–8]. Non-cardiogenic pulmonary oedema appears to result in accelerated clearance of ^{99m}Tc-DTPA as compared with cardiogenic pulmonary oedema [5,9].

METHOD OF MEASUREMENT OF DTPA TRANSFER

Lung ^{99m}Tc-DTPA transfer (permeability, clearance) relies on the inhalation of an aerosol of ^{99m}Tc-DTPA (particle size of approximately 1 µm or less) for as short a period as possible, usually less than 1 minute. The patient is often positioned supine or semi-recumbent for this inhalation, and is then scanned in that posture, since there is less likelihood of movement. The camera head is situated posteriorly, or occasionally anteriorly, and data can be acquired using a gamma-camera equipped with a high-sensitivity collimator and linked to an on-line computer. Dynamic acquisition of 30-second or 1-minute duration frames are obtained over a period of 20–60 minutes. The acquisition protocol varies from centre to centre. If background activity correction is used, then an intravenous injection of ^{99m}Tc-DTPA is given to allow the background region activity to be related to the lung regions. From the resultant time-activity curves, the half-time or clearance rate can be derived (with or without background correction).

A discussion on the need for background correction is beyond the scope of this chapter; however, the need for background subtraction will increase with the faster transit rates in the more diseased lungs [6,10–16]. The permeability is measured in terms of either a half-time (T) of transfer (expressed in minutes) or a clearance rate, k, (expressed as % per minute reduction in initial activity). The two values are easily related by the formula: $T_{1/2} = 0.693/k$.

ADULT RESPIRATORY DISTRESS SYNDROME

The American Thoracic Society and the European Society of Intensive Care Medicine define acute lung injury as 'a syndrome of inflammation and increasing permeability that is associated with a constellation of clinical, radiological and pathophysiological abnormalities that cannot be explained by, but may coexist with, left atrial or pulmonary capillary hypertension', and the adult respiratory distress syndrome (ARDS) as 'a more severe form of acute lung injury'. The link is therefore between structural change and pathophysiological changes resulting in the clinical syndrome. The ARDS has been evaluated with lung permeability measurements, both of the vascular endothelium and the epithelial surfaces. These techniques reflect the structural damage that can be done to the lung membranes. The movement of proteins from the vascular space into the interstitium and airspace through the endothelium and the epithelium is the most appropriate measurement to make. The measurements have included epithelial permeability measurements using ^{99m}Tc-DTPA, as well as in-

haled charged dextrans or intravenously administered tracers including [113m]In-transferrin, ^{68}Ga-transferrin, ^{18}F and ^{99m}Tc-labelled dextrans. Most assessments in ARDS would be performed using intravenously administered tracers; however, lung ^{99m}Tc-DTPA transfer has been shown to have a fast transfer-rate [9]. The amount of damage to the endothelium has also been shown to be severe using [113m]In-transferrin accumulation within the lung [17]. Braude *et al.* [18] demonstrated a correlation between ^{99m}Tc-DTPA transfer and the [113m]In-transferrin measurement in patients with ARDS. The degree of structural damage has been assessed using PET techniques in humans [19,20] and dogs [21,22] by measuring the changes in blood flow using ^{15}O-H_2O, protein flux using ^{68}Ga-transferrin, and blood volume using ^{15}O-CO measurements. The measurements made include the transcapillary escape rate and the normalized slope index, which are mathematically equivalent. One may question the clinical role of these measurements, since the damage to the lung can be assessed by blood gas measurements, right heart pressure measurements and the chest X-ray evaluation. However, bed-side permeability measurements can be used to define the severity of the disease and linked to the degree of lung injury. These measurements can then be used to monitor therapy, to help understand how the disease process progresses, and to provide requisite information for developing various therapeutic strategies.

GRANULOMATOUS DISEASES OF THE LUNG

There are a number of hypotheses as to the formation of granulomas within the lung – varying between the sensitization of lymphocytes by antigens producing lymphokines that attract monocytes and inhibit macrophages, to theories that propose agents that activate macrophages which then secrete factors that attract monocytes. Whatever the aetiology, there are a variety of granulomatous diseases affecting the lung that may be infective in origin (e.g. mycobacterial infection), possibly immune complex (e.g. Wegener's granulomatosis, Churg–Strauss syndrome), foreign body-induced (e.g. talc granulomatosis) or undetermined cause (e.g. sarcoidosis) [23]. [67]Ga scanning has been demonstrated to have increased uptake in these conditions. The primary role of scanning is to define the disease activity as well as the extent of the disease. The most investigated disease is sarcoidosis.

SARCOID

Sarcoidosis is a multisystem inflammatory granulomatous disease with an incidence varying between 2 to 18 per 100 000 of the world population. The disease predominantly affects the pulmonary system, but almost any organ can be affected. The conventional classification of the disease using the chest X-ray (CXR) is: stage 0, normal CXR; stage I, bilateral hilar lymphadenopathy; stage II, bilateral hilar lymphadenopathy and lung changes; and stage III, lung changes alone. However, the CXR is highly insensitive, and up to 60% of patients with granulomas in the parenchyma may have a normal CXR. With a predominant hilar and mediastinal adenopathy, the differential diagnosis is essentially between lymphoma and sarcoidosis – unless the patient has underlying malignancy or immunosuppression. The differential diagnosis is weighted towards sarcoid if the patient is black or of Irish descent. Computed tomography (CT) and high-resolution CT show abnormalities not present on CXR, with reports that a first-choice diagnosis of sarcoid was provided with 57% of radiographic findings and 76% of CT scan readings. CT was superior to MRI in the assessment of parenchymal disease; although the correlation be-

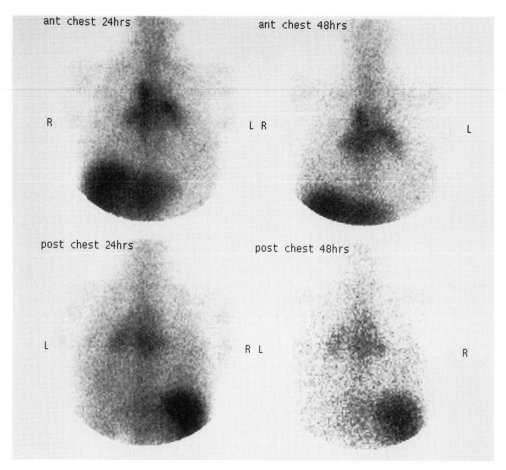

Figure 7.12 ^{67}Ga scan in a patient with sarcoidosis, demonstrating increased gallium accumulation in the hilar lymph nodes and the mediastinal lymph nodes at 24 and 48 hours post-injection. There is no parenchymal lung uptake.

tween the CT abnormality and the pulmonary function was good, there was no correspondence with the degree of alveolitis, and therefore prediction of disease response was poor (for reviews, see Clarke *et al.*, 1994).

Using the ^{99m}Tc-DTPA technique (as discussed above), lung permeability has also been shown to be increased in pulmonary sarcoidosis. Increased ^{99m}Tc-DTPA flux across the epithelial membrane of the lung has been observed in types I, II and III pulmonary sarcoidosis [24–26]. There is increased permeability associated with a deterioration in pulmonary function, which can be decreased by treating patients with steroids [24]. This increased permeability is likely to be related to the degree of inflammation associated with sarcoidosis. The rate of ^{99m}Tc-DTPA transfer has no definite relationship to the serum angiotensin converting enzyme levels, or to the lymphocyte amounts in bronchoalveolar lavage fluid.

Radionuclide assessment of sarcoidosis has normally involved the use of ^{67}Ga, but more recently the disease has been assessed using ^{18}F-fluorodeoxyglucose (FDG) and ^{111}In-octreotide. Gallium scanning at 24, 48 and 72 hours has been performed nominally injecting 110 MBq ^{67}Ga and imaging over the thorax and the head. Diffuse uptake in the lung can be seen in sarcoid involving the lung parenchyma, and this may be associated with intense uptake in the mediastinum and the

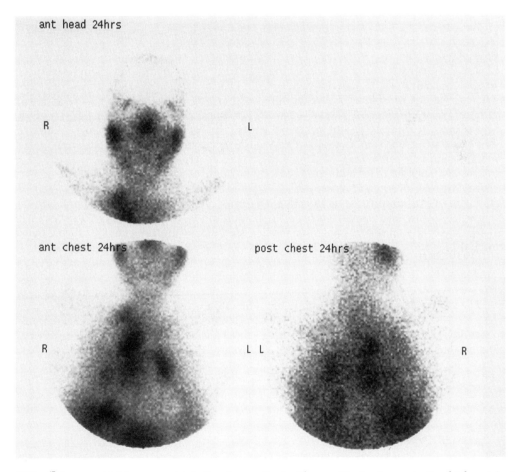

Figure 7.13 ^{67}Ga scan at 24 hours post-injection in a patient with sarcoidosis, demonstrating high uptake in the parotid glands, nasal area and low uptake in the lachrymal glands. Increased uptake is also seen in the mediastinum and the hilar nodes and a right supraclavicular node. There is also diffuse low-grade increased uptake in the lung parenchyma with a negative cardiac silhouette seen on the anterior view.

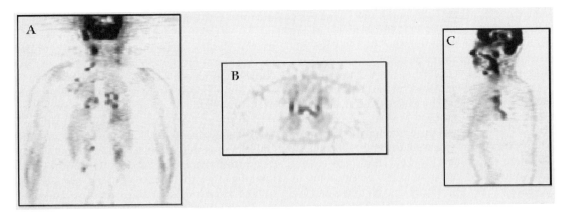

Figure 7.14 An ^{18}F-fluorodeoxyglucose PET scan in a patient with sarcoidosis. The scan appearances show increased uptake in the hilar regions, the supra- and infra-clavicular lymph nodes and the cervical chain as well as the mediastinum. The coronal (A), transaxial (B) and the sagittal (C) sections are shown.

hilum when these nodes are involved (Figures 7.12 and 7.13). The intensity of uptake in the lung relates to disease activity [27]. Uptake patterns have been described as the 'lambda' distribution (mediastinal and hilar uptake) and 'panda' pattern when there is increased uptake in the lachrymal, parotid and nasal areas. The combination is likely to be pathognomonic of sarcoidosis [28,29]. ^{67}Ga imaging is seen as a method of following the activity of disease in response to therapy [30,31]. Quantitation has been attempted using ^{67}Ga to assess response of diffuse parenchymal uptake to therapy [32]. The combination of a negative gallium scan and biochemical markers is predictive of the absence of active sarcoidosis. Sarcoidosis in muscle or skin will only be detected by gallium if large areas are involved; gallium scanning should be reserved for atypical cases or to determine sites for biopsy.

^{111}In-octreotide has also been used to image granulomatous diseases (including sarcoidosis), but no direct comparison with gallium has been performed [33]. Abnormal uptake in the lung parenchyma as well as in lymph nodes has been observed. ^{111}In-octreotide was found to be more sensitive than radiological imaging. The uptake does fall with response to treatment, but this was only seen in two out of five patients who were followed-up; the other three remained positive with apparent failure of response to therapy by other parameters. A novel approach to imaging sarcoidosis is the development of macrophage-targeted glycolipeptide J001 [34], though the usefulness of this agent remains to be seen.

PET imaging in sarcoidosis has been attempted, and owing to the non-specific accumulation of FDG into inflammatory cells [35], the disease can be visualized [36]. The uptake is high in both lymph nodes and lung parenchyma, as might be expected (Figure 7.14) [36,37]. Regional glucose metabolism per gram of lung tissue can be calculated using FDG; this has been shown to be elevated in sarcoidosis with these abnormal levels returning to normal during treatment with steroids [38]. The improvement in glucose metabolism was reflected by an improvement in the level of serum angiotensin converting enzyme and was thought to reflect 'disease activity'.

The use of PET radiotracers in the lung presents the ability not only to assess tumours, but also inflammation and infection. The variety of tracers allow the assessment of regional metabolism in disease, regional blood volume and flow as well as permeability measures. Interest is also advancing in the measurement of receptors in the lung, their site and distribution as well as their abundance, using labelled β-receptor agonists and ACE inhibitors.

REFERENCES

1. O'Doherty, M.J. and Miller, R.F. (1993) Aerosols for therapy and diagnosis. *Eur. J. Nucl. Med.*, **20**, 1201–13.

2. Staub, N.C., Hyde, R.W. and Crandall, E. (1990) Workshop on techniques to evaluate lung alveolar-microvascular injury. *Am. Rev. Respir. Dis.*, **141**, 1071–7.

3. Taplin, G.V., Chopra, S.K. and Uszler, J.M. (1978) Imaging experimental pulmonary ischaemic lesions after inhalation of a diffusible radioaerosol. Recent experience and further developments. *J. Nucl. Med.*, **19**, 567–8.

4. Jones, J.G., Minty, B.D., Lawler, P., Hulands, G., Crawley, J.C.W. and Veall, N. (1980) Increased epithelial permeability in cigarette smokers. *Lancet*, **i**, 66–8.

5. Barrowcliffe, M.P. and Jones, J.G. (1989) Pulmonary clearance of 99mTc-DTPA in the diagnosis and evolution of increased permeability pulmonary oedema. *Anaesth. Intens. Care*, **17**, 422–32.

6. Jefferies, A.L., Coates, G. and O'Brodovich, H. (1984) Pulmonary epithelial permeability in Hyaline-Membrane disease. *N. Engl. J. Med.*, **311**, 1075–80.

7. O'Doherty, M.J., Page, C.J., Bradbeer, C.S. *et al.* (1987) Alveolar permeability in HIV patients with *Pneumocystis carinii* pneumonia. *Genitourin. Med.*, **63**, 268–70.

8. O'Doherty, M.J., Page, C.J., Bradbeer, C.S. *et al.* (1989) The place of lung 99mTc DTPA aerosol transfer in the investigation of lung infections in HIV positive patients. *Resp. Med.*, **83**, 395–401.

9. Mason, G.R., Effros, R.M., Uszler, J.M. *et al.* (1985) Small solute clearance from the lungs of patients with cardiogenic and noncardiogenic pulmonary edema. *Chest*, **88**, 327–34.

10. Oberdorster, G., Utell, M.J., Weber, D.A., Ivanovich, M., Hyde, R.W. and Morrow, P.E. (1984) Lung clearance of inhaled 99m-Tc DTPA in the dog. *J. Appl. Physiol.*, **57**, 589–95.

11. Langford, J.A., Lewis, C.A., Gellert, A.R., Tolfree, S.E.J. and Rudd, R.M. (1986) Pulmonary epithelial permeability: vascular background effects on whole lung and regional half-time values. *Nucl. Med. Commun.*, **7**(3), 183–90.

12. Kohn, H., Kohn, B., Klech, H., Pohl, W. and Mostbeck, A. (1990) Urine excretion of inhaled technetium-99m-DTPA: an alternative method to assess lung epithelial transport. *J. Nucl. Med.*, **31**(4), 4419.

13. Groth, S. and Pedersen, M. (1989) Pulmonary permeability in primary ciliary dyskinesia. *Eur. Respir. J.*, **2**, 64–70.

14. Barrowcliffe, M. P., Otto, C. and Jones, J.G. (1988) Pulmonary clearance of ^{99m}Tc-DTPA: influence of background activity. *J. Appl. Physiol.*, **64**(3), 1045–9.

15. O'Doherty, M.J., Page, C.J., Croft, D.N. and Bateman, N.T. (1985) Lung ^{99m}Tc DTPA transfer: a method for background correction. *Nucl. Med. Commun.*, **6**, 209–15.

16. O'Doherty, M.J., Page, C.J., Croft, D.N. and Bateman, N.T. (1985) Regional lung 'leakiness' in smokers and nonsmokers. *Nucl. Med. Commun.*, **6**, 353–7.

17. Basran, G.S., Byrne, A.J. and Hardy, J.G. (1985) A noninvasive technique for monitoring lung vascular permeability in man. *Nucl. Med. Commun.*, **3**, 3–10.

18. Braude, S., Apperley, J., Krausz, T., Goldman, J.M. and Royston, D. (1985) Adult Respiratory Distress Syndrome after allogeneic bone marrow transplantation: evidence for a neutrophil independent mechanism. *Lancet*, **i**, 1239–42.

19. Kaplan, J.D., Calandrino, F.S. and Schuster, D.P. (1991) A positron emission tomographic comparison of pulmonary vascular permeability during the adult respiratory distress syndrome and pneumonia. *Am. Rev. Respir. Dis.*, **143**, 150–4.

20. Velazquez, M., Weibel, E.R., Kuhn, C. *et al.* (1991) PET evaluation of pulmonary vascular permeability: a structure-function correlation. *J. Appl. Physiol.*, **70**, 2206–16.

21. Mintun, M.A., Dennis, D.R., Welch, M.J., Mathias, C.J. and Schuster, D.P. (1987) Measurements of pulmonary vascular permeability with PET and gallium-68-transferrin. *J. Nucl. Med.*, **28**, 1704–16.

22. Mintun, M.A., Warfel, T.E. and Schuster, D.P. (1990) Evaluating pulmonary vascular permeability with radiolabeled proteins: an error analysis. *J. Appl. Physiol.*, **68**, 1696–706.

23. Bekerman, C., Hoffer, P.B., Bitran, J.D. and Gupta, R.G. (1980) Gallium-67 citrate imaging studies of the lung. *Semin. Nucl. Med.*, **10**, 286–301.

24. Chinet, T., Jaubert, F., Dusser, D., Danel, C., Chretien, J. and Huchon, G.J. (1990) Effects of inflammation and fibrosis on pulmonary function in diffuse lung fibrosis. *Thorax*, **45**, 675–8.

25. Dusser, D.J., Collignon, M.A., Stanislas-Leguern, G., Barritault, L.G., Chretien, J. and Huchon, G.J. (1986) Respiratory clearance of 99mTc DTPA and pulmonary involvement in sarcoidosis. *Am. Rev. Respir. Dis.*, **134**, 493–7.

26. Watanabe, N., Inoue, T., Oriuchi, H., Suzuki, H., Hirano, T. and Endo, K. (1995) Increased pulmonary clearance of aerosolised ^{99m}Tc-DTPA in patients with a subset of stage I sarcoidosis. *Nucl. Med. Commun.*, **16**, 464–7.

27. Line, B.R., Hunninghake, G.W., Keogh, B.A. *et al.* (1981) Gallium-67 scanning to stage the alveolitis of sarcoidosis: correlation with clinical studies, pulmonary function studies and bronchoalveolar lavage. *Am. Rev. Respir. Dis.*, **123**, 440–6.

28. Sulavik, S.B., Spencer, R.P., Palestro, C.J. *et al.* (1993) Specificity and sensitivity of distinctive chest radiographic and/or ^{67}Ga images in the noninvasive diagnosis of sarcoidosis. *Chest*, **103**, 403–9.

29. Sulavik, S.B., Spencer, R.P., Weed, D.A., Shapiro, H.R., Shiue, S. and Castriotta, R.J. (1990) Recognition of distinctive patterns of gallium-67 distribution in sarcoidosis. *J. Nucl. Med.*, **31**, 1909–14.

30. Baughman, R.P., Fernandez, M. and Bosken, C. (1984) Comparison of gallium-67 scanning, bronchoalveolar lavage and serum angiotensin-converting enzyme levels in pulmonary sarcoidosis: predicting response to therapy. *Am. Rev. Respir. Dis.*, **129**, 676–81.

31. Lawrence, E.C., Teague, R.B. and Gottlieb, M.S. (1983) Serial changes in markers of disease activity with corticosteroid treatment in sarcoidosis. *Am. J. Med.*, **74**, 747–56.

32. Alberts, C. and Van der Schoot, J.B. (1988) Standardized quantitative 67Ga scintigraphy in pulmonary sarcoidosis. *Sarcoidosis*, **5**, 111–18.
33. Vanhagen, P.M., Krenning, E.P., Reubi, J.C. *et al.* (1994) Somatostatin analogue scintigraphy in granulomatous disease. *Eur. J. Nucl. Med.*, **21**, 497–502.
34. Diot, R., Lemarie, E., Baulie, J.L. *et al.* (1992) Scintigraphy with J001 macrophage targeting glycolipeptide. A new approach for sarcoidosis imaging. *Chest*, **102**, 670–6.
35. Kubota, R., Yamada, S., Kubota, K., Ishiwata, K., Tamahashi, N. and Ido, T. (1992) Intratumoral distribution of fluorine-18-fluorodeoxyglucose in vivo: high accumulation in macrophages and granulocytes studied by microautoradiography. *J. Nucl. Med.*, **33**, 1972–80.
36. Lewis, P.J. and Salama, A. (1994) Uptake of fluorine-18-fluorodeoxyglucose in sarcoidosis. *J. Nucl. Med.*, **35**, 1647–9.
37. Valind, S.O., Rhodes, C.G., Paltin, C., Suzuki, T. and Hughes, J.M.B. (1984) Measurements of pulmonary glucose metabolism in patients with cryptogenic fibrosing alveolitis and pulmonary sarcoidosis. *Am. Rev. Respir. Dis.*, **129**, A53.
38. Brudin, L.H., Valind, S.O., Rhodes, C.G. *et al.* (1994) Fluorine-18 deoxyglucose uptake in sarcoidosis measured with positron emission tomography. *Eur. J. Nucl. Med.*, **21**, 297–305.

FURTHER READING

Clarke, D., Mitchell, A.W.M., Dick, R. and James, G.D. (1994) The radiology of sarcoidosis. *Sarcoidosis*, **11**, 90–9.
O'Doherty, M.J. and Peters, A.M. (1997) Pulmonary technetium-99m diethylene triamine pentaacetic acid aerosol clearance as an index of lung injury. *Eur. J. Nucl. Med.*, **24**, 81–7.

CHAPTER 8

Musculoskeletal

P. J. Ryan and I. Fogelman

INTRODUCTION

Patients with a wide variety of musculoskeletal disorders can be usefully investigated by nuclear medicine techniques, particularly through bone scintigraphy. This aspect of nuclear medicine work is on the increase and forms a large part of the current workload of most departments. The bone scan is performed with ^{99m}Tc-labelled bisphosphonates and has an exquisite sensitivity for the detection of skeletal pathology. Although bone scan appearances may be non-specific, the patterns of abnormality allow a diagnosis to be made in most circumstances. The principal conditions that can be imaged are metastatic bone disease, osteomyelitis, and a variety of benign conditions including fractures and their sequelae, avascular necrosis, reflex sympathetic dystrophy syndrome, enthesopathies and biomechanical stress lesions, inflammatory arthropathies, metabolic bone disease and miscellaneous bone conditions such as costochondritis. Single-photon emission tomography (SPECT) has provided new indications for bone scintigraphy such as the evaluation of spondylolysis and facet syndrome in the spine, and meniscal tears and ligamental lesions in the knee.

PATHOPHYSIOLOGY OF BISPHOSPHONATE UPTAKE

The bone scan provides information that reflects skeletal metabolic activity. The exact mechanism(s) involved in bisphosphonate uptake are not completely understood, but it is thought that they react through the phosphorous group by chemiabsorption onto the calcium of hydroxyapatite in bone, i.e. the bisphosphonate molecule is adsorbed onto the surface of bone. The major factors which affect this adsorption are thought to be osteoblastic activity and skeletal vascularity with preferential uptake at sites of active bone formation [1]. The bone scan therefore reflects the metabolic reaction to a disease process. Because of its ability to detect functional change, the bone scan can often be strongly positive, well before the structural X-ray changes occur. Although the bone scan is more sensitive than conventional radiology, the findings are relatively non-specific, and for optimal interpretation needs to be assessed with all the relevant clinical information and correlated with corresponding X-rays.

EQUIPMENT

Bone scanning is invariably performed with the gamma-camera. Most studies are acquired using single or multiple static 'spot' images. This enables the camera head to be positioned as close to the patient as possible, improving resolution. Many modern cameras allow a continuous scanning mode that enables a more rapid acquisition and the production of a whole-body skeletal image (rather than multiple overlapping views), but at the expense of resolution. Dual-headed cameras are increasing, and allow the simultaneous acquisition of anterior and posterior images, reducing the time needed to complete a study. Some camera systems

Clinical Nuclear Medicine, 3rd edn. Edited by M.N. Maisey, K.E. Britton and B.D. Collier. Published in 1998 by Chapman & Hall, London. ISBN 0 412 75180 1

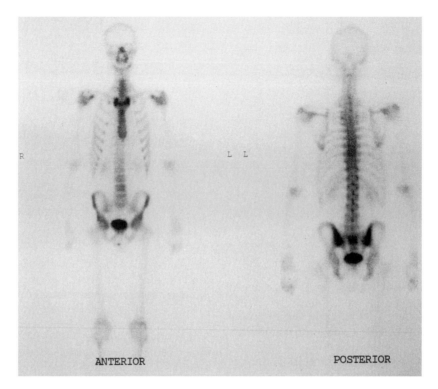

Figure 8.1 Normal whole-body bone scan. Note tracer in bladder due to normal excretion of bisphosphonate via the renal tract.

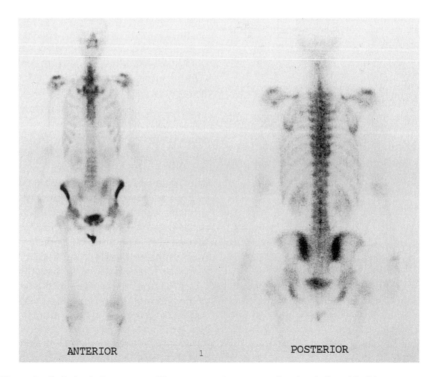

Figure 8.2 Normal whole-body bone scan. Note some urine contamination below bladder, a common finding.

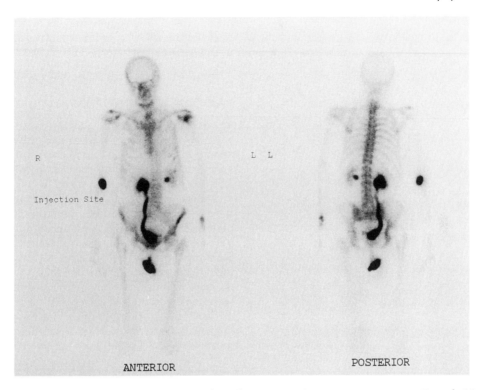

Figure 8.3 There is marked retention of tracer in the right kidney and ureter, suggesting significant hold-up at the pyeloureteric joint level. Also note non-skeletal activity at injection site, a common incidental finding.

offer body-contouring, which helps to improve resolution when using the scanning mode.

THE NORMAL BONE SCAN

A familiarity with the normal appearances and normal variations is vital for interpreting bone scans. The most important feature of a normal bone scan is symmetry about the mid-line in the sagittal plane. The left and right halves of the skeleton should be virtually mirror images of each other. There should be uniform uptake of tracer throughout the skeleton, although there is greater activity at sites of highest metabolic activity such as the joint margins and areas rich in trabecular bone such as the spinal vertebral bodies (Figures 8.1 and 8.2). Bisphosphonate not taken up by the skeleton is excreted via the urinary tract. In a normal patient, tracer is visualized in kidneys and bladder (Figure 8.3). A variety of non-skeletal abnormalities may be detected ' incidentally' on a bone scan and many of these will relate to abnormalities of

kidney or bladder. Uptake of bone scanning agents can also occur in soft tissues, indicating significant abnormalities (Figure 8.4). Assessment of the bone scan therefore requires careful examination of soft tissue and renal tract as well as the skeleton.

'THREE-PHASE' BONE SCAN

In some circumstances a three-phase bone scan will provide additional valuable information regarding the vascularity of a lesion. This involves an initial dynamic flow study (1st phase) with rapid sequential images obtained every 2–3s for 30s. This is followed by a blood pool image at 5 minutes (2nd phase) when the radiopharmaceutical is still predominantly within the vascular compartment, although some will already have been taken into bone. A delayed static image or images can be obtained between 2 and 4 hours (3rd phase), with earlier imaging more suitable in children where there is greater skeletal extraction of tracer, and later imaging in the elderly where skel-

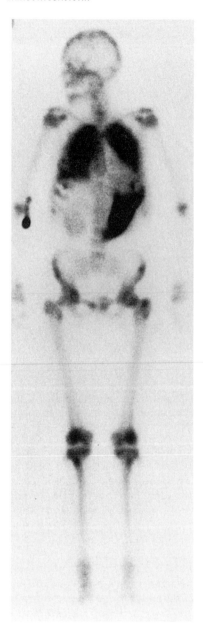

Figure 8.4 Soft tissue activity in lungs and stomach due to presumed ectopic calcification.

etal uptake is less. The longer the delay between injection and imaging, the greater the contrast between the lesion and the bone. For the diagnosis of osteomyelitis, the three-phase bone scan is typically used. In some situations, a four-phase bone scan is performed by acquiring a delayed 24-hour image – where there may be improved contrast despite a lower count rate. This has proved useful for imaging osteomyelitis in the extremities [2].

PATTERN RECOGNITION

The evaluation of a bone scan requires familiarity with the normal appearances and the variety of abnormal appearances. While abnormal bone scan activity may be non-specific, the distribution and pattern of uptake usually enables the diagnosis to be made. On some occasions, the bone scan will need to be combined with other imaging investigations, and rarely a biopsy will be necessary to establish the diagnosis. Examples of typical patterns of abnormality include metastases where there are often multiple lesions randomly distributed throughout the axial skeleton (Figures 8.5 and 8.6), rib fractures where there are foci in a linear pattern (Figure 8.7), and osteomyelitis where there is intense uptake on all three phases of a bone scan, usually confined to one side of a joint (Figure 8.8).

THE BONE SCAN IN MALIGNANCY

The detection of metastatic skeletal disease remains the most important indication for performing a bone scan. The common cancers that metastasise to the bone are those of the prostate, breast and lung. However, all malignant tumours may metastasise to bone and can be detected by bone scintigraphy. The most characteristic feature of metastases is irregular focal lesions in a pattern that does not correspond to any single anatomical structure. Lesions are mostly confined to the axial skeleton although less commonly they may involve the non-marrow-containing skeleton.

In general, metastases must generate an osteoblastic response in order to be detected on the bone scan. False-negative results may occur but are rare [3]. Metastases can on occasion produce an area of decreased uptake (cold lesion) reflecting bone destruction and failure to stimulate a 'healing' response (Figure 8.9). This is most often seen in myeloma or renal carcinoma.

An important variant to recognize is the 'superscan' of malignancy [4]. This arises when focal lesions are so extensive that they coalesce to produce a relatively diffuse image. Due to very

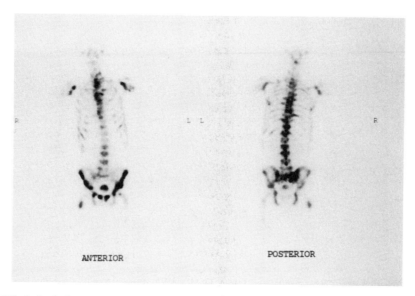

ANTERIOR   POSTERIOR

Figure 8.5 Whole-body bone scan with multiple sites of increased tracer uptake due to skeletal metastases.

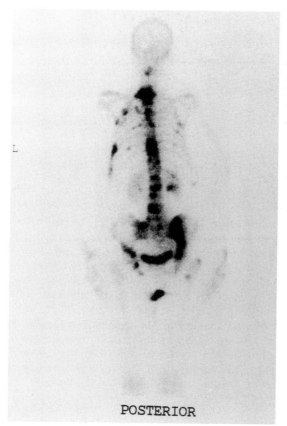

POSTERIOR

Figure 8.6 Posterior image. Multiple skeletal metastases.

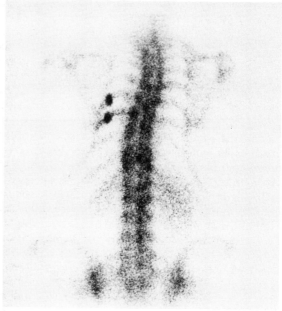

Figure 8.7 Bone scan. Posterior image. Patient with rib fracture, left 8th and 9th ribs.

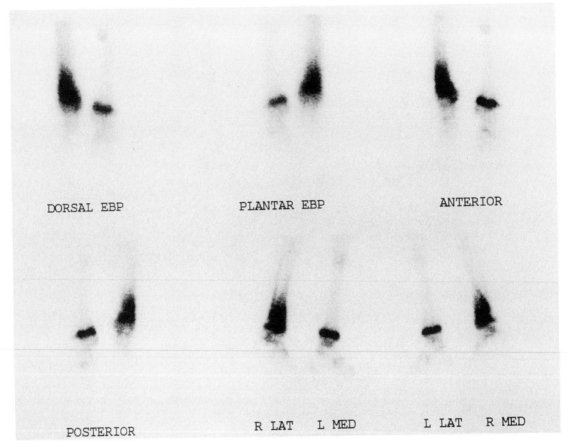

DORSAL EBP   PLANTAR EBP   ANTERIOR

POSTERIOR   R LAT   L MED   L LAT   R MED

Figure 8.8   Osteomyelitis, right lower tibia. Illustration shows increased uptake on second and third phase of bone scan.

high skeletal uptake with heightened contrast between bone and soft tissue, the initial impression is that the scan is 'too good to be true'. The renal images are not visualized due to increased contrast, and because less tracer is excreted via the renal tract (Figure 8.10). Usually, there is still some irregularity of tracer uptake with focal lesions apparent in ribs, humeri or femora. Where there is doubt about a superscan of malignancy, a single X-ray of the pelvis will clarify the issue, as it is always abnormal in such cases. If there is any diagnostic uncertainty, a bone scan should be followed by more specific investigations directed to the site of abnormality. A useful diagnostic pathway is shown in Figure 8.11. In patients with X-ray evidence of metastases, the bone scan will often provide valuable additional information on the

extent of disease. Bone SPECT is also particularly valuable in the spine where only one or two lesions are present. The improved localization of activity may enable the separation of benign and malignant patterns of uptake. Metastases most commonly show uptake in the vertebral body and pedicle, or diffuse uptake throughout the vertebral body. Different uptake patterns are seen in benign disease, in particular, activity in the facetal joints or focal vertebral body activity are rarely found in metastases [5].

BONE SCAN VERSUS MRI IN MALIGNANCY

There is now good evidence that magnetic resonance imaging (MRI) is very sensitive for the detection of metastatic tumour involvement of the

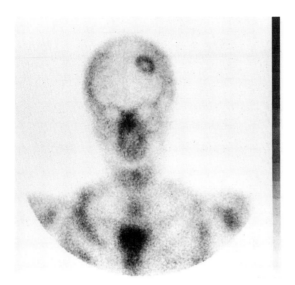

Figure 8.9 Metastasis of the skull. There is a central photon-deficient area with a rim of increased osteoblastic activity.

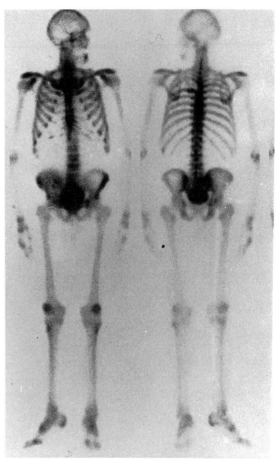

Figure 8.10 Superscan. Note the focal abnormal uptake left 6th rib posteriorly and right pelvis, including probable metastases.

bone marrow. In the spine, MRI will detect lesions not visualized on the bone scan, although the bone scan can also detect lesions not identified on MRI [6]. The bone scan carries many advantages over MRI such as an ability to easily visualize the entire skeleton, faster imaging and lower costs. In general, it remains the best method to detect skeletal metastases, with the MRI being used in the spine where there is a negative or equivocal scan and high clinical suspicion or a positive scan and low clinical suspicion. MRI may also be useful to distinguish benign from malignant vertebral collapse and to monitor response to therapy [7].

BONE SCANNING IN THE MANAGEMENT OF MALIGNANCY

The bone scan is often used for staging for a malignancy at presentation. Metastases may be present in an asymptomatic individual and even in a patient with a suspected metastasis because of bone pain, more extensive disease may be found when the bone scan is undertaken. The bone scan is invaluable where a patient is clinically suspected of having metastases for, if confirmed, this will determine the direction of therapy. This may be more aggressive chemotherapy or hormonal therapy, or specific palliative measures such as local radiotherapy, hemi-body radiation or radionuclide therapy. Patients with hypercalcaemia can commonly have metastases and the bone scan will form an important component of management.

The bone scan can be helpful in monitoring response to therapy. Reliance on symptoms can be misleading and radiological evidence of healing has a low sensitivity, is slow and not possible in the presence of sclerotic metastases. The use of the bone scan to assess the response to therapy is not always straightforward. In some patients there may be a reduction in the number of lesions with reduced scan intensity, indicating successful treat-

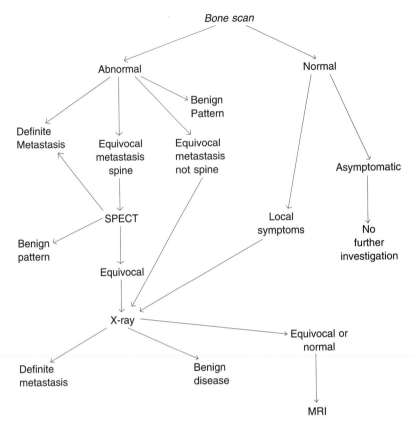

Figure 8.11   Diagnostic pathway for skeletal malignancy.

ment. In others there may be an increase in the number of lesions, indicating progression. However, it is not uncommon to find improvement or disappearance of some lesions with also the appearance of new lesions, making interpretation difficult. It is also recognized there may be a transient worsening of scan findings in response to treatment in the first few months after therapy. This is known as the flare response and reflects activation of the osteoblasts as part of the healing process. The flare response usually produces an increase in intensity of lesions but new lesions can also be seen. The flare response is not usually seen more than 6 months after starting therapy [8].

The detection of disease at potential sites of fractures is important, as prophylactic surgery may be worthwhile. The patient's quality of life in the last few months will be considerably worse if a fracture occurs, particularly if complicated. Long bone involvement, especially in the femur, should be noted on the bone scan, and if relevant, the possible need for prophylactic surgery mentioned.

It is worth noting that metastases should only rarely demonstrate anything more than mild uptake on the first and second phase of bone scan images and this can be helpful in distinguishing them from primary bone tumours. A delayed 24-hour image may be helpful to separate malignant from benign bone lesions. Malignant lesions mostly show a higher lesion-to-background ratio at 24 hours than at 4 hours, whereas in benign lesions it is unchanged [9].

INDIVIDUAL TUMOURS

BREAST CANCER

Bone scanning remains an important part of staging in breast cancer patients, although this is now largely only performed in those with recurrent or more advanced disease (large tumours or lymph node involvement). In early breast cancer, the pick-up rate of metastases is low, about 3% in stage II disease [10]. However, some surgeons still feel the bone scan has a useful role as a baseline study in reducing the number of equivocal studies due to uncertainty about confounding benign disease on later bone scans. In more advanced disease, at presentation the pick-up rate of metastases is high with a mean figure of 28%. An abnormal bone scan carries a mean survival of 2–3 years, and is clearly of prognostic importance [11].

PROSTATE CANCER

In prostate cancer there is a higher incidence of metastases at presentation than in breast cancer. This is around 38% and increases in more advanced disease. There is therefore a good case for bone scans in all patients at presentation for staging. This is reinforced by the prognostic value with a 45% mortality at 2 years with an abnormal scan versus a 20% mortality for a normal scan [12]. There has been recent interest in the use of prostate-specific antigen (PSA) to detect patients with or without metastases. There is a high negative predictive value of low levels of PSA (<20 ng/ml), but measurements above this do not necessarily predict disease [13]. Although patients with an elevated PSA should have a bone scan, there is still a good case to perform a bone scan in those with low levels, as it is not uncommon in clinical practice to find patients with normal PSA but who still have skeletal metastases. It should be remembered that, in patients who have had androgen deprivation therapy, PSA is unreliable for the detection of metastases [14]. The bone scan can help in the stratification of advanced prostate cancer as patients with one or two involved skeletal areas have a longer disease-free interval that those with three or four areas [15]. Recent work has suggested that a PSA cut-off level of 20 ng/ml may be too high for initial staging, as seven of 35 patients with a level less that this had metastases, although none had a PSA less than 10 ng/ml [16].

LUNG CANCER

Most patients with lung cancer have a poor prognosis at presentation. The bone scan is important in such patients where surgery is considered to exclude skeletal metastases, as this would imply disseminated disease. It is of course essential to identify the nature of scan abnormalities and find the precise cause so that patients are not excluded from surgery on the basis of a false-positive scan. The prognosis in patients with carcinoma of the lung who have skeletal metastases is poor, with an 87% mortality at 6 months [17]. However, if metastases are suspected it is of clinical importance to identify them as palliation can be considered.

Imaging of the distal limbs can be useful in patients with suspected hypertrophic pulmonary osteoarthropathy (HPOA) where the bone scan shows increased tracer uptake in the lateral aspect of the long bones – the tram-line sign – due to periosteal activity. Although the low frequency of HPOA in lung cancer does not warrant imaging the distal limbs in all patients, it is worthwhile where there is clinical suspicion, as a positive diagnosis can then be made. Multiple myelomatosis with skeletal involvement will usually produce a positive bone scan. However, false-negative scans may occur when disease is purely lytic and no osteoblastic response occurs [18]. The bone scan may underestimate the extent of disease in multiple myelomatosis, and cannot replace a full skeletal survey.

PRIMARY BONE TUMOURS

A wide variety of benign and malignant tumours can be investigated with bone scintigraphy although in clinical practice nuclear medicine techniques are only infrequently required. Of the malignant tumours, osteosarcomas, Ewing's tumours and giant cell tumours usually show increased tracer uptake on both blood pool and delayed images. The latter may be more intense at the periphery than at the centre, producing a 'doughnut' appearance. Primary lymphomas of bone, although rare, also characteristically show a pattern of tracer uptake peripherally and a relatively cold area centrally. In addition, skeletal angiomatosis can show increased early activity and decreased delayed activity, although increased at the rim.

For malignant primary bone tumours the bone scan is most useful to investigate the extent of skeletal metastases in Ewing's sarcoma. For this tumour there is a good case for having a bone scan at initial diagnosis, whereas in osteosarcoma the role of bone scan is less clear as metastases to bone are rare at presentation [19]. It should be noted that non-osseous metastases, particularly in the lung, may take up bone scanning tracers, most probably due to uptake of tracer associated with microcalcification in the lesion. This situation is most commonly found in osteosarcoma. It is of interest that a high sensitivity for primary breast cancer has been found on bone scanning and therefore breast activity should be commented on as possibly representing malignancy if visualized [20]. A number of studies have examined the value of thallium and technetium MIBI to evaluate primary bone tumours and identify whether or not they are malignant. This appears worthwhile where there is clearly low or high tracer uptake, but there is an overlap of benign and malignant patients in situations of moderate tracer uptake [21]. [18]FDG-PET has also been evaluated as a means of grading malignant tumours and has produced promising results.

Among the benign bone tumours, bone scanning is most useful for detecting osteoid osteoma, as radiographs are commonly normal and the bone scan has a characteristic appearance. The lesion is most often found in adolescents and young adults, and it is not generally seen after the age of 30 years [22]. The tibia and femur account for 50% of cases but any bone may be involved. Patients usually present with pain which characteristically is severe, worse at night and relieved by aspirin. If positive, the radiograph shows a small round focus with a radiolucent central nidus surrounded by reactive sclerosis. The bone scan is more sensitive than X-rays and there is typically an intense discrete focal lesion in the cortex of the bone with an increased blood pool. Activity can be found within diffuse uptake where there is local reaction to a lesion. Osteoid osteomas can usually be distinguished from a healing fracture with less uptake on blood pool, osteomyelitis with more diffuse uptake on blood pool and in the spine from spondylolysis with no increased blood pool [23]. A normal bone scan essentially excludes the diagnosis of osteoid osteoma. Osteoblastomas and chondroblastomas also show increased activity on both blood pool and delayed images but have characteristic X-ray appearances.

TRAUMA

FRACTURES

The majority of fractures will be detected radiographically, although certain sites such as the sternum, sacrum and scapula are difficult to visualize on X-ray; in such cases the bone scan may be particularly helpful. The bone scan is also useful where there may be a delay before typical radiographic features appear; for example, the scaphoid, pelvis, talar dome, or proximal femur in the elderly or osteoporotic patients. Clinical practice shows that most fractures will be detected on bone scan within hours of injury. Data from Matin [24] show that 95% of all fractures in those under 65 years of age were detected by 24 hours, and 95% of fractures in those over 65 by 72 hours. However, recent work by Spitz *et al.* [25] has suggested that axial fractures may on occasions take as long as 12 days to become apparent. Three stages of scintigraphic patterns in fractures have been described. The acute phase is characterized by diffuse increased uptake at the fracture site for 2–4 weeks after injury, although a distinct fracture line may be seen at this stage. Increased activity is usually also seen on the dynamic images (Figure 8.12). For the next 8–12 weeks there is a well-defined linear abnormality at the fracture site. Subsequently, there is a gradual reduction in intensity of tracer uptake until the scan returns to normal. Around 60% of fractures heal scintigraphically by 1 year and 90% by 2 years. However, around 80% of rib fractures heal by 1 year. On occasion, activity may persist at the fracture site for many years and even decades. This is most likely where there is a pathological fracture due to malignancy or poor apposition of bone ends or in the elderly. External fixation devices will delay the return of the bone scan to normal with less than 50%, having normalized by 3 years. Work from our own unit has shown that localization of activity due to a fracture can be improved by registration with X-rays (Figure 8.13). Registration further allows activity within a hand or foot bone to be distinguished from activity arising from the joints. Another fracture that may be difficult to diagnose on X-ray but where the bone scan can assist is the Lisfrank mid-foot fracture dislocation, where there is a band of increased activity across multiple tarsometatarsal joints on the bone scan. Insufficiency fractures of the pelvis are also notoriously

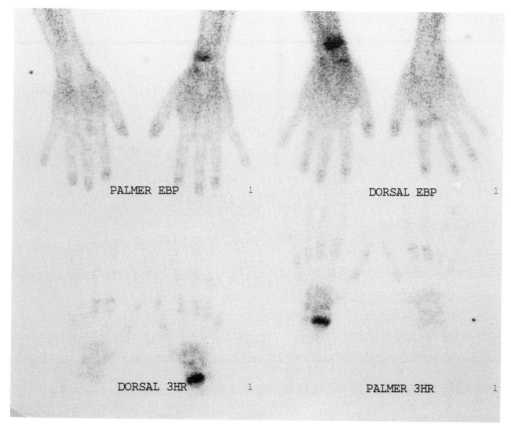

Figure 8.12   Distal radius fracture. Discrete uptake at the fracture site on blood pool and delayed images.

difficult to diagnose on X-ray, but can be reliably demonstrated on a bone scan. Sacral fractures typically show increased vertical activity medial to the sacroiliac joints with a horizontal line across the sacrum just below the inferior margin of the sacroiliac joints – an H-shaped pattern. Incomplete H-patterns may occur with one or two limbs missing. Other sites of pelvic insufficiency fractures include the para-symphysial region, iliac blades and the supra-acetabular region.

NON-UNION

The distinction between delayed healing and non-union is not always possible, as definition of the terms is imprecise and both may show increased scintigraphic activity. However, the latter is commonly defined as failure of a fracture to heal 6–8 months following injury [26]; and when time of injury and other clinical data such as movement at the fracture site, pain on stressing the fracture site or tenderness over the site are combined with the scintigraphic findings, it is possible to separate delayed from non-union. The latter term applies to about 5% of fractures with the most common sites being the tibia and femur. Non-union is more likely when fractures are compound, comminuted, immobilized for an insufficient length of time, or poorly fixed. Infection, impaired blood supply to the fracture site or poor nutrition may also contribute. Atrophic non-union is characterized by reduced or absent bone scan activity at the fracture site; and this group of patients respond poorly to pulsed electromagnetic field stimulation and require surgical exploration. The absent or reduced activity is either due to inability of cells at

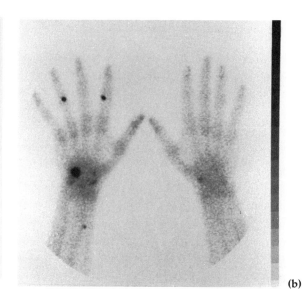

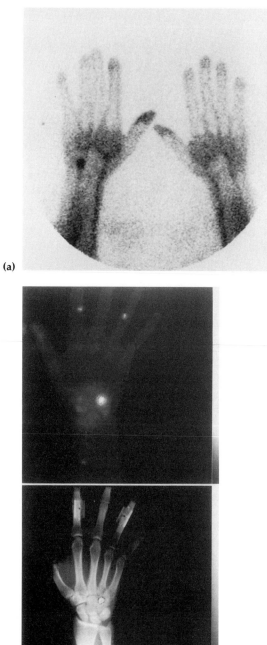

(a)

(b)

(c)

Figure 8.13   Hook of hamate fracture. Registration of bone scan with X-ray improves localization. (a) Increased blood pool; (b) increased delayed activity; (c) registration image.

the fracture surfaces to respond appropriately to injury due to a pseudoarthrosis, interposition of soft tissue, infection or an interrupted blood supply. A more frequent scintigraphic pattern of non-union is that of increased activity, presumably implying a degree of callus formation, and this group responds well to pulsed electromagnetic field stimulation [27].

BONE GRAFTS

Bone scintigraphy may be useful in the evaluation of bone grafts. Radiological investigation does not reveal viability for several weeks after surgery, but bone scintigraphy can do so quickly by demonstrating increasing uptake, or conversely non-viability with absent uptake. The addition of SPECT can be valuable, particularly if there is a requirement to separate soft tissue activity from the bone graft and if metallic appliances such as plates have been used to hold the graft together. Blood flow and blood pool imaging improve the reliability of the bone scan for this indication and studies on vascular grafts should ideally be performed less than a week post-operatively to avoid false-positive results for viability. Free cancellous grafts may show evidence of revascularization by 2–3 weeks in the nose, although 4–8 weeks is probably the optimum time for imaging for iliac or split rib grafts to other sites. It should be remembered that infection can produce increased activity on all three phases of the bone scan as well as a normal graft with post-operative hyperaemia.

MUSCLE INJURY

Bone-imaging agents will localize in muscle in certain pathological conditions. These include electrical burns, myositis ossificans and idiopathic rhabdomyolysis. The mechanism for uptake of bisphosphonate is uncertain, but probably requires microcalcification related to the injury with localization onto calcium phosphate or hydroxyapatite. However, bisphosphonates can complex to myofibril and other factors such as hyperaemia, absorption onto soft tissue, or calcium binding to damaged protein or collagen may be relevant. Uptake can occur into the damaged muscles of marathon runners, which is usually most intense by 24–48 hours after injury and starts resolving by one week. Traumatic myositis may appear as increased activity on the first two phases of the bone scan with only mild reactive change in the adjacent bone on the third phase.

PAEDIATRIC ORTHOPAEDIC CONDITIONS

In infants and young children with occult fractures of the tibia and femur, in the first week after injury there may be diffuse uptake along the entire length of the injured bone on both blood pool and

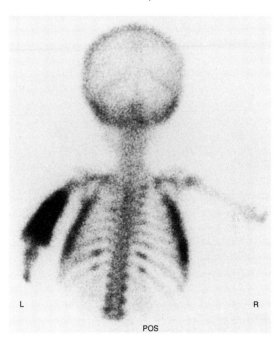

Figure 8.14 Non-accidental injury. Bone scan shows fracture of the ribs and left humerus.

delayed images. In some cases early images may show focal uptake with a diffuse picture on delayed views [28]. Imaging plays an important role in evaluating skeletal trauma especially in cases of child abuse (Figure 8.14). Where clinical examination does not give direct evidence of a skeletal lesion, bone scintigraphy should be performed with radiographs of affected areas. Bone scintigraphy should not be performed until at least 2 days after injury [29]. If examination reveals a bone injury, X-rays are usually performed first and bone scintigraphy later. Skull X-rays should always be taken, as fractures at this site are commonly negative on bone scan.

A common clinical situation where the bone scan is useful is the child presenting with acute leg pain where a variety of orthopaedic conditions may be suspected such as bone or soft tissue trauma, infection and avascular necrosis. Fractures of the small bones of the ankle and foot, especially calcaneus or cuboid [30], and non-displaced spiral fractures of the tibia, are most common between the ages of 2 and 4 years, and are readily detected by bone scintigraphy. From 5–10 years, greenstick and epiphyseal plate fractures

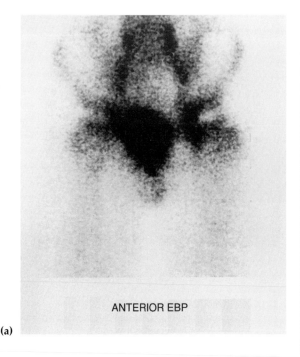

ANTERIOR EBP

(a)

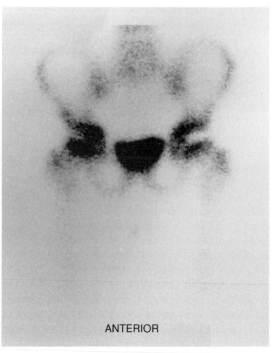

ANTERIOR

(b)

Figure 8.15 Perthes' disease. (a) Left femoral head. Note the reduced activity on the blood pool. (b) Delayed images.

are common, and also occur in older children. Fractures related to sports are increasingly being recognized; for example, pars fractures of the spine or avulsion fractures of the ischial tuberosities in gymnasts. At the hip, the bone scan is useful to help distinguish transient synovitis from septic synovitis and Perthes' disease. In the former, the bone scan is usually normal although it may show slightly increased uptake at the acetabulum on delayed views or slightly reduced bone uptake with reduced blood pool activity [31]. In septic arthritis, there are usually typical changes on bone scan (increased uptake on dynamic and delayed views), although reduced uptake in the femoral head due to vascular spasm or vascular compression can occur. Perthes' disease is usually found in boys between the ages of 4 and 8 years. Bilateral disease is uncommon, and it is rare for both hips to be affected at the same time. A 'cold' femoral head on bone scan is the typical feature of Perthes' disease, but it should be noted that this can also occur with transient synovitis, trauma and septic arthritis where there is a large joint effusion (Figure

8.15). Slipped femoral epiphysis is usually found in children aged 10–15 years. Bone scintigraphy shows abnormal increased accumulation in the growth plate and is particularly helpful in the identification of avascular necrosis of the femoral head. Bone scintigraphy of the spine is useful to detect benign bone tumours, discitis and exclude vertebral disease as a cause of pain. In discitis there is typically increased uptake in the vertebral endplates and findings are apparent within 2 days of the onset of symptoms.

INFLAMMATORY ARTHROPATHIES

The role of nuclear medicine in the evaluation of major arthropathies has been limited, but it is a field that is growing and warrants further research. The most promising possibility is in the investigation of rheumatoid arthritis (RA). Bone scanning will demonstrate increased activity on both the dynamic and static phases in active disease, and uptake parallels other markers of disease activity [32]. However, the bone scan is non-

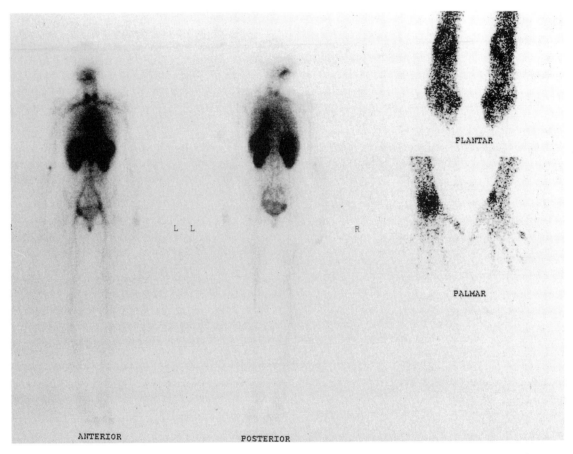

PLANTAR

PALMAR

L L

R

ANTERIOR

POSTERIOR

Figure 8.16 Whole-body HIg images with SPECTs of the hands and feet. There is increased activity in the wrists and metatarsophalangeal joints, indicating active disease.

specific and cannot always separate active rheumatoid arthritis from osteoarthritis, which may have a significant inflammatory component. It is nevertheless potentially helpful to decide which joints require therapy – for example, those with chronic inflammation not responsive to usual treatments and where aggressive therapy with intra-articular yttrium-90 synovectomy may be of value. It is also of note that joints with absent or minimal bone scan activity in patients with newly diagnosed RA do not appear to erode and erosions are more likely to appear in joints with persistent and high scintigraphic activity [33].

Labelled white cell imaging appears a more specific test for joint inflammation: the reduction of activity following intra-articular steroids parallels the pain response. At present, in clinical practice,

joint inflammation is assessed by symptoms, signs and crude indices such as erythrocyte sedimentation rate (ESR) or C-reactive protein (CRP). Both isotope bone and labelled white cell imaging could be used as an adjunct to other measurements to assess the level of disease activity and the requirement for monitoring second-line therapies. However, further research is required to demonstrate the value of this approach.

Recent studies with ^{99m}Tc-labelled human immunoglobulin (HIg) have also shown it to be useful to image rheumatoid arthritis (Figure 8.16) [34], and it is more sensitive and specific than the bone scan. HIg scintigraphy reflects individual variation in disease activity in RA [35], and is more sensitive than physical examination in the detection of histologically determined synovitis

[36]. It appears to reflect only local inflammation and not other aspects of destructive arthritis. It probably binds to intra-articular proteins in inflamed joints [37], and may be more sensitive and specific for active joints than labelled white cells.

Current in-progress studies are examining the role of labelled antibodies such as ^{99m}Tc-CD3 and CD4 lymphocyte antibodies, and E selectin antibodies, and the results from the initial work have been promising. Labelled cytokines have also been investigated.

The value of scintigraphy in osteoarthritis (OA) is even less well defined than in RA. It is rarely performed for primary diagnosis, with clinical and radiological findings being adequate. However, it has been shown that scan activity may precede radiographic changes and can also predict radiographic change. Joints that are inactive on scan show little or no progression, implying a prognostic role for the bone scan [38]. With the advent of chondroprotection therapy, bone scintigraphy may have an enhanced role in selecting patients for treatment. In the knees, the bone scan can be helpful in determining whether there is disease in one or both weight-bearing compartments. This is important as it can guide the appropriate operative intervention (osteotomy, uni or bicompartmental joint replacement). Although planar scintigraphy is less sensitive for the identification of OA in the patella/femoral compartment than the medial and lateral compartments, this is markedly improved with SPECT.

The bone scan has been used for many years in investigation of ankylosing spondylitis (AS). There are two main diagnostic issues where scintigraphy may be helpful in this condition. Firstly, at presentation the diagnosis may be uncertain; secondly, later in the disease process the cause of non-inflammatory chronic back pain may be unclear. For diagnosis, quantitative sacroiliac joint (SIJ) uptake has been used for almost two decades. The rationale for this is that in early disease there will be increased SIJ activity due to inflammation, which predates X-rays changes. The most common technique has been to derive a profile of tracer uptake over the SIJs and sacrum, and to establish an SIJ-to-sacral ratio from the peaks. Initial studies were promising and showed good separation from other causes of back pain, although later studies were less conclusive and it is

now apparent that other conditions such as RA, lumbosacral spondylitis or excessive physical activity can also produce elevated SIJ-to-sacral ratios. It is also recognized that the sacrum may be involved in AS, and improvements can be achieved by comparing SIJ activity to other bony areas or a trough of activity between the sacrum and the SIJ. Provided that other causes of elevated SIJ-to-sacral ratios are excluded, the test remains a valuable tool to identify patients who require further investigation or follow-up [39]. The value of bone scintigraphy in chronic back pain associated with long-standing disease has only received limited attention. However, one study in 1984 using SPECT suggested that sites of abnormal uptake could be identified. Recent work from our own unit has shown that many patients with AS have uptake in the facet joints and this may well be relevant with regard to identifying the cause of pain in some cases [40].

Most other arthropathies, with the exception of infection, have not been investigated in detail by nuclear medicine techniques. However, it has been shown that gout can mimic an infected joint clinically, and may show increased activity on the three-phase bone scan as well as gallium and white cell scans.

OSTEOMYELITIS

The use of bone scintigraphy for osteomyelitis has become an established routine procedure. Early work recognized that there was a hyperaemic pattern on blood pool images. A three-phase bone scan can distinguish osteomyelitis from cellulitis, which typically shows increased activity in the first two phases that is usually diffuse with normal or faintly diffuse increased uptake in the third phase. Uptake in osteomyelitis is usually focal and present in all three phases (Figure 8.17). On occasion, a 24-hour image or fourth-phase view has proved useful, particularly in the extremities where bone detail may be poor at 3–4 hours post-injection [2]. A bone scan will often show increased activity about 2 weeks before an X-ray becomes positive, and in adults with normal X-rays, the three-phase bone scan has a sensitivity and specificity around 95%. In neonates and infants, the sensitivity of the three-phase bone scan may be less, and infection on the bone scan can appear as a cold defect; however, recent work has demonstrated high sensitivity [41]. Where there is

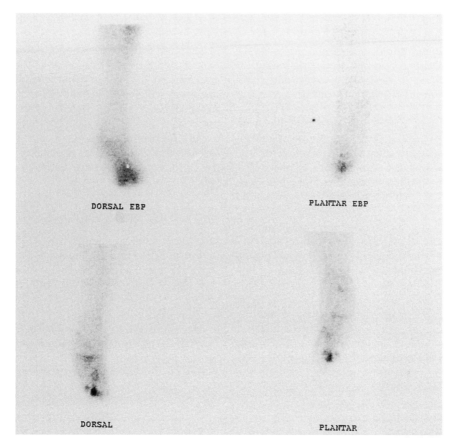

DORSAL EBP

PLANTAR EBP

DORSAL

PLANTAR

Figure 8.17 Osteomyelitis involving the fourth toe. Increased uptake is visualized on blood pool and delayed image.

a strong clinical suspicion but a normal three-phase bone scan, a gallium scan may be performed.

In complicated osteomyelitis (e.g. following surgery, fracture or insertion of a joint prosthesis) and in certain conditions such as sickle cell disease or diabetic Charcot joints, the sensitivity of the three-phase bone scan remains high but specificity is poor. To overcome this, ^{67}Ga citrate or labelled white cell scans are used. Gallium citrate, however, suffers from the problem of increased uptake at sites of bone remodelling, poor resolution and the disadvantages of having to wait 24–48 hours after injection for imaging to be performed. Attempts to define criteria for diagnosis of infection on gallium imaging such as requiring either disparate uptake compared with the bone scan or increased activity compared

with the bone scan have improved specificity [42].

Labelled white cell imaging is generally preferred in complicated osteomyelitis, although in the bone marrow-containing axial skeleton, 'cold' defects due to marrow replacement may be seen, and in vertebral osteomyelitis gallium still has a useful role [43]. Photon-deficient areas on white cell imaging can represent osteomyelitis, but are non-specific and may occur in other conditions such as fractures and metastases. Nevertheless, a high sensitivity and specificity has been found for labelled white cells in osteomyelitis complicating fracture, non-union and diabetic feet. The combined bone and indium-labelled white cell scan can usually distinguish soft tissue from bone infection, although even this combination may not always be able to separate a diabetic Charcot joint from osteomyelitis. Increased uptake of labelled white cells into joints and bones can be caused by other conditions such as rheumatoid arthritis, healing fractures, non-infective prostheses or metastases, but it is usually faint and with healing fractures is only seen for a few weeks after injury.

Different combinations of scans and the introduction of new agents have recently been investigated for osteomyelitis. Improvement in the specificity of imaging in the marrow-containing skeleton in complicated osteomyelitis has been shown with a combination of ^{99m}Tc nanocolloid bone marrow scan and ^{111}In-labelled white cell imaging, with any incongruity of the imaging considered significant [44]. The investigators also considered this the approach of choice in complicated osteomyelitis of the bone marrow-containing skeleton. It can also be a useful combination in chronic osteomyelitis as indium white cells accumulate in active marrow. In the non-marrow-containing skeleton, the combined bone and white cell scan is probably preferable in both acute and chronic complicated osteomyelitis. ^{99m}Tc-HMPAO has recently become available for white cell imaging and appears to give similar results to ^{111}In-labelled white cells. It has the advantages that greater doses of radioactivity can be used, with improved resolution, and earlier results may be obtained with 1- and 4-hour images. There is also greater availability of technetium and a lower radioisotope cost. The principal disadvantages are loss of the option to perform a combined white cell scan with bone or bone marrow scans at the same time, as they all use technetium as the radioisotope, and poorer target-to-background activity at 24 hours compared with indium-white cell imaging. Several recent studies have also demonstrated the value of indium- and technetium-labelled HIg for the diagnosis of infection. ^{99m}Tc-HIg has advantages in availability, but has more rapid washout from the target and background than indium, and may be of less value in low-grade infection. The clinical role of HIg in osteomyelitis is at present unclear, with its overall sensitivity less than white cell imaging. However, one attractive application is for imaging patients with insufficient white cells for labelling. Attempts have also been made to image osteomyelitis with technetium nanocolloid, with some work suggesting that the results obtained are comparable with the white cell scans [45]. Nonetheless, the clinical place of this agent

remains undefined. Recent studies have also examined the value of antibodies labelled with technetium and indium. Although the results appear promising, the studies reported so far suggest that a significant number of false-positives and false-negatives will occur, particularly in the spine [46]. Research has also been directed at labelling antibiotics such as ciprofloxacin to detect infection, called 'infection' imaging. A recent study showed improved sensitivity and specificity for bacterial infection compared with labelled white cells [47].

METABOLIC BONE DISEASE

The bone scan in osteoporosis is useful for the detection and ageing of fractures, particularly of the vertebrae. Acute vertebral collapse is associated with a characteristic pattern of intense linear uptake corresponding to the site of fracture. Activity fades over the ensuing 6–18 months, which allows the intensity of uptake to enable assessment of the age of fracture [48]. Hence, it is possible to determine (using the bone scan) that a radiological vertebral collapse is recent and is the likely cause of acute back pain, or whether an alternative cause of pain should be sought.

The bone scan itself may suggest other causes of back pain such as rib fracture, metastases, Paget's disease or infection, and can help distinguish osteomalacia from osteoporosis. In patients with chronic back pain and osteoporotic vertebral collapse, a SPECT study can detect coexistent facet joint syndrome as a cause of pain [49]. The detection of suspected fracture(s) when X-rays are negative or equivocal is another important role of the bone scan. Unrecognized fractures of the pelvis and sacrum detected by the bone scan have been described, as well as at other sites such as the humerus, scapula, ribs and the neck of femur. The bone scan can also help in the diagnosis of regional migratory osteoporosis and transient osteoporosis of the hip where there is typically intense uptake in the femoral head and greater trochanter.

Paget's disease is characterized by an initial phase of bone resorption followed by an intense osteoblastic response seen in the formation of woven bone. The disease is usually polyostotic but in 20% of cases it is monostotic. Typically, the bone scan shows markedly increased tracer activity evenly distributed through the affected bone

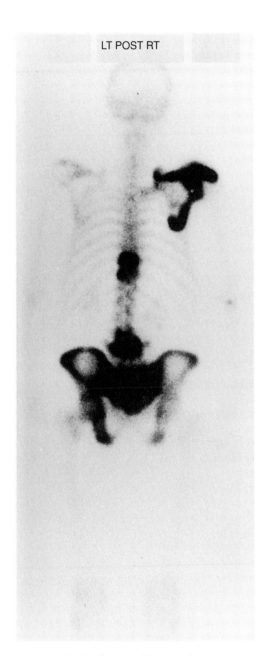

LT POST RT

Figure 8.18 Multiple sites of Paget's disease.

abnormal bone. In the appendicular skeleton there is commonly a progression from the articular end of the shaft, with the distal end having a sharp edge corresponding to the flame-shaped resorption front seen on X-ray. In clinical practice, the bone scan is the imaging technique of choice to evaluate the extent of the disease, with advantages over radiology of being able to rapidly assess the whole skeleton and having better sensitivity. In the patient with an incidentally raised serum alkaline phosphatase the bone scan will resolve whether Paget's disease is the explanation. The bone scan is also valuable where X-rays are equivocal or in a patient with unexplained bone pain or deformity. Atypical expansion of a lesion or a photon-deficient area in an involved site, should alert the physician to the presence of sarcomatous change, but this is rare. Scan appearances may show dramatic change following bisphosphonate therapy, particularly with the more powerful bisphosphonates now being used to treat Paget's disease.

It should be noted that individual lesions on a bone scan vary in their response to therapy and may change from diffuse involvement of bone to more focal appearance which can cause confusion with metastases [50,51]. Metabolic activity may persist at an involved site on the bone scan following bisphosphonate therapy despite normalization of biochemistry, suggesting that the bone scan may be an important parameter when assessing suppression of disease activity, particularly in patients with monostotic disease where the serum alkaline phosphatase is within the normal range. Evidence suggests that the bone scan can help predict the requirement for further therapy.

SPORTS MEDICINE

Some sports medicine injuries involving the skeleton are either difficult to diagnose on X-rays or may not produce radiological change for some days or weeks, but can be easily detected on the bone scan. These include periosteal injuries, stress fractures, shin splints and some ligamental/tendon injuries.

Trained athletes undergoing strenuous training and non-athletes undertaking new forms of exercise are particularly prone to develop stress fractures; the most common sites being the tibiae and fibulae, but they can occur in almost any bone. There is a spectrum of severity ranging from a

(Figure 8.18), an exception being osteoporosis circumscripta where tracer uptake is most intense at the margins of the lesion. The bone scan in Paget's disease shows preservation or even enhancement of the normal anatomical configuration of bone and clear delineation of normal and

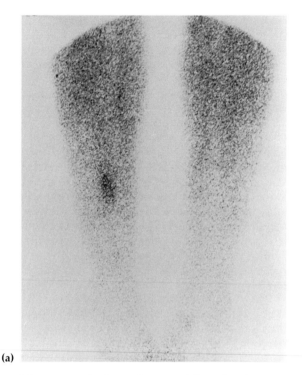

(a)

Figure 8.19 (a) Stress fracture of the right tibia. Note the focal increased uptake on blood pool. (b) Delayed images in the same patient.

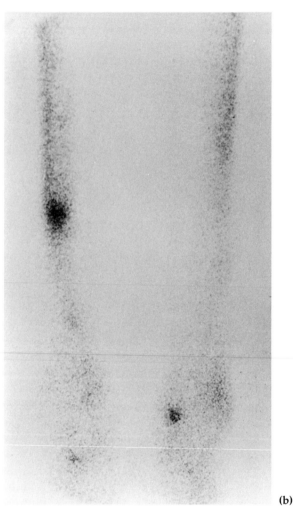

(b)

mild periosteal reaction through to a stress fracture and a full thickness fracture. Differentiation requires lateral views in addition to anterior and posterior views of the relevant bone to assess the percent thickness involved. Stress fractures usually show increased vascularity that may help to distinguish them from shin splints with normal vascularity. Resolution of scan changes in stress fractures may occur by 2–3 months if mild but may take up to 6 months if more severe.

The classic appearance in shin splints or tibial stress syndrome is increased activity of moderate intensity extending along the medial border of the posterior portion of the tibia. It is important to distinguish shin splints from stress fractures, with

the former carrying no risk of fracture. The two conditions can usually be distinguished with activity in shin splints, superficial, extending along cortical surfaces and of moderate intensity, while the stress fracture lesion is more localized, uniform and intense (Figure 8.19(a,b)). Also, shin splints are rarely associated with increased blood pool.

Enthesopathies may also be usefully imaged with the bone scan and are sometimes detected as incidental findings. Activity is typically focal at the relevant site, but can be associated with increased blood flow and blood pool that may be more diffuse. Examples are abductor tendonitis of the hip, osteitis pubis, plantar faciitis and Achilles tendonitis [52]. Bursitis, such as greater trochanteric bursitis and retro-calcaneal bursitis, can also be identified by bone scintigraphy. The distinction of bursitis and stress fractures from enthesopathies may be difficult and obtaining optimal views and careful correlation of scan results with clinical findings is important.

Other lesions due to long-standing or chronic low-level repetitive stress that may lead to a positive bone scan may be found in such conditions as facet syndrome, os trigonum syndrome, and tibiotalar impingement syndrome and talar coalitions. The os trigonum syndrome is due to an accessory ossicle of the posterior margin of the talus, and abnormal activity on delayed images can help in the decision regarding the need for removal. Similar use of the bone scan can be found for a bipartite patella and lesions predisposing to degenerative change such as an accessory navicular bone. The tibio-talar impingement syndrome is due to a bony spur of the anterior lip of the tibia and is found in athletes who drive off the planted foot. Increased activity at this site suggests that the spur is the cause of pain. In talar coalition this activity is commonly not found in the fusion site, but in the posterior sub talar joint or anterior superior talus, predominantly due to abnormal biomechanics.

AVASCULAR NECROSIS

Bony infarction is a recognized complication of fracture although it may occur in other conditions such as in patients on steroids or in sickle cell disease. Early diagnosis is important to prevent complications. The bone scan appearances are initially those of reduced uptake due to diminished blood supply but when reparative processes begin, increased uptake occurs, and at this stage the diagnosis is more difficult. Investigation should be performed as soon as possible after suspicion of such a diagnosis. SPECT of the hip can sometimes allow identification of a photon-deficient centre in an area of increased activity which is not apparent on planar imaging. Delayed imaging of the hip can be useful to assess whether patients will require hip replacement [53].

REFLEX SYMPATHETIC DYSTROPHY SYNDROME (RSDS)

Bone scintigraphy is increasingly being recognized as having an important role in the diagnosis of RSDS, a condition which although uncommon, can complicate fractures, particularly those of the hand, wrist, foot and ankle. It is also associated with a wide range of other conditions such as stroke or malignancy. High sensitivity and specificity for the bone scan has been found in several studies compared with a relative poor sensitivity for X-ray. Sensitivity is greater on the static images although there is usually increased blood flow and blood pool. It should be recognized that on rare occasions there is reduced rather than increased activity. Recently it has been demonstrated that increased activity in RSDS in the extremities is not confined to the periarticular areas, but occurs throughout the bones in the hands and feet in the region affected by the disorder [54].

PROSTHESES

Bone scans have been used for many years for the investigation of pain following the insertion of joint prostheses, particularly at the hip. The typical feature of loosening of the femoral component is increased tip uptake or lesser trochanter uptake but without increased dynamic activity, in contrast to infection where there is increased uptake in all three phases (Figures 8.20 and 8.21). A high degree of accuracy for loosening and infection can be achieved with a bone scan, although some uptake around the femoral component can persist for a year and in the acetabular component for 2 years after insertion of the prosthesis [55]. Infection can be excluded by a normal bone scan or minor focal uptake. Diffuse uptake usually implies infection, although where activity is modest on the initial phases specificity can be improved by the addition of gallium citrate or labelled white cell imaging. False-positive diagnosis of infection can occur with white cell imaging due to the presence of islands of residual bone marrow, particularly at the hip. This is a potential although uncommon source of confusion. It is, however, advised that bone marrow scans should be obtained at the same time as a white cell scan. Imaging cementless hip prostheses may cause difficulty, as prolonged activity can persist in both components following insertion of the prosthesis. However, this is usually in the acetabulum and greater trochanter of the femoral component (Figure 8.22), and knowledge of this normal pattern of uptake usually enables the diagnosis to be made.

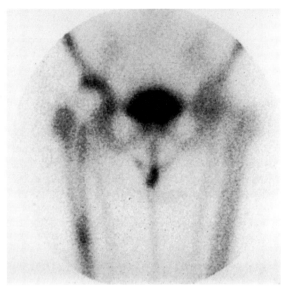

Figure 8.20 Increased activity at the tip of the femoral component of a right hip prosthesis, typical for loosening.

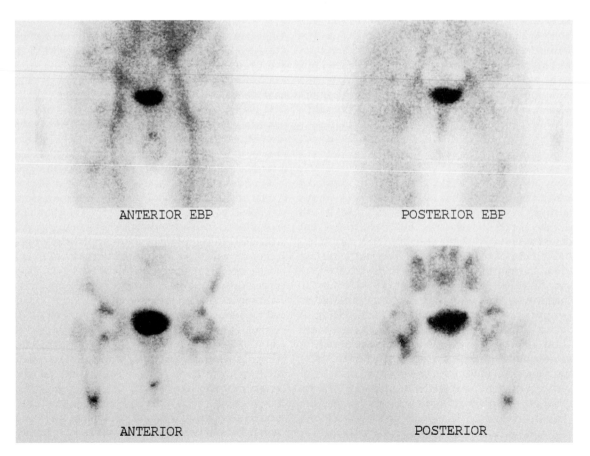

ANTERIOR EBP

POSTERIOR EBP

ANTERIOR

POSTERIOR

Figure 8.21 Loosening of a right hip prosthesis. Note the focal uptake at the tip of the femoral component and lesser trochanter. There is also uptake of the acetabulum, which could imply acetabular loosening. Activity of the left hip is typical for marked degenerative change.

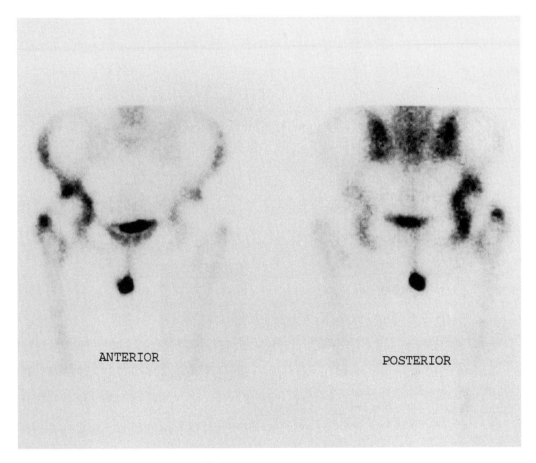

ANTERIOR   POSTERIOR

Figure 8.22   Normal variant right hip prosthesis.

MISCELLANEOUS CONDITIONS

Bone scintigraphy may assist in the diagnosis of costochondritis (Tietze's syndrome) with typical features being increased activity in the sternal or costochondral junctions. This condition may also be associated with increased gallium activity. Findings are non-specific but other conditions can usually be excluded by the clinical presentation or radiographic findings. Rheumatoid arthritis, gout, pyogenic infection and RSDS should be considered. There may be confusion with condensing osteitis of the clavicle and Freidrich disease of the clavicle, but these conditions are confined to the clavicle, the latter being found in children or teenagers. Sternoclavicular hyperostosis (arthro-osteitis) should also be considered; although it is mainly a disease of the sternoclavicular joints it can affect the costosternal junction. However, it is often associated with plantar pustulosis and sometimes ankylosing spondylitis or peripheral arthritis and the ESR and white cell count are usually raised. Bone scintigraphy may be of value in osteopetrosis to demonstrate fractures or osteomyelitis, although increased uptake can occur as part of the disease process in the epiphyses and metaphysis of the long bones and spine. Increased activity on the bone scan can also be visualized in fibrous dysplasia where scintigraphy is helpful to assess the full extent of the disease. Where multiple bones are involved, the pattern may resemble metastases. Other conditions that can cause confusion includes Schmorl's nodes in the spine with focal increased uptake, or an interosseous ganglia where there may be increased uptake on all three phases of the bone scan with appearances resem-

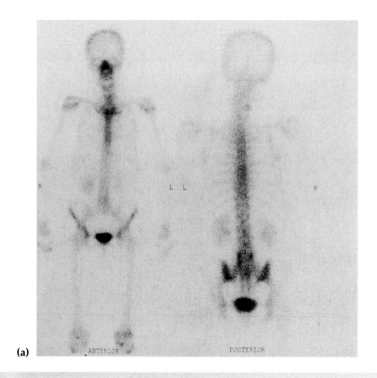

(a)

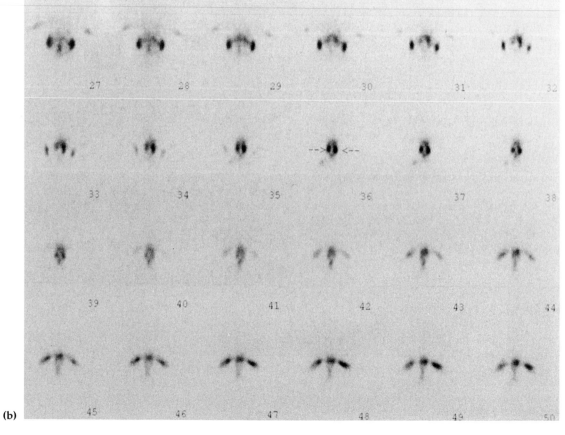

(b)

bling an osteoid osteoma. In osteopoikilosis, the radiographic findings may resemble osteoblastic metastases, but a normal bone scan can be invaluable in excluding the diagnosis.

SPECT

Bone SPECT has proved particularly useful in imaging complex bony structures where it allows the removal of overlying and underlying activity from the areas of interest [56]. The widest applications are in the spine, hips and knees, although other sites such as the skull base, temporomandibular joint, nasal sinuses and mandibular condyles have been usefully imaged. Various studies have shown improved lesion detection and localization. In addition to the improved target-to-background ratio, SPECT also allows display of multiple planes and more specific anatomical mapping. For example, in the spine, a transaxial view enables a separate examination of activity in the vertebral body, pedicle, articular process, pars interarticularis and spinous process. The greatest application of bone SPECT has been in the spine. Several studies have shown improved lesion detection in benign disease, particularly in the posterior elements of a vertebra [57]. Lesion specificity is also improved because of more accurate localization – for example, a lesion localized to the facet joint is almost certainly due to osteoarthritis or a mechanical stress syndrome (Figures 8.23(a,b)). Lesions at this site are not found with metastases, fracture or discitis [58]. Specific applications of bone SPECT in the lumbar spine are for detection of symptomatic spondylolysis and occult fracture which can then provide a guide to therapy [59]. In young people with stress fractures of the pars interarticularis, if there is uptake on SPECT, they will heal by conservative treatment, but if SPECT is negative, operative repair is required.

Bone SPECT is also useful in detection of facet syndrome to enable selection of patients for corticosteroid injection or radiofrequency denervation [60]. It is also valuable in the diagnosis of back pain following lumbar fusion. In patients with underlying malignancy and only one or two spinal lesions on bone scan, a SPECT study can help distinguish a benign from a malignant process. The other major applications are imaging the hips and knees. Avascular necrosis of the hips shows improved specificity with SPECT, as discussed earlier [61]. However, other artefacts such as severe degenerative change in the acetabulum producing an apparent ring of activity in the femoral head may on occasion cause confusion. SPECT imaging of the knees is valuable for the detection of meniscal tears (Figure 8.24), but can also be useful for the detection of ligament injuries (e.g. anterior cruciate ligament, posterior cruciate ligament and collateral ligament tears) [62,63] and avascular necrosis. SPECT is also valuable for the detection of disease within the patellofemoral compartment, e.g. chondromalacia patellae, osteochondritis, avascular necrosis and stress lesions such as jumper's knee. In the skull, SPECT has been shown to be successful in identifying skull base involvement in nasopharyngeal carcinoma when it is superior to planar imaging [64] and also for the detection of necrotizing otitis externa [65].

QUANTITATIVE MEASUREMENT

Bisphosphonate uptake in the skeleton reflects metabolic activity. In situations of diffusely altered skeletal metabolism, slight increases in bisphosphonate uptake will not be apparent from subjectively examining the bone scan images. Bisphosphonate uptake is a measure of skeletal metabolism and, if accurately quantified, can be of clinical value. Such techniques have been mostly applied in the field of metabolic bone disease, although there is also some limited evidence of value in more focal conditions to assess clinical response.

LOCAL MEASUREMENT

Uptake of bisphosphonate can be quantified in focal disease with the count-rate in an area-of-interest compared with that in adjacent soft tissue or normal bone. An uptake ratio is therefore obtained rather than an absolute count-rate. Uptake ratios are obtained from computerized bone scan images most often by drawing a region-of-interest around the areas being studied or by obtaining a count profile across the area. The region-of-

Figure 8.23 (a) Planar scan demonstrating increased uptake lumbar spine bilaterally L4/5 and left L5/S1. (b) SPECT shows marked uptake in facet joints (arrowed).

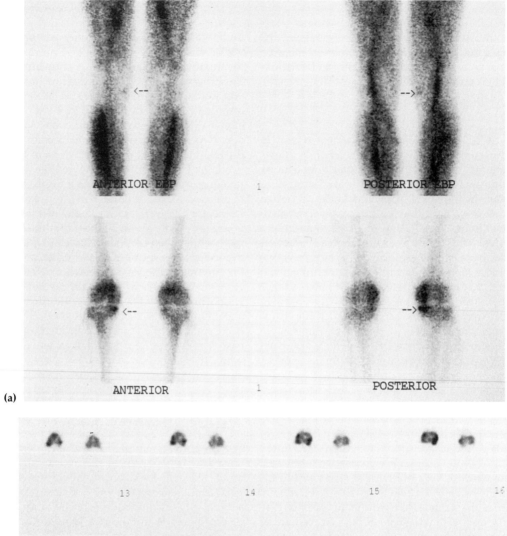

(a)

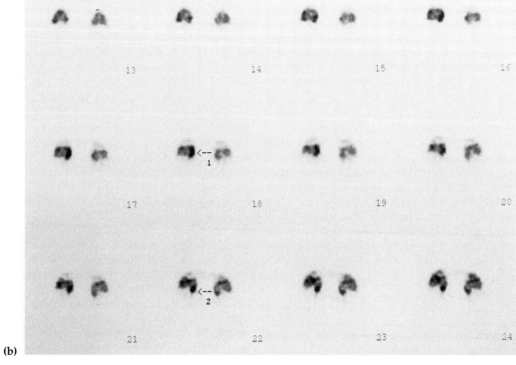

(b)

interest technique has been used successfully in Paget's disease particularly in measuring response to therapy in patients with a normal serum alkaline phosphatase before treatment [65]. Count profiles have been used for example to detect sacroiliitis (see earlier).

WHOLE-BODY MEASUREMENT

The most commonly employed technique is to measure the 24-hour whole-body retention (WBR) of technetium-labelled bisphosphonates, which is a sensitive means of identifying increased bone turnover in a variety of metabolic bone disorders [66]. This is the most sensitive method for assessing total skeletal metabolism, as the whole skeleton rather than a small area is used. The method is based on the theory that, while most of the injected bisphosphonate is taken up by the skeleton, the remainder is excreted by the urinary tract. Thus, by 24 hours after injection, most of the soft tissue activity has been excreted and the great majority of bisphosphonate remaining in the body is within the skeleton. Small amounts of ^{99m}Tc-bisphosphonate can be injected, and by using a whole-body counter, the activity following injection and at 24 hours is obtained. WBR is only valid as an index of skeletal metabolism in the presence of normal renal function. It has no role to play in the presence of renal osteodystrophy [67]. An elevated WBR is diagnostic of altered skeletal metabolism, but is non-specific and can be found in osteomalacia, Paget's disease and primary hyperparathyroidism. Most patients with osteoporosis have normal values of WBR, although in some it is raised and it is possible that WBR could have a role in identifying high-turnover disease in the future.

An indirect method of quantification is provided by measuring the bone clearance of bisphosphonate by the ^{51}Cr-EDTA / ^{99m}Tc-MDP ratio. This relies on the assumption that ^{51}Cr-EDTA is cleared only by the kidneys, whereas ^{99m}Tc-MDP

is removed from the plasma both by renal excretion and bone uptake. Thus, by injecting a combination of both radiopharmaceuticals and measuring the ratio of the two in a single plasma sample (at 4 h), an indirect measure of bone uptake can be obtained [68]. This technique has been carefully applied in Paget's disease to assess the therapeutic dose of pamidronate needed to suppress biochemical markers [69,70].

MEASUREMENT OF BONE MASS

There is a wide variety of non-invasive techniques available for the measurement of bone mass. Some, such as radiogrammetry and radiographic photodensitometry, are now virtually obsolete due to poor precision and being confined to the peripheral skeleton. Others, such as neutron activation analysis, have failed to find widespread implementation due to high cost and technical complexity. Until comparatively recently, the most widely available techniques were those of single-photon absorptiometry (SPA) and dual-photon absorptiometry (DPA). However, these have mostly been superseded by dual X-ray absorptiometry (DXA) and transmission quantitative computerized tomography (QCT). The clinical utility of bone mass measurements has increased rapidly in the recent years, as their application in the management of osteoporosis has become clear. The measurement of bone mass has long been within the scope of nuclear medicine – since the development of photon absorptiometry and many nuclear medicine departments today continue to perform bone densitometry using the newer X-ray-based techniques.

SPA, still performed in some centres, was first described by Cameron and Sorenson [71] and involves measuring the transmission of a mono-energetic photon beam generated by an ^{125}I source through bone and soft tissue. The low photon energy enables maximum contrast between bone and soft tissue to be achieved, but unfortunately the attenuation of the beam limits the use of the technique to appendicular body sites. The total thickness of soft tissue has to be constant over the scanning path, which is achieved by surrounding the limb with soft tissue equivalent (a water bath). Given that the attenuation of the beam within the bone is exponential, bone mass can be computed. Modern instruments incorporate automatic detection of the width of the inter-osteo

Figure 8.24 (a) Increased blood pool and delayed activity of the right medial joint line, in a patient with a medical meniscal tear. (b) SPECT shows a crescent of uptake medial tibial plateau (1) and focal posterior femoral condyle activity (2); these are typical findings in a meniscal tear.

space between the radius and the ulna and regions-of-interest are positioned and scanned in relation to some selected value (e.g. 8 mm gap). In general, most authors report that accuracies of 4–5% and precision of 1–2%.

Dual-photon absorptiometry developed in the late 1970s allowed measurement of bone mass at the clinically more important sites of spine and hip. In order to overcome the problem of variable soft tissue thickness, the commercial instruments incorporated gadolinium-153 as the radiation source because its energy spectrum has discrete emissions of 44 and 100 keV. Simultaneous transmission measurements are made at the two energies and the thickness of soft tissue and the amount of bone mineral in the beam path can then be computed. This technique does not demand constant soft tissue thickness. A determination of bone mineral density is made by point-by-point scanning of the region-of-interest and estimating the total bone mineral content by summation. Scanning data collection and processing are controlled by microcomputer. A bone edge-detection algorithm is used to define bone and soft tissue. Although the technique measures aerial density, it closely correlates with volumetric density. The accuracy of DPA is around 3–6% for the spine (short-term precision around 2%) and 3–4% for the femoral neck [72].

The most recent advance in absorptiometry has been the introduction of DXA. This technique uses an X-ray tube rather than a radionuclide source to produce the photon beam. X-rays of two photon energies are generated either by rapid switching of a generator voltage between the high and low keV in synchrony with the mains supply, or by using a constant potential generator with a rare earth filter with a K absorption edge of around 45 keV. The latter splits the polyenergetic X-ray spectrum into high- and low-energy components. The X-ray tube produces a much higher photon flux than gadolinium-153, enabling the radiation beam to be highly collimated and resulting in high-resolution images and consequent improved precision, scanning times and reduced radiation dose. The expense of regular replacement of the gadolinium-153 source is also obviated. DXA has now largely replaced DPA and become the most widely used technique for measurement of bone mass in the UK. In addition to being able to measure spine and hip, DXA scanners can be used to measure forearm, lateral spine and total body images. Software is also available to measure hand bone density and bone mass around prostheses [73].

QCT can also be used for the measurement of bone mass, although this is less widely available than DXA. Most measurements are performed at the spine where tomographic imaging techniques allow spatial separation of the cortical and metabolically more active trabecular bone. Peripheral sites are now starting to be imaged with QCT, although this is not widely undertaken in the UK. QCT also requires a higher radiation dose than DXA [74].

Ultrasound has received a great deal of recent interest. Most devices measure the ultrasonic attenuation and speed of sound at the heel. However, ultrasound is now also being applied to other sites such as the patella, tibia and fingers. The technique has the advantage of equipment that is cheap, portable and does not cause exposure to radiation, but unfortunately is unable to be used at the sites of greatest clinical interest, i.e. the spine and hip. In addition, bone density measurements of these sites directly remain superior for the assessment of risk of spinal and hip fractures. There is some evidence that ultrasound can provide information on bone quality as well as bone mass, but this remains subject to controversy [75].

Bone densitometry is now widely used to assess the risk of osteoporotic fractures [76]. Bone strength has been shown to correlate strongly with bone mass. There have been a large number of prospective studies demonstrating the predictive value of bone density measurements for osteoporotic fractures. Early data emerged from forearm measurements, but more recent studies of spine and hip measurements show more powerful predictive power for bone density than previously realized. Bone mass is normally distributed in the population, and cut-off values that determine whether osteoporosis is present are arbitrary. However, for practical purposes a bone mass of more than 2.5 standard deviations below the mean values for the young adults (T < 2.5) is widely used to define osteoporosis. This cut-off will include the majority of patients who will fracture. This value, however, only applies to Caucasian women and it is not clear at present whether such cut-off values can be applied to men and individuals of other races [77].

The risk of fracture approximately doubles for every standard deviation decrease in bone mass. This knowledge enables patients with conditions predisposing to osteoporosis to be detected early and advice on prophylactic therapy to be given. There are a large number of predisposing factors to osteoporosis, including oestrogen deficiency, family history of osteoporosis, use of oral corticosteroids, and a wide variety of other conditions such as malabsorption, chronic inflammatory diseases, hypogonadism and myeloma. Whether bone density should be used for whole population screening is controversial and at present is not advocated.

Bone mass measurements are also used in diagnosis. In clinical practice it is important to establish whether osteoporosis has developed and whether a fracture is due to osteoporosis or some other cause. The detection of a sufficiently low bone mass to produce osteoporotic fractures is therefore an important contribution to present day management. Bone density is also widely used to evaluate X-ray-identified osteopenia and establish its severity, as X-rays are poorly discriminatory for osteoporosis and lack a quantitative analysis. Bone density is also valuable for clinical management to assess the severity of disease and also to monitor the effect of therapy. The most widely used osteoporosis therapies, such as hormone replacement therapy and the bisphosphonates, are largely resorption inhibitors, and in most patients produce a modest rise in bone mass, particularly at the spine. This can be detected with repeat bone mass measurements. Some patients appear not to respond to these types of therapies and this can be detected at an early stage with bone densitometry. Recently, it has been realized that other factors are important in determining the risk of fracture such as hip axis length, bone turnover as assessed by biochemical markers, and the propensity to fall. However, these factors are less powerful than measurement of bone mass, which will continue to be widely used as the best indicator of fracture risk.

REFERENCES

1. Fogelman, I. (1980) Skeletal uptake of bisphosphonate: a review. *Eur. J. Nucl. Med.*, **3**, 224–5.
2. Alazraki, N., Dries, F., Datz, F., Lawrence, P., Greenberg, E. and Taylor, A., Jr. (1985) Value of 24 hour image (Four phase bone scan) in assessing osteomyelitis in patients with peripheral vascular disease. *J. Nucl. Med.*, **26**, 711–17.
3. Pistenna, D.A., McDougall, I.R. and Kriss, J.P. (1975) Screening for bone metastases: are only scans necessary? *JAMA*, **231**, 46–50.
4. Constable, A.R., and Cranage, R.W. (1981) Recognition of the super scan in prostatic bone scintigraphy. *Br. J. Radiol.*, **54**, 122–6.
5. Evan Sapir, E., Martin, R.H., Barnes, D.C., Pringle, C.P., Iles, S.F. and Mitchell, M.J. (1993) Role of SPECT in differentiating malignant from benign lesions in the lower thoracic and lumbar vertebrae. *Radiology*, **187**, 193–8.
6. Gosfield, E., Alavi, A. and Kneeland, B. (1993) Comparison of radionuclide bone scans and MRI in the detection of spinal metastases. *J. Nucl. Med.*, **34**, 2191–8.
7. Cunningham, D. (1995) Other imaging in bony metastases. *Nucl. Med. Commun.*, **16**, 313–16.
8. Van Schelven, W.D. and Pauwels, E.K.J. (1994) The flare phenomenon; far from fair and square. *Eur. J. Nucl. Med.*, **21**, 377–80.
9. Guan, L.S., Hwang, W.S. and Shan, W.L. (1990) The differential diagnosis of benign from malignant bony lesions in bone scanning using the ratio of uptake at different times. *Clin. Nucl. Med.*, **6**, 424–7.
10. Coleman, R.E., Rubens, R.P. and Fogelman, I. (1988) Reappraisal of the baseline bone scan in breast cancer. *J. Nucl. Med.*, **29**, 1045–9.
11. McKillop, J.H., Blumgart, L.H., Wood, C.B. *et al.* (1978) The prognostic and therapeutic implications of the positive radionuclide bone scan in clinically early breast cancer. *Br. J. Surg.*, **65**, 649–52.
12. Lund, F., Smith, P.J. and Suciu, S. (1984) Do bone scans predict prognosis in prostatic cancer. *Br. J. Urol.*, **56**, 58–63.
13. Chybowski, F.M., Keller, J.J., Bergstralh, E.J. *et al.* (1991) Predicting radionuclide bone scan findings in patients with newly diagnosed untreated prostate cancer. Prostate specific antigen is superior to all other clinical parameters. *J. Urol.*, **145**, 313–18.
14. Leo, M.E., Bilhartz, D.L., Bergstralh, E.J. *et al.* (1991) Prostate specific antigen in hormonally treated stage 2 prostate cancer. Is it an accurate indication of disease status? *J. Urol.*, **145**, 802–6.
15. Knuchan, G., Grieves, G., Lopez Majano, V. *et al.* (1991) Bone scan as a stratification variable in advanced prostate cancer. *Cancer*, **68**, 316–20.
16. Rudoni, M., Anronini, G., Farro, M. *et al.* (1993) The clinical value of prostate specific antigen and bone scintigraphy in the staging of patients with newly diagnosed pathologically proven prostate cancer. *Eur. J. Nucl. Med.*, **22**, 207–11.
17. Graventein, S., Peltz, M.A. and Poreis, W. (1979) How ominous is an abnormal scan in bronchogenic carcinoma? *JAMA*, **241**, 2523–4.
18. Wahner, H.W., Kyle, R.A. and Beebout, J.W. (1980) Scintigraphic evaluation of the skeleton in multiple myeloma. *Mayo Clin. Proc.*, **55**, 232–6.
19. Goldstein, H., McNeil, B.J., Zufall, E. and Treves, S. (1980) Is there still a place for bone scanning in Ewing's sarcoma? *J. Nucl. Med.*, **21**, 10–12.

20. Piccolo, S., Lastoria, S., Mainolfi, C., Muto, P., Bazzicalupo, L. and Salvatore, M. (1995) Technetium 99m methylene disphosphonate scintomammography to image primary breast cancer. *J. Nucl. Med.*, **36**, 718–24.

21. Caluner, C.I., Abdel-Dayem, H.M., Macapinlac, H.A. *et al.* (1994) The value of thallium and three-phase bone scans in the evaluation of bone and soft tissue sarcomas. *Eur. J. Nucl. Med.*, **21**, 1198–205.

22. Lichenstein, L. (1977) *Bone Tumours*, 5th edn, Mosby, St Louis.

23. Weeks, R.G., Miller, J.H. and Sty, J.R. (1987) Scintigraphic pattern in osteoid osteoma and spondylolysis. *Clin. Nucl. Med.*, **12**, 39.

24. Matin, P. (1979) The appearance of bone scans following fractures, including immediate and long term studies. *J. Nucl. Med.*, **20**, 1227–31.

25. Spitz, J., Louner, I., Tittal, K. and Weigard, H. (1993) Scintimetric evaluation of remodelling of the bone fractures in man. *J. Nucl. Med.*, **34**, 1403–9.

26. Matin, P. (1983) Bone scintigraphy in the diagnosis and management of traumatic injury. *Semin. Nucl. Med.*, **13**, 104–22.

27. Gunalp, B., Ozguven, M., Oztrak, E. and Bayhan, H. (1992) Role of bone scanning in the management of non-united fractures: a clinical study. *Eur. J. Nucl. Med.*, **19**, 845–7.

28. Park, H.M., Kernek, C.B. and Robb, J.A. (1988) Early scintigraphic findings of occult femoral and tibial fractures in infants. *Clin. Nucl. Med.*, **13**, 271–5.

29. Piepsz, A., Gordon, I. and Hahn, K. (1991) Paediatric nuclear medicine. *Eur. J. Nucl. Med.*, **18**, 41–6.

30. Englaro, E.E., Gelfand, M.J. and Paliel, H.J. (1992) Bone scintigraphy in preschool children with lower extremity pain of unknown origin. *J. Nucl. Med.*, **33**, 351–4.

31. Minkel, J., Sty, J. and Simons, F. (1983) Segmental radionuclide imaging in avascular paediatric hip conditions. *Clin. Orthopaed.*, **175**, 202–8.

32. Park, H.M., Terman, S.A., Ridolfo, A.S. and Wellman, H.N. (1977) A quantitative evaluation of rheumatoid arthritis activity with Tc99m HEDP. *J. Nucl. Med.*, **18**, 973–6.

33. Mottonen, T.T., Hannannen, P., Toivanen, J. *et al.* (1988) Value of joint scintigraphy in the prediction of erosiveness in early rheumatoid arthritis. *Ann. Rheum. Dis.*, **47**, 183–9.

34. Van der Lubbe, P.A.H.M., Arndtt, J.W., Calame, W. *et al.* (1991) Measurement of synovial inflammation in rheumatoid arthritis with technetium 99m labelled human polyclonal immunoglobulin. *Eur. J. Nucl. Med.*, **18**, 119–23.

35. de Bois, M.H.W., Westedt, M.L., Arndt, J.W. *et al.* (1995) Technetium 99m labelled polyclonal human immunoglobulin G scintigraphy before and 26 weeks after initiation of parenteral gold treatment in patients with rheumatoid arthritis. *J. Rheumatol.*, **22**, 1461–5.

36. de Bois, M.H.W., Tak, P.P., Arndt, J.W. *et al.* (1995) Joint scintigraphy for quantification of synovitis with 99mTc labelled human immunoglobulin G compared to histologic examination. *Clin. Exp. Rheumatol.*, **13**, 155–9.

37. de Bois, M.H.W., Welling, M.L., Vewey, C.L. *et al.* (1996) Tc99m HIG accumulates in the synovial tissues of rats with adjuvant arthritis by binding to extra cellular matrix proteins. *Nucl. Med. Commun.*, **17**, 54–9.

38. Dieppe, P., Cushnaghan, J., Young, P. and Kirwan, J. (1993) Prediction of the progression of joint space narrowing in osteoarthritis of the knee by bone scintigraphy. *Ann. Rheum. Dis.*, **52**, 567–63.

39. Ryan, P.J. and Fogelman, I. (1993) Sacroiliac quantitative bone scintigraphy. *Nucl. Med. Commun.*, **14**, 719–20.

40. Ryan, P.J., Chicanza, I., Gibson, T. *et al.* (1995) Single photon emission computed tomography and the source of lumbar pain in advanced ankylosing spondylitis. *J. Clin. Rheumatol.*, **1**, 323–7.

41. Aigner, R.M., Fueger, G.E. and Ritter, G. (1996) Results of three phase bone scintigraphy and radiography in 20 cases of neonatal osteomyelitis. *Nucl. Med. Commun.*, **17**, 20–1.

42. Schauwecher, D.S., Mock, B.H. *et al.* (1984) Evaluation of complicating osteomyelitis with Tc99m MDP, In-111 granulocytes and Ga-67 citrate. *J. Nucl. Med.*, **25**, 849–53.

43. Jacobson, A.F., Gilles, C.P. and Cergueira, M.D. (1992) Photopaenic defects in marrow-containing skeleton on Indium 111 leucocyte scintigraphy. Prevalence at sites of suspected osteomyelitis as an incidental finding. *Eur. J. Nucl. Med.*, **19**, 858–64.

44. Palestro, C.J., Roumanas, P., Kim, C.K. *et al.* (1991) Improved accuracy for diagnosing osteomyelitis using combined In-111 leucocyte and Tc99m sulfur colloid imaging. *J. Nucl. Med.*, **32**, 962–3 (abstract).

45. Ang, E.S., Sundram, F.X., Goh, A.S.W. *et al.* (1993) 99m Tc polyclonal and 99m Tc nanocolloid scans in orthopaedics; a comparison with conventional bone scan. *Nucl. Med. Commun.*, **14**, 419–32.

46. Hotze, A.L., Briele, B. and Overbeck, B. (1992) Technetium 99m labelled antigranulocyte antibodies in suspected bone infection. *J. Nucl. Med.*, **33**, 526–31.

47. Vinjamuri, S., Hall, A.V., Solonki, K. *et al.* (1996) Comparison of 99m Tc infecton imaging with radiolabelled white cell imaging in the evaluation of bacterial infection. *Lancet*, **347**, 233–5.

48. Fogelman, I. and Carr, D. (1980) A comparison of bone scanning and radiology in the evaluation of patients with metabolic bone disease. *Clin. Radiol.*, **31**, 321–6.

49. Ryan, P.J., Evans, P.A., Gibson, T. *et al.* (1992) Osteoporosis and chronic back pain. A study with single photon emission computed bone scintigraphy. *J. Bone Min. Res.*, **7**, 1455–9.

50. Ryan, P.J., Gibson, T. and Fogelman, I. (1992) Bone scintigraphy following Pamidronate therapy for Paget's disease of bone. *J. Nucl. Med.*, **33**, 1589–93.

51. Ryan, P.J. and Fogelman, I. (1994) Five years follow up after Pamidronate therapy. *Br. J. Rheumatol.*, **33**, 98–9.

52. Intenzo, C.M., Wapner, K.L., Park, C.M. *et al.* (1991) Evaluation of plantar faciitis by three phase bone scintigraphy. *Clin. Nucl. Med.*, **15**, 105–6.

53. Alberts, K.A., Dahlborn, M., Glas, C.E. *et al.* (1984) Radionuclide scintigraphy for the diagnosis of com-

plications following femoral neck fractures. *Acta Orthop. Scand.*, **55**, 606–11.

54. Atkins, R.M., Tindale, W. and Bickerstaff, D. (1993) Quantitative bone scintigraphy in reflex sympathetic dystrophy. *Br. J. Rheumatol.*, **32**, 41–5.

55. Rubello, D., Borsato, N. and Chierichetti, F. (1995) Three phase bone scintigraphy pattern of loosening in uncemented hip prosthesis. *Eur. J. Nucl. Med.*, **22**, 299–301.

56. Ryan, P.J. (1994) SPECT bone scanning in the 1990s. *Appl. Radiol.*, **5**, 30–7.

57. Ryan, P.J., Fogelman, I. and Gibson, T. (1992) The identification of spinal pathology in chronic back pain using single photon emission computed tomography. *Nucl. Med. Commun.*, **13**, 497–502.

58. Rees, D., Mayer, P. and Crine, J.S. (1995) Assessment and treatment of stress fractures of the lumbar spine in elite young sports people. *Nucl. Med. Commun.*, **16**, 230–1.

59. Dolan, A., Ryan, P., Arden, N. *et al.* (1995) SPECT scanning can predict successful facet joint injection. *Br. J. Rheumatol.*, **34**, 71.

60. Collier, B.D., Carrera, G.F. and Johnson, R.P. (1985) Detection of femoral head avascular necrosis in adults by SPECT. *J. Nucl. Med.*, **26**, 929.

61. Ryan, P.J., Taylor, M., Grevitt, M. *et al.* (1995) Bone SPECT in recent meniscal tears 'An assessment of diagnostic criteria'. *Eur. J. Nucl. Med.*, **20**, 703–7.

62. Cook, G.J.R., Ryan, P.J., Clarke, S.E.M. *et al.* (1995) Anterior cruciate ligamental tear. Findings on SPECT bone scintigraphy of the knee. *Nucl. Med. Commun.*, **16**, 231.

63. Lee, C.H., Wang, P.-W., Chen, H.-Y. *et al.* (1995) Assessment of skull bone involvement in nasopharyngeal carcinoma. Comparison of single photon emission tomography with planar bone scintigraphy and X-ray computed tomography. *Eur. J. Nucl. Med.*, **22**, 514–20.

64. Hardoff, R., Gips, S., Uri, N. *et al.* (1994) Semiquantitative skull planar and SPECT bone scintigraphy in diabetic patients. Differentiation of necrotising (malignant) external otitis from severe external otitis. *J. Nucl. Med.*, **35**, 411–15.

65. Patel, S., Pearson, D. and Hosking, D.J. (1995) Quantitative bone scintigraphy in the management of monostatic Paget's disease of bone. *Arthritis Rheum.*, **38**, 1506–12.

66. Fogelman, I., Bessent, R.G., Turner, J.G., Citrin, D.L., Boyle, I.T. and Greig, R.G. (1978) The use of whole body retention of Tc99m disphosphonate in the diagnosis of metabolic bone disease. *J. Nucl. Med.*, **19**, 270–5.

67. Fogelman, I. and Bessent, R.G. (1982) Age-related alterations in skeletal metabolism; 24 hour whole body retention of disphosphonate in 250 normal

subjects: concise communication. *J. Nucl. Med.*, **23**, 296–300.

68. Nisbet, A.P., Edwards, S. and Lazarus, C.R. (1984) Chromium 51 EDTA/technetium 99m MDP plasma ratio to measure total skeletal function. *Br. J. Radiol.*, **57**, 667–80.

69. Evans, A., Pertiun, A., Wastie, M., Stone, M. and Hosking, D. (1991) The disphosphonate space: a useful quantitative index of disease activity in patients undergoing hexamethylene disphosphonate (HMPD) bone imaging for Paget's disease. *Eur. J. Nucl. Med.*, **18**, 757–9.

70. Stone, M.D., Marshall, D.H., Hosking, D.J., Perkin, A.C., Evans, A.J. and Wastie, M.L. (1992) Bisphosphonate space measurement in Paget's disease of bone treated with APD. *J. Bone Min. Res.*, **7**, 295–301.

71. Cameron, J.R. and Sorenson, J. (1963) Measurement of bone mineral in vivo: an improved method. *Science*, **142**, 230–2.

72. Wahner, H.W., Dunn, W.L. and Riggs, B.L. (1983) Non invasive bone mineral measurements. *Semin. Nucl. Med.*, **13**, 282–9.

73. Genant, H.K., Engelke, K., Fuerst, T. *et al.* (1996) Non-invasive assessment of bone mineral and structure: state of the art. *J. Bone Min. Res.*, **6**, 707–30.

74. Yu, W., Glucer, C.C., Grampp, S., Jergas, M., Feurst, T., Wu, C.Y., Lu, Y., Far, B. and Genant, H.K. (1995) Spinal bone mineral assessment in post menopausal women: a comparison between dual X-ray absorptiometry and quantitative computed tomography. *Osteoporosis Int.*, **5**, 433–9.

75. Herd, R.J.M., Ramalingham, T., Ryan, P.J., Blake, G.M. and Fogelman, I. (1992) Measurement of broad band ultrasound attenuation in the calcaneum in pre and post menopausal women. *Osteoporosis Int.*, **2**, 247–51.

76. Compston, J.F., Cooper, C. and Kanis, J.A. (1995) Bone densitometry in clinical practice. *Br. Med. J.*, **310**, 1507–10.

77. Kanis, J.A., Devogelaer, J.P. and Gerrari, C. (1996) Practical guide for the use of bone mineral measurements in the assessment of treatment of osteoporosis: a position paper of the European foundation for osteoporosis and bone disease. *Osteoporosis Int.*, **6**, 256–61.

FURTHER READING

Ryan, P.J. and Fogelman, I. (1994) The role of nuclear medicine in orthopaedics. *Nucl. Med. Commun.*, **15**, 341–60.

Ryan, P.J. and Fogelman, I. (1995) The bone scan: where are we now? *Semin. Nucl. Med.*, **XXV**(2), 76–91.

CHAPTER 9

Neuropsychiatric

Tracers

L. S. Pilowsky

INTRODUCTION

Imaging with radiolabelled tracers has revolutionized our understanding of brain chemistry, blood flow and metabolism. These powerful techniques now allow testing of neurochemical and clinical hypotheses in living human subjects.

Two main strategies have been developed for functional imaging of the CNS. The first evaluates cerebral blood flow (CBF) or metabolism, and assumes that these parameters are tightly coupled to and, thus reflect, neuronal activity [1]. These studies may be performed in the resting state or following some intervention designed to activate the cortex in a particular fashion (e.g. visual stimulation of the occipital cortex or regional cerebral activation by drug challenge). The second strategy estimates brain chemistry directly: for example, by imaging of receptors located on nerve-cell surfaces and neurotransmitter reuptake sites, and measurement of neurotransmitter or amino acid uptake and breakdown rates.

Both strategies are important research tools. Blood flow and metabolism studies have transferred most successfully to the clinical arena, but the neurochemical studies are catching up and are beginning to demonstrate clinical usefulness in some disorders (e.g. epilepsy and movement disorders).

This chapter will focus mainly on the use of tracers to measure neurochemical parameters, specifically using the positron emission tomography (PET) and single-photon emission computed tomography (SPECT) techniques. These methods follow similar physical and mathematical principles (detection and mapping the path of injected radiolabelled tracers in the brain), and evidence is accumulating to suggest data obtained by either method is highly correlated [2,3].

IMAGING BLOOD FLOW AND METABOLISM

Cerebral function is supported primarily by oxidative metabolism. As the brain is unable to store either oxygen or glucose, it is thought that regional blood flow is continuously regulated to supply those substrates locally. In 1980, Roy and Sherrington [4] were the first to propose that the blood supply changes in response to alterations in the level of functional activity. Subsequently, many studies of cerebral glucose utilization and blood flow in animal and human models have supported this notion [5–7]. Importantly, it is recognized that local variations in neuronal activity are closely mirrored by altered regional blood supply. The capacity of the radionuclide tracers to measure this function *in vivo* opens the way to understanding of the brain function in health and disease.

Tracers for blood flow imaging can be grouped into two main categories: (i) those that remain intravascular; and (ii) those that diffuse into

Clinical Nuclear Medicine, 3rd edn. Edited by M.N. Maisey, K.E. Britton and B.D. Collier. Published in 1998 by Chapman & Hall, London. ISBN 0 412 75180 1

cerebral tissue. Substances suitable for either method should be affordable, non-toxic, metabolically inert, and remain physiologically and biochemically stable without any intrinsic effect(s) on blood flow or any other relevant parameter during the period of the study [8].

XENON

In 1948, Kety and Schmidt [9] developed the first paradigm for measuring CBF in humans by using the inert gas nitrous oxide, measured in a peripheral artery and the jugular vein. By applying Fick's method for calculating cardiac output from arterial–venous differences in O_2 and CO_2 concentration, whole-brain blood flow could be estimated. Subsequent researchers modified the technique to obtain indices of regional cerebral blood flow (rCBF) by intracarotid bolus injection of a radioactive inert gas (^{85}Kr) and recording its clearance rate by using an external radiation detector [10]. Later, with the introduction of the ^{133}Xe inhalation rCBF technique [11], this simple and inexpensive method entered into wide use.

^{133}Xe permits quantification of rCBF, and due to its rapid washout, it is possible to perform several studies in a single session. However, its use is complicated by several factors including contamination by extracerebral areas, recirculation of the isotope, difficulty in maintaining a reliable gas-tight seal and problems in imaging deep cortical structures [8]. When fast-rotating detector systems became available, the ^{133}Xe technique was adapted [12], but its rapid washout and poor imaging properties prevented high-resolution imaging.

RCBF TRACERS FOR SPECT

The development of tracers that are retained in brain tissue overcame many problems associated with the use of xenon. These tracers are invariably small and highly lipophilic molecules, which cross the blood–brain barrier in proportion to blood flow [13]. A high extraction efficiency and retention in the brain with fixed distribution permit reliable image acquisition. Tracers that exhibit these characteristics (in order of development) include ^{123}I-IMP (*N*-alpha-methylethyl-*p*-iodoamphetamine), ^{99m}Tc-HMPAO (hexamethyl-propyleneamineoxime) and ^{99m}Tc-ECD (ethylene-cysteine-dimer); Table 9.1 outlines

the characteristics of each ligand. In general, relative or semi-quantification of rCBF is performed in SPECT by normalizing regional signals to whole brain.

The compound HMPAO, a demethylated derivative of the lipophilic amine PnAO, is capable of carrying ^{99m}Tc across the intact blood–brain barrier. Following this, it is rapidly converted to a less-lipophilic form, becomes trapped in the brain and remains in a stable distribution for many hours. Thus a 'freeze-frame' image of blood flow corresponding to the time of injection can be imaged several hours later, with negligible loss of cerebral activity except through physical decay of the isotope [13]. The major advantage of technetium-labelled tracers is the economy and simplicity of production of the radioisotope by generators available in nuclear medicine departments [14]. Further novel tracers are under development, including ^{99m}Tc-ECD, which is now commercially available (see Table 9.1).

PET CEREBRAL BLOOD FLOW AND METABOLISM TRACERS

Methods used to study rCBF by PET are based on the principles of inert freely diffusible tracers [15]. $H_2^{15}O$ is most extensively used, and is administered in several forms including bolus injection and constant infusion or inhalation of $C^{15}O_2$. The very short half-life (2 min) of ^{15}O allows rapid and repeated rCBF mapping in the same individual. Absolute quantification of rCBF may also be performed by PET. It is also possible to compute regional cerebral oxygen metabolism after injection of $^{15}O_2$ by combining measures of rCBF with the oxygen extraction fraction (by the tissues from the arterial blood) [16]. Measurement of brain glucose metabolism is obtained by ^{18}F-fluorodeoxyglucose PET (FDG-PET). After injection, ^{18}F-FDG crosses the blood–brain barrier, is transported into most cells by facilitated diffusion, phosphorylated to FDG-6-PO$_4$, and trapped intracellularly [17]. The tracer has been used to image the brain in many neurological and psychiatric disorders, and for the study of cerebral tumours. Due to its longer half-life (109.6 min), it is less suitable than ^{15}O for multiple or serial studies in the same individual, and so is less applied to cognitive activation experiments with PET. Though the resolution obtained with ^{15}O is slightly lower than that with ^{18}F-FDG, it

Table 9.1 SPECT rCBF tracers

Tracer	Physical Half-life	Administration	Usual dose	Advantages	Drawbacks
[133]Xe	5–6 days	Inhalatory or intravenous	110–250 MBq/l or 350–750 MBq (i.v.)	• Inexpensiveness • ready availability • quantitation possible • multiple scans in one session possible	• poor physical properties • poor spatial resolution • high incidence of artifacts
^{123}I-IMP	13 hours	Intravenous	110–185 MBq	• high brain uptake	• expensiveness • cyclotron needed • tracer not readily available • long half-life • radiation doses have to be limited • early tracer redistribution (1 hour post injection) • absolute quantitation not possible
^{99m}Tc-HMPAO	6 hours	Intravenous	500–600 MBq	• inexpensiveness • ready availability • high brain uptake • distribution stable for several hours	• unstable *in vitro* • rCBF underestimation in highly perfused areas • absolute quantitation not possible
^{99m}Tc-ECD	6 hours	Intravenous	500–600 MBq	• same as HMPAO plus • rapid blood clearance – good image contrast • rapid renal excretion – low radiation exposure • high stability *in vitro*	• early wash-out from the brain • absolute quantitation not possible • limited data available to date

is felt that rCBF more accurately reflects neural activity than cerebral glucose metabolism.

FDG-PET is mainly useful for studying patterns of cerebral activity associated with stable mental states, or relatively slowly changing pharmacological effects.

IMAGING BRAIN CHEMISTRY WITH TRACERS

RECEPTOR THEORY

In 1878, Langley formulated the concept of 'receptive substances' in the tissues, which mediated drug response [18]. The idea was elaborated by subsequent researchers [19,20] who proposed surface groups on cells that interacted with toxin molecules, and exhibited great chemical specificity in their interactions. These surface groups were named receptors, and through many careful studies, their role was clarified [21]. Receptors are now believed to be protein or glycoprotein macromolecules located on the surface of the cell membrane [20]. Specific neurotransmitters or drugs (called ligands) are

recognized by and bind to these structures (by weak, non-covalent binding), thereby altering their configuration. A cascade of intracellular events mediated by second messenger systems ensue, and may result in flow of currents that affect the physiological response to the drug or neurotransmitter or importantly, the ligand–receptor interaction may have no functional result at all.

IN VIVO RECEPTOR MEASUREMENT

As receptors are the targets of drugs, the ability to measure their density and evaluate the effects of drugs at these sites is crucial. By incubating tissue preparations with the radionuclide-labelled ligand probes (i.e. tracers), the degree and distribution of ligand-binding to receptors was measured by detection of radioactivity emitted by the decaying isotope. The binding of tracers by receptor populations in post-mortem tissue was initially studied using autoradiographic or radioassay techniques. Mathematical or graphical ways of relating the amount of ligand detected in the tissue to the number of receptors available for binding have been reviewed in detail [20,22]. Many of these principles are still being applied very closely to the visualization and measurement of *in vivo* neuroreceptor function using PET and SPECT [23].

After injection, the distribution of the tracer in the brain is detected and mapped by PET and SPECT detectors. In general, areas with high receptor density (i.e. high specific binding to the receptor populations of interest) show relatively longer time-to-peak activity with delayed natural washout, but rapid clearance following a specific displacer (for example, displacement of ^{123}I-IBZM binding to striatal D2 receptors by antipsychotic drugs) (Figure 9.1). Areas with low receptor density (i.e. mainly non-specific binding to blood proteins, capillary walls, fat and connective tissue) show short time-to-peak activity, a rapid natural washout and no effect of displacer on the natural washout rate.

Mathematical modelling of the radioligand uptake and clearance rates during scanning experiments attempt precisely to quantify receptor binding in terms of classical binding parameters, affinity and density (K_d / B_{max}), influx constants, volumes of distribution or specific rate constants [24]. Several assumptions are necessary for these approaches. Methodological problems include: difficulty of correctly assuming that all the photons detected emerge from the region under investigation; suitable attenuation correction; scatter; and correction for volume averaging or partial volume effects [25].

PET AND SPECT TRACERS: GENERAL PRINCIPLES

It is generally agreed that selection of tracers suitable for PET and SPECT imaging is dependent on several factors including ligand specificity, biodistribution, mechanism of ligand binding, blood–brain barrier permeability, ligand metabolism and tracer synthesis [24,26,27].

The ideal ligand would be easily and economically synthesized, show high selectivity and affinity for the targeted receptor, cross the blood–brain barrier with ease, be metabolically stable with a low accumulation of active metabolites, clear rapidly from the non-specific binding sites and the blood pool, and should have no clinical effects at receptor-saturating doses.

Many radioligands have now been prepared and evaluated. Comprehensive reports on the range of synthesized compounds for SPECT and PET are available [15,27,28]. Table 9.2 provides a summary of some of the ligands in fairly wide research or clinical use for a variety of neurotransmitter systems.

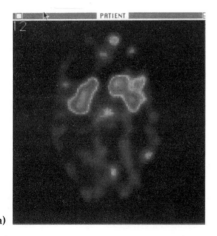

(a)

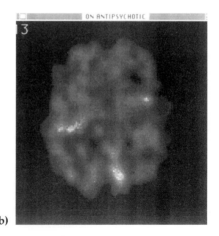

(b)

Figure 9.1 The SPECT images show displacement of ^{123}I-IBZM from dopamine D2 receptors in the striata of a patient receiving typical antipsychotic treatment. (a) The patient is completely free of medication and ^{123}I-IBZM binding to D2 receptors is clearly seen as two 'hot' areas in the striatal regions. (b) The patient is receiving high dose conventional medication (>500 mg chlorpromazine equivalents), there is almost complete blockade of D2 binding by the antipsychotic treatment, ^{123}I-IBZM is displaced from the receptor, and very little signal is seen in striatal regions.

Table 9.2 Some PET and SPECT radioligands in use in human subjects

Neurotransmitter system	PET ligands	SPECT ligands
Cholinergic presynaptic neuron	^{11}C choline	
Nicotinic	^{11}C nicotine	
Muscarinic	^{11}C QNB	^{123}I QNB
	^{11}C dexetimide	^{123}I iododexetimide
Serotonergic		
5HT reuptake transporter	^{11}C β-CIT	^{123}Iβ-CIT
$5HT_{1a}$		
$5HT_{2a}$	^{11}C WAY-100635	
	^{11}C MDL 100907	^{123}I R-91150
	^{18}F altanserin	
	^{18}F setoperone	
	^{11}C NMSP	
Dopaminergic	^{11}C β-CIT and derivatives	^{123}I β-CIT and derivatives
dopamine reuptake site	(CFT)	(CFT)
	^{11}C nomifensine	^{99m}Tc-0-861R
		(technepine)
dopamine synthesis	^{18}F-fluoro-L-DOPA	
D1	^{11}C-SCH 23390	
D2	^{11}C NMSP	^{123}I IBZM
	^{11}C raclopride	^{123}I IBF
	^{11}C epidepride	^{123}I epidepride
GABA/benzodiazepine	^{11}C flumazenil	^{123}I iomazenil
(GABAa/BZ) complex		^{123}I NNC 13-8241
Opioid	^{11}C diprenorphine	
Histamine	^{11}C doxepin	
Somatostatin		^{111}In octreotide

RECEPTOR IMAGING IN DRUG EVALUATION AND DEVELOPMENT

Before the development of PET and SPECT neuroreceptor imaging, the effects of drugs on brain receptors and enzymes in humans had to be deduced from studies in animals or in the test tube. Now it is possible to directly examine the impact of many drugs on the brain. By correlating the physiological effects of drugs at receptors with their behavioural consequences in living subjects, long-held hypotheses of drug action can at last be tested.

FUNCTIONAL IMAGING OF ANTIPSYCHOTIC DRUG ACTION

Many theorists propose, from post-mortem and other indirect research, that antipsychotic drugs (vital in the treatment of major mental illness) act through occupancy of dopamine D2 receptors, since they are potent antagonists of this receptor class [29]. As previously stated, simple blockade of a receptor by an antagonist may have no functional result at all, and to test the hypothesis that antipsychotic drug action is mediated through D2 receptors, functional imaging studies are necessary.

With ^{11}C-raclopride PET, Farde *et al.* [30] indeed confirmed that ten chemically distinct classes of typical antipsychotics occupy striatal D2 receptors (in the range 65–85%), and this was taken as important evidence in support of the D2 blockade hypothesis of antipsychotic drug action. However, to test critically whether striatal D2 occupancy by antipsychotics mediates their clinical efficacy, it is necessary to correlate the degree of blockade with measures of clinical response. Paradoxically, some schizophrenic patients have high levels of D2 blockade on antipsychotics but respond very poorly to the drugs [31,32]. Furthermore, the highly effective antipsychotic drug clozapine had only a 45% occupancy of D2 receptors, and a high level of occupancy of D1 receptors (42%) compared with five other classical antipsychotics. Clozapine also had a decreased propensity to produce parkinsonian side-effects [33]. Pilowsky *et al.* [34], by using ^{123}I-IBZM SPECT, proved that a marked clinical improvement on clozapine (in patients previously unresponsive to typical antipsychotics) was associated with decreased occupancy of D2 receptor binding, and this was quantitatively and qualitatively obvious (Figure 9.1). These findings are the opposite of what would be predicted if the classical D2 blockade hypothesis were correct. Functional imaging has shown that the mode of action of antipsychotic drugs is less clear than was once supposed.

Recent investigations suggest that other receptor systems may also be important in antipsychotic drug action. Nordstrom *et al.* [35] and Nyberg *et al.* [36] showed that clozapine and risperidone have a high occupancy of $5HT_2$ receptors (84–90% and 60% respectively) with ^{11}C-NMSP PET, which may presumably account for the unique treatment profile of clozapine. It is now possible to study $5HT_{2a}$ receptors with more selective ligands, including ^{18}F-setoperone PET [37] and ^{123}I-R91150 SPECT [38]. SPECT with ^{123}I-R91150 demonstrates a relatively high uptake in frontal cortex (a $5HT_{2a}$ receptor-rich area) and washout from cerebellum ($5HT_{2a}$ receptor-poor area) [38].

In vivo probes that are selective for the recently cloned D2 receptor subtypes, D3 and D4 [39,40], are not yet available. These receptors are of very great interest in antipsychotic drug development, given their distribution in the mesolimbic regions, which are clearly disrupted in schizophrenia. Recently, the highly selective D2/D3 receptor antagonist, epidepride has been radiolabelled with ^{123}I for SPECT [41], which images these receptors both in striatal, and in highly relevant extrastriatal brain regions (e.g. temporal cortex, thalamus). Studies have begun to test whether clozapine selectively targets extrastriatal D2 receptor populations, and spares striatal D2 receptors, which could explain its unique clinical profile.

FUNCTIONAL IMAGING OF ANXIOLYTIC/SEDATIVE DRUG ACTION

Benzodiazepines (BZ) are probably the most commonly prescribed class of drugs in psychiatric and general clinical practice, yet the way in which these drugs exert their multiple effects is little un-

derstood. ^{123}I-Iomazenil has been used as a SPECT probe of the BZ receptor to measure occupancy by agonists and antagonists. The potency of these drugs (in terms of the degree of receptor occupancy required to produce a clinical effect) may be evaluated and compared. Innis *et al.* [43] calculated the ED_{50} (the dose of drug required to displace 50% of brain ^{123}I-Iomazenil activity) of BZ agonists and antagonists, and found the following rank order of potency: iomazenil > flumazenil > clonazepam > alprazolam > diazepam. Seibyl *et al.* [42] assessed receptor occupancy of the highly potent BZ lorazepam (by a clinically relevant dose) and showed that at doses which produce sedation in humans, lorazepam occupies <4% of BZ receptors. Receptor imaging has confirmed the massive functional reserve of central GABAergic pathways, in that dramatic physiological effects occur at very low occupancy of receptors by agonists.

PAIN

The neurochemical mechanisms of pain response are being evaluated with PET using the opiate receptor ligand ^{11}C-diprenorphine. Jones *et al.* [44] scanned rheumatoid arthritis patients during a flare-up of their disease and in the pain-free state. Global increases in ^{11}C-diprenorphine binding were found in relation to pain reduction. Specific regional increases over the global activity were noted in the prefrontal, orbital, cingulate and temporal cortices. The hypothesis that inflammatory pain results in production of endogenous opiate peptides is reinforced by these data, which enlightens research into the functional anatomy of pain.

MOVEMENT DISORDERS

Functional imaging of brain chemistry has begun to contribute to the clinical management of movement disorders by assessing the severity of nigrostriatal deterioration, by helping predict response to therapy, and by monitoring of novel therapies including foetal tissue transplants (Table 9.3).

Patterns of nigrostriatal disruption in movement disorder

^{18}F-DOPA uptake into dopaminergic neurones reflects the functional integrity of nigrostriatal

Table 9.3 The use of receptor imaging in Parkinson's disease

Ligand	PET and SPECT findings	Comments
^{18}F-DOPA PET	Decreased binding in caudate and putamen (caudate > putamen)	Correlates with severity of disease, and with asymmetrical severity Can differentiate between movement disorders
[123]I-β-CIT SPET ^{11}C WIN 35428	Decreased putamen and caudate binding	Early prediction of disease and disease staging. Monitoring integrity of foetal transplants
[123]I IBZM SPET ^{11}C raclopride pET	No difference in binding compared with controls Decreased binding after LDOPA treatment, decreased in patients resistant to LDOPA	Prediction of response to LDOPA treatment Can differentiate between movement disorders

dopamine projections. The rate of uptake in living patients correlates with nigral cell counts at necropsy [45]. In sporadic levodopa-responsive Parkinson's disease (PD), a characteristic pattern of striatal ^{18}F-DOPA is seen, consistent with disruption of ventrolateral nigral projections to the putamen, found in Parkinson's tissue at postmortem examination. Putamen uptake is decreased by 40% and caudate 80% of normal [46]. In other disorders – for example, progressive supranuclear palsy (where nigrostriatal projections are uniformly affected) – ^{18}F-DOPA PET shows equally severe loss of uptake in anterior and posterior putamen, and caudate nuclei [47]. Interestingly, correlations are found between movement asymmetries, ^{18}F-DOPA and ^{11}C-nomifensine uptake asymmetries in the putamen, but not the caudate [46]. This suggests a more critical role for the putamen in movement control.

Predictive markers: staging severity of movement disorder

The SPECT and PET pre-synaptic dopamine transporter ligands are sensitive markers for dopaminergic nerve terminals in the striatum. PD patients show loss of pre-synaptic dopamine transporter sites in the caudate and putamen to 20–39% of control values, measured by ^{123}I-β-CIT SPECT [48]; and 48% and 55% decreases in dopamine transporter binding in the anterior and posterior putamen respectively, measured by ^{11}C-WIN 35428 PET [49]. Dopamine transporter ligands may therefore be useful both in diagnosis and in screening populations of 'at-risk' individ-

uals, particularly by SPECT, which is less costly and more widely available. Many more ligands, highly selective for the dopamine transporter, are under investigation, and this may well prove a vitally useful clinical and research tool.

Assessing and predicting response to treatment

The beneficial effects of dopamine agonist treatment for PD are mediated through post-synaptic D2 receptors [50]. In untreated PD, patients have similar D2 binding values to controls as measured by ^{11}C-raclopride PET and ^{123}I-IBZM SPECT [50–52]. Relative up-regulation of putamen D2 receptors in PD has been found contralateral to more affected limbs, though this was not necessarily consistent [53,54]. Levodopa treatment results in a decrease in D2 receptor availability for binding to ^{123}I-IBZM SPECT [52]. Patients with Parkinsonism due to other causes (multiple system atrophy; MSA) show marked reduction in post-synaptic D2 receptors measured by ^{123}I-IBZM SPECT with no overlap compared with controls [55]. This group is also distinguishable from idiopathic PD by the pattern of opioid receptor binding measured by ^{11}C-diprenorphine PET. PD patients show similar values to controls, but MSA patients, in whom loss of enkephalinergic neurones is found at post-mortem, show a significant decrease in binding [56]. Huntington's disease, associated with severe degeneration of the caudate nuclei, shows bilaterally decreased D2 binding [52] and loss of GABAergic binding sites compared with controls [57]. Sawle *et al.* [58] recently combined ^{18}F-DOPA and ^{11}C-raclopride

PET measures in nine patients diagnosed as having PD, and demonstrated post-synaptic D2 receptor up-regulation consequent on diminished pre-synaptic DOPA uptake. One patient did not show this pattern, showing a decrease in both pre- and post-synaptic markers, and later developed MSA.

Therapeutic responsivity can be predicted by assessing the functional status of D2 receptors *in vivo*. This is usually done by examining response to the apomorphine challenge test. In one study, patients with positive responses to apomorphine challenge showed significantly higher striatal D2 binding on ^{123}I-IBZM SPECT than those with a negative outcome. ^{11}C-raclopride PET studies find chronically treated PD patients with fluctuating resistance to levodopa have a uniform reduction in D2 binding sites in caudate and putamen [50,59,60].

MONITORING THERAPEUTIC INTERVENTIONS

Neuroligand PET and SPECT can help to monitor and develop therapeutic interventions. Peripheral decarboxylation of DOPA is a problem in the drug treatment of PD. Ruottinen *et al.* [61] found that peripheral COMT inhibition by drugs such as nitecapone and entacapone increases the bioavailability of ^{18}F-DOPA into the brain. The progress of neural cell transplantation has been monitored by ^{18}F-DOPA PET, and increased uptake of the ligand at the transplant site correlated with clinical improvement [62].

PET and SPECT clearly have a place in the differential diagnosis of movement disorders, in screening at risk individuals, predicting and monitoring response to dopamine agonist treatment, and elucidating neurochemical mechanisms underlying these conditions.

FUTURE DIRECTIONS

Brain PET and SPECT tracer development is moving rapidly. The availability, variety and selectivity of tracers to examine neurochemical systems is perpetually expanding. Novel instrumentation and data analysis greatly enhance information from classical tracer studies and increase the power of these tools accordingly. A tracer for the dopamine transporter labelled with [99mm]Tc has been synthesized [63], and could herald a new era in the

design of more accessible, economic SPECT tracers. Functional magnetic resonance imaging techniques, which can image brain blood flow without recourse to ionizing radiation may supersede PET and SPECT measures of regional cerebral blood flow. There are no such alternatives for neurochemical estimation, and undoubtedly research with PET and SPECT nuclear medicine techniques will continue to define their place in the clinic.

REFERENCES

1. Frackowiack, R.S.J., Lenzi, G.L., Jones, T. and Heather, J.D. (1980) Quantitative measurement of regional cerebral blood flow and oxygen metabolism in man using [15]O and positron emission tomography: theory, procedure and normal values. *J. Comput. Assist. Tomogr.*, **4**, 727–36.
2. Westera, G., Buck, A., Burger, C., Leenders, K.L., von-Schultess, G.K. and Schubiger, A.P. (1996) Carbon-11 and iodine-123 labelled iomazenil: a direct PET-SPET comparison. *Eur. J. Nucl. Med.*, **23**, 5–12.
3. Lasagne, N. (1996) A reappraisal of the relative merits of SPET and PET in the quantitation of neuroreceptors: the advantage of a longer half life (editorial). *Eur. J. Nucl. Med.*, **23**, 1–4.
4. Roy, C.S. and Sherrington, C.S. (1890) On the regulation of the blood supply of the brain, *J. Physiol. Lond*, **11**, 85–100.
5. Raichle, M.E. (1987) Circulatory and metabolic correlates of normal brain function in humans, in *The Nervous System: Higher Functions of the Brain* (ed. F. Plum), American Physiological Society, Bethesda, pp. 643–74.
6. Sokoloff, L. (1981) Localisation of functional activity in the central nervous system by measurement of glucose utilisation with radioactive deoxyglucose. *J. Cereb. Blood Flow Metab.*, **1**, 7–36.
7. Madsen, P.L. (1993) Cerebral blood flow(CBF) and cerebral metabolic rate (CMR) during sleep and wakefulness. *Acta Neurol. Scand. (Suppl.)*, 88.
8. Merrick, M.V. (1994) Xenon, red cell and transit time methods for cerebral blood flow and perfusion reserve measurement, in *Nuclear Medicine in Clinical Diagnosis and Treatment*, vol. 1 (eds I.P.C. Murray and P.J. Ell), Churchill Livingstone, pp. 535–49.
9. Kety, S.S. and Schmidt, C.F. (1948) The nitrous oxide method for the quantitative determination of cerebral blood flow in man; theory, procedure and normal values. *J. Clin. Invest.*, **27**, 107–19.
10. Ingvar, D.H. and Lassen, N.A. (1963) Regional cerebral blood flow of the cerebral cortex determined by 85-krypton. *Acta Physiol. Scand.*, **54**, 325–38.
11. Veall, N. and Mallett, B.L. (1965) The two compartment model using 133Xe inhalation and external counting. *Acta Neurol. Scand.*, **14** (suppl), 83–4, 325–38.
12. Lassen, N.A., Sveindottir, E., Kanno, I., Stokeley, E.M. and Rommer, P. (1972) A fast moving, single

photon emission tomography for regional cerebral blood flow studies in man. *J. Comput. Assist. Tomogr.*, **2**, 661–2.

13. Costa, D.C. (1990) Single Photon Emission Tomography (SPET) with 99Tcm-hexamethyl-propyleneamineoxime (HMPAO) in research and clinical practise – a useful tool. *Vasc. Med. Rev.*, **1**, 179–201.

14. Perkins, A.C. (1995) The nature of nuclear medicine procedures, in *Nuclear Medicine; Science and Safety*, John Libbey & Co. Ltd, pp. 22–47.

15. Maziere, B. and Maziere, M. (1994) PET tracers for brain scanning, in *Nuclear Medicine in Clinical Diagnosis and Treatment*, vol. 1 (eds I.P.C. Murray and P.J. Ell), Churchill Livingstone. pp. 519–21.

16. Herscowitch, P., Mintun, M.A. and Raichle, M.E. (1985) Brain oxygen utilisation measured with oxygen-15 radiotracers and positron emission tomography. *J. Nucl. Med.*, **26**, 416–17.

17. Phelps, M.E., Huang, S.C. and Hoffman, E.J. (1979) Tomographic measurements of local cerebral glucose metabolism in humans with (F-18)-2-fluoro-2-deoxy-D-glucose: validation of method. *Ann. Neurol.*, **6**, 371–88.

18. Langley, J.N. (1878) On the physiology of salivary secretion II. On the mutual antagonism of atropin and pilocarpin having special reference to their relations in the submaxillary gland of the cat. *J. Physiol.*, **1**, 339–69.

19. Erlich, P. (1900) On immunity with special reference to cell life. Croonian Lecture. *Proc. R. Soc. London*, **66**, 424–48.

20. Dean, P.M. (1991) *Molecular Foundations of Drug–Receptor Interaction*, Cambridge University Press, Cambridge.

21. Taylor, P. and Insel, P.A. (1990) Molecular basis of pharmacological selectivity, in *Principles of Drug Action: the Basis of Pharmacology* (eds W.B. Pratt and P. Taylor), Churchill Livingstone, London, pp. 1–103.

22. Kerwin, R.W. and Pilowsky, L.S. (1995) Traditional receptor theory and its application to neuroreceptor measurements in functional imaging. *Eur. J. Nucl. Med.*, **22**, 699–710.

23. Pilowsky, L.S. and Kerwin, R.W. (1994) Nuclear medicine and drug studies in the brain, in *Nuclear Medicine in Clinical Diagnosis and Treatment*, Vol. 1 (eds I.P.C. Murray, P.J. Ell and H.W. Strauss), Churchill Livingstone, London, pp. 629–43.

24. Dolan, R., Bench, C. and Friston, K. (1990) Positron emission tomography in psychopharmacology. *Int. Rev. Psychiatry*, **2**, 427–39.

25. Woods, S.W., Pearsall, H.R., Seibyl, J.P. and Hoffer, P.B. (1991) The Quinn Essay: single photon emission computed tomography in neuropsychiatric disorders, in *The Year Book of Nuclear Medicine* (ed. P.B. Hoffer), Mosby Year Book, St. Louis, XIII–XIVii.

26. Young, A.B., Frey, K.A. and Agranoff, B.W. (1986) Receptor assays, in vitro and in vivo, in *Positron Emission Tomography and Autoradiography: Principles and Applications for the Brain and Heart* (eds M.E. Phelps, J.C. Mazziotta and H.R. Schelbert), Raven Press, New York, pp. 73–113.

27. Stocklin, G. (1992) Tracers for metabolic imaging of brain and heart: radiochemistry and radio-pharmacology. *Eur. J. Nucl. Med.*, **19**, 527–51.

28. Verhoeff, N.P.L.G. (1994) Ligands for neuroreceptor imaging by single photon emission tomography (SPET) or positron emission tomography (PET), in *Nuclear Medicine in Clinical Diagnosis and Treatment*, vol. 1 (eds I.P.C. Murray and P.J. Ell), Churchill Livingstone, London, pp. 483–519.

29. Peroutka, S.J. and Snyder, S.H. (1980) Relationship of neuroleptic drug effects at brain dopamine, serotonin, alpha adrenergic and histamine receptors to clinical potency. *Am. J. Psychiatry*, **137**, 1518–22.

30. Farde, L., Weisel, F.-A., Nordstrom, A.-L. and Sedvall, G. (1989) D1 and D2 dopamine receptor occupancy during treatment with conventional and atypical neuroleptics. *Psychopharmacology*, **99**, S28–31.

31. Pilowsky, L.S., Costa, D.C., Ell, P.J., Murray, R.M., Verhoeff, N.P.L.G. and Kerwin, R.W. (1993) Antipsychotic medication, D2 dopamine receptor blockade and clinical response – a ^{123}I IBZM SPET (single photon emission tomography) study. *Psychol. Med.*, **23**, 791–9.

32. Cambon, H., Baron, J.C., Boulenger, J.P., Loc, C., Zarifian, E. and Maziere, B. (1987) In vivo assay for neuroleptic receptor binding in the striatum. *Br. J. Psychiatry*, **151**, 824–30.

33. Farde, L., Nordstrom, A.L., Wiesel, F.-A. *et al.* (1992) Positron emission tomographic analysis of central D1 and D2 receptor occupancy in patients treated with classical neuroleptics and clozapine. *Arch. Gen. Psychiatry*, **49**, 538–44.

34. Pilowsky, L.S., Costa, D.C., Ell, P.J., Murray, R.M., Verhoeff, N.P.L.G. and Kerwin, R.W. (1992) Clozapine, single photon emission tomography and the D2 dopamine receptor blockade hypothesis of schizophrenia. *Lancet*, **340**, 199–202.

35. Nordstrom, A.-L., Farde, L. and Halldin, C. (1993) High 5HT2 receptor occupancy in clozapine treated patients demonstrated by PET. *Psychopharmacology*, **110**, 365–7.

36. Nyberg, S., Farde, L., Eriksson, L., Halldin, C. and Eriksson, B. (1993) 5HT2 and D2 dopamine receptor occupancy in the living human brain. *Psychopharmacology*, **110**, 265–72.

37. Trichard, C., Paillere-Martinot, M.L., Attar-Levy, D., Recassens, C., Monnet, F., Blin, J. and Martinot, J.L. (1996) 5HT2 receptor measurement in schizophrenia by PET. *Eur. Psychiatry*, **11** (suppl. 4), S232.

38. Busatto, G.F., Pilowsky, L.S., Costa, D.C. *et al.* (1997) Initial evaluation of 123I-5-I-R91150, a selective 5-HT_{2a} ligand for single photon emission tomography (SPET) in healthy human subjects. *Eur. J. Nucl. Med.*, **24**, 119–25.

39. Sokoloff, P., Giros, B., Martres, M.P. *et al.* (1990) Molecular cloning and characterization of a novel dopamine receptor (D3) as a target for neuroleptics. *Nature*, **347**, 146–51.

40. Van Tol, H.H.M., Bunzow, J.R., Guan, H.C., Sunahara, R.K., Seeman, P., Niznik, H.B. and Civelli, O. (1991) Cloning of the gene for a human dopamine

D4 receptor with high affinity for the antipsychotic clozapine. *Nature*, **350**, 610–14.

41. Kessler, R.M., Mason, N.S., Votaw, J.R., De Paulis, T.D., Clanton, J.A., Sib Ansari, M., Schmidt, D.E., Manning, R.G. and Bell, R.L. (1992) Visualisation of extrastriatal dopamine D2 receptors in the human brain. *Eur. J. Pharmacol.*, **223**, 105–7.

42. Seibyl, J., Sybirska, E., Bremner, D. *et al.* (1993) [I-123] Iomazenil SPECT brain imaging demonstrates significant benzodiazepine receptor reserve in human and nonhuman primate brain. *J. Nucl. Med.*, **34**, 102P.

43. Innis, R.B. (1992) Neuroreceptor imaging with SPECT. *J. Clin. Psychiatry*, **53** (suppl. 11), 29–34.

44. Jones, A.K.P., Cunningham, V.J., Ha-Kawa, S. *et al.* (1993) Increases in central opioid receptor binding with relief of inflammatory pain in man demonstrated by PET and [^{11}C]diprenorphine. *J. Cereb. Blood Flow Metab.*, **13** (suppl. 1), S792.

45. Snow, B.J., Tooyama, I., McGeer, E.G. and Calne, D.B. (1993) Premortem [18F] fluorodopa uptake correlates with post-mortem dopaminergic cell counts and striatal dopamine in humans. *J. Cereb. Blood Flow Metab.*, **13** (suppl. 1), S251.

46. Leenders, K.L., Salmon, E.P., Tyrrell, P., Perani, D., Brooks, D.J., Sager, H., Jones, T., Marsden, C.D. and Frackowiack, R.S.J. (1990) The nigrostriatal dopaminergic system assessed in vivo by positron emission tomography in healthy volunteer subjects and patients with Parkinson's disease. *Arch. Neurol.*, **47**, 1290–8.

47. Brooks, D.J., Ibanez, V., Sawle, G.V. *et al.* (1990) Differing patterns of striatal 18F DOPA uptake in Parkinson's disease, multiple system atrophy and progressive supranuclear palsy. *Ann. Neurol.*, **28**, 547–55.

48. Innis, R.B., Seibyl, J.P., Wallace, E. *et al.* (1993) SPECT imaging demonstrates loss of dopamine transporters in Parkinson's disease. *J. Nucl. Med.*, **34**, 31P.

49. Frost, J.J., Rosier, A.M., Reich, S., Smith, J., Ehlers, M., Snyder, S.H., Ravert, H.T. and Dannals, R.F. (1993) PET imaging of dopamine reuptake sites in Parkinson's disease by C-11- WIN 35 428 and PET. *J. Nucl. Med.*, **34**, 31P.

50. Brooks, D. (1991) PET: its clinical role in neurology. *J. Neurol. Neurosurg. Psychiatry*, **54**, 1–5.

51. Tatsch, K., Schwarz, J., Oertel, W.H. and Kirsch, C.-M. (1992) I-123 IBZM SPECT for imaging dopamine D2 receptors in idiopathic Parkinson syndrome, Parkinsonian-like syndromes and Wilson's disease, in *Nuclear Medicine; Nuclear Medicine in Research and Practice* (eds H.A.E. Schmidt and R. Höfer), Schattauer, Stuttgart, New York, pp. 406–10.

52. Brucke, T., Podrecka, I., Angelberger, P., Wenger, S., Topitz, A., Kufferle, B., Muller, Ch. and Deecke, L.

(1991) Dopamine D2 receptor imaging with SPECT: studies in different neuropsychiatric disorders. *J. Cereb. Blood Flow Metab.*, **11**, 220–8.

53. Sawle, G.V., Brooks, D.J., Ibanez, V. and Frackowiack, R.S.J. (1990) Striatal D2 receptor density is inversely proportional to dopa uptake in untreated Parkinson's disease. *J. Neurol. Neurosurg. Psychiatry*, **53**, 177.

54. Rinne, U.K., Laihinen, A., Rinne, J.O. *et al.* (1990) Positron Emission Tomography demonstrates dopamine D2 receptor supersensitivity in the striatum of patients with early Parkinson's disease. *Movement Disorders*, **5**, 55–9.

55. Van Royen, E.A., Verhoeff, N.P.L.G., Speelman, J.D., Wolters, E.Ch., Kuiper, M.A. and Janssen, A.G.M. (1993) Diminished striatal dopamine D2 receptor activity in multiple system atrophy and progressive supranuclear palsy demonstrated by 123I IBZM SPECT. *Arch. Neurol.*, **50**, 513–16.

56. Burn, D.J., Mathias, C.J., Cunningham, V.J., Waters, S., Quinn, N., Marsden, C.D. and Brooks, D.J. (1993) Striatal opiate receptor binding in Parkinson's disease and multiple system atrophy: a ^{11}C diprenorphine study. *J. Cereb. Blood Flow Metab.*, **13**, S367.

57. Holthoff, V.A., Koeppe, R.A., Frey, K.A., Penney, J.B., Markel, D.S., Kuhl, D.E. and Young, A.B. (1993) Positron emission tomography measures of benzodiazepine receptors in Huntington's disease. *Ann. Neurol.*, **34**, 76–81.

58. Sawle, G.V., Playford, E.D., Brooks, D.J., Quinn, N. and Frackowiack, R.S.J. (1993) Asymmetrical presynaptic and post-synaptic changes in the striatal dopamine projection in dopa naive parkinsonism. *Brain*, **116**, 853–67.

59. Hierholzer, J., Cordes, M., Schelosky, L., Schrag, A., Richter, W., Poewe, W., Semmeir, W. and Felix, R. (1993) Functional receptor testing in patients with iodiopathic Parkinson's syndrome versus Parkinson's plus syndrome. *J. Nucl. Med.*, **34**, 31P.

60. Schwarz, J., Tatsch, K., Arnold, G., Gasser, T., Trenkwalder, C., Kirsch, C.M. and Oertel, W.H. (1992) 123I iodobenzamide-SPECT predicts dopaminergic responsiveness in patients with *de novo* parkinsonism. *Neurology*, **42**, 556–61.

61. Ruottinen, H., Rinne, J.O., Laihinen, A., Rinne, U.K., Oikenen, V., Ruotsalainen, U., Bergman, J. and Solin, O. (1993) The effect of COMT inhibition with entacapone on 18F-6-fluorodopa PET in Parkinson's disease. *J. Cereb. Blood Flow Metab.*, **13**, S359.

62. Sawle, G. and Myers, R. (1993) Combined PET and MRI studies following neural cell transplantation for Parkinson's disease. *J. Cereb. Blood Flow Metab.*, **13**, S366.

Epilepsy

H. A. Ring

INTRODUCTION

Epilepsy was described by Hughlings Jackson in 1886 as involving 'sudden, excessive, rapid and local discharges of the grey matter' of the brain. This simple definition remains a useful summary of the phenomenon. Epilepsy is relatively common. In both the UK and the USA, studies suggest that five out of each thousand people will suffer from the condition. The incidence is highest in childhood and lowest in middle life. It has been estimated that approximately 5% of the population will have at least one seizure at some time in their life.

A diagnosis of epilepsy describes a syndrome characterized by the tendency to have recurrent seizures. The condition may be considered as the symptom of a primary pathology. However, in about two-thirds of people with epilepsy, no aetiology can be found. In the remaining one-third of cases, the most common cause is hippocampal sclerosis, often resulting from prolonged febrile convulsions in infancy. Other relatively common aetiologies include birth injury, traumatic (particularly penetrating) brain injury, encephalitis, cerebrovascular and neurodegenerative diseases and cerebral tumours. It is important to distinguish epilepsy itself from the occurrence of a seizure, which may be a symptom of many disease states.

The diagnosis of epilepsy may be considered at two levels: first, at the level of whether an episodic disturbance of functioning is indeed a seizure associated with recognized electroencephalographic (EEG) findings (Table 9.4); and second, once the episode has been established as a seizure, whether it is part of a syndrome of idiopathic epilepsy or of another state (Table 9.5), for instance alcohol withdrawal. In clinical practice, the diagnosis of epilepsy is based on an evaluation of the clinical phenomena, with supportive evidence coming from EEG findings.

CLASSIFICATION OF EPILEPSIES AND SEIZURES

For many years, the classification of epilepsy was a complex area, in which misunderstandings were common, and in which aetiological and phenomenological categorizations were confused. In 1981 and 1989, new schemes were introduced by the International League Against Epilepsy, and this system has now become the accepted approach. An abbreviated classification of epilepsies is given in Table 9.6. In Table 9.7, an abbreviated classification of seizures, based on seizure phenomenology, is given.

THE ROLE OF NUCLEAR MEDICINE IN PATIENTS WITH SEIZURES

Epilepsy is a clinical diagnosis. The 'gold standard' with respect to investigations into the pathophysiology of the condition, and with respect to providing a pathophysiological confirmation of the clinical diagnosis, has for many years been, and continues to be, EEG measurement. However, interictal scalp EEG recording may show epileptiform phenomena in those without epilepsy and conversely, may fail to reveal epileptic activity in those with epilepsy, particularly in those with a focus in deep temporal or orbitofrontal regions. Although intracranial recording avoids these limitations, this is an invasive and expensive procedure with some associated morbidity. Hence the possibility of non-invasive imaging techniques that will complement the information obtained from EEG recording has been eagerly accepted by those working with patients with epilepsy.

ICTAL AND INTERICTAL STUDIES

Clinically and electrophysiologically, three distinct periods may be defined in association with a seizure. The **ictus** is the fit itself. This may last from a few seconds to a few minutes or longer. If the ictus continues for longer than perhaps 10 minutes, then medical intervention to terminate the seizure is indicated. The **post-ictal** period describes the time after the end of the seizure itself

Clinical Nuclear Medicine, 3rd edn. Edited by M.N. Maisey, K.E. Britton and B.D. Collier. Published in 1998 by Chapman & Hall, London. ISBN 0 412 75180 1

Table 9.4 Differential diagnoses of episodic disturbance of functioning

Neurological disorders
  Transient ischaemic attack
  Migraine
  Transient global amnesia
  Gilles de la Tourette's syndrome

Sleep disorders
  Physiological myoclonus
  Enuresis
  Nightmares
  Sleep apnoea

Psychiatric states
  Non-epileptic seizures
  Panic attacks
  Dissociative states
  Rage attacks
  Brief psychotic states

Medical disorders
  Syncope
  Cardiac arrhythmias
  Metabolic disorders (e.g. hypoglycaemia)
  Hypertensive crisis

Table 9.5 Causes of seizures

Epilepsy
  Idiopathic
  Symptomatic (e.g. hippocampal sclerosis)

Infective
  Encephalitis (e.g. herpes simplex, neurosyphilis)
  Cerebral abscess

Neurodegenerative
  Alzheimer's disease
  Tuberose sclerosis
  Spongiform encephalopathies

Neurovascular
  Infarction
  Intracranial haemorrhage
  Arteriovenous malformations
  Cerebral aneurysms

Space-occupying lesions
  Tumours

Metabolic disturbances
  Hepatic failure
  Renal failure
  Hypoglycaemia

Haematological conditions
  Polycythaemia
  Leukaemia

Exogenous toxins
  Alcohol
  Heavy metals
  Barbiturate toxicity

Table 9.6 ILAE* Classification of epilepsies (abbreviated)

1. Generalized
  Idiopathic generalized epilepsies – with age-related onset
    Benign neonatal convulsions
    Childhood absence epilepsy
    Juvenile myoclonic epilepsy
    Other idiopathic generalized epilepsies
  Cryptogenic or symptomatic generalized epilepsies
    West's syndrome
    Lennox–Gastaut syndrome
  Symptomatic generalized epilepsies with non-specific aetiology

2. Localization-related
  Idiopathic with age-related onset
    Benign epilepsy with centrotemporal spikes
  Symptomatic
    Epilepsia partialis continua
    Temporal lobe epilepsies
    Frontal lobe epilepsies
    Parietal lobe epilepsies
    Occipital lobe epilepsies

3. Epilepsies and syndromes undetermined as to whether focal or generalized

4. Special syndromes
  Febrile convulsions
  Seizures occurring only when there is an acute metabolic or toxic event related to e.g. alcohol, eclampsia.

*International League Against Epilepsy.

Table 9.7 ILAE* Classification of epileptic seizures (abbreviated)

I. Focal (partial, local) seizures
  A. Simple partial seizures
    with motor symptoms
    with somatosensory or special sensory symptoms
    with autonomic symptoms or signs
  B. Complex partial seizures
    with simple onset followed by impairment of consciousness
    with impairment of consciousness at onset
  C. Partial seizures evolving to secondarily generalized seizures (may be tonic–clonic, tonic, or clonic)

2. Generalized seizures
  A. Absence seizures
  B. Myoclonic seizures
  C. Clonic seizures
  D. Tonic seizures
  E. Tonic–clonic seizures
  F. Atonic seizures

*International League Against Epilepsy.

when post-ictal EEG changes may be seen and during which patients may be drowsy or disorientated. This period normally lasts for a few minutes to less than an hour, but after severe or prolonged seizures may be considered to persist for longer than this. The **interictal** period describes the rest of the time, i.e. all the time except the ictal or post-ictal periods.

It has been determined that in patients with focal epilepsy (i.e. with seizures originating from one or more localized areas of dysfunctional brain), the ictal and interictal periods may have fairly characteristic abnormalities of regional cerebral perfusion and metabolism. During the ictal phase, there is an increase in local cerebral blood flow and metabolism, in the region of the epileptic focus. At the end of the seizure, the hyperperfusion may persist for up to a minute into the post-ictal period, but for most of the post-ictal period the activity at the site of the focus falls greatly, and the focus may be observed to be even more hypoperfused than it is during interictal scans.

During the interictal phase, there is localized hypoperfusion in an area extending well beyond the epileptogenic region [1]. Because of this relatively extensive hypoperfusion, the localizing value of interictal SPECT scans is limited. Useful information regarding the lateralization of the focus may however be obtained. Initially, there was considerable scepticism about the clinical value of interictal scans, as the early studies were of low resolution and the correlations with EEG findings were imprecise. The SPECT scans were observed to be more likely to show hypoperfusion when the MRI image was also abnormal, than when it was normal. Figures on the sensitivity of interictal focus detection of SPECT in the literature range from 40% to 80% [2,3]. These patterns of disordered cerebral activity can be difficult to detect, representing a challenge to the technical limitations of the imaging techniques used. Recently, attention has been paid to optimizing imaging paradigms to increase the chance of detecting abnormalities. Hence, with respect to SPECT imaging, increased rates of detection of interictal abnormalities have been reported for studies that have used brain-dedicated multi-headed scanners. Detection of disturbances in hippocampal regions may be aided by orienting the transverse planes parallel to the long axis of the temporal lobe. It is also important to be aware of the risks of

using methods of relative quantification that involve regions-of-interest, which though distant from the presumed seizure focus, may nevertheless have disturbed functioning related to the focus (e.g. the cerebellum, as a result of diaschisis). Using brain-dedicated multi-headed camera systems, the sensitivity of SPECT is comparable to ^{18}F-fluorodeoxyglucose (FDG) positron emission tomography (PET) [4].

What is not clear from the literature is the meaning of the often-reported finding that PET and SPECT functional abnormalities are more extensive than the EEG findings. It has been suggested that the actual relationship between interictal hypometabolic areas and ictal foci will remain undetermined until data on a large group of surgical resections, from appropriately characterized patients, are available. The extent of hypometabolism is not simply related to the degree of gliosis [5]. Perfusion deficits associated with focal lesions such as gliomas may not be as extensive as those seen with hippocampal sclerosis. The particular association of structural and functional changes in the hippocampus has been further defined in a group of patients with epilepsy originating from a medial temporal focus. In this study, it was observed that temporal hypometabolism, measured using high-resolution FDG-PET, correlated with hippocampal atrophy (as defined by volumetric MRI). However, atrophy in other temporal regions was not reliably associated with hypometabolism [6].

In summary, although interictal SPECT scans are easier to perform than ictal studies, unless optimal scanning techniques are used, the data obtained are rarely sensitive and reliable enough to be considered as more than an occasional adjunct to other modes of investigation. Ictal studies, while logistically demanding, provide valuable information that generally justifies the effort expended in collecting it.

SPECIFIC CLINICAL APPLICATIONS

The clinical indications for nuclear medicine applications in the management of epilepsy can largely be subsumed under two main headings: first, contributing to the diagnosis of an apparent seizure disorder; and second, identifying the site of the seizure focus in patients with partial epilepsy being considered for surgical excision of the focus.

Although the majority of patients scanned have been adults, a number of studies have demonstrated valuable roles for emission tomography in children with epilepsy [7,8], both in aiding diagnosis and in focus localization before surgical treatment.

Diagnosis of deep foci

The majority of partial seizures originate from a focus in the temporal lobe, and the associated clinical manifestations are relatively well recognized. However, in recent years, 20–30% of partial seizures have been recognized as being of frontal lobe origin [9]. These seizures may be associated with unusual clinical presentations, which together with the limited value of the scalp EEG in recording the activity of deep frontal foci, often lead to difficulties in diagnosis. In a study of 22 patients with seizure behaviours and ictal plus interictal EEG recordings suggesting a frontal focus, the localizing value of MRI, CT and FDG-PET were compared [10]. Overall, in 64% of the patients, FDG-PET demonstrated areas of focal hypometabolism; in 45%, MRI was informative; and CT abnormalities were seen in 32%. However, considering the PET data, although the extent of the abnormalities seen varied from focal to hemispheric, it was only the more localized focal frontal or contiguous frontal and temporal findings, seen in 27% of the patients, which correlated significantly with the electroclinical focus localization. In the majority of patients with PET abnormalities, these extended further than predicted from the electroclinical analysis.

Diagnosis of non-epileptic seizures

SPECT in epilepsy has mainly been confined to the imaging of regional cerebral blood flow (rCBF). Currently, ^{99m}Tc-HMPAO is the most widely used tracer for cerebral perfusion SPECT. Recently, HMPAO-SPECT has been used to help in the distinction between patients with non-epileptic seizures (NES) associated with a psychiatric condition and patients with epilepsy. This distinction may be difficult to make clinically with confidence. Patients with NES are generally resistant to anticonvulsant medication. Because of this apparent resistance to treatment, they often undergo many investigations and may be prescribed large doses of anticonvulsant medication. Therefore, an improvement in the diagnostic accuracy will protect these patients from unhelpful, potentially harmful and often expensive intervention. A recent study [11] scanned 10 patients with non-epileptic seizures and a further matched control group of 10 patients with epilepsy characterized by complex partial seizures (CPS). All subjects were scanned at rest during an interictal period because, for assessing the clinical utility of this diagnostic technique, these are the easiest circumstances in which to scan subjects. It was found that in those with NES, 70% of scans were normal, while in those with CPS, 80% of scans showed the predicted abnormality in the rCBF. The authors anticipate that these results will be of significant value in directing clinical practice in resolving the differential diagnosis of patients presenting with seizure disorders of uncertain origin or in association with psychiatric disorders.

Use of functional neuroimaging in the preparation of patients for epilepsy surgery

Approximately 25% of patients with epilepsy have intractable seizures, which cannot be fully controlled with anticonvulsant medication. In this group, alternative treatment strategies must be considered. In patients with focal epilepsy where the responsible focus can be clearly identified, and where anatomical considerations such as site of the lesion do not exclude it, surgical excision of the focus is an alternate treatment. This is a specialist treatment requiring combined surgical, electrophysiological, neuropsychological and psychiatric expertise. However, it is an increasingly popular approach with more units being developed around the world. Currently, there are about half a dozen such centres in the UK. Historically, pre-surgical localization of the seizure focus often involved intracerebral EEG recording. However, this is a process with associated morbidity and occasional mortality. Therefore, the possibility of obtaining reliable localizing information from non-invasive functional neuroimaging techniques has been explored by several centres. Both ictal and interictal studies have been performed and PET and SPECT techniques have been evaluated. The aim of these studies was to assess the value of these techniques in identifying the location and extent of the seizure focus, checking for existence of multiple foci and providing a guide for stereotactic placement of intracerebral electrodes where it is still felt that these are indicated.

The easiest and most available approach has been to use interictal SPECT with ^{99m}Tc-HMPAO. In a study of 31 patients, selected because the epileptic focus had been clearly defined (in 29 patients by invasive foramen ovale EEG recording and in two patients by MRI), who subsequently underwent selective amygdalohippocampectomy, interictal ^{99m}Tc-HMPAO-SPECT correctly identified the lateralization of the primary epileptogenic area in 48% [12]. The zones of decreased rCBF were much larger than the foci as identified by EEG or MRI. Pre-operative MRI identified structural lesions in 65% of the patients. In only 12 of 31 patients (39%) did both SPECT and MRI correctly identify the EEG-defined, and subsequently surgically proven focus. In the 20 patients with pathological MRI findings, corresponding SPECT abnormalities were noted in 65%. The authors concluded from their study that while interictal SPECT was a useful way of increasing the confidence of EEG findings, its value was not sufficient to reduce the need for invasive focus–localization procedures.

Although precise focus–localization is necessary for surgery, it is also of value to determine in which hemisphere the epileptic focus resides, particularly in patients with a frontotemporal dysfunction. This is because if the focus is in the dominant hemisphere, then surgery may be ruled out because of the proximity of the focus to speech centres. Hence, even if interictal SPECT cannot identify the precise location of the focus, information regarding laterality is useful at an early stage of the pre-surgical assessment in order to help indicate whether the patient is likely to be a suitable candidate for epilepsy, before more invasive investigations. In a recent meta-analysis of studies using interictal SPECT in partial epilepsy, the sensitivity (defined as the fraction of unifocal or multifocal ipsilateral SPECT findings among all unilateral EEGs) was 58% [13].

Interictal PET studies, most commonly using ^{18}F-FDG to measure regional glucose metabolism, have also been investigated for their value as non-invasive focus-localizing techniques. In a study that correlated surgical findings at temporal lobectomy in 26 patients with intractable epilepsy with pre-surgical observations obtained using EEG, MRI, CT and PET, it was found that FDG-PET showed a region of focal interracial hypometabolism corresponding to the EEG localization of seizure onset in 21 cases [14]. MRI agreement with the EEG findings was observed in five patients, while CT was abnormal in three. Three of the patients who were found to have tumours at surgery were all detected with MRI, while PET identified focal hypometabolism in two of these. The PET findings were non-specific and could not distinguish focal gliosis from tumour.

In one study, the value of interictal FDG-PET in surgical planning was assessed using a blind prospective comparison of PET with surface and subdural EEG recording [15]. All 53 patients in the study, with uncontrolled temporal lobe epilepsy, were investigated using video-EEG telemetry and PET, and 46 of these also received an MRI scan. Visual inspection of the PET scans suggested a trend to a correlation between temporal hypometabolism and a good outcome to surgery. (Good surgical outcome was taken as proof that the identified area had indeed been the seizure focus.) Using a template-based region-of-interest analysis of the PET scans, it was found that the presence of temporal hypometabolism of at least 15% was significantly correlated with a good outcome after temporal lobectomy. In addition, asymmetry-indices were calculated for the lateral and medial temporal regions. There were no significant differences between these values, and only the figure for the lateral temporal area correlated with the surgical outcome. The failure to find the expected focus-related abnormalities may have been due to greater partial volume effects confounding the measurements of the medial temporal region, this being smaller than the lateral temporal area. The authors concluded that FDG-PET was superior in focus localization to T2-weighted MRI, but they were unable to make clear recommendations about the role of interictal FDG-PET in focus localization, although they did conclude that while the technique lacked the spatial resolution of intra-operative cortical mapping, it could be used to guide the placement of invasive EEG electrodes.

It has been possible for some centres to develop routine peri-ictal imaging protocols using SPECT. The distribution of ^{99m}Tc-HMPAO in the brain is largely complete within about 2 minutes after injection, and subsequently remains fixed for several hours. If the radioisotope is injected during or shortly after an epileptic seizure, scanning can be carried out post-ictally, without any problems due to involuntary movements. Post-ictal and ictal SPECT is more sensitive than interictal SPECT, and typically shows hyperperfusion ipsilateral to the epileptogenic focus. A study of 77 seizures in 51 patients with temporal lobe epilepsy using post-ictal injection of ^{99m}Tc-HMPAO (with a mean delay from the seizure onset to injection of 4.3 ± 4.5 min), observed increased focal uptake predominantly confined to the ipsilateral anteromesial temporal region. This was observed in 83% of the patients, and rapidly declined as the delay between the end of the seizure and the injection of the tracer moved towards 5 minutes [2]. However, in most patients seizures develop unpredictably and are of relatively short duration (e.g. about 1 minute). In general, it is considered unsafe to allow a more prolonged seizure to continue for more than 10 minutes at the most without attempting to terminate it (e.g. using intravenous or rectal diazepam). Performing ictal scans can therefore be logistically demanding, requiring ongoing EEG monitoring and rapidly available ^{99m}Tc-HMPAO. It has been reported that in patients with temporal lobe epilepsy, hyperperfusion of the anterior temporal lobe persists for up to 60 seconds into the immediate post-ictal period. Hence, ^{99m}Tc-HMPAO injected in the very early post-ictal period (as defined by EEG), will still result in an ictal appearance on scanning [16]. This somewhat eases the logistical difficulties that exist in obtaining an ictal scan. The use of derivatives of HMPAO with a longer 'shelf-life' may aid more rapid response. The benefits of ictal, as opposed to interictal scanning, have been clearly demonstrated in a study that examined ictal and interictal scans in 119 patients with known unilateral temporal lobe epilepsy [17]. These authors found that ictal scans gave correct localization in 97% of the patients, while later post-ictal scans provided 71% correct and interictal scans only 48% correct localization.

Ictal PET studies employing ^{15}O-labelled tracers or ^{18}F-FDG to measure rCBF or metabolism are difficult. The short half-life of the ^{15}O positron-emitting radioisotope requires it to be made at the time of administration which, given the need for rapid scanning when a seizure occurs, is technically demanding as it requires a cyclotron already to be producing it. Although the labelled FDG has a longer radioactive half-life, it has a 30–45 minute uptake period, which means, since seizures would

normally terminate or be terminated in considerably less time than this, that the data obtained would include post-ictal as well as ictal events, with the result weighted in favour of events occurring soon after injection of the isotope [18].

Given the greater expense and the relative rarity of PET scanning, an important question concerns the relative values of SPECT and PET techniques in localizing the epileptic focus in patients being considered for neurosurgical treatment. In one study comparing interictal FDG-PET with ictal HMPAO-SPECT in 35 patients with well-lateralized temporal lobe epileptic foci it was found that, based on the SPECT scans, two observers correctly identified the laterality of the foci with certainty in 89% of subjects. Considering the PET data, foci were correctly lateralized with certainty in 63% and with less confidence in a total of 83%. In patients with no regional abnormalities noted on structural MRI, correct identification of laterality of the focus was greater in the ictal SPECT than in the interictal PET scans [19]. Hence, considering the two most commonly used tracers in PET and SPECT studies, ictal SPECT scans appear to provide more useful data than do interictal PET scans. However, although SPET scans are cheaper and more widely available than PET scans, the logistics of reliably obtaining ictal or even peri-ictal studies are demanding, and currently routine in only a few specialist centres around the world.

USE OF BENZODIAZEPINE RECEPTOR RADIOLIGANDS

It has been well established that in several brain regions inhibitory activity mediated by the neurotransmitter gamma aminobutyric acid (GABA) is anticonvulsant, while an excess of excitatory activity, related to excitatory amino acid neurotransmitters, mainly glutamate, may be proconvulsant. There has therefore been interest in finding ways of assessing the nature of local inhibitory activity in epileptic brain regions. The benzodiazepine binding sites that are associated with and modulate the activity of GABA receptors have been imaged by SPECT (using ^{123}I-iomazenil) and PET (using ^{11}C-flumazenil). Decreased flumazenil binding, of the order of approximately 30%, has been observed in patients with epilepsy in the region of the epileptic focus. In theory, measures of flumazenil binding will provide a more accurate visualization of epileptogenic sites than measures of cerebral perfusion or metabolism. A study of quantitative autoradiography on anterior and mesial temporal specimens removed at surgery from patients undergoing surgical excision of their epileptic focus reported that the predominant source of PET-demonstrated decreases in ^{11}C-flumazenil binding in patients with medial temporal lobe surgery is a specific pathological process of hippocampal sclerosis, rather than a more general down-regulation of central benzodiazepine binding sites on surviving hippocampal neurones [20]. However, in general, results from scans in epileptic subjects have not shown more localized abnormalities than those observed on the perfusion studies. It has been suggested that more localized abnormalities will be observed using higher-resolution cameras with optimal scan orientation.

^{123}I-Iomazenil binding measures were able to detect a normalization of benzodiazepine receptor site binding after successful treatment of seizures with an anticonvulsant agent in one case [21]. It is possible that future research work in radioligand binding may help in treatment selection.

REFERENCES

1. Holman, B.L. and Devous, M.D. (1992) Functional Brain SPECT: the emergence of a powerful clinical method. *J. Nucl. Med.*, **33**, 1888–904.
2. Rowe, C.C., Berkovic, S.F., Austin, M.C., McKay, W.J. and Bladin, P.F. (1991) Patterns of post-ictal cerebral blood flow in temporal lobe epilepsy: qualitative and quantitative analysis. *Neurology*, **41**, 1096–103.
3. Biersack, H.J., Stefan, H., Reichmann, K. *et al.* (1987) HM-PAO SPECT and epilepsy. *Nucl. Med. Commun.*, **8**, 513–18.
4. Andersen, A.R., Waldemar, G., Dam, M., Fuglson-Frederitsen, A., Herning, M. and Kruse-Larsen, C. (1990) SPECT in the presurgical evaluation of patients with temporal lobe epilepsy – a preliminary report. *Acta Neurochirurgica Suppl.*, **50**, 80–3.
5. Hajek, M., Antonini, A., Leenders, K.L. and Wieser, H.G. (1993) Mesiobasal versus lateral temporal epilepsy: metabolic differences in the temporal lobe shown by interictal ^{18}F-FDG positron emission tomography. *Neurology*, **43**, 79–86.
6. Semah, F., Baulac, M., Hasboun, D. *et al.* (1995) Is interictal temporal hypometabolism related to mesial temporal sclerosis? A positron emission/magnetic resonance confrontation. *Epilepsia*, **36**, 447–56.
7. Cummings, T.J., Chugani, D.C. and Chugani, H.T. (1995) Positron emission tomography in pediatric epilepsy. *Neurosurg. Clin. North Am.*, **6**, 465–72.
8. Cross, J.H., Gordon, I., Jackson, G.D. *et al.* (1995) Children with intractable focal epilepsy: ictal and interictal 99Tcm HMPAO single photon emission computed tomography. *Dev. Med. Child Neurol.*, **37**, 673–81.
9. Swartz, B.E. and Delgado-Escueta, A.V. (1987) Complex partial seizures of extratemporal origin, in *The Epileptic Focus. Current Problems in Epilepsy, Vol. 3* (eds H. Wieser and E.J. Speckmann), John Libbey, London.
10. Swartz, B.E., Halgren, E., Delgado-Escueta, A.V. *et al.* (1989) Neuroimaging in patients with seizures of probable frontal lobe origin. *Epilepsia*, **30**, 547–58.
11. Varma, A.R., Moriarty, J., Costa, D.C. *et al.* (1996) HMPAO SPECT in non-epileptic seizures – preliminary results. *Acta Neurol. Scand.* (in press)
12. Hajek, M., Siegel, A.M., Haldemann, R., von Schulthess, G.K. and Wieser, H.G. (1991) Value of HM-PAO SPECT in selective temporal lobe surgery for epilepsy. *J. Epilepsy*, **4**, 43–51.
13. Devous, M.D., Thisted, R., Rowe, C.C., Leroy, R.F. and Morgan, G.F. (1994) SPECT brain imaging in epilepsy: a meta-analysis. *J. Nucl. Med.*, **35**, 31P (abstract)
14. Theodore, W.H., Katz, D., Kufta, C. *et al.* (1990) Pathology of temporal lobe foci: correlation with CT, MRI, and PET. *Neurology*, **40**, 797–803.
15. Theodore, W.H., Sato, S., Kufta, C., Balish, M.B., Bromfield, M.B. and Liederman, D.B. (1992) Temporal lobectomy for uncontrolled seizures: the role of positron emission tomography. *Ann. Neurol.*, **32**, 789–94.
16. Newton, M.R., Berkovic, S.F., Austin, M.C., Rowe, C.C., McKay, W.J. and Bladin, P.F. (1992) Postictal switch in blood flow distribution and temporal lobe seizures. *J. Neurol., Neurosurg. Psychiatr*, **55**, 891–4.
17. Newton, M.R., Berkovic, S.F., Austin, M.C., Rowe, C.C., McKay, W.J. and Bladin, P.F. (1995) SPECT in the localization of extratemporal and temporal seizure foci. *J. Neurol., Neurosurg. Psychiatry*, **59**, 26–30.
18. Theodore, W.H. (1992) MRI, PET, SPECT: interrelations, technical limits, and unanswered questions, in *Surgical Treatment of Epilepsy* (Epilepsy Research, Suppl. 5) (ed. W.H. Theodore), Elsevier Science Publishers B.V., Amsterdam, pp. 127–34.
19. Ho, S.S., Berkovic, S.F., Berlangieri, S.U. *et al.* (1995) Comparison of ictal SPECT and interictal PET in the presurgical evaluation of temporal lobe epilepsy. *Ann. Neurol.*, **37**, 738–45.
20. Burdette, D.E., Sakurai, S.Y., Henry, T.R. *et al.* (1995) Temporal lobe central benzodiazepine binding in unilateral mesial temporal lobe epilepsy. *Neurology*, **45**, 934–41.
21. Staedt, J., Stoppe, G., Kogler, A. and Steinhoff, B.J. (1995) Changes in central benzodiazepine receptor density in the course of anticonvulsant treatment in temporal lobe epilepsy. *Seizure*, **4**, 49–52.

FURTHER READING

Dierckx, R.A., Vandevivere, J., Melis, K. *et al.* (1992) Single photon emission computed tomography using perfusion tracers in seizure disorders. *Epilepsy Res.,* **12**, 131–9.

Duncan, J.S., Shorvon, S.D. and Fish, D.R. (1995) *Clinical Epilepsy*, Churchill Livingstone, New York.

Engel, J. Jr (ed.) (1993) *Surgical Treatment of the Epilepsies*, 2nd edn, Raven Press, New York.

Sperling, M.R. (1993) Neuroimaging in Epilepsy. *Neurol. Clin.*, **11**, 883–903.

Dementia

D. C. Costa

INTRODUCTION

The term dementia is often used to describe chronic, irreversible and progressive development of multiple cognitive deficits that include memory impairment (Criterion A1) and at least one of the following other cognitive abnormalities (Criterion A2): aphasia, apraxia, agnosia, or a disturbance in executive functioning [1,2]. These cognitive deficits must be severe enough to produce impairment in occupational or social functioning (Criterion B) and there must be a clear-cut decline from previously higher levels of functional capacity. The nature and degree of impairment are variable and often influenced by the social setting and sometimes also by the cultural environment. Approximately one-third of patients initially presenting with dementia have reversible syndromes at their final diagnosis [3]. Therefore, we have to define dementia more precisely as a clinical syndrome of acquired and persistent impairment of intellect with compromised function in multiple spheres of mental activity (e.g. memory, language, visuospatial skills, emotion or personality and cognition) [4]. However, dementia may also occur at a younger age, in which case there is a more rapid deterioration of the clinical condition.

Advances in public health measures throughout the world, particularly vaccines and sanitation, have led to a significant shift in the population growth towards the elderly. The average life expectancy in Europe and the United States has risen from around 47 years in the late 1890s to more than 75 years in 1993. Investment in improved nutrition, medical technology and public health explain an average life expectancy of more than 76 years for men and 83 years for women in Japan [5]. Developing countries seem to follow this trend towards the elderly – considered by some as 'one of the greatest triumphs of humanity'. The burden of this population growth must not be underestimated. While there is some debate about the normal life expectancy limit – 85 or 95 or 100 years –

there is no doubt that with an increase in elderly population there is a dramatic rise in the incidence of dementia. It has been estimated that 1–3% of the population aged 65 years and over, and as many as 10% of the over-75 age group, have cognitive deficits compatible with dementia [6]. In 1987, the US Congress, Office of Technology Assessment, projected an increase in the number of severely demented Americans to 60% and 100% by the years 2000 and 2020 respectively [7].

This chapter will focus on the role of radionuclide brain imaging with single-photon (SPECT) and positron (PET) emitters in the evaluation of patients with dementia.

AETIOLOGY

According to the aetiology, dementia syndromes may be subclassified into: degenerative, vascular, myelinoclastic, traumatic, neoplastic, hydrocephalic, inflammatory, infection-related, toxic, metabolic and other psychiatric disorders. Among the degenerative, there are two main diagnostically useful categories of dementing disorders: (i) cortical, consisting of dysfunction of the cerebral cortex manifested by amnesia (memory impairment), aphasia, apraxia and agnosia – Alzheimer's disease being the classical example; and (ii) subcortical, caused by dysfunction of the deep grey matter nuclei (basal ganglia, thalamus, brainstem nuclei, and projections from the frontal lobe to these deep structures) and deep white matter structures. The most characteristic examples of subcortical dementias are those due to Parkinson's, Huntington's and Wilson's diseases. Because injury to the subcortical structures frequently produces abnormalities in arousal circuits (e.g. motivation, concentration/attention and information processing), patients with these types of dementia are often depressed, apathetic, show signs of other mood and personality disorders and generally reveal psychomotor retardation.

CLINICAL EVALUATION AND DIAGNOSTIC DILEMMAS

The most important aspect in the clinical assessment of a patient presenting with dementia is the

Clinical Nuclear Medicine, 3rd edn. Edited by M.N. Maisey, K.E. Britton and B.D. Collier. Published in 1998 by Chapman & Hall, London. ISBN 0 412 75180 1

clinical history, often from a relative. It is paramount to exclude diseases causing acute confusional states. Clinical evaluation alone may contribute to differential diagnosis within the dementias. Alzheimer's disease (AD) is classically manifested as a progressive, gradual and steady cognitive decline. Multi-infarct dementia (MID) is often abrupt in onset with a 'stepwise' deterioration; AD may coexist with MID.

Operational criteria have been developed to enable greater accuracy both for clinical diagnosis and for the selection of homogeneous patient samples for research. Among the most important are those of the Diagnostic and Statistical Manual (DSM-IV) [2], and specifically for AD, the National Institute and Communicative Disorders and Stroke (NINCDS) criteria [8]. The NINCDS criteria allow a diagnosis of 'probable', 'possible' or 'definite' AD. 'Definite' AD requires histopathological evidence from biopsy or post-mortem.

In the diagnosis of MID, the Ischaemia Scale (IS), also known as Hachinski ischaemia scores [9,10], is the most commonly used criterion. Although these scores help to differentiate AD from MID [11], they will not differentiate MID from MID plus AD [12]. In addition, they are only partially successful in the *in vivo* diagnosis of subjects with dementia. The accuracy of NINCDS-ADRDA, Alzheimer's Disease and Related Disorders Association, criteria can be as low as 80% in comparison with post-mortem studies [13]. Up to 50% of patients with an *in vivo* diagnosis of MID are found at post-mortem to have AD or mixed AD and MID [14]. These difficulties led to the incorporation of structural imaging techniques such as computerized tomography (CT) and magnetic resonance imaging (MRI) in the work-up of patients with dementia, particularly when using the NINCDS–ADRDA criteria.

Functional imaging techniques such as SPECT and PET have shown characteristic patterns that are significantly different from age-matched normal controls. These abnormal patterns correlate with the severity of cognitive impairment, and appear to be more or less specific to some types of dementia when compared with neuropsychological testing, the 'gold standard' of cognitive function assessment. The commonly used neuropsychological tests include: (i) Mini-Mental State Examination (MMSE) [15], which comprises 19 separate items with a maximum (intact) score of 30; (ii) Blessed Dementia Scale (BDS) [16] is used as a severity score, which measures

functional ability and has a maximum (most disabled) score of 32; and (iii) the CAMCOG, which is more rigorous and part of a larger clinical assessment, the CAMDEX [17,18]. CAMCOG has 67 items including eight subscales: orientation, comprehension, expression, language, memory (remote, recent, learned and total), attention, praxis, calculation, abstraction and perception. It also includes items from the MMSE and has a maximum (intact) score of 107.

Other tests using discriminant function analysis have been studied [19] and several others recently reviewed [20]. It is clear that the most problematic to diagnose are the cases with early dementia presenting mainly with memory impairment. An early diagnosis will become increasingly essential with the development of new therapeutic agents to slow the progression of dementia. In addition to the differential diagnosis between MID and AD, another dilemma deserving particular attention is the association between Alzheimer's disease, Parkinson's disease and motor neurone disease. Although the clinical and pathological overlap in these conditions may suggest a common genetic and environmental background [21], the label 'neurodegenerative' often used to describe these diseases may have distinct clinical and therapeutic implications. Parkinson's disease patients are more likely to develop dementia [22] and patients with Alzheimer's disease seem to be at greater than expected risk of increased extrapyramidal signs with variable frequency from 28% to 92% [23]. It has been recently discovered that there is a strong association of the apolipoprotein E e4 allele with increased risk of Alzheimer's disease, cortical Lewy body dementia (LBD), and bulbar onset motor neurone disease [24,25]. There appears to be no such association with Parkinson's disease, at least in the absence of dementia [26]. The spectrum of disorders with similar pathological findings is widening. For instance, patients with Lewy body disorders present with clinical symptoms and signs that reflect the distribution of Lewy bodies in the cerebral cortex and brainstem regardless of clinical diagnosis. There is an increasing concern about this new entity – LBD accounts for at least 20% of the cases of dementia [27]. Extrapyramidal symptoms are initially less severe than in Parkinson's disease and respond to L-dopa. There is mild nigrostriatal degeneration and marked psychotic symptoms, mainly visual hallucinations. In addition to cortical Lewy bodies (eosinophilic intracellular inclusions smaller than in Parkinson's disease), it is hypothesized that there is a degeneration of dopaminergic neurones. Future research studies including comparison between clinical presentation, imaging features and post-mortem diagnosis may help in furthering our understanding of these disorders.

RADIONUCLIDE IMAGING IN THE EVALUATION OF DEMENTIA

Radionuclide brain imaging will be helpful if it can aid in: (i) the differential diagnosis between different types of dementia; (ii) the assessment of extent and severity of brain involvement; (iii) the longitudinal follow-up of patients with dementia, either to understand the spontaneous evolution of the disease or to evaluate the response to well-established or new therapeutic regimens; (iv) the identification of the neurotransmitter systems involved and possibly responsible for the clinical presentation; (v) therapeutic decision making; and (vi) in prognostic assessment.

The image patterns expected with normal aging, cortical and subcortical dementias will be discussed and the observations pertinent to other types of dementias will be mentioned briefly.

NORMAL AGING

Memory impairment in the normal elderly seems to be different from the impairment found in patients with dementia [28]. Many elderly people develop small areas of ischaemia, which are more frequent in the white matter. The accepted idea that neuronal number loss with age is a normal finding, seen as grey matter atrophy, particularly well demonstrated by high-resolution structural imaging, is now under debate [29]. Some authors have reported that atrophic changes mainly occur in the white matter, while the grey matter is relatively preserved [30]; unfortunately, these data relate to animal studies on primates.

The regional distribution of radiotracers that depict glucose utilization, oxygen consumption and blood flow in the brain shows some differences between the young and elderly people. The same is true for the regional distribution of neuroreceptor ligands. After an initial rise in the rate of glucose utilization to the third year of age, there is almost no change from 3 to 7 years, which is followed by progressive decline [31]. Later in life, there is an age-related reduction in all of these

physiological parameters of brain function [32–35]. The changes in cerebral blood flow are well demonstrated on brain perfusion studies with SPECT using either HMPAO or ECD. They consist mainly of slight reduction of the radioactivity ratios (using the cerebellum as reference region) bilaterally, slightly more marked in the left hemisphere and in the frontal lobes [36]. However, the most important and significant finding is the appearance of larger irregularities and areas with marked asymmetry of the radioactivity ratios between the hemispheres with increasing age [36]. This is apparent in Figure 9.2, which shows representative graph plots of brain perfusion maps in two populations of normal volunteers: Figure 9.2(a) refers to young people with ages from 21 to 59, and Figure 9.2(b) to elderly volunteers with ages from 61 to 84 years [37]. The mean radioactivity ratio for each brain region is shown along the full line and the 95% confidence limits (±2 S.D.) are within the grey area. The grey area is larger in the elderly population, mainly because of the more marked asymmetries and irregularities of the distribution of the perfusion ratios within this population in comparison with the young volunteers. Figure 9.3(a,b) which accompanies the graphs shows transverse, coronal and sagittal slices of brain perfusion SPECT studies of two normal volunteers – a young (45-year-old female) subject in Figure 9.3(a), and an elderly (70-year-old male) subject in Figure 9.3(b). The main differences are the less well-defined cortical grey matter outline (on black) in the elderly male with more heterogeneous tracer distribution than the younger female.

In the elderly volunteer, asymmetries are mainly seen in the frontal, parietal and temporal lobes. The images show: transverse slices in the top row (from left to right – cerebellum and brainstem, basal ganglia, mid-ventricular level and supraventricular white matter); coronal cuts in the middle row (frontal to occipital, from left to right); and sagittal slices in the bottom row (right hemisphere in the first two and left hemisphere in the next two slices; one cut through the temporal lobe and a para-medial cut through the basal ganglia plane for each hemisphere).

CORTICAL DEMENTIAS

Among the entire spectrum of dementing diseases, Alzheimer's disease is by far the most frequent. Other types of cortical dementias are Lewy

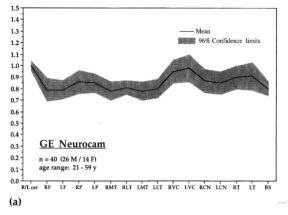

(a)

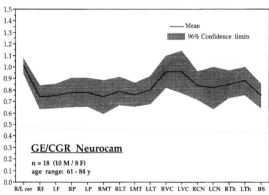

(b)

Figure 9.2 Graph plots of distribution of radioactivity ratios in the brain of normal volunteers. R, right; L, left; cer, cerebellum; F, frontal; P, parietal; MT, mesial temporal; LT, lateral temporal; VC, visual cortex; CN, caudate nucleus; Th, thalamus; BS, brainstem.
(a) Graph plot for a population of 40 young normal volunteers; (b) graph plot for a population of 18 elderly normal volunteers.

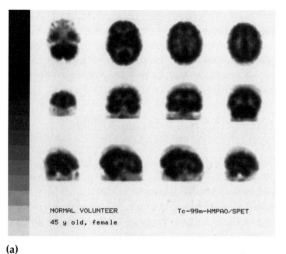

(a)

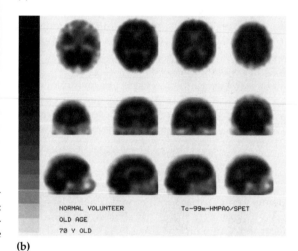

(b)

Figure 9.3 Distribution of the brain perfusion tracer (^{99m}Tc-HMPAO) uptake in the brain of a young (a) and elderly (b) normal volunteer. See text for orientation, which is kept the same for all the figures with images. The text describes these images in detail.

body disease, Pick's disease and the frontal lobe degeneration of non-Alzheimer type.

Alzheimer's disease

Alzheimer's disease (AD) is the most common cause of dementia. It was first reported in 1907 by Alois Alzheimer as a 'peculiar disease of the cerebral cortex' in a 51-year-old woman. AD accounts for approximately 50% of patients clinically presented with progressive cognitive decline. It is characterized by cortical atrophy, enlarged ventricles and widened sulci. In addition there are non-specific abnormal white matter signals

in MR imaging [38]. The neuropathology is mainly characterized by neuronal loss, presence of neurofibrillary tangles, neuritic plaques, granulovacuolar degeneration and abnormal amyloid deposition.

The majority of studies in the literature agree on the most frequent patterns of abnormalities found in AD patients on PET and/or SPECT. There is usually bilateral reduction of regional cerebral blood flow (rCBF), perfusion and metabolism in the temporal cortex and posterior parietal lobe. In more advanced stages of the disease, these abnormalities extend into the frontal lobes. PET studies have mainly used ^{15}O-oxygen [39] and ^{18}F-FDG [40]. Quantitative analysis helps to discriminate patients with mild degree of dementia from healthy controls, with more severe abnormalities found in the association neocortex, than in sensorimotor and calcarine (visual cortex) regions. Some of these metabolic abnormalities precede cognitive deficits, e.g. neocortical metabolic abnormalities can be seen before clinical detection of attention deficits and abstract reasoning by 8–16 months [41]. In a longitudinal study of 26 patients with memory impairment, bilateral parietal hypometabolism preceded the clinical definition of probable AD according to the NINCDS–ADRDA criteria by a period of 13 months [42].

Early SPECT studies of brain perfusion/rCBF were carried out by ^{123}I-IMP, which has now been almost completely replaced by ^{99m}Tc-labelled radiopharmaceuticals such as HMPAO and ECD.

The perfusion deficits on SPECT are very similar to the previously reported PET abnormalities of oxygen and glucose utilization rates. There is a clear reduction of perfusion to the temporal and posterior parietal lobes, bilateral but not always symmetrical (Figures 9.4 and 9.5). In later stages of the disease, the abnormalities are seen to extend into the frontal lobes (Figure 9.6). The wider availability of SPECT instrumentation and tracers have led to studies of relatively large numbers

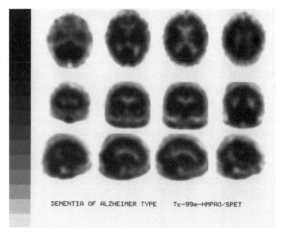

Figure 9.5 Another patient with Alzheimer's disease. In this case there are bilateral but asymmetrical perfusion deficits in the temporal and posterior parietal cortices.

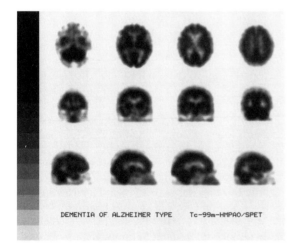

Figure 9.4 Bilateral and symmetrical reduction of brain perfusion in the mesial cortex of the temporal lobes, less marked in the posterior parietal and frontal lobes of a patient with Alzheimer's disease. There is some ventricular dilatation with cortical atrophy seen as enlargement of the anterior and posterior interhemispheric grooves.

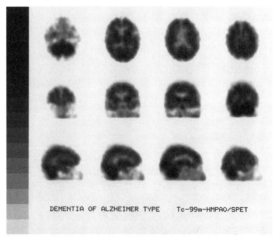

Figure 9.6 This brain perfusion SPECT study is from a patient with advanced Alzheimer's disease. The perfusion deficits are seen throughout the cerebral cortex, bilateral and almost symmetrical. Note the preserved perfusion ratios to the visual cortex, cerebellum and basal ganglia. This is a clear-cut case of cortical dementia of the Alzheimer type.

of patients. It is apparent that this affordable radionuclide procedure can be useful not only for differentiating the various types of dementia, but also perhaps in aiding the diagnosis of suspected dementia [43]. A prospective study of 132 patients with memory loss and/or cognitive deficits showed SPECT abnormalities to be predictive of AD: only 19% of those with apparently normal perfusion (visual analysis only with predefinition of pattern abnormalities) developed AD during the follow-up, as compared with 77% of those with bilateral temporoparietal reduction of perfusion [44]. The perfusion abnormalities correlate with neuropsychiatric deficits [45,46], and there appears to be a progression of the perfusion abnormalities from the mesial into the lateral cortex of the temporal and posterior parietal lobes, with progression of the cognitive impairment from simple memory loss to presence of apraxia and visuospatial deficits [47]. Although there are no significant data on therapeutic efficacy evaluation in Alzheimer's disease, a relatively large sample study of correlation with post-mortem neuropathology [48] has demonstrated that brain perfusion studies with SPECT drastically reduced the number of false-positive diagnoses.

A small number of studies have described the potential use of radiotracers to evaluate the pre- and post-synaptic sites of cholinergic neurotransmission (muscarinic and nicotinic), as well as benzodiazepine and serotonin receptors in the central nervous system (CNS). However, there are as yet insufficient data available to extract messages about their real application in the understanding of disease processes in patients with dementia of the Alzheimer type.

Lewy body disease

Lewy body disease or dementia (LBD) accounts for approximately 20% of dementia cases in patients over 70 years of age [27]. These figures are from post-mortem examination of patients with several dementia syndromes diagnosed in life. The clinical presentation is a reflection of the distribution of Lewy bodies throughout the cortex and brainstem. Lewy bodies are eosinophilic intracellular inclusions usually observed in the basal ganglia and substantia nigra of patients with Parkinson's disease. The Lewy bodies found in the cortex and subcortical structures of LBD patients are similar but smaller, and can be

demonstrated by immunocytochemistry which identifies the protein ubiquitin [49]. Short-term memory impairment, depression, psychosis and extrapyramidal symptoms, less severe than in Parkinson's disease, are the main complaints. LBD patients tend not to tolerate antipsychotic medication and can develop severe extrapyramidal symptoms.

Very little is known about radionuclide imaging in this new disease. However, the perfusion abnormalities that may be found in the brain of LBD patients are not specific and sometimes resemble the distribution found in patients with AD. The dopamine hypothesis led to studies of the dopamine receptors in the CNS, which showed reduction of the D2 dopamine neuroreceptors [studied with ^{123}I-iodobenzamide (IBZM)] in the striatum, with inversion of the caudate-to-putamen ratio [50]. This may indicate up-regulation at the putamen. Further studies with comparison against PD patients are necessary to elucidate the true meaning of these findings. In addition, the use of pre-synaptic dopaminergic ligands (e.g. ^{123}I-β-CIT and ^{123}I-FP-CIT) [51] will be of further help to demonstrate neurodegeneration in the striatum, or otherwise.

Frontal lobe dementias (FLD) or frontotemporal dementias (FTD)

These include Pick's disease and other frontal lobe degenerations of non-Alzheimer type and account for 13% to 16% of dementias in some studies [1]. Around 20% of the cases fulfil the neuropathological criteria for Picks' disease, while the other 80% have to be called FLD of the non-Alzheimer type. The inclusion of temporal by some authors is due to the involvement of the temporal lobes at some stage of the disease. The two main types of FLD are clinically indistinguishable and patients present with marked personality changes often preceding obvious cognitive decline (usually by at least 2 years). Frontal lobe atrophy is not apparent on CT or MRI until late in the evolution of the disease. Both PET and SPECT show the characteristic bilateral and almost symmetrical reduction of rCBF, oxygen and glucose utilization rates, as well as perfusion in the frontal lobes (Figure 9.7) [52]. One of the temporal lobes is frequently involved early in the disease. Later both temporal lobes show reduced perfusion. These findings are useful in differentiating between FLD and AD patients [53].

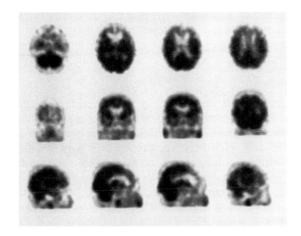

Figure 9.7 The images show sequential slices in frontal lobe dementia: top row, transverse; middle row, coronal; bottom row, sagittal. Reduction in uptake in the frontal lobes is evident. For description, see text.

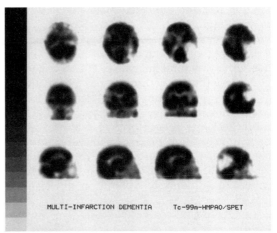

Figure 9.8 Clear-cut case of multi-infarct dementia. Large wedge-shaped perfusion deficits are clearly seen in the cortex, demonstrative of relatively large vessel occlusive disease.

SUBCORTICAL DEMENTIAS

This group includes Parkinson's disease, Huntington's disease, progressive supranuclear palsy, spinocerebellar degenerations, idiopathic basal ganglia calcification, striatonigral degeneration [corticobasal degeneration (CBD)], Wilson's disease and thalamic dementia.

Although cortical abnormalities are observed, the most clinically important radionuclide imaging features can be found with neurotransmitter studies: ^{18}F-DOPA for PET, ^{123}I-IBZM (post-synaptic D2 dopamine), ^{123}I-β-CIT and ^{123}I-FP-CIT (dopamine transporter system) for SPECT (Plate 17); these studies are of great value in the differential diagnosis of several Parkinsonian syndromes. ^{18}F-DOPA and both ^{123}I-β-CIT and ^{123}I-FP-CIT are able to aid the early diagnosis of patients with Parkinsonism. ^{18}F-DOPA has been used to demonstrate improvement in the pre-synaptic neuronal performance post-therapy with implants. However, brain perfusion SPECT studies may demonstrate changes between the 'On' and 'Off' periods of PD patients [45,47] and in response to therapy. In Huntington's and Wilson's disease, the most characteristic findings are reduction of perfusion and ^{123}I-IBZM uptake in the basal ganglia, particularly the caudate nucleus. This is due to the atrophic changes in Huntington's disease and deposition of copper in Wilson's disease.

The findings in CBD are very interesting [53]. There are reductions in brain perfusion, confined not only to the basal ganglia, but also to cortical territories, where structural imaging modalities may demonstrate no significant abnormality, mainly atrophy; Plate 18 is an illustration of this. It shows large perfusion abnormalities in the cortex of both parietal lobes, more marked in the right hemisphere, as well as reduced perfusion to both caudate nuclei and the right temporal lobe. MRI showed mild atrophy in the right parietal cortex with no other visible abnormality. Plate 19 shows the distribution of the D2 dopamine neuroreceptors in the CNS of the same patient confirming reduced dopaminergic transmission. The uptake of ^{123}I-IBZM in the basal ganglia was reduced in both hemispheres with specific-to-nonspecific ratios of 1.6 and 1.4, respectively on the right and the left (normal > 1.9).

VASCULAR DEMENTIAS

This category includes the groups of patients with multiple large vessel occlusions, multiple subcortical infarctions (lacunar infarcts), Binswanger's disease (white matter ischaemic small vessel disease) and mixed cortical and subcortical infarctions. Once again, the radionuclide image findings on PET or SPECT are very similar, and cortical infarcts are seen as multiple and almost wedge-shaped deficits in the cortex (Figure 9.8).

In cases of lacunar infarcts and Binswanger's disease, radionuclide modalities are significantly inferior to structural imaging – CT and in particular MRI – which are considered the 'gold standard' techniques for demonstrating multiple foci of white matter disease and small cortical and subcortical infarctions. However, they are less efficient in separating patients with MID from patients with AD [54]. In addition to the ability to separate MID from AD patients according to the pattern of distribution of perfusion abnormalities [55], PET and/or SPECT studies with rCBF tracers depict abnormalities of blood flow that correlate with the severity of disease and neuropsychiatric performance [54].

In summary, patients with MID show brain perfusion maps with deficits related to the distribution of the major arterial network. AD patients have reduced perfusion in the temporal and posterior parietal cortex (bilateral but not always symmetrical). Brain perfusion studies in FLD patients demonstrate characteristic reduction in the blood flow to the frontal lobes (bilateral and al-most symmetrical) with possible involvement of one or both temporal lobes (Figure 9.7).

OTHER DEMENTIAS

In this group, a large variety of dementia syndromes of diverse aetiology may be included. The most important are the diseases with a strong immunological background such as multiple sclerosis and HIV-positive dementia complex. The former, because it is a demyelinating disease, is best suited for high-resolution MRI. The latter will be discussed in a later section, 'Infection/ Oncology', together with other infections and tumours.

A final reference must be made to the potential clinical benefits of radionuclide imaging of the brain to distinguish between dementia and depression, particularly in the elderly. In depression, there is reduced perfusion/rCBF in the frontal lobes and temporal lobes part of the limbic system, apparently responsible for the development of mood disorders. The reduction in perfusion ratios is less marked than in FLD. More importantly, the reduction appears more marked in the prefrontal cortex [56,57] and improves dramatically with adequate therapy with accompanying improvement in symptomatology (Figure 9.9).

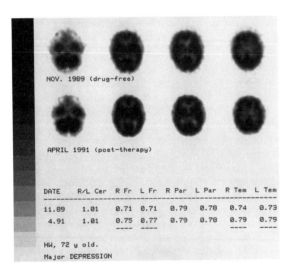

Figure 9.9 Similar transverse slices of a longitudinal study, pre- and post-therapy follow-up of a patient with major depression. In the first study (November, 1989) when the patient was drug-free there was reduced perfusion to both frontal and temporal lobes, but less marked than in FLD (Figure 9.7). Quantitative analysis confirmed the findings and the improvement after treatment (April, 1991) with a course of tricyclic antidepressants.

REFERENCES

1. Hales, R.E., Yudofsky, S.C. and Talbott, J.A. (eds) (1994) *The American Psychiatric Press Textbook of Psychiatry*, 2nd edn, The American Psychiatric Press, Inc., Washington, DC, London.
2. American Psychiatric Association (1994) *Diagnostic and Statistical Manual of Mental Disorders*, 4th edn, American Psychiatric Association, Washington, DC.
3. Rabins, P.V. (1983) Reversible dementia and the misdiagnosis of dementia: a review. *Hospital Community Psychiatry*, **34**, 830–35.
4. Cummings, J.L., Benson, D.F. and LoVerme, S. Jr (1980) Reversible dementia. *JAMA*, **243**, 2434–9.
5. Oshima, S. (1996) Live Long and Prospect? *Science*, **273**, 42–5.
6. Ineichen, B. (1987) Measuring the rising tide: how many dementia cases will there be by 2001? *Br. J. Psychiatry*, **150**, 193.
7. US Congress (1987) Office of Technology Assessment: Losing a Million Minds: Confronting the Tragedy of Alzheimer's Disease and Other Dementias (OTA-BA-323). Washington, DC, US Government Printing Office.
8. McKhann, G., Drachman, D., Folstein, M. *et al.* (1984) Clinical diagnosis of Alzheimer's disease: report of the NINCDS–ADRDA Work Group under the aus-

pices of the Department of Health and Human Services Task Force on Alzheimer's disease. *Neurology*, **34**, 939–44.

9. Hachinski, V.C., Iliff, L.D., Zilhka, E. *et al.* (1975) Cerebral blood flow in dementia. *Arch. Neurol.*, **32**, 632–7.

10. Hachinski, V.C. (1987) Multi-infarct dementia, in *Dementia*, Churchill Livingstone, Edinburgh.

11. Rosen, W.G., Terry, R.D., Fuld, P.A. *et al.* (1980) Pathological verification of ischaemic score in differentiation of dementias. *Ann. Neurol.*, **7**, 486–8.

12. Erkinjuntti, T., Haltia, M., Palo, J. *et al.* (1988) Accuracy of the clinical diagnosis of vascular dementia: a prospective clinical and post-mortem neuropathological study. *J. Neurol. Neurosurg. Psychiatry*, **51**, 1037–44.

13. Joachim, C.L., Morris, J. and Selkoe, D.J. (1986) Autopsy neuropathology in 76 cases of clinically diagnosed Alzheimer's disease. *Neuropathology*, **36**(suppl. 1), 226.

14. Davis, K.L. (1992) The scintigraphic appearance of Alzheimer's disease: a prospective study using technetium-99m-HMPAO SPECT [editorial]. *J. Nucl. Med.*, **33**, 312.

15. Folstein, M.F., Folstein, S.E. and McHugh, P.R. (1975) Mini-mental state': a practical method for grading the cognitive state of patients for the clinician. *J. Psychiatr. Res.*, **12**, 189–98.

16. Blessed, G., Tomlinson, B.E. and Roth, M. (1968) The association between quantitative measures of dementia and of senile change in the cerebral grey matter of elderly subjects. *Br. J. Psychiatry*, **114**, 797–811.

17. Roth, M., Tym, E., Mountjoy, C.Q. *et al.* (1986) CAMDEX. A standardized instrument for the diagnosis of mental disorders in the elderly with special reference to the early detection of dementia. *Br. J. Psychiatry*, **149**, 698–709.

18. Roth, M., Huppert, F.A., Tym, E. *et al.* (1988) *CAMDEX: The Cambridge examination for mental disorders of the elderly*. Cambridge University Press, Cambridge.

19. Beardsall, L. and Huppert, F. (1991) A comparison of clinical, psychometric and behavioural memory tests: findings from a community study of the early detection of dementia. *Int. J. Geriatric Psychiatry*, **6**, 295–306.

20. Albert, M.S. (1992) Neuropsychology: detection of dementia using rating scales and psychometric testing. *Curr. Opin. Psychiatry*, **5**, 543–7.

21. Appel, S.H. (1981) A unifying hypothesis for the cause of ALS, parkinsonism and Alzheimer disease. *Ann. Neurol.*, **10**, 499–503.

22. Brown, R.G. and Marsden, C.D. (1984) How common is dementia in Parkinson's disease. *Lancet*, **i**, 1262–5.

23. Hamil, R.W., Caine, E., Eskin, T. *et al.* (1988) Neurodegenerative disorders and aging. Alzheimer's disease and Parkinson's disease – common ground. *Ann. N. Y. Acad. Sci.*, **515**, 411–20.

24. Harrington, C.R., Louwagie, J., Rossau, R. *et al.* (1994) Influence of apolipoprotein E genotype on senile dementia of the Alzheimer and Lewy body types. *Am. J. Pathol.*, **145**, 1472–84.

25. Al-Chalabi, A., Anayat, Z.E., Bakker, M.C. *et al.* (1996) Association of apolipoprotein E e4 allele with bulbar-onset motor neuron disease. *Lancet*, **347**, 159–60.

26. Marder, K., Maestre, G., Cote, L. *et al.* (1994) The apolipoprotein e4 allele in Parkinson's disease with and without dementia. *Neurology*, **44**, 1330–1.

27. Perry, R.H., Irving, D., Blessed, G. *et al.* (1990) Senile dementia of the Lewy body type. *J. Neurol. Sci.*, **95**, 119–39.

28. Crook, T., Bartus, R.T., Ferris, S.H. *et al.* (1986) Age-associated memory impairment: proposed diagnostic criteria and measures of clinical change – report of a National Institute of Mental Health work group. *Dev. Neuropsychiatry*, **2**, 261–76.

29. Wickelgren, I. (1996) The aging brain – for the cortex, neuron loss may be less than thought. *Science*, **271**, 48–50.

30. Peters, A. *et al.* (1994) The effects of aging on area 46 of the frontal cortex of the rhesus monkey. *Cerebral Cortex*, **6**, 621.

31. Chugani, H.T. and Phelps, M.E. (1986) Maturational changes in cerebral function in infants determined by [18]FDG positron emission tomography. *Science*, **231**, 840–3.

32. Hoffman, J.M., Guze, B.H., Hawk, T.C. *et al.* (1988) Cerebral glucose metabolism in normal individuals: effects of aging, sex, and handedness. *Neurology*, **38**(suppl.1), 371.

33. Yoshii, F., Barker, W.W., Chang, J.Y. *et al.* (1988) Sensitivity of cerebral glucose metabolism to age, gender, brain volume, brain atrophy, and cerebrovascular risk factors. *J. Cereb. Blood Flow Metab.*, **8**, 654–61.

34. Waldemar, G., Hasselbalch, S.G., Andersen, A.R. *et al.* (1991) 99mTc-d,l-HMPAO and SPECT of the brain in normal aging. *J. Cereb. Blood Flow Metab.*, **11**, 508–21.

35. Amenta, F., Zaccheo, D. and Collier, W.L. (1991) Neurotransmitters, neuroreceptors and aging. *Mech. Ageing Dev.*, **61**, 249–73.

36. Markus, H.S., Ring, H., Kouris, K. and Costa, D.C. (1993) Alterations in regional cerebral blood flow, with increased temporal interhemispheric asymmetries, in the normal elderly: an HMPAO SPECT study. *Nucl. Med. Commun.*, **14**, 628–33.

37. Costa, D.C., Tannock, C. and Brostoff, J. (1995) Brainstem perfusion is impaired in patients with myalgic encephalomyelitis/chronic fatigue syndrome. *Q. J. Med.*, **88**, 767–73.

38. Constans, J.M., Meyerhoff, D.J., Gerson, J. *et al.* (1995) H-1 MR spectroscopic imaging of white matter signal intensities: Alzheimer disease and ischaemic vascular dementia. *Radiology*, **197**, 517–23.

39. Frackowiak, R.S.J., Pozzilli, C., Legg, N.J. *et al.* (1981) Regional cerebral oxygen supply and utilization in dementia. A clinical and physiological study with oxygen-15 and positron tomography. *Brain*, **104**, 753–78.

40. Kumar, A., Schapiro, M.B., Grady, C. *et al.* (1991) High-resolution PET studies in Alzheimer's disease. *Neuropsychopharmacology*, **4**, 35–46.

41. Grady, C., Haxby, J., Horwitz, B. *et al.* (1988) Longitudinal study of the early neuropsychological and

cerebral metabolic changes in dementia of the Alzheimer type. *J. Clin. Exp. Neuropsychol.*, **10**, 576–96.

42. Kuhl, D.E., Small, G.W., Riege, W.H. *et al.* (1987) Cerebral metabolic patterns before the diagnosis of probable Alzheimer's disease. *J. Cereb. Blood Flow Metab.*, **7**(suppl.), S406.

43. Launes, J., Sulkava, R., Erkinjuntti, T. *et al.* (1991) 99Tcm-HMPAO SPECT in suspected dementia. *Nucl. Med. Commun.*, **12**, 757–65.

44. Holman, B.L., Johnson, K.A., Gerada, B. *et al.* (1992) The scintigraphic appearance of Alzheimer's disease: a prospective study using technetium-99m-HMPAO SPECT. *J. Nucl. Med.*, **33**, 181–5.

45. Costa, D.C., Ell, P.J., Burns, A. *et al.* (1988) CBF tomograms with [99mTc]-HM-PAO in patients with dementia (Alzheimer type and HIV) and Parkinson's disease – initial results. *J. Cereb. Blood Flow Metab.*, **8**, S109–15.

46. Burns, A., Philpot, M., Costa, D.C. *et al.* (1989) The investigation of Alzheimer's disease with single photon emission tomography. *J. Neurol. Neurosurg. Psychiatry*, **52**, 248–53.

47. Costa, D.C. (1989) *A study of the first 99Tcm-labelled radiopharmaceutical for the investigation of cerebral blood flow in man.* PhD Thesis, University of London.

48. Jobst, K.A., Smith, A.D., Barker, C.S. *et al.* (1992) Association of atrophy of the medial temporal lobe with reduced blood flow in the posterior parietotemporal cortex in patients with a clinical and pathological diagnosis of Alzheimer's disease. *J. Neurol. Neurosurg. Psychiatry*, **55**, 190–4.

49. Lennox, G., Lowe, J., Morrell, K. *et al.* (1989) Diffuse Lewy body disease using correlative neuropathology anti-ubiquitin immunocytochemistry. *J. Neurol. Neurosurg. Psychiatry*, **52**, 1236–47.

50. Costa, D.C., Walker, Z. and Katona, C.L.E. (1995) Lewy body dementia – dopamine D2 neuroreceptor availability studied with single photon emission tomography. *Eur. J. Nucl. Med.*, **22**, 823.

51. Costa, D.C., Walker, S., Waddington, W. *et al.* (1996) Pharmacokinetics and dosimetry of FP-CIT a new ligand to study the pre-synaptic transporter system. *Nucl. Med. Commun.*, **17**, 287.

52. Neary, D., Snowden, J.S., Northen, B. *et al.* (1988) Dementia of the frontal lobe type. *J. Neurol. Neurosurg. Psychiatry*, **51**, 353–61.

53. Miller, B.L., Cummings, J.L., Villanueva-Meyer, J. *et al.* (1991) Frontal lobe degeneration: clinical, neuropsychological, and SPECT characteristics. *Neurology*, **41**, 1374–82.

54. Markus, H.S., Lees, A.J., Lennox, G., Marsden, C.D. and Costa, D.C. (1995) Patterns of regional cerebral blood flow in corticobasal degeneration studied using HMPAO SPECT; comparison with Parkinson's disease and normal controls. *Movement Disorders*, **10**, 179–87.

55. Butler, R.E., Costa, D.C., Greco, A. *et al.* (1995) Differentiation between Alzheimer's disease and multi-infarct dementia: SPECT vs MR imaging. *Int. J. Geriatric Psychiatry*, **10**, 121–8.

56. McKeith, I.G., Bartholomew, P.H. and Irvine, E.M. (1993) Single photon emission computerised tomography in elderly patients with Alzheimer's disease and multi-infarct dementia. regional uptake of technetium-labelled HMPAO related to clinical measurements. *Br. J. Psychiatry*, **163**, 597–603.

57. Sackheim, H.A., Prohovnik, I., Moeller, J.R. *et al.* (1993) Regional cerebral blood flow in mood disorders. II. Comparison of major depression and Alzheimer's disease. *J. Nucl. Med.*, **34**, 1090–101.

Cerebrovascular disease

J. Patterson and D. J. Wyper

INTRODUCTION

There are several causes of stroke, but common to all is a critical reduction in cerebral blood flow, resulting in a focal neurological deficit. The presumption that functional imaging, particularly of cerebral perfusion, should therefore have a major role to play in the management of this disorder was contradicted initially by a relatively indifferent attitude to these techniques. A clearer definition of the true value of the technique has now emerged confirming that SPECT has much to offer. This chapter gives an outline of the potential benefits, which can result from a knowledge of regional cerebral perfusion: in the acute post-stroke period where exciting new therapies targeted at limiting the neurological damage are under trial; in the later stages when the main effort lies in rehabilitation; and in the vital 'warning' stages in patients with carotid artery disease who are at greatest risk of suffering a stroke.

ACUTE STROKE

Rapid advances in the understanding of the pathophysiology of cerebral ischaemia have been made in recent years. The likelihood of tissue infarction following a reduction in cerebral perfusion is dependent on the degree and duration of the ischaemic insult. The more profound the drop in perfusion, the faster the tissue progresses to irreversible damage and the less is the time available for therapeutic intervention [1]. When flow almost ceases, the time-scale is so short that intervention is impractical in all but rare cases. In any stroke, perfusion within the affected area is heterogeneous and some tissue, especially in the postulated penumbral region, will remain in a potentially salvageable but parlous haemodynamic state for several hours. For this tissue, there appears to be a 'window of opportunity' [2], within which time measures to restore perfusion or improve collateral circulation may salvage the tissue. Delayed beyond this point, therapy would not only be ineffective but may also be harmful.

As long as tissue remains ischaemic, many processes conspire to shift the precarious balance towards infarction. Blood pressure, glucose and electrolyte levels, and fluid balance are among the factors that need to be carefully controlled. It is now also recognized that a cascade of secondary processes within the brain are fundamental to the development of ischaemic damage. In particular, the high level of intracellular calcium resulting from ischaemia triggers several events that lead to cell death. Siesjo et al. [3] have recently emphasized that much of the cellular calcium influx follows directly from the release of neuroactive chemicals such as the excitatory amino acid, glutamate, an agonist that opens ion channels in the cell membrane. Also implicated in the mechanism of ischaemic damage are acidosis and the release of highly reactive and toxic free radicals.

Two distinct strategies for acute therapeutic intervention therefore present themselves: manoeuvres designed to restore perfusion [4], and pharmacological intervention to provide neuronal protection [2,5]. In each case, the therapeutic time-window is finite. Although most evidence points to a period of 3–6 hours, recent data not only challenge the concept of a rigid time-window [6], but also demonstrate that some benefit might be obtained even beyond 24 hours [7]. Conceptually, there may be merit in considering any stroke as having an individual 'map' of varying time-windows, with the shortest value being in the densely ischaemic centre.

In acute stroke, diagnostic imaging has a role to play only if it can provide useful information within the short time-scale relevant to therapeutic intervention. Computed tomography (CT) is guaranteed such a role by its ability to detect haemorrhage associated with the stroke. However, neither CT nor routine MRI can reliably detect ischaemic tissue in the crucial early stages [8], since only minimal structural changes occur at this time. In marked contrast to this, the SPECT cerebral perfusion scan is

Clinical Nuclear Medicine, 3rd edn. Edited by M.N. Maisey, K.E. Britton and B.D. Collier. Published in 1998 by Chapman & Hall, London. ISBN 0 412 75180 1

abnormal from the moment the blood supply is disrupted.

An illustration of the inherent advantage of SPECT is given in Plate 20. Whereas the CT at 7 hours shows no clear abnormality, the SPECT study performed 4 hours earlier confirms the clinical impression of a right middle cerebral artery stroke. At this time there is some preservation of perfusion in the head of caudate and in the lateral temporal region. By 24 hours the infarct is apparent on the CT and shows little change in the size of the abnormal region over the next 10 days. But on SPECT, the profound perfusion deficit expands to include the head of caudate plus more of the temporal region by 24 hours, and covers almost the entire temporal lobe on the 11th day. Although the mere presence of perfusion does not necessarily indicate viability, there is no doubt that this SPECT study provides additional information, which is consistent with the current concepts of stroke pathophysiology. First, as expected, SPECT exhibits a significant perfusion deficit at a time when the CT is still completely normal [9–12]. Second, the SPECT scan also demonstrates that the perfusion deficit may enlarge over the first 24 hours [13], i.e. over a time-scale similar to the postulated therapeutic time-window when secondary damage may be taking place. In this patient, active pharmacological intervention may well have prevented progression of the infarcted area. Finally, and most surprising, is the change in perfusion deficit between 24 hours and 11 days, which lends support to the recent evidence that the therapeutic time-window may extend beyond 24 hours in some cases and that reperfusion therapy, even when delayed, may improve the clinical outcome [4].

Angiography and Doppler ultrasound [4,14] are used to assess the reopening of larger blood vessels, but the ultimate test of reperfusion therapy must be the effect on cerebral tissue, for which SPECT is the most appropriate method of assessment. Baird *et al.* [11,15] performed ^{99m}Tc-HMPAO-SPECT within 8 hours of stroke onset and repeated the scans at 24 hours to assess reperfusion. In both studies reperfusion was associated with a better outcome. Interestingly, in the latter study, which compared patients who had no treatment with those who had streptokinase thrombolytic therapy, an improvement in perfusion was seen in 65% of the patients who received streptokinase, but this also happened in 52% of patients who received no active treatment. Therefore, spontaneous reperfusion appears to be a common occurrence after stroke. The outcome was again better in patients with evidence of reperfusion, regardless of whether this occurred with streptokinase or spontaneously. A dramatic illustration of spontaneous reperfusion is in the syndrome known as the 'spectacular shrinking deficit' [13] where SPECT changes parallel the clinical features. Hanson *et al.* [10] have issued a cautionary note that there may be a threshold in the initial perfusion deficit beyond which reperfusion may have a high likelihood of inducing oedema or haemorrhage. A very large perfusion deficit is likely to include a significant area which has been irreversibly damaged within a very short time period, and for which there is no therapeutic window. Efforts to reperfuse that area could result in catastrophic haemorrhage.

A number of recent papers have examined the ability of SPECT to provide prognostic information in acute stroke. It is essential to recognize that this is an elusive aim for three main reasons. First, for many patients, the outcome in acute stroke is as likely to be determined by their general management and by non-cerebral events as by the cerebral infarct itself. Second, estimates of prognosis may vary with the time after onset because of the changing nature of the acute ischaemic insult over the first day or so, during which it may progress or disappear altogether (as portrayed by the 'spectacular shrinking deficit' syndrome). Third, an estimate of prognosis delayed beyond 48 hours suffers from the complicating factors of non-nutritional hyperperfusion and tracer hyperfixation that appear in the subacute stage as described below. By this time, CT also generally depicts the infarct.

It is almost certainly for the last reason that so many of the early SPECT studies in 'acute' stroke inevitably concluded that perfusion imaging had little prognostic value, as they were all performed days after the onset. Now that studies have been published where SPECT has been carried out within the first 6–12 hours, it is apparent that SPECT provides prognostic information that correlates with long-term outcome [10,12] and which may complement clinical rating scales such as the Canadian Neurological Scale [12].

The most important predictive information which SPECT can provide is in the first few hours after the onset, when decisions on clinical management and selection for clinical trials are being made. Marchal *et al.* [16] classified PET cerebral blood flow and oxygen consumption images acquired 5–18 hours after the onset of stroke into three categories and compared the scan results with the clinical outcome. In category I, with profoundly reduced perfusion, the outcome was consistently poor, whereas in category III, where perfusion was increased, the outcome was excellent. The category II patients with mild to moderate perfusion compromise had a variable outcome. The authors postulated that acute therapy would be too late in category I and ineffective in category III, and suggested that such patients be excluded from clinical trials. They concluded that SPECT would be preferable from a practical point of view. Now that the capability of SPECT has been confirmed [10,11,13], it should be adopted as an integral part of all acute stroke trials.

It is worth noting that one feature of SPECT which gives it an advantage over PET scanning is that when using perfusion tracers which are chemically trapped (e.g. ^{99m}Tc-HMPAO or ECD) it can effectively be the first investigation carried out on a stroke patient. If the radiopharmaceutical is administered immediately on admission, other essential procedures can then be carried out before the patient need be taken to the SPECT scanner. Since there is little redistribution of tracer, the scan corresponds to the perfusion pattern at the time of radiopharmaceutical administration.

SUBACUTE STROKE

The interpretation of SPECT images becomes more difficult in the subacute stage – approximately between 48 hours and 28 days following the stroke. During this time, the so-called 'luxury perfusion', i.e. an over-abundant cerebral blood flow relative to the metabolic needs of the tissue, can sometimes appear [17]. This relative increase in flow (not necessarily hyperperfused compared with normal tissue), relies on at least some recanalization of previously obstructed vessels, but occurs at a time too late to aid recovery, and is indicative of tissue damage. The rise in flow is probably caused by substances released by the damaged tissue and gradually declines again over the next 2–3 weeks, until it reaches an equilibrium level compatible with metabolism. At this point,

the perfusion pattern will resemble that seen in the acute stage.

Fundamental differences between the perfusion tracers are highlighted by the luxury perfusion phenomenon, which is detected by IMP and HMPAO but not by ECD [18]. This inability of ECD to reflect a true rise in perfusion is probably linked to a disturbance within the damaged tissue of the enzyme activity necessary for the trapping of ECD. The HMPAO trapping mechanism therefore appears to be more robust. It has been argued that the metabolically limited uptake of ECD may be beneficial in depicting tissue viability more directly than HMPAO [19], although the difficulty in interpreting the data, in a transient condition with known uncoupling of flow and metabolism, cannot be ignored.

During the early subacute period, blood-brain barrier disruption also becomes established, allowing polar molecules to enter the tissue and oedema to form. This is one of the possible causes of the hyperfixation phenomenon shown by Sperling and Lassen [20] to occur only in subacute stroke many days after onset and to appear only in areas destined for infarction. Although as yet only reported for HMPAO, this is likely to apply to all perfusion tracers, and results in an enhancement of the uptake in an area of the brain that is already hyperperfused.

An example of subacute imaging is illustrated in Plate 21. Ten days following a middle cerebral artery stroke, the HMPAO-SPECT scan shows a very high tracer uptake representing non-nutritional luxury perfusion, although a component of hyperfixation may also be present. At day 13, the uptake has reduced slightly and by day 24, the uptake is below the normal contralateral hemisphere. At day 170, the completed infarct is now well visualized. In this case, reperfusion has been achieved in the subacute stage, several days post ictus, by which time tissue damage has occurred. The hyperperfusion is non-nutritional and tissue is not salvageable.

Some clues as to the viability of tissue within the context of this complicated picture have been described. Infeld and colleagues [21] report that if reduced perfusion is seen in the cerebellum contralateral to a hyperperfused area (a phenomenon known as crossed cerebellar diaschisis), this is evidence of a reduction in afferent input to the cerebellum from the site of the affected tissue and therefore indicates non-viable tissue. The washout of tracer is also thought to be relevant. Costa and Ell [22] found that viable tissue has a high uptake of HMPAO with a long retention time, whereas non-viable tissue washed out at a much higher rate – the late images therefore give a better indication of tissue viability.

Later in the subacute stage, once hyperperfusion has resolved, it is generally accepted that tissue damage is complete, and the main effort is directed towards devising rehabilitation strategies. During this period, the damaged parts of the brain may regain functional activity or brain 'plasticity' may lead to a partial restoration of activity by functional reorganization within the brain [23]. SPECT has been advocated as a tool for the prediction of recovery to ensure efficient use of resources targeted at long-term rehabilitation. Mountz *et al.* [24] compared CT with HMPAO-SPECT, and by using a quantitative index showed that the recovery of neurological deficits was greatest in strokes where the SPECT abnormality was much larger than the completed infarct on CT – similar to the image shown in Plate 21(d), where reduced perfusion is seen anterior and posterior to the MRI-defined infarct. The SPECT 'penumbra' presumably represents areas of the brain with the potential for revival. Further evidence of the recoverability of this tissue may be demonstrated by a normal or even increased response [9] to cerebrovascular reactivity testing using acetazolamide. Dam *et al.* [25] showed that a mild perfusion asymmetry on HMPAO-SPECT scans at 3 months, was a good predictor of recovery one year later, even in patients with unfavourable clinical parameters.

STROKE PREVENTION

A role for perfusion imaging is also indicated in patients at risk of developing a stroke, particularly in carotid artery disease. A number of major clinical trials have proven beyond doubt that endarterectomy for a symptomatic carotid stenosis >70% is an effective procedure compared with aggressive medical management. The risk of major or fatal stroke within the following 2 years is reduced from 13% to <4% [26]. In patients with asymptomatic stenoses, the benefits of operative intervention are less certain due to the lower intrinsic stroke risk.

Selection of patients for endarterectomy is determined by the precise criteria indicated in the clinical trials and involves accurate identification of the extent of stenosis in the artery. SPECT has no role to play in that particular process. The impressive statistical benefits of endarterectomy cannot, however, disguise the fact that only one person will gain these substantial benefits for every ten operations performed. The ratio is even higher for asymptomatic or lower degrees of stenoses. Refinement of the selection procedure and identification of particular patient subgroups would increase the effectiveness of the procedure.

While most perfusion studies in acute and subacute stroke are performed under resting conditions, in carotid artery disease, the sensitivity of perfusion measurements is poor unless the circulation is stressed. This can be achieved either by the inhalation of 5–7% carbon dioxide (which can be uncomfortable but is rapidly reversible), or by the administration of acetazolamide, a carbonic anhydrase inhibitor that increases the local carbon dioxide concentration in the brain. A comparison of the resting and stressed scans produces an estimate of the cerebral perfusion reserve (CPR), normalizing tracer uptake in each region to the cerebellum or total brain [27,28]. Findings in SPECT are consistent with other techniques of assessing blood flow, and show reduced CPR in a large but variable proportion of patients with carotid artery disease, provided that the degree of stenosis is greater than 50–70% [29]. The importance of assessing the cerebral circulation rather than the carotid artery is illustrated by the poor correlation between the degree of carotid stenosis and the ipsilateral CPR [29,30]. This highlights the vital role played by the collateral circulation in the brain, especially in the presence of haemodynamic compromise. Following endarterectomy, the CPR improves [31], and the improvement also extends into the contralateral side.

The predictive ability of CPR measurements in patients with symptomatic disease has been demonstrated in several reports [32,33]. Poor CPR is an important predictor of impending infarction, with a ten-fold difference in stroke risk between patients with good reactivity and those with a poor response [33]. Although gross indicators of cerebral perfusion and CPR, such as Doppler ultrasound, have been used in some studies, the importance of heterogeneity of cerebral haemodynamics has been emphasized [34]. An example of CPR evaluation is illustrated in Plate 22, which shows the CT and HMPAO-SPECT images of a 60-year-old female patient with severe bilateral carotid disease. The CT is relatively normal, with no gross evidence of infarction, and the resting perfusion scan shows only a slight deficit in the right parietal region. Perfusion in the right parietal and occipital regions is unable to respond to the stimulus provided by acetazolamide, indicating haemodynamic instability on this side. The patient was scheduled for carotid artery surgery, but before that could be carried out she developed a massive right hemisphere stroke.

SPECT can identify patients with haemodynamically significant carotid artery disease, and is ideally placed to aid in the selection of patients for endarterectomy. The technique can be extended to other cerebrovascular diseases such as moyamoya [27] and arteritis where therapeutic approaches should be based as much on the assessment of end-organ perfusion as on large vessel changes.

BEYOND PERFUSION

Imaging of perfusion is of undoubted value, but clearly can address only some of the pathophysiological issues in stroke. Other biochemical processes, however, are also amenable to investigation by SPECT, and these may provide a more revealing insight into the mechanisms of ischaemic damage.

Nitroimidazoles are compounds which are preferentially retained in hypoxic tissue and are therefore capable of demarcating viable but at-risk tissue. They have been labelled with technetium-99m, and the initial distribution is highly dependent on blood flow. This provides a powerful combination of early and late images representing perfusion and tissue viability respectively [35].

In cerebral ischaemia, there is a marked elevation of the extracellular concentration of glutamate, irrespective of the nature and primary cause of the ischaemic episode. This is known to be neurotoxic as a consequence of the extreme activation of the NMDA glutamate receptor subtype which opens membrane ion channels with a high calcium permeability and leads to a lethal influx of calcium [36]. There are a number of distinct sites within the NMDA receptor ion channel complex at which drugs may act to attenuate the effects of glutamate, and therefore are also open to binding by a suitable radiotracer. Agents such as dizocipline (MK-801) interact with a site within the ion channel itself to produce non-

competitive agonist-dependent blockade of the actions of glutamate. In experimental animals with focal cerebral ischaemia, the initial (5–15 min) uptake of radiolabelled (^{3}H or ^{125}I) MK-801 reflects cerebral blood flow, but at later times (60–240 min), the retention of the tracer is enhanced in the ischaemic territory, reflecting putatively the elevated glutamate levels and the active opening of the ion channels. Production of (+)-3-^{123}I-Iodo-MK-801 has enabled SPECT imaging of NMDA receptor activation to be performed in living humans [37]. The utility of (+)-3-^{123}I-Iodo-MK-801 as a SPECT ligand for assessing modest alterations in NMDA receptor activity may however be limited by its lipophilicity (and consequent high nonspecific binding); improved agents with lower lipophilicity are currently being developed in order to allow imaging of this active ischaemic process.

The benzodiazepine (BZ) receptor ligand ^{123}I-iomazenil, provides an alternative approach to the assessment of tissue damage. Central-type BZ receptors are located principally on neuronal synapses and are part of the GABAergic inhibitory system, which is widely distributed in the cerebral cortex. The concentration of these receptors equates with the number of synapses and is hence an indication of the intactness of the cortical neurones [7]. A limitation of iomazenil is that it gives no information on the central grey matter structures of the basal ganglia and thalamus because of the sparsity of BZ receptors in these structures. In comparative studies with HMPAO, iomazenil showed less of a decrease in the acute stroke phase than HMPAO, suggesting presence of viable but underperfused tissue [38]. The opposite picture is seen in the chronic phase and is consistent with the notion of incomplete infarction advanced by Garcia *et al.* [7]. A disadvantage of all of the above compounds is the late imaging time (an average of 2–3 hours after administration), which may be too long to influence the vital decisions that have to be taken as early as possible in acute stroke.

REFERENCES

1. Jones, T.H., Morawetz, R.B., Crowell, R.M., Marcoux, F.W., Fitzgibbon, S.J., DeGirolami, U. and Ojemann, R.J. (1981) Thresholds of focal cerebral ischaemia in awake monkeys. *J. Neurosurg.*, **54**, 773–82.
2. Camarata, P.J., Heros, R.C., Latchaw, R.E., Piepgras, D.G., Whisnet, J.P. and Smith, R.R. (1994) 'Brain

Attack': the rationale for treating stroke as a medical emergency. *Neurosurgery*, **34**, 144–58.

3. Siesjo, B.K., Zhao, Q., Pahlmark, K., Siesjo, P., Katsura, K.I. and Folbergrova, J. (1995) Glutamate, calcium, and free radicals as mediators of ischemic brain damage. *Ann. Thorac. Surg.*, **59**, 1316–20.

4. Von Kummer, R., Holle, R., Rosin, L., Forsting, M. and Hacke, W. (1995) Does arterial recanalization improve outcome in carotid territory stroke? *Stroke*, **26**, 581–7.

5. Asplund, K. (1995) Stroke therapy – time for a clinical breakthrough: introduction. *J. Int. Med.*, **237**, 73–8.

6. Baron, J.C., von Kummer, R. and del Zopo, G.J. (1995) Treatment of acute ischemic stroke: challenging the concept of a rigid and universal time window. *Stroke*, **26**, 2219–21.

7. Garcia, J.H., Lassen, N.A., Weiller, C., Sperling, B. and Nakagawara, J. (1996) Ischemic stroke and incomplete infarction. *Stroke*, **27**, 761–5.

8. Mohr, J.P., Biller, J., Hilal, S.K. *et al.* (1995) Magnetic resonance versus computed tomography imaging in acute stroke. *Stroke*, **26**, 807–12.

9. Mountz, J.M., Deutsch, G. and Khan, S.H. (1993) Regional cerebral blood flow changes in stroke imaged by Tc-99m HMPAO SPECT with corresponding anatomic image correlation. *Clin. Nucl. Med.*, **18**, 1067–82.

10. Hanson, S.K., Grotta, J.C., Rhoades, H., Tran, H.D., Lamki, L.M., Barron, B.J. and Taylor, W.J. (1993) Value of single-photon emission-computed tomography in acute stroke therapeutic trials. *Stroke*, **24**, 1322–9.

11. Baird, A.E., Donnan, G.A., Austin, M.C., Fitt, G.J., Davis, S.M. and McKay, W.J. (1994) Reperfusion after thrombolytic therapy in ischemic stroke measured by single-photon emission computed tomography. *Stroke*, **25**, 79–85.

12. Laloux, P., Richelle, F., Jamart, J., De Coster, P. and Laterre, C. (1995) Comparative correlations of HMPAO SPECT indices, neurological score and stroke subtypes with clinical outcome in acute carotid infarcts. *Stroke*, **26**, 816–21.

13. Baird, A.E., Donnan, G.A., Austin, M.C. and McKay, W.J. (1995) Early reperfusion in the 'spectacular shrinking deficit' demonstrated by single photon emission computed tomography. *Neurology*, **45**, 1335–9.

14. Zanette, E.M., Roberti, C., Mancini, G., Pozzilli, C., Bragoni, M. and Toni, D. (1995) Spontaneous middle cerebral artery reperfusion in ischemic stroke. *Stroke*, **26**, 430–3.

15. Baird, A.E., Donnan, G.A., Sperling, B. and Lassen, N.A. (1993) Increased ^{99m}Tc-HMPAO uptake in ischemic stroke (2). *Stroke*, **24**, 1261–2.

16. Marchal, G., Serrati, C., Rioux, P. *et al.* (1993) PET imaging of cerebral perfusion and oxygen consumption in acute ischaemic stroke: relation to outcome. *Lancet*, **341**, 925–7.

17. Moretti, J.L., Defer, G. and Cinotti, L. (1990) Luxury perfusion with ^{99m}Tc-HMPAO and ^{123}I-IMP SPECT during the subacute phase of stroke. *Eur. J. Nucl. Med.*, **16**, 17–22.

18. Lassen, N.A. and Sperling, B. (1994) ^{99m}Tc-bicisate reliably images CBF in chronic brain diseases but fails to show reflow hyperemia in subacute stroke: report of a multicenter trial of 105 cases comparing ^{133}Xe and ^{99m}Tc-bicisate (ECD, neurolite) measured by SPECT on same day. *J. Cereb. Blood Flow Metab.*, **14**, S44–8.

19. Moretti, J.L., Caglar, M. and Weinmann, P. (1995) Cerebral perfusion imaging tracers for SPECT: which one to choose? *J. Nucl. Med.*, **36**, 359–63.

20. Sperling, B. and Lassen, N.A. (1993) Hyperfixation of HMPAO in subacute ischemic stroke leading to spuriously high estimates of cerebral blood flow by SPECT. *Stroke* **24**, 193–4.

21. Infeld, B., Davis, S.M., Lichtenstein, M., Mitchell, P.J. and Hopper, J.L. (1995) Crossed cerebellar diaschisis and brain recovery after stroke. *Stroke*, **26**, 90–5.

22. Costa, D.C. and Ell, P.J. (1989) Tc-99m HMPAO washout in prognosis of stroke. *Lancet*, **i**(8631), 213–14.

23. Weiller, C., Chollet, F., Friston, K.J., Wise, R.J.S. and Frackowiak, R.S.J. (1992) Functional reorganization of the brain in recovery from striatocapsular infarction in man. *Ann. Neurol.*, **31**, 463–72.

24. Mountz, J.M., Modell, J.G., Foster, N.L., DuPree, E.S., Ackermann, R.J., Petry, N.A., Bluemlein, L.E. and Kuhl, D.E. (1990) Prognostication of recovery following stroke using the comparison of CT and Tc-99m HMPAO SPECT. *J. Nucl. Med.*, **31**, 61–6.

25. Dam, M., Tonin, P., Casson, S. *et al.* (1996) Technetium-99m HMPAO SPECT predicts long term recovery after stroke. *Neurology*, **46**, A338–9.

26. North American Symptomatic Carotid Endarterectomy Trial Collaborators (NASCET) (1991) Beneficial effect of carotid endarterectomy in symptomatic patients with high grade carotid stenosis. *N. Engl. J. Med.*, **325**, 445–53.

27. Hoshi, H., Ohnishi, T., Jinnouchi, S., Futami, S., Nagamachi, S., Kodama, T., Watanabe, K. Ueda, T. and Wakisaka, S. (1994) Cerebral blood flow study in patients with moyamoya disease evaluated by IMP SPECT. *J. Nucl. Med.*, **35**, 44–50.

28. Oku, N., Matsumoto, M., Hashikawa, K. *et al.* (1994) Carbon dioxide reactivity by consecutive Technetium-99m-HMPAO SPECT in patients with chronically obstructed major cerebral artery. *J. Nucl. Med.*, **35**, 32–40.

29. Powers, W.J. (1991) Cerebral hemodynamics in ischemic cerebrovascular disease. *Ann. Neurol.*, **29**, 231–40.

30. Asenbaum, S., Reinprecht, A., Bricke, T., Wenger, S., Podreka, I. and Deecke, L. (1995) A study of acetazolamide-induced changes in cerebral blood flow using ^{99m}Tc HMPAO SPECT in patients with cerebrovascular disease. *Neuroradiology*, **37**, 13–19.

31. Cikrit, D.F., Burt, R.W., Dalsing, M.C., Lalka, S.G., Sawchuk, A.P., Waymire, B. and Witt, R.M. (1992) Acetazolamide enhanced single photon emission computed tomography (SPECT) evaluation of cerebral perfusion before and after carotid endarterectomy. *J. Vasc. Surg.*, **15**, 747–54.

32. Yonas, H., Smith, H.A., Durham, S.R., Pentheny, S.L. and Johnson, D.W. (1993) Increased stroke risk pre-

dicted by compromised cerebral blood flow reactivity. *J. Neurosurg.*, **79**, 483–9.

33. Webster, M.W., Makaroun, M.S., Steed, D.L. *et al.* (1995) Compromised cerebral blood flow reactivity is a predictor of stroke in patients with symptomatic carotid artery occlusive disease. *J. Vasc. Surg.*, **21**, 338–45.

34. Duncan, D.B., Fink, G.R., Wirth, M., Lottgen, J., Pawlik, G. and Heiss, W.D. (1996) Heterogeneity of cerebral haemodynamics in carotid artery disease. *J. Nucl. Med.*, **37**, 429–32.

35. DiRocco, R.J., Kuczynski, B.L., Pirro, J.P. *et al.* (1993) Imaging ischemic tissue at risk of infarction during stroke. *J. Cereb. Blood Flow Metab.*, **13**, 755–62.

36. McCulloch, J., Bullock, R. and Teasdale, G.M. (1991) Excitatory amino acid antagonists: opportunities for the treatment of ischaemic brain damage in man, in *Excitatory Amino Acid Antagonists* (ed. B.S. Meldrum), Blackwell Scientific Publications, London, pp. 287–326.

37. McCulloch, J., Owens, J., Patterson, J., Brown, D.R.P., Teasdale, G.M. and Wyper, D.J. (1994) Imaging NMDA receptor activation in cerebral ischaemia in man with ^{123}I-MK-801 and SPECT, in *Pharmacology of Cerebral Ischemia* (eds H. Krieglstein and H. Oberpichler-Schwenk), Wissenschaftliche Verlagsgesellschaft, Stuttgart, pp. 233–8.

38. Matsuda, H., Tsuji, S., Kuji, I., Shiba, K., Hisada, K. and Mori, H. (1995) Dual tracer autoradiography using ^{125}I-iomazenil and ^{99m}Tc-HMPAO in experimental brain ischaemia. *Nucl. Med. Commun.*, **16**, 581–90.

Infection and oncology

D. C. Costa and P. J. Ell

INTRODUCTION

The brain is protected from internal and external injury by special and specific physiological barriers. These are of three main types: (i) the blood–brain barrier (BBB) that separates the blood from the brain parenchyma; (ii) the blood–CSF barrier between the blood and the cerebrospinal fluid (CSF); and (iii) the CSF–brain barrier separating the CSF from the brain parenchyma [1].

Only when the BBB and/or the blood–CSF barriers are disrupted may aggressive pathogens pass through the meninges into the brain tissue and cause, for example, meningitis, encephalitis and other conditions.

The first steps in radionuclide imaging in the clinical area of brain infection and oncology were made in the early 1970s with the so-called classical BBB radiotracers. At that time, and before the advent of CT scanning, ^{99m}Tc-pertechnetate, ^{99m}Tc-DTPA, and later ^{99m}Tc-glucoheptonate, were highly successful in the localization of a disrupted BBB. These techniques were used in the diagnosis of extra- and intra-dural haematomas and intracranial abscesses, as well as of primary and secondary tumours. Even with the advent of CT scanning, the overall sensitivity of BBB radiotracers with SPECT in comparison with morphological imaging was sufficiently good [2].

Nowadays, the greatest value of BBB-SPECT is confined to the evaluation of patients with claustrophobia and others reluctant to enter the CT scanning suite or the MR imaging tunnel – apart from long waiting lists. More recently, brain perfusion radiotracers (e.g. ^{99m}Tc-HMPAO and ^{99m}Tc-ECD) and potassium analogues (e.g. ^{201}Tl, ^{99m}Tc-MIBI and ^{99m}Tc-Tetrofosmin) play a much more important role. The former is used to demonstrate regional cerebral blood flow abnormalities in patients with encephalitis (Herpes simplex, HIV-positive patients and myalgic encephalomyelitis/chronic fatigue syndrome); the latter is used to aid the differential diagnosis between tumour recurrence and post-irradiation necrosis, as well as between intracerebral lymphoma and toxoplasma infection.

HERPES SIMPLEX VIRAL ENCEPHALITIS

Although not a frequent condition, Herpes simplex viral encephalitis is difficult to diagnose, and has a poor outcome if not treated early; indeed, the earlier the diagnosis, the better the outcome. The final diagnosis is made either by the demonstration of abnormal CSF with high viral titres, or by biopsy. Brain perfusion SPECT studies demonstrate focal increase of the perfusion ratios in one or both temporal lobes during the acute phase (within 1 week) of the viral infection. Later in the evolution of the disease (more than 3 weeks) there is reduced perfusion, which can be almost absent in the same site of the initial hyperperfusion. These abnormalities are more frequently located in the mesial cortex of the temporal lobe. MRI shows some degree of gliosis in the same region [3,4].

MYALGIC ENCEPHALOMYELITIS/CHRONIC FATIGUE SYNDROME

There is some reluctance among neurologists and psychiatrists to accept myalgic encephalomyelitis/chronic fatigue syndrome (ME/CFS) as an independent disease entity. Depression is often considered as the main explanation for patients' complaints. ME/CFS is a major cause of absenteeism. All patients complain of significant lack of concentration and extreme fatigue, which may sometimes be severely disabling, leading to career disadvantage and often job loss. The discrepancy between patients' symptoms and objective findings on physical and neuropsychiatric examination has given rise to long debates in the peer-reviewed literature [5–7]. Although patients present with distinctive clinical features, no single causative agent has so far been identified. Neuropsychiatric manifestations of the disease include impairment of short-term memory, loss of concentration, excessive irritability, nominal dysphasia, hypersomnia, insomnia, recurrent vertigo and/or tinnitus. Their nature and severity

Clinical Nuclear Medicine, 3rd edn. Edited by M.N. Maisey, K.E. Britton and B.D. Collier. Published in 1998 by Chapman & Hall, London. ISBN 0 412 75180 1

raises the possibility of an organic component in the evolution of ME/CFS. Several groups have demonstrated widespread perfusion abnormalities throughout the cerebral cortex [8,9]. However, only one group has so far shown marked reduction of the perfusion to the brainstem of these patients, which is significantly different from normals and other patients with depression [10]. The findings were based on quantitative analysis. Figure 9.10 shows transverse slices of the brainstem of a patient with ME/CFS in comparison with a normal control and another patient with major depression. All the slices are at a similar level to show the brainstem, mainly composed of the upper part of the spinal cord, the pons and the lower part of the hypothalamus.

It remains to be seen if other researchers can confirm this pattern of brainstem hypoperfusion, and more importantly, how specific is this finding in this group of patients. Further studies should address the investigation of the natural course of the disease and the SPECT clinical correlates in response to either any available or newly developed therapeutic approach.

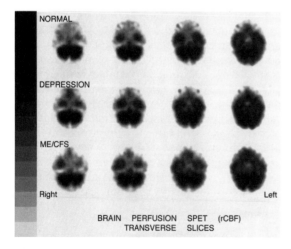

Figure 9.10 Each row shows four consecutive transverse slices through the brainstem (from left to right, the upper spinal cord, the pons and the lower hypothalamus are included). The brainstem is identified as the small round area almost in the centre of each slice, just ahead of the cerebellar hemispheres (dark) and pedunculi (white).

HUMAN IMMUNODEFICIENCY VIRUS (HIV) DISEASES

Infection with the type-1 human immunodeficiency virus (HIV-1), may produce a wide variety of central nervous system (CNS) symptoms and signs. CNS involvement in patients with the acquired immunodeficiency syndrome (AIDS), is frequently manifested by a dementing illness. However, focal infection and tumour infiltration are of significant concern in patient management – due to the difficulty in differentiating lymphoma infiltration from toxoplasma infection in the brain.

Several brain perfusion studies have demonstrated cortical perfusion deficits in patients with HIV encephalopathy. The first description in 1987 of abnormal perfusion deficits in HIV-positive patients reported two cases of cortical perfusion abnormalities, resembling those seen in patients with dementia of the Alzheimer type [11]. One of the patients, a 40-year-old homosexual male, presented with increasing lethargy, a tendency to fall to the left, and marked impairment of memory. Psychometric testing confirmed severe dementia with learning and memory deficits as well as marked apathy. A CT scan showed some cortical atrophy with enlarged lateral ventricles. Brain perfusion studies with ^{99m}Tc-HMPAO demonstrated bilaterally reduced perfusion to the temporoparietal region, and to the right frontal lobe. The second case presented with features of early encephalopathy, with minor atrophy on the CT scan. The brain perfusion study showed left parieto-occipital and bilateral temporal lobe perfusion abnormalities. Brain perfusion deficits correlate well with clinical presentation and increasing severity of clinical involvement [12]. Some patients were studied more than once and clinical progression of their dementia was shown to parallel the progression of abnormalities in the brain perfusion studies. Sometimes the abnormalities found in AIDS patients with dementia cannot be distinguished from those observed in other types of dementia [13,14]. Comparative studies between clinical presentation, brain perfusion using SPECT and structural imaging demonstrate the superiority of SPECT for the identification of cortical deficits, even in patients with unremarkable structural findings [15]. Furthermore, SPECT consistently demonstrates more perfusion abnormalities than the structural deficits observed with CT and/or MRI. However, MRI continues to be the modality of choice to study the white matter and its involvement in AIDS patients, where brain perfusion studies are practically of no help. Brain perfusion scintigraphy is more sensitive than CT and MRI in defining abnormalities during the early stages of clinical involvement. Therefore, its use in the management of patients with HIV encephalopathy appears to be important during the early phases of clinical involvement when structural imaging techniques may show little or no abnormalities. Unfortunately, there are no prospective studies assessing response to therapy.

Interestingly, in early HIV encephalopathy there appears to be relative hypermetabolism, and this has been demonstrated in the basal ganglia and thalamus of less severely affected patients by FDG-PET. It is followed in the later stages by hypometabolism, which can be either cortical or subcortical [16]. Metabolic rates in the white matter do not correlate with the severity of dementia. The most frequent finding is diffuse hypometabolism with some changes towards normal metabolic rates of glucose during therapy with zidovudine [17].

OPPORTUNISTIC INFECTIONS AND CNS NEOPLASMS

AIDS patients are susceptible to a wide variety of opportunistic infections and neoplasms, *Toxoplasma gondii* being one of the most common organisms. This infection is usually treated with pyrimethamine and either sulfadiazine or clindamycin. The diagnosis is based on the demonstration of simple or multiple intracerebral mass lesions, which may show a pattern of diffuse or ring enhancement on MRI. When anti-toxoplasma therapy fails, other diagnoses are likely and cerebral biopsy is considered. Brain biopsy of the patients with clinical 'toxoplasma' who did not respond to therapy confirms the continued presence of toxoplasma in 30% of the cases. However, the majority of the other 60% have intracerebral lymphoma. Primary intracerebral lymphoma occurs in the absence of extracranial disease. The majority are B-cell lymphomas. However, a few are primary T-cell lymphomas of the CNS. Approximately 2% of the entire AIDS population develop primary intracranial lymphoma. CNS lymphoma has a poor prognosis with a median survival time of less than 1 year, usually not greater than 7 months. There is an initial response to radiotherapy but recurrence and progression of the disease is fatal. The lesions are commonly single, and located in the periventricular brain tissue. However, 20–40% are multifocal, and difficult to distinguish from lesions due to toxoplasma [18,19]. It is not possible to establish the diagnosis, even with spectroscopic analysis [20]. In addition, serology is unhelpful in the diagnosis of toxoplasma. CSF cytology is only positive for lymphoma in one-third of the cases. CSF Epstein–Barr virus DNA detection shows highest yield in lymphoma, but lumbar puncture cannot always be performed as it is not safe in patients with raised intracranial pressure. MRI is sensitive but shows poor specificity.

Radionuclide imaging studies have been used to try and overcome these difficulties in the differential diagnosis between toxoplasma abscess(es) and lymphoma in patients with AIDS. The radionuclide of choice is ^{201}Tl thallous chloride, used either for planar gamma-camera imaging or SPECT. The rationale for the use of ^{201}Tl is based on the findings of previous studies that demonstrated the value of this radionuclide in the identification of intracerebral neoplasms and the differential diagnosis between tumour-recurrence and post-irradiation necrosis [21]. Abnormal focal increase of ^{201}Tl uptake can be demonstrated in patients with toxoplasmosis and subjects with confirmed lymphoma. However, tumour-to-background radioactivity ratios help differentiate between these two groups: ratios greater than 2.5 are likely to represent lymphoma, whereas a ratio of less than 2.0 favours a diagnosis of toxoplasmosis [22]. Figures 9.11 and 9.12 show examples of toxoplasma abscess and intracerebral lymphoma respectively. FDG-PET studies also demonstrate good separation of the two entities, with high uptake in lymphoma and low or normal uptake at sites of toxoplasma infection.

CEREBRAL TUMOUR RECURRENCE VERSUS RADIATION NECROSIS

After radiotherapy, clinical deterioration due to either recurrence of the tumour or radiation necrosis is not rare [23]. High-resolution structural imaging (CT, MRI and cerebral angiography) has been unable to provide a clear distinction between these conditions. Either tumour-recurrence or radiation necrosis may show contrast enhancement [24,25].

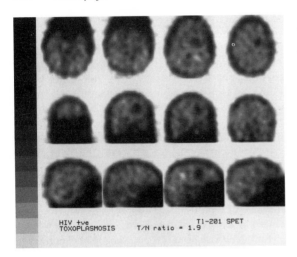

Figure 9.11 Transverse (top row), coronal (middle row) and sagittal (bottom row) slices of a ^{201}Tl study of a patient with intracerebral toxoplasma abscesses. Multiple small foci of increased tracer uptake are seen in the sites demonstrated by MR imaging. One of them, in the deep left frontoparietal area shows more intense tracer uptake than the others. However, the tumour-to-background radioactivity ratio is 1.9, indicative of *Toxoplasma* abscess and not lymphoma.

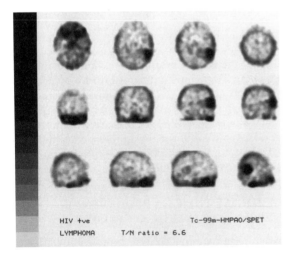

Figure 9.12 With similar orientation to Figure 9.11, this demonstrates the characteristic appearance of lymphoma infiltration of the brain in a HIV-positive patient. There is a single focus of marked increase of the ^{201}Tl uptake in the left posterior temporoparietal area with a tumour-to-background radioactivity ratio equal to 6.6, clearly indicative of intracerebral lymphoma.

Radionuclide imaging, due to its physiological behaviour, is the most likely tool to assist the differential diagnosis between metabolically active tumour (primary or recurrent) and post-irradiation necrosis. Based on the suggestion that tumours have higher rates of aerobic glycolysis (lactate production) than normal tissues [26], ^{18}F-deoxyglucose (FDG) has been used to measure the degree of malignancy in brain tumours [27]. In addition to grading malignant neoplasms *in vivo* [28], FDG has been able to distinguish between tumour recurrence and post-irradiation necrosis [29,30]. Other tracers labelled with positron emitters (e.g. ^{18}F, ^{11}C or ^{13}N) have been suggested for the evaluation of brain tumours. They include sugar derivatives, amino acids, putrescine and receptor ligands. Among these, the amino acid ^{11}C-methionine appears to be the most promising [31]. It shows good correlation with histopathological grades, and tumour delineation is more accurate with ^{11}C-methionine PET than with CT scanning. The major function of SPECT is to find practical methods, which may be much more widely available and affordable than PET. Indeed, one SPECT tracer, ^{201}Tl thallous chloride, has already shown potential in the differential diagnosis of tumour-recurrence and post-irradiation necrosis [32].

Promising results have also been obtained with ^{123}I-L-AMT (3-iodo-alpha-methyl-L-tyrosine), an amino acid labelled with a single-photon emitter. ^{201}Tl is useful in the pre-operative localization of brain tumours, or after surgery for detecting recurrence or neoplastic residue. It differentiates between low- and high-grade tumours [33,34]. Low-grade gliomas show reduced or absent ^{201}Tl uptake, whereas in contrast, the high-grade gliomas always demonstrate markedly increased tracer concentration in the tumour as compared with the normal brain tissue. However, ^{201}Tl may be taken up by brain abscesses [35], presumably due to the presence of intensive reactive gliosis and endothelial proliferation observed around the abscess. The combination of ^{201}Tl and brain perfusion SPECT with HMPAO may prove even more helpful in the evaluation of brain tumours pre- and post-surgically, and in the distinction between tumour-recurrence and post-irradiation necrosis. In fact, this approach was used in a group of 15 consecutive patients (seven patients with solid tumour and eight with post-irradiation necrosis – all confirmed on biopsy) with suspected post-irradiation recurrence of high-grade gliomas. All seven patients with confirmed foci of solid tumour had increased ^{201}Tl uptake, classified as moderate in three and high in four; five of the eight patients with no tumour had moderate ^{201}Tl uptake. The discriminative power was substantially improved by a combination of ^{201}Tl and HMPAO uptake patterns. The HMPAO uptake in all of the seven patients with tumour-recurrence was either similar to or more than the normal brain tissue [32]. This novel approach deserves further evaluation using a larger study sample.

The other potassium analogue radiotracers are also likely to have similar characteristics and potential for the evaluation of primary tumours, and would allow distinction between tumour recurrence and areas of radiation necrosis with poor tracer uptake.

REFERENCES

1. Costa, D.C. (1994) The blood-brain barrier, in *Nuclear Medicine in Clinical Diagnosis and Treatment* (eds I.P.C. Murray and P.J. Ell), Churchill Livingstone, Edinburgh, pp. 449–55.
2. Morgan, G.F. and Costa, D.C. (1993) Radiopharmaceuticals for conventional blood–brain barrier and brain perfusion studies, in *New Trends in Nuclear Neurology and Psychiatry* (eds D.C. Costa, G.F. Morgan and N.A. Lassen), John Libbey and Company Ltd, London, pp. 65–84.
3. Schmidbauer, M., Podreka, I., Wimberger, D. *et al.* (1991) SPECT and MR Imaging in Herpes Simplex Encephalitis. *J. Comput. Assist. Tomogr.*, **15**, 812–15.
4. Henkes, H., Huber, C., Hierholzer, J. *et al.* (1991) Temporal-medial hot spot in HMPAO/SPET: key finding in acute herpes encephalitis. *Radiology*, **18**(P), 173.
5. Kendell, R.E. (1991) Chronic fatigue, viruses, and depression. *Lancet*, **337**, 160–2.
6. Palca, J. (1991) On the track of an elusive disease. *Science*, **254**, 1726–8.
7. Ray, C. (1991) Chronic fatigue syndrome and depression: conceptual and methodological ambiguities. *Psychol. Med.*, **21**, 1–9.
8. Ichise, M., Salit, I., Abbey, S. *et al.* (1992) Assessment of regional cerebral perfusion by 99Tcm-HMPAO/SPECT in Chronic Fatigue Syndrome. *Nucl. Med. Commun.*, **13**, 767–72.
9. Schwartz, R.B., Komaroff, A.L., Garada, B.M. *et al.* (1994) SPECT Imaging of the brain: comparison of findings in patients with Chronic Fatigue Syndrome, AIDS Dementia Complex, and major unipolar depression. *Am. J. Radiol.*, **162**, 943–51.
10. Costa, D.C., Tannock, C. and Brostoff, J. (1995) Brainstem perfusion is impaired in patients with myalgic encephalomyelitis/chronic fatigue syndrome. *Q. J. Med.*, **88**, 767–73.
11. Ell, P.J., Costa, D.C. and Harrison, M. (1987) Imaging cerebral damage in HIV infection. *Lancet*, **ii**, 569–70.
12. Pohl, P., Vogl, G. and Fill, H. (1988) Single-photon emission computed tomography in AIDS dementia complex. *J. Nucl. Med.*, **29**, 1382–6.
13. Costa, D.C., Ell, P.J., Burns, A. *et al.* (1988) CBF tomograms with [99mTc]-HM-PAO in patients with dementia (Alzheimer type and HIV) and Parkinson's disease – Initial results. *J. Cereb. Blood Flow Metab.*, **8**, S109–15.
14. Tatsch, K., Schielke, E., Einhaulp, K.M. *et al.* (1989) 99mTc-HMPAO-SPECT in patients with HIV infection: a comparison with neurological, CT and MRI findings. *Eur. J. Nucl. Med.*, **15**, 418.
15. Maini, C.L., Pigorini, F., Pau, F.M. *et al.* (1989) 99mTc-HM-PAO brain SPECT in acquired immunodeficiency syndrome (AIDS). *Eur. J. Nucl. Med.*, **15**, 418.
16. Rottenberg, D.A., Moeller, J.R., Strother, S.C. *et al.* (1987) The metabolic pathology of the AIDS dementia complex. *Ann. Neurol.*, **22**, 700–6.
17. Brunetti, A., Berg, G., DiChiro, X. *et al.* (1989) Reversal of brain metabolic abnormalities following treatment of AIDS dementia complex with 3'-azido-2',3'-thymidine AZT, zidovudine: a PET-FDG study. *J. Nucl. Med.*, **30**, 581–90.
18. Ramsey, R.G. (1994) Central nervous system infections in the immunocompromised and immunocompetent patient, in *Syllabus: Special Course in Neuroradiology – Clinical Approach and Management for Diagnostic Imaging* (eds G. Forbes, R.M. Quencer and H.R. Hansberger), Radiological Society of North America, pp. 181–9.
19. Naidich, T.P. (1994) Pathology of adult intracranial neoplasms: useful interpretation of mass, in *Syllabus: Special Course in Neuroradiology – Clinical Approach and Management for Diagnostic Imaging* (eds G. Forbes, R.M. Quencer and H.R. Hansberger), Radiological Society of North America, pp. 83–95.
20. Chinn, R.J.S., Wilkinson, I.D., Hall-Craggs, M. *et al.* (1994) Spectroscopic tissue diagnosis of CNS mass lesions in HIV infection, in *Proceedings of The Society of Magnetic Resonance*, 2nd Meeting, vol. 1, 133.
21. O'Malley, J.P., Ziessman, H.A., Kumar, P.N. *et al.* (1994) Diagnosis of intracranial lymphoma in patients with AIDS: value of 201-Tl single-photon emission computed tomography. *Am. J. Roentgenol.*, **163**, 417–21.
22. Costa, D.C., Gacinovic, S. and Miller, R.F. (1995) Radionuclide brain imaging in Acquired Immunodeficiency Syndrome (AIDS). *Q. J. Nucl. Med.*, **39**, 243–9.
23. Loeffler, J.S., Siddon, R.L., Wen, P.Y. *et al.* (1989) Stereotactic radiosurgery of the brain using a standard linear accelerator: a study of early and late effects. *Radiother. Oncol.*, **17**, 311–21.
24. Burke, J.W., Podrasky, A.E. and Bradley, W.G. (1990) Meninges: benign postoperative enhancement on MR images. *Radiology*, **174**, 99–102.
25. Dischino, D.D., Welch, M.J., Kilbourn, M.R. and Raichle, M.E. (1983) Relationship between lipophilicity and brain extraction of C-11-labelled radiopharmaceuticals. *J. Nucl. Med.*, **24**, 1030–8.

26. Warburg, O. (1930) *The Metabolism of Tumours*, Arnold Constable, London, pp. 75–327.
27. Reivich, M., Kuhl, D., Wolf, A. *et al.* (1979) The (18F)fluorodeoxyglucose method for the measurement of local cerebral glucose utilization in man. *Circ. Res.*, **44**, 127–37.
28. Di Chiro, G. (1986) Positron emission tomography using [18F]fluorodeoxyglucose in brain tumours: a powerful diagnostic and prognostic tool. *Invest. Radiol.*, **22**, 360–71.
29. Glantz, M.J., Hoffman, J.M., Coleman, R.E. *et al.* (1991) Identification of early recurrence of primary central nervous system tumours by [18F] Fluorodeoxyglucose positron emission tomography. *Ann. Neurol.*, **29**, 347–55.
30. Valk, P.E., Budinger, T.F., Levin, V.A. *et al.* (1988) PET of malignant cerebral tumours after interstitial brachytherapy: demonstration of metabolic activity and correlation with clinical outcome. *J. Neurosurg.*, **69**, 830–8.
31. Mosskin, M., Von Holst, H., Bergstrom, M. *et al.* (1987), Positron emission tomography with ^{11}C-methionine and computed tomography of intracranial tumours compared with histopathologic examination of multiple biopsies. *Acta Radiol.*, **28**, 505–9.
32. Schwartz, R.B., Carvalho, P.A., Alexander, E., III *et al.* (1992) Radiation necrosis versus high-grade recurrent glioma: differentiation by using dual-isotope SPECT with ^{201}Tl and ^{99m}Tc-HMPAO. *Am. J. Nucl. Radiol.*, **12**, 1187–92.
33. Kim, K.T., Black, K.L., Marciano, D. *et al.* (1990) Thallium-201 SPECT imaging of brain tumours: methods and results. *J. Nucl. Med.*, **31**, 965–9.
34. Maier-Hauff, K., Barzen, G.S. and Gottschalk, H. (1991) Value of Tl-201 imaging in cerebral lesions: emission CT with autoradiography. *Radiology*, **185**(P), 232.
35. Krishna, L., Slizofski, W.J., Katsetos, C.D. *et al.* (1992) Abnormal intracerebral thallium localization in a bacterial brain abscess. *J. Nucl. Med.*, **33**, 2017–19.

FURTHER READING

Costa, D.C., Morgan, G.F. and Lassen, N.A. (eds) (1993) *New Trends in Nuclear Neurology and Psychiatry*, John Libbey, London.
Harrison, M.J.G. and McArthur, J.C. (eds) (1995) *AIDS and Neurology*, Churchill Livingstone, Edinburgh.
Wise, M.G. and Gray, K.F. (1994) Delirium, Dementia, and Amnestic Disorders, in *The American Psychiatric Press Textbook of Psychiatry*, 2nd edn (eds R.E. Hales, S.C. Yudofsky and J.A. Talbott), American Psychiatric Press, Inc. Washington, DC and London, pp. 313–53.

Psychiatric disorders

A. Lingford-Hughes

INTRODUCTION

The nuclear medicine techniques of positron emission tomography (PET) and single-photon emission tomography (SPECT) are powerful tools for the *in vivo* elucidation of the neurochemistry and aetiology of neuropsychiatric disorders. Both have played a major role in the advancement of psychopharmacology of psychiatric disorders. It is now over 20 years since functional neuroimaging (using ^{133}Xe inhalation) first contributed to the debate about pathophysiological mechanisms in schizophrenia [1]. Since then, there has been a plethora of studies in neuropsychiatry, with the PET and SPECT techniques playing a central role. New techniques such as multiple organs coincidence counter [2], and ligands for specific receptor subtypes, are likely to increase the application of nuclear medicine in the development of new pharmacotherapies. PET has been described as 'the most specific and sensitive means for quantitatively imaging molecular pathways and molecular interactions within tissues of man' [3]. Although SPECT has been considered 'the poor man's PET scanner', because of its wider availability and with the recent technological advances in equipment along with the continuing development and use of new single-photon emitting radionuclides, the SPECT technique no longer lags far behind PET. Clinically though, there is limited diagnostic application for PET and SPECT, but this is likely to change. This chapter aims to give an overview of some of the PET and SPECT studies to illustrate their potential in exploring the pathophysiological mechanisms that underlie psychiatric disorders. Neuropsychological and pharmacological challenges during scanning are strategies that add to the power of PET and SPECT for *in vivo* hypothesis testing. These are primarily illustrated in reference to studies in schizophrenia.

SCHIZOPHRENIA

Schizophrenia is a common severe mental illness, affecting 1% of the population, and is associated with high morbidity and mortality. Although most patients respond to treatment, side effects or partial responsivity to medication creates further problems in a proportion of the affected subjects. Schizophrenia is generally described in terms of positive (e.g. hallucinations and delusions) and negative (e.g. apathy and social withdrawal) symptoms. Positive symptoms, which are thought to result from overactivity within the dopaminergic mesolimbic system, usually characterize the acute phase of the illness and respond to antipsychotic medication. Negative symptoms presumed secondary to dysfunction within the frontal lobes characterize the more chronic phase of the illness and generally do not improve significantly with antipsychotics.

REGIONAL CEREBRAL BLOOD FLOW (RCBF) AND METABOLISM

Frontal lobes

Ingvar and Franzen [1], using ^{133}Xe to study cerebral blood flow, were the first to show that patients with schizophrenia had relatively lower rCBF in the anterior as compared with the posterior regions of the frontal lobes, a reversal of the normal physiological pattern. This phenomenon, known as 'hypofrontality' has been replicated by a number of groups [4,5], but not consistently [6,7], and some studies have even shown hyperfrontality [8–10], particularly in unmedicated patients [9,10]. There are many factors that may contribute to the observed variabilities. An important factor contributing to the conflicting reports is the medication status, both past and current. In early studies showing hypofunction, the patients were invariably chronically medicated. Even in the studies on unmedicated patients, the subjects were drug-free rather than drug-naive. Although antipsychotic treatment reportedly results in decreased cortical metabolism [11], hypofrontality has also been observed in drug-naive patients [6]. Furthermore, in studies show-

Clinical Nuclear Medicine, 3rd edn. Edited by M.N. Maisey, K.E. Britton and B.D. Collier. Published in 1998 by Chapman & Hall, London. ISBN 0 412 75180 1

ing 'hyperfrontal' patterns in schizophrenia, no changes were seen after treatment [9,12]. However, the influence of medication is complex, since the effects vary depending on the antipsychotic drug used, with increases, decreases or no change being reported [12,13]. Thus, it appears that hypofrontality is a primary characteristic of schizophrenia, and that medication may have secondary effects.

Apart from medication, other confounding variables include the patient's symptom profile, the presence of negative symptoms, and mental activity state. Although hypofrontality and the chronicity of disease seem unrelated, there is an apparent association with the presence of negative symptoms [6,10]. Schizophrenics perform neuropsychological tasks involving frontal lobe activation poorly; however, variability in the mental activity at the time of the scan may also contribute to the inconsistencies. Therefore, to address this issue, the effect of neuropsychological activation on cerebral blood flow/metabolism has been investigated. The first such report used the Wisconsin Card Sort Test (WCST) for activating the dorsolateral prefrontal cortex (DLPFC) to study the rCBF using ^{133}Xe inhalation [14]. The schizophrenic patients and the normal controls had similar resting blood flow; however, compared with the normal controls, the schizophrenic patients had lesser increase in the blood flow failed to the DLPFC during the WCST. There was an association between WCST performance and blood flow – with those patients performing better, showing a greater increase in blood flow. Medication status, attention and severity of psychotic symptoms were shown not to influence the findings [15]. Importantly, similar results have been obtained in drug-naive patients, showing that failure to activate is not a consequence of treatment. Poorer performance was associated with more prominent negative symptoms, supporting the hypothesis that frontal lobe dysfunction underlies these symptoms [6].

A critical problem with these early studies is an inability to exclude the possibility of the subject's poor performance as a cause of the reduced activation. Frontotemporal dysfunction, particularly within the superior temporal gyrus (STG), has been implicated in schizophrenia [16]. To address this, recently Frith *et al.* [16], using a paced verbal fluency task, showed equivalent frontal activation in chronic schizophrenics and controls with similar performance. However, unlike the control subjects, the schizophrenic patients failed to reduce blood flow in the STG. This study also illustrates how PET can map functional connectivity between regions of the brain. This information can be valuable, as dysfunction within such network connectivity may underlie the pathophysiology of schizophrenia, rather than deficits in one particular region(s) of the brain.

More recently, a pharmacological challenge has been used with PET to explore the neurochemistry underlying frontal dysfunction. Apomorphine, a dopaminergic agonist, was seen to reverse the failure of the 'paced verbal fluency tasks' to increase rCBF in the anterior cingulate cortex in the schizophrenic patients compared to controls [17]. This study lends support to the hypotheses on the causation of schizophrenia, which propose that an abnormal processing within the anterior cingulate region in schizophrenia with decreased dopamine release results in an up-regulation of post-synaptic dopamine receptors.

Basal ganglia

The dopamine-rich basal ganglia have attracted much attention in neuroimaging. Some studies on unmedicated schizophrenics tended to show decreased metabolism within the basal ganglia that normalizes with treatment and improvement in psychosis [18–20]. However, other studies in unmedicated schizophrenic patients have shown increased blood flow/metabolism in parts of the basal ganglia including the left globus pallidus and right lenticular nucleus [10,21].

Interestingly, Buchsbaum *et al.* [19] found that those patients with low striatal metabolism were more likely to improve clinically with haloperidol treatment, than those with normal or high metabolic rates. In the responders, haloperidol treatment increased the metabolic rate towards the normal range, while there was no change in the non-responders. These results emphasize the importance of medication as a confounder, and also suggest that a characteristic metabolic rate/blood flow pattern reflects specific symptoms and/or pathophysiological processes. The study also suggests the possibility of a future clinical application of PET in predicting the clinical response of a patient to a particular antipsychotic, thus avoiding unnecessary morbidity.

Temporal lobe

The temporal lobe, particularly the medial temporal region, has long been the focus of attention in schizophrenia. Many neurochemical and structural abnormalities have been found. Early functional neuroimaging studies have reported decreased activity within the temporal lobe [23], which is in conflict with a recent study reporting increased activity in this region [22]. Further, rCBF within the parahippocampal gyrus has been shown to correlate with the severity of psychopathology [24]. Neuropsychological activation has been performed during scanning procedures to try and identify temporal lobe abnormalities in schizophrenia. Busatto *et al.* [25] used ^{99m}Tc-HMPAO-SPECT and a verbal memory task to activate the left medial temporal lobe. Despite their significantly poor performance at this task, left medial temporal lobe activation in schizophrenics was not different from controls. Hence, impaired memory does not necessarily result in alteration of blood flow.

SYMPTOMATOLOGY

As already described, schizophrenia is commonly discussed in terms of positive and negative symptoms with correlations between these and the temporal and frontal lobe respectively. However, based on segregation analysis of symptoms, Liddle *et al.* [26] using $^{15}O_2$ PET found three distinct syndromes – psychomotor poverty, disorganization and reality distortion. Each syndrome was characterized by a distinctive perfusion pattern: reality distortion (hallucination and delusions) was associated with increased rCBF in the left medial temporal lobe; psychomotor poverty with decreased blood flow in the frontal region – results consistent with previous studies; and the disorganization syndrome was associated with hypoperfusion in particular frontal regions and relative hypoperfusion in Broca's area. This distribution of altered blood flow is consistent with the predictions regarding the particular neural networks that are dysfunctional in schizophrenic syndromes. These results have been replicated [10].

There have been several studies exploring activity associated with hallucinations. Generally, an increase in activity in the left medial temporal lobe has been shown [26]. McGuire *et al.* [28] scanned patients while they were hallucinating (Plate 23) and again later when they were not hallucinating. Hallucinations were associated with significant increased perfusion within Broca's area, and a trend toward increased perfusion in the left anterior cingulate cortex and left temporal lobe. These findings are consistent with the hypothesis that auditory hallucinations are a failure of schizophrenics to recognize their own thoughts, regarding them as alien. More recently, Silbersweig *et al.* [29] examined cerebral blood flow using $^{15}O_2$ PET in schizophrenic patients who experienced hallucination intermittently during the single scanning procedure. The duration of the hallucinations was shown to be associated with activation in the left medial temporal lobe, anterior cingulate, thalamus and striatum. Bilaterally decreased metabolism in the superior temporal gyrus (including Wernicke's area) has also been reported, with a positive correlation between hallucinations and the reduction of metabolism in the anterior cingulate cortex and striatum [27].

NEURORECEPTOR IMAGING

PET and SPECT neuroreceptor imaging in schizophrenia has been an extremely fruitful area of research. Not only has the classical dopaminergic hypothesis been tested *in vivo*, but also PET and SPECT are involved in drug evaluation and development.

Neurochemical pathology

As already described, abnormalities in the dopaminergic system have long been implicated in the pathophysiology of schizophrenia. The hypothesis that D2 receptor levels were increased in schizophrenia was supported by early studies of striatal D2 receptors [30,31]. However, later studies failed to replicate this finding [32,33]. It is now generally accepted that there is no increase of D2 receptors within the striatum of schizophrenics. More subtle changes are seen, however, with a lack of age-related decline [33], and a greater asymmetry of D2 receptors with higher levels in the left than right putamen but not caudate [32], particularly in males [34]. Negative symptoms, such as blunted affect and alogia, are negatively related with striatal D2 receptors [35].

How do these results fit in with the classical dopamine hypothesis proposed? First, the studies visualize dopamine receptors within the striatum and the hypothesis refers to dysfunction within mesolimbic pathways. Compared with the striatum, the level of D2 receptors is much lower in the mesolimbic cortex, making them more difficult to image adequately. In addition, there are two families of dopamine receptors, the D1-like (D1 and D5 subtypes) and D2-like (D2, D3 and D4 subtypes). Ligands previously described as D2 ligands also have affinity at other dopamine receptors, e.g. raclopride binds to both the D2 and D3 subtypes. Thus, conflicting results from different ligands may be due to their pharmacological profile at particular subtypes. Specific PET and SPECT ligands for these receptor subtypes (with the exception of D1) are awaited. In addition to the dopamine receptors, some of the ligands also have an affinity for other neurotransmitter receptors; for example, spiperone binds to the $5HT_2$ receptor. Neuroanatomically, the $5HT_2$ and D2 receptor are separated, with the former present in high levels in the neocortex where there are few D2 receptors. Hence, ^{11}C-*N*-methylspiperone (^{11}C-NMS) activity in the neocortex and striatum reflect $5HT_2$ and D2 receptors respectively.

Drug development

Clinically, the potency of antipsychotic drugs was thought to be related to their D2 affinity. Farde *et al.* [32], using ^{11}C- raclopride PET, first showed that treated schizophrenic patients had 84–90% occupancy of the D2 receptor in the putamen, and later went on to report 65–85% occupancy by several different classes of typical antipsychotics [36]. The degree of D2 occupancy has been correlated with clinical improvement in schizophrenic patients [37].

About 30% of schizophrenic patients do not fully respond to antipsychotic medication. Comparing responders and non-responders, PET and SPECT studies using a variety of D2 ligands, have shown that the poor response is not due to low D2 receptor occupancy by antipsychotics as one might have expected [34,38]. Rather, some antipsychotic drugs, such as clozapine, have been shown to result in clinical improvement with low (38–63%) D2 occupancy [39,40]. Thus, in regard to developing new antipsychotics, high D2 occupancy is not an absolute requirement for clinical efficacy (Figure 9.13).

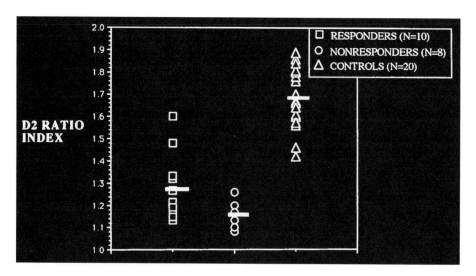

Figure 9.13   D2 binding indices and response to typical antipsychotic medication. Scatter-plots of individual D2 binding indices [basal ganglia/frontal cortex ratio of ^{123}I-iodobenzamide (IBZM) uptake] in schizophrenic patients treated with typical antipsychotic medication. The higher the index, the lower the occupancy by the antipsychotic medication and hence the more D2 receptors available for ^{123}I-IBZM uptake. Both groups of patients showed occupancy of D2 receptors by their medication, with those who were non-responsive having a greater degree of occupancy. (Courtesy of Dr L.S. Pilowsky.)

Clozapine is one of a group of antipsychotics, called 'atypical' due to their low propensity to induce extrapyramidal side effects (EPSE). There is no single underlying pharmacological mechanism, which results in the atypical profile, and it may be due to activity at a number of different receptors including dopaminergic (D1), muscarinic and serotonergic. Such EPSE are common with more traditional antipsychotics (e.g. haloperidol and chlorpromazine), and can be as devastating as schizophrenia itself. EPSE are related to the degree of D2 occupancy in the striatum with a threshold of about 70–80% [37]. Since antipsychotic effects are seen at lower levels of occupancy, increasing the dose of typical antipsychotics may result in debilitating EPSE and yet not confer any additional therapeutic effect. Therefore, PET and SPECT can be used to optimize drug dosages.

Of the atypical neuroleptics, clozapine has attracted the most attention due to its efficacy in treating non-responsive schizophrenic patients. PET and SPECT neuroreceptor imaging has played a central role in determining its *in vivo* pharmacology that results in minimal EPSE. This has been crucial in developing other antipsychotics. The serotonergic system has attracted the most attention. Clozapine treatment results in above 80% occupancy of $5HT_2$ receptors [41]. Other atypical antipsychotics also display high levels of occupancy of this receptor. In healthy volunteers, risperidone (1 mg) resulted in 60% occupancy of neocortical $5HT_2$ receptors and 50% of striatal D2 receptors using ^{11}C-NMS-PET [42]. In schizophrenics receiving clinical doses of risperidone (4–14 mg), an ^{123}I-IBZM study showed a level of occupancy of the D2 receptor comparable with those on typical antipsychotics and much greater than that seen on clozapine [43] (Figure 9.14). Hence, according to previous findings by Farde *et al.*, one would expect EPSE to be present with such degrees of occupancy. It has been suggested that it is the presence of high $5HT_2$ occupancy which is protective of D2-inducing-EPSE in drugs such as risperidone.

DEPRESSION

Although it has been recognized for centuries that there are many different types of depression, functional neuroimaging has greatly enhanced our ability to delineate depressive syndromes, their

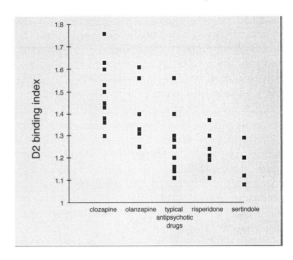

Figure 9.14 Dopamine D2 binding index: typical and atypical antipsychotics. Scatterplots of individual D2 binding indices (basal ganglia: frontal cortex ratio of ^{123}I-iodobenzamide (IBZM) uptake) in schizophrenic patients treated with a variety of antipsychotic medication. The higher the index the lower the occupancy by the antipsychotic medication and hence the more D2 receptors that are available for ^{123}I-IBZM uptake. (Courtesy of Dr L.S. Pilowsky.)

aetiology and treatment. Depressive symptoms such as disturbed sleep, reduced appetite and poor concentration are very common. At the more severe end of the spectrum, major depression and bipolar disorder occur in up to 5% of the population. Current classification systems use symptom profile and length of illness as criteria for diagnosis; hence, the underlying pathophysiological mechanisms may be different and may help explain the conflicting results reported.

REGIONAL CEREBRAL BLOOD FLOW AND METABOLISM

Generally, studies revealed that depression is associated with reduced glucose metabolism. As in schizophrenia, frontal hypometabolism is also seen in depressed bipolar and unipolar patients [44]. Other regions that show reduced metabolism include the right temporal lobe [45], the head of the caudate [46] and the parietal lobe [47]. That the observed reduction reflects the depressed state rather than a trait marker, is supported by the findings that as patients became euthymic or manic, glucose metabolism increased [46]. In addition, hypometabolism occurs in different diagnostic categories, namely bipolar or unipolar depression, dysthymia and obsessive compulsive disorder with depression [48,49]. Although some studies have revealed no changes [50,51], specific patients did show hypometabolism. Arguably, this might be a reflection of different aetiological factors. In general, although no differences have been shown between the different diagnostic categories, the numbers are often too small for definitive analysis.

The possibility of a relationship between particular symptoms and rCBF patterns has been explored. Generally, the more severe the depression, the greater the reduction of blood flow/metabolism [52]. Anxiety symptoms correlate positively with blood flow in the posterior cingulate cortex and the inferior parietal lobe [53]. Depressed mood and psychomotor retardation has been shown to correlate negatively with blood flow in the left dorsolateral prefrontal cortex and the inferior parietal lobe [53]. However, in subjects with prominent endogenous symptoms, a relative increase has been found in frontal and cingulate cortex [52]. Gender differences have also been shown with higher [54] and lower [49] blood flow in female compared with male depressed patients.

Clinically, depression results in an impairment of cognitive tasks. Cognitive function has been shown to correlate with decreased rCBF in the medial prefrontal cortex in depressed patients [53]. Using activation paradigms as described previously for schizophrenia, Gur *et al.* [54] first showed that blood flow tended to normalize during cognitive testing, more so in males than females.

NEURORECEPTOR IMAGING

Neurochemical hypotheses concerning the aetiology of depression involve depletion of 5HT and noradrenergic systems. There have been fewer neuroreceptor ligand studies than in schizophrenia to test this hypothesis, but with the development of 5HT ligands this is likely to change. Pre-synaptic function in patients with unipolar depression has been studied by measuring uptake of dopamine and serotonin precursors, using ^{11}C-L-DOPA and ^{11}C-5-hydroxytryptophan ([11]C-5HTP) respectively [55]. Decreased uptake of both

precursors across the blood–brain barrier, with increased utilization of [11]C-5HTP but not ^{11}C-L-DOPA was seen in the inferomedial prefrontal cortex.

In the dopaminergic system, reduced D1 receptor binding in the frontal cortex has been reported using SCH 23390 PET [56]. No changes were seen in D2 receptor levels in the striatum in people with bipolar disorder using ^{11}C-NMS-PET [57]. However, an increased D2 striatum/cerebellar ratio in unipolar depressives has been found with ^{123}I-IBZM-SPECT [58]. The dopaminergic system has also been studied in sleep deprivation, which has been used for many years to treat depression. In responsive depressed patients, reduced levels of D2 receptors was found using ^{123}I-IBZM-SPECT, suggesting enhanced dopamine release [59].

Regarding the serotonergic system, an ^{123}I-ketanserin SPECT study reported higher 5HT$_2$ receptors in the parietal cortex and a greater right-to-left asymmetry in the inferofrontal region in depressed patients [60].

ADDICTION

The prevalence and cost of drug and alcohol abuse is immense, both on a personal and societal level. Determining its neurobiological basis is crucial in developing treatment and prevention strategies. Broadly speaking, addiction to a particular drug, including alcohol, may be separated into two components. The first involves a specific effect of a drug on a neurotransmitter system and the second concerns their positive reinforcing properties, which may be common across different substances and involves the dopaminergic mesolimbic system.

DRUG DEPENDENCY

Studies of the effects of drugs, other than cocaine and alcohol, on blood flow/metabolism are somewhat limited, but generally show acute and chronic use results in reduced metabolism [61]. Apart from ligands available to image the catecholaminergic system, few other systems can currently be visualized.

Cocaine

rCBF and metabolism Acute administration of cocaine has been shown to result in global reduction in glucose metabolism which correlates with its euphorigenic effects [62]. In recently abstinent chronic cocaine abusers, decreased metabolism, particularly in the prefrontal cortex, is seen [63]. These deficits could be due to cocaine's sympathomimetic effect, resulting in vasoconstriction and/or a direct effect on catecholaminergic neuronal activity.

Acutely after withdrawal from cocaine, glucose metabolism is increased [64]. In particular, metabolism was greater in the orbitofrontal cortex and basal ganglia. This was hypothesized to be due to changes in dopaminergic activity, since the orbitofrontal area receives dopaminergic projection of the mesocortical system and the basal ganglia is rich in dopamine receptors. Interestingly, changes in the cortical region were related to craving, a poorly understood aspect of addiction that is involved in relapse and continued use. However, more prolonged abstinence is associated with hypometabolism, persisting for up to 4 months [65], correlating with the dose and duration of cocaine use.

Buprenorphine, a mixed opioid agonist/antagonist, has been shown to reduce the number of perfusion defects in cocaine polydrug users in a dose-dependent manner, which is in addition to the improvement seen with abstinence [66]. Clinically however, it remains unclear whether this gives any further benefits.

Neuroreceptor studies That cocaine does specifically affect the dopamine system has been shown by a number of studies. Delineating this interaction is important in understanding the considerable positive reinforcing properties of this drug and how to intervene in treatment. This is likely to be applicable to other drugs of abuse.

Reduced levels of D2 receptors in the striatum have been found within the first week of abstinence. However, levels at 1 month were comparable with those in control subjects [67]. Studies of the dopaminergic system after detoxification in chronic cocaine abusers revealed a decrease in ^{18}F-DOPA, suggesting reduced dopamine uptake and synthesis [68]. Decreased D2 receptor levels have also been shown with ^{18}F-NMS, which were maintained for 4 months and were associated with a specific decrease in frontal cortex metabolism [69]. These studies support the hypothesis that dopamine depletion may be involved in craving and dependence.

Alcohol

rCBF and metabolism Chronic use and abuse of alcohol leads to deleterious effects in the brain, manifested as structural and functional changes. The underlying pathological process and whether effects are global or specific, remains unclear.

Acutely, alcohol increases cerebral blood flow in cortical regions and reduction within the cerebellum, which likely accounts for muscular incoordination [61]. The regional pattern of reduction in glucose metabolism correlates with the distribution of the benzodiazepine receptor [70]. Interestingly, in alcoholics, greater reductions in glucose metabolism were seen than in control subjects. It was hypothesized that this reflected differential sensitivity of the benzodiazepine receptor. Further support for such a hypothesis came from a study of the effects of lorazepam on glucose metabolism: those subjects with a positive family history had lower baseline glucose metabolism and the response to lorazepam was blunted in the cerebellum [71].

In abstinent chronic alcoholics, widespread reductions in blood flow or glucose metabolism have been reported, though not consistently for any particular region. Alcoholics have globally lower cerebral metabolism [72], with regional reductions in frontal and parietal areas [73,74]. Inconsistent results may be due to different age groups, severity of alcohol abuse, or structural changes. In some studies although there is a poor relationship with age, only older alcoholics showed reductions [72,73]. Increasing severity of alcoholism is associated with more pronounced reductions [73]. Atrophy secondary to alcohol abuse is a well-recognized phenomenon, and although greater impairment is seen in those with atrophy, subjects with only mild or no structural changes also show altered blood flow/metabolism [74].

In the first few weeks of abstinence, changes are seen in brain structure and function, and thus the timing of any neuroimaging is critical when comparing studies. Berglund *et al.* [73] found that blood flow improved with abstinence within the first week in younger (<45 years) alcoholics, but took up to 7 weeks in older subjects. Volkow *et al.* [75] similarly showed that glucose metabolism increases predominantly between 2–4 weeks of abstinence, with little further improvement in the second month. The frontal cortex showed the largest increase in metabolism with significantly impaired metabolism persisting in the parietal cortex and basal ganglia.

Although many studies are inconclusive, generally where blood flow/metabolism is reduced, there is impairment in tasks requiring activation of that area [73]. Higher metabolic rates in the frontal lobes are associated with better performance [76].

Neuroreceptor imaging As described previously, dopaminergic mechanisms are intimately involved with addictive processes. ^{11}C-raclopride-PET revealed reduced striatal/cerebellar ratios in alcoholics, though absolute levels in these regions were not different [77]. Using β-CIT-SPECT to image striatal dopamine re-uptake sites, differences have been found between abstinent alcoholics and controls [78]. Lower levels were seen in nonviolent alcoholics, and the reverse in violent alcoholics. This intriguing finding has yet to be extended looking at violent behaviour in other disorders.

As described above, the benzodiazepine receptor is thought to be involved in mediating the central effects of alcohol. Alcohol has no acute effect on ^{11}C-flumazenil binding [79]. In a small study of abstinent alcoholics, levels of ^{11}C-flumazenil uptake differed from control subjects, with two having higher and three lower levels in a number of cortical regions. Interestingly, characteristics of their alcohol history correlated with the receptor level [80].

ANXIETY DISORDERS

Anxiety disorders are among the most common psychiatric disorders and involve high rates of morbidity. There have been many studies into the effect of anxiety and blood flow, but their interpretation is often difficult [81]. For example, in normal subjects, an inverted U-shaped curve was found for blood flow, with mild and severe anxiety associated with reduced blood flow, compared with increased blood flow with moderate anxiety [82]. On the other hand, no such association was seen with metabolism, with only severe anxiety resulting in reduced metabolism. Thus, the effect of anxiety on blood flow/metabolism is complex

and depends on its level. Studies where anxiety is induced are inconclusive [81].

Anxiety disorders are comprised of several different components, which need to be taken into consideration. In obsessive compulsive disorder (OCD) for instance, obsessions, compulsions and low mood, are associated with reduced blood flow in frontocortical regions, whereas anxiety and avoidance correlated with increases in other cortical regions and basal ganglia [83].

OCD was one of the first psychiatric disorders to be studied with PET and SPECT. Blood flow/metabolism studies have reported dysfunction within frontal–subcortical circuits with increased activity within the orbitofrontal cortex bilaterally, dorsal parietal region and decreased activity in the head of the caudate [84]. Studies examining the effect of either pharmacological (serotonin re-uptake inhibitors) or behavioural treatment on activity within this network found both treatments led to a decrease in activity within the right caudate nucleus, which correlated with reduction in symptoms [85]. Thus, behavioural treatment can normalize brain activity.

Benzodiazepines are commonly prescribed in anxiety disorders, but there have been few PET or SPECT studies looking at the GABA-benzodiazepine receptor *in vivo* and the findings are inconclusive.

REFERENCES

1. Ingvar, D.H. and Franzen, G. (1974) Abnormalities of cerebral blood flow in patients with chronic schizophrenia. *Acta Psychiatr. Scand.*, **50**, 425–62.
2. Malizia, A., Forse, G., Haida, A. *et al.* (1995) A new human (psycho)pharmacology tool: the multiple organs coincidences counter (MOCC). *J. Psychopharmacol.*, **9**, 294–306.
3. Jones, T. (1996) The role of PET within the spectrum of medical imaging. *Eur. J. Nucl. Med.*, **23**, 207–11.
4. DeLisi, L.E., Buchsbaum, M.S., Holcomb, H.H. *et al.* (1985) Clinical correlates of decreased antero-posterior metabolic gradients in positron emission tomography (PET) of schizophrenic patients. *Am. J. Psychiatry*, **142**, 78–81.
5. Wolkin, A., Angrist, B., Wolf, A.P. *et al.* (1988) Low frontal glucose utilization in chronic schizophrenia: a replication study. *Am. J. Psychiatry*, **145**, 251–3.
6. Andreasen, N.C., Rezai, K., Alliger, R. *et al.* (1992) Hypofrontality in neuroleptic naive patients and in patients with chronic schizophrenia. *Arch. Gen. Psychiatry*, **49**, 943–58.
7. Sheppard, G., Gruzelier, J., Manchanda, R. *et al.* (1983) ^{15}O Positron emission tomographic scanning

in predominantly never-treated acute schizophrenic patients. *Lancet*, **ii**, 1448–52.

8. Szechtman, H., Nahmias, C., Garnett, S. *et al.* (1988) Effect of neuroleptics on altered cerebral glucose metabolism in schizophrenia. *Arch. Gen. Psychiatry*, **45**, 523–32.

9. Cleghorn, J.M., Garnett, E.S., Nahmias, C. *et al.* (1989). Increased frontal and reduced parietal glucose metabolism in acute untreated schizophrenia. *Psychiatry Res.*, **28**, 119–33.

10. Ebmeier, K.P., Blackwood, D.H.R., Murray, C. *et al.* (1993) Single photon emission tomography with 99mTc-exametazine in unmedicated schizophrenia patients. *Biol. Psychiatry*, **33**, 487–95.

11. Gur, R.E., Resnick, S.M., Alavi, A. *et al.* (1987) Regional brain function in schizophrenia. *Arch. Gen. Psychiatry*, **44**, 119–29.

12. Volkow, N.D., Brodie, J.D., Wolf, A.P. *et al.* (1986) Brain metabolism in patients with schizophrenia before and after acute neuroleptic administration. *J. Neurol. Neurosurg. Psychiatry*, **49**, 1199–202.

13. Wolkin, A., Sanfilipo, M., Duncan, E. *et al.* (1996) Blunted change in cerebral glucose utilization after haloperidol treatment in schizophrenic patients with prominent negative symptoms. *Am. J. Psychiatry*, **153**, 346–54.

14. Weinberger, D.R., Berman, K.F. and Zec, R.F. (1986) Physiologic dysfunction of dorsolateral prefrontal cortex in schizophrenia. I. Regional cerebral blood flow evidence. *Arch. Gen. Psychiatry*, **43**, 114–24.

15. Berman, K.F., Zec, R.F. and Weinberger, D.R. (1988) Physiologic dysfunction of dorsolateral prefrontal cortex in schizophrenia. *Arch. Gen. Psychiatry*, **43**, 126–35.

16. Frith, C.D., Friston, K.J., Herold, S. *et al.* (1995) Regional brain activity in chronic schizophrenic patients during the performance of a verbal fluency task. *Br. J. Psychiatry*, **167**, 343–9.

17. Dolan, R.J., Fletcher, P., Frith, C.D. *et al.* (1995) Dopaminergic modulation of impaired cognitive activation in the anterior cingulate cortex in schizophrenia. *Nature*, **378**, 180–2.

18. Buchsbaum, M.S., Haier, R.J., Potkin, S.G. *et al.* (1992) Fronto-striatal disorder of cerebral metabolism in never medicated schizophrenics. *Arch. Gen. Psychiatry*, **49**, 935–42.

19. Buchsbaum, M.S., Potkin, S.G., Siegel, B.V. *et al.* (1992) Striatal metabolic rate and clinical response to neuroleptics in schizophrenia. *Arch. Gen. Psychiatry*, **49**, 966–74.

20. Resnick, S.M., Gur, R.E., Alavi, A. *et al.* (1988) Positron emission tomography and subcortical glucose metabolism in schizophrenia. *Psychiatry Res. Neuroimaging*, **24**, 1–11.

21. Early, T.S., Reiman, E.M., Raichle, M.E. and Spitznagel, E.L. (1987) Left globus pallidus abnormality in never-medicated patients with schizophrenia. *Proc. Natl. Acad. Sci. USA*, **84**, 561–3.

22. DeLisi, L.E., Buchsbaum, M.S., Holcomb, H.H. *et al.* (1989) Increased temporal lobe glucose use in chronic schizophrenic patients. *Biol. Psychiatry*, **25**, 835–51.

23. Wolkin, A., Jaeger, J., Brodie, J.D. *et al.* (1985) Persistence of cerebral metabolic abnormalities in chronic schizophrenia as determined by positron emission tomography. *Am. J. Psychiatry*, **142**, 564–71.

24. Friston, K.J., Liddle, P.F., Frith, C.D. *et al.* (1992) The left medial temporal region and schizophrenia. *Brain*, **115**, 367–82.

25. Busatto, G.F., Costa, D.C., Ell, P.J. *et al.* (1994) Regional cerebral blood flow (rCBF) in schizophrenia during verbal memory activation: a 99mTc-HMPAO single photon emission tomography (SPET) study. *Psychol. Med.*, **24**, 463–72.

26. Liddle, P.F., Friston, K.J., Frith, C.D. *et al.* (1992) Patterns of cerebral blood flow in schizophrenia. *Br. J. Psychiatry*, **160**, 179–86.

27. Cleghorn, J.M., Franco, S., Szechtman, B. *et al.* (1992) Toward a brain map of auditory hallucinations. *Am. J. Psychiatry*, **149**, 1062–9.

28. McGuire, P.K., Shah, G.M.S. and Murray, R.M. (1993) Increased blood flow in Broca's area during auditory hallucinations in schizophrenia. *Lancet*, **342**, 703–6.

29. Silbersweig, D.A., Stern, E., Frith, C. *et al.* (1995) A functional neuroanatomy of hallucinations in schizophrenia. *Nature*, **378**, 176–9.

30. Wong, D.F., Wagner, H.N., Tune, L.E. *et al.* (1986) Positron emission tomography reveals elevated D2 dopamine receptors in drug-naive schizophrenics. *Science*, **234**, 1558–63.

31. Tune, L.E., Wong, D.F., Pearlson, G. *et al.* (1993) Dopamine D2 receptor density estimated in schizophrenia: a positron emission tomography study with ^{11}C-N-methylspiperone. *Psychiatry Res.*, **49**, 219–37.

32. Farde, L., Eriksson, L., Blomqvist, G. and Halldin, C. (1989) Kinetic analysis of central [11C] raclopride binding to D2 dopamine receptors studied by PET – A comparison to the equilibrium analysis. *J. Cereb. Blood Flow Metab.*, **9**, 696–708.

33. Martinot, J.L., Peron Magnan, P., Huret, J.D. *et al.* (1990) Striatal D2 dopaminergic receptors assessed with positron emission tomography and [76]Br] bromospiperone in untreated schizophrenic patients. *Am. J. Psychiatry*, **147**, 44–50.

34. Pilowsky, L.S., Costa, D.C., Ell, P.J. *et al.* (1994) D2 receptor binding in the basal ganglia of antipsychotic free schizophrenic patients – a ^{123}I IBZM single photon emission tomography (SPET) study. *Br. J. Psychiatry*, **164**, 16–26.

35. Martinot, J.L., Paillere-Martinot, M.L., Loc'h, C. *et al.* (1994) Central D2 receptors and negative symptoms of schizophrenia. *Br. J. Psychiatry*, **164**, 27–34.

36. Farde, L., Nordstrom, A.-L., Wiesel, F.-A. *et al.* (1992). Positron emission tomographic analysis of central D1 and D2 dopamine receptor occupancy in patients treated with classical neuroleptics and clozapine. *Arch. Gen. Psychiatry*, **49**, 538–44.

37. Nordstrom, A.-L., Farde, L., Wiesel, F.-A. *et al.* (1993) Central D2 dopamine receptor occupancy in relation to antipsychotic drug effects: a double blind PET study of schizophrenic patients. *Biol. Psychiatry*, **33**, 227–35.

38. Coppens, H.J., Sloof, C.J., Paans, A.M.J. *et al.* (1991). High central D2-dopamine receptor occupancy as assessed with positron emission tomography in medicated but therapeutic resistant schizophrenic patients. *Biol. Psychiatry*, **29**, 629–34.

39. Pilowsky, L.S., Costa, D.C., Ell, P.J. *et al.* (1992) Clozapine, single photon emission tomography and the dopamine D2 receptor blockade hypothesis of schizophrenia. *Lancet*, **340**, 199–202.

40. Farde, L. and Nordstrom, A.-L. (1992) PET analysis indicates atypical central dopamine receptor occupancy in clozapine-treated patients. *Br. J. Psychiatry*, **160**(suppl.17), 30–3.

41. Nordstrom, A.L., Farde, L. and Halldin, C. (1993) High 5HT$_2$ receptor occupancy in clozapine treated patients demonstrated by PET. *Psychopharmacology*, **110**, 365–7.

42. Nyberg, S., Farde, L., Eriksson, L. *et al.* (1993) 5-HT$_2$ and D2 dopamine receptor occupancy in the living brain. A PET study with risperidone. *Psychopharmacology*, **110**, 265–72.

43. Busatto, G.F., Pilowsky, L.S., Costa, D.C. *et al.* (1995) Dopamine D2 receptor blockade in vivo with the novel antipsychotics risperidone and remoxipride – an ^{123}I-IBZM single photon emission tomography (SPET) study. *Psychopharmacology*, **117**, 55–61.

44. Buchsbaum, M.S., DeLisi, L.E., Holcomb, H. *et al.* (1984) Anteroposterior gradients in cerebral glucose use in schizophrenia and affective disorders. *Arch. Gen. Psychiatry*, **41**, 1159–66.

45. Post, R.M., DeLisi, L.E., Holcomb, H.H. *et al.* (1987) Glucose utilization in the temporal cortex of effectively ill patients: positron emission tomography. *Biol. Psychiatry*, **22**, 545–53.

46. Baxter, L.R., Phelps, M.E., Mazziotta, J.C. *et al.* (1985) Cerebral metabolic rates for glucose in mood disorders. *Arch. Gen. Psychiatry*, **42**, 441–7.

47. Sackheim, H.A., Prohovnik, I., Moeller, J.R. *et al.* (1990) Regional cerebral blood flow in mood disorders. *Arch. Gen. Psychiatry*, **47**, 60–70.

48. Baxter, L.R., Schwartz, J.M., Phelps, M.E. *et al.* (1989) Reduction of prefrontal cortex glucose metabolism common to three types of depression. *Arch. Gen. Psychiatry*, **46**, 243–50.

49. Thomas, P., Vaiva, G., Samaille, E. *et al.* (1993) Cerebral blood flow in major depression and dysthymia. *J. Affective Disord.*, **29**, 235–42.

50. Maes, M., Dierckx, R., Meltzer, H.Y. *et al.* (1993) Regional cerebral blood flow in unipolar depression measured with Tc-99m-HMPAO single photon emission computed tomography: negative findings. *Psychiatry Res.: Neuroimaging*, **50**, 77–88.

51. Kling, A.S., Metter, E.J., Riege, W.H. and Kuhl, D.E. (1986) Comparison of PET measurement of local brain glucose metabolism and CAT measurement of brain atrophy in chronic schizophrenia and depression. *Am. J. Psychiatry*, **143**, 175–80.

52. Austin, M.P., Dougall, N., Ross, M. *et al.* (1992) Single photon emission tomography with ^{99m}Tc-exametazine in major depression and the pattern of brain activity underlying the psychotic/neurotic continuum. *J. Affective Dis.*, **26**, 31–44.

53. Bench, C.J., Friston, K.J., Brown, R.G. *et al.* (1993) Regional cerebral blood flow in depression measured by positron emission tomography: the relationship with clinical dimensions. *Psychol. Med.*, **23**, 579–90.

54. Gur, R.C., Skolnick, B.E., Gur, R.E. *et al.* (1984) Brain function in psychiatric disorders. *Arch. Gen. Psychiatry*, **41**, 695–9.

55. Agren, H. and Reibring, L. (1994) PET studies of presynaptic monoamine metabolism in depressed patients and healthy volunteers. *Pharmacopsychiatry*, **27**, 2–6.

56. Suhara, T., Nakayama, K., Inoue, O. *et al.* (1992) D1 dopamine receptor binding in mood disorders measured by positron emission tomography. *Psychopharmacology*, **106**, 14–18.

57. Wong, D.F., Wagner, H.N., Pearlson, G. *et al.* (1989) Dopamine receptor binding of C-11-3-*N*-methylspiperone in the caudate in schizophrenia and bipolar disorder: a preliminary report. *Psychopharmacol. Bull.*, **21**, 595–8.

58. D'Haenen, H.A. and Bossuyt, A. (1994) Dopamine D2 receptors in depression measured with single photon emission computed tomography. *Biol. Psychiatry*, **35**, 128–32.

59. Ebert, D., Fiestel, H., Kaschka, X. *et al.* (1994) Single photon emission computerized tomography assessment of cerebral dopamine D2 receptor blockade in depression before and after sleep deprivation-preliminary results. *Biol. Psychiatry*, **35**, 880–5.

60. D'Haenen, H., Bossuyt, A., Mertens, J. *et al.* (1992) SPECT imaging of serotonin 2 receptors in depression. *Psychiatry Res.: Neuroimaging*, **45**, 227–37.

61. Mathew, R.J. and Wilson, W.H. (1991) Substance abuse and cerebral blood flow. *Am. J. Psychiatry*, **148**, 292–305.

62. London, E.D., Cascella, N.G., Wong, F. *et al.* (1990) Cocaine induced reduction of glucose utilization in human brain. *Arch. Gen. Psychiatry*, **47**, 587–94.

63. Volkow, N.D., Mullani, N., Gould, K.L. *et al.* (1988) Cerebral blood flow in chronic cocaine users. *Br. J. Psychiatry*, **152**, 641–8.

64. Volkow, N.D., Fowler, J.S., Wolf, A.P. *et al.* (1991) Changes in brain glucose metabolism in cocaine dependence and withdrawal. *Am. J. Psychiatry*, **148**, 621–6.

65. Volkow, N.D., Hitzemann, R., Wang, G.J. *et al.* (1992) Long-term frontal brain metabolic changes in cocaine abusers. *Synapse*, **11**, 184–90.

66. Levin, J.M., Mendelson, J.H., Holman, B.L. *et al.* (1995) Improved regional cerebral blood flow in chronic cocaine polydrug users treated with buprenorphine. *J. Nucl. Med.*, **36**, 1211–15.

67. Volkow, N.D., Fowler, J.S., Wolf, A.P. *et al.* (1990) Effects of chronic cocaine abuse on postsynaptic dopamine receptors. *Am. J. Psychiatry*, **147**, 719–24.

68. Baxter, L.R., Schwartz, J.M., Phelps, M. *et al.* (1988) Localisation of neurochemical effects of cocaine and other stimulants in the human brain. *J. Clin. Psychiatry*, **49**, 23–6.

69. Volkow, N.D., Fowler, J.S., Wang, G.-J. *et al.* (1993) Decreased dopamine D2 receptor availability is

associated with reduced frontal metabolism in cocaine abusers. *Synapse*, **14**, 169–77.

70. Volkow, N.D., Hitzemann, R., Wolf, A.P. *et al.* (1990) Acute effects of ethanol on regional brain glucose metabolism and transport. *Psychiatry Res.*, **35**, 39–48.

71. Volkow, N.D., Wang, G.J., Begleiter, H. *et al.* (1995) Regional brain metabolic response to lorazepam in subjects at risk for alcoholism. *Alcoholism: Clin. Exp. Res.*, **19**, 510–16.

72. Sachs, H., Russell, J.A.G., Christman, D.R. and Cook, B. (1987) Alteration of regional cerebral glucose metabolic rate in non-Korsakoff chronic alcoholism. *Arch. Neurol.*, **44**, 1242–51.

73. Berglund, M., Hagstadius, S., Risberg, J. *et al.* (1987) Normalization of regional cerebral blood flow in alcoholics during the first 7 weeks of abstinence. *Acta Psychiatr Scand.*, **75**, 202–8.

74. Volkow, N.D., Hitzemann, R., Wang, G.J. *et al.* (1992) Decreased brain metabolism in neurologically intact healthy alcoholics. *Am. J. Psychiatry*, **149**, 1016–22.

75. Volkow, N.D., Wang, G.J., Hitzemann, R. *et al.* (1994) Recovery of brain glucose metabolism in detoxified alcoholics. *Am. J. Psychiatry*, **151**, 178–83.

76. Adams, K.M., Gilman, S., Koeppe, R.A. *et al.* (1993) Neuropsychological deficits are correlated with frontal hypometabolism in positron emission tomography studies of older alcoholic patients. *Alcohol: Clin. Exp. Res.*, **17**, 205–10.

77. Hietala, J., West, C., Syvalahti, E. *et al.* (1994) Striatal D2 dopamine receptor binding characteristics in vivo in patients with alcohol dependence. *Psychopharmacology*, **116**, 285–90.

78. Tiihonen, J., Kuikka, J., Bergstrom, K. *et al.* (1995) Altered striatal dopamine reuptake site densities in habitually violent and non-violent alcoholics. *Nature Med.*, **1**(7), 654–7.

79. Pauli, S., Liljequist, S., Farde, L. *et al.* (1992) PET analysis of alcohol interaction with the brain disposition of [11C] flumazenil. *Psychopharmacology*, **107**, 180–5.

80. Litton, J.-E., Neiman, J., Pauli, S. *et al.* (1993) PET analysis of [11C] flumazenil binding to benzodiazepine receptors in chronic alcohol dependent men and healthy controls. *Psychiatry Res.: Neuroimaging*, **50**, 1–13.

81. Mathew, R.J. and Wilson, W.H. (1990) Anxiety and cerebral blood flow. *Am. J. Psychiatry*, **147**, 838–49.

82. Gur, R.C., Gur, R.E., Resnick, S. *et al.* (1987) The effect of anxiety on cortical cerebral blood flow and metabolism. *J. Cereb. Blood Flow Metab.*, **7**, 173–7.

83. Lucey, J.V., Costa, D.C., Blanes, T. *et al.* (1995) Regional cerebral blood flow in obsessive-compulsive disordered patients at rest. *Br. J. Psychiatry*, **167**, 629–34.

84. Insel, T.R. (1992) Toward a neuroanatomy of obsessive-compulsive disorder. *Arch. Gen. Psychiatry*, **49**, 739–44.

85. Baxter, L.R., Schwartz, J.M., Bergman, K.S. *et al.* (1992) Caudate glucose metabolic rate changes with both drug and behaviour therapy for obsessive-compulsive disorder. *Arch. Gen. Psychiatry*, **49**, 681–9.

CHAPTER 10

Endocrine

Thyroid

M. N. Maisey

INTRODUCTION

The prevalence of diseases of the thyroid is high. In 1956, Perlmutter and Slater [1] estimated that 4–12% of the population of the USA had palpable thyroid nodules of which 2–5% were probably malignant. In a population study of north-east England, Tunbridge *et al.* [2] reported that in adult females, the prevalence of hyperthyroidism was 1.9–2.7%, of overt hypothyroidism 1.4–1.9%, of subclinical hypothyroidism 7.5%, and of non-toxic goitres 8.6%; however, the prevalence of these conditions was much lower in males. The classification of thyroid diseases is shown in Table 10.1.

The correct management of thyroid diseases depends on accurate diagnosis, appropriate treatment and careful monitoring. Radionuclides have always played a leading part in all aspects of the management of thyroid diseases: radioimmuno-assay techniques revolutionized the investigation of thyroid dysfunction while radionuclide scanning has long been the main method of investigating the thyroid *in vivo*. The role of thyroid scanning in clinical practice has expanded with the introduction of new radiopharmaceuticals (see Table 10.2). The increasing use of other diagnostic imaging techniques including ultrasound, computed tomography (CT) and magnetic resonance imaging (MRI), all have had an impact on the way

we use radioisotopes in the investigation of thyroid disease, but have not significantly detracted from the importance of radionuclide scanning. Radioactive iodine is established as a simple, cheap and effective method of treating thyrotoxicosis, and in most cases represents the treatment of choice.

In this chapter we discuss systematic and practical approaches to the management of the most important clinical problems in thyroid disease with emphasis on the role of nuclear medicine techniques.

DIAGNOSIS OF THYROID DYSFUNCTION

PATHOPHYSIOLOGY

A knowledge of the changes that occur in hyperthyroidism and hypothyroidism is fundamental to an understanding of the laboratory investigations of these conditions. The basic abnormality in hyperthyroidism and hypothyroidism is an increased or decreased concentration of circulating free thyroid hormones with a corresponding change in the total serum concentration of these hormones.

In hyperthyroidism, both serum thyroxine (T4) and triiodothyrorine (T3) are usually raised, and therefore it is not necessary to measure both hormones routinely for diagnosis, but in a proportion of hyperthyroid patients (about 10%), serum total T3 concentration may be abnormally raised at presentation when serum T4 lies within the normal range; elevated serum T4 with normal T3 has rarely been reported. These discrepancies occur

Clinical Nuclear Medicine, 3rd edn. Edited by M.N. Maisey, K.E. Britton and B.D. Collier. Published in 1998 by Chapman & Hall, London. ISBN 0 412 75180 1

Table 10.1   Classification of thyroid disease

I.   *Diseases primarily characterized by euthyroidism*
    A. Non-toxic diffuse goitre
        1. Sporadic
        2. Endemic
        3. Compensatory, following subtotal
            thyroidectomy
    B. Non-toxic uninodular goitre
        1. Functional nodule
        2. Non-functional
    C. Non-toxic multinodular goitre due to causes
        under IA
        1. Functional nodules
        2. Non-functional nodules
        3. Functional and non-functional nodules
    D. Tumours
        1. Adenoma and teratoma
        2. Carcinoma
        3. Lymphoma
        4. Sarcoma
    E. Acute thyroiditis
        1. Suppurative
        2. Subacute, non-suppurative
    F. Chronic thyroiditis
        1. Lymphocytic (Hashimoto's)
        2. Invasive fibrous (Riedel's)
        3. Suppurative
        4. Non-suppurative
    G. Degeneration or infiltration
        1. Haemorrhage or infarction
        2. Amyloid
        3. Haemochromatosis
    H. Congenital anomaly
II.   *Diseases primarily characterized by hyperthyroidism*
    A. Toxic diffuse goitre (Graves', Basedow's disease)
        1. With eye changes (ophthalmopathy)
        2. With localized dermopathy or acropachy
        3. Neonatal or congenital
        4. With incidental non-functional nodule(s)
        5. With euthyroidism and eye changes
    B. Toxic uninodular goitre
    C. Toxic multinodular goitre
        1. Functional nodules, non-functional
            parenchyma
        2. Functional nodules, functional parenchyma
    D. Nodular goitre with hyperthyroidism due to
        exogenous iodine (Jod–Basedow)
    E. Exogenous thyroid hormone excess
        1. Thyrotoxicosis factitia
        2. Thyrotoxicosis medicamentosa
    F. Tumours
        1. Adenoma of thyroid, follicular
        2. Carcinoma of thyroid, follicular
        3. Thyrotrophin-secreting tumours
III.   *Diseases primarily characterized by hypothyroidism*
    A. Idiopathic hypothyroidism
        1. Myxoedema
        2. Cretinism
    B. Iatrogenic destruction
        1. Surgery
        2. Radioiodine
        3. X-ray
    C. Thyrotrophin deficiency
        1. Isolated
        2. Panhypopituitarism
    D. Thyrotrophin-releasing factor (TRF) deficiency
        due to hypothalamic injury or disease

Modified from Werner (1969).

less often with free T3 (fT3) and free T4 (fT4) measurements. Other factors beside hyperthyroidism such as a coexisting severe non-thyroidal illness, which impairs peripheral conversion of T4 to T3, may also account for disparities in hormone concentrations. For most patients with hyperthyroidism, the rise in serum T3 is much greater than that of serum T4. It is clear from these observations that measurement of serum T3 is a more sensitive and reliable investigation for hyperthyroidism than serum T4.

In hypothyroidism, there is a greater and earlier fall in serum T4 compared with serum T3, which may often remain within the normal range. Thus, while serum T3 is the investigation of choice for hyperthyroidism, serum T4 is a better screening test for hypothyroidism. Thyroid failure may be a primary abnormality of the thyroid gland, or rarely may be secondary to impaired secretion of thyroid-stimulating hormone (TSH) by the pituitary gland. In primary hypothyroidism, the low serum T4 is accompanied by a raised serum TSH; whereas in secondary hypothyroidism the low serum T4 is associated with a low serum TSH. Measurement of serum TSH is therefore essential for distinguishing between primary and secondary hypothyroidism. A low serum TSH is not always sufficient to confirm hypothyroidism due to pituitary failure, and it may be necessary to show that serum TSH concentration is unresponsive to thyrotrophin-releasing hormone (TRH) stimulation. Lately, TSH assays have increased in sensitivity, and low suppressed levels of serum TSH that occur in hyperthyroidism can be distinguished from normal levels. Ultrasensitive TSH assays have consequently been used as a primary investigation of hyper- and hypothyroidism.

Changes in serum total T3 (tT3) and T4 (tT4) levels may be due not only to altered thyroid function but also to altered concentrations of carrier proteins, especially thyroxine-binding globulin (TBG) in the absence of any thyroid dysfunction. Since over 99% of the total circulating thyroid hormones are bound to serum proteins, an increase or decrease in serum TBG is accompanied by a corresponding increase or decrease in bound and total serum T3 and T4 in the presence of normal concentrations of free hormones. In such cases, serum total T3 and T4 levels may not reflect the patient's true thyroid status. Serum TBG should therefore be measured in any condition that is

Table 10.2 Radiopharmaceuticals used in the investigation of thyroid diseases

Radiopharmaceutical	Application(s)
^{99m}Tc-pertechnetate	Routine thyroid scanning
^{123}I sodium iodide	Thyroid scanning when a radioisotope of iodine is required
^{131}I sodium iodide	The investigation of thyroid cancer
^{127}I (stable) iodide	Investigation of thyroid nodules and suppressed tissue
^{67}Ga citrate	Investigation of thyroid lymphoma, silent thyroiditis, thyroid infection and amyloid
^{201}T1 thallous chloride	Investigation of thyroid cancer, thyroid nodules, demonstration of suppressed thyroid tissue
^{99m}Tc-labelled pentavalent DMSA	Investigation of medullary thyroid carcinoma
^{131}I / ^{123}I-MIBG	Investigation of medullary thyroid carcinoma
^{18}F-FDG	All forms of thyroid cancer

Table 10.3 Factors that affect serum TBG concentration

Increased TBG	Decreased TBG
1. Contraceptive pill and other oestrogens	1. Androgens and anabolic steroids
2. Pregnancy	2. Severe illness
3. Hypothyroidism	3. Hyperthyroidism
4. Inherited disorders of TBG production	4. Inherited disorders of TBG production
	5. Chronic diseases, especially liver disease, nephrotic syndrome, malnutrition/malabsorption

known to alter its concentration (Table 10.3), and whenever the serum tT3 or tT4 is close to the limits of the normal range or does not correspond to the clinical status of the patient. Artefactual changes in the total serum T3 and T4 concentrations can also occur if the binding of these hormones to TBG is interfered with by drugs such as salicylates, sulphonylureas and phenytoin in the absence of any change in the TBG concentration. However, the widespread use of free hormone measurements has made these considerations of less importance.

CLINICAL SITUATIONS

Hyperthyroidism

The single most reliable test for hyperthyroidism is a sensitive TSH measurement, which will demonstrate TSH suppressed below the normal range (0.3–3 mU/l). A serum total or free T3 level will provide increased diagnostic certainty, and in the absence of an available sensitive TSH assay, the T3 measurement is the primary test for hyperthyroidism. Rarely, the serum T4 will be elevated when the serum T3 is normal, but when a normal T3 is found with a suppressed TSH, and if

the ultra-sensitive TSH assay is used and T4 measured, this should not be a problem. The TRH stimulation test remains a useful discriminating test when results are equivocal, but is much less frequently used now that low levels of TSH can be routinely measured. If total hormone assays are being used, the measurement of TBG may be helpful when discrepantly high or low total hormone levels are discovered.

Hyperthyroid patients receiving treatment

β-Blockers Propranolol or other β-blocking drugs that are used for symptomatic treatment of hyperthyroidism may slightly lower serum T3 concentrations, probably by interfering with peripheral conversion of T4 to T3. However, the fall is quantitatively minimal, and does not account for the main therapeutic effect of the drugs, and is therefore unlikely to cause confusion in the laboratory assessment of thyroid function.

Antithyroid drugs Patients receiving treatment with antithyroid drugs should have serum T3 and T4 levels measured regularly to assess whether they are being under- or overtreated, as it is may be difficult to assess the clinical status. During treatment, there is a tendency for an earlier and greater fall in serum T4 compared with serum T3, and measurement of one hormone may be misleading. A persistently raised serum T3 with raised or normal serum T4 means that the patient is still hyperthyroid. A normal serum T3 and T4, or a borderline high serum T3 with normal or borderline low T4, indicates that the patient is euthyroid. A low serum T4 with normal or low serum T3 suggests that the patient is becoming hypothyroid. The dose of antithyroid drugs will be adjusted in the light of the thyroid function results and the patient's clinical state. The TSH level may be helpful in indicating excess treatment if it is elevated, but the reverse does not apply – the patient may be euthyroid or hypothyroid with a persistently suppressed TSH level.

Radioiodine and subtotal thyroidectomy Both serum T3 and TSH should be routinely measured during the first few months (usually at 6-weekly intervals) following radioidine treatment or subtotal thyroidectomy, to determine whether the patient remains hyperthyroid, or is becoming euthyroid or hypothyroid. When the T3 has become normal, the TSH and T4 measurements are used to detect developing hypothyroidism. Hypothyroidism occurring within the first 6 months of radioiodine or surgical treatment may be transient and revert spontaneously, especially when the fall in T4 is not accompanied by a rise in TSH. On the other hand, late onset hypothyroidism is usually permanent. Early asymptomatic or mild hypothyroidism may be left untreated and followed up with TSH measurements to allow recovery to occur. If the patient becomes symptomatic, thyroid replacement should not be withheld but it may be advisable to stop treatment for 4–6 weeks at the end of the first year to confirm that hypothyroidism is permanent. All patients who have been treated with ^{131}I or had surgery for hyperthyroidism due to Graves' disease must have long-term follow-up to detect late hypothyroidism. In the absence of any specific symptoms or signs, an annual serum T4 estimation is the best and easiest routine follow-up investigation for screening. If T4 is below normal, hypothyroidism can be confirmed by measurement of serum TSH on the same sample. If recurrent hyperthyroidism is suspected clinically, serum T3 should be estimated. The addition of a sensitive TSH measurement to the follow-up

protocol improves the effectiveness of the assessment but increases the cost.

Block/replacement regime The best tests for assessing the effectiveness of a thyroid hormone replacement therapy regime where antithyroid drugs and thyroid hormones are given together will depend on which thyroid hormone (T3 or T4) is given in combination with the antithyroid drug. The TSH level should ideally be maintained in the normal range during treatment. If T4 is given, both the T3 and T4 should be measured and maintained in the normal range; however, a better regime is to give T3 as the replacement hormone, and keep the TSH and T3 in the normal range. Under these circumstances, the T4 level should be almost undetectable and will establish whether the antithyroid drug-blocking effect is complete.

Hypothyroidism – diagnosis

When hypothyroidism is suspected clinically, laboratory investigations should be performed not only to confirm the diagnosis but also to differentiate between primary and secondary thyroid failure. The distinction is important as in addition to thyroid replacement secondary hypothyroidism requires further investigation for the diagnosis and subsequent management of the underlying cause.

Serum T4 is usually the initial investigation of choice as it is a more sensitive and reliable test of hypothyroidism than serum T3; better results are obtained if this is combined with TSH, which should always be measured when T4 levels are found to be low.

Normal serum T4 If the serum T4 is within the normal range, the diagnosis of hypothyroidism is practically excluded and no further investigation is necessary unless the clinical suspicion of thyroid failure remains high, when further confirmatory investigations should be performed.

Low or borderline low serum T4 If the serum T4 is below or near the lower limit of the normal range, serum TSH concentration should be measured on serum stored from the same blood specimen. Raised serum TSH and low or borderline low serum T4 confirms mild primary hypothyroidism. It is useful to measure serum thyroid microsomal **auto-antibodies** in these patients, as their presence in significant titres indicates primary hypothyroidism due to autoimmune thyroiditis (Hashimoto's disease), which usually requires life-long thyroid replacement. This should be distinguished from the transient hypothyroidism, which may be associated with De Quervain's thyroiditis, radioiodine therapy or subtotal thyroidectomy.

If the TSH is not elevated in spite of a low T4, the patient may either have secondary hypothyroidism or, if total T4 has been measured, may be euthyroid and have a low serum TBG. A low TBG should be excluded by measuring serum TBG or free T4. A TRH stimulation test may be performed to confirm or exclude pituitary hypothyroidism. An absent TSH response to TRH with a low serum T4 will confirm pituitary hypothyroidism. Further investigations including full pituitary function tests and radiographs and CT of the pituitary fossa should be carried out to establish the nature and extent of the pituitary abnormality.

Hypothyroidism – treatment

Thyroid function tests should be used to monitor thyroid hormone replacement in hypothyroid patients. L-Thyroxine (T4) is the usual preparation used and the normal replacement dose is 0.1–0.2 mg daily (100–200 µg). A low dose is used initially (0.05 mg T4 daily), increasing gradually by small increments every 2–4 weeks until the full replacement dose is achieved. In elderly patients, and subjects with prolonged hypothyroidism or associated heart disease, the starting dose should be even lower – 0.025 mg (25 µg) daily, and increased very slowly every 4 weeks, to avoid the risk of precipitating tachycardia and/or myocardial ischaemia.

The dose of thyroid hormone is adjusted until the elevated serum TSH has fallen to normal levels, but not suppressed below the normal range. It is important to remember that the TSH levels may continue to fall for several weeks after a change of dose; thyroid function tests should not be performed until the patient has been on the same dose of thyroxine for at least 4 weeks. When the serum TSH has returned to normal, serum T4 is usually found to be in the upper normal range or slightly elevated, whereas T3 is usually in the mid-normal range. In all patients receiving thyroid replacement, it is advisable to check the serum TSH concentration once a year, in order to ensure that their requirements have not changed.

With pituitary hypothyroidism, since serum TSH is not elevated, serum T4 estimations are used to monitor the dose of thyroid replacement, which is increased until the serum T4 concentration is within the upper normal range.

It may be necessary to assess whether thyroxine treatment need be continued in patients who were started on hormone replacement without a definitive diagnosis of hypothyroidism. Thyroid medication is withheld for 4–6 weeks and serum T4 and TSH measured. If the patient is unwilling to withhold the full treatment dose for the test, the dose is halved for 6 weeks and serum T4 and TSH are measured. If the patient is found biochemically to be hypothyroid on half doses, medication can then be withheld completely and the tests repeated.

Neonatal hypothyroidism

Congenital hypothyroidism is an important cause of severe mental retardation, with an estimated incidence of one in every 3000–6000 live births in non-endemic areas. Early diagnosis and treatment significantly affects the prognosis for mental development. Routine biochemical screening of all newborn babies for congenital hypothyroidism is now considered essential for the early diagnosis and treatment of this condition.

Commercial radioimmunoassay kits are now available for T4 or TSH estimation on dried capillary blood collected on filter paper. Screening is carried out on capillary blood collected on filter paper at 4–6 days after birth. This enables samples to be mailed to a central laboratory. Alternatively, cord blood collected at the time of delivery can be used, but is less suitable for dispatch.

Measurement of serum T4 alone will miss many cases of neonatal hypothyroidism, including particularly those with 'compensated hypothyroidism', i.e. normal T4 and high TSH at or shortly after birth, which may occur with ectopic thyroids. If the condition is not diagnosed and remains untreated, frank hypothyroidism and associated mental retardation may develop subsequently. Measurement of serum TSH alone is a more sensitive screening test than serum T4 but will miss secondary hypothyroidism, which contributes only 3–5% of all cases of congenital hypothyroidism. Measurement of serum T4 and TSH both will detect all cases, but the increased workload and cost make it a less practical proposition, particularly since the detection rate is only improved by 3–5% over that of screening with serum T4 or TSH alone.

It is intended that the screening programme will permit the diagnosis of congenital hypothyroidism to be made as quickly as possible after birth, preferably within 2 weeks so that patients can be recalled for assessment and further testing if necessary and treatment started with minimum delay. It has also been shown that hypothyroidism may be transient in about 10% of cases, so that the need to continue permanent thyroid replacement should be reviewed at a suitable time when treatment may be safely withheld for a few weeks for repeat thyroid function tests.

Pregnancy and oestrogen therapy

Due to high circulating oestrogen concentrations, pregnant women and those on the contraceptive pill or other oestrogen preparations have raised serum TBG concentrations, which may spuriously increase serum tT3 and tT4 levels, even when they are euthyroid. Therefore, free thyroid hormones should always be used to assess thyroid function in this group of patients; however, if total T3 and T4 are used, serum TBG need to be measured, and the serum T3 and T4 results interpreted carefully in the light of the serum TBG value. Sensitive serum TSH measurements are the most useful measurements together with the free hormones.

Elderly sick patients

Serum T3 falls slightly but significantly in old age, even in the absence of any thyroid dysfunction. On the other hand, serum T4 either remains unchanged or shows a comparatively lesser age-related decrease. The fall in serum T3 becomes more marked in elderly patients who are seriously ill for whatever reason, probably due to failure of peripheral conversion of T4 to T3. Consequently, the serum concentration of these hormones, particularly serum T3, may not reflect the true thyroid status. Serum TSH estimation and its response to TRH may be necessary to confirm or exclude thyroid dysfunction in elderly sick patients, particularly since clinical diagnosis is often difficult in this age group. Alternatively, serum T3 or T4 can be reassessed when the patient has recovered from the acute illness and compared with the normal range for this age group.

HYPERTHYROIDISM

The diagnosis of hyperthyroidism is incomplete without establishing the cause, since the choice of management and prognosis will depend on the underlying cause. A brief discussion of the aetiology and mechanism of hyperthyroidism is important for understanding the method(s) of investigation and diagnosis. Table 10.4 lists the most important causes of hyperthyroidism.

Most commonly, excess thyroid hormone secretion is associated with the presence of an abnormal 'thyroid-stimulating immunoglobulin' (TSI or TSab) directed against the TSH receptor. This thyroid stimulator is found in patients with a toxic diffuse goitre (Graves' disease), and results in diffuse hyperplasia of the thyroid tissue that is capable of responding. If the gland contains pre-existing non-functioning nodular areas, cysts or scars, only the paranodular tissue will be stimulated and the gland may be nodular. The cause of hyperthyroidism is then Graves' disease superimposed on a previous nodular goitre, i.e. Graves' disease with incidental non-functioning nodules.

Hyperthyroidism may also occur if a localized area of the thyroid has changed in such a way that the follicular cells secrete thyroid hormones independently of TSH control. This is an autonomous functioning nodule, and as the nodule grows in size, it may secrete sufficient hormones to exceed the physiological requirements and the patient becomes hyperthyroid. The rest of the gland may

Table 10.4 Causes of hyperthyroidism

1. Graves' disease (diffuse or nodular variants)
2. Solitary or multiple toxic autonomous nodules (toxic adenoma, Plummer's disease)
3. Thyroid hormone 'leakage'
   (a) Subacute (De Quervain's) thyroiditis
   (b) Painless (silent) thyroiditis
   (c) Hashimoto's thyroiditis
   (d) Post-partum thyroiditis
4. Iodide-induced hyperthyroidism (Jod–Basedow's phenomenon)
5. Excess thyroid hormone ingestion
6. Rare causes including:
   (a) Pituitary TSH-dependent hyperthyroidism
   (b) Ectopic TSH-secreting tumour
   (c) Extensive functioning differentiated thyroid cancer
   (d) Trophoblastic tumour
   (e) Struma ovarii

be normal but have function suppressed due to secondary suppression of TSH. The gland may also contain pre-existing non-functioning nodules, if the autonomous change has occurred in a pre-existing nodular goitre. Hyperthyroidism caused by one or more such autonomous functioning nodules is also referred to as single or multiple toxic adenomas (or Plummer's disease), and sometimes, toxic nodular goitre. The last terminology is the least satisfactory and should be avoided, as it is a descriptive clinical term for a nodular goitre associated with hyperthyroidism, which may be due to either autonomous functioning nodules or non-functioning nodules in a diffuse toxic goitre as discussed above.

Hyperthyroidism may occur if stored hormones leak out of the thyroid due to an inflammatory process which damages the follicles. This may be related to recent viral infection, subacute De Quervain's thyroiditis or an autoimmune process, Hashitoxicosis, post-partum thyroiditis or the cause may be unknown (painless thyroiditis). In each case, hyperthyroidism is usually mild and transient. Hyperthyroidism may be precipitated by excess iodide or thyroid hormone ingestion and very rarely may be due to extensive functioning papillary or follicular thyroid carcinoma or excess TSH production. In practice, Graves' disease and single or multiple autonomous toxic nodules (uninodular or multinodular Plummer's disease) account for the majority of cases of thyrotoxicosis. Nevertheless, the remaining causes are clinically important and should always be borne in mind because their management and clinical course is different.

DIAGNOSIS OF THE CAUSE OF HYPERTHYROIDISM

The history and physical examination will often suggest the cause of hyperthyroidism in patients with Graves' disease, but a clinical diagnosis can only be made with certainty in the presence of pathognomonic ocular or cutaneous signs, i.e. exophthalmos or other infiltrative eye signs, localized pretibial myxoedema and acropachy. However, this classical presentation of Graves' disease is uncommon, and investigations are usually necessary to confirm or establish the aetiology. A diffuse goitre although most commonly associated with Graves' disease is not by itself diagnostic of

the condition as it may occur in patients with subacute or painless thyroiditis or in those who are ingesting excessive thyroid hormones for a non-toxic goitre.

The finding of a thyroid nodule or a multinodular goitre in a hyperthyroid patient does not establish the cause of hyperthyroidism since the diagnosis may be either Plummer's disease or variants of Graves' disease (as discussed above). In a proportion of hyperthyroid patients, the thyroid gland is not palpable, which may make the clinical diagnosis of the underlying cause even more difficult. The patient should be carefully questioned for the possibility of iodide or thyroid hormone-induced hyperthyroidism, but most commonly the cause of hyperthyroidism is found on investigation to be a small diffuse toxic goitre or a non-palpable toxic nodule.

Hyperthyroidism associated with subacute thyroiditis typically presents with a short history of painful tender goitre often accompanied by fever, anorexia and other constitutional symptoms. The clinical picture is often atypical, and in most cases investigations are necessary to confirm or establish the diagnosis. Painless thyroiditis as a cause of hyperthyroidism can only be diagnosed by appropriate investigations, although a proportion of these occurring in epidemics have been shown to be due to the incorporation of beef thyroid into hamburger meat. It is thus apparent that investigations are usually necessary to establish the cause of hyperthyroidism.

DIAGNOSIS AND MANAGEMENT OF THYROTOXICOSIS

The appropriate management of patients with hyperthyroidism depends in many instances on an accurate initial diagnosis; and the thyroid scan has an important role in thyrotoxicosis [4]. The radionuclide scan has three main uses in managing hyperthyroidism: (i) establishing the cause of thyrotoxicosis; (ii) the measurement of tracer uptake and gland size for the selection of an appropriate ^{131}I therapy regime; and (iii) for the follow-up of patients after treatment.

Establishing the cause of thyrotoxicosis

There are a large number of patients in whom the diagnosis cannot be made clinically, and without the thyroid scan an incorrect diagnosis may often be assumed. This can result in inappropriate treatment; in a review, we found that 22% of patients with toxic nodules (Plummer's disease) had received long-term antithyroid medication before the correct diagnosis was established and appropriate treatment instituted [5].

The solitary thyroid nodule and thyrotoxicosis When a patient with thyrotoxicosis is found to have a solitary thyroid nodule on clinical examination, this is usually due to an autonomous toxic nodule (Figure 10.1). However, clinical examination is unreliable, in up to one-third of patients. Other causes may be identified by subsequent investigations, for example, a solitary non-functioning nodule in a patient with Graves' disease (Figure 10.2), an asymmetrically enlarged thyroid (Figure 10.3), or diffuse enlargement of a single lobe with agenesis of the other lobe, may all simulate a toxic nodule. It may not always be possible to differentiate between these on the initial scan: for example, differentiating a large toxic nodule with complete suppression of the other lobe from

agenesis of a lobe in a patient with Graves' disease may require further investigations; and repeating the scan after stimulation with exogenous TSH will demonstrate suppressed tissue, or a repeat scanning with ^{201}Tl may often show uptake in tissue that is not accumulating ^{99m}TcO$_4$ or ^{123}I/^{131}I (Figure 10.4); ultrasound will demonstrate a lobe which is present but not taking up tracer, or a hypoplastic or aplastic lobe; and the use of fluorescent X-ray will establish the presence of ^{127}I-containing tissue on the contralateral side. Even a simple method of shielding the active nodule with lead on routine thyroid scintigraphy may be sufficient to show the other lobe. The importance of making the correct diagnosis lies in the choice of treatment and subsequent follow-up. Patients with toxic nodules respond well to radioiodine treatment, and the nodule usually decreases in size to 50–60% of the original volume, with complete cure being the normal outcome and hypothyroidism a rare sequel [6,7], whereas a single lobe with Graves' disease will usually be treated in a conventional manner – initially with antithyroid drugs, and is followed by ablative radioiodine therapy only when a relapse occurs. However, some centres prefer to treat these nodules surgically; but this now represents a minority view. Children with toxic nodules will still usually be treated surgically. A patient with Graves' disease who has an incidental non-functioning nodule on the radionuclide scan is usually treated by subtotal thyroidectomy in order to identify possible malignancy, which has an incidence similar to a cold nodule in a normal gland. An alternative approach is fine needle aspiration cytology examination of the nodule followed by radioiodine treatment of the toxic diffuse goitre, after which

Figure 10.1 A typical left-sided thyroid toxic nodule with complete suppression of the right lobe.

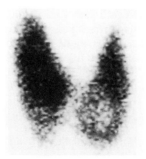

Figure 10.2 Scan of a patient with a diffuse toxic goitre (Graves' disease) and an incidental cold nodule in the left lower pole.

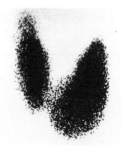

Figure 10.3 Graves' disease presenting with an asymmetrical goitre simulating a single nodule on clinical examination.

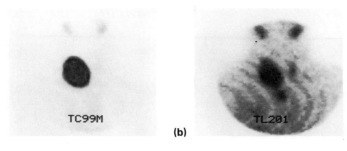

(a)   **(b)**

Figure 10.4 (a) ^{99m}Tc-pertechnetate scan with virtually no uptake on the left side. (b) ^{201}Tl scan shows the presence of metabolically active thyroid tissue on the left.

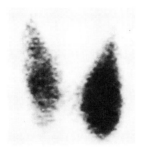

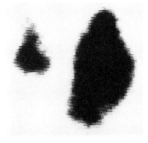

Figure 10.5 The non-functioning nodule in Figure 10.2 is now taking up the tracer: the Marine–Lenhart syndrome.

Figure 10.6 Confluent nodules in a patient with multiple autonomous toxic thyroid nodules.

some non-functioning nodules that are TSH-dependent (Marine–Lenhart syndrome), will function following resolution of disease (Figure 10.5). These nodules probably do not require surgical treatment.

Nodular goitre associated with thyrotoxicosis When thyrotoxic patients present with a multinodular goitre, they are often labelled as having a toxic nodular goitre. However, there are three possible causes for this: (i) multiple toxic nodules developing in a long-standing multinodular goitre (Plummer's disease); (ii) Graves' disease occurring in a patient with a previous non-toxic multinodular goitre; and (iii) a patient with Graves' disease in whom the enlarged gland has become nodular. The latter two can be differentiated by the presence or absence of a previous history of nodular goitre. The scan appearances of Plummer's disease may vary from a single toxic nodule to multiple clearly defined nodules throughout the gland. Occasionally, the nodules appear almost confluent when the scan

may be difficult to differentiate from Graves' disease in a multinodular gland (Figure 10.6). Most often, the diagnosis can be made from the scan, although appearances do overlap and further investigations may be necessary. These include the measurement of serum thyroid-stimulating antibody, the use of repeat scans after TSH to demonstrate stimulation of suppressed tissue – this may also be achieved when the serum TSH rises with antithyroid drugs [8]. Alternatively, a diagnosis may be established retrospectively when patients are re-scanned after radioiodine treatment (Figure 10.7). As mentioned previously for the single nodule, ^{201}Tl can be used to demonstrate tissue in which the uptake function but not the metabolic activity is suppressed and may demonstrate the suppressed perinodular thyroid tissue.

The impalpable gland and thyrotoxicosis If the thyroid is small it may be difficult to palpate and when it is not obviously enlarged in thyrotoxicosis, a thyroid scan should always be performed. In a series of patients with toxic nod-

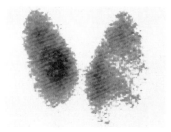

Figure 10.7 After treatment with ^{131}I of the patient whose scan is shown in Figure 10.6, there is a quite different distribution of uptake, confirming the original diagnosis.

Table 10.5 Causes of low tracer uptake in hyperthyroidism

Subacute thyroiditis
Iodine-induced thyrotoxicosis (Jod–Basedow)
Amiodarone-induced thyrotoxicosis
Ectopic thyroid tissue
Thyrotoxicosis factitia (excess thyroid hormone
  administration)
Recent high iodine load (due to dilutional effects)

ules, 10% were impalpable and some of these nodules could not be palpated even after identification on the scan [5]. The scan may demonstrate any of the recognized patterns associated with thyrotoxicosis such as diffuse uptake, low uptake or functioning nodules. This is particularly important in elderly patients with atrial fibrillation, who should have a scan to detect toxic nodules that may not be producing obvious clinical disease, as these can be easily treated with radioiodine.

Low tracer uptake and thyrotoxicosis The thyroid scan in patients with thyrotoxicosis may have low uptake. This finding may indicate a cause for thyrotoxicosis, which could be self-limiting and avoid unnecessary and ineffective administration of radioiodine. These conditions are shown in Table 10.5.

Amiodarone, an iodine-rich drug, has recently been recognized to be a frequent cause of thyrotoxicosis through a number of mechanisms, and is almost always associated with low uptake of tracer and non-visualization of the thyroid on the scan. In an early review of 35 patients with amiodarone-induced thyrotoxicosis [9], 24-hour ^{131}I uptake was less than 4% in 12 patients who had

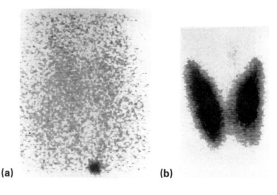

(a) **(b)**

Figure 10.8 (a) Subacute thyroiditis causing thyrotoxicosis. (b) With resolution of the hyperthyroidism the scan returns to normal.

no palpable abnormality but was more than 8% in the 17 patients with goitres.

Ectopic tissue may occasionally cause hyperthyroidism with non-visualization of the 'normal' thyroid on routine scanning. This may be due to thyrotoxicosis caused by metastatic follicular cancer, or a retrosternal goitre with a toxic nodule, or an intrathoracic goitre causing Graves' thyrotoxicosis. In each case, the cervical thyroid uptake was low or absent, either due to suppression or absence of tissue. In females, a scan in such cases should include the pelvis to identify the rare struma ovarii. Post-partum thyroiditis is being increasingly recognized and may be associated with both hypo and hyperthyroidism (or occasionally both), which is usually transient. In both situations, the scan reveals low tracer uptake.

Subacute thyroiditis continues to be a regular cause of transient hyperthyroidism. This is usually diagnosed clinically in a patient with a painful thyroid and a low technetium or iodine uptake on the scan (Figure 10.8). Occasionally, the diagnosis may be more difficult, and cases of subacute thyroiditis have been demonstrated while being investigated for pyrexia of unknown origin (PUO), and the cause of the PUO and hyperthyroidism was identified with intense ^{67}Ga scan uptake in the thyroid. While subacute thyroiditis is occasionally painless, what was initially thought to be a mini-epidemic of such cases was shown to result from the addition of bovine thyroid tissue to hamburgers – the so-called 'hamburger thyrotoxicosis'.

TREATMENT OF HYPERTHYROIDISM

The diagnosis of hyperthyroidism should be confirmed biochemically and its cause established (as discussed in preceding sections) before specific therapy is advised. While awaiting laboratory investigations, provided there are no contraindications such as asthma, a β-adrenergic blocking drug such as propranolol may be prescribed to relieve sympathetic symptoms such as sweating, tremors, palpitations or irritability. An adequate adult dose is 40 mg of propranolol two or three times daily, or a single 160 mg daily dose of a long-acting preparation. Specific treatment can subsequently be instituted when the diagnosis is confirmed.

The importance of diagnosing the cause of hyperthyroidism is stressed as it determines the choice of therapy, the clinical course of the condition and the likelihood of hypothyroidism or recurrent hyperthyroidism. The tendency of some physicians to initiate therapy with antithyroid drugs routinely in every patient with hyperthyroidism is open to criticism as they may be ineffective in certain types of hyperthyroidism, such as that associated with thyroiditis, or may not represent the treatment of choice in other cases, such as elderly patients or those with Plummer's disease.

Graves' disease (toxic diffuse goitre)

The conventional treatments for hyperthyroidism due to Graves' disease include antithyroid drugs, subtotal thyroidectomy and radioactive iodine. The advantages and disadvantages of each form of therapy are summarized in Table 10.6, and should always be weighed against each other when selecting the most appropriate treatment for an individual patient. The treatment of choice for a particular patient depends on several factors: the patient's age; the presence of any associated cardiovascular problems such as atrial fibrillation, heart failure, ischaemic heart disease or other major medical problems; a previous history of hyperthyroidism and the type of treatment received; local medical facilities such as the availability of an experienced thyroid surgeon or an adequately equipped nuclear medicine department; the physician's personal experience and preference, and the patient's willingness to undergo the particular form of therapy advised.

For a young patient with uncomplicated Graves' disease, the conventional treatment is a course of antithyroid drug therapy for 6 months to 2 years. Drugs such as propylthiouracil and carbimazole or methimazole are effective in reducing thyroid hormone production and release, but in at least 50% of patients there is an early relapse or later recurrence of hyperthyroidism when treatment is stopped even after a prolonged course. Side-effects of antithyroid drugs are uncommon and usually become manifest within a few weeks of starting treatment. Allergic skin reactions are the most common, but the most serious is agranulocytosis, which has been reported in 0.2–0.3% of patients.

Subtotal thyroidectomy offers a higher chance of cure in a much shorter time but requires admission, an experienced thyroid surgeon and the patient's fitness and willingness to undergo surgery. Complications of subtotal thyroidectomy depend on the surgeon's experience and the adequacy of the patient's pre-operative preparation. They include post-operative haemorrhage, recurrent laryngeal nerve palsy and transient or permanent hypoparathyroidism; the morbidity ranges between 0.2% and 1%. It is now used only for patients with very large goitres where there is a suspicion of malignancy or when the patient is particularly keen to avoid radioiodine therapy.

Radioactive iodine provides the highest rate of cure, approaching 100%, although the effective

Table 10.6 Treatment of Graves' disease: advantages and disadvantages of each type of treatment

	Drugs	*Surgery*	*Radioiodine*
Relapse or recurrence	High	Low	Low (dose-related)
Hypothyroidism	Low	Intermediate	High (dose-related)
Complications	Rare	Low but significant mortality and morbidity	Rare
Ease of treatment and cost	Intermediate	Least favourable	Simple and cheap
Onset of therapeutic effect	Moderate (1 or 2 weeks)	Rapid after pre-op. preparation	Slow (few weeks)

dose is variable and more than one treatment dose may be necessary. Radioiodine has the advantage of being a very simple and cheap form of therapy. In the past, radioiodine treatment has been confined entirely to hyperthyroid patients over the reproductive age, owing to the fear of radiation-induced cancer or genetic complications. As experience with radioiodine treatment has increased, many thyroidologists now feel that the use of ^{131}I need no longer be restricted but may be extended to younger adults and children. The major disadvantage of radioiodine therapy for Graves' disease is the high incidence of post-treatment hypothyroidism. With moderate doses of ^{131}I the incidence of hypothyroidism is about 20% in the first year of treatment, with an additional annual increase of 3% over subsequent years, and by 10 years up to 50% of treated patients may be hypothyroid. The risk of hypothyroidism is less with smaller doses of radioiodine but the chance of successful therapy is also reduced. Large single doses of [131]I (e.g. 15 mCi), achieve a high cure rate in Graves' hyperthyroidism, with 70–90% requiring T4 replacement.

Choice of therapy for hyperthyroidism

Children and adolescents Antithyroid drugs are the treatment of choice in very young patients with Graves' disease, but the duration of therapy may be a problem. The aim of therapy is to continue with antithyroid drugs in yearly courses as necessary until the patient has reached the late teens or early twenties. Clinical and biochemical evidence of persistent or recurrent hyperthyroidism is sought at the end of each course of antithyroid drugs before resuming a new course of treatment.

Adults In general, a course of antithyroid drugs for 6 months to 2 years is recommended for most adults with newly diagnosed Graves' disease. At the end of the course of treatment, if the disease is still active or if it recurs subsequently, they are referred for ^{131}I therapy. In a small proportion of patients, hyperthyroidism is not satisfactorily controlled with a regular maintenance dose of antithyroid drugs. The problem can usually be overcome by keeping these patients on a 'block-replace' regime, which consists of a full dose of antithyroid drugs to completely block endogenous thyroid hormone production, supplemented by a replacement dose of exogenous

thyroid hormone, e.g. 20–40 μg of T3 or 0.1–0.2 mg of T4 daily. Replacement with exogenous T3 is preferred so that the block of endogenous hormone production can be assessed by measuring serum T4 which comes only from endogenous secretion and should be very low. Patients with associated disease such as cardiac disease or diabetes are best treated with [131]I.

Pregnancy and lactation The whole issue of thyroid disease and pregnancy is complex and has been reviewed [10,11]. Radioiodine treatment or investigation is absolutely contraindicated during pregnancy and lactation owing to irradiation of the foetus or newborn, from radioiodine transferred across the placenta and in the milk as well as from indirect exposure from the radioiodine in the mother. The choice of treatment therefore lies between surgery and antithyroid drugs. Surgery should in any case be avoided during the first and third trimester of pregnancy owing to the risk of abortion or premature labour. The middle trimester is thus the safest period for thyroidectomy if considered necessary. Hypothyroidism after surgery should be detected and treated as soon as possible as it increases the risk of spontaneous abortion and foetal death. Many clinicians recommend that thyroxine therapy should routinely be given after surgery and the dose subsequently adjusted rather than wait until the patient is hypothyroid.

The preferred treatment during pregnancy is antithyroid drugs but it is essential to avoid over treatment, which may increase foetal mortality from maternal hypothyroidism, and as antithyroid drugs cross the placenta they may induce foetal goitre and hypothyroidism particularly when used in larger doses. It is therefore safer to maintain the mother in a slightly hyperthyroid state using the smallest possible dose of antithyroid drugs. Thyroid function tests including serum T3, T4 and TSH should be carried out frequently.

Iodide treatment and propranolol should be avoided during pregnancy. The former crosses the placenta, blocks the foetal thyroid and may induce goitre or hypothyroidism; the latter increases uterine muscle tone, which may result in a small placenta and growth retardation of the foetus. Propranolol can also induce bradycardia in the newborn baby, hypoglycaemia and impaired response to hypoxia.

As antithyroid drugs are secreted in breast milk, they should either be stopped whenever possible if the mother wishes to breast-feed, or if treatment needs to be continued artificial feeding should be advised. It is essential to check babies born of mothers with Graves' disease for neonatal hyperthyroidism or hypothyroidism, which is usually transient (due to placental transfer of maternal thyroid-stimulating immunoglobulins) and may be prolonged. When treatment of the baby is indicated, it usually involves antithyroid drugs and propranolol but great care should be taken to avoid hypothyroidism in the newborn child owing to the risk of subsequent mental and physical retardation.

Thyrotoxicosis in the elderly Hyperthyroidism in the elderly constitutes a more serious problem, with an increased mortality and morbidity rate, particularly due to cardiovascular complications such as heart failure and atrial fibrillation, with the added risk of arterial embolism. The aim of treatment in these patients is to cure hyperthyroidism promptly and permanently, when they first present, in order to avoid or reverse any cardiovascular problems and prevent recurrence of the hyperthyroid state, and its associated complications. In view of the increased risk of surgery in this age group and the high relapse rate after antithyroid drugs, this is best achieved with radioiodine. Elderly patients and those with cardiac complications or other associated serious medical problems, irrespective of age, should be treated with a short course (usually 4–8 weeks) of antithyroid drugs in full dosage, until they are clinically and biochemically euthyroid. The drug is then stopped for 48–72 hours, after which the patient is given a single large oral dose of ^{131}I (e.g. 550 MBq), which will result in a 70–90% cure rate of Graves' hyperthyroidism, albeit at the risk of permanent hypothyroidism. It is advisable to resume the antithyroid drug at a suitable dosage 2–3 days after the radioiodine drink for another 4–6 weeks to cover the period before the ^{131}I has its full therapeutic effect. Patients under the age of 65 years with atrial fibrillation may also be anticoagulated prophylactically against thromboembolism, but this remains controversial. Digoxin and/or β-blockers may be used to control the heart rate, and diuretics may be needed to control heart failure. Treated in this way, many patients with atrial fibrillation will revert to sinus

rhythm spontaneously while being treated. Those who are still in atrial fibrillation after having become euthyroid or hypothyroid should be advised DC cardioversion, which will often restore sinus rhythm. Anticoagulants and digoxin may be stopped if sinus rhythm is maintained for a few weeks after the patient has become euthyroid or hypothyroid.

The thyroid scan before ^{131}I treatment

One of the major factors involved in calculating the radiation from a therapeutic dose of ^{131}I is the measurement of thyroid mass. There have been a number of formulae proposed for calculating the thyroid mass derived from the thyroid scan, which make assumptions about the geometry of the lobe. Thyroid volume is best calculated using a combined radionuclide and ultrasound method. However, with regard to calculating the dose for ^{131}I for therapy, the functional tissue volume as opposed to the total tissue volume is likely to be much more important. Positron emission tomography (PET) may be the optimal technique for this although the more widely available single-photon emission computed tomography technique may be able to achieve this.

The second important factor in dose calculation is the peak uptake of ^{131}I. At the present time, no careful studies have been performed comparing the early ^{99m}Tc uptake (which can be routinely obtained) with the 24-hour ^{131}I uptake, although the clinical diagnostic accuracy is equal, and ^{123}I uptake measured at 4–5 hours, using a gamma-camera, can replace the ^{131}I uptake. However, it is not certain that in the absence of detailed measurements of ^{131}I turnover and possibly some measure of tissue sensitivity the results from these measurements can significantly improve upon the results achieved using the much more convenient approach of an arbitrary choice of dose.

It has been suggested that the thyroid scan, together with an uptake measurement, may be used to assess thyroid activity during antithyroid drug treatment to provide an indication as to the likelihood of a relapse when the patient discontinues treatment. However, the ^{99m}Tc uptake is a poor predictor of relapse in patients with Graves' disease. Turner *et al.* [12] in a detailed study of 76 patients with Graves' disease using 21 clinical, biochemical, scan and tracer-kinetic parameters, concluded that no single or combination of treatment variables was able to predict outcome from ^{131}I treatment.

Treatment of toxic autonomous nodules (Plummer's disease)

Treatment of hyperthyroidism caused by single or multiple autonomous nodules is similar, but differs in several important aspects from that of Graves' disease. First, long-term antithyroid drugs should not be used to treat Plummer's disease, as functioning nodules rarely go into spontaneous remission. Second, hyperthyroidism due to Plummer's disease is more resistant to radioiodine and usually requires larger therapeutic doses, but despite this, post-radiation hypothyroidism is rarely observed. This is explained on the basis that in Graves' disease, the whole of the gland concentrates radioiodine and becomes irradiated, which subsequently leads to hypothyroidism. In contrast, in Plummer's disease, radioiodine concentrates only in the autonomous nodules, which are destroyed, while the suppressed extranodular tissue takes up little radioiodine and returns to normal function after the nodules have been destroyed. It is important to note that this is only true if at the time of radioiodine treatment, the extranodular tissue has not been stimulated by a rise in TSH as a result of preceding antithyroid drug therapy. Radioiodine has the added advantage that it also destroys functioning micronodules and thus prevents recurrence of hyperthyroidism. Patients who refuse ^{131}I may be treated with surgery.

It is important to obtain a thyroid scan before giving radioiodine for treating autonomous toxic nodules (Plummer's disease); particularly in those who have received antithyroid drug therapy, because in order to prevent subsequent hypothyroidism it is important to ensure that the normal thyroid tissue is fully suppressed at the time of ^{131}I administration. When patients with toxic nodules are treated in this way, the likelihood of hypothyroidism is very low. In a series of 48 patients treated with 500 MBq of ^{131}I, not a single patient developed hypothyroidism in the follow-up period (mean 37 months) [7]. The only patients who are likely to become hypothyroid have received antithyroid drugs before treatment without first establishing that the normal tissue was suppressed and the TSH was not elevated. If the normal thyroid tissue is not fully suppressed because the TSH has risen during treatment, then a further

period of time off antithyroid drugs is required, or alternatively thyroid hormone replacement therapy may be instituted, if clinically acceptable, and the thyroid scan repeated before giving ^{131}I dose.

Radioiodine treatment usually consists of a single large dose of [131]I (standard adult dose, 400–500 MBq). Unless the patient is seriously ill with thyrocardiac complications such as heart failure or atrial fibrillation, pre-treatment with antithyroid drugs should be avoided, as it increases the risk of post-radioiodine hypothyroidism. A course of propranolol for 2–4 weeks may be helpful in providing symptomatic relief until the radioiodine starts to have a therapeutic effect. If the patient has received antithyroid drugs, these should be stopped and radioiodine treatment postponed for 4 weeks (Figure 10.9). If exogenous TSH has been given, radioiodine administration is deferred for at least a week to restore suppression of the extranodular tissue.

After radioiodine treatment, patients are usually reviewed at 1, 3, 6, 9 and 12 months. A repeat thyroid scan is carried out after 6 months, at which time most patients with Plummer's disease will be clinically and biochemically euthyroid and have a normal TSH. The thyroid scan can be used to establish that radioiodine therapy has been completely successful in destroying autonomous nodule(s) (Figure 10.10). Successfully treated nodules will be non-functional on the scan by 6 months after treatment, but those with a liability to relapse will retain some functional activity. The

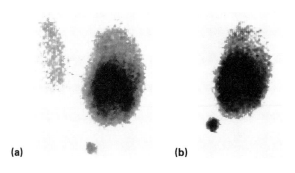

(a)   (b)

Figure 10.9 Patient with thyrotoxicosis who has received treatment with antithyroid drugs. (a) The use of these drugs has permitted some tracer uptake into the normally suppressed perinodular tissue. (b) After discontinuing the drugs for a few weeks, there is a return to the suppressed state.

Figure 10.10 Complete destruction of the toxic nodule shown in Figure 10.1 has resulted in a return to normal function of the previously suppressed tissue.

scan at 6 months can thus be valuable as an indicator of prognosis because residual activity in the nodule predisposes to a subsequent relapse of thyrotoxicosis and these patients should be followed up. Those who are not cured at 6 months, are given a second dose of ^{131}I and followed as before. Once the patient is cured annual examination is sufficient since post-radiation hypothyroidism is quite rare.

Treatment of other types of hyperthyroidism

The management of hyperthyroidism due to causes other than Graves' disease and Plummer's disease depends on the underlying condition, but in general, treatment with antithyroid drugs, subtotal thyroidectomy or radioiodine, is not applicable to these conditions.

Subacute thyroiditis and Hashimoto's thyroiditis Hyperthyroidism is usually mild, transient and requires no specific therapy, except possibly symptomatic treatment with a β-sympathetic blocking drug such as propranolol. Since the raised serum hormones in these conditions are due to leakage of stored thyroid hormones accompanying the inflammatory process rather than excess production, the conventional treatment for Graves' disease is ineffective. In subacute thyroiditis and occasionally with Hashimoto's thyroiditis, pain and tenderness over the neck, with or without constitutional symptoms, may require symptomatic relief with an anti-inflammatory analgesic such as salicylate. In more severe cases, steroid treatment in moderate doses, for a few weeks, may be necessary. Subacute thyroiditis is a self-limiting condition and complete recovery after a few weeks or months is the rule. Mild hypothyroidism may occur in the recovery stage

but this is usually transient. On the other hand, permanent hypothyroidism is common with Hashimoto's thyroiditis, and long-term thyroid replacement is usually necessary.

Hyperthyroidism associated with excess iodide Hyperthyroidism precipitated by acute excess iodide such as administration of radiological contrast media is also usually mild and remits spontaneously without any specific treatment. Rarely, if the condition is severe, a course of antithyroid drugs may be necessary, but surgery and radioiodine treatment are not used. The low uptake of radioiodine in this condition, as in thyroiditis, precludes the use of radioiodine. In the case of chronic excess iodide ingestion, appropriate dietary advice should also be given to avoid persistence of the condition. One of the most common causes of iodine-induced hyperthyroidism is now the anti-arrhythmic cardiac drug, amiodarone. Initial treatment with antithyroid drugs together with withdrawal of amiodarone, and followed by ^{131}I when the uptake is high enough, is generally advised. Ideally, this will result in hypothyroidism, enabling the patient to restart amiodarone.

Hyperthyroidism associated with excess thyroid hormone If the patient is on an excessive dose of thyroid hormone for documented hypothyroidism, the dose should be adjusted until the patient is clinically and biochemically euthyroid. The usual therapeutic dose of thyroxine is 100–200 μg daily. Occasionally, a patient may have been put on thyroid replacement for unrecognized transient hypothyroidism, and may subsequently produce adequate or even excess endogenous hormone; therefore, in such cases thyroid hormone medication should be stopped and the patient's thyroid status assessed to determine the need for continuation of thyroid hormone replacement. Patients taking excess thyroid hormones of their own accord should also be advised to discontinue the drug, and their thyroid status should be reassessed clinically and biochemically. Some of these patients may also need psychiatric assessment and advice.

Hyperthyroidism associated with thyroid cancer This is a rare complication of extensive metastatic functioning papillary or follicular thyroid cancer, which may secrete excess endogenous thyroid hormones due to the large mass of functioning tumour. The management is essentially that of the underlying carcinoma, involving large ablation doses of radioiodine. If hyperthyroidism is severe, treatment with antithyroid drugs and β-blockers may be necessary. Exogenous thyroid hormone medication should not be given while hyperthyroidism from tumour secretion persists.

Hyperthyroidism may also occur if patients with thyroid cancer are put on excess suppressive doses of thyroid hormone. The optimal dose is that which suppresses the TSH below normal – in the average patient this is 150–300 µg of thyroxine daily. Patients with functioning metastases producing significant amounts of endogenous hormones will of course need smaller doses of thyroid hormone.

Hyperthyroidism associated with pituitary or ectopic TSH hypersecretion, trophoblastic tumours and ectopic thyroid tissue in ovarian tumours is exceedingly rare, and will be treated by removing the primary cause.

SOLITARY THYROID NODULES

This is a common clinical problem, and as many as 15.5% of the population may have palpable nodules [2], with a 3.2% incidence of solitary nodules in women and 0.8% in men in England. In the USA, the incidence of thyroid nodules has been reported at 4–7% [13]. The various causes of solitary thyroid nodules are shown in Table 10.7.

The likelihood of malignancy occurring in a single nodule is 2–10%, but varies considerably from series to series, depending on selection criteria. The problem is compounded by the frequency with which nodules are found in normal adults (up to 50% in those over 50 years of age) [14]. There is an increased risk of thyroid cancer associated with previous external radiation to the head or neck, although the clinical course of the cancer is the same as thyroid cancers found in other settings. Schneider *et al.* [15] identified 318 cases of thyroid cancer in 5379 patients given radiotherapy for benign conditions of head, neck and upper thoracic area. Metastases frequently occur in the thyroid, but rarely present clinically as thyroid nodules.

The clinical problem is how to detect the small number of solitary thyroid nodules due to cancer, without the need to perform unnecessary operations on the other 90%, and it has been this goal, i.e. to identify benign disease with a high degree of accuracy without loss of sensitivity in detecting cancer, that has driven the diagnostic developments in this area. Certain clinical features increase the probability of malignancy in a solitary nodule.

1. The presence of an invasive tumour may be suggested by hoarseness, fixation and hardness of the nodule, rapid or painful enlargement, cervical lymphadenopathy or distant metastases. These clinical features are usually absent at the time of presentation of most differentiated thyroid carcinomas.
2. A previous history of irradiation to the head or neck should be specifically asked for, as this will increase the likelihood of malignancy in a solitary nodule.
3. Symptoms and signs that are characteristic of a medullary thyroid carcinoma, such as diarrhoea, mucosal neuromas, a marfanoid appearance, a history or suspicion of associated phaeochromocytoma or hyperparathyroidism, and a known family history of any of these conditions.
4. Age and sex of the patient; e.g. a solitary nodule in a man over 40 years has a higher probability of being malignant than in a young woman.

INVESTIGATION AND MANAGEMENT OF SOLITARY NODULES

The thyroid scan has been the most widely used method for investigating a thyroid nodule, on the basis that finding a solitary cold nodule increases the probability of malignancy, whereas finding a functioning nodule or a simple multinodular goitre without a single dominant nodule decreases the chance of malignancy to low levels.

Ultrasound provides a valuable tool for demonstrating thyroid abnormalities, and in particular for discriminating between solid and cystic lesions

Table 10.7 Causes of solitary thyroid nodules

Thyroid cyst
Local subacute thyroiditis
Local Hashimoto's disease
Functioning adenoma (hot nodule)
Benign adenoma
Colloid nodule
Thyroid cancer
Metastatic deposit

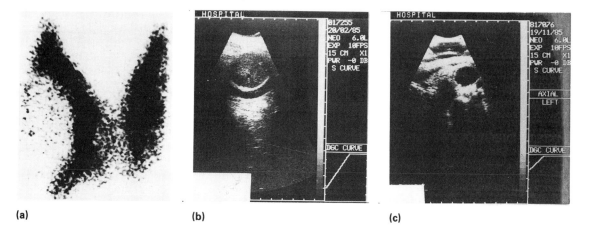

(a)   **(b)**   **(c)**

Figure 10.11 Non-functioning nodule in the right lobe (a) shown to be solid on ultrasound (b) compared with a cyst on ultrasound (c).

(Figure 10.11). It can be used to measure thyroid volumes and to detect nodules. Sonographically, most malignancies are hyperechogenic, but ultrasound cannot differentiate between functioning and non-functioning nodules, and even cystic lesions seen on ultrasound may be functional on a radionuclide scan.

The most important adjunct to imaging is fine needle aspiration (FNA) of a nodule for cytological examination, and this is now widely available [16,17]. Several groups have shown a reduction in surgery rate for nodules as a consequence of routine FNA of cold nodules; for example, Al Sayer *et al.* [18] found a 25% reduction in surgery with an increased surgical detection rate of malignancy – from 31% to 50%, and Reeve *et al.* [19] reported a 60% reduction with FNA and selective surgery.

Christensen *et al.* [20], in a prospective study of 100 consecutive patients, selected for surgical treatment of a clinically solitary thyroid nodule who had FNA confirmed that all 12 cases that appeared hot on the scan were benign.

The thyroid scan can be regarded as a supplement to physical examination and serving as a guide to FNA in pre-operative selection of patients. The problem of non-diagnostic or suspicious lesions will probably always remain. In a review of the Mayo Clinic experience, it was found that 20% of the results were non-diagnostic, and on follow-up of these cases about one-fifth of them were found malignant [21].

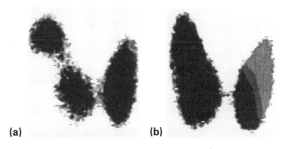

(a)   **(b)**

Figure 10.12 Patient who presented with a cold nodule in the right lobe (a) due to a cyst. A follow-up scan after aspiration (b) confirms complete aspiration with no recurrence.

It has been suggested that all patients with a solitary nodule should have FNA as their initial investigation and a thyroid scan is not required. However, clinical examination may fail to detect that the 'clinically solitary nodule' is the more easily palpable nodule of a multinodular goitre. The combination of FNA and thyroid scan is an efficient method for detecting cancer in patients who have a cold nodule on the thyroid scan (Figure 10.12). The thyroid scan is of value in the follow-up of patients who have had thyroid cysts aspirated.

Other methods are used to reduce the surgical rate for thyroid nodules. X-ray fluorescence, which measures ^{127}I, is accurate for the identification of benign disease with a reported sensitivity of 63% and specificity of 99% [22], but the technique is not widely available. More controversial is the use of ²⁰¹Tl or ⁹⁹ᵐTc-MIBI or ¹⁸F-FDG for evaluating the thyroid nodule. While these tracers are taken up into malignant nodules they may also accumulate in benign lesions, and do not separate these entities sufficiently.

It is generally agreed that the correct management of a non-functioning nodule is hemithyroidectomy and not suppressive therapy with thyroxine as has been used in the past.

Functioning 'hot' nodule

If the thyroid scan shows the solitary nodule to be functioning or 'hot', the probability of malignancy is reduced to less than 1%, since most hot nodules are benign autonomously functioning adenomas; however, there have been occasional reports of malignancy. Ashcroft and Van Herle [23], in their early review of the literature, reported a 9% incidence of malignancy in 'warm' and 'hot' nodules. Nagai *et al.* [24] reported three cases of malignancy in hot nodules on ¹²³I scans, and Evans [25] found that 44% of patients with thyroid malignancy presented with warm nodules. Three problems can be identified from these reports. The first is that some malignancies, while they do not organify the isotopes, do trap ⁹⁹ᵐTc-pertechnetate and iodine, and appear as hot or warm nodules on ⁹⁹ᵐTc scans or early ¹²³I scans. If we only consider those nodules that suppress TSH or remain hot on a ¹²³I scan after a perchlorate discharge test or delayed imaging as

'functioning', then the likelihood of malignancy remains very low. The second consideration is that nodules often occur in multinodular glands and the 'hot nodule' may be close to an 'incidentally' found malignancy, which may behave differently from the cancers that present clinically. Third, many adenomas and carcinomas have a good blood supply and it is the blood volume which 'creates' a 'warm' nodule rather than the true uptake of tracer.

Walfish *et al.* [26] reviewed their experience of 12 FNA cases of functioning nodules to evaluate the consequences of not obtaining a radionuclide scan first. They concluded that not performing a scan to diagnose a functioning nodule could expose some unprepared patients with thyrotoxicosis to surgical morbidity and might induce hyperthyroidism in patients with functioning nodules if they were treated with suppression therapy. FNA was not able to differentiate a functioning from a non-functioning adenoma.

There is no consensus on the investigation of this common clinical problem. Routine removal of all clinically apparent thyroid nodules no longer seems justified, and results in a great deal of unnecessary surgery. A reasonable policy (Figure 10.13) remains that of a ⁹⁹ᵐTc or ¹²³I scan in the first instance, which is a cheap, accurate and widely available test. Functioning nodules are identified and these patients should have a sensitive TSH to confirm true biological function with subsequent follow-up and treatment for thyrotoxicosis as necessary. The evidence for any significant likelihood

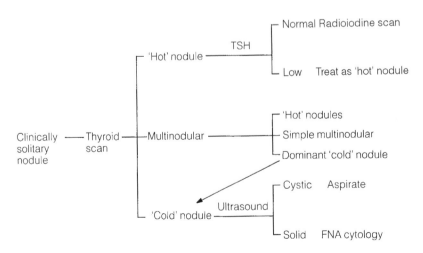

Figure 10.13 Scheme for the investigation of thyroid nodules.

of malignancy in this group is not convincing. If reliable cytology is available then all non-functioning solitary nodules should have FNA cytology because of the well-documented reduction in unnecessary surgery. Ultrasound is only necessary as an adjunct to the scan when FNA is not available; simple cysts can then be aspirated and recurrences may be considered for injection with sclerosants. ^{201}Tl, ^{99m}Tc-MIBI or ^{18}F-FDG can be used when there is a relative contraindication to surgery, and when a negative or positive scan will help in making a decision, but it is probably not justified otherwise.

Multinodular goitre

A proportion of patients who are thought to have a solitary nodule on palpation are shown to have a multinodular goitre on scanning. The frequency with which this is noted depends on the experience of the clinician in palpating the thyroid, the ease with which the patient's thyroid can be palpated and the technique of the scan. Approximately 30–40% of clinically diagnosed solitary nodules can be shown to be multiple on scan; an even higher percentage has been found at operation or autopsy [27]. It is often possible to palpate previously unsuspected nodules in the light of the scan findings.

The scintigraphic finding of a multinodular goitre, when a solitary nodule was suspected clinically, considerably decreases the probability of thyroid cancer in the absence of any clinical suspicion. Probably less than 1% of all multinodular goitres are malignant. Unless there is clinical suspicion of malignancy or local symptoms, a solitary nodule that is found to be part of a multinodular goitre on scanning does not need surgical excision.

The presence of a dominant cold nodule (Figure 10.14) in a gland with otherwise generally irregular uptake on scanning does not reduce the probability of malignancy to that of a typical multinodular goitre. Such dominant cold nodules should therefore be investigated with ultrasound and FNA cytology as for a solitary nodule, and excised if indicated.

PAINFUL GOITRE

Pain originating from the thyroid associated with palpable enlargement may be due to one of the following conditions.

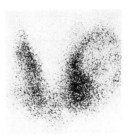

Figure 10.14 An example of a dominant non-functioning nodule in the left lobe of a multinodular gland.

1. Subacute (De Quervain's) thyroiditis.
2. Subacute or acute onset of Hashimoto's thyroiditis.
3. Haemorrhage into a thyroid nodule or cyst.
4. Thyroid cancer, particularly anaplastic carcinoma.
5. Acute suppurative thyroiditis (rare).

A careful history and clinical examination will often suggest the diagnosis, but should always be supplemented with appropriate investigations for confirmation. The most useful investigations include a full blood count and erythrocyte sedimentation rate (ESR), thyroid function tests, a radionuclide thyroid scan with ^{99m}Tc or ^{123}I, a perchlorate discharge test and serum thyroid microsomal antibodies. Rarely, a biopsy may be necessary. Sudden onset of pain in the thyroid is most often caused by haemorrhage in a thyroid nodule or cyst, which may either be solitary or part of a multinodular goitre; thyroid function tests are normal and the thyroid scan shows a solitary cold nodule or a multinodular goitre with one or more cold nodules. Pain due to haemorrhage into a thyroid nodule usually lasts only a few days, and the nodule appears very rapidly, usually over a few hours. The nodule gets smaller and may disappear completely after a few weeks. The patient should therefore be reviewed after two or three months and the thyroid scan repeated to confirm resolution or reduction of the nodule. If symptoms persist and the nodule enlarges, excision is advisable to exclude malignancy.

Subacute onset of pain over the neck, often described as a sore throat by the patient, associated with a recent upper respiratory infection, fever, malaise, anorexia and a tender diffuse goitre, are characteristic of subacute thyroiditis. However, similar features may sometimes be caused by subacute onset of Hashimoto's thyroiditis. Investigations will establish the correct diagnosis. A mild leucocytosis and moderately elevated ESR may occur in both conditions, but subacute thyroiditis is characterized by mild biochemical hyperthyroidism in the early stages, a diffusely low uptake on ^{99m}Tc scan and absence of thyroid antibodies or only a transient rise. On the other hand, in Hashimoto's thyroiditis, thyroid function tests usually show frank or compensated hypothyroidism (high TSH with low or low–normal serum T4); thyroid scan characteristically, though not always, shows a high ^{99m}Tc uptake but a low radioiodine uptake, indicating trapping of iodine without organic binding. This can also be shown by a perchlorate discharge test, which will have an increased discharge of radioiodine. Hashimoto's thyroiditis may occasionally be associated with a normal or raised radioiodine uptake. Thyroid microsomal antibodies are present in high titres and persist in Hashimoto's thyroiditis. The differential diagnosis of Hashimoto's and subacute thyroiditis is important because their clinical course is quite different. In subacute thyroiditis, the thyroid usually recovers spontaneously after a few weeks or months without any sequelae, whereas Hashimoto's thyroiditis usually results in permanent hypothyroidism requiring long-term thyroid replacement.

It is important to distinguish atypical cases of thyroiditis with minimal or absent constitutional symptoms and a painful goitre, from a rapidly enlarging anaplastic thyroid carcinoma. The latter condition usually affects older patients and is often associated with evidence of local invasion such as hoarseness, Horner's syndrome, upper respiratory or oesophageal obstruction, or distant metastases. The goitre is usually asymmetrical and hard, and the thyroid scan shows a focal area of low uptake with areas of normal uptake. Thyroid function tests are usually normal.

Acute suppurative thyroiditis due to bacterial or tuberculous infection is rare. The patient is very ill with marked constitutional symptoms, high fever and a very tender goitre. Biopsy may be necessary to establish the diagnosis and provide culture material for antibiotic sensitivity. Confusion may be caused when subacute thyroiditis involves only one lobe with the characteristic low uptake in that lobe only on the scan. This may then resolve and the other lobe may be affected; this may occur in as many as 20% of the cases.

NON-TOXIC GOITRES

INVESTIGATION AND TREATMENT OF NON-TOXIC GOITRES

The goitre may be diffuse or multinodular on examination, although occasionally it may be difficult to describe it clearly as one type or the other. Outside endemic areas of iodine deficiency, the main causes of a non-toxic goitre and the scan appearances are shown in Table 10.8.

Certain points in the history and clinical examination of the patient are helpful in the diagnosis. They include the age of onset and duration of the goitre, a family history of goitre (suggesting Hashimoto's thyroiditis or familial dyshormonogenesis), the regular ingestion of goitrogens or a low iodine intake, the presence of nerve deafness in the patient (Pendred's syndrome) and the type of goitre on palpation (e.g. a soft diffuse simple colloid goitre, a simple multinodular goitre with several discrete nodules, or a bosselated firm goitre of Hashimoto's thyroiditis). Recent rapid enlargement of a long-standing goitre should raise a suspicion of malignancy, especially lymphoma or anaplastic carcinoma.

The basic investigations of a non-toxic goitre consist of thyroid function tests, particularly serum T4 and TSH, estimation of serum thyroid microsomal or thyroglobulin antibodies, and a thyroid scan with quantitative uptake. Further investigations that may be necessary include a perchlorate discharge test *in vivo*, studies of iodine kinetics and a thyroid biopsy.

Simple colloid goitre and simple multinodular goitre

These are the most common causes of a sporadic diffuse or nodular non-toxic goitre. The exact cause of these goitres is uncertain, but they are thought to represent different stages of the same pathological process. Thyroid function tests including TSH are usually normal and thyroid antibodies are usually absent or in low titre. Uptake of ^{99m}Tc or radioiodine is normal. The distribution of uptake on the scan is diffuse in a simple colloid goitre, but markedly irregular often with discrete areas of diminished uptake in a multinodular goitre. Oblique views may be helpful. Occasionally, the goitre may contain one or more areas of increased uptake indicating developing autonomous functioning nodules. The TSH level will be suppressed and an impaired TSH

Table 10.8 The thyroid scan in the assessment of goitre

Scan findings	Cause	Comment
Diffuse, normal uptake of tracer	Diffuse non-toxic (simple) goitre	
Diffuse, with high uptake of tracer	Diffuse toxic goitre (Graves' disease)	May be first indication of hyperthyroidism
	Lymphocytic thyroiditis (Hashimoto's disease)	Occurs in early disease
	Iodine deficiency	
	Organification defects (inherited or goitrogens)	May be difficult to distinguish
Diffuse, low uptake of tracer	Subacute thyroiditis (De Quervain's)	
	Iodine-induced goitre	May be indistinguishable on the scan but presentation is entirely different
	Hashimoto's disease	
	Lymphoma	
Multifocal irregularity	Simple multinodular	Detection of autonomous nodule is important
Normal uptake of tracer	Hashimoto's disease	Diagnosis by antibodies
Irregular replacement of thyroid tissue	Diffuse cancer	Usually clinically apparent, but may be confused with multinodular goitre

From Fogelman and Maisey (1988).

response to TRH injection may be seen in spite of normal serum T3 and T4 concentration. These autonomous nodules may give rise to frank hyperthyroidism (Plummer's disease) as the disease progresses.

No specific treatment is usually necessary for asymptomatic simple colloid or multinodular goitres. A large multinodular goitre causing tracheal or oesophageal compression, as shown by radiography of the thoracic inlet or a barium swallow, should be resected; however, some of these patients may be treated with [131]I [28]. Thyroid hormone therapy in suppressive doses is rarely helpful in reducing goitre size, but may be tried in moderate-sized goitres if serum TSH is elevated. Multinodular goitres with autonomous nodules should be followed up regularly for signs of developing hyperthyroidism, which should then be treated with radioiodine or surgery. Recent rapid enlargement of a long-standing multinodular goitre should raise the possibility of malignancy and an aspiration biopsy or ^{201}Tl scan should be performed, followed by surgical excision if indicated.

The appearance of two symmetrical solitary nodules in a goitre should raise the suspicion of a medullary thyroid cancer (Figure 10.15) (although this is an uncommon tumour) and will further increase the likelihood of it being the familial type

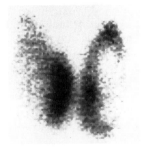

Figure 10.15 A patient discovered by family screening to have a medullary thyroid cancer, showing the symmetrical cold areas due to bilateral medullary cancers.

that has arisen from symmetrically distributed C-cell hyperplasia. Serum calcitonin measurement in addition to FNA cytology may be helpful in making a pre-operative diagnosis as may uptake of ^{99m}Tc-labelled pentavalent DMSA or ^{123}I/^{131}I-MIBG [29]. This will be of particular value in cases of multiple endocrine neoplasia, and clearly phaeochromocytoma must be identified prior to initial surgery. First-degree family screening is undertaken in all patients with diagnosed medullary thyroid cancers to establish whether or not it is the inherited type. When an elevated calcitonin is detected in a relative of the patient investigation of the thyroid is necessary. Because most surgeons prefer to know if there is a nodule present rather than simply perform a prophylactic total thyroidectomy, it will also be necessary to use the radionuclide thyroid scan and ultrasound or CT.

A thyroid lymphoma may develop spontaneously, with the patient usually presenting with a rapidly enlarging diffuse goitre, or may occur in a patient with Hashimoto's disease where there is recognized to be an increased risk of lymphoma. A radionuclide thyroid scan is not helpful because in the latter situation the patient will be hypothyroid and receiving thyroxine treatment, and in the former case the scan will usually show diffuse enlargement with an overall low uptake due to the diffuse infiltration. In these instances it is usual to proceed directly to surgical biopsy but there are clinical circumstances, e.g. if the patient is too anxious or has other pathology, when this is not advised and then a gallium-67 or ^{18}F-FDG PET scan, which shows avid accumulation in lymphoma, may provide valuable information (Figure 10.16). Finally, De Quervain's subacute thyroiditis if it is localized or initially involves only one lobe may simulate a malignant lesion [30]. Repeat thyroid scans show recovery of function in one area with appearance of the typical low uptake in the other lobe, confirming the diagnosis of thyroiditis and not malignancy.

Hashimoto's thyroiditis

The diagnosis of this condition depends on three main features: first, the presence of a goitre which is typically bosselated and firm on palpation; second, subclinical or frank hypothyroidism, i.e. raised TSH with borderline low or low serum T4;

and third, serum thyroid microsomal antibodies which are usually strongly positive although they have been reported to be negative in a small proportion of biopsy-proven Hashimoto's thyroiditis. Other investigations are of limited diagnostic value, e.g. thyroid scan may show high, normal or low uptake of radionuclide with varying distribution (uniform, irregular or nodular) according to the degree of fibrosis. We have reviewed 32 cases, and a wide variety of scan patterns were obtained [31]. The most common scan appearances were either of an enlarged gland with diffusely increased tracer uptake similar to Graves' disease or those of a multinodular gland. However, other scans appeared normal, or showed a focal defect, or reduced tracer uptake throughout one lobe, or generally low-uptake by the whole gland. Perchlorate discharge test shows excess discharge of radioiodine in most of the cases. Cytology or biopsy may be helpful in equivocal cases.

Hashimoto's thyroiditis is treated with long-term suppressive doses of thyroid hormones (e.g. thyroxine 100–200 mg daily). If treatment is started in the early stages of the condition considerable reduction in size of the goitre can be expected, whereas if diagnosis is made late, when considerable fibrosis is present in the gland, little or no improvement in goitre size may occur.

Dyshormonogenesis

This refers to a group of genetic abnormalities, each involving a specific enzyme defect in the metabolic pathway of thyroid hormones. Most are transmitted by autosomal recessive inheritance and are rare. The best known and least rare is Pendred's syndrome, in which a familial goitre is associated with nerve deafness. Familial dyshormonogenesis should be considered in the differential diagnosis of goitre in the younger patient with a family history of goitre, absent thyroid antibodies and subclinical or frank hypothyroidism.

From the point of view of clinical investigation, dyshormonogenesis may be divided into three groups.

1. Abnormality of iodide transport into the thyroid cell. This condition is characterized by a very low iodine uptake in the thyroid as well as in the salivary glands, which share the same iodide trapping mechanism. The salivary glands should therefore be included in the

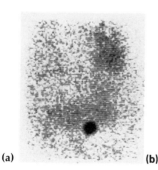
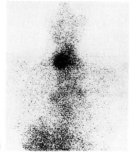

(a)   (b)

Figure 10.16 Scans of a patient with lymphoma with markers (a) shows a large gland with low uptake (^{99m}TcO$_4$), but the ^{67}Ga scan (b) shows avid accumulation.

field-of-view when the thyroid scan is performed.

2. Abnormality of organification of iodine to tyrosine. This defect is characterized by a normal iodine uptake in the gland but the perchlorate discharge test reveals an excess discharge of unorganified iodide. The best-known and most common condition in this group is Pendred's syndrome. The organification defect is usually only partial, as indicated by normal or slightly low serum T4 with raised serum TSH and excess radioiodine discharge on perchlorate discharge test.

3. Other enzyme defects. Familial goitres with a normal or high iodine uptake and normal perchlorate discharge may result from an abnormality in the metabolic pathway beyond the organification stage of iodine. Various types have been described, all of which are rare and depend on more detailed biochemical investigation for diagnosis.

ECTOPIC THYROID

Thyroid tissue may occur in other than the normal anatomical positions, when it may constitute a diagnostic or therapeutic problem. The most common places are at the back of the tongue (lingual thyroid), in the mid-line position of the upper neck (sublingual or subhyoid thyroid), inside the thoracic cavity (anterior or posterior mediastinal goitre) and in ovarian tumours (struma ovarii).

LINGUAL AND SUBLINGUAL THYROID

Failure or incomplete descent of the thyroid gland from its embryological mid-line position at the back of the tongue results in a lingual or sublingual thyroid. Either may contain the whole or only part of the patient's thyroid tissue. These ectopic thyroids usually present as a mid-line swelling at the back of the tongue or upper neck or as congenital hypothyroidism. Failure to recognize and diagnose a lingual or sublingual thyroid swelling may lead to inadvertent excision and permanent hypothyroidism requiring life-long thyroid replacement.

A midline swelling at the back of the tongue or upper neck should therefore always be investigated for the possibility of an ectopic thyroid before excision. The presence or absence of a normally situated thyroid gland should also be confirmed. The sublingual or subhyoid ectopic thyroid is particularly likely to be mistaken clinically for a thyroglossal cyst or other non-thyroid swelling.

Thyroid function tests are performed to assess the patient's thyroid status and a radionuclide scan is carried out. ^{123}I is better because of the higher uptake which avoids confusion with saliva and salivary glands on a ^{99m}Tc scan. The radiation dose with either radionuclide is small compared with ^{131}I, and the scan can therefore be used in infants, children or adolescents. The whole area from the mouth to the sternal notch should be imaged and reference markers placed on any palpable nodule and appropriate anatomical landmarks (e.g. the sternal notch). In the case of a lingual thyroid, a lateral view is important for accurate three-dimensional localization. Radionuclide uptake in the nodule confirms the presence of ectopic thyroid whereas other types of nodule (e.g. a thyroglossal cyst) appear cold. The presence or absence of a normal thyroid is also established at the same time. Rarely, if the normal thyroid is not visualized the scan should be repeated after TSH stimulation to exclude the possibility that its function may be suppressed.

A nodule that shows no uptake of ^{99m}Tc or ^{123}I can be excised. A functioning ectopic thyroid nodule can also be excised if the scan confirms the presence of a normal thyroid in addition in the normal site. However, a sublingual thyroid that contains the entire functioning thyroid tissue should be preserved. For cosmetic reasons the ectopic thyroid can be divided and relocated.

In patients who have undergone previous thyroid surgery, congenital remnants of thyroid tissue along the thyroglossal tract may hypertrophy to produce a mid-line swelling in the upper neck, particularly with recurrence of Graves' disease. This can be confirmed on a thyroid scan.

INTRATHORACIC (MEDIASTINAL) GOITRES

A normally situated thyroid gland may enlarge downward into the anterior mediastinum to produce a retrosternal goitre, or less commonly it may extend downwards behind the trachea and oesophagus, as a posterior mediastinal goitre. These intrathoracic goitres are most commonly caused by non-toxic nodular goitres. Rarely, they are congenitally ectopic glands which have migrated with the primitive heart into the mediastinum. They may be asymptomatic and come to light incidentally in the differential diagnosis of an upper mediastinal opacity noted on routine chest radiography, or they may cause symptoms due to compression of the trachea, oesophagus or superior vena cava. Occasionally, a large diffuse toxic goitre or toxic nodule may extend retrosternally or in the posterior mediastinum and cause similar symptoms in addition to those of hyperthyroidism.

Most retrosternal goitres are associated with palpable enlargement of the cervical thyroid and the diagnosis of retrosternal goitre can be inferred if the lower border of the goitre cannot be felt in the neck.

To confirm the intrathoracic goitre and assess its extent, a radiograph of the thoracic inlet and a thyroid scan with ^{123}I or ^{131}I should be performed. Although the presence of radioiodine uptake below the sternal notch confirms the diagnosis of intrathoracic goitre, its absence does not exclude a non-functioning intrathoracic goitre. In such cases, mediastinoscopy and tissue biopsy or a formal thoracotomy may be necessary to confirm the diagnosis. Mediastinal CT or MRI may be necessary to assess the extent and to evaluate tracheal compression.

Retrosternal or posterior intrathoracic goitres should be removed surgically if there is evidence of increasing tracheal or oesophageal compression as the goitre enlarges. If the patient is also thyrotoxic, initial treatment with antithyroid drugs until the patient is euthyroid, followed by surgery, is usually advised. However, if the patient is considered a poor surgical risk, antithyroid drugs followed by radioiodine therapy under close supervision in hospital may be preferable.

NEONATAL HYPOTHYROIDISM

If congenital hypothyroidism remains undiscovered, the neurological and skeletal sequelae can be irreversible and devastating. Over the past decade, the usefulness of the introduction of widespread screening programmes for the detection of neonatal hypothyroidism has been confirmed. The incidence of disease in most countries is about 1 in 4000 with a female preponderance of around 4:1. The diagnosis of primary congenital hypothyroidism is based on the finding of a low thyroxine together with an elevated TSH level. This however, fails to distinguish between the

presence of an ectopic or hypoplastic thyroid, athyreosis, dyshormonogenesis and transient hypothyroidism. Neonatal hypothyroidism represents a spectrum of disease ranging from transient underactivity to complete absence of a thyroid gland. It is in this context that the question of the role of the thyroid scan in the investigation and management of these patients continues to be discussed.

The thyroid scan accurately delineates the anatomy in infants with congenital hypothyroidism, and in addition provides functional information. A scan should be obtained before commencing treatment with thyroxine. The anatomical findings may be broadly characterized into four groups based on scan findings:

- a normal gland;
- ectopic location;
- no detectable thyroid activity; and
- normal location with increased size of gland or increased tracer uptake.

An ectopic thyroid gland is found in approximately 45% of cases and athyreosis in 35%. Some 10% will have a normal gland and 10% other abnormalities [32]. In the latter cases it is presumed that there is a disorder of thyroid hormonogenesis and a number will have defects of thyroid hormone synthesis. A perchlorate discharge test will identify those cases with an organification defect. Two cases of a congenital defect in iodide trapping have been reported where the scan showed absence of not only thyroid but also gastric uptake [33]. There is some controversy as to the role of inhibitive immunoglobulins ('blocking' antibodies) as these may cause transient hypothyroidism. Further, the scan findings in isolation are misleading in terms of prognosis as there is no tracer uptake by the thyroid and will suggest athyreosis. The role of transplacental passage of maternal immunoglobulins may be important in the pathogenesis of sporadic congenital hypothyroidism, but it remains controversial.

The thyroid scan has prognostic significance as those with anatomical defects will have permanent hypothyroidism. Information obtained from a scan may also aid in genetic counselling as an ectopic thyroid or athyreosis occurs spontaneously while impaired biosynthesis of thyroid hormones implies an inherited defect. Thyroid scan data presented in a form that patients find easy to understand and accept is important with long-term therapy, as good patient compliance is required [32]. Where an ectopic thyroid is present, a scan may avoid an unnecessary operation for a base of tongue swelling.

While in the great majority of cases of neonatal hypothyroidism the disease is permanent, some will have transient hypothyroidism, and clearly it is desirable to identify these cases. It has however, been found that those with an anatomical defect or a secondary rise in TSH after the TSH has been initially suppressed by thyroxine therapy have permanent hypothyroidism. Thus, only approximately one-third of cases will qualify for a trial off therapy. Thyroxine should be discontinued for a 3-week period after 3 years of age, and this is adequate and safe to confirm that hypothyroidism is permanent. Only 1–2% of newborn cases of hypothyroidism identified on screening will have transient disease.

REFERENCES

1. Perlmutter, M. and Slater, S.L. (1956) Which nodular goiters should be removed? A physiologic plan for the diagnosis and treatment of nodular goiter. *N. Engl. J. Med.*, **255**, 65–71.
2. Tunbridge, W.M.G., Evered, D.C., Hall, R. *et al.* (1977) The spectrum of thyroid disease in a community: the Wickham survey. *Clin. Endocrinol.*, **7**, 481–93.
3. Werner, S.C.J. (1969) Classification of thyroid disease. Report of the Committee on Nomenclature: American Thyroid Association. *J. Clin. Endocrinol.*, **29**, 860–2.
4. Fogelman, I., Cooke, S.G. and Maisey, M.N. (1986) The role of thyroid scanning in hyperthyroidism. *Eur. J. Nucl. Med.*, **11**, 397–400.
5. Cooke, S.G., Ratcliffe, G.E., Fogelman, I. and Maisey, M.N. (1986) Prevalence of inappropriate drug treatment in patients with hyperthyroidism. *Br. Med. J.*, **291**, 1491–2.
6. Ratcliffe, G.E., Fogelman, I. and Maisey, M.N. (1986) The evaluation of radioiodine therapy for thyroid patients using a fixed dose regime. *Br. J. Radiol.*, **59**, 1105–7.
7. Ratcliffe, G.E., Cooke, S., Fogelman, I. and Maisey, M.N. (1986) Radioiodine treatment of solitary functioning thyroid nodules. *Br. J. Radiol.*, **59**, 385–7.
8. Reschini, E. and Peracchi, M. (1993) Thyroid scintigraphy during antithyroid treatment for autonomous nodules as a means of imaging extranodular tissue. *Clin. Nucl. Med.*, **18**, 597–600.
9. Martino, E., Aghini Lombardi, F., Lippi, F. *et al.* (1985) Twenty-four hour radioactive iodine uptake in 35 patients with amiodarone associated thyrotoxicosis. *J. Nucl. Med.*, **26**, 1402–7.
10. Becks, G.P. and Burrow, G.N. (1991) Thyroid disease and pregnancy. (Review). *Med. Clin. North Amer.*, **75**, 121–50.
11. Lazarus, J.H. and Othman, S. (1991) Thyroid disease in relation to pregnancy. (Review). *Clin. Endocrinol.*, **34**, 91–8.
12. Turner, J., Sadler, W., Brownlie, B. and Rogers, T. (1985) Radioiodine therapy for Graves' disease: mutli-variate analysis of pre-treatment parameters and early outcome. *Eur. J. Nucl. Med.*, **11**, 191–3.
13. Rojeski, M.T. and Gharib, H. (1985) Nodular thyroid disease evaluation and management. *N. Engl. J. Med.*, **313**, 428–36.
14. Horlocker, T.T., Hay, I.D., James, E.M. *et al.* (1986) in *Frontiers in Thyroidology*, Vol. 1 (eds G. Neto and E. Gaitan), Plenum Press, New York, pp. 1309–12.
15. Schneider, A.B., Recant, W., Pinsky, S.M. *et al.* (1986) Radiation-induced thyroid carcinoma: clinical course and results of therapy in 296 patients. *Ann. Intern. Med.*, **105**, 405–12.
16. Gharib, H. (1994) Fine-needle aspiration biopsy of thyroid nodules: advantages, limitations, and effect. (Review). *Mayo Clin. Proc.*, **69**, 44–9.
17. Woeber, K.A. (1995) Cost-effective evaluation of the patient with a thyroid nodule. (Review). *Surg. Clin. North Am.*, **75**, 357–63.
18. Al Sayer, H.M., Krukowski, Z.H., Williams, V.M.M. *et al.* (1985) Fine needle aspiration cytology in isolated thyroid swellings: a prospective two year evaluation. *Br. Med. J.*, **290**, 1490–2.
19. Reeve, T.S., Delbridge, L., Sloan, D. and Crummer, P. (1986) The impact of fine needle aspiration biopsy on surgery for single thyroid nodules. *Med. J. Aust.*, **145**, 308–11.
20. Christensen, S.B., Bondesson, L., Ericsson, U.B. and Lindholm, K. (1984) Prediction of malignancy in the solitary thyroid nodule by physical examination, thyroid scan, fine needle biopsy and serum thyroglobulin: a prospective study of 100 surgically treated patients. *Acta Chir. Scand.*, **150**, 433–9.
21. Gharib, J., Goellner, J.R., Zunsmeister, A.R. *et al.* (1984) Fine needle aspiration biopsy of the thyroid: the problem of suspicious cytological finding. *Ann. Intern. Med.*, **10**, 25–8.
22. Patton, J.A., Sandler, M.P. and Partain, C.L. (1985) Prediction of benignancy of the solitary 'cold' thyroid nodule by fluorescent scanning. *J. Nucl. Med.*, **26**, 461–4.
23. Ashcroft, M.W. and Van Herle, A.J. (1981) Management of thyroid nodules II: scanning techniques, 64 thyroid suppressive therapy and fine needle aspiration. *Head Neck Surg.*, **3**, 297–322.
24. Nagai, G.R., Pitts, W.C., Basso, L. *et al.* (1987) Scintigraphic hot nodules and thyroid carcinoma. *Clin. Nucl. Med.*, **12**, 123–7.
25. Evans, D.M. (1978) Diagnostic discriminants of thyroid cancer. *Am. Surg.*, **153**, 569–70.
26. Walfish, P.G., Strawbridge, J.T. and Rosen, I.B. (1985) Management implications from routine needle biopsy of hyperfunctioning thyroid nodules. *Surgery*, **98**, 1179–88.

27. Maisey, M.N., Moses, D.C., Hurley, P.J. and Wagner, N.H., Jr (1973) Improved methods for thyroid scanning. *JAMA*, **223**, 761–3.
28. Huysmans, D.A., Hermus, A.R., Corstens, F.H., Barentsz, J.O. and Kloppenborg, P.W. (1994) Large, compressive goiters treated with radioiodine. *Ann. Intern. Med.*, **121**, 757–62.
29. Clarke, S.E.M., Lazarus, C.R., Wraight, P. *et al.* (1988) Pentavalent (^{99m}Tc)DMSA, (^{131}I)MIBG, and (^{99m}Tc)MDP: an evaluation of three imaging techniques in patients with medullary carcinoma of the thyroid. *J. Nucl. Med.*, **29**, 33–8.
30. Ramtoola, S. and Maisey, M.N. (1988) Subacute (De Quervain's) thyroiditis. *Br. J. Radiol.*, **61**, 515–16.
31. Ramtoola, S., Maisey, M.N., Clarke, S.E.M. and Fogelman, I. (1988) The thyroid scan in Hashimoto's thyroiditis: the great mimic. *Nucl. Med. Commun.*, **9**, 639–45.
32. Brooks, P.T., Archard, N.D. and Carty, H.M.L. (1988) Thyroid screening in congenital hypothyroidism: a review of 41 cases. *Nucl. Med. Commun.*, **9**, 613–17.
33. Leger, F.A., Doumith, R., Courpotin, C. *et al.* (1987) Complete iodine trapping defect in two cases with congenital hypothyroidism: adaptation of thyroid to huge iodine supplementation. *Eur. J. Clin. Invest.*, **17**, 249–55.

FURTHER READING

De Groot, L.J. (1993) Effects of irradiation on the thyroid gland. (Review). *Endocrinol. Metab. Clin. North Am.*, **22**(3), 607–15.
Dworkin, H.J., Meier, D.A. and Kaplan, M. (1995) Advances in the management of patients with thyroid disease. (Review). *Semin. Nucl. Med.*, **25**(3), 205–20.
Fisher, D.A. (1996) Physiological variations in thyroid hormones: physiological and pathophysiological considerations. (Review). *Clin. Chem.*, **42**(1), 135–9.
Freitas, J.E. and Freitas, A.E. (1994) Thyroid and parathyroid imaging. (Review). *Semin. Nucl. Med.*, **24**(3), 234–45.
Gharib, H. (1994) Fine needle aspiration biopsy of thyroid nodules: advantages, limitations, and effect. (Review). *Mayo Clin. Proc.*, **69**(1), 44–9.
Hopkins, C.R. and Reading, C.C. (1994) Thyroid and parathyroid imaging. (Review). *Ultrasound, CT and MRI*, **16**(4), 279–95.
Reiners, C. (1992) Imaging methods for medullary thyroid cancer. (Review). *Rec. Results Cancer Res.*, **125**, 125–45.
Reinhart, M.J. and Moser, E. (1996) An update on diagnostic methods in the investigation of diseases of the thyroid. (Review). *Eur. J. Nucl. Med.*, **23**(5), 587–94.

Adrenal

R. T. Kloos, F. Khafagi, M. D. Gross and B. Shapiro

INTRODUCTION

The adrenal glands are paired retroperitoneal organs which lie superomedial to each kidney, the right adrenal gland usually being more cephaloposterior compared with the left. Each gland consists of an outer cortex and an embryologically, histologically and functionally distinct medulla. The cortex is derived from the posterior coelomic mesoderm (the urogenital ridge). The adrenal cortex can be considered as two organs: (i) the subcapsular zona glomerulosa, which synthesizes mineralocorticoids (principally aldosterone), primarily under the control of the renin-angiotensin system; and (ii) the deeper zona fasciculata and reticularis that elaborate glucocorticoids (principally cortisol), and weak androgens [dehydroepiandrosterone (DHEA), its sulphate (DHEA-S), and androstenedione] and oestrogens primarily under the control of adrenocorticotrophic hormone (ACTH) from the anterior pituitary (Figure 10.17). The adrenal medulla shares its neural crest origin with the sympathetic ganglia, paraganglia and other adrenergic tissues. Like those organs, it synthesizes and stores noradrenaline (norepinephrine), but its ability to convert noradrenaline to adrenaline (epinephrine) is unique.

Excess secretion of adrenal hormones may give rise to well-known clinical syndromes (Table 10.9). Collectively, these syndromes may result from benign or malignant adrenal tumours, adrenal hyperplasia, or least frequently, from extra-adrenal disease. Differentiating among these possibilities is often impossible on clinical or biochemical grounds alone. The non-invasive evaluation of adrenal anatomy was revolutionized by the advent of X-ray computed tomography (CT) and the subsequent development of magnetic resonance imaging (MRI), both of which can reliably detect tumours greater than 0.5–1 cm in diameter. However, CT and MRI are relatively insensitive for smaller lesions, for recognizing contour changes of bilateral hyperplasia, and for localizing extra-adrenal disease; they may be difficult to interpret post-operatively, particularly in the presence of surgical clips. Moreover, the functional significance of anatomical abnormalities cannot be determined by CT or MRI. Further, the widespread use of thoracic and abdominal anatomical imaging has led to the frequent finding of unanticipated adrenal masses (incidentalomas). The complete differential diagnosis of these lesions is extensive and includes hypersecreting and non-hypersecreting, as well as benign and malignant lesions. Incorporation of specific radiopharmaceuticals into the normal or abnormal tissues, or onto their surface receptors, allows scintigraphic localization and functional characterization with a high degree of efficacy in each of the adrenal disorders outlined above. Thus, adrenal scintigraphy can direct and complement anatomical studies obviating the need for invasive diagnostic procedures in most cases.

ADRENAL CORTEX

PHYSIOLOGY AND RADIOPHARMACOLOGY

Cholesterol is the precursor for steroid hormone biosynthesis. The major source of adrenal cholesterol is circulating cholesterol carried by low-density lipoprotein (LDL). Adrenal cortical cells bear specific, high-affinity cell membrane receptors for LDL. After the receptor–LDL complex is internalized, cholesterol is liberated, and that which is surplus to requirements for cell membrane maintenance is re-esterified by acyl-CoA:cholesterol acyltransferase (ACAT) and stored.

Cholesterol labelled with iodine-131 (^{131}I-19-iodocholesterol) was the first clinically successful adrenocortical scintigraphic agent [1]. It has been superseded by the cholesterol analogues ^{131}I-6β-iodomethyl-19-norcholesterol (NP-59) [2] and ^{75}Se-6β-selenomethyl-19-norcholesterol (SMC, Scintadren®) [3], both of which have greater affinity for the adrenal cortex and more favourable target-to-background activity ratios. Normal adrenocortical radiopharmaceutical uptake is roughly symmetrical, with a normal right:left

Clinical Nuclear Medicine, 3rd edn. Edited by M.N. Maisey, K.E. Britton and B.D. Collier. Published in 1998 by Chapman & Hall, London. ISBN 0 412 75180 1

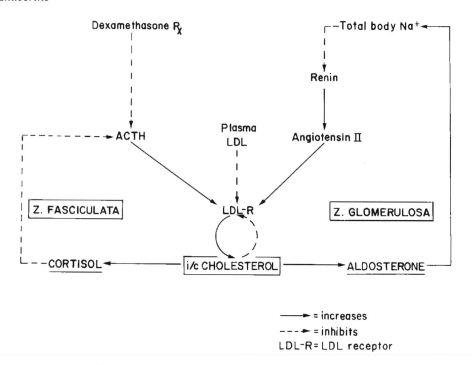

Figure 10.17   Regulation of the adrenocortical intracellular (i/c) cholesterol pool and hormone biosynthesis.

Table 10.9   Syndromes of adrenal hormone excess

Organ	Zone	Hormone	Syndrome
Cortex	Glomerulosa and outermost fasciculata	Aldosterone	Primary aldosteronism
	Fasciculata (and reticularis less importantly)	Cortisol	Cushing's syndrome
	Fasciculata and reticularis	Androgens	Masculinization
		Oestrogens	Congenital adrenal hyperplasia
			Feminization
Medulla		Adrenaline and noradrenaline	Phaeochromocytoma
Paraganglia		Noradrenaline	Extra-adrenal phaeochromocytoma

adrenal uptake ratio on the posterior scintiscan (corrected for background) of 0.9–1.2. The slight right dominance is due to the slightly more posterior (superficial) right adrenal gland location. Following uptake, the radiocholesterol analogues may be esterified by ACAT but are not significantly further metabolized. The major pathway of radiocholesterol excretion is hepatobiliary.

Both NP-59 and SMC appear to behave virtually identically *in vivo*. Potential advantages and disadvantages of each tracer are listed in Table 10.10. Radiocholesterol analogue adrenocortical uptake

parallels that of cholesterol (Figure 10.17). Thus, ACTH stimulation enhances radiocholesterol uptake; conversely, complete acute suppression of endogenous ACTH secretion by dexamethasone reduces adrenal radiocholesterol uptake by 50% [4]. Similarly, sodium loading with resultant extracellular volume expansion inhibits renin secretion and angiotensin II production, and reduces adrenal radiocholesterol uptake by a further 10%. Thus, 40% of adrenocortical radiocholesterol uptake appears independent of either ACTH or angiotensin II stimulation. Hyper-

Table 10.10 Techniques of adrenal scintigraphy

	Radiopharmaceutical				
	NP-59	SMC	131I-MIBG	123I-MIBG*	111In-pentetreotide
Thyroid blockade† (SSKI 1 drop or Lugol's 2 drops in beverage t.i.d.)	Start 2 days before injection and continue for 14 days	Not required	Start 2 days before injection and continue for 6 days	Start 2 days before injection and continue for 4 days	Not required
Adult Dose (i.v.)	37 MBq	9.25 MBq	18.5 MBq–37 MBq	370 MBq	222 MBq
Shelf-life	2 weeks; frozen	6–8 wks; room temp.	2 weeks; 4°C	24 h; 4°C	6 h; room temp.
% Uptake/adrenal	0.07–0.26%	0.07–0.30%	0.01–0.22%	0.01–0.22%	–
Dosimetry (cGy/dose)			From package insert	From package insert	
Adrenal	28–88	6.1	0.38–0.75	8–28	1.51
Ovaries	8.0	1.9	0.14–0.27	0.35	0.98
Liver	2.4	3.5	1.45–2.90	0.32	2.43
Kidneys	2.2	–	0.16–0.32	–	10.83
Spleen	2.7	–	1.10–2.20	–	14.77
Urinary bladder	–	–	1.40–2.80	–	6.05
Thyroid	150‡	0.43‡	0.17‡–0.33‡	17.7‡	1.49
Whole body	1.2	1.4	–	0.29	–
Effective dose equivalent	–	–	0.35–0.70	–	2.61
Beta emission	Yes	No	Yes	No	No
Laxatives (e.g. bisacodyl 5–10 mg p.o. bid)	Begin 2 days before and continue during imaging	No	Begin post-injection	Begin post-injection	Begin post-injection.
Imaging interval post-radiotracer administration (optional additional imaging times)	Non-DS: one or more days 5, 6, or 7 post-injection. DS: one or more early: (3), 4 and one or more late: 5, 6, or 7 days post-injection	7 (14) days post-injection (No published experience with DS scans)	24, 48 (72) hours post-injection	2–4, 24 (48) hours post-injection	4–6, 24, (48) hours post-injection
Collimator	High-energy, parallel-hole	Medium-energy, parallel-hole	High-energy, parallel-hole	Low-energy, parallel-hole	Medium-energy, parallel-hole
Principal photopeak (abundance)	364 keV (81%)	137 keV (61%), 265 keV (59%), 280 keV (25%)	364 keV	159 keV	172 keV (90%), 245 keV (94%)
Window	20% window	20% window	20% window	20% window	20% window
Imaging time/counts (per view)	20 min/100K	20 min/200K (±SPECT)	20 min/100K	10 min (at 3h); 20 min/1M (±SPECT)	Head and neck: 10–15 min/300K (at 4–24h) and 15 min/200K (at 48h) Chest and abdomen: 10 min/500K (±SPECT)

* 0–1.4% 125I contamination.
† Patients allergic to iodine may be given potassium perchlorate 200 mg every 8 h after meals or triiodothyronine 20 mg every 8 h.
‡ No thyroid blockade (can be reduced to 1–2% by iodide administration).
DS, dexamethasone suppression; K, thousand counts; M, million counts.

cholesterolaemia, by diluting radiocholesterols in the expanded extracellular cholesterol pool and down-regulating LDL receptors, reduces adrenal radiocholesterol uptake and enhances hepatobiliary excretion [5].

It follows that several drugs may modify the uptake of adrenocortical scintigraphic agents (Table 10.11). Clinically, these effects are only important in the setting of primary aldosteronism and syndromes of sex hormone excess when the timing of adrenocortical visualization under dexamethasone suppression (DS) is important to scan interpretation. Medications that increase adrenal radiocholesterol uptake may lead to bilateral early adrenal visualization and falsely suggest a bilateral process (e.g. hyperplasia). In most cases, the drug effect can be predicted from its known actions on the simplified schema in Figure 10.17. Important exceptions are spironolactone (a mainstay of therapy for primary aldosteronism and masculinization) and the combination oral contraceptive pill (OCP). Spironolactone, in addition to its well-known aldosterone antagonism, inhibits aldosterone biosynthesis in aldosterone-producing adenomas (APA), at least in the first month of therapy [6,7]. The combination OCP also has dual effects: the oestrogen increases hepatic synthesis of the renin substrate angiotensinogen and increases plasma renin, while the progestagen induces a natriuresis which further promotes

renin secretion; the net result is an increase in angiotensin II levels [8]. It is not known if the currently marketed low-dose OCPs cause a similar phenomenon. Clearly, proper adrenocortical scintiscan interpretation is critically dependent not only on a secure biochemical diagnosis, but also on a careful drug history and their exclusion when relevant.

Radiocholesterols are dissolved in an alcoholic vehicle containing Tween-80 and should be injected intravenously over 2–3 minutes to avoid extremity pain or discomfort. Repeated flushing of the syringe ensures complete delivery of the dose. Iodine-containing preparations are given to block thyroidal uptake of free iodine-131 derived from *in vivo* deiodination (Table 10.10). A laxative is used to decrease bowel background radioactivity (Table 10.10). Images are obtained by a gamma-camera interfaced with a dedicated, digital computer (>50 000 counts/image) after an appropriate delay post radiotracer injection (Tables 10.10 and 10.12). Additional images may be obtained daily or on alternate days for several weeks, but rarely are more than 1–2 days of imaging necessary. The posterior view affords the best adrenal gland visualization and is often the only image necessary. The normal posterior image demonstrates equal or slightly greater and cephalad radiotracer accumulation in the right adrenal gland compared with the left. A lateral view may assist in differen-

Table 10.11   Clinically important modifiers of adrenocortical uptake of radiocholesterol analogues

Drug	Effect on uptake	Mechanism	Drug withdrawl interval
Dexamethasone/glucocorticoids	Decrease (zona fasciculata/reticularis)	ACTH suppression	None*
Spironolactone	Increase (zona glomerulosa)	Naturesis, decrease aldosterone action (±secretion) causes PRA and AII increases	4–6 weeks
Diuretics	Increase (zona glomerulosa)	Naturesis causes PRA and AII increases	4–6 weeks
Oral contraceptives	Increase (zona glomerulosa)	Naturesis and increased angiotensinogen causes PRA and AII increases	4–6 weeks
Cholestyramine and other lipid-lowering drugs	Increase (all zones)	Decreased plasma cholesterol decreases radiotracer dilution and up-regulates LDL receptors	4–6 weeks
Minoxidil/Hydralazine	Increase (zona glomerulosa)	Vasodilatation causes PRA and AII increases	1–2 weeks

*Studies may be intentionally performed with dexamethasone suppression.
PRA, plasma renin activity; AII, angiotensin II.

Table 10.12 Summary of scintigraphic findings in adrenocortical disorders

Disorder	Pathology	Scintigraphy
Cushing's syndrome	Adenoma	Concordant, unilateral increased uptake, normal suppressed
	Hyperplasia	Bilateral increased uptake (may be asymmetrical)
	Carcinoma	Bilateral non-visualization, or very rarely concordant, unilateral increased uptake
Primary aldosteronism*	Adenoma	Concordant, unilateral adrenal imaging before day 5
	Hyperplasia	Bilateral adrenal imaging before day 5 (may be asymmetrical)
	Carcinoma (very rare)	Discordant image day 5 or later, or concordant, unilateral adrenal image before day 5
Masculinization*	Adrenal adenoma	Concordant, unilateral adrenal imaging before day 5
	Adrenal carcinoma	Discordant image day 5 or later, or concordant, unilateral adrenal image before day 5
	Adrenal hyperplasia	Bilateral adrenal imaging before day 5 (may be asymmetrical)
	Ovarian	Ovarian visualization
Incidental adrenal mass	Non-hypersecretory benign adenoma	Concordant, increased uptake
	Non-adenoma (e.g. metastasis or primary adrenal carcinoma)	Discordant, decreased uptake

*Dexamethasone suppression imaging with 1 mg orally four times per day starting 7 days before radiotracer administration and continuing through the 'eary visualization' imaging period (see Table 10.10).

tiating adrenal gland radiotracer accumulation from hepatic activity, or right adrenal gland accumulation from gallbladder activity. An anterior pelvic view should be obtained in cases of suspected ovarian or testicular hypersecretion. NP-59 and/or [^{75}Se]-selenomethyl-norcholesterol is widely commercially available world-wide as a routine imaging agent. In the United States, NP-59 is available as an investigational new drug (IND) and can be obtained from the University of Michigan Nuclear Pharmacy after filing an abbreviated Physician Sponsored IND Application with the US Food and Drug Administration.

CUSHING'S SYNDROME

Cushing's syndrome (CS) is due to excessive glucocorticoid secretion, usually associated to a greater or lesser extent with androgen excess. The syndrome may arise from several possible disorders: bilateral, generally symmetrical adrenocortical hyperplasia due to ACTH stimulation from the anterior pituitary (Cushing's disease) or from an extrapituitary benign or malignant neoplasm (ectopic ACTH and/or corticotrophin releasing hormone); or it may be due to a benign or malignant adrenocortical tumour autonomously secreting excess cortisol.

Rarely, CS results from autonomous cortical nodular hyperplasia (CNH) which, although bilateral, is often asymmetrical. ACTH-secreting pituitary tumours are responsible for two-thirds of CS cases. Ectopic ACTH secretion accounts for about 15% of cases, half of which are due to small-cell lung carcinoma and the remainder are due to carcinoids, medullary thyroid carcinomas, phaeochromocytomas, and other neuroendocrine tumours. Adrenal cortical adenomas account for 10% of CS cases, and adrenal carcinomas and CNH each account for approximately 5%.

Irrespective of its pathogenesis, CS is characterized biochemically by excess cortisol secretion with loss of the diurnal variation in plasma cortisol levels. The diagnosis is best established by measuring the 24-hour urinary free cortisol (UFC) level and/or the 8:00 am serum cortisol response to an overnight 1 mg dexamethasone suppression test (Table 10.13). If diagnostic uncertainty persists, then a low-dose dexamethasone suppression test may be helpful. Once the diagnosis of CS is certain, a baseline plasma ACTH level and a high-dose dexamethasone suppression test are used to determine the aetiology of CS (Table 10.13). Suppression after high-dose but not low-dose dexamethasone with a mid- to upper-normal or elevated ACTH level is characteristic of Cushing's

Table 10.13 Diagnostic testing in Cushing's syndrome

Test	Diagnostic value	Sensitivity (%)	Specificity (%)	Reference
For diagnosis of Cushing's syndrome				
24-hour UFC	>120 μg/day (331 nmol/day)	94	97	[9]
Overnight 1 mg dexamethasone suppression test (dose between 11 p.m. and midnight)	8 a.m. plasma cortisol >3–5 μg/dl (83–138 nmol/l)	100	88	[9]
Low-dose dexamethasone suppression test (0.5 mg every 6 h for 2 days)	Plasma cortisol >5 μg/dl (138 nmol/l)*, or urinary 17-OHCS >2.5–4 mg/day (6.9–11 μmol/d)[†], or UFC >10–20 μg/day (28–55 nmol/day)[†]	100	88	[10,11]
To differentiate the aetiology of Cushing's syndrome[‡]				
High-dose dexamethasone suppression test (2 mg every 6 h for 2 days)	Urinary 17-OHCS suppressed by ≥40–50% from baseline[†]	87	88	[11]
High-dose dexamethasone suppression test (2 mg every 6 h for 2 days)	Urinary 17-OHCS suppressed by ≥64% from baseline[†] or UFC suppressed by ≥90% from baseline[†]	83	100	[11]
Overnight 8 mg dexamethasone suppression test (dose between 11 p.m. and midnight)	8 a.m. plasma cortisol suppressed by ≥50% from baseline	90	92	[11]

*Plasma cortisol level measured at 8 a.m. on the morning of the third day, or at 4 p.m. on the second day.
[†]24-h urine is collected on the second day.
[‡]Sensitivity and specificity for the diagnosis of Cushing's disease.
UFC, urinary free cortisol.

disease. Failure to suppress on either dose indicates either ACTH-independent CS (adrenal adenoma, carcinoma or CNH) or ectopic ACTH secretion. ACTH serum levels will be suppressed in ACTH-independent CS, whereas they will be high in the ectopic ACTH syndrome.

The scintigraphic patterns of radiocholesterol uptake in the various forms of CS reflect the underlying pathophysiology (Figure 10.18 and Table 10.12). In ACTH-dependent adrenal hyperplasia, radiocholesterol uptake is bilaterally increased, and the degree of uptake correlates closely with the 24-hour UFC excretion [12]; thus, uptake in the ectopic ACTH syndrome is generally higher than in Cushing's disease. An autonomous adrenal cortical adenoma will demonstrate avid unilateral uptake; the suppression of pituitary ACTH secretion inhibits tracer uptake by the contralateral adrenal cortex (and the ipsilateral normal cortical tissue). Similarly, inhibition of contralateral radiocholesterol uptake occurs with functioning adrenal carcinomas; however, because cholesterol

uptake per gram of tissue in these tumours is usually very low [13], the primary tumour itself is typically not visualized. Other causes of 'bilateral non-visualization' such as severe hypercholesterolaemia and subcutaneous extravasation of the radiotracer dose must be excluded in such cases. Radiocholesterol uptake by both primary and metastatic adrenocortical carcinoma has rarely been reported. Finally, ACTH-independent CNH produces bilaterally but usually asymmetrically increased radiocholesterol uptake.

In clinical practice, adrenal cortical scintigraphy for CS is indicated only in patients with ACTH-independent CS [14]. Once the biochemical diagnosis of the condition is made, abdominal CT is usually performed to locate the disease and define the surgical anatomy. In tumours without clear-cut CT signs of malignancy, scintigraphy will be helpful since bilateral non-visualization will indicate the malignant nature of the tumour and allow appropriate surgical planning. More importantly, scintigraphy will reliably distinguish between

CUSHING' SYNDROME (CS)   SCAN PATTERN

A. ACTH – DEPENDENT – CS
   1. Bilateral hyperplasia
      (hypothalamic, pituitary,
      ectopic)

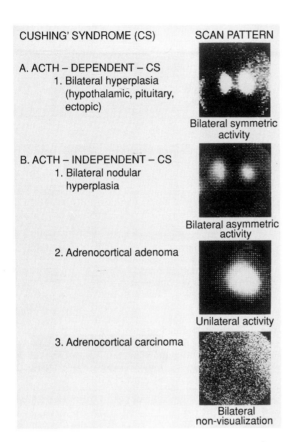

Bilateral symmetric
activity

B. ACTH – INDEPENDENT – CS
   1. Bilateral nodular
      hyperplasia

Bilateral asymmetric
activity

   2. Adrenocortical adenoma

Unilateral activity

   3. Adrenocortical carcinoma

Bilateral
non-visualization

Figure 10.18 Patterns of adrenocortical scintigraphy in CS (NP-59 posterior scintiscans, no dexamethasone suppression). (Reproduced from [78] with permission.)

adenoma and CNH. CNH should be suspected if CT has identified no tumour, only a small tumour, more than one tumour, any suggestion of a contralateral adrenal abnormality; in children and the young; when CS is associated with blue nevi, pigmented lentigines, myxomas, acromegaly, or testicular or other tumours; and in the very rare patient with intermittent or cyclical CS. In patients whose CS has relapsed after bilateral adrenalectomy for primary or secondary adrenocortical hyperplasia, scintigraphy is valuable for locating the functioning remnant(s) [15].

PRIMARY ALDOSTERONISM
(CONN'S SYNDROME)

Excess aldosterone secretion by an adrenal cortical tumour (almost always benign and <2 cm) or by diffuse or nodular hyperplasia of the zona glomerulosa is characterized by hypertension and usually hypokalaemia. Adenomas (aldosteronomas) account for little more than half of all cases. High circulating aldosterone levels result in kaliuresis, sodium retention and expansion of extracellular fluid volume with secondary inhibition of renin release. It is essential to exclude more common causes of hypokalaemia among hypertensive patients, such as overt or covert use of diuretics and laxatives. The diagnosis of primary aldosteronism is confirmed by the demonstration of suppressed plasma renin activity (PRA) with an elevated plasma or urinary aldosterone level, regardless of the presence of drugs which may interfere with the renin-angiotensin system. However, because many drugs interfere with this system, it is imperative to stop all potentially interfering medications for an appropriate interval before proceeding with diagnostic testing, or to at least know how they may alter the results so that the tests may be interpreted appropriately [16]. If antihypertensive therapy cannot be interrupted, peripheral alpha- and beta-blocking agents and clonidine are generally acceptable [16]. Primary aldosteronism can also be confirmed in the settings of a low PRA with a mid-to-upper range aldosterone level or with a lower-normal PRA with an upper-normal to elevated aldosterone level, but only when the aldosterone level cannot be suppressed by saline loading or by inhibition of the angiotensin converting enzyme [17,18]. Adherence to these diagnostic criteria (e.g. hypertension, unexplained or easily provoked hypokalaemia, suppressed PRA, non-suppressible aldosterone) will exclude the much more common cases of 'low-renin essential hypertension' (in whom potassium and aldosterone levels are normal) and secondary aldosteronism (elevated PRA), and the much rarer cases of mineralocorticoid hypertension not mediated by aldosterone [congenital adrenal hyperplasia, deoxycorticosterone (DOC) excess, and others] in which aldosterone levels are low [19].

The vexing distinction between an aldosterone-producing adenoma (APA) and bilateral adrenal hyperplasia (BAH) as the cause of primary aldosteronism is important, since the treatment is primarily surgical in the former and medical in the latter. Clues which favour one cause over the other are listed in Tables 10.12 and 10.14. Each of these diagnostic tests offer accuracy rates of 70–85%, except for bilateral adrenal vein catheterization

Table 10.14 Diagnostic tests to differentiate an aldosterone-producing adenoma (APA) from bilateral adrenal micro- or macronodular hyperplasia (BAH) as the cause of primary aldosteronism

Diagnostic test	Findings which suggest APA	Findings which suggest BAH	Reference
PA	≥53 ng/dl (1470 pmol/l)	≤42 ng/dl (1650 pmol/l)	[20]
PA/PRA ratio	PA (ng/dl)/PRA (ng angiotensin/ml/90 min)>80, or PA (ng/dl)/PRA [(ng angiotensin/ml/h) = (μg/l/h)] >120	No adequately specific value	[20]
CT or MR	>1 cm unilateral single mass with a normal contralateral gland	Bilateral normal or abnormal adrenal glands	[19,21]
Recumbent 8 a.m. plasma 18-OHB	>50–100 ng/dl	<50–100 ng/dl	[18,19]
Postural studies*	Decrease in PA and serum cortisol from 8 a.m. to mid-day	≥33% rise in PA and a fall in serum cortisol from 8 a.m. to mid-day	[21]
Serum potassium	<3.0 mEq/l (3.0 mmol/l)	No adequately specific value	[22]
Saline infusion test[†]	18-OHB/plasma cortisol ratio rises, and is >3.0 after infusion. PA/plasma cortisol ratio rises and is >2.2 after infusion	18-OHB/plasma cortisol ratio is constant or falls, and is <3.0 after infusion. PA/plasma cortisol ratio is <2.2 after infusion	[18]
Ipsilateral/contralateral adrenal vein PA ratio	>10:1 and a symmetric ACTH-induced cortisol response with a suppressed contralateral adrenal vein PA level	<10:1 with a symmetric ACTH-induced cortisol response and non-suppressed adrenal vein PA levels [normal 100–600 ng/dl (2774–16664 pmol/l)]	[19,22]
DS adrenocortical scintigraphy	Concordant, unilateral adrenal imaging before day 5	Bilateral adrenal imaging before day 5 (may be asymmetrical)	[4]

*Measure plasm aldosterone and serum cortisol at 8 a.m. after ≥1 h in the supine position and again in the standing position after 4 h of upright/ambulatory posture. [†]The patients is supine for ≥1 h then the PA, 18-OHB (ng/dl), and cortisol (μg/dl) are measured before and after intravenous infusion of 1250 ml 0.9% saline solution at a rate of 16.7 ml/min for the first 30 min and then 8.3 ml/min for the final 90 min, beginning at 8 a.m.
DS, Dexamethasone suppression; PA, plasma aldosterone; PRA, plasma renin activity; 18-OHB, 18-hydroxycorticosterone.

whose accuracy is 95% when both adrenal veins are entered [19,21,22]. However, selective adrenal vein sampling is invasive, technically demanding with a 26% rate of failure to enter the right adrenal vein, and may be associated with adrenal haemorrhage or infarction, and adrenal or iliac vein thrombosis. Adrenal venography adds no further diagnostic information and is to be avoided given its high incidence (10%) of corticomedullary haemorrhage and infarction due to the volume of contrast material required [19,21,22].

As anticipated from the autonomous pathophysiology of primary aldosteronism, patients with APA have increased radiocholesterol uptake in the affected adrenal and nearly normal uptake on the unaffected side, since ACTH-dependent uptake by the zona fasciculata and reticularis is unaffected. In BAH, radiocholesterol uptake is increased bilaterally, and often asymmetrically. However, since ACTH-dependent tissue normally accounts for 50% of adrenal radiocholesterol up-

take (see above) and the normal range of radiocholesterol uptake is broad, there is a significant overlap between quantitative uptake in normals and in patients with primary aldosteronism due to BAH [4]. The dexamethasone suppression (DS) adrenal scan was introduced to suppress the ACTH-dependent component of radiocholesterol uptake. In normal individuals, oral dexamethasone (1 mg every 6 hours) for 7 days before injection of NP-59 and throughout the imaging period, inhibits visualization of normal adrenals until at least 5 days after injection [23]. Visualization at or beyond 5 days presumably reflects the 50% of normal radiocholesterol uptake that is ACTH-independent. Unilateral or bilateral visualization earlier than 5 days after injection under DS in biochemically proven primary aldosteronism suggests adenoma or hyperplasia, respectively (Figure 10.19; Table 10.12). Drugs which increase adrenal radiocholesterol uptake must be discontinued for an appropriate time in-

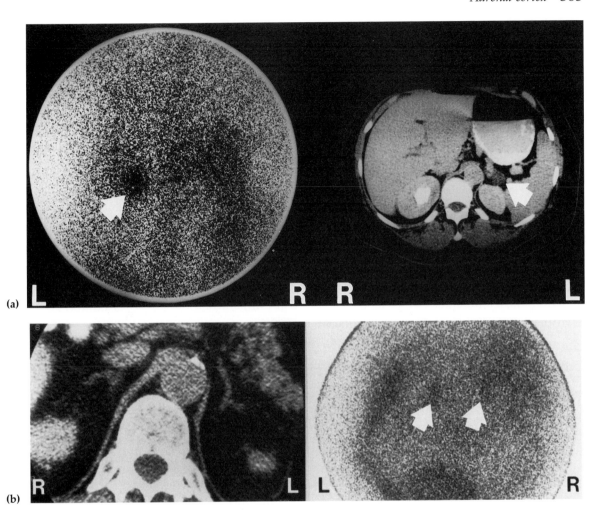

Figure 10.19 Dexamethasone suppression adrenocortical scans in primary aldosteronism (NP-59 posterior scintiscans 4 days after injection). (a) 2 cm left aldosteronoma (arrows) on NP-59 (left panel) and CT images (right panel). Right adrenal NP-59 uptake is suppressed by dexamethasone. (b) Bilateral adrenal hyperplasia. The adrenals appeared morphologically normal on CT (left panel). Bilateral early uptake of NP-59 (right panel, arrows) despite dexamethasone.

terval before scintigraphy as discussed above (Table 10.11). While quantification of NP-59 uptake on the DS adrenal scan has been shown to correlate with 24-hour urinary aldosterone excretion [24], the qualitative endpoint of early unilateral or bilateral visualization better separates APA from BAH, since hyperplasia can produce such marked asymmetry of quantitative uptake as to suggest unilateral disease [25]. In the rare, autosomal dominant variant, glucocorticoid-remediable aldosteronism, early adrenal visualization will not occur and the biochemical (high PA and low PRA) and physiological (hypertension) manifestations resolve with DS.

If a convincing majority of non-invasive evidence suggests a unilateral adenoma, adrenalectomy can proceed without recourse to adrenal vein sampling. However, it has been stated that patients with APA do not benefit from adrenalectomy when their hypertension does not respond to a 3-week trial of high-dose spironolactone (400 mg/day) [19].

HYPERANDROGENISM

Apparent disorders of sex hormone excess (androgens and oestrogens) are not uncommon clinical problems. Symptoms of masculinization are more common than feminization and will be addressed here. While the differential diagnosis of feminization is distinct from that of masculinization, many of the principles discussed would be applicable.

Excessive androgens in women cause masculinization (e.g. hirsutism, menstrual disturbances, etc.) with frank virilization in more severe cases (e.g. clitoromegaly, male body habitus, voice deepening, fronto-temporal balding). The differential diagnosis of masculinization is extensive [26]. However, pathological conditions associated with morbidity and mortality make up <10% of cases. While the social and psychological consequences of masculinization should not be underestimated, most cases likely reflect one end of the normal female physiological spectrum (e.g. 'idiopathic' hirsutism). The initial goal should be to separate benign forms of masculinization from more serious causes. Currently, this is best accomplished with a careful history and physical examination, followed by biochemical testing. Benign forms of hirsutism typically begin around the time of puberty, progress slowly, and are associated with a positive family history. The rapid onset of severe masculinization should suggest an androgen-secreting tumour. Anatomical and functional imaging is reserved for the very small minority of patients whose history, examination, or biochemical testing suggests a tumour.

The major ovarian androgen is androstenedione, whereas the adrenal cortex secretes both androstenedione and DHEA-S. These weak androgens are converted to testosterone in peripheral tissues. In general, the more marked the clinical degree of masculinization, the higher the levels of testosterone and/or androstenedione and the greater the likelihood of significant underlying ovarian pathology, while an elevated DHEA-S level suggests an adrenal aetiology. The 24-hour urinary excretion of 17-ketosteroids (17KS) provides an integrated measure of daily androgen secretion, but does not distinguish between ovarian and adrenal androgens.

One approach to the biochemical investigation of masculinized women is to measure serum testosterone (total ± free), DHEA-S, thyroid-stimulating hormone, prolactin and follicle-stimulating hormone (in the presence of abnormal menses), 1 mg overnight dexamethasone suppression test (Table 10.13), and a Cortrosyn stimulation test for 17-hydroxyprogesterone (17OHP), 17-hydroxypregnenolone, 11-deoxycortisol, and cortisol to exclude congenital adrenal hyperplasia (CAH). Patients with normal results are highly unlikely to harbour a tumour. An androgen-secreting tumour should be suspected in patients with total testosterone values >150–200 ng/dl or DHEA-S >700 μg/dl, and CAH and Cushing's syndrome are absent [27].

Patients with a suspected androgen-secreting tumour undergo further biochemical testing and/or anatomical testing, neither of which is without pitfalls. Anatomical imaging should not be performed without careful consideration of the differential diagnosis, the biochemical investigation, and a strong suspicion of a neoplastic process. The incidence of occult benign non-hypersecretory adrenal adenomas ('incidentalomas') rises after 30 years of age, they are common in CAH, and are more prevalent in obesity and diabetes mellitus. These latter two features are common in women with polycystic ovarian disease [28]. Further, unilateral adrenal enlargement, or significant asymmetrical enlargement, is well recognized in bilateral adrenal diseases such as Cushing's disease, ACTH-independent Cushing's syndrome and CAH [26]. Misinterpretation of these findings may falsely suggest a unilateral neoplastic adrenal process. If an androgen-secreting adrenal tumour is strongly suspected, then a thin-cut adrenal CT with contrast or MRI study should be performed. Suspected ovarian neoplasms should prompt a transvaginal ultrasound, although small tumours may still be missed. Ovarian and adrenal vein catheterization is occasionally helpful; however, its performance and interpretation require special expertise. In general, selective venous sampling studies should be reserved for those cases with equivocal findings on non-invasive testing [29].

The ovaries take up cholesterol as a precursor for steroid hormone biosynthesis in a similar fashion to the adrenal glands. The ratio of ovarian to adrenal uptake is increased by glucocorticoid suppression of adrenal cortical uptake. Thus, in women with hyperandrogenism, radiocholesterol scintigraphy may be performed using the same dexamethasone suppression regimen with the exclusion of potential modifiers of radiocholesterol uptake as described for primary aldosteronism (Tables 10.11 and 10.12). Dexamethasone suppression scintigraphy has also been useful for defining the functional significance of ovarian enlargement discovered by ultrasonography or CT during the evaluation of hyperandrogenism. Indeed, the limited comparative data available indicates that DS scintigraphy may be more accurate than either CT or selective adrenal/ovarian vein sampling in the differential diagnosis of hyperandrogenism [29].

The most common identifiable disorder in hyperandrogenic, oligomenorrhoeic or amenorrhoeic women is the polycystic ovary (Stein–Leventhal) syndrome (PCOS). The pathogenesis of PCOS is obscure, and abnormal adrenal androgen metabolism has frequently been demonstrated, however, the majority of evidence favours the ovary as the primary source of androgen excess [30,31]. Adrenal radiocholesterol uptake (without dexamethasone suppression) tends to be bilaterally increased in these patients, with the mean uptake being similar to that found in patients with Cushing's disease [32].

Adrenal radiocholesterol uptake is increased bilaterally in glucocorticoid under-treated CAH, but is normal in patients who have received adequate long-term replacement. 'Accessory' adrenal tissue in the broad ligament near the ovary and in the epididymis have been found scintigraphically in patients with CAH.

THE 'INCIDENTAL' ADRENAL MASS

The incidental adrenal mass has become a common clinical problem due to the widespread use of high-resolution abdominal imaging (MRI, CT and ultrasound) which identify an asymptomatic adrenal mass in approximately 0.35–5% of patients imaged for reasons other than suspected adrenal pathology [33]. In the absence of a known extra-adrenal malignancy, 70–94% of these masses are non-hypersecretory benign adenomas [28]. Benign adenomas are more common with advancing age, hypertension, Blacks compared with Whites, diabetes mellitus (2- to 5-fold), obesity, heterozygote carriers of CAH, multiple endocrine neoplasia, and the McCune–Albright syndrome [16,28]. In the setting of a known extra-adrenal malignancy the incidence of adrenal masses approximately doubles, with roughly 50% being adrenal metastases. Further, in this setting, malignancy rates in adrenal masses <3 cm are from 0% to 50%,

while in adrenal masses >3 cm malignancy rates have ranged from 43% to 100% [28]. The adrenal is a frequent site of metastasis, particularly for carcinomas of the lung, breast, stomach, ovary and kidney, as well as leukaemias, lymphomas and melanomas. The distinction between a metastasis and other causes of adrenal masses may be critical in patients who may benefit from curative surgery if the primary malignancy is not disseminated.

It is suggested that hormonal hypersecretory states be initially excluded; the benign versus malignant nature of those deemed non-hypersecretory can then be investigated. Hypersecretory masses usually require surgical excision; however, adrenalectomy is not generally indicated for CAH, primary aldosteronism due to bilateral adrenal hyperplasia, or ACTH-dependent Cushing's syndrome with secondary macronodular adrenal hyperplasia. History and physical examinations must consider hypersecretion of cortisol, androgens, oestrogen, mineralocorticoids and catecholamines. However, the need for biochemical screening of all adrenal masses lacking an obvious radiological diagnosis – regardless of the history and physical examination – cannot be overemphasized, as clinically silent hypersecretory lesions are common [16,28]. Partially cystic lesions also warrant complete evaluations of their secretory status and malignant potential.

The prevalence of phaeochromocytoma in patients with classic symptoms of episodic headache, palpitations, and diaphoresis is similar to the 0–11% incidence of phaeochromocytomas among adrenal incidentalomas [28]. Up to 80% of patients with unsuspected phaeochromocytoma who underwent surgery or anaesthesia have died [28]. Some 65% of phaeochromocytomas overlap with adrenal metastases in relative signal intensity on T2-weighted spin-echo MRI, and percutaneous adrenal biopsy of phaeochromocytoma may precipitate hypertensive crisis, severe retroperitoneal bleeding and death [28]. Plasma or urinary catecholamines and metanephrines, and urinary vanillylmandelic acid (VMA) are of approximately equal diagnostic utility; however, the latter may be the least sensitive [28,34]. An understanding of the factors which may result in false-negative and false-positive tests is required for proper test selection, performance, and interpretation (Table 10.15). Pharmacological stimulation or suppression tests may occasionally be helpful

Table 10.15   Drug interactions with phaeochromocytomas and their diagnosis*

Drug	Contraindicated with possible phaeochromocytoma	Increase catecholamines and metabolites	Reduce MIBG uptake	Interval of drug withdrawl before MIBG imaging
Acute clonidine or alcohol withdrawal, β-blockers, minoxidil, hydralazine	Yes	Yes	No	None
Phenoxybenzamine, phentolamine, prazosin, doxazosin, diuretics, spironolactone, amiloride, levodopa, methyldopa	No	Yes	No	None
Cocaine, sympathomimetics	Yes	Yes	Yes	1 week
Dopamine, dopaminergic drugs	Yes	Yes	Possible	1 week
Clonidine, ACE inhibitors	No	No	No	None
Butyrophenones, amphetamines	No	Yes	Possible	1 week
Labetalol	No	Yes	Yes	4 weeks
Guanethidine, guanadrel	Yes	No	Possible	1 week
Phenothiazines	Possible	Variable	Possible	1 week
Tricyclic antidepressants	No	Variable	Yes	4 weeks
Calcium-channel blockers	No	No	Possible	1 week
Methylglucamine (component of iodinated contrast)	No	False normal up to 72h	No	None
Reserpine	No	No	Yes	4 weeks

*Reproduced with permission from Kloos, R., Korobkin, M., Thompson, N.W., Francis, I.R., Gross, M.P. and Shapiro, B. (1997) Incidentally discovered adrenal masses, in *Endocrine Neoplasms* (ed. A. Arnold), Kluwer Academic Publishers.

[35,36]. When the diagnosis is strongly suspected in the face of equivocal biochemistry results, measurement of plasma catecholamines basally in the fasting, unstressed, recumbent state and again 2–3 hours after a single 300 mg oral dose of clonidine may be diagnostic [36]. In normal subjects and essential hypertensives, central α-stimulation by clonidine produces a reduction in peripheral neuronal catecholamine release; in patients with phaeochromocytoma, in whom catecholamine levels reflect excess hormone secretion from the autonomous tumour, levels will not be suppressed by clonidine. Clonidine decreases plasma aldosterone concentration (PAC) and plasma renin activity (PRA) in normal and hypertensive subjects, but has little effect in primary aldosteronism [16]. Thus, clonidine may be the antihypertensive agent of choice in patients with adrenal incidentalomas in whom antihypertensive therapy must be continued during diagnostic investigations. Meta-iodobenzylguanidine (MIBG) scintigraphy for further evaluation of suspected phaeochromocytoma when biochemical screening tests are abnormal is discussed below.

Given the 0–18% prevalence of Cushing's and pre-Cushing's syndrome (biochemical evidence of Cushing's syndrome without physical stigmata) among adrenal incidentalomas, it is suggested that the cortisol secretory status be investigated with an overnight dexamethasone (1 mg) suppression test (DST) [16].

Blood pressure and serum potassium should be measured to exclude mineralocorticoid excess. In the absence of hypertension, it is not necessary to pursue mineralocorticoid excess if the serum potassium is normal (>3.5 mmol/l). Spontaneous or easily provoked hypokalaemia (<3.5 mmol/l), or diuretic-induced hypokalaemia (<3.0 mmol/l) should prompt further investigation [28]. In patients with hypertension, paired upright (>2h since supine) PAC and PRA are advised. These determinations are most accurate after interfering medications have been discontinued for an appropriate interval [16]. Suppressed PRA and PAC values with hypokalaemia suggest non-aldosterone-mediated mineralocorticoid hypertension (e.g. DOC).

Dehydroepiandrosterone sulphate (DHEA-S) should always be measured as a marker of adrenal androgen excess (e.g. virilizing adenomas, adrenocortical carcinomas and CAH). Low DHEA-S values may represent suppression of normal adrenal androgen secretion by autonomous cortisol hypersecretion, and thus DHEA-S should not be measured concomitantly with the overnight DST. A low DHEA-S value may also suggest primary adrenal insufficiency. Testosterone or oestradiol determinations are not necessary in asymptomatic patients.

The CT appearance of most adrenal incidentalomas is non-specific (e.g. no clear evidence of spread beyond the adrenal to indicate malignancy, or the presence of a simple thin-walled cyst, haemorrhage or myelolipoma). Further, although some CT morphological features are more common in malignancies, no single feature – or combination of features – can reliably distinguish a metastasis from an adenoma. Malignancies tend to be large, less well-defined, have inhomogeneous attenuation, and a thick irregular enhancing rim. Adenomas tend to be smaller with a homogeneous density. However, even when >6 cm in maximal diameter, adenomas are more common than non-adenomatous lesions in the absence of a known extra-adrenal malignancy [28]. Because morphologic CT features alone do not usually allow an unequivocal differentiation of adrenal adenoma from malignancy, recent attention has centred on the value of CT densitometry. Using a threshold value of <10 Houndsfield Units (HU), there is a 73% sensitivity and 96% specificity for the diagnosis of adrenal adenoma by unenhanced CT. At <0 HU, specificity is 100% but sensitivity is reduced to 33–47% [28,37]. Unlike unenhanced CT attenuation values, immediate post-injection contrast enhanced CT values cannot accurately differentiate adrenal adenomas from non-adenomas [37].

There has been extensive investigation of MRI features of benign and malignant adrenal lesions, with initial studies demonstrating a diagnostic overlap in about 20–30% of cases. The most promising of the MRI approaches is chemical shift imaging. Taking advantage of the different hydrogen atom resonant frequency peaks in water and triglyceride (lipid) molecules, this technique demonstrates a decreased signal intensity (SI) of tissue containing both lipid and water compared with tissue without lipid. This technique was described by Mitchell *et al.* [38] to detect the significant amount of lipid often present in adrenal adenomas and typically absent in most metastases and other non-adenomatous adrenal masses. Korobkin *et al.* [39] compared quantitative to qualitative assessment of opposed-phase images: only adenomas showed a visible decrease in relative signal intensity ratio (100% specificity), with a sensitivity of 81%; with a quantitative relative SI loss of 12% compared with liver, specificity was 100% and sensitivity was 84% [39].

The incidental adrenal mass is one of the best clinical applications of adrenal scintigraphy as the currently available data suggest it has the highest accuracy and lowest cost in this setting [40]. Adrenal scintigraphy is comparable to thyroid scanning for characterizing lesions as non-functioning ('cold', and possibly malignant) versus functioning ('hot', and probably benign) [28]. However, unlike thyroid scanning, the majority of adrenal images offer a diagnostic result without need for further investigation. Non-adenomas demonstrate decreased, distorted, or absent radiocholesterol uptake in the affected adrenal gland (discordant image; Figure 10.20(a)). Hormonally non-hypersecretory adrenal adenomas demonstrate increased NP-59 accumulation (concordant image; Figure 10.20(b)). With over 25 years of experience to date, in the setting of a normal biochemical screening evaluation and the absence of interfering medications, NP-59 avidity has been a 100% accurate predictor of benignity, while discordant imaging has been a 100% accurate predictor of a non-adenomatous lesion [28]. Similar accuracy has been reported with [75Se]-selenomethyl-norcholesterol [42]. Symmetrical bilateral NP-59 uptake (normal, or non-lateralizing scan pattern) is seen in all peri-adrenal and pseudo-adrenal masses. Unfortunately, non-lateralizing scans also occur in some patients harbouring either benign or malignant adrenal masses <2 cm. Non-hypersecretory masses ≤1 cm, and >1 to ≤2 cm have yielded diagnostic (e.g. lateralizing) images in 52% and 89% of patients, respectively. Non-adenomatous lesions, including malignancies, ≤1 cm, >1 to ≤2 cm and >2 to ≤3 cm were present in 0%, 9% and 10% of patients, respectively [43].

As with scintigraphic imaging of functioning thyroid nodules, unilateral non-hypersecretory adrenal adenomas produce a range of patterns in remaining normal tissue from clear visualization to absent uptake [28]. It is likely that NP-59 uptake in normal tissue is reduced in these latter cases due to ACTH suppression (albeit incomplete or partial) by the functioning adenoma, suggesting autonomy and relative hypersecretion despite normal biochemistry based upon simple screening tests (such as the 24-hour UFC and 1 mg overnight DST). Currently, there is no evidence that these

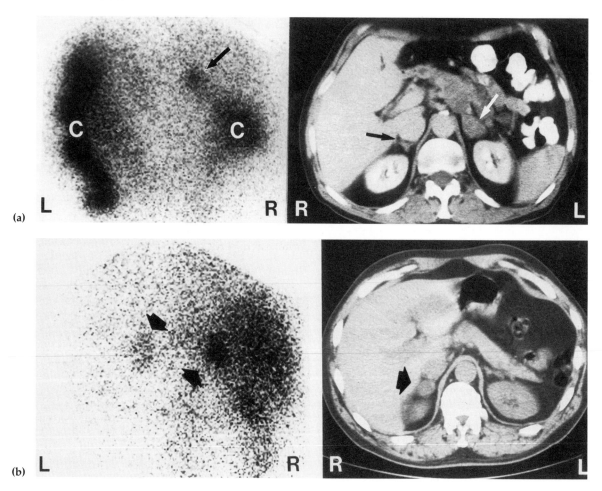

Figure 10.20 Incidental adrenal masses (NP-59 posterior scintiscans 5 days after injection, no dexamethasone suppression). (a) Discordant scintigraphy (left panel) with less NP-59 uptake on the side of the left adrenal mass seen on CT (right panel, white arrow) relative to the morphologically and scintigraphically normal right adrenal (black arrows). CT-guided biopsy diagnosed metastatic adenocarcinoma. (C, NP-59 in colon). (b) Concordant scintigraphy (left panel) with greater NP-59 uptake on the side of the 2 cm right adrenal mass seen on CT (right panel, arrow) than on the side of the morphologically normal left adrenal gland. No biochemical evidence of adrenocortical dysfunction (including adrenal vein sampling). (Reproduced from [41] with permission.)

patients benefit from adrenalectomy unless clear biochemical evidence of Cushing's syndrome (with or without clinical features) develops.

Adrenal masses are bilateral in 11–16% of incidentaloma cases [16]. NP-59 uptake equal to or greater than the contralateral adrenal gland and/or liver (as a normal reference tissue) by visual inspection is compatible with a benign process, while NP-59 uptake markedly less than the contralateral adrenal gland and/or liver is compatible with a non-adenomatous lesion. In this setting, Gross *et al.* [44] reported that NP-59 scintigraphy may identify bilateral benign adrenal masses, as well as the gland toward which further evaluation should be directed. Clinical and biochemical evaluations in this setting are critical given the probable increased incidence of CAH, and the rare occurrence of primary adrenal insufficiency from bilateral adrenal destruction by metastases, haematological malignancy, haemorrhage, infection or granulomatous diseases.

Positron emission tomography (PET) with 2-[fluorine-18]-fluoro-2-deoxy-D-glucose (FDG) has also been used to characterize adrenal masses in 20 patients with cancer [45]. PET tumour-to-background ratios (standardized uptake value, SUV) correctly differentiated benign (0.2–1.2 SUV) from all malignant lesions (2.9–16.6 SUV). However, adrenal masses <1.5 cm were excluded, and the estimated spatial resolution is 1 cm (possibly less for lesions with intense FDG uptake). This remarkable separation of benign from malignant tumours has not yet been replicated.

Percutaneous adrenal biopsy is commonly used to evaluate adrenal masses detected by CT in patients with a known primary neoplasm and either no other evidence of metastatic disease or no other lesions more amenable to biopsy. As with many endocrine tissues, histological distinction between benign and well-differentiated primary malignancy of the adrenal gland is often difficult, with a reported cytological sensitivity of only 54–86% [28]. Bleeding and pneumothorax are the most common complications. Less commonly observed are pain, fever, bacteraemia, abdominal discomfort and nausea, needle track metastasis and severe acute pancreatitis. Overall complication rates range from 8–12.7% when mild and self-limited events are included, and are closer to 3% when only major complications requiring hospitalization or therapeutic intervention are included [16]. The overall accuracies of fine-needle aspiration biopsy of adrenal masses range from 80–100%, and with experienced cytopathologists the positive predictive value approaches 100% [28]. Non-diagnostic aspiration biopsy rates range from 6% to 12% [16]. Overall, the procedure may be best utilized to further characterize an adrenal mass deemed non-adenomatous, or suspicious, by a non-invasive technique in a patient with a potentially resectable extra-adrenal primary malignancy without evidence of other metastatic foci.

SUMMARY

Adrenocortical scintigraphy is of proven value in the evaluation of ACTH-independent CS, primary aldosteronism and the incidental adrenal mass. It may be helpful in difficult cases of hyperandrogenism or feminization. It is, however, essential for the optimal performance and interpretation of these studies that the clinical, biochemical and anatomical findings be reviewed before the scan is performed. Currently, adrenocortical scintigraphy remains an underutilized technique. The need for several visits is inconvenient, and the dosimetry, although by no means unacceptable, is less favourable than is usual for nuclear medicine studies. The multidisciplinary complexity and unfamiliar biochemical evaluations required by these patients demand greater physician input than do most nuclear medicine studies. Nevertheless, time and effort devoted to the proper evaluation of the patient is well spent. To perform mistakenly a unilateral adrenalectomy in a patient with bilateral disease is a gross disservice, and it is precisely this type of patient who is most likely to benefit from adrenocortical scintigraphy.

ADRENAL MEDULLA

PHYSIOLOGY

Catecholamines are derived from the amino acid L-tyrosine. The first committed (and rate-determining) step in the catecholamine biosynthetic pathway is the hydroxylation of tyrosine to dihydroxyphenylalanine (dopa), catalysed by tyrosine hydroxylase. Dopa is decarboxylated in the cytosol to dopamine, which is taken up into the catecholamine storage vesicles, where it is hydroxylated to noradrenaline (norepinephrine). This pathway is common to both adrenergic neurones and the adrenal medulla. The major blood supply to the adrenal medulla is via an adrenal portal system which is derived from the cortical sinusoidal plexus. The resulting high medullary level of cortisol induces and maintains the activity of phenylethanolamine-N-methyltransferase (PNMT), which catalyses the methylation of noradrenaline to adrenaline (epinephrine). Noradrenaline and adrenaline are stored in membrane-bound storage vesicles in association with soluble proteins (chromogranins) and nucleotides. Stimulation of the adrenal medulla by the preganglionic, cholinergic splanchnic nerves or by other secretagogues (angiotensin, serotonin, histamine, bradykinin) releases the vesicle contents by exocytosis. Some of the released catecholamines diffuse from the medullary interstitium (or, in the case of adrenergic neurones, from the synaptic cleft) into the general circulation. However, most of the catecholamines are inactivated locally by reuptake via a stereospecific, sodium- and energy-dependent, saturable pathway (uptake-1), following which they are stored or, if unstored, are rapidly degraded by monoamine oxidase (MAO) to dihydroxymandelic acid. Circulating catecholamines are inactivated predominantly in extra-neuronal, extra-adrenal tissues by uptake via a non-specific, sodium-independent mechanism (uptake-2), rapidly followed by metabolism by catechol-*O*-methyltransferase (COMT) to metanephrines [normetadrenaline (normetanephrine) and metadrenaline (metanephrine)]. Dihydroxymandelic acid and the metanephrines are both metabolized further (by COMT and MAO, respectively) to 3-methoxy-4-hydroxymandelic acid (vanillylmandelic acid, VMA). Dopamine undergoes a similar metabolic sequence to homovanillic acid (HVA).

PHAEOCHROMOCYTOMA

Phaeochromocytomas are neoplasms arising from mature adrenal medullary cells (phaeochromocytes). They produce a well-described syndrome of hypertension associated with a classical triad of paroxysmal headache, palpitations (with relative bradycardia) and sweating attributable to episodic hypersecretion of catecholamines. The same syndrome can be produced by catecholamine-secreting tumours arising from the extra-adrenal paraganglia (functioning paragangliomas, 'extra-adrenal phaeochromocytomas') which include the organ of Zuckerkandl (caudal to the origin of the inferior mesenteric artery) and the 'chemoreceptor' organs such as the carotid bodies.

While hypertension is a virtually constant feature of the phaeochromocytoma syndrome, it is paroxysmal in fewer than half of the cases. Most patients have sustained hypertension with or without further paroxysmal increases. A high index of suspicion is essential, since these tumours have potentially life-threatening cardiovascular effects and their resection is curative. Important clinical clues include orthostatic hypotension in an untreated hypertensive, hypertension resistant to standard therapy (including exacerbation by β-blockers due to unopposed α-adrenergic peripheral vasoconstriction), and failure of the blood pressure to fall at night. The diagnosis can be established biochemically in most cases of phaeochromocytoma, as described above under incidental adrenal masses.

More recently, an increased number of phaeochromocytomas have come to clinical attention as adrenal incidentalomas. This is consistent with the fact that the classic phaeochromocytoma syndrome is present in an estimated 0.1% of hypertensive patients and yet, an estimated 0.1% of the general population is found at autopsy to harbour a phaeochromocytoma [28]. These tumours demonstrate biochemical profiles ranging from normal to only several-fold elevations as opposed to the typical >5 to 10-fold elevations seen with classically symptomatic phaeochromocytomas.

Most phaeochromocytomas arise in the adrenal medulla. However, this condition has been referred to as 'the 10% disease' since approximately 10% of adrenal tumours are bilateral, 10% are extra-adrenal, and 10% are malignant (defined by local invasion or distant metastases). Some 10% of cases are associated with one of the following autosomal dominant syndromes: multiple endocrine neoplasia (MEN) type 2a (Sipple's syndrome) or 2b (the mucosal neuroma syndrome); neurofibromatosis (von Recklinghausen's disease); von Hippel–Lindau disease (angioma of the retina, cerebellar haemangioblastoma, renal-cell carcinoma, pancreatic cysts, and epididymal cystadenoma); or the syndrome of familial phaeochromocytomas with or without paragangliomas. Finally, 10% of phaeochromocytomas occur in children, among whom bilaterality, multiplicity and malignancy are more frequent than in adults. Bilateral phaeochromocytomas should always raise the strong suspicion of a familial syndrome and prompt a search for medullary thyroid carcinoma (MTC), characteristic of MEN-2a and 2b, as well as screening of family members for MEN, phaeochromocytoma and MTC. The recent discovery of RET proto-oncogene mutations associated with MEN-2a, 2b and familial medullary thyroid cancer have led to improved genetic counselling for these families [46].

The first successful scintigraphic demonstration of phaeochromocytomas in humans was reported in 1981 using ^{131}I-meta-iodobenzylguanidine (MIBG) [47]. Since that report, extensive worldwide experience with this agent in large series of patients has shown uniformly high sensitivity (87%) and specificity (97%) of ^{131}I-MIBG for locating adrenal (Figure 10.21) and extra-adrenal

(Figure 10.22) tumour sites and metastases of malignant phaeochromocytoma (Figure 10.23) [50]. Whereas the sensitivity of CT approaches 100% for adrenal tumours >2 cm in diameter, ^{131}I-MIBG has greater specificity and has clearly superior sensitivity for smaller tumours and extra-adrenal sites. It can also detect pre-neoplastic adrenal medullary hyperplasia in asymptomatic affected relatives of patients with MEN-2a or 2b [51].

RADIOPHARMACOLOGY

MIBG is an aralkylguanidine which structurally resembles noradrenaline sufficiently to be recognized by the uptake-1 mechanism and to be stored in the catecholamine storage vesicles [52]. Whereas unstored noradrenaline is rapidly degraded, the halogenated benzyl ring of MIBG confers resistance to COMT while its guanidino side-chain is resistant to MAO. After intravenous injection of ^{131}I-MIBG, approximately 50% of the administered radioactivity appears in the urine by 24 hours and 70–90% is recovered within 4 days; 75–90% of the urinary activity is in the form of unaltered MIBG, with *meta*-iodohippuric acid and free iodide accounting for most of the remainder. There is thus little *in vivo* metabolism of MIBG [53].

Uptake of MIBG is inhibited both *in vitro* and *in vivo* by uptake-1 inhibitors (Table 10.15).

Phenylpropanolamine and other sympathomimetics are frequent constituents of non-prescription 'decongestants', cough remedies, and anorectic 'diet aids', the use of which should be specifically ruled out before radiotracer administration.

MIBG should be slowly injected intravenously over 2–3 minutes. If tracer uptake is to be quantified, the activity in the syringe should be measured before and after injection for accurate calculation of the administered dose. ^{131}I-MIBG is normally taken up by liver, spleen, myocardium, salivary glands, colon and occasionally lungs and brain [50,54,55]. Thyroid uptake of liberated radioiodide will occur unless blocked with stable iodide (Table 10.10). The normal adrenal glands are usually not seen, but faint uptake may be visible 48–72 hours after injection in up to 16% of cases. Laxative administration decreases intraluminal colonic radiotracer activity seen in 15–20% of cases, which may mimic or obscure tumour activity (Table 10.10). Splenic, myocardial and salivary gland uptake reflect the rich sympathetic innervation of these organs – thus, salivary gland uptake cannot be blocked by perchlorate or iodide, but is reduced on the affected side in patients with Horner's syndrome or stellate ganglion blockade. The degree of myocardial uptake (and, to a lesser extent, salivary gland uptake) is inversely related to circulating noradrenaline levels

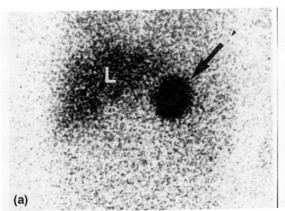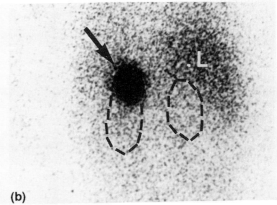

Figure 10.21 Left adrenal phaeochromocytoma (arrows). (a) Anterior and (b) posterior ^{131}I-MIBG scintiscans 48 hours after injection. The renal outlines are transferred from a ^{99m}Tc-DTPA renal scan. Note the displacement of the left kidney. L, liver.

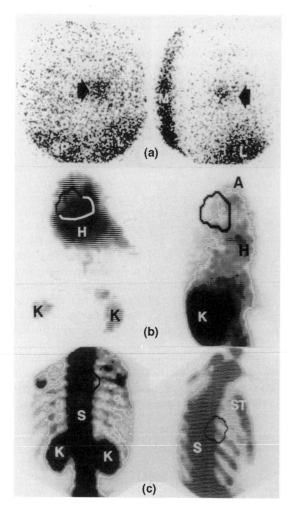

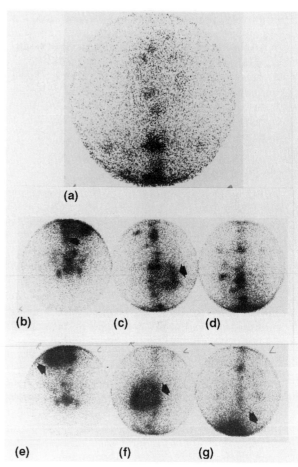

Figure 10.22 Left atrial phaeochromocytoma. Previous thoracic CT and exploratory thoracotomy were negative. (a) Posterior (left) and right lateral (right) ^{131}I-MIBG scintiscans of chest, with area of abnormal uptake (arrow). M, marker on spine; L, liver; SP, spleen. (b) ^{99m}Tc-labelled red cell blood pool images [anterior (left) and right lateral (right) views], with region of abnormal ^{131}I-MIBG uptake superimposed. A, aortic arch; H, cardiac blood pool; K, kidney. (c) ^{99m}Tc-MDP bone scan [posterior (left) and right posterior oblique (right) views], with region of abnormal ^{131}I-MIBG uptake superimposed. K, kidney; S, spine; ST, sternum. (Reproduced from [48] with permission.)

[56], so that cardiac uptake is frequently reduced or absent in patients with phaeochromocytomas.

Dosimetric considerations limit the dose of ^{131}I-MIBG for diagnostic studies (Table 10.10). This,

Figure 10.23 Malignant phaeochromocytoma. Widespread skeletal metastases demonstrated with ^{131}I-MIBG. (a) Anterior head and neck; (b) posterior pelvis; (c) posterior abdomen; (d) posterior chest; (e) anterior pelvis; (f) anterior abdomen; (g) anterior chest. Arrows indicate right adrenal primary – note photopenic, necrotic centre. (Reproduced from [49] with permission.)

coupled with the low detection efficiency of gamma-cameras for the 364 keV photon of ^{131}I, led to the introduction of ^{123}I-MIBG. The 159 keV photon of iodine-123 is efficiently detected, and the 20-fold larger dose yields sufficiently high counting statistics to improve spatial resolution, permit single photon emission computed tomography (SPECT), and improve lesion detection [57] (Figure 10.24). The shorter imaging time is beneficial, especially in children. In spite of high circulating catecholamines, the normal adrenal medullary

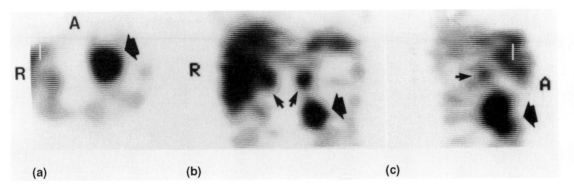

Figure 10.24 Paraganglioma of left renal hilum (large arrow) demonstrated by ^{123}I-MIBG SPECT. (a) Transverse; (b) coronal; (c) sagittal sections. The normal adrenals are clearly seen (small arrows). A, anterior; R, right; l, liver uptake.

output of catecholamines is not suppressed [58]. The normal adrenal medulla, lacrimal glands and even the uterus [59] are more frequently visualized with ^{123}I-MIBG compared with ^{131}I-MIBG images (Figure 10.24). The disadvantages of ^{123}I-MIBG are its cost, limited availability, and limited shelf-life.

In spite of these difficulties, ^{123}I-MIBG is the ideal imaging agent for phaeochromocytoma. A sensitivity of 93% and specificity of 100% for ^{123}I-MIBG compared with 86% and 100%, respectively, for X-ray CT was reported in a comparative study [60]. It is proposed that, after the initial biochemical investigation for a suspected phaeochromocytoma, the first imaging screen should be with ^{123}I-MIBG. In those with equivocal clinical and biochemical findings, a negative ^{123}I-MIBG excludes the need for further investigation. If there is strong clinical or biochemical evidence and a negative ^{123}I-MIBG scan, then X-ray CT or MRI of the neck, chest, abdomen and pelvis should be performed. A positive ^{123}I-MIBG scan for a primary tumour showing no metastases may lead to a tailored X-ray CT of the site to accurately delineate the mass and help plan the appropriate surgical intervention. Where ^{123}I-MIBG shows metastatic disease, X-ray CT is mainly helpful when considering surgical debulking.

^{123}I-MIBG permits quantification of the percentage uptake of the injected dose (ID) in each adrenal medulla and in the tumours [61]. A direct correlation has also been shown between the percentage ID in tumour and the number of positive neurosecretory granules seen on electron microscopy [62]. Lack of uptake in some APUDomas (see p. 377) such as carcinoid, and

variation in uptake between metastases may thus be related to the paucity of neurosecretory granules, presence of atypical granules, and intervening stroma in a tumour. Altered permeability and necrosis of tumour cells can also affect this uptake. The quantitative approach has also been used to assess the integrity and function of the adrenergic system in humans [63,64]. Impaired uptake and rapid clearance from the heart and liver is seen in patients with autonomic neuropathies and phaeochromocytomas.

Because MIBG is excreted in the urine, normal bladder activity may obscure pelvic or bladder tumour foci. Thus, pelvic views are best obtained immediately after the patient has voided. Alternatively, simultaneous dual-window data acquisition following the injection of 74 MBq of ^{99m}Tc-DTPA with subsequent computer-assisted subtraction of urinary tract activity may be used. The same principle, using the appropriate ^{99m}Tc-labelled radiopharmaceutical, has been used to clarify the relationship of abnormal MIBG uptake to bone, liver or cardiac blood pool (Figure 10.22).

Somatostatin is a naturally occurring neuropeptide with a wide range of physiological actions and a short half-life of 2–3 minutes. A high concentration of somatostatin receptors (of which there are at least five subtypes) has been demonstrated on many neuroendocrine tumours and these may be exploited for imaging (Figure 10.25) with the long-acting somatostatin peptide analogue ^{111}In-pentetreotide (OctreoScan®). Unlike MIBG, ^{111}In-pentetreotide does not have an extensive list of potentially interfering medications. It is recommended that concurrent Octreotide therapy be discontinued 24–48 hours before radiotracer

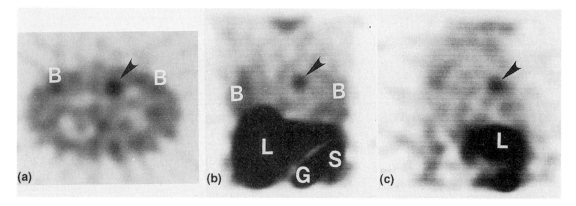

Figure 10.25 ^{111}In-pentetreotide SPECT images 24 hours post-radiotracer injection in patient with a retrosternal pulmonary phaeochromocytoma metastasis (arrow), status post-left adrenalectomy and nephrectomy. (a) transverse; (b) coronal; (c) sagittal sections. B, breast; L, liver; G, gut; S, spleen.

administration, so as to not saturate the receptors. However, pre-treatment with Octreotide in a small group of patients has been reported to improve visualization of hepatic metastases [65]. After binding, the somatostatin–receptor complex may become internalized with subsequent somatostatin detachment and removal from the cell. While binding properties of ^{111}In-pentetreotide to somatostatin receptors are similar to those of somatostatin, they are not identical. ^{111}In-pentetreotide is cleared rapidly from the blood with 68-85% excreted unaltered in the urine by 24 hours [50]. Normal tissue accumulation of ^{111}In-pentetreotide includes intense uptake in the spleen, liver and kidneys, with more modest uptake in the pituitary, thyroid, urinary bladder, colon, breast (variable), and occasionally the gallbladder (Figure 10.25). ^{111}In-pentetreotide imaging lacks specificity for neuroendocrine tumours as a number of non-neuroendocrine tumours, granulomatous diseases, autoimmune diseases and inflammatory conditions may also be imaged. ^{123}I- or ^{131}I-MIBG and ^{111}In-pentetreotide detect phaeochromocytomas almost equally. MIBG offers the advantages of absent or minimal confounding of normal renal and hepatic radiotracer accumulation, and the potential for therapy should the tumour be malignant [50,66]. Some data suggest that ^{123}I- or ^{131}I-MIBG and ^{111}In-pentetreotide may serve complementary roles [28,67].

PET imaging with 2-[fluorine-18]-fluoro-2-deoxy-D-glucose (FDG) and ^{11}C-hydroxy-ephedrine has been used to localize phaeochromocytomas [68,69]. As described earlier, adrenaline is an endogenous substrate for the uptake-1 mechanism. PET imaging with ^{11}C-adrenaline suggests that most phaeochromocytomas accumulate the radiotracer; however, it appears that MIBG and ^{11}C-adrenaline are not handled identically, as one tracer may locate tumours when the other does not [70].

NEUROBLASTOMA AND OTHER 'NEUROENDOCRINE' TUMOURS

Neuroblastomas are highly malignant neural crest tumours. They are the most common tumour in infants <1 year of age, the second most common solid malignancy of childhood, and 97% of cases occur before the age of 10 years. The overall incidence from birth to age 15 is 8.7 per million per year in the USA, with a male and non-Hispanic white predominance [71]. Approximately 50% of the primary tumours arise in the adrenals, 25% from abdominal sympathetic ganglia, and 15% in the posterior mediastinum. They are locally invasive and metastasize to liver, skin, lymph nodes, bone and bone marrow. Long-term survival for stage IV disease is less than 15%. Common presentations are pain (primary tumour, focal osseous metastasis or bone marrow involvement), an abdominal mass, malaise and weight loss, anorexia, irritability, haematuria, paraspinal mass or cord compression, fever of unknown origin, anaemia or pathological fracture. Less common presentations include neck mass, Horner's syndrome, and paraneoplastic syndromes such as watery diarrhoea or acute cerebellar encephalopathy. Although they secrete catecholamines (mainly dopamine), these are extensively metabolized within the tumour itself, so that urinary levels of VMA and HVA are disproportionately elevated and hypertension is unusual. Other circulating biochemical markers of disease activity and prognostic value include carcinofoetal isoferritins (detected as high serum ferritin), lactate dehydrogenase, number of copies of the gene for the oncogene NMYC, cytogenetics, DNA index, and neurone-specific enolase.

Prognosis and appropriate treatment are critically dependent on accurate staging, which generally includes abdominal and thoracic CT or MRI scans to assess the extent of primary disease, bone scan, and bilateral bone marrow examinations. Neuroblastomas and their metastases regularly show MIBG uptake (Figure 10.26) with 92% sensitivity compared with 77% for ^{111}In-pentetreotide [50]. MIBG uptake in the extremities is a more sensitive index of skeletal involvement than conventional ^{99m}Tc-labelled MDP bone scans (Figure 10.26), bone marrow aspiration and biopsy, and plain radiographs [73]. PET imaging with ^{11}C-hydroxyephedrine has also been used to localize neuroblastoma [74].

A number of tumours other than phaeochromocytomas and neuroblastomas image with MIBG and ^{111}In-pentetreotide with varying frequencies. MIBG appears to be more sensitive to detect ganglioneuroma (100%), Schwannoma, and retinoblastoma [50]. ^{111}In-pentetreotide appears more sensitive for carcinoid tumours (86% versus 70%), medullary thyroid cancer (66% versus 35%), endocrine pancreatic tumours (70% versus 60%), paraganglioma (97% versus 89%), small cell lung cancer (95% versus 15%), Merkel cell tumours (80% versus 50%), and several pituitary tumour types (GH, TSH and non-secretory) [50]. Although several of these tumours do not actively secrete catecholamines, they originate from the neural crest and retain the mechanisms for Amine Precursor Uptake and Decarboxylation (hence, 'APUDomas') and have typical dense core neurosecretory granules on electron microscopy. Uptake of MIBG by these tumours is likely to be via a mechanism similar or identical to uptake-1.

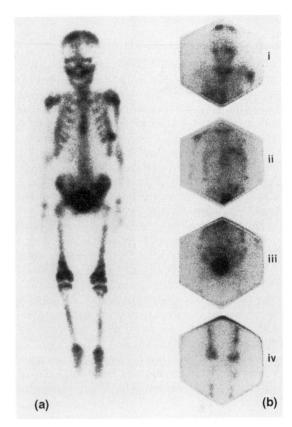

Figure 10.26 Metastatic neuroblastoma. (a) ^{99m}Tc-labelled MDP bone scan showing multiple skeletal metastases. (b) ^{131}I-MIBG scan showing more extensive skeletal and bone marrow involvement than suggested by the bone scan. i, anterior head and neck; ii, anterior chest and abdomen; iii, anterior pelvis and proximal femurs; iv, anterior lower limbs. (Reproduced from [72] with permission.)

THERAPY WITH ^{131}I-MIBG

Following the demonstration of ^{131}I-MIBG uptake by metastases of neural crest-derived tumours, it was hypothesized that MIBG would be a useful therapeutic agent for these conditions. The cautious optimism raised by early reports [75,76] has been borne out for a minority of malignant phaeochromocytomas and paragangliomas, which are relatively radioresistant tumours. Currently, therapy with high doses (e.g. 7.4 GBq per dose) of ^{131}I-MIBG is indicated only in patients with progressive disease who have failed conventional therapy or with intractable bone pain from skeletal metastases, and only if a previous dosimetric study has predicted a delivered tumour dose of >0.5 cGy/MBq. The degree of MIBG uptake cannot be predicted from the biochemistry of the tumour as assessed by plasma or urinary levels of catecholamines or their metabolites. An improved method for calculating tumour dosimetry has recently been described [77]. Total tumour doses in excess of 200 Gy are probably necessary to achieve a therapeutic effect, and bone marrow toxicity is the limiting factor. In a cumulative experience of 116 patients with malignant phaeochromocytoma, three were reported to have achieved complete remission, with an objective response attained in 56% [50].

Neuroblastomas are inherently more radiosensitive than malignant phaeochromocytomas. The cumulative experience in 276 neuroblastoma patients indicated a complete remission in 6% and an overall objective response in 35%. Most of these patients were stage IV and received ^{131}I-MIBG in the setting of progressive disease following the failure of chemotherapy and conventional teleradiotherapy [50].

Therapy with ^{131}I-MIBG has been used in a small number of medullary thyroid cancer patients with a 5% complete remission rate, 32% objective response rate, and a 50% palliation rate. Similarly, a 4% complete remission rate, 15% objective response rate, and a 65% palliation rate has been reported in carcinoid tumours [50].

SUMMARY

In the relatively brief period since its development, MIBG has proved to be a safe, sensitive and highly specific agent for the location of phaeochromocytoma and neuroblastoma. Its use is clearly indicated in the evaluation of patients suspected of harbouring these diseases, whether or not CT scanning has been positive. ^{123}I-MIBG should be considered the radiopharmaceutical of choice for imaging purposes, if available. Although MIBG uptake has been demonstrated by a variety of other tumours of neural crest origin, its routine use in these situations is not warranted. The role of ^{131}I-MIBG in the therapy of malignant neural crest tumours shows promise, but remains to be clarified. ^{111}In-pentetreotide has demonstrated relatively high sensitivity for many neural crest tumours with relatively lower specificity. ^{111}In-pentetreotide is an excellent alternative to MIBG imaging when MIBG is not available, when drugs known to interfere with MIBG imaging cannot be withdrawn, and for some APUDomas other than phaeochromocytoma and neuroblastoma.

ACKNOWLEDGEMENTS

Partial support for this manuscript was provided by the Cancer Research Training in Nuclear Medicine Grant NCI 2 T32 CA09015-19, and the Department of Veterans Affairs.

REFERENCES

1. Beierwaltes, W.H., Lieberman, L.M., Ansari, A.N. *et al.* (1971) Visualization of human adrenal glands in vivo by scintillation scanning. *JAMA,* **216,** 275–7.
2. Sarkar, S.D., Cohen, E.L., Beierwaltes, W.H. *et al.* (1977) A new and superior adrenal imaging agent, ^{131}I-6-beta-iodomethyl-19-nor-cholesterol (NP-59): evaluation in humans. *J. Clin. Endocrinol. Metab.,* **45,** 353–62.
3. Hawkins, L.A., Britton, K.E. and Shapiro, B. (1980) Selenium 75 selenomethyl cholesterol: a new agent for quantitative functional scintigraphy of the adrenals: physical aspects. *Br. J. Radiol.,* **53,** 883–9.
4. Gross, M.D., Valk, T.W., Swanson, D.P. *et al.* (1981) The role of pharmacologic manipulation in adrenal cortical scintigraphy. *Semin. Nucl. Med,* **11,** 128–48.
5. Lynn, M.D., Gross, M.D., Shapiro, B. *et al.* (1986) The influence of hypercholesterolaemia on the adrenal uptake and metabolic handling of ^{131}I-6-beta-iodomethyl-19-norcholesterol (NP-59). *Nucl. Med Commun.,* **7,** 631–7.
6. Conn, J.W. and Hinerman, D.L. (1977) Spironolactone-induced inhibition of aldosterone biosynthesis in primary aldosteronism: morphological and functional studies. *Metabolism,* **26,** 1293–307.
7. Kater, C.E., Biglieri, E.G., Schambelan, M. *et al.* (1983) Studies of impaired aldosterone response to spironolactone-induced renin and potassium elevations in adenomatous but not hyperplastic primary aldosteronism. *Hypertension,* **5,** V115–21.
8. Cain, M.D., Walters, W.A. and Catt, K.J. (1971) Effects of oral contraceptive therapy on the renin-angiotensin system. *J. Clin. Endocrinol. Metab.,* **33,** 671–6.
9. Meikle, A.W. (1993) A diagnostic approach to Cushing's syndrome. *The Endocrinologist,* **3,** 311–20.
10. Orth, D.N. (1995) Cushing's syndrome. *N. Engl. J. Med.,* **332,** 791–803. [Published erratum appears in *N. Engl. J. Med.* (1995) **332**(22):1527].
11. Miller, J. and Crapo, L. (1994) The biochemical diagnosis of hypercortisolism. *The Endocrinologist,* **4,** 7–16.
12. Gross, M.D., Valk, T.W., Freitas, J.E. *et al.* (1981) The relationship of adrenal iodomethylnorcholesterol uptake to indices of adrenal cortical function in Cushing's syndrome. *J. Clin. Endocrinol. Metab.,* **52,** 1062–6.

13. Seabold, J.E., Haynie, T.P., DeAsis, D.N. *et al.* (1977) Detection of metastatic adrenal carcinoma using ^{131}I-6-beta-iodomethyl-19-norcholesterol total body scans. *J. Clin. Endocrinol. Metab.*, **45**, 788–97.

14. Fig, L.M., Gross, M.D., Shapiro, B. *et al.* (1988) Adrenal localization in the adrenocorticotropic hormone-independent Cushing syndrome. *Ann. Intern. Med.*, **109**, 547–53.

15. Shapiro, B., Britton, K.E., Hawkins, L.A. *et al.* (1981) Clinical experience with ^{75}Se selenomethyl-cholesterol adrenal imaging. *Clin. Endocrinol., Oxford*, **15**, 19–27.

16. Kloos, R.T., Korobkin, M., Thompson, N.W. *et al.* (1997) Incidentally discovered adrenal masses, in *Endocrine Neoplasms* (ed. A. Arnold), Kluwer Academic Publishers, Boston, pp 263–92.

17. Bunnag, P. and Tuck, M.L. (1995) Captopril test in the evaluation of primary aldosteronism. *The Endocrinologist*, **5**, 253–7.

18. Arteaga, E., Klein, R. and Biglieri, E.G. (1985) Use of the saline infusion test to diagnose the cause of primary aldosteronism. *Am. J. Med.*, **79**, 722–8.

19. Melby, J.C. and Azar, S.T. (1993) Adrenal steroids and hypertension: new aspects. *The Endocrinologist*, **3**, 344–51.

20. Weinberger, M.H. and Fineberg, N.S. (1993) The diagnosis of primary aldosteronism and separation of two major subtypes. *Arch. Intern. Med.*, **153**, 2125–9.

21. Young, W.F., Jr, Hogan, M.J., Klee, G.G. *et al.* (1990) Primary aldosteronism: diagnosis and treatment. *Mayo Clin. Proc.*, **65**, 96–110.

22. Bravo, E.L. (1993) Primary aldosteronism: new approaches to diagnosis and management. *Cleve. Clin. J. Med.*, **60**, 379–86.

23. Gross, M.D., Freitas, J.E., Swanson, D.P. *et al.* (1979) The normal dexamethasone-suppression adrenal scintiscan. *J. Nucl. Med.*, **20**, 1131–5.

24. Gross, M.D., Shapiro, B., Grekin, R.J. *et al.* (1983) The relationship of adrenal gland iodomethylnorcholesterol uptake to zona glomerulosa function in primary aldosteronism. *J. Clin. Endocrinol. Metab.*, **57**, 477–81.

25. Gross, M.D., Shapiro, B. and Freitas, J.E. (1985) Limited significance of asymmetric adrenal visualization on dexamethasone-suppression scintigraphy. *J. Nucl. Med.*, **26**, 43–8.

26. Kloos, R.T., Khafagi, F. and Shapiro, B. (1996) Four case histories of androgen excess: pitfalls of diagnosis. *The Endocrinologist*, **6**, 1–13.

27. Mechanick, J.I. and Dunaif, A. (1990) Masculinization: a clinical approach to the diagnosis and treatment of hyperandrogenic women, in *Advances in Endocrinology and Metabolism* (eds E.L. Mazzaferri, R.S. Barr and R.A. Kreisberg), Mosby Year Book, St. Louis, vol. **1**, pp. 129–73.

28. Kloos, R.T., Gross, M.D., Francis, I.R. *et al.* (1995) Incidentally discovered adrenal masses. *Endocrine Reviews*, **16**, 460–84.

29. Taylor, L., Ayers, J.W., Gross, M.D. *et al.* (1986) Diagnostic considerations in virilization: iodomethylnorcholesterol scanning in the localization of androgen secreting tumors. *Fertil. Steril.*, **46**, 1005–10.

30. Soulez, B., Dewailly, D. and Rosenfield, R.L. (1996) Polycystic ovarian syndrome: a multidisciplinary challenge. *The Endocrinologist*, **6**, 19–29.

31. Franks, S. (1995) Polycystic ovary syndrome. *N. Engl. J. Med.*, **333**, 853–61. [Published erratum appears in *N. Engl. J. Med.* (1995) **333**(21), 1435.]

32. Gross, M.D., Wortsman, J., Shapiro, B. *et al.* (1986) Scintigraphic evidence of adrenal cortical dysfunction in the polycystic ovary syndrome. *J. Clin. Endocrinol. Metab.*, **62**, 197–201.

33. Kloos, R.T., Shapiro, B. and Gross, M.D. (1995) The adrenal incidentaloma. *Curr. Opin. Endocrinol. Diabetes*, **2**, 222–30.

34. Lenders, J.W., Keiser, H.R., Goldstein, D.S. *et al.* (1995) Plasma metanephrines in the diagnosis of pheochromocytoma. *Ann. Intern. Med.*, **123**, 101–9.

35. Bravo, E.L. (1994) Evolving concepts in the pathophysiology, diagnosis, and treatment of pheochromocytoma. *Endocr. Rev.*, **15**, 356–68.

36. Bravo, E.L. and Gifford, R.W., Jr (1984) Current concepts. Pheochromocytoma: diagnosis, localization and management. *N. Engl. J. Med.*, **311**, 1298–303.

37. Korobkin, M., Brodeur, F.J., Yutzy, G.G. *et al.* (1996) Differentiation of adrenal adenomas from nonadenomas using CT attenuation values. *Am. J. Roentgenol.*, **166**, 531–6.

38. Mitchell, D.G., Outwater, E.K., Matteucci, T. *et al.* (1995) Adrenal gland enhancement at MR imaging with Mn-DPDP. *Radiology*, **194**, 783–7.

39. Korobkin, M., Lombardi, T.J., Aisen, A.M. *et al.* (1995) Characterization of adrenal masses with chemical shift and gadolinium-enhanced MR imaging. *Radiology*, **197**, 411–18.

40. Dwamena, B.A., Kloos, R.T., Fendrick, A.M. *et al.* (1996) The adrenal incidentaloma: decision and cost-effectiveness analyses of diagnostic management strategies (abstract 692). *J. Nucl. Med.*, **37**, 158P.

41. Gross, M.D., Shapiro, B., Bouffard, J.A. *et al.* (1988) Distinguishing benign from malignant euadrenal masses. *Ann. Intern. Med.*, **109**, 613–18.

42. Dominguez-Gadea, L., Diez, L., Bas, C. *et al.* (1994) Differential diagnosis of solid adrenal masses using adrenocortical scintigraphy. *Clin. Radiol.*, **49**, 796–9.

43. Kloos, R.T., Gross, M.D., Shapiro, B. *et al.* (1997) The diagnostic dilemma of small incidentally discovered adrenal masses: a role for ^{131}I-β-iodomethyl-norcholesterol (NP59) scintigraphy. *World. J. Surg.*, **21**, 36–40.

44. Gross, M.D., Shapiro, B., Francis, I.R. *et al.* (1995) Incidentally discovered bilateral adrenal masses. *Eur. J. Nucl. Med.*, **22**, 315–21.

45. Boland, G.W., Goldberg, M.A., Lee, M.J. *et al.* (1995) Indeterminate adrenal mass in patients with cancer: evaluation at PET with 2-[F-18]-fluoro-2-deoxy-D-glucose. *Radiology*, **194**, 131–4.

46. Hofstra, R.M., Landsvater, R.M., Ceccherini, I. *et al.* (1994) A mutation in the RET proto-oncogene associated with multiple endocrine neoplasia type 2B and sporadic medullary thyroid carcinoma. *Nature*, **367**, 375–6.

47. Sisson, J.C., Frager, M.S., Valk, T.W. *et al.* (1981) Scintigraphic localization of pheochromocytoma. *N. Engl. J. Med.*, **305**, 12–17.

48. Shapiro, B., Sisson, J., Kalff, V. *et al.* (1984) The location of middle mediastinal pheochromocytomas. *J. Thorac. Cardiovasc. Surg.*, **87**, 814–20.

49. Shapiro, B., Sisson, J.C., Lloyd, R. *et al.* (1984) Malignant phaeochromocytoma: clinical, biochemical and scintigraphic characterization. *Clin. Endocrinol., Oxford.*, **20**, 189–203.

50. Hoefnagel, C.A. (1994) Metaiodobenzylguanidine and somatostatin in oncology: role in the management of neural crest tumours. *Eur. J. Nucl. Med.*, **21**, 561–81.

51. Valk, T.W., Frager, M.S., Gross, M.D. *et al.* (1981) Spectrum of pheochromocytoma in multiple endocrine neoplasia. A scintigraphic portrayal using ^{131}I-metaiodobenzylguanidine. *Ann. Intern. Med*, **94**, 762–7.

52. Tobes, M.C., Jaques, S., Jr, Wieland, D.M. *et al.* (1985) Effect of uptake-one inhibitors on the uptake of norepinephrine and metaiodobenzylguanidine. *J. Nucl. Med.*, **26**, 897–907.

53. Mangner, T.J., Tobes, M.C., Wieland, D.W. *et al.* (1986) Metabolism of iodine-131 metaiodobenzylguanidine in patients with metastatic pheochromocytoma. *J. Nucl. Med.*, **27**, 37–44.

54. Nakajo, M., Shapiro, B., Copp, J. *et al.* (1983) The normal and abnormal distribution of the adrenomedullary imaging agent m-[I-131]iodobenzylguanidine (I-131 MIBG) in man: evaluation by scintigraphy. *J. Nucl. Med.*, **24**, 672–82.

55. Shapiro, B., Copp, J.E., Sisson, J.C. *et al.* (1985) Iodine-131 metaiodobenzylguanidine for the locating of suspected pheochromocytoma: experience in 400 cases. *J. Nucl. Med.*, **26**, 576–85.

56. Nakajo, M., Shapiro, B., Glowniak, J. *et al.* (1983) Inverse relationship between cardiac accumulation of meta- [131I]iodobenzylguanidine (I-131 MIBG) and circulating catecholamines in suspected pheochromocytoma. *J. Nucl. Med.*, **24**, 1127–34.

57. Lynn, M.D., Shapiro, B., Sisson, J.C. *et al.* (1985) Pheochromocytoma and the normal adrenal medulla: improved visualization with I-123 MIBG scintigraphy. *Radiology*, **155**, 789–92.

58. Bomanji, J., Bouloux, P.M., Levison, D.A. *et al.* (1987) Observations on the function of normal adrenomedullary tissue in patients with phaeochromocytomas and other paragangliomas. *Eur. J. Nucl. Med.*, **13**, 86–9.

59. Bomanji, J. and Britton, K.E. (1987) Uterine uptake of iodine-123 metaiodobenzylguanidine during the menstrual phase of uterine cycle. *Clin. Nucl. Med.*, **12**, 601–3.

60. Bomanji, J., Conry, B.G., Britton, K.E. *et al.* (1988) Imaging neural crest tumours with ^{123}I-metaiodobenzylguanidine and X- ray computed tomography: a comparative study. *Clin. Radiol.*, **39**, 502–6.

61. Bomanji, J., Flatman, W.D., Horne, T. *et al.* (1987) Quantitation of iodine-123 MIBG uptake by normal adrenal medulla in hypertensive patients. *J. Nucl. Med.*, **28**, 319–24.

62. Bomanji, J., Levison, D.A., Flatman, W.D. *et al.* (1987) Uptake of iodine-123 MIBG by pheochromocytomas, paragangliomas, and neuroblastomas: a histopathological comparison. *J. Nucl. Med.*, **28**, 973–8.

63. Nakajo, M., Shimabukuro, K., Miyaji, N. *et al.* (1985) Rapid clearance of iodine-131 MIBG from the heart and liver of patients with adrenergic dysfunction and pheochromocytoma. *J. Nucl. Med.*, **26**, 357–65.

64. Sisson, J.C., Shapiro, B., Meyers, L. *et al.* (1987) Metaiodobenzylguanidine to map scintigraphically the adrenergic nervous system in man. *J. Nucl. Med.*, **28**, 1625–36.

65. Dorr, U., Rath, U., Sautter-Bihl, M.L. *et al.* (1993) Improved visualization of carcinoid liver metastases by indium-111 pentetreotide scintigraphy following treatment with cold somatostatin analogue. *Eur. J. Nucl. Med.*, **20**, 431–3.

66. Pujol, P., Bringer, J., Faurous, P. *et al.* (1995) Metastatic phaeochromocytoma with a long-term response after iodine-131 metaiodobenzylguanidine therapy. *Eur. J. Nucl. Med.*, **22**, 382–4.

67. Tenenbaum, F., Lumbroso, J., Schlumberger, M. *et al.* (1995) Comparison of radiolabeled octreotide and meta-iodobenzylguanidine (MIBG) scintigraphy in malignant pheochromocytoma. *J. Nucl. Med.*, **36**, 1–6.

68. Shulkin, B.L., Wieland, D.M., Schwaiger, M. *et al.* (1992) PET scanning with hydroxyephedrine: an approach to the localization of pheochromocytoma. *J. Nucl. Med.*, **33**, 1125–31.

69. Shulkin, B.L., Koeppe, R.A., Francis, I.R. *et al.* (1993) Pheochromocytomas that do not accumulate metaiodobenzylguanidine: localization with PET and administration of FDG. *Radiology*, **186**, 711–15.

70. Shulkin, B.L., Wieland, D.M., Shapiro, B. *et al.* (1995) PET epinephrine studies of pheochromocytoma. *J. Nucl. Med.*, **36**, 229P.(abstract)

71. Matthay, K.K. (1995) Neuroblastoma: a clinical challenge and biologic puzzle. *CA: Cancer J. Clin.*, **45**, 179–92.

72. Geatti, O., Shapiro, B., Sisson, J.C. *et al.* (1985) Iodine-131 metaiodobenzylguanidine scintigraphy for the location of neuroblastoma: preliminary experience in ten cases. *J. Nucl. Med.*, **26**, 736–42.

73. Gelfand, M.J. (1993) Meta-iodobenzylguanidine in children. *Semin. Nucl. Med.*, **23**, 231–42.

74. Shulkin, B.L., Wieland, D.M., Baro, M.E. *et al.* (1996) PET hydroxyephedrine imaging of neuroblastoma. *J. Nucl. Med.*, **37**, 16–21.

75. Sisson, J.C., Shapiro, B., Beierwaltes, W.H. *et al.* (1984) Radiopharmaceutical treatment of malignant pheochromocytoma. *J. Nucl. Med.*, **25**, 197–206.

76. Fischer, M., Winterberg, B., Zidek, W. *et al.* (1984) [Nuclear medical therapy of pheochromocytoma]. *Schweiz. Med. Wochenschr.*, **114**, 1841–3.

77. Shulkin, B.L., Sisson, J.C., Koral, K.F. *et al.* (1988) Conjugate view gamma camera method for estimating tumor uptake of iodine-131 metaiodobenzylguanidine. *J. Nucl. Med.*, **29**, 542–8.

78. Gross, M.D., Thompson, N.W. and Beierwaltes, W.H. (1981) Scintigraphic approach to the localization of adrenal lesions causing hypertension. *Urol. Radiol.*, **3**, 241–4.

Parathyroid

A. J. Coakley and C. P. Wells

INTRODUCTION

Hyperparathyroidism is the disease state associated with overproduction of parathormone (PTH), the biologically active hormone of the parathyroids. While some patients with hyperparathyroidism are managed medically, the only curative treatment is removal of the abnormal gland or glands.

The varying anatomical siting of the parathyroid means that their localization at operation can be difficult, and a strong case can be made for parathyroidectomy to be performed only by surgeons with specialized training and experience in the procedure. A wide variety of pre-operative localizing techniques have been described to assist the surgeon find the glands, particularly if these are at ectopic sites or when the patient has had previous neck surgery. This chapter gives an account of the available radionuclide and other pre-operative localization techniques, and indicates their role in the management of hyperparathyroidism.

ANATOMY AND PHYSIOLOGY

There are normally four parathyroid glands, situated in close proximity to the thyroid; 5% of patients have more than four glands, and another 5% only three. The complicated embryological development of the parathyroids results in a number of variations in the normal anatomy, and glands may be sighted in a number of ectopic sites in the neck or upper mediastinum.

Parathormone is the active peptide produced by the parathyroid. It acts by raising ionized calcium in the blood by increasing calcium release from bone, promoting re-absorption from the renal tubules, and increasing synthesis of the active compound 1,25-dihydroxycholecalciferol. Both primary and secondary hyperparathyroidism are recognized. In primary hyperparathyroidism there is endogenous hypersecretion of PTH which may be due to:

1. A parathyroid adenoma (80% of cases); rarely there may be more than one adenoma.
2. Hyperplasia involving more than one gland, usually with all four glands being involved; this occurs in 10–15% of primary cases.
3. Parathyroid carcinoma occurs in 3–4% of cases.

Secondary hyperparathyroidism occurs when there is a tendency to hypocalcaemia, resulting in increased stimulation of the parathyroid glands which increase PTH production. The most common clinical cause is renal failure, but the condition can occasionally be seen with malabsorption or renal tubular disorder. In some cases of secondary hyperparathyroidism one or more of the glands can become autonomous, so that even when the primary disease is treated the glands continue to hypersecrete PTH – this is termed tertiary hyperparathyroidism.

RADIONUCLIDE LOCALIZING TECHNIQUES

Historically, a large number of techniques have been employed in an attempt to localize glands in hyperparathyroidism [1]. Most of these techniques had only limited success, and few were widely adopted. A major breakthrough came with the recognition that thallium-201, in the form of thallous chloride, was taken up by overactive parathyroid glands and could be utilized for localization of parathyroid adenomas. More recently, scanning with ^{99m}Tc-sestamibi has been demonstrated to be a suitable technetium-labelled alternative to thallium, and with a number of associated advantages. Several other agents are under investigation. Many of these radiopharmaceuticals are taken up by the thyroid as well as the parathyroid, and techniques are needed to separate the two types of gland. One method is by using subtraction techniques, and with the technetium agents increasing interest is being shown in utilizing the different kinetics of the tracers in thyroid and parathyroid tissue as a means for distinguishing these glands.

Clinical Nuclear Medicine, 3rd edn. Edited by M.N. Maisey, K.E. Britton and B.D. Collier. Published in 1998 by Chapman & Hall, London. ISBN 0 412 75180 1

THALLIUM SCANNING

Following the initial description by Ferlin *et al.* [2], thallium-201/^{99m}Tc-pertechnetate subtraction scanning became established as the standard radionuclide technique for localizing parathyroid glands. Thallium is taken by the thyroid and parathyroid, and so either ^{99m}Tc-pertechnetate or iodine-123 are given to outline the thyroid, and by subtraction allow localization of the parathyroid gland. There was considerable debate as to the precise techniques used, and especially over the optimal sequence of radiopharmaceutical administration [3,4]. However, successful results have been described with a variety of techniques. A vital part of the procedure is to examine whether patient movement has taken place during acquisition and, if so, to correct for this. There are several causes of false-positive scans, but the main problem occurs with coexisting solid thyroid nodules which can take up thallium and be indistinguishable from parathyroid adenomas.

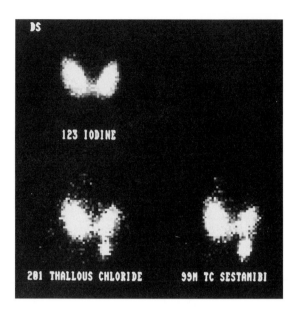

Figure 10.27 Parathyroid adenoma sited caudally to the inferior pole of the left lobe of thyroid.

^{99m}Tc-SESTAMIBI SCANNING

[99m]Tc-sestamibi is a cationic complex developed as an alternative to thallium for studying myocardial blood flow. It was also found to localize in parathyroid adenomas, and could be used in a similar fashion to thallium [5] (Figure 10.27). As with thallium, false-positives can be seen with thyroid nodules (Figure 10.28(a,b)). Investigation showed important differences between the two agents [6]. Uptake per gram of parathyroid tissue is lower than with thallium, but the parathyroid-to-thyroid ratio is higher. The kinetics are different in the two tissues – after initial uptake, sestamibi levels in the parathyroid remain almost constant, probably due to mitochondrial binding of the agent. In contrast, there is washout of sestamibi from the thyroid cells, thus resulting in an increasing parathyroid-to-thyroid ratio with time.

The original description of sestamibi relied on a subtraction technique, using iodine-123. Others have described success with using ^{99m}Tc-pertechnetate as the subtraction agent [7]. The differences in kinetics of sestamibi in the thyroid and parathyroid have resulted in the development of a two-phase technique following a single injection of sestamibi [8]. Images are acquired after 30 min-

utes and 2 hours (or later) and by comparing these the parathyroid can be distinguished from the thyroid gland (Figure 10.29). Few direct comparisons have been made between subtraction and two-phase techniques. The two-phase technique appears to produce more variable results and a slightly lower sensitivity [9,10], but more data are needed to confirm this.

CLINICAL RESULTS FROM RADIONUCLIDE PARATHYROID IMAGING

The sensitivity of detection depends on the type of hyperparathyroidism under investigation and the agent used. The most widely investigated agent has been thallium-201 [11], and for primary adenomas sensitivity of detection rates vary between 42% and 96%, with a mean of 72%. The detection rate is lower for secondary hyperparathyroidism, varying from 32% to 81% with a mean of 43%. The sensitivity in re-operative cases has varied from 26% to 100% with a mean of 45%. It is clear that the highest sensitivity of detection is with primary adenomas before the first operation. Further, there is marked variation of detection rates between different centres. Reasons for these variations in sensitivity have been much

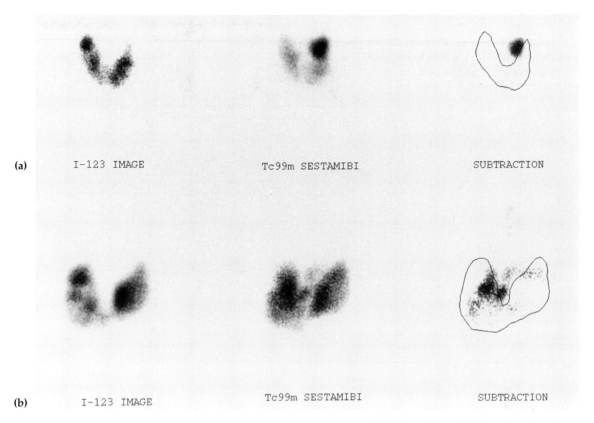

Figure 10.28 (a) Images with parathyroid adenoma at upper pole of left lobe of thyroid. Note thyroid nodule at upper pole of right lobe on I-123 image only. (b) Cold nodule in right lobe of thyroid in iodine image demonstrating sestamibi uptake.

discussed, but the precise explanation remains obscure [1,12].

Sensitivity of gland detection is higher with sestamibi than with thallium, and again is higher for adenomas than other causes of hyperparathyroidism. One review using pooled data gave an overall sensitivity for sestamibi of 87% compared with 71% for thallium [9]. These are global figures, since they include different types of hyperparathyroidism and imaging protocols obtained from different centres. However, sestamibi appears consistently superior to thallium in investigating re-operative cases [13,14].

Sestamibi has now largely taken over from thallium for parathyroid localization, mainly because of its improved sensitivity of detection, lower radiation dose to the patient, and convenience of the ^{99m}Tc radiolabel.

NEWER RADIONUCLIDE TECHNIQUES

A number of radiopharmaceuticals and associated techniques are under investigation [1], including the use of monoclonal antibodies. The most promising area comes from the continuing development of new agents with different kinetics in the thyroid and parathyroid. Like sestamibi, some are being developed for myocardial perfusion studies, and one such agent, ^{99m}Tc-tetrofosmin, has also been shown to localize in parathyroid glands [15]. The kinetics of tetrofosmin in thyroid and parathyroid tissues has not yet been fully investigated, and its optimal imaging protocol is still to be determined. Clinical comparison with sestamibi is awaited.

Positron emission tomography (PET) is providing an increasing range of potentially useful

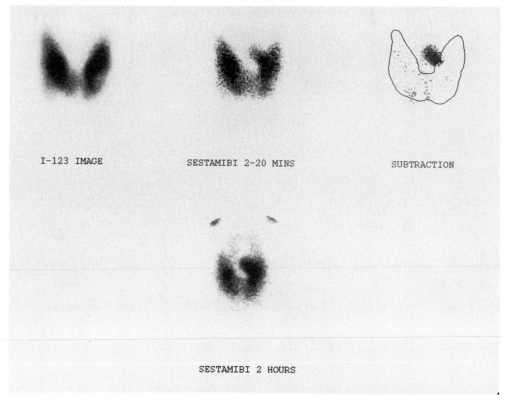

I-123 IMAGE   SESTAMIBI 2-20 MINS   SUBTRACTION

SESTAMIBI 2 HOURS

Figure 10.29   Upper row of images show conventional scan. Lower image shows 2-h sestamibi scan acquired on different day showing higher parathyroid-to-thyroid uptake than the early image.

radiopharmaceuticals. Of these 18-fluoro-2-deoxy-D-glucose (FDG) has been utilized, but with one exception [16], the reports are disappointing [17,18]. ^{11}C-Methionine has also been used (Figure 10.30) and has shown some promise [19]. Because of its present limited availability, the clinical application of PET is likely to be confined to the most difficult re-operative cases.

OTHER IMAGING TECHNIQUES

Although a wide range of imaging techniques have been utilized to localize parathyroid glands [1], all have shown marked variations in sensitivity of detection (Table 10.16). The reasons for this are unclear, but local interest and expertise must be at least one factor.

The sensitivity of ultrasound for localizing parathyroid glands varies from 38% to 92%. Ultrasound cannot detect mediastinal disease, and has a lower sensitivity after neck exploration when the vascular anatomy and relationship to tissue plains have been altered. As with scintigraphy, ultrasound cannot distinguish between parathyroid and thyroid nodules. When diffuse thyroid enlargement is present, the posteriorly placed parathyroid glands can be more difficult to identify with the high-resolution transducers used. Ultrasound has been used together with fine-needle aspiration in selected cases, and also for ablation of parathyroids by ethanol injection – this technique is not without side effects.

Despite the high resolution of computed tomography (CT), results for parathyroid localization have been generally disappointing. The sensitivity of detection appears higher for upper mediastinal glands than elsewhere in the neck, and again problems are encountered with coexisting thyroid disease. Magnetic resonance imaging (MRI), while not having the intrinsic resolution of

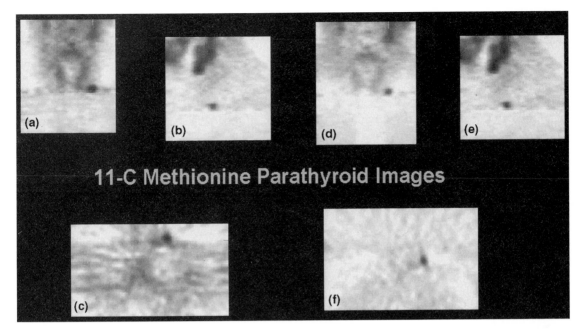

Figure 10.30 ^{11}C-Methionine parathyroid images. Left three images show (b) sagittal, (a) coronal and (c) transverse sections with attenuation correction. Right three images show (d) sagittal, (e) coronal and (f) transverse sections without attenuation correction. (Images reproduced with kind permission of Dr G. Cook.)

Table 10.16 Detection rates in adenomas, hyperplasia and re-operative cases*

Modality	No. of publications	No. of patients	Sensitivity (%)	% False-positive
Primary hyperparathyroidism: adenoma				
Nuclear medicine	60	1785	72 (1280/1780)	11 (144/1275)
Ultrasound	42	1724	63 (1145/1805)	18 (244/1374)
Computed tomography	22	507	65 (343/524)	16 (61/387)
Magnetic resonance imaging	13	243	74 (184/247)	14 (29/203)
Primary hyperparathyroidism: hyperplasia				
Nuclear medicine	20	140	43 (131/303)	8 (6/77)
Ultrasound	15	84	30 (72/243)	12 (7/58)
Computed tomography	2	11	45 (18/40)	0 (0/11)
Magnetic resonance imaging	5	11	40 (10/25)	0 (0/3)
Hyperparathyroidism at re-operation				
Nuclear medicine	22	316	45 (141/315)	10 (24/241)
Ultrasound	23	606	60 (374/620)	13 (53/407)
Computed tomography	16	408	48 (198/411)	10 (24/238)
Magnetic resonance imaging	6	85	66 (57/86)	14 (8/57)

*Data reproduced with permission from [11].

CT has fewer streak artefacts and superior soft tissue contrast. The potential of MRI in parathyroid localization has not yet been fully explored, but it seems likely the technique will prove superior to CT, particularly for re-operative cases.

Selective venous sampling, with or without prior arteriography, has the advantage of high specificity and can allow parathyroid glands to be distinguished from thyroid nodules. This is an invasive technique available in only a few specialized centres; it has now been largely replaced by other methods, but is still occasionally used for reoperative cases.

CLINICAL ROLE OF PARATHYROID LOCALIZATION

Parathyroid-localizing tests have no role to play in establishing the diagnosis of hyperparathyroidism – this is done biochemically. The techniques described are used to help the surgeon by localizing the gland(s) pre-operatively, and their use will be determined by their value to the surgeon.

There are a number of important considerations here. Firstly, it is well established that an experienced parathyroid surgeon will localize the gland in 90–95% of cases. When there is a failed parathyroidectomy, it has been shown that this is commonly due to the initial operation being carried out by a relatively inexperienced parathyroid surgeon. The abnormal gland(s) is frequently in the neck, or is accessible from it, and often in normal anatomical sites [20]. It has been said that the best localization test that can be performed is to localize a good parathyroid surgeon! Equally, concern has been expressed that the availability of pre-operative localizing tests may encourage the inexperienced surgeon to try his or her hand at the procedure.

The attitude of parathyroid surgeons to pre-operative localization varies. Many will point out that with the high detection rate at operation, the need for pre-operative localization, which is both expensive and less accurate, is of dubious value [21]. This is particularly true in secondary hyperparathyroidism when pre-operative tests have lower sensitivity and there is exploration of all four glands. Other surgeons find pre-operative localization helpful, and have demonstrated that it can significantly shorten the operating time [22]. A number now practice a more limited neck exploration for excision of the offending gland [23]. This approach appears to be finding increasing favour among surgeons, but does require a reliable method of predicting the site of the abnormal gland.

In patients undergoing re-operation, whether because of a failed primary operation or because of recurrence of hyperparathyroidism, there is a strong case for pre-operative localization. This is because second operations have a higher morbidity and a lower chance of establishing normocalcaemia. Some surgeons would advise that the localization should be confirmed by at least two techniques [24].

The choice of a pre-operative localizing technique depends on a number of factors, including local availability and expertise. There is increasing evidence that of the radionuclide techniques sestamibi is now the radiopharmaceutical of choice, and most of the published data show it to have a higher sensitivity of detection than the other commonly used imaging techniques.

REFERENCES

1. Coakley, A.J. (1995) Parathyroid imaging. *Nucl. Med. Commun.*, **16**, 522–33.
2. Ferlin, G., Borsato, N., Camerani, M. *et al.* (1983) New perspectives in localising enlarged parathyroids by technetium-thallium subtraction scan. *J. Nucl. Med.*, **24**, 438–41.
3. Fogelman, I., McKillop, J.H., Bessent, R.G. *et al.* (1984) Successful localisation of parathyroid adenomata by thallium-201 and technetium-99m subtraction scintigraphy: description of an improved technique. *Eur. J. Nucl. Med.*, **9**, 545–7.
4. Sandrock, D., Dunham, R.G. and Neumann, R.D. (1990) Simultaneous dual energy acquisition for ^{201}Tl/^{99m}Tc parathyroid subtraction scintigraphy: physical and physiological considerations. *Nucl. Med. Commun.*, **11C**, 503–10.
5. Coakley, A.J., Kettle, A.G., Wells, C.P., O'Doherty, M.J. and Collins, R.E.C. (1989) ^{99m}Tc-sestamibi new agent for parathyroid imaging. *Nucl. Med. Commun.*, **10**, 791–4.
6. O'Doherty, M.J., Kettle, A.G., Wells, P.C., Collins, R.E.C. and Coakley, A.J. (1992) Parathyroid imaging with technetium-99m-sestamibi: preoperative localisation and tissue uptake studies. *J. Nucl. Med.*, **33**, 313–18.
7. Geatti, O., Shapiro, B., Orsolon, P.G. *et al.* (1994) Localization of parathyroid enlargement: experience with Tc-99m MIBI and thallium-201 scintigraphy, ultrasonography and computerised tomography. *Eur. J. Nucl. Med.*, **21**, 17–22.
8. Taillefer, R., Boucher, Y., Potvin, C. *et al.* (1992) Detection and localization of parathyroid adenomas in

patients with hyperparathyroidism using a single radionuclide imaging procedure with technetium-99m-sestamibi (double-phase study). *J. Nucl. Med.*, **33**, 1801–7.

9. McBiles, M., Lambert, A.T., Cote, M.G. *et al.* (1995) Sestamibi parathyroid imaging. *Semin. Nucl. Med.*, **XXV**, no 3, 221–34.

10. Chen, C.C., Skarulis, M.C., Fraker, D.L. *et al.* (1995) Technetium-99m-sestamibi imaging before re-operation for primary hyperparathyroidism. *J. Nucl. Med.*, **36**(12), 2186–91.

11. Price, D.C. (1993) Radioisotopic evaluation of the thyroid and the parathyroids (review). *Radiol. Clin. North Am.*, **31**(5), 991–1015.

12. Sandrock, D., Merino, M.J., Norton, J.A. and Neumann, R.D. (1990) Parathyroid imaging by Tc/Tl scintigraphy. *Eur. J. Nucl. Med.*, **16**, 607–13.

13. Bugis, S.P., Berno, E., Rusnak, C.H. *et al.* (1995) Technetium-99m-sestamibi scanning before initial neck exploration in patients with primary hyperparathyroidism. *Eur. Arch. Otol. Rhinol. Laryngol.*, **252**(3), 149–52.

14. Caixas, A., Berna, L., Piera, J. *et al.* (1995) Utility of 99mTc-sestamibi scintigraphy as a first line imaging procedure in the pre-operation evaluation of hyperparathyroidism. *Clin. Endocrinol.*, **43**(5), 525–30.

15. Giordano, A., Meduri, G. and Marozzi, P. (1996) Parathyroid imaging with Tc99m-tetrofosmin. *Nucl. Med. Commun.*, **17**(8), 706–10.

16. Neumann, D.R., Esselstyn, C.B., Jr, MacIntyre, W.J. *et al.* (1994) Primary hyperparathyroidism: pre-operative parathyroid imaging with regional body FDG PET. *Radiology*, **192**(2), 509–12.

17. Sisson, J.C., Thompson, N.W., Ackerman, R.J. *et al.* (1994) Use of 2-(F-18)-Flouro-2-deoxy-D-glucose PET to locate parathyroid adenomas in primary hyperparathyroidism. *Radiology*, **192**, 280.

18. Melon, P., Luxen, A., Hamoir, E. *et al.* (1995) Flourine-18-flourodeoxyglucose positron emission tomography for pre-operative parathyroid imaging in primary hyperparathyroidism. *Eur. J. Nucl. Med.*, **22**(6), 556–8.

19. Hellman, P., Ahlstrom, H., Bergstrom, M. *et al.* (1994) Positron emission tomography with ^{11}C-methionine in hyperparathyroidism. *Surgery*, **116**(6), 974–81.

20. Edis, A.J., Sheedy, P.F., Beahrs, O.H. and van Heerden, J.A. (1978) Results of re-operation for hyperparathyroidism, with evaluation of pre-operative localisation studies. *Surgery*, **84**, 384–93.

21. Consensus Development Conference Panel (1991) Diagnosis and management of asymptomatic primary hyperparathyroidism: consensus development conference statement. *Ann. Intern. Med.*, **114**(7), 593–7.

22. Wei, J.P. and Burke, G.J. (1995) Analysis of savings in operative time for primary hyperparathyroidism using localization with technetium 99m sestamibi scan. *Am. J. Surg.*, **170**(5), 488–91.

23. Davis, R.K., Hoffmann, J., Dart, D. *et al.* (1990) Unilateral parathyroidectomy. *Otolaryngol. Head Neck Surg.*, **102**, 635–8.

24. Miller, D.L. (1991) Preoperative localization and interventional treatment of parathyroid tumours: when and how ? *World J. Surg.*, **15**, 706–15.

FURTHER READING

Parathyroid imaging (review). *Radiol. Clin. North Am.*, 1993, **31**(5), 967–1028. A comprehensive series of review articles on techniques for parathyroid imaging.

CHAPTER 11

Kidney and urinary tract

Renal disease

K. E. Britton and M. N. Maisey

INTRODUCTION

The fundamental purpose of nephrourology is the preservation and improvement of renal function. The contribution that renal radionuclide studies makes to this goal is increasing in parallel with the developments in renal radiological techniques. This is through the application of renal 'stress' tests: frusemide-induced diuresis and captopril-enhanced determination of renovascular disorder; and because the sets of renal images are increasingly used as windows to analysis programs. These give objective measurements of two important renal functions: **uptake function**, the ability of each kidney to take up compounds from the blood leading to measurements of total and relative renal functions; and **transit function**, the time dependency of nephron transport which is utilized in the assessment of obstructive nephropathy and renovascular disorder. As outcome analysis of therapeutic interventions or surgery becomes a key feature of evidence-based medicine and essential to the individual, so will there be growth in the applications of objective non-invasive measurements with their small and explicit errors. Renal radionuclide studies are well set for the future.

The easiest way to locate the kidneys is to feel for the lumbar spine and the costal margins fol-lowing the line of the ribs medially and cranially. A disc 10 cm in diameter may then be set with its medial edge towards the lumbar spine and the lowest rib overlying a quarter of its upper surface. The kidneys move with respiration and with change of posture, falling forward in the prone and sitting forward positions, so investigations are best performed with the patient reclining. In this position the two kidneys are at approximately equal depths, less than 1 cm difference in 75% of cases. The actual depth of the kidney in any individual varies from 4 to 11 cm; therefore, it is usual to calculate individual renal function as a fraction or percentage of the total, and measure the total function separately to avoid the need to measure the absolute radiotracer content of each kidney. To correct for tissue attenuation, renal depth may be estimated directly or indirectly.

In each kidney there are about 1 million nephrons, each composed of a glomerulus, proximal tubule, loop of Henle and distal tubule connected to the collecting duct. It is not known exactly how the kidneys work but it is clear that the physical arrangement of the filters, tubes and loops made up of living cells is important; that the interaction of physical phenomena – forces, resistances, filtration, diffusion, osmosis, pressure gradients and flows with active transport mechanisms – enable the system to work; and that a hierarchy of control systems – the cell and intercellular channels, tubuloglomerular balance, nephron autoregulation, the juxtaglomerular apparatus, intrarenal flow distribution and hormonal interactions – maintain not only the

Clinical Nuclear Medicine, 3rd edn. Edited by M.N. Maisey, K.E. Britton and B.D. Collier. Published in 1998 by Chapman & Hall, London. ISBN 0 412 75180 1

functioning kidney but also conserve and support the internal environment of the body. The maintenance of salt and water balance and the control of osmolality and acidity of the body and the levels of plasma potassium, calcium and phosphate ions are essential functions. Important substrates such as glucose and amino acids are retained while unnecessary metabolites such as uric acid, urea, sulphate, creatinine and guanidine derivatives are excreted. The kidney also produces and responds to a range of hormones.

TECHNIQUE AND INTERPRETATION

The patient requires hydration with about 300 ml fluid at least 30 minutes before the test so that the urine flow during the test is 1–4 ml/minute. The patient should receive a reassuring explanation of the test before entering the renography room. The patient should be studied reclining, for example in a modified dental chair. The supine position may be preferred since the kidneys are less likely to descend, but positioning of the camera is difficult. The sitting position, particularly sitting forward, and the standing position, allow the kidneys to drop and move anteriorly, making positioning and quantitation less reliable. The reclining position is a suitable compromise.

The gamma-camera is positioned so that its face is set back about 20° off the vertical plane. The patient sits on a comfortable backless chair with side-arms and reclines back against the camera face. With the arm abducted, the injection of the chosen radiopharmaceutical is given in less than 1 ml, rapidly into a deep antecubital vein. Alternatively, a 'butterfly' needle with a sterile extension tube and three-way tap may be used. The injectate is introduced into the extension tube and flushed in using 10–20 ml saline. This system also allows access for a subsequent injection of frusemide for the diuresis technique. Data are collected for 20 minutes, or longer if the pelvis is not visualized and for at least 10 minutes after an injection of frusemide if that technique is used. Frusemide (40 mg) should be injected before 20 minutes have elapsed in the adult, but it may be necessary to wait for 30 minutes in a child (0.5 mg/kg body weight administered).

Images on transparent film (analogue images) are usually collected at 30-second intervals for the first 180 seconds; and then at 5-minute intervals for the remainder of the study. Image data are transferred to the computer with a 10-second frame rate. The following features should be noted:

- the heart, the length of time the activity in the left ventricular cavity is visible – prolonged with renal impairment;
- the patency and tortuosity of the aorta and possible aneurysm;
- whether the times of arrival and tracer distribution are equal in the two kidneys – prolongation on one side may occur with an inflow disorder;
- the site and position of the kidneys relative to the liver and spleen – possible space-occupying lesion between;
- whether the cortical outline of each kidney is complete – possible scar due to infection, infarction or tumour;
- whether there are any defects in the parenchyme – possible tumour, cyst or parenchymal infection or scar.

A dilated calyx should fill at the pelvic retention stage, but not if it contains a stone. A cyst in the parenchyme will not show any tracer uptake, whereas a vascular tumour may show initial tracer activity which may persist for longer than that in adjacent normal tissue and be followed by a focal defect in the distribution of activity due to the absence of normal nephrons.

Corticopelvic transfer will normally be seen to occur as the tracer moves from parenchyme to pelvis as the lateral edge of the kidney, noted on the 1- to 2-minute frames, appears to move medially as the test progresses. Pelvic, calyceal and/or ureteric retention of tracer occurs when the capacity of these structures has increased through dilation but cannot be used to distinguish whether obstruction is or is not present. The ureter should not be considered to have retained tracer unless its whole length or that down to a block can be seen to persist over several images. Blobs of activity in the ureter are of no significance and do not mean ureteric hold up. The bladder is usually visualized at the end of the test. A ureterocele or a diverticulum of the bladder may be observed.

On visual inspection a normal pair of renal activity–time curves – 'renograms' – are characterized by their symmetry. A normal renogram curve has a steeply rising part usually lasting 20–30 seconds and ending with an apparent discontinuity of the slope. This is called the **first phase** and is absent in the renogram when it is corrected for tissue and blood background. The renogram then rises over the next few minutes towards peak and this is called the **second phase**. If there is no peak to the renogram as is the case in certain diseases, it can be said that the second phase continues to rise. After the second phase is the peak which, if the chart specification is correct, should be sharp. The record descends after the peak in the normal and this is called the **third phase**. If there is no peak (in disease) then there is no third phase.

An abnormal renogram is characterized by loss of the sharpness of the peak and alteration of either the second or third phase, or both of these. Absence of the second phase does not necessarily mean absence of renal function; absence of the third phase certainly does not necessarily mean obstruction to outflow. Differences in peak time between two renograms of over 1 minute are of clinical significance only if either the second or third phase of the renogram with the delayed peak is impaired.

Small, rapid fluctuations seen in the second or third phases are statistical in nature. When there are fluctuations in renal blood flow, for example due to anxiety, sudden noise or discomfort, an unsteady state occurs and larger irregularities occur. These last over 2 minutes and return to the line of the third phase. Since ureteric peristalsis is about six contractions per minute and since increase in resistance to flow in the ureter leads to a rise in distending pressure and reduced force but increased frequency of peristalsis, these irregularities are *not* due to ureteric 'spasm', which does not occur in man [1]. Hydronephrosis or reflux of urine may also be associated with large alterations of the third phase, with irregularities descending below the line of the third phase.

The report of an abnormal renogram should be in two parts, the description and the interpretation in the individual clinical context. After describing the images the abnormal renogram is reported. The first phase should be ignored. The second phase may be called 'absent', 'impaired', 'normal' and/or 'continuing to rise' when no peak occurs. The third phase may be called 'absent', 'impaired' or 'normal'. The time to peak varies non-linearly with the state of hydration and urine flow. It is indirectly related to the rate of salt and water reabsorption by the nephrons and to the state of the pelvis. It is a crude index of the tracer transit through the parenchyme and pelvis. Normal peak

times vary from 2.0–4.5 minutes with a mean of 3.7 minutes at a urine flow of 1 ml/minute.

If renograms without third phases are symmetrically abnormal, pre-renal or renal parenchymal disorder is the most likely explanation. If the renograms without third phases are asymmetrical, then bilateral renovascular or outflow disorder is more likely. In the context of bilateral outflow obstruction, the kidney that should be operated upon first to relieve the outflow obstruction is that with the better uptake function [2]. A successful operation is followed by an improvement in the rate of rise of the second phase; however, the third phase may remain absent for weeks or even months after successful operation. Apparent retention in the pelvis may also be overcome by standing the patient up and then repositioning. A pre- and post-micturition image of the lower urinary tract is recommended.

RENAL MODELS

There are two types of measurement, 'descriptive' and 'physiological', that can be made from renal radionuclide studies. There are at least 20 different points or times that have been taken from the renogram, such as the time for the curve to fall from peak to half its height, the height of the curve at the end of the first phase, and so on. Such measurements are descriptive, and enable one to classify the shape of the curve and to compare one curve with another. It should not be expected that such values have inherent physiological significance. This has to be demonstrated empirically by clinical observation and correlation with other tests applied to the kidney. This is true of the classification technique called principal component analysis. Secondly, there are those measurements that relate directly to the physiology and pathophysiology of the kidney through a 'physiological model'.

It is crucial to understand that the application of mathematics or a mathematical model to the analysis of data depends on the physiological model that represents as simply and truly as possible the reality of the clinical situation. A crude example is the statement that blood is in a space (compartmental) and that the kidney is made up of tubes (linear). The more anatomically and physiologically acceptable (isomorphic) the physiological model is, the more is one able to understand deviations from normal data obtained in pathological situations. Conversely, data analysis based on an incorrect physiological model, while appearing correct in the original test system, may well give uninterpretable or wrongly interpreted results in pathophysiological situations. Just as there are rules for mathematics so there are for physiology and each model has its own rules and assumptions. Thus, a conceptually isomorphic model gives both the physiological basis for interpreting a particular measurement and allows one to appreciate the biological assumptions and sources of error that are inherent in such an interpretation in the context of renal disorders. These are in addition to the more readily documented random and systematic measurement errors due to the physical basis of the external counting technique.

Two different models are typically used in assessing dynamic studies: the compartmental model and the linear system model.

THE COMPARTMENTAL MODEL

The compartmental model is most often isomorphic to fluid collections, for example, the interchange of tracer between blood and extracellular fluid. If a tracer that is only taken up by the organ under study is chosen, the rate of loss from, for example, blood plasma will equal the rate of uptake by the chosen organ which may be termed the **uptake function** of the organ.

The uptake function may also be determined relatively in paired organs, in parts of organs and in sites of suspected pathology. The popularity of compartmental models led to their attempted and incorrect use in the kidney, in which they are not isomorphic. As well as all the assumptions required by indicator dilution theory, an important feature of a compartmental model is that the rate of mixing in one compartment is rapid compared with the rate of exchange between compartments. This situation is clearly reasonable for a tracer introduced into the blood, but hardly likely to occur in a kidney made up of tubes of nephrons which show no cross-mixing of their contents.

Provided that a compartmental model is justified as for plasma clearance, then the results of compartmental analysis of the data may be applied to the compartments. Compartmental (exponential) analysis may be applied to curves obtained from many different sites. It is only when they are obtained from a site with which a compartmental model is isomorphic that the results of the compartmental analysis may be meaningfully related to the model and to the clinical problem.

LINEAR SYSTEM

A linear system has and requires the assumptions of **stationarity:** if an input at a single time gives a particular response, then the same input at a later time will give the same response; and **linearity** that the sum of all the inputs will give a response which is the total of all of the individual responses to all the individual inputs. Looking at the kidneys from the point of view of these two models, it is evident that the compartmental model may be applied to the extracellular fluid, plasma and renal uptake, but it cannot realistically apply to the outer cortex, inner cortex and medulla because there is no mixing between the contents of the nephrons in these regions. Because the nephrons are tubes there has to be a tube model and the model that deals best with tubes is the linear system. Compounds are taken up and move progressively forward along the tubes. Thus, the linear system is applicable to the nephrons of the kidney. There is a very short delay due to the tubular uptake of MAG3 or hippuran and or filtration of DTPA less than a second. There is a longer delay in the cortical nephron (about 3 minutes) and for the juxtamedullary nephron (about 5.5 minutes). There is a short delay in the normal pelvis (about 20 seconds).

The appropriate mathematics for a linear system is called **deconvolution analysis**. This is conceptually quite simple. Arthur Milne described the game of 'Pooh sticks' where you all stand on a bridge over a river and you all drop sticks in together. You all rush to the other side to see which stick is the winner. To understand that simple game as a child is to understand deconvolution analysis. There was a spike input into the system, the simultaneous entry of sticks. The system has responded in some way so that there was an output response which is the distribution of sticks coming out from under the bridge. This implies a distribution of pathways, or a distribution of path lengths, some long and some short, and thus a distribution of path times. If the input is known and also the output you can work out what has happened in that river, that is the distribution of path times, and so you have undertaken deconvolution analysis. If you know the input and output you can find the transit time distribution. Alternatively if the bridge was made of glass and you had a helicopter flying above it you could actually watch the cumulative effect of all these sticks moving. That is in fact what happens with an activity–time curve from the kidney from a gamma-camera over it. You are looking at all the sticks as packets of activity moving through the kidney. As there are multiple paths the input, which was a spike input, will be distributed in time at the output. In other words, if a bolus were injected into the renal artery you would get a distribution of output times. If you know input and total content curve, the renogram, or input and output, or total content and output, you can work out the transit times through the kidney by deconvolution and it is not that difficult.

How is it done in practice? The blood clearance curve obtained from the region of interest over the left ventricle is considered as a series of little spike inputs, decreasing in size over time. The renogram is considered to be the sum of all the responses to this complex input. Deconvolution analysis gives the single response that would have been obtained from a spike injection into the renal artery. Therefore, deconvolving the blood clearance curve and the renogram shows that the renogram is made up of all those similar impulse response functions, also called retention functions, resulting from that input. Thus, from this content curve (the renogram), deconvolution gives the response that would have been obtained from a direct injection of a spike of activity into the renal artery. The beauty of this technique for all of nuclear medicine is that although the injection is given to the patient through an easily accessible vein, it allows the determination non-invasively of what would have been obtained if the injection had been directly and invasively into an artery supplying the organ of interest.

This **impulse retention function** is quite complicated (Figure 11.1). After the input there are renal artery to vein transit times. After this short falling portion of the impulse response with time there is a plateau as the activity goes along all the nephrons. Then there is a shoulder to the impulse response and that point defines a minimum transit time that is common to all nephrons. This minimum transit time can be functionally related to the collecting ducts which are common to all nephrons (20 collecting ducts for a million

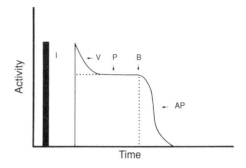

I. Impulse deconvolved from the blood clearance curve;
V. Vascular contribution;
P. Plateau of impulse retention function;
B. Shortest transit time;
AP. Area of retention function indicating the longer transit times.

Figure 11.1 Parenchymal impulse retention function. The plateau P is extrapolated to the vertical axis to exclude the vascular component V. B gives the time of change from the plateau to a falling activity and delineates the minimum transit time. The mean parenchymal transit time is given by the area divided by the height of the impulse retention function and for the parenchymal transit time index the area AP for transit times longer than the minimum divided by the height of the impulse retention function. The transit times are measured in seconds.

nephrons). The distribution of transit times just after the shoulder is called the parenchymal transit time index.

Time is a fundamental biological variable which is determined by nuclear medicine techniques, which radiology conventionally does not consider. Time can be measured accurately, is easily understood and is universal. For deconvolution there should be a good bolus of high activity for good statistics because these impulse retention functions are rather noisy. A 10-second frame rate must be used. The input is obtained from the left ventricle region of interest, and the content curve from the whole kidney or from a region of interest from the parenchyme excluding any pelvis or calyceal elements. Note that any part of the parenchyme is representative of the whole because it is time not counts that is the variable.

Deconvolution becomes straightforward only where a protocol is used to ensure stability and robustness of the solution given the statistical noise in the data obtained. The choice of pre-processing, filtering and the inclusion of a prior knowledge in the form of mathematical constraints is important. These include monotonicity, which means curves which must have only one peak and be without major irregularities in them, so there is a need for a quiet and content patient; and non-negativity: if there are negative deviations these are removed [3]. The curves should not be smoothed because that will cause data loss. The first value should be the maximum which should be so if the patient has been given a bolus input. If not so, then use the maximum input value and adjust the time base. For the impulse retention function, the shoulder is defined visually or with a gradient operator or by differentiation, and extrapolated back to give the plateau. That shoulder point separates the minimum transit time and the parenchymal transit times index. The main prob-

lems with deconvolution are a poor bolus, an anxious patient (or doctor), human error since the program is interactive, too little parenchyme, or too little left ventricle in the chosen regions of interest and computer failure. Nowadays the computers are stable and the main requirement is to obtain the data in a form that appropriately meets the constraints.

TRANSIT TIMES

The nephron can be divided into its transit times (Figure 11.2). The mean whole kidney transit time is related to the peak of the renogram. It is non-discriminatory, partly parenchyme, partly pelvis and related to the peak of the renogram. When the pelvis is separated out, the pelvic transit time and

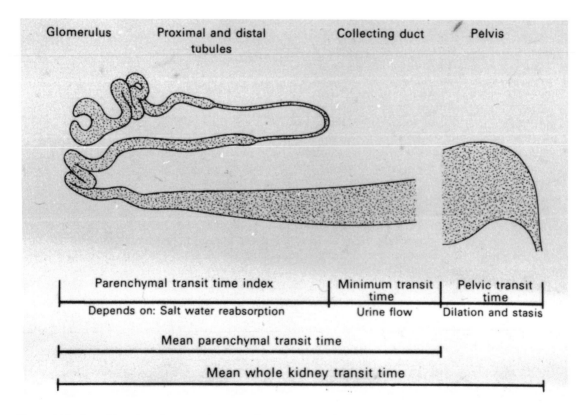

Figure 11.2   Renal functions from transit times. The mean parenchymal transit time excludes the pelvic transit time and is best for evaluating renovascular disorder. The minimum transit time common to all nephrons is related to the flow in the collecting ducts common to all nephrons and is subtracted from the mean parenchymal transit time to give the parenchymal transit time index (PTTI), which is best for obstructive nephropathy evaluation. (Reproduced courtesy of the *British Journal of Urology*.)

the mean parenchymal transit time (MPTT) are obtained. (MPTT is used to determine the presence of renovascular disorder.) MPTT is divided into the minimum transit time and the residue, called the parenchymal transit time index (PTTI). This PTTI is the transit time representing mainly activity in the proximal nephron and is most dependent on salt and water and is used to tell whether the patient has an obstructive nephropathy or not. The pelvic transit time is the time through the pelvis and is prolonged if the pelvis is enlarged, whatever the cause such as dilation without obstruction. This is because there will be eddying and mixing in an enlarged pelvis. The renal transit times can be summarized as follows. The very short time for ^{99m}Tc-labelled DTPA to pass the glomerular filter and the slight difference in timing between this and the secretion of ^{99m}Tc-labelled MAG3 or ^{123}I-labelled OIH into the proximal tubular lumen are quite lost in consideration of the nephron transit times when the usual data sampling interval is 10 seconds. The whole kidney transit time (WKTT) is given by the total transit time through renal parenchyme and pelvis. The mean parenchymal transit time (MPTT) is that through the whole of the parenchyme and added together with the pelvic transit time (PVTT) equals WKTT. The mean parenchymal transit time is made up of a minimum transit time (minTT) common to all nephrons, and parenchymal transit time index (PTTI). The whole kidney transit time corrected for the minimum transit time is called the whole kidney transit time index (WKTTI). Thus

$$WKTT = MPTT + PVTT$$

$$MPTT = MinTT + PTTI$$

$$WKTT = MinTT + WKTTI$$

Normal ranges are: PTTI = 10–156 seconds; MPTT 100–240 seconds; WKTTI = 20–170 seconds.

When first published [4], the transit times were given in 2-second intervals and compared with the antegrade perfusion pressure measurements. In those patients where there was outflow obstruction according to the criterion of a resistance increasing the pressure to over 20 cm of water pressure, then the parenchymal transit time index was over 160 seconds. However, in a few patients with pelvic outflow disorder with no evidence of a positive pressure response to the antegrade perfusion measurements, the PTTI value was up

to 142 seconds. The normal value was taken as 156 seconds and below.

It is necessary to separate the pelvis from the parenchyme. Often it is obvious and a region of interest can be drawn. A reliable way when the separation is not obvious is to make a mean time image. The 2-minute image of the kidney has no pelvis or calyceal activity because nothing has reached there yet. This is the first template. At 15 minutes, if the border between pelvis or calyces and parenchyme cannot be drawn, then the matrix of pixels and the activity–time curve in each pixel is obtained. This is representative of a mean time by an area over height method for each pixel. If it is a parenchymal pixel it will have a short mean time. If it is a calyceal pixel it will have at least 2 minutes before activity appears and therefore it will have a long mean time. If the mean time image is obtained and colour-coded so that any pixel that has a short mean time has a low intensity and any pixel with a long mean time has a high intensity, a generous region of interest can be drawn around the pelvicalyceal system. The parenchymal region is thus separated, from which the parenchymal activity–time curve is obtained for deconvolution with the blood clearance curve. From the intact nephron hypothesis, a part of the kidney parenchyme is representative of the whole, unless there is a calyceal obstruction in one calyx, in which case the kidney divides into two regions and each is treated separately.

UPTAKE AND OUTPUT COMPONENTS

The activity–time curve recorded over a kidney using an externally placed detector or gamma-camera represents the variation with time of the quantity of radiation arriving at the detector from radioactive material within its field of view. When the organ of interest is the kidney and a probe detector is used then the activity–time curve has been called the 'renogram' and the technique 'renography'. When the gamma-camera is used, the term renal radionuclide study is preferred for the technique and 'renogram' is used loosely for the activity–time curve recorded from a region of interest taken to include the kidney.

This 'renal' activity–time curve is a complex and composite curve, $R(t)$. One component is the curve representing the variation with time of the quantity of activity in non-renal tissue in the chosen region of interest, mainly in front of and behind the kidney; another is the component representing activity in the renal vasculature not taken up by the kidney; and the important component of interest is how the amount of radiotracer activity taken up by the kidney varies with time, which is called the kidney activity–time curve, $K(t)$. This may be considered to have been derived or obtained theoretically as in an idealized situation free of blood and tissue background activity. In practice, the kidney curve is obtained as the resultant activity–time curve after appropriate assumptions or corrections have been applied to the composite activity–time curve $R(t)$, obtained from the gamma-camera, for tissue and blood background activity, depth, attenuation and size of region of interest. The supply curve, i.e. the blood clearance curve $B(t)$ which is usually obtained from a region of interest posteriorly over the left ventricle in the field-of-view of the camera, decreases with time as the radiopharmaceutical is taken up by the kidneys.

Since the non-renal blood and tissue component of the composite externally recorded activity–time curve, $R(t)$, is proportional to the blood clearance curve, the relationship between $R(t)$ and $K(t)$ is given by

$$R(t) = K(t) + F\int B(t)\mathrm{d}t \qquad (11.1)$$

where F is a constant called the blood background subtraction factor. For probe renography the factor F was calculated using a prior injection of radiolabelled human serum albumin [5,6].

The kidney activity–time curve, $K(t)$ – also called the kidney content curve – is itself complex and it can be separated into uptake and removal components [5,6]. Such a separation not only aids an understanding of the underlying physiology but also leads to new ways of analysis for determining renal blood flow [7–9] and for determining the radiotracer output curve and response to frusemide [10,11].

Taking ^{99m}Tc-labelled MAG3 as an example, it is evident that before any MAG3 leaves the kidney parenchyme to enter the pelvis in urine, the amount of MAG3 in the kidney depends on the amount which has been supplied to it in the blood and the renal extraction efficiency. The early part of the kidney activity–time curve during the minimum time of transit of MAG3 from its tubular uptake site along the nephron, and before any urinary loss of MAG3 activity occurs, represents the accumulation with time of MAG3 in the kidney.

The kidney is in effect integrating the uptake of the supplied and extracted MAG3. The MAG3 supplied to the kidney in renal arterial blood can take one of two paths: either it remains in the intrarenal blood circulation returning via the renal vein, or it is taken up by the tubules (with a few percent filtered at the glomerulus). The renal artery to renal vein transit time is of the order of 4 seconds with a range of about 3–20 seconds. The renal uptake of MAG3, the fraction of blood activity taken up per second, designated $U(t)$ (the uptake constant), will be proportional to the blood activity, and the total uptake (during the period of the minimum parenchymal transit time, t) will be proportional to the integral of the blood curve $\int B(t).\mathrm{d}t$.

This is the uptake component $Q(t)$ of $K(t)$:

$$Q(t) = U(t).\int B(t)\mathrm{d}t \qquad (11.2)$$

Then, combining Equations 11.1 and 11.2, during minimum transit time, t, when $K(t) = Q(t)$:

$$R(t) = U(t).\int B(t)\mathrm{d}t + FB(t) \qquad (11.3)$$

Alternatively, dividing both sides of the equation by $B(t)$:

$$\frac{R(t)}{B(t)} = \frac{U(t).\int B(t)\mathrm{d}t}{B(t)} + F. \qquad (11.4)$$

This is in the form y = mx + c, the equation of a straight line. The intercept F and the slope $U(t)$ can be obtained by plotting the actual externally detected renal $R(t)$ divided by the actual background $B(t)$ data against the integral of $B(t)$, $\int B(t)$ divided by $B(t)$. This approach to the measurement of the background component and the individual kidney (IK) uptake constant (i.e. IKGFR for DTPA and IKERPF for radio-iodinated OIH) has been developed by Rutland [7], and applied not only to renal events but also to the renal arterial inflow and outflow. The same logic has been applied to the separate determination of the extravascular and intravascular components of the non-renal activity in the renal region of interest by Peters et al. [9], in selecting the most appropriate region for the background correction of $R(t)$ to give $K(t)$.

Since during the minimum transit time period, $K(t)$ is proportional to $\int B(t)\mathrm{d}t$, consider a situation where no activity appears in the urine for a long time, as with complete outflow obstruction; then the kidney continues to integrate the supply for as long as this period and $K(t)$ becomes the uptake component, $Q(t)$, a 'zero output' curve. Therefore one considers the curve of the integral of the blood clearance curve $\int B(t)dt$ as a representation of the kidney curve that would have been obtained if no activity had left the kidney. Then, by fitting (using a least-squares technique) the integral of the blood clearance curve to the uptake phase of a particular normal or abnormal kidney curve that decreases with time after a delay period, the difference between the two curves (fitted $\int B(t)dt$ and $K(t)$) gives the cumulative output, also called the removal or output component, $O(t)$, (Figure 11.3). Differentiation of the removal component gives the tracer output curve, which is the variation with time of the quantity of tracer leaving the kidney. This should act as a reminder that the falling phase (third phase) of a kidney activity–time curve is not an 'excretory' phase, but an 'amount of tracer left behind in the kidney' phase. Only by deriving the tracer output curve in this way can the true 'excretory' activity–time curve be obtained.

By comparing the removal component with the uptake component an estimate of the efficiency of the process of excretion can be made. An isotope removal factor can be calculated for a series of renal transit times in order to make this compari-

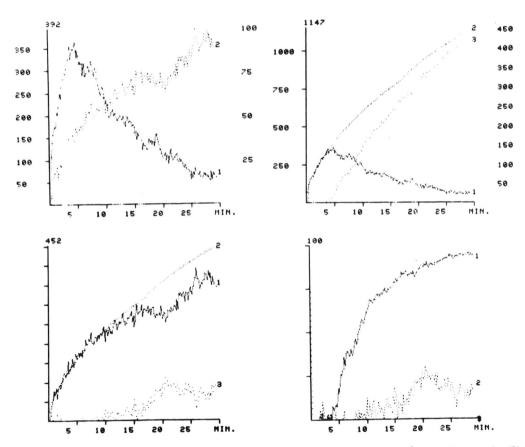

Figure 11.3 Outflow efficiency. Top left shows a normal renogram (1) and a renogram that continues to rise (2). Top right shows the production of the cumulative output curve (3) by subtracting the renogram curve (1) from the integral of the blood clearance curve (2) fitted to the second phase of the renogram. The cumulative output is similar to the cumulative input and the outflow efficiency is over 90%. Bottom left the renogram with a rising curve has the integral of the blood clearance curve fitting to it (2). The difference between the two is the poor cumulative output (3). Bottom right shows the two cumulative outputs. For (1), the cumulative output is normal. For (2), the cumulative output has an outflow efficiency of less than 25% confirming an obstructing uropathy.

son. For example, a kidney recovering after operation for pelviuretic junction obstruction would show progressive improvement of the isotope removal factor with time [5,6]. This approach has been developed by Chaiwatanarat *et al.* [11] to determine the appropriateness of the renal response to frusemide, particularly when renal function is impaired. The output component $O(t)$ is expressed as a percentage of the uptake component $Q(t)$ to give the output efficiency $OE(t)\%$.

$$OE(t)\% = [Q(t)/O(t)] \times 100.$$

The output efficiency may be calculated both before and after frusemide. The normal range of $OE(t)\%$ post-frusemide in patients with a dilated pelvis is better than 78% and similar to the normal range in patients with no outflow disorder. This means that over 78% of that which entered the kidney has left the kidney by 30 minutes. An inappropriately impaired response to frusemide gives a value below 78%.

A general discussion of these analysis methods is given by Britton and Brown [5,6], Peters [12,13] and Rutland [14].

RENAL RADIOPHARMACEUTICALS

The main agents are shown in Table 11.1.

^{99m}Tc-LABELLED MAG3

The disadvantages of the current renal imaging agents ^{99m}Tc-labelled DTPA and radio-iodinated OIH have led many workers to search for a better agent. The properties of an ideal substitute for radio-iodinated OIH are as follows. It should be labelled with ^{99m}Tc. It should have an extraction efficiency at least three times greater than ^{99m}Tc-labelled DTPA, i.e. over 60%, and preferably better than radio-iodinated OIH. It should be a stable compound easily prepared from a robust kit, cheap to purchase and easy to use. It should show weak or no protein binding to improve glomerular filtration and tubular secretion.

Compounds based on a linking of three nitrogens and one sulphur atom with ^{99m}Tc, N3-S were developed by Fritzberg *et al.* [15], leading to MAG3, mercaptoacetyltriglycine, which was shown to be tubular secreted by probenecid inhibition studies and equivalent to radioiodinated OIH. The three nitrogens and the sulphur of MAG3 are in a ring structure which is able to bind reduced technetium in a stable way. It also contains the appropriate combination of polar and non-polar groups that make it suitable for proximal tubular uptake, anionic transport and secretion, as a technetium-99m labelled replacement for OIH. The MAG3 kit preparation contains a benzoyl group to protect the ring structure and this must be displaced by a boiling step to enable the binding of technetium-99m in to the ring. MAG3 is supplied in the form of white powder in sealed glass vials. A lead-shielded water bath is prepared and brought to the boil. About 185 MBq (5 mCi) of ^{99m}TcO4 is eluted in the standard way from a technetium generator. Volume dilution of the pertechnetate stock to give the required activity should be only with physiological 0.9% saline.

Table 11.1 Comparison of renal radiopharmceuticals for gamma-camera studies

	^{99m}Tc DTPA	^{99m}Tc MAG3	^{99m}Tc EC	^{123}I-OIH
ERPF, fraction of	0.2	0.67	0.75	1
Dose (MBq)	300	100	80	60
Kidney count rate	low	high	high	high
Background	high	low	low	low
Extraction efficiency	20%	58%	65%	87%
Weak protein binding	<5%	90%	50%	70%
Fraction filtered	100%	2%	10%	6%
volume of distribution	large	small	moderate	large
Availability	Routine	routine	No	weekly
Boiling step	No	yes	No	No
Impurities	Rare	lipophilic, avoided by 'cold' MAG3	?	Free iodine Iodobenzate
Cost	Low	Moderate	–	High

An amount should be calculated so that the volume to be added to the vial of MAG3 is not less than 4 ml and not more than 10 ml. The vial is then placed in the boiling water and left there for 10 minutes. It is then removed and cooled under running tap water or by immersion in cold water. Investigations of this method of preparation have shown that a number of modifications may be made to improve its convenience in routine use. First, the addition of ^{99m}Tc to the MAG3 powder may take place at a time convenient to the radiopharmacist at the time of elution of the generator for routine dispensing. Up to 4 hours may be allowed to elapse before the boiling step. It is, however, important to avoid the entrance of air into the system and to keep the product cold. After boiling for 10 minutes the kit is cooled and can be divided into four portions in four sterile syringes. Each is capped and frozen at 4°C – the 'cold' MAG3 method. When the patient arrives, the syringe is thawed under a table lamp and used. By spreading this arrangement through the day, eight renal studies can be prepared using two MAG3 vials. Radiochromatography shows that the impurities increase with time after the boiling step at room temperature. At 1 hour, less than 5% of non-tubularly secreted MAG3 is present, made up of three or more components, two of which are lipophilic and slowly taken up by the liver and excreted in the bile and intestine. The amount of this hepatic-excreted contaminant depends on the preparation conditions and the length of time between boiling and injection, and not on the level of renal function. The 'cold' MAG3 method reduces this liver contaminant a hundred fold [16]. Delayed imaging and or poor renal function will show stomach, intestinal and colonic activity with time.

Accidental omission of the boiling step leaves benzoyl MAG3, which is a ^{99m}Tc-labelled DTPA-like renal agent. By 5 hours without boiling, much of the benzoyl group has dissociated and 90% is in the form of ^{99m}Tc-labelled MAG3. No adverse effects, either clinical or biochemical, have been demonstrated using ^{99m}Tc-labelled MAG3. ^{99m}Tc-labelled MAG3 shows between 78% and 93% of weak protein binding, which reduces its glomerular filtration in the same way but to a greater extent than radio-iodinated OIH.

The clearance studies showed that ^{99m}Tc-MAG3 had a 65% smaller volume of distribution than ^{131}I-labelled hippuran and a similar blood clearance half-life (slow component ratio ^{99m}Tc-labelled MAG3 : ^{123}I-labelled hippuran is 1.09 : 1). The clearance relationship is:

$$\text{ERPF hippuran} = 1.5 \times \text{ERPF } ^{99m}\text{Tc-labelled} \\ \text{MAG3} + 40\,\text{ml/min} \\ (\text{SEM} = 8\%).$$

Although its clearance had a linear relationship with effective renal plasma flow, ^{99m}Tc-labelled MAG3 is not yet proposed as a substitute for the absolute measurement of glomerular filtration rate (GFR) or ERPF by the appropriate agents [17,18]. The reproducibility of ^{99m}Tc MAG3 studies is assessed by Klingensmith *et al.* [19].

Clinical studies performed have shown it to be a successful radiopharmaceutical for routine renal work, combining the physiological advantages of OIH with the benefits of using ^{99m}Tc label [20,21]. At an administered activity of 100 MBq (2.5 mCi) it is better than 400 MBq (10 mCi) DTPA and equivalent to 80 MBq (2 mCi) of ^{123}I-OIH for routine renal imaging, for relative function measurements, for renal transit time analysis and for frusemide diuresis studies. It is suitable for use for renal transplants and for the measurement of the intrarenal plasma flow distribution.

^{99m}Tc-EC (ETHYLENE DICYSTEINE)

This agent, although not yet commercially in Western Europe may replace ^{99m}Tc-MAG3 because it does not require a boiling step and has a greater extraction efficiency: 75% of that of hippuran. It may be used for the full range of renal radionuclide studies [22–25]. It has a volume of distribution similar to that of hippuran, but lower protein binding (Table 11.1).

^{99m}Tc-DACH (DIAMINOCYCLOHEXANE)

This agent is cationically transported through tubules, a property in common with thiamine, cyclosporin and cisplatinum, as well as being glomerular filtered. It may have a role in assessing cyclosporin toxicity [26–28].

^{99m}Tc-LABELLED DMSA (DIMERCAPTOSUCCINIC ACID)

[99m]Tc-labelled DMSA is a representative of a class of compounds that are taken up and fixed by the kidneys with less than 5% being excreted. In order

to avoid urinary excretion and liver uptake attention to detail is required in their preparation. It is necessary to keep air (oxygen) out of the vials and to use the compound within 30 minutes of preparation. Poor preparations show high urinary loss which may interfere with the measurement of renal function. The compound binds to plasma proteins and then is glomerular filtered [29] and taken up by the kidney tubules. If renal function is poor, uptake by the liver is seen. Acidosis also affects renal uptake [30]. A total of 100 MBq (2.7 mCi) is administered intravenously and static images are taken at 1 hour if renal function is good, or 3 or 6 hours if renal function is poor. Single-photon emission computed tomography (SPECT) studies with DMSA have indicated that they may have advantages over planar studies [31].

^{51}Cr-EDTA

^{51}Cr-EDTA is used for GFR measurement through serial blood samples.

Although many other radiopharmaceuticals have been used to evaluate renal function, those described above will meet all routine clinical requirements.

RENAL CLEARANCE

MEASUREMENT OF INDIVIDUAL RENAL FUNCTION

When a restorative operation on a kidney or nephrectomy is about to be performed electively it is essential to know the contribution that that kidney makes to total renal function. In an adult with a total GFR of over 50 ml / minute, in the presence of obstructive nephropathy or renovascular disorder a kidney contributing less than 7% of total function is usually not worth preserving, but a kidney contribution over 16% is worth preserving by a restorative operation; between 7% and 16% the decision will be affected by other factors: pain, tuberculosis, surgical difficulty, etc. A kidney with better than 20% function may need nephrectomy for tumour or bleeding, for example. Generally kidneys work better than their radiological assessments would suggest and too many kidneys contributing substantial renal function have been removed unnecessarily in the past, particularly in the context of obstructive nephropathy. This was because intravenous urography (IVU) is designed

to give resolution of the anatomical and pathological detail of the cortical outline, calyces and outflow system. If urography had a 'grey scale' representing function levels, it would by its very nature obscure such detail by loss of contrast. The advances in urography have been to improve the demonstration of detail by high-contrast infusion and / or tomography when glomerular filtration is impaired, rather than to improve the measurement of the degree of impairment of GFR. Cortical thickness is also an unreliable guide to function since it varies so much from pole to pole. IVU and CT contrast techniques have been proposed to measure individual renal function but they fail to meet the assumptions of the tracer principle.

It must be made clear, however, that there is no non-invasive method, based on the use of radionuclides, for obtaining a precise estimate of the absolute measure of any function from each kidney in humans. This is because the organ of interest is not the sole organ in the field of view of the radiation detector, the uptake of radionuclide is time-dependent, and the distance of the organ from the detector varies from patient to patient.

The relative contribution of each kidney to total function can be reliably determined as follows. From the regions of interest over the two kidneys, activity–time curves are generated. These are each corrected for the effects of tissue background using the data from superior or C-shaped background regions of interest (ROIs). From these it can be seen that a normal peak occurs at about 150–180 seconds, at which time the initial bolus of tracer entering the kidney starts to leave the kidney. Therefore, no analysis of percentage function can be taken after this time. During the first 90 seconds or so there are unstable conditions with mixing effects and therefore it is best to limit the consideration of relative renal function to that period when uptake is unaffected by these factors, usually between 90 and 150 seconds in kidneys without outflow disorder. The time period may be later, e.g. 3–4 minutes, in kidneys that have outflow disorder. The specified time period can be determined from the time period where the ratio $Q_L / (Q_L + Q_R)$ is a constant. The quantity in a kidney at such a time $Q(t)$ is given by the supply rate, which is RPF × plasma concentration, $P(t)$. This product is multiplied by the extraction efficiency, E, of the tracer. For radioiodinated OIH, RPF × E is called the 'effective renal plasma flow' (ERPF). Thus,

$$Q(t) = \text{ERPF} \times P(t).$$

For ^{99m}Tc-labelled DTPA, $Q(t) = \text{RPF} \times$ the filtration fraction $\times$ the plasma concentration.

The filtration fraction is given by GFR divided by RPF and so this cancels down to the quantity in the kidney being equal to GFR $\times$ the plasma concentration.

Then for the left and right kidneys, the following apply:

For OIH

$$Q_L = \text{ERPF}_L \times P(t)$$

$$Q_R = \text{ERPF}_R \times P(t)$$

For DTPA

$$Q_L = \text{GFR}_L \times P(t)$$

$$Q_R = \text{GFR}_R \times P(t)$$

Since, over a small time interval, $P(t)$ is the same for each kidney and $\text{FF}_L = \text{FF}_R$, then by division:

$$Q_L / Q_R = \text{ERPF}_L / \text{ERPF}_R = \text{GFR}_L / \text{GRF}_R$$

By rearrangement

$$\frac{Q_L}{Q_L + Q_R} = \frac{\text{ERPF}_L}{\text{ERPF}_L + \text{ERPF}_R} = \frac{\text{ERPF}_L}{\text{Total ERPF}}$$

or

$$\frac{\text{GFR}_L}{\text{Total GFR}}$$

Thus, if Q_L and Q_R are measured, the percentage contributions of each kidney to total renal uptake function may be obtained. The problem then is to estimate $Q(t)$, the quantity of OIH or DTPA in each kidney at a given time, in order to obtain $Q_L / (Q_L + Q_R)$.

It is obtained using the regions of interest selected from the gamma-camera as above. $Q(t)$ can be obtained by measuring the relative uptake components of each kidney using the techniques previously described [7,9,32].

The potential errors in measuring $Q(t)$ are not negligible. The most important assumption is that the kidneys are at equal depth so that the attenuation of ^{99m}Tc or radio-iodine may be considered to be equal. With the patient reclining, 75% of kidneys have less than 1 cm difference in depth and the count rate loss is about 10% per cm for ^{99m}Tc or ^{123}I. Such a loss leads to an error of about +3.5% for the measured percentage relative function. Corrections for depth may be undertaken using true lateral views of the kidney [33–35], ultrasound [36] or from a height–weight formula [37].

Errors due to variation of distribution of the radiopharmaceutical in the kidney are probably small: counting errors due to Poisson statistics re-

quire the use of ^{123}I-OIH rather than ^{131}I-OIH, with the gamma-camera giving on average a 20-fold increase in count rate and a five-fold reduction in absorbed dose for the same administered activity. Reduction of non-renal background activity by ROI selection does not eliminate the contribution from anterior and posterior to the kidney, but for ^{99m}Tc and ^{123}I, unlike ^{131}I, the mean effective equivalent source of background is posterior to the kidneys, from the largely symmetrical muscle bulk. Background ROIs for conventional correction should be taken from C-shapes around the cortex of each kidney or from two separate areas above and below each kidney [9]. These ROIs should not include aorta or renal hilum. Testing the chosen background ROI using patients with unilateral nephrectomy is wise since differences in equipment, particularly collimation and data processing, give slightly differing results. It is not ideal since the intrarenal blood pool is missing. The alternative approach is by interpolative background subtraction [38,39]. This gives reliable results in moderately well-functioning kidneys but may lead to gross errors when one kidney's contribution is less than 15% of total function – the very circumstances when such a correction is required.

The normal range for relative uptake function determined in practice and thus incorporating both biological variation and physical sources of error is 42.5–57.5% for one kidney's contribution. The accuracy of a particular figure depends on the overall renal function and the number of nephrons in a kidney, but the standard error ranges from 4.5% at 40% of total uptake with a creatinine clearance of 90 ml/minute to 7.5% at 20% of total uptake at a creatinine clearance of 20 ml/minute. Nevertheless, this accuracy is sufficient for most clinical applications since the usual decision is whether to perform nephrectomy or a restorative operation.

In order to obtain the flow to each kidney in millilitres per minute, the percentage relative function is applied to the total GFR or ERPF as appropriate. Because of the arguments set out above and the intact nephron hypothesis, the same equations apply to the relative function determined by ^{99m}Tc-labelled MAG3 [20,40], or by the use of ^{99m}Tc-labelled DMSA [41]. The preferred method for determining relative function (RF) with ^{99m}Tc-labelled DMSA is to use the geometric mean of background corrected anterior (A) and posterior (P), left (L) and right (R) renal counts (C), taken between 2 and 3 hours after injection [42]:

$$RF_L\% = \frac{\sqrt{(C_{LP} \times C_{LA})}}{\sqrt{(C_{LP} \times C_{LA})} + \sqrt{(C_{RP} \times C_{RA})}} \times 100\%$$

The percentage uptake should rise gradually after successful treatment to one kidney to relieve inflow or outflow disorder assuming unchanging function in the other. The rate of improvement will depend on many factors, such as the length of time that an obstruction has been there before its successful relief.

The uptake function is made up of two components. First, an irreversible component which depends on the number of nephrons present and which can only change for the worse when there is destruction of nephrons as, for example, by infection or tumour. Second, a reversible component in which nephron function such as ERPF or GFR falls as a physiological control response to some pathological process, to rise again when such a process is corrected. To take an example, a stone obstructing the renal outflow tract will lead to a reduction in GFR through its normal autoregulatory response to a rise in resistance to outflow, but when the stone is removed this resistance falls and GFR returns towards normal. However, if the obstructing stone is associated with infection in the kidney then the infection may cause nephron damage and thereby loss of functioning nephrons. Such a loss of nephrons will not be made up when the infection is treated by removal of the stone and by antibiotics, and that component of uptake function will not improve.

In the context of bilateral outflow obstruction – for example due to bilateral stone disease – Sreenevasan [2] showed that, in deciding which kidney should have its obstruction relieved, measurement of relative uptake function was crucial. The kidney with the better uptake function as demonstrated by renography was the kidney on which to operate first. Its better initial function would lead to a quicker recovery from obstruction and thus the clinical situation would be stabilized sooner.

HYPERTENSION

INTRODUCTION

For the patient, the taking of treatment for hypertension is essentially the paying of the premium of an insurance policy, in that long-term reduction of blood pressure reduces the incidence of the complications of heart failure, stroke and renal impairment. The incidence of myocardial infarction also falls if other risk factors are controlled at the same time. Depending on the selection of patients attending the general practitioner or the special clinic, and their age, so the incidence of causes for hypertension varies between 1 in 20 and 1 in 8. The most common cause is bilateral renal disease. Depending on further selection, between 1% and 5% of hypertensives can be shown to have a renal or adrenal disorder whose correction by surgery will lead to amelioration of hypertension. Since virtually all hypertension responds to the right combination of drugs, the question is whether the pursuit of these few is worthwhile. This depends on whether the clinical tests demonstrating those likely to benefit from surgery are sufficiently simple, non-invasive, reliable and cost effective; and whether the patient should be denied the right to choose a possibility of cure, whether by surgery or angioplasty as an alternative to a life-time of drug taking. For those that answer these questions affirmatively the search for these few may be considered as a five stage process:

1. Identification of the hypertensives in the population.
2. Selection of hypertensives that possibly have correctable lesions.
3. Demonstration of those with the functional pattern of renovascular disorder.
4. Definition of the surgical anatomy.
5. Making the choice between angioplasty, a restorative operation and nephrectomy.

What is required is an evaluation of what each technique can and cannot do, and the scientific basis for its use; and for each hospital to outline a strategy of investigation and management. This will be different for different hospitals, partly because of the differing prevalence of renovascular hypertension, partly because of different availability of equipment, and partly because of differing expertise in the use and interpretation of results obtained with such equipment. Thus, as in most of medicine, there is no one right way of solving a diagnostic or patient management problem (Table 11.2).

In essential hypertension, the renal images are of similar size, the renograms are symmetrical, relative functions and peak times are also similar.

Table 11.2 Hypertension: assessment of renovascular hypertension

Hypertension: case finding for renovascular disorder
1. Renal radionuclide study – baseline
                             – captopril intervention
2. Positive study – large-vessel or small-vessel disease?
    Small vessel:
        clinical, urine: infection, casts, proteins, sugar, etc.
        renal function, glomerulonephritis, diabetes, etc.
    Large vessel:
        Doppler US, MRI?
3. Positive study
    Is control of blood pressure good?
        Serial renal readionuclide studies
4. Positive study
    Is control of blood pressure poor or deterioration in renal function?
5. Renal artery stenosis
    Angioplasty, surgery or nephrectomy if relative function is less then 7% of total.
6. Improvement in hypertension
    Serial renal radionuclide studies to demonstrate improvement in renal function and to detect return of renovascular disorder, e.g. due to restenosis.

Hypertension: alternative approaches
1. (a) Small kidney or not?
        US (IVU, XCT, MRI)
  (b) Reduced flow or not?
        Doppler US (MRI)
  (c) Renal artery stenosis, incidental on angiography, e.g. for peripheral vascular disease.
2. Proceed to assessment of presence of renovascular disorder:
    renal radionuclide studies:
    base line + captopril or captopril intervention alone.

The mean parenchymal transit times are normal. Cortical nephron flow is reduced equally in each kidney and may be improved by angiotensin converting enzyme inhibitors [43,44].

RENOVASCULAR HYPERTENSION

In renovascular hypertension the crucial clinical problem is whether successful correction of an arterial stenosis to one kidney is likely to relieve the hypertension. Renovascular hypertension may be defined as being present in those patients in whom an occlusive lesion (or lesions) of the large or small arteries or arterioles is associated with a particular pattern of renal function and in whom angioplasty, surgical repair of the lesion, or nephrectomy is likely to relieve the hypertension.

If no corrective procedure is undertaken to be followed by prolonged relief of hypertension, the diagnosis of renovascular hypertension remains in doubt, although the pattern of disordered renal function may be typical. Five statements may be made about renal radionuclide studies in renovascular hypertension.

1. Renovascular disorder is not renal artery stenosis.
2. Renovasular disorder is most commonly due to small-vessel disease, usually bilateral.
3. Renal radionuclide studies do not distinguish small-vessel from large-vessel disease as the cause of renovascular hypertension.
4. Angiographic renal artery narrowing is common particularly in the elderly. Only the renographic demonstration of the characteristic functional abnormality shows that there is renovascular disorder causing hypertension. Proof is only given when correction of the renovascular disorder (or nephrectomy) gives prolonged correction of the hypertension and returns the functional abnormality to normal.
5. It is not uncommon to find a small kidney on one side in hypertensive patients. Homer Smith [45] stated if all small kidneys in this situation

were excised, about 25% of patients would recover from hypertension. His challenge was how to tell which 25%.

The other kidney is important. It must not have renovascular disorder for relief of a contralateral renal artery stenosis to improve hypertension.

This functional pattern has three features relevant to radionuclide studies. First, there is an increased proximal tubular water and salt reabsorption related to the slight relative reduction in peritubular capillary pressure due to the occlusive arterial or arteriolar lesions. A non-reabsorbable solute such as ^{99m}Tc-MAG3 will therefore become relatively concentrated within a pool of fluid that travels more slowly along the nephron. The time to peak of the renogram which represents a crude measure of the mean transit time of MAG3 entering and leaving the kidney will be prolonged as compared with a normal kidney. A reduction of the perfusion pressure is associated with a reduction of medullary blood flow whose consequence is an improvement in the concentration gradient in the medulla with increased reabsorption of water from the collecting duct, and a slowing of flow in it with further prolongation of the time of transit of a non-reabsorbable solute. Thus, the MPTT of a non-reabsorbable solute, whether it be OIH, DTPA, MAG3, EC, or whatever, will be increased. In the absence of outflow system disorder and in a normally hydrated person this explains why a difference of over a minute between peak times in the two renograms is an indicator of prolonged MAG3 transit [46]. Similarly, the corticopelvic transfer time is prolonged over 190 seconds [47]. Second, the blood supply and therefore delivery of the radiopharmaceutical to the kidney with renovascular disorder is reduced below normal due to the occlusive arterial or arteriolar lesions. An uptake function less than 42% of total function is abnormal, and the second phase of the renogram of the affected usually smaller kidney is impaired. It should, however, be noted that renal artery stenosis is not an all-or-none phenomenon and in the early 'unstable' stage only a difference in peak time may be seen, without reduction in function. The third requirement is that the 'non-affected' kidney has not itself undergone small vessel renovascular disorder as a consequence of hypertension. This may be demonstrated by the normality of the renogram from the unaffected kidney. A non-affected kidney should have an ERPF of at least 300 ml/minute.

The selection from hypertensive patients of those that might have a renovascular disorder used to be most simply undertaken by probe renography [48,49]. These authors showed that 99.4% of 980 essential hypertensives with normal renograms were correctly assumed to be free of significant unilateral renal parenchymal or renovascular disease. They found no benefit in pursuing further investigations for renovascular disorder in hypertensives with normal results of renography. Taking angiographic demonstration of renal artery stenosis as the gold standard, Britton and Brown [5] showed that 90% of patients with a 'false-positive' probe renogram had elevated peripheral renins, indicating the likelihood of small-vessel disorder causing 'high-renin' essential hypertension. Renal radionuclide studies do not and cannot in principle distinguish small-vessel from large-vessel causes of renovascular disorder. Nordyke *et al.* [50] found that 15% of their hypertensive patients had abnormal findings from standard probe renography, and in one-third of these after further tests, surgery for renovascular disorder was undertaken and ameliorated hypertension.

These findings may be contrasted with the use of rapid sequence IVU. One in four patients with successfully corrected renovascular disorder have an undiagnostic rapid sequence IVU; hypertension *per se* is no longer an indication for an IVU. Ultrasound is used by some as a screen for unequal renal size and will also demonstrate pelvic dilatation, but it gives no functional information. Doppler ultrasound is an approach to demonstrating the presence of a renal artery stenosis causing an increased pressure gradient through change in the wave form and time characteristics of the response. It is cost-effective when carried out by an expert, but there is a 17% failure rate [51].

Using a conventional gamma-camera technique, different authors place different emphases on the features that are extractable from the study. A conventional region of interest around each kidney and a C-shaped background for each kidney are used to obtain whole kidney background-corrected activity–time curves. Rapid recording of the initial arrival of activity at the kidney using 2-second frames and with a ROI over the left ventricle or aorta demonstrates the aortic to renal 'appearance time', which may be prolonged if renal plasma flow is reduced. However, the technique is not reliable in diagnosis of renovascular disorders, because of the arrival of activity in vascular underlying and overlying tissue such as the gastrointestinal tract.

The distribution of uptake in the kidneys at 2 minutes is important and will be decreased in significant renovascular disorders. Reduction of size is typical of but not specific for renovascular disorder and a normal-sized kidney does not exclude it. Parenchymal defects such as infarct, small or large cystic disease and pyelonephritic scars may be noted. Functionally significant branch artery stenosis may be identified as delayed parenchymal uptake at one pole of a kidney and this may also be noted with the patchy microangiopathy sometimes associated with use of the contraceptive pill. Such appearances are due to local prolongation of the tracer's mean parenchymal transit time. Duplex kidneys may be shown, one moiety of which is ischaemic.

Asymmetry of renal uptake function is the first step towards the demonstration of stable, unilateral, functionally significant renovascular disorder.

MEAN PARENCHYMAL TRANSIT TIME

The second requirement is the demonstration of an abnormally prolonged mean parenchymal transit time which reflects the second disorder of renal function in the ischaemic kidney: that of increased salt and water reabsorption due to a tiny reduction of peritubular capillary pressure relative to the intratubular luminal pressure in the proximal tubules. Thirdly there is also an increase in medullary concentrating ability through the reduction in juxtamedullary (JM) nephron flow. JM nephrons cannot autoregulate in response to the fall in perfusion pressure and their efferent arteriolar tone is heightened by the increased circulating angiotensin II. The flow of fluid in the collecting ducts is thus reduced. In consequence, the MPTT is prolonged in renovascular disorder because of both the prolonged minimum transit time and a prolonged PTTI. The separation of the pelvis from the parenchyme for the calculation of MPTT is important since it obviates the effect of changes in pelvic transit time by which the specificity of the WKTT or peak time of activity–time curve is reduced. Thus, in renovascular hypertension, the MPTT of a non-reabsorbable

solute, whether it be hippuran, DTPA, MAG3 or EC will be increased. This is usually reflected as a delayed peak to the renogram.

In a normal hydrated hypertensive patient, a mean parenchymal transit time over 240 seconds or, in a small kidney, over 1 minute should lead to a captopril intervention study. Taken together with an uptake function of less than 42%, this is strongly suggestive of functionally significant renovascular disorder. Such finding does not distinguish between large-vessel and small-vessel disease. Normals (kidney donors) showed equal percentage relative function (RF%) of $50 \pm 8\%$, and MPTT of 171 ± 43 seconds. Hypertensive patients with radiologically significant unilateral renal artery stenosis showed RF% less than 30% and a prolonged MPTT of 344 ± 76 seconds. The contralateral unaffected kidney showed a normal MPTT of 186 ± 32 seconds, similar to that of hypertensive patients without renal artery stenosis (222 ± 87 seconds). The prolonged MPTT in unilateral renal artery stenosis was significantly different from the other groups [52]. Bilaterally prolonged MPTT was seen in patients with impaired renal function due to small-vessel disease. Bilateral functionally significant renal artery stenosis is rare and causes bilateral prolongation of MPTT. Renal activity–time curves and MPTT findings more usually demonstrate that one stenosis is significant at the time of the study when arteriography shows bilateral stenoses.

Congenitally small kidney and the small kidney due to pyelonephritis unilaterally will have a normal parenchymal transit time if they are an incidental occurrence in a hypertensive patient. The unilaterally small pyelonephritic kidney with a prolonged mean parenchymal transit time may be considered usually to have renovascular disorder and contributing to hypertension. Smith [53] and Luke *et al.* [54] showed that only about one-quarter of nephrectomies for unilaterally small kidneys in hypertensives would relieve hypertension.

It should also be noted that the demonstration of a renal artery stenosis incidentally in a hypertensive patient, for example undergoing aortography for peripheral vascular disease, does not mean it is necessarily contributing to hypertension, particularly in the elderly. Essential hypertension and atheroma are both common and less than 1% of all hypertension is due to renal artery stenosis. Fibromuscular hyperplasia is typically found in the artery of a mobile kidney usually on the right side in a tall or thin woman and it may be due to the artery taking on a support function for the kidney. It is a correctable cause of renovascular disorder.

One can summarize the functional changes of renovascular disorder as the following:

1. Loss of autoregulation of cortical nephrons, due to maximal arteriolar dilation in response to the fall in perfusion pressure.
2. Increased passive reabsorption of salt and water in the proximal tubule due to a slight relative reduction of peritubular capillary pressure as compared with intraluminal pressure.
3. Increased urinary concentration in the medulla due to reduced medullary blood flow.
4. Prolonged parenchymal transit time of non-reabsorbable solutes such as DTPA, OIH and MAG3 causing a prolongation of MPTT, typically giving rise to a delayed peak to the renogram.
5. Renin production and release into the circulation.
6. Increased efferent arteriolar tone of the JM nephrons due to the increased circulating angiotensin II.

Significant renovascular disorder can occur with normal peripheral and renal vein renins. Renal size is not a reliable indication of relative renal function. The presence of renovascular disorder may be found in the presence of normal renal arteries on angiography in the situation of, for example, glomerulonephritis, pyelonephritis, diabetic or interstitial nephritis.

THE CAPTOPRIL RENAL
RADIONUCLIDE STUDY

The difference between essential hypertension and renovascular disorder can be enhanced by the use of an angiotensin converting enzyme (ACE) inhibitor such as captopril. The enhancement of the functional abnormality of renovascular disorder is through the following mechanisms.

1. It will tend to reduce blood pressure and thus reduce the perfusion pressure to cortical and juxtamedullary nephrons. However, it is not the reduction of blood pressure that is the important stimulus. Reduction of blood

pressure can be obtained by many other hypotensive agents which do not have the characteristics of ACE inhibitors in improving the diagnosis of renovascular disorder. So small, non-blood pressure-lowering doses of captopril (e.g. 25 mg) are to be preferred to larger doses.
2. Angiotensin II has a vasoconstrictor effect on efferent arterioles. In the human kidney the efferent arterioles of cortical nephrons have virtually no muscle in them, and therefore there is very little, if any, effect of circulating angiotensin II on the efferent arterioles of cortical nephrons (their control is through the afferent arterioles). However, the JM nephrons have thick muscular efferent arterioles which control their blood flow. Circulating angiotensin II is an important vasoconstrictor for these. ACE inhibition causes a fall in circulating angiotensin II and thus a loss of constriction of the efferent arterioles of the JM nephrons. This lack of resistance causes a dramatic fall in JM nephron glomerular filtration rate, which is one of the features of captopril intervention.
3. Captopril will inhibit the intrarenal angiotensin II activity in the juxtaglomerular apparatus. Thus, if an afferent arteriole of a cortical nephron is not fully vasodilated in an autoregulatory response to the arterial or arteriolar narrowing, then it will dilate further, tending to increase the flow through a cortical nephron. In essential hypertension where afferent arterioles of cortical nephrons are vasoconstricted to a greater extent than normal, their vasodilation due to captopril [43] is the main reason for the improvement in MPTT.
4. Angiotensin II has an activity on tubular function which will be affected by ACE inhibitors, prolonging further the transit time of non-reabsorbable solutes. In essential hypertension this effect will not be seen.

TECHNIQUE OF CAPTOPRIL INTERVENTION
AND INTERPRETATION

^{99m}Tc-DTPA is only suitable for the test if renal function is good. ^{123}I-Hippuran, ^{99m}Tc-MAG3 or ^{99m}Tc-EC [25] are to be preferred if renal function is poor, or if there is a small kidney.

The data should be recorded from the start in 10-second frames from ROIs over the left ventricular cavity and over the two kidneys. The left ventricular cavity activity time curve gives a good input function for subsequent deconvolution. The baseline curve normally has an impaired second phase, a delayed peak and sometimes an impaired third phase in functionally significant renovascular disorder. The delayed peak time is a crude reflection of the prolonged MPTT. After captopril, the second phase may or may not become more impaired. The peak time will be further delayed and the third phase may not be seen at all. There is a deterioration of the curve, depending on to what extent the blood flow and glomerular filtration rate have fallen. The MPTT should be obtained by deconvolution of the input function and the parenchymal activity–time curve to give the MPTT whose normal value is less than 240 seconds with a borderline range of 220–240 seconds. In functionally significantly renovascular disorder due to large- or small-vessel disease, this is typically prolonged greater than 240 seconds [52], and with the captopril test it is prolonged even further [55]. Whether a baseline renal radionuclide study is required as well as the captopril intervention will depend on the referral pattern of patients to the department. Primary or secondary referral will require it, whereas tertiary referral may not.

If one kidney appears smaller than the other, but its activity–time curve is normal or MPTT is borderline, captopril intervention may be recommended.

For captopril intervention, the patient should be off diuretics for 3 days, off captopril for 2 days, and off other ACE inhibitors for 7 days. The patient should be normally hydrated and reclining against the gamma-camera. Blood pressure should be monitored before and at 5- to 10-minute intervals after oral administration of captopril (25 mg). The renal radionuclide study should start if the diastolic pressure falls 10 mmHg or at 1 hour. ^{99m}Tc-MAG3 (100 MBq; up to 3 mCi) is given as a bolus and recordings made at a 10-second frame rate for 30 minutes. A baseline study when renal function is fair may be followed 2 hours later by captopril intervention on the same day, provided that the patient is properly prepared.

The interpretation of the response to captopril should be based on both visual and numerical criteria.

The images may show an increased corticopelvic transfer time. The activity–time curve changes were classified by Oei [56]. Typically, a normal-shaped renogram shows change from a reduction in second phase and a further delay in peak time at least over 60 seconds to a rising curve without a peak. The poorer the initial renogram, the less the visual change with captopril intervention. The relative function typically shows a 5% reduction on the affected side. These criteria were used for the successful European multicentre trial of captopril intervention [57]. Using ^{99m}Tc-DTPA, angiography sensitivity for unilateral renal artery stenosis was 73% and for bilateral stenosis 91%. Taking the overall population, specificity was 84% for unilateral and 92% for bilateral stenosis, and prediction of reduction of hypertension was 93% for unilateral and 88% for bilateral stenosis. A 5% reduction in relative function may not be seen and this lack of change should not exclude a positive response, if other criteria are positive and the MPTT is prolonged. A greater than 10% reduction in relative function with ACE inhibitor is fairly specific. Nally *et al.* [58] proposed probabilistic criteria for interpretation.

- Low probability: normal findings or improvement in abnormal base line findings after ACE inhibition. (This is typical of essential hypertension.)
- Indeterminate probability: abnormal baseline unchanged by ACE inhibition. Specificity for renal artery stenosis is poor since such features may be due to small-vessel disease. MPTT helps to evaluate this population. Prolongation of MPTT from borderline to abnormal indicated renovascular disorder is present due to small- or large-vessel disease, but from abnormal to very prolonged is likely to be due to critical renal artery stenosis [55]. No change or improvement in MPTT makes renovascular disorder unlikely.
- High probability: marked deterioration of the renogram with ACE inhibition.

Taylor and Nally [59] have reviewed published studies and a consensus report on ACE inhibitor renography recommends good practice [60].

Once the combination of unilaterally reduced uptake, prolonged MPTT, a positive captopril test, and a contralateral normal kidney is found in a hypertensive patient – particularly if blood pressure is difficult to control – the next step, after considering that small-vessel disease is unlikely, is renal arteriography (Table 11.1). The patient's blood pressure must be controlled as well as possible. This procedure should include a free aortic injection as well as selective catheterization to check the renal ostium and the number of renal arteries.

Selective renal vein sampling for plasma renin activity is still practised in some centres. As well as the renal vein samples, a low inferior vena cava (IVC) sample must be obtained. It should be noted that over three-quarters of the renin that leaves by the renal vein entered by the renal artery, so the correct estimation of renin output is given by individual kidney plasma flow × the renin arteriovenous difference. However, a renal vein renin activity twice that from the non-affected kidney has been used as an indicator of renovascular disorder [61].

The decision to carry out nephrectomy or not depends partly on the contribution that the affected kidney makes to total uptake function. A nephrectomy is indicated if this is less than 7% and a restorative operation if it is more than 16% of total function. Between these limits, the decision depends on other factors such as the complexity of the surgical anatomy, the overall renal function, and the clinical state of the patient. In bilateral renal artery stenosis it is usual that only one is functionally significant. Angioplasty may be appropriate and it is an unwise surgeon who attempts to revascularize both renal arteries at the same time, as the morbidity and mortality even in the best hands outweigh any likely benefits. The success of the captopril intervention and MPTT measurement in predicting the outcome of angioplasty of the renal artery stenosis and the importance of using MPTT in the follow-up to detect restenosis have been demonstrated.

Finally, to answer Homer Smith's original question: if 100 hypertensive patients with a small kidney on one side and a normal kidney on the other side have all the small kidneys excised, about 25% of these patients will lose their hypertension. How to choose the 25%? The answer is by identifying the typical findings of a renovascular disorder on baseline and captopril renal radionuclide studies. If the shape of the renogram and/or the MPTT are normal on the side of the small kidney, it is not causing renovascular disorder.

In conclusion, the renal radionuclide study, with baseline and captopril intervention provide the appropriate cost-effective way of demonstrating renovascular disorder in hypertension [51]. The techniques of IVU, ultrasound, X-ray, CT and MRI may demonstrate that a kidney is small or has a reduced blood flow but are unable to demonstrate the particular functional disorder of renovascular hypertension. Demonstration of a narrowed renal artery and its anatomy is required before angioplasty and surgery, but does not show whether it is functionally significant. The renal radionuclide study shows the presence or absence of renovascular disorder both before and after correction of a renal artery stenosis.

A captopril intervention study enables one to evaluate whether ACE inhibition is of benefit or is detrimental to renal function in patients with renal impairment [62–64].

Recently, aspirin – as an inhibitor of prostaglandin-mediated vasodilation in the kidney – has been proposed as an alternative to captopril for intervention [65].

OBSTRUCTIVE NEPHROPATHY

INTRODUCTION

In obstructive nephropathy, definitions are important:

- **Obstructive uropathy**: this is a change in the outflow tract which is suggestive of an obstructing process being present, such as pelvic dilatation seen on ultrasound. Dilatation does not mean obstruction.
- **Obstructing uropathy**: this is a change in the outflow tract due to an increased resistance to flow above normal. 'Obstructing' instead of 'obstructive' uropathy indicates confirmation of the presence of an obstructing process.
- **Obstructive nephropathy**: this is the effect of an obstructing process on the kidney.
- **Diuresis renography**: this is the use of a pharmacologically active diuretic before, during or after injection of the radionuclide labelled agent excreted by the kidney. The convention is to use minus time e.g. –15 (minutes), 0, or plus time e.g. +18 (minutes) to indicate the timing of the injection of the diuretic to that of the radionuclide [66].
- **Obstructing process**: this is an increase above normal of the resistance to outflow and this has a number of different consequences. Acute obstruction is the province of intravenous urography, IVU and ultrasound. Chronic

obstruction to outflow means chronically increased resistance to outflow. There is still fluid flowing down the ureter in the presence of a chronically increased resistance to outflow.

The causes of the chronic obstruction include pelviureteric junction disorder, stones, malignancies of various sorts, benign strictures and other benign causes of narrowing of the outflow tract such as retroperitoneal fibrosis. A clinical history and an examination must be performed. Normally, intravenous urography or ultrasound is done in this situation to see if there is an obstructive uropathy – in other words, dilatation of the outflow tract. A renal radionuclide study follows to show if there is an increased resistance to outflow, an obstructing uropathy causing an obstructive nephropathy. Antegrade perfusion pressure measurements, antegrade or retrograde contrast studies might follow.

Direct antegrade perfusion of the pelvis with pressure measurements is the technique of Whitaker [67], who showed that, if under local anaesthetic one punctures into the pelvis (through the cortex of the kidney in order to hold the needle steady), then the pelvis can be perfused with saline at different rates, typically 10 ml/minute. A pressure transducer system records if there is a rising pressure due to this high flow. If there is no change in pressure, the flow rate is increased to 20 ml/minute and if there is still no pressure rise, then there is no resistance to outflow. In other words, although the pelvis is dilated there is no obstructing uropathy. On the other hand, if there is an increasing pressure that exceeds 15 cm of water or 13 mmHg, there is a resistance to flow. This was used as a standard. The disadvantages are that it is an invasive technique, and if there is leakage around the needle there will fail to be a pressure rise in the patient with an obstructing uropathy. Alternatively, the IVU can be used with a diuresis with frusemide at 20 minutes. The dilated pelvis 15 minutes later has changed in size. If it increases in size by over 22% on planimetry, that would be an indication of an obstructing uropathy [68]. If it does not increase in size, or increases by no more than 10%, then that is taken as the normal response to frusemide. In the past many patients were operated on because of loin pain and dilated pelvis on the urogram on the side of the pain, but with no evidence of resistance to outflow. Just looking at a dilated pelvis on ultrasound or urography cannot distinguish an increased resistance to outflow from normal.

The renal radionuclide study gives a whole range of events: images, activity–time curves, relative function, the response to frusemide, the outflow efficiency, and measurements of transit times including the PTTI. It shows the responses of the kidney to the obstructing process, the obstructive nephropathy. The reason that a surgeon wants to operate on the outflow tract is not to make it look more normal, but actually to improve or prevent the deterioration of renal function as well as relieving pain. A set of images with ^{99m}Tc-MAG3 which show retention in the pelvis may or may not respond to frusemide given at 18–20 minutes. Either the diuretic caused no response and the response is considered 'obstructive', or there is a 'normal' response which is considered 'non-obstructive'. The problem is that there is an important group which is often wrongly called 'partial obstruction' – wrongly because partial obstruction is no answer to the problem. The surgeon cannot reach for half a knife to do half an operation. He or she must make the decision to operate or not and this depends on whether there is an increased resistance to outflow causing an obstructive nephropathy or not. This weakness of the frusemide response when it is indeterminate, often occurs in the 'difficult' patients, particularly if renal function is impaired [69].

In a patient with hydronephrosis, the activity–time curve is usually a rising curve, even when the relative function of the two kidneys is the same. Clearly, there is a function of the kidney which is different between the hydronephrotic and the normal kidney, and it is the time that it is taking for the activity that was taken up by the kidney to move through the nephrons, the pelvis and out of the system. It is called the **transit time**. The uptake function, giving the total and relative function, and the transit times are two independent variables that can be used to evaluate an obstructive nephropathy.

FORCE, RESISTANCE AND TIME

The physical basis of obstructive nephropathy should be understood. The **force** comes first from cardiac output and the force acts on a **resistance** and this give rise to a **pressure**. Pressure may be measured as the consequence of a force acting on a resistance. If there is a pressure difference between two points there is a **pressure gradient**, and if there is fluid in the system there will be **flow** from the higher to the lower pressure. If there is flow between two points there will be a **time** taken for a tracer flowing between those points. The time it takes to go from one point to the other is the **transit time**. In chronic outflow obstruction the force is the same, the heart is still beating and filtration is going on, but the resistance is increased. The pressure gradient changes from the source of the force to the site of the resistance. So, there is not just a pressure change in the pelvis because for example, there is a pelviureteric junction resistance, there is a pressure change all through the kidney from the force which is at the site of glomerular filtration right to the point of resistance. There is no such thing as 'back pressure' on the kidney. Pressure is equal and opposite in all directions. If the pressure gradient increases in the tubules, then there will be increased salt and water reabsorption by that kidney in the proximal tubules and therefore the flow in the lumens of the nephrons will be reduced. Therefore, the time it takes to go from the glomerulus to the site of the obstruction will be prolonged and non-reabsorbable solutes, such as MAG3, DTPA, Hippuran or whatever, will take longer to transit the kidney. The resistance to flow is transduced to a prolongation of the renal transit time.

Micropuncture studies have shown that if there is an increase in the pressure in the lumen of the tubule relative to the peritubular capillary by fractions of 1 mmHg, then increased reabsorption occurs passively between tubule cells through the so-called 'tight' junctions (which are loose) of salt and water and other electrolytes into the peritubular capillaries. This is the basis of the increased transit time of the non-reabsorbable solutes. To summarize: an increased resistance to outflow gives a slightly increased pressure in the lumen of the tubule. Increased salt and water reabsortion decreases fluid flow in the lumen of the tubule and therefore there is a prolonged transit time of the non-reabsorbable solutes. Therefore, an abnormal parenchymal transit time will be an indicator of obstructive nephropathy.

The PTTI (p. 394) will work in patients who have poor renal function, when deconvolution is performed properly, whereas the frusemide response may differ. The frusemide response may be normal if there is a very stiff pelvis in spite of there being an increased resistance to outflow causing the parenchymal transit index time to be prolonged. Alternatively, if the kidney has very good uptake function, a mild but abnormal resistance may be overcome by a high diuresis. The transit times may be normal and the response to frusemide may be impaired if the renal function is much reduced; or, if there is a very large hydronephrosis and or mega/ureter, into which the discharged activity is diluted.

One must highlight the fact that two different kidney functions can be measured with radionuclides, for example, in a patient with renal stone disease. The stone could be just in the kidney and there is normal uptake and normal transit times so there is no obstructive nephropathy; or else normal uptake and a prolonged transit time so that there is an obstructive nephropathy but it has not yet altered the kidney function; or else reduced uptake and a normal transit time so that there is a reduced nephron population perhaps due to infection around the stone but there is no obstructive nephropathy; or else a reduced uptake and a prolonged transit time giving evidence of a reduced nephron population and an obstructive nephropathy. These uptake and transit functions are independent of each other. The PTTI is more accurate than the frusemide response judged visually as evaluated by outcome analysis [70].

PELVIC DILATATION OR OBSTRUCTING UROPATHY

Consider the question of outflow dilatation. Dilatation does not mean obstruction and this is the problem for the overenthusiastic ultrasound reader. Lack of dilatation also does not mean lack of obstruction. In an oliguric renal transplant there may be no dilatation of the pelvis associated with a low urine flow, and yet there may be an obstructive nephropathy present because of increased resistance to flow.

The frusemide response can be evaluated in a number of ways and there are various visual classifications of the responses into types 1, 2, 3 or A, B, C, etc. [68–72]. Visual criteria may be interpreted as normal or non-obstructive, obstructive and indeterminate.

Consider an alcoholic trying to get the last drop of alcohol out of the bottle. He has learned that if there is no alcohol in the bottle he cannot get any out. Alternatively if the bottle were full, he could get plenty out of it. If the bottle was half-full and there was a cork which only had a very small hole in it, then he might know that he might be able to get something out of it but he cannot get it out quickly enough to satisfy him. Thus, what comes out depends on what is in there. This is fundamentally obvious, but when it is applied to the kidney somehow this principle is forgotten. Consider the frusemide response: if only a little goes in then the correct response is only a little coming out. If a lot goes in then you must expect a lot to come out. If nothing goes in, nothing will come out and that is not an abnormal response, that is normality. Thus, in evaluating the response from the activity–time curves, instead of saying that the responses are good or bad, what should be said is that the responses are appropriate or not appropriate. Take a normal curve which is rising and then falling after giving the frusemide, $t_{1/2}$ is 5 minutes (Figure 11.4). Another curve with poor uptake had a poor response with a $t_{1/2}$ of 15 minutes. Another curve showed good uptake and a poor output, with a $t_{1/2}$ of 15 minutes. The first one is an appropriate response in that with only a little going in, there is only a little going out, whereas the second one is certainly inappropriate as there is a lot going into the kidney and only a little coming out. Thus, you cannot distinguish frusemide response by looking at the post-frusemide curve or by measuring a $t_{1/2}$ or a 20-minute percent fall, or an excretion index, or whatever. What goes out of the kidney must be related to what went into it before. Visually, the response to frusemide should be reported as appropriate or inappropriate to the second phase of the renogram. Finally, nil in and nil out is totally appropriate.

OUTFLOW EFFICIENCY

There is now a method whereby response can be corrected for the level of renal function and that is called the **outflow efficiency** (see p. 398). Consider the kidney curve that would be obtained if the kidney was totally obstructed; nothing would come out and therefore the kidney is acting as an integrator. Each package of activity in the blood going to the kidney is taken up and held. Therefore, the curve that is found with a zero output is in fact the integral of the blood clearance curve. If the integral of the blood clearance curve from the left ventricle is fitted to the second phase of the renogram, then one sees what that kidney's curve would have looked like if the kidney had been

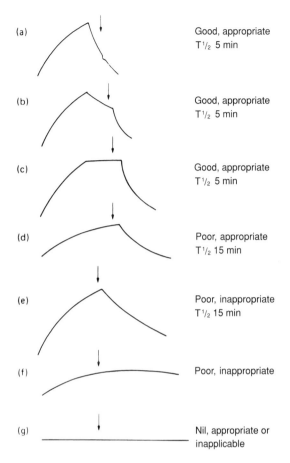

Figure 11.4 Responses to frusemide. Curves a, b, and c have good responses to frusemide (arrowed) with a $t_{\frac{1}{2}}$ of the post-frusemide curve of 5 minutes. Curve d shows an impaired second phase and a poor response to frusemide, $t_{\frac{1}{2}}$ 15 minutes, but it can be seen that the response is appropriate to the second phase. Curve e shows a normal second phase and a poor response to frusemide ($t_{\frac{1}{2}}$ 15 minutes). Here the response is inappropriate to the second phase, indicating an obstructing uropathy. Curve f shows a very impaired second phase with an even more impaired third phase indicating an inappropriate response and an obstructing uropathy. Curve g shows that if nothing goes in it is appropriate that nothing comes out of the kidney.

totally obstructed. However, as it was not totally obstructed, the difference between what was actually obtained and what would have been obtained if it had been totally obstructed is the cumulative output. If the cumulative output is differentiated, the true output curve is obtained. The so-called excretory or third phase of the renogram is actually the 'left-behind-in-the-kidney-curve'. The third phase falls because of reducing input to the kidney as well as excretion. The method is to take the integral of blood clearance curve and fit it to the second phase of the actual kidney curve, and subtract the actual kidney curve from the fitted integral to give the cumulative output. The outflow efficiency is obtained by taking the cumulative output as a percentage of the cumulative input (the fitted integral of the blood clearance curve equivalent to zero output) curve. This calculation is straightforward and it relates what comes out to what goes in [11].

Controlled studies show that, in the absence of an obstructing process, 82–98% of what went in comes out in 30 minutes – whatever the level of renal function. If activity enters 100 nephrons, 100 nephrons' worth comes out and that gives an output efficiency of 100%. The lower limit of normal is 78%.

Considering the data on validating the output efficiency, 11 kidneys with obstructive uropathy had a mean output efficiency of 56%. In a series of patients, normal outflow efficiency in 53 out of 54 had no obstructive uropathy in the final diagnosis. In the one patient who had an obstructive uropathy, the condition was thought to be due to a stone moving from being non-obstructive to being obstructive at operation 4 days after the test. The outflow efficiency has been compared with the visual response for 65 kidneys. In seven kidneys with an indeterminate frusemide response, the outflow efficiency was abnormal in five (subsequently confirmed to be obstructing uropathy), but not confirmed in two with very poor renal function. When the frusemide response was normal visually, all the kidneys had a normal outflow efficiency. When the visual response was interpreted as obstructive, the outflow efficiency was in fact abnormal in nine out of the 10. From outcome analysis giving true positive and true negative outcomes, outflow efficiency had an accuracy of 94% and the visual frusemide response an accuracy of 86% [11]. Outflow efficiency is not perfect, but it does consider the basic pathophysiology so that what comes out of the kidney is related to what went in before.

Do not report that it was a good frusemide response, a poor response or an indeterminate response – report that it was appropriate or not appropriate to what went in (from the second phase). The output efficiency is a useful addition to the frusemide response which corrects the response quantitatively for the level of renal function. It does not correct the other problems associated with the use of frusemide, such as the effects of a stiff pelvis, a large pelvis, a mega ureter or a poor injection. A consensus on the conventional use of frusemide diuresis during a renal radionuclide study is given by O'Reilly et al. [66].

In summary, the distinction between obstructive nephropathy and a dilated pelvis that is not obstructed, has a number of particular features: the PTTI is prolonged, the pelvic transit time is prolonged, the outflow efficiency after frusemide is impaired and the response to frusemide is inappropriate; as compared with the non-obstructed dilated pelvis which has a normal outflow efficiency, and a normal PTTI but a long pelvic transit time because of eddying of activity in the pelvis. Figures 11.5 and 11.6 show that measurements have advantages over images and curves, but all should be considered together.

DISTRIBUTION OF RENAL FUNCTION – CLINICAL USES

The theoretical basis for the measurement of regional distribution of function within the kidney is the same as that for the distribution of function between the two kidneys as previously described. Measurement of the uptake function of the radiopharmaceutical at the appropriate time, i.e. ^{99m}Tc-labelled DMSA at 1–3h, or ^{99m}Tc-labelled DTPA, ^{99m}Tc-labelled MAG3 and ^{123}I-labelled hippuran at 90–150 seconds, have been shown in a large number of studies to correlate well with GFR and RPF using conventional invasive methods. Thus, the distribution of uptake function of these renal localizing radiopharmaceuticals in different areas of the kidney presents a functional image of the distribution of renal parenchyma. It must be emphasized that we are not considering the regional distribution of function in terms of parts of the nephron but simply the distribution of 'functioning renal parenchyma' as measured by GFR and RPF. It is essential that all assessments of distribution of function either within or between kidneys must be made in the light of a measurement of total renal function, usually ^{51}Cr-labelled EDTA measurement of GFR, without which serious errors may be made. No other method of renal investigation gives this functional information so

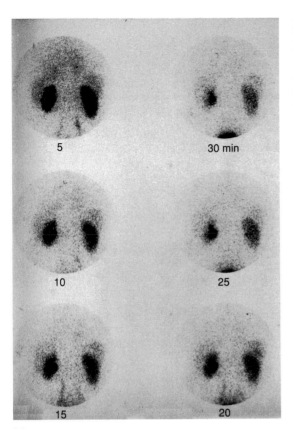

Figure 11.5 Pelvic dilatation. (a) A series of ^{99m}Tc-MAG3 images. Frusemide was given at 18 minutes and there is some slight response visually. (b) Activity–time curves: the left kidney (*) shows an impaired second phase and a somewhat more impaired third phase which is difficult to assess visually. The outflow efficiency however was 94% and the PTTI 61 seconds – both normal – indicating no obstructive nephropathy or obstructing uropathy. The right kidney (+) is normal.

(a)

```
Percentage Left Renal Uptake =      32.9  %


Background_Subtracted_Curves

1     +
1     +
1    +
1
1        +
1  +    +
1        +
1        +
1+        +*******
1     ***++      *****
1   **       ++       *** *
1    *          +        ** **
1 **          ++         *****
1             ++++++          *******
1 *              +++++ +   +++      ****
1                   + +++   +++++++++   **
1*                              +++++++++++++
1                                     ****++
+                                          *
*
-----------------------------------------------------
 L kidney (BBS):  *   R kidney (BBS):  +
 L kidney OUTF%:  *  94.%  R kidney OUTF%:  +  96.%

 Kidney Transit Times in units of one second
         PTTI    WKTTI    MIN PTT    MEAN PTT    MEAN WTT
 Left:    61     409      100        161         509
 Right:   36      58      100        136         158
 NORMAL RANGE
         <156    <170                <270
```

(b)

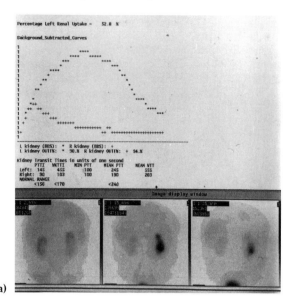

(a)

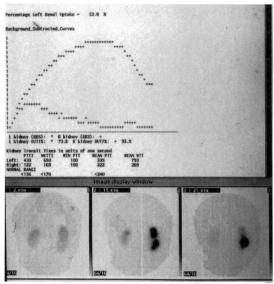

(b)

Figure 11.6   Progression of obstructive nephropathy. (a) ^{99m}Tc-MAG3 study, 12.11.92. The left kidney curve (*) rises to a delayed peak and falls. The third phase appears appropriate to the second phase. Outflow efficiency 90% PTTI 145 seconds close to the upper range of normal. (b) ^{99m}Tc-MAG3 study, 17.11.93. The left kidney curve looks similar to that of 12.11.92 with a rounded delayed peak and a third phase that appears appropriate to the second phase. There has been no change in relative function. However, the left kidney outflow efficiency has fallen to 73% and the PTTI has risen to 439 seconds, confirming the presence of obstructive nephropathy and obstructing uropathy. This diagnosis could not have been made on assessment of the curves and images alone.

the radionuclide studies are always complementary and never competitive with the structural studies of ultrasound or IVU. The clinical situation in which knowledge of distribution of renal function is helpful in the management of the patient will be considered.

Reflux nephropathy

The measurement of divided renal function is now an essential part of the investigation and follow-up of the patient with ureteric reflux as decisions about surgical management may depend on serial measurements of renal function. Urinary reflux may differentially affect parts of a single kidney, for example where there is a duplex system with reflux up one ureter only with consequent damage to that renal moiety (usually the lower moiety) of a duplex system. In this situation it is essential to know what proportion of function there is in each of the two moieties in order to make rational decisions about the need for partial nephrectomy, total nephrectomy or reconstructive surgery. A

^{99m}Tc-DMSA scan performed at 3 hours after injection will clearly display the regional variations in functional damage brought about by reflux and associated infection (Figure 11.7), and is currently the most sensitive method to show renal scarring [76].

Calculous disease

The measurement of the contribution of each kidney to total function should always be performed in the assessment and follow-up of patients with intrarenal stone formation. Knowledge of the distribution of function within the kidney will be additionally helpful before surgical treatment to enable the surgical approach to be planned in such a way as to minimize surgical damage to the residual renal tissue and also to decide between total and partial nephrectomy or simple stone removal. Post-operative repeat assessment will be used to determine how successful the operation has been in preserving renal function and subsequent progress of the disease. Large masses of calcium

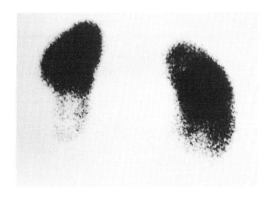

Figure 11.7 ^{99m}Tc-DMSA scan showing the effect of reflux into a lower moiety of a duplex kidney on the left, and a lower pole scar in the right kidney.

lying between the kidney and the gamma-camera may result in misinterpretation of the distribution of function, so it is advisable to make anterior in addition to routine posterior images.

Hypertension due to local ischaemia

Renal scanning with DMSA, DTPA, OIH or MAG3 may be helpful in defining an abnormal renal segment with poor function which is responsible for hypertension and which can be treated by partial nephrectomy or segmental angioplasty. The delayed DMSA scan (Figure 11.8) will show a focal area of decreased function and the DTPA or MAG3 scan may show an early uptake defect at 2 minutes with an increase later due to local delayed transit times secondary to local ischaemia and water reabsorption. This assessment will usually be performed together with regional venography for the measurement of segmental renin secretion and arteriography. The theoretical basis for these abnormalities are as described under renovascular hypertension.

Renal localization

Although renal localization before biopsy is routinely performed under X-ray fluoroscopy control, occasionally localization using ^{99m}Tc-labelled DMSA may be preferable, for example when renal function is impaired so that contrast media localization is poor or when there is a particular region of the kidney which is functionally abnormal. It may also be valuable to localize the renal outline on the skin surface when planning radiotherapy of the abdomen in order to avoid unnecessary renal radiation.

Pyelonephritic scarring

Pyelonephritis is one of the most common causes of end-stage renal failure and in children is often associated with reflux and/or asymptomatic bacteriuria. To follow-up and treat these children and young adults appropriately with long-term antibiotics or ureteric reimplantation it is necessary to identify the presence or absence and progress of renal parenchymal scarring.

The identification of scar using urography is good when there is impeccable technique and good preparation, especially with nephrotomography. However, frequently bowel gas complicates the picture, too low a dose of contrast is used, and nephrotomography is not employed. Radionuclide imaging with ^{99m}Tc-DMSA has a sensitivity of 96% and a specificity of 98%. Renal scanning, therefore, is an important adjunct in the identification of scars as well as in the measurement of divided function in children and young adults with reflux or urinary infections [77]. Care must be taken in the presence of current infection as focal 'scars' may be due to focal nephritis and resolve with time, whereas true scars cannot resolve (Figure 11.9).

Congenital abnormalities

Renal imaging with ^{99m}Tc-DMSA is valuable for the proper assessment of many congenital abnormalities affecting the renal tract (Figure 11.10). Reflux and duplex kidneys with 'seesaw' reflux have already been mentioned; other examples include the assessment of horseshoe kidneys where the function of the 'bridge' can often be assessed very much more easily than with urography; ectopic kidneys, for example pelvic kidney, can usually be more easily identified and investigated because once the radiopharmaceutical has been given, a whole-body search can be undertaken if necessary, whereas a small pelvic kidney, especially if it is poorly functioning, cannot always be seen against the background of the pelvic bone. Renal abnormalities and the assessment of divided function associated with neurological abnormalities such as meningomyelocele can easily be documented.

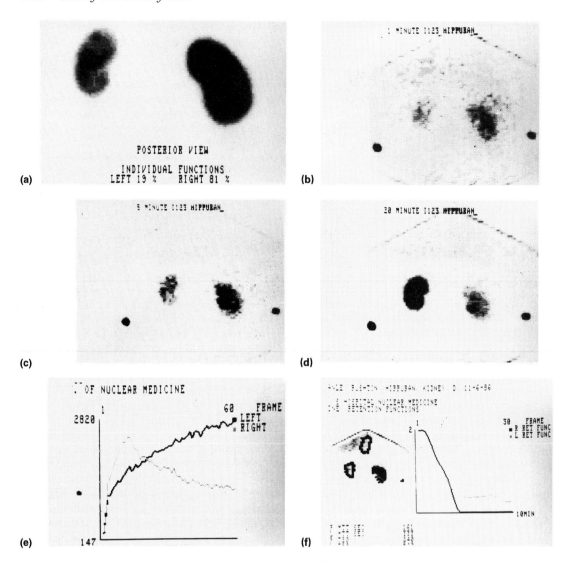

Figure 11.8 An example of left renal artery stenosis. (a) The ^{99m}Tc-DMSA scan shows decreased uptake of the left kidney. (b-d) The ^{123}I-hippuran study shows decreased uptake on the left, with prolonged parenchymal transit. Activity–time curves from the hippuran study (e) show delayed renogram peak on the left and the deconvolution study (f) a prolonged transit time (333 versus 161 seconds).

RENAL FAILURE

Renal failure is present when the urine output of metabolites and waste products is insufficient to maintain the normal body composition without alteration in body fluids. This may be a chronic process resulting in progressive renal insufficiency or it may be an acute clinical presentation.

It is important to appreciate the role radionuclide studies may have in these conditions.

ACUTE RENAL FAILURE

Acute renal failure is frequently complicating another medical or surgical condition. There is usu-

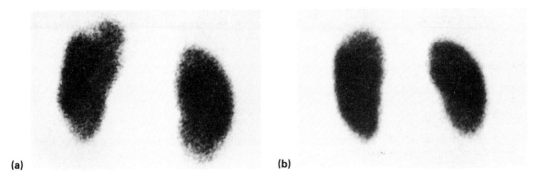

Figure 11.9 (a) Focal loss of function at the upper pole of the left kidney on a DMSA scan during an infection. (b) The infection is resolved a few months later, with no scar formation.

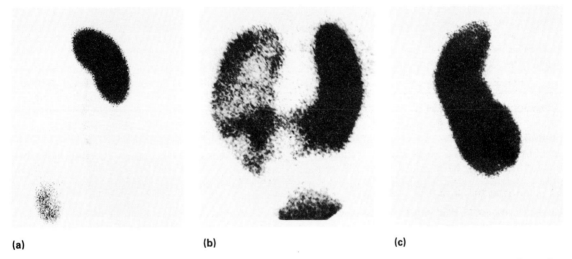

Figure 11.10 ^{99m}Tc-DMSA scans showing: (a) posterior view of a pelvic kidney; (b) anterior view of a horseshoe kidney; (c) posterior view of crossed renal ectopia.

ally a rapid rise in blood urea and creatinine, the rate of rise depending on the degree of failure and associated catabolism or muscle damage, but is normally in the order of 10mg/100ml per day of urea and 0.5mg/100ml per day of creatinine. Oliguria is usually present, although non-oliguric acute renal failure occurs in up to one-third of cases of acute renal failure and may frequently cause considerable diagnostic confusion. There is no clear definition of oliguria, but less than 400ml/day of urine is generally accepted as indicating oliguria and less than 50ml/day represents anuria. The causes of acute renal failure are multiple and occur in all branches of medical sub-

specialities but broadly may be classified as shown in Table 11.3.

The mechanism of acute tubular necrosis is controversial and indeed probably should not be called acute tubular necrosis because it is now well established that necrosis is by no means always present or always necessary for the clinical picture of acute tubular necrosis (ATN). The initial insult in all cases is probably decreased renal perfusion which results in a decrease in renal blood flow and renal ischaemia. As GFR is acutely dependent on renal blood flow so the GFR falls, resulting in a decrease in urine flow (oliguria). The renal ischaemia is then in some way self-perpetuating,

Table 11.3   Classification of acute renal failure

1. Post-renal – obstruction, e.g. from calculi, prostate, urethral valves
2. Pre-renal
   (a) Hypovolaemia, e.g. haemorrhage, diarrhoea and vomiting, burns
   (b) Cardiac, e.g. heart failure, infarction
   (c) Vascular, e.g. sepsis, anaphylaxis, hypotension
3. 'Acute tubular necrosis' (ATN)
   (a) Post-ischaemia secondary to 2
   (b) Pigment precipitation, e.g. intravascular haemolysis, trauma, acute myositis
   (c) Nephrotoxins, e.g. heavy metals, ethylene glycol, drugs, radiographic contrast media
4. Parenchymal renal disease
   (a) Glomerulonephritis
   (b) Interstitial nephritis
   (c) Acute pyelonephritis and papillary necrosis
   (d) Intratubular precipitates, e.g. myeloma, sulphonamides
   (e) Vasculitis
   (f) Hepatorenal syndrome
5. Vascular
   (a) Arterial, e.g. thrombosis, embolus, aneurysm
   (b) Venous, e.g. IVC thrombosis, renal vein thrombosis

possibly by arteriolar vasoconstriction due to angiotensin, obstruction to microcirculation due to swelling of the vascular endothelium, or possibly a decrease in secretion of intrarenal vasodilators such as prostaglandins. Certainly if the ischaemia is severe or nephrotoxins are present actual tubular cell necrosis will occur, with consequent back-leakage of filtrate and also tubule obstruction by debris. Whatever the mechanism may be, recognition of the clinical picture is important. With ATN as with other causes of acute renal failure, correct recognition with appropriate vigorous treatment usually results in a return to normal renal function, even though this may take up to one year. On the other hand, a wrong diagnosis or inappropriate treatment may result in chronic renal failure, the need for long-term supportive treatment or death.

CLINICAL AND DIAGNOSTIC EVALUATION

In most instances a careful history and physical evaluation will elicit the cause. For example, exposure to toxin or drug, recent surgery with hypotension, heart failure or sore throat. However, in a significant number of patients no cause of acute renal failure is ever established. Basic urine and serum biochemistry is also helpful in a number of cases but there are no formulae for classifying every case. Urine analysis may be helpful; anuria is not usual in ATN; intermittent changes in urine output suggest obstruction; tubular casts may be present in ATN and red cells and red cell casts are frequently found in acute glomerular nephritis. Urine composition may help to differentiate pre-renal oliguria from ATN and thereby allow the possibility of preventing progression of one to the other.

History, examination and other simple measures may not permit a firm diagnosis and therefore further imaging measures are required, including urography, ultrasound, renal biopsy and radionuclide investigations.

Ultrasound examinations should always be performed early and will provide essential information about renal size, and may exclude obstruction as a cause of renal failure.

Intravenous urography with high dosage and early nephrotomography may be used, although the disadvantages of a high osmolar load, possible sensitivity to contrast, high sodium content and nephrotoxicity must be weighed against the diagnostic information needed. In cases which might have a vascular basis, angiography may be required to demonstrate the anatomical lesion but this also carries the risk of further renal damage, even though the modern contrast media are superior in this respect to the older ones. A combination of ultrasound examination and radionuclide functional study will usually provide all the necessary information for clinical management, without the associated toxicity and further deterioration of renal function which may be associated with contrast agents. A dynamic ^{99m}Tc-DTPA or ^{99m}Tc-MAG3 scan is the method of choice, possibly with the addition of a ^{99m}Tc-labelled complex radiopharmaceutical such as DMSA.

The radionuclide study provides information about renal perfusion (first-pass), the handling of the glomerular-filtered agent and, if there is sufficient urine flow, the collecting systems. Radionuclide imaging also provides prognostic information concerning eventual recovery. The single most useful role of the dynamic radionuclide scan is to make a firm diagnosis of ATN, which has a good prognosis given adequate dialysis. Well-perfused kidneys which have a typical ATN pattern are likely to return to adequate function given adequate supportive treatment, including dialysis.

It may also be possible to differentiate the early onset phase of ATN which may be reversible by fluid and electrolyte correction from the established phase of ATN. The typical images seen in ATN (Figure 11.11) using ^{99m}Tc-DTPA are: a practically normal perfusion phase during the first transit followed by a moderately good visualization of the kidneys at 90–180 seconds which represents a blood pool image of the kidneys; as the tracer diffuses into the larger extracellular space from the vascular space the renal image diminishes without the appearance of tracer into the collecting system. Early signs of recovery are:

- increasing retention of tracer in the kidney, as the GFR returns to normal and is superimposed on the blood pool image;
- progressive concentration as glomerular filtration continues to improve but intrarenal transit remains grossly prolonged; and
- excretion as at the onset of the diuretic phase of ATN.

These progressive appearances are shown diagrammatically in Figure 11.12.

The findings associated with acute obstruction are a decreased perfusion image during first transit and poor early uptake image with progressive parenchymal accumulation due to the grossly delayed intrarenal transit. Dilated calyces are frequently seen on the early images as negative photon-deficient areas which then progressively accumulate tracer over several hours. These findings, although characteristic, should be confirmed with ultrasound before surgical treatment and the absence of evidence of obstruction on a ^{99m}Tc-DTPA scan should never be used to exclude it without ultrasound confirmation.

Pre-renal failure associated with acute oliguria due to, for example, dehydration or hypovolaemia but before the established phase of ATN, is identical to phase 2 or 4 of the ATN recovery pattern, i.e. well-perfused kidneys with a significant secretory peak representing glomerular filtration, markedly delayed parenchymal transit but with some excretion of tracer which may only appear in the calyces towards the end of the normal 20- to 30-minute period of imaging.

Acute nephritis and most other renal parenchymal diseases usually show significantly worse perfusion as compared with ATN, with markedly decreased uptake at 2 minutes with either no accumulation or slow progressive accumulation in the renal parenchyma but without significant excretion.

In addition to these patterns representing the majority of cases of acute renal failure, other causes may be diagnosed, such as acute loss of perfusion unilaterally associated with renal artery embolus. In aortic obstruction (Figure 11.13) there will be lack of visualization of the aorta as well as grossly diminished renal perfusion; aneurysm if associated with a large lumen will be identified as

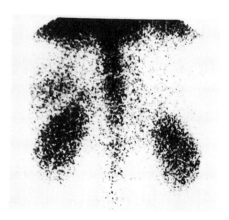

(a)

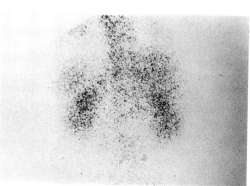

(b)

Figure 11.11 ^{99m}Tc-DTPA scan in a patient with acute tubular necrosis. In (a), there is good perfusion to both kidneys, but DTPA is not concentrated. In (b), the image fades as the tracer distributes into the larger extracellular space.

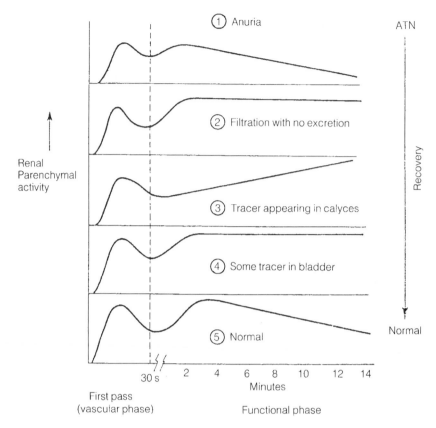

Figure 11.12 ^{99m}Tc-DTPA renal parenchymal activity–time curves during phases of recovery from acute tubular necrosis.

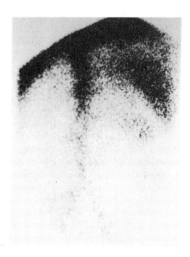

Figure 11.13 An example of severe loss of perfusion, which is complete on the left and almost complete on the right, due to vascular complications during aortic surgery for aneurysm.

a large abdominal blood pool; venous thrombosis decreases perfusion but to a lesser extent than arterial occlusion.

When the visualization is very poor or absent with ^{99m}Tc-DTPA or ^{99m}Tc-MAG3, a repeat image following ^{99m}Tc-DMSA usually demonstrates better visualization and may possibly be a better guide to eventual prognosis. However, no systematic studies are available at the present time to answer this important question.

CHRONIC RENAL FAILURE

Chronic renal insufficiency is usually the result of progressive renal disease, the most common being chronic pyelonephritis, malignant hypertension, chronic glomerulonephritis, diabetic nephropathy and polycystic disease. In many cases an exact diagnosis beyond end-stage contracted kidneys is not possible and frequently the exact diagnosis is not of great importance in management, which consists essentially of delaying the effects of renal failure to excrete waste products and metabolites before supportive treatment with chronic dialysis or renal transplantation. Chronic obstruction is an obvious exception where relief and drainage may restore a very useful amount of renal function.

Ultrasound examination remains the best initial investigation in chronic renal failure and may indicate the aetiology, for example irregularly scarred kidneys of pyelonephritis or reflux, the enlarged kidneys of polycystic disease, the small uniformly contracted kidneys of chronic glomerulonephritis, and the dilated ureters, collecting system and enlarged kidneys of chronic obstruction. Radionuclide investigations certainly visualize chronically damaged kidneys in this situation and to a very limited extent predict the degree of recoverable function. Only occasionally would radionuclide imaging be of any clinical value and then is best performed with ^{123}I-hippuran, ^{99m}Tc-MAG3 or ^{99m}Tc-DMSA.

RENAL MASS LESIONS

When renal parenchyma is replaced by a space-occupying lesion, whether it is a tumour, cyst, infarct or scar, it can be identified by a loss of functioning renal tissue compared with the surrounding normal renal parenchyma, together with the presence or absence of changes in local perfusion during the angiographic phase. This is the basis for the use of radionuclide methods. Early studies with ^{99m}Tc-DTPA and ^{99m}Tc-DMSA concentrated on the detection of tumours and cysts of the kidney, but with the development of improved structural imaging techniques (high-dose nephrotomography, ultrasonography and CT scanning) together with a more widespread use of diagnostic cyst puncture with cytological examination, the role of nuclear medicine techniques has changed.

In the vast majority of cases there is no real problem and most patients receive the appropriate investigative sequence and treatment. ^{99m}Tc-DMSA scans may be used when the ultrasound examination does not confirm a mass lesion or is equivocal. This is not often a problem, but when it does arise the renal scan is the next best investigation to confirm or exclude a tumour. The renal scan may also help to answer the related question 'is it a single or multiple lesion?' Lateral and oblique views of the kidney are often helpful and should always be performed. These images should be reviewed in conjunction with the IVU in order to correlate the abnormality on the IVU with the scan and to identify the site and size of the calyces on the renal scan, because with current high-resolution images of the renal parenchyma normal calyces may be confused with a space-occupying lesion.

The second situation when renal scanning may be helpful is in the further evaluation of a definite lesion on IVU which is solid on ultrasound but could possibly be a pseudo-tumour. In this situation, if it is possible to demonstrate that the 'tumour' is functionally normal renal tissue without resorting to arteriography, that is an advantage. Examples of pseudo-tumours are the lump from splenic pressure, foetal lobulation, compensatory hypertrophy, and prominent columns of Bertin.

Occasionally, when arteriography and surgery are contraindicated for other reasons, the renal scan with particular emphasis on the first-pass arteriographic phase may help to establish the diagnosis. Increased blood flow in the lesion indicates a high probability of tumour; no flow in a large lesion increases the likelihood of a cyst, but there are a significant number of cases in which the tumour has a relatively poor supply and the differentiation of benign and malignant is not possible. Finally, it must be emphasized that this is a small part of the investigation of such patients and the radionuclide scan must not be used as just one more test to document the lesion when it is not going to influence the management of the patient.

REFERENCES

1. Kiil, F. (1957) *The Function of the Ureter and Renal Pelvis. Pressure Recordings and Radiographic Studies of the Normal and Diseased Upper Urinary Tract of Man*, W.B. Saunders & Co., Philadelphia.
2. Sreenevasan, G. (1974) Bilateral renal calculi. *Ann. R. Coll. Surg. Engl.*, **55**, 3–12.
3. Nimmon, C.C., Lee, T.Y., Britton, K.E. *et al.* (1981) Practical application of deconvolution techniques to dynamic studies, in *Medical Radionuclide Imaging*, Vol. I, International Atomic Energy Agency Vienna, pp. 367–88.
4. Britton, K.E., Nimmon, C.C., Whitfield, H.N. *et al.* (1979) Obstructive nephropathy: successful evaluation with radionuclides. *Lancet*, **i**, 905–7.
5. Britton, K.E. and Brown, N.J.G. (1971) *Clinical Renography*, Lloyd Luke, London.

6. Britton, K.E. and Brown, N.J.G. (1971) The value in obstructive nephropathy of the hippuran output curve derived by computer analysis of the renogram, in *The Proceedings of the International Symposium on Dynamic Renal Studies with Radioisotopes in Medicine*, Vienna, International Atomic Energy Agency, pp. 263–75.

7. Rutland, M.D. (1985) A comprehensive analysis of renal DTPA studies. I. Theory and normal values. *Nucl. Med. Commun.*, **6**, 11–20.

8. Rutland, M.D. and Stuart, R.A. (1986) A comprehensive analysis of renal DTA studies II. Renal artery stenosis. *Nucl. Med. Commun.*, **7**, 879–85.

9. Peters, A.M., Gordon, I., Evans, K. *et al.* (1987) Background in the 99mTc-DTPA renogram: analysis of intravascular and extravascular components. *Am. J. Physiol. Imaging*, **2**, 66–71.

10. Nimmon, C.C., Britton, K.E., Bomanji, J.B. *et al.* (1988) in *Proceedings of the European Nuclear Medicine Congress* (eds H.A.E. Schmidt and L. Csernay), Schattauer Verlag, Stuttgart, pp. 472–6.

11. Chaiwatanarat, T., Padhy, A.K., Bomanji, J.B. *et al.* (1993) Validation of renal output efficiency as an objective quantitative parameter in the evaluation of upper urinary tract obstruction. *J. Nucl. Med.*, **34**, 845–8.

12. Peters, A.M. (1993) A unified approach to quantification by kinetic analysis in nuclear medicine. *J. Nucl. Med.*, **34**, 706–13.

13. Peters, A.M. (1994) Graphical analysis of dynamic data the Patlak–Rutland plot. *Nucl. Med. Commun.*, **15**, 669–72.

14. Rutland, M.D. (1995) Tracer flows and difficult organs. *Nucl. Med. Commun.*, **16**, 31–7.

15. Fritzberg, A.R., Sudhaker, K., Eshima, D. *et al.* (1986) Synthesis and biological evaluation of Tc-99m MAG3 as a hippuran replacement. *J. Nucl. Med.*, **17**, 111–16.

16. Solanki, K.K., Al Nahhas, A. and Britton, K.E. (1989) Cold Tc-99m MAG3, in *Trends and Possibilities in Nuclear Medicine* (eds H.A.E. Schmidt and G.L. Buraggi), Schattauer Verlag, Stuttgart, pp. 443–6.

17. Bubeck, B., Brandau, W., Weber, E. *et al.* (1990) Pharmacokinetics of technetium-99m-MAG3 in humans. *J. Nucl. Med.*, **31**, 1285–93.

18. Rehling, M., Nielsen, B.V., Pedersen, E.B. *et al.* (1995) Renal and extra renal clearance of ^{99m}Tc-MAG3: a comparison with ^{125}I-OIH and ^{51}Cr-EDTA in patients representing all levels of glomerular filtration rate. *Eur. J. Nucl. Med.*, **22**, 1379–84.

19. Klingensmith, W.C., Briggs, D.E. and Smith, W.I. (1994) Technetium-99m MAG3 renal studies; normal range and reproducibility of physiologic parameters as a function of age and sex. *J. Nucl. Med.*, **35**, 1612–17.

20. Jafri, R.A., Britton, K.E., Nimmon, C.C. *et al.* (1988) 99m-Tc MAG3: a comparison with I-123 and I-131 orthoiodohippurate in patients with renal disorder. *J. Nucl. Med.*, **29**, 147–58.

21. Al-Nahhas, A.A., Jafri, R.A., Britton, K.E. *et al.* (1988) Clinical experience with ^{99m}Tc-MAG3, mercaptoacetyltriglycine and a comparison with ^{99m}Tc-DTPA. *Eur. J. Nucl. Med.*, **14**, 453–62.

22. Van Nerom, C., Bormans, C., Bauwens, J. *et al.* (1992) Comparative evaluation of Tc-99m LL ethylene dicysteine and Tc-99m MAG3 in volunteers. *Eur. J. Nucl. Med.*, **33**, 551–7.

23. Ozker, R., Onsel, C., Kabasakal, L. *et al.* (1994) Technetium-99m-*N, N* Ethylene dicysteine: a comparative study of renal scintigraphy with Technetium-99m MAG3 and iodine-131-OIH in patients with obstructive renal disease. *J. Nucl. Med.*, **35**, 840–5.

24. Gupta, N.K., Bomanji, J.B., Waddington, W., Lui, D., Costa, D.C. and Verbruggen, A.M. (1995) Technetium-99m-L-L ethylene dicysteine scintigraphy in patients with renal disorders. *Eur. J. Nucl. Med.*, **22**, 617–24.

25. Kostadinova, I. and Simeonova, A. (1995) The use of ^{99m}Tc-EC captopril test in patients with hypertension. *Nucl. Med. Commun.*, **16**, 128–31.

26. Padhy, A.K., Solanki, K.K., Bomanji, J.B. *et al.* (1993) Clinical evaluation of ^{99m}Tc Diaminocyclohexane, a renal agent with cationic transport: results in healthy normal volunteers. *Nephron*, **65**, 294–8.

27. Sonmezoglu, K., Demir, M., Erdil, T.Y. *et al.* (1995) Evaluation of renal function in patients with psoriasis on low dose cyclosporin regimen by using Tc-99m Diamino-cyclohexane (DACH). *Eur. J. Nucl. Med.*, **22**, 834.

28. Datseris, I., Boletis, J., Papadakis, E. *et al.* (1995) ^{99m}Tc-Diamino cyclohexane (DACH), a renal tubular agent with cationic transport excretion in renal transplant patients. *Eur. J. Nucl. Med.*, **22**, 835.

29. Peters, A.M., Jones, D.H., Evans, K. and Gordon, I. (1988) Two routes for 99m-Tc-DMSA uptake into the renal cortical tubular cell. *Eur. J. Nucl. Med.*, **14**, 555–61.

30. Yee, C.A., Lee, H.B. and Blaufox, M.D. (1981) ^{99m}Tc DMSA renal uptake: influence of biochemical and physiological factors. *J. Nucl. Med.*, **22**, 1054–8.

31. Williams, E., Parker, D. and Roy, R. (1986) Multiple-section radionuclide tomography of the kidney: a clinical evaluation. *Br. J. Radiol.*, **59**, 975–83.

32. Delcourt, E., Franken, P., Motte, S. *et al.* (1995) Measurement of glomerular filtration rate by means of a ^{99m}Tc DTPA complex and a scintillation camera: a method based on the kinetics of the distribution volume of the tracer in the kidney area. *Nucl. Med. Commun.*, **6**, 787–94.

33. Duffy, G.J., Casey, M. and Barker, F. (1982) in *Radionuclides in Nephrology* (eds A.M. Joekes, A.R. Constable, N.J.G. Brown and W.N. Tauxe), Academic Press, London, pp. 101–6.

34. Lee, T.Y., Constable, A.R. and Cranage, R.W. (1982) in *Radionuclides in Nephrology* (eds A.M. Joekes, A.R. Constable, N.J.G. Brown and W.N. Tauxe), Academic Press, London, pp. 107–12.

35. Rutland, M.D. (1983) Glomerular filtration rate without blood sampling. *Nucl. Med. Commun.*, **4**, 425–33.

36. Shone, R.M., Koff, S.A., Mentser, M. *et al.* (1984) Glomerular filtration rate in children: determination from the Tc-99m DTPA renogram. *Radiology*, **151**, 627–33.

37. Tonnesen, K.H., Munck, O., Hald, T. *et al.* (1975) in *Radionuclides in Nephrology* (eds K. Zum Winkel, M.D. Blaufox and J.L.F. Brentano), Georg Thieme, Stuttgart, pp. 79–86.

38. Goris, M.L., Daspit, S.G., McLaughlin, R. and Kriss, J.P. (1976) Interpolative background subtraction. *J. Nucl. Med.*, **17**, 744–7.

39. Brown, N.J.G. (1982) in *Radionuclides in Nephrology* (eds A.M. Joekes, A.R. Constable, N.J.G. Brown and W.N. Tauxe), Academic Press, London, pp. 113–18.

40. Russell, C.D., Thorstad, B.L., Yester, M.B. *et al.* (1988) Quantitation of renal function with technetium–99m MAG3. *J. Nucl. Med.*, **29**, 1931–3.

41. Nimmo, M.J., Merrick, M.V. and Allan, P.L. (1987) Measurement of relative renal function: a comparison of methods and assessment of reproducibility. *Br. J. Radiol.*, **60**, 861–4.

42. Wujanto, R., Lawson, R.S., Prescott, M. *et al.* (1987) The importance of using anterior and posterior views in the calculation of differential renal function using ^{99m}Tc DMSA. *Br. J. Radiol.*, **60**, 869–72.

43. Britton, K.E. (1981) Essential hypertension: a disorder of cortical nephron control? *Lancet*, **ii**, 900–2.

44. Al-Nahhas, A., Nimmon, C.C., Britton, K.E. *et al* (1990). The effect of ramipril, a new angiotensin converting enzyme inhibitor on cortical nephron flow and effective renal plasma flow in patients with essential hypertension. *Nephron*, **54**, 47–52.

45. Smith, H.W. (1951) *The Kidney: Structure and Function in Health and Disease*, Oxford University Press, Oxford.

46. Russell, C.D., Japanwalla, M., Khan, S., Scott, J.W. and Dubovsky, E.V. (1995) Techniques for measuring renal transit time. *Eur. J. Nucl. Med.*, **22**, 1372–8.

47. Makoba, G.I., Nimmon, C.C., Kouykin, V. *et al.* (1996) Comparison of a corticopelvic transfer index with renal transit times. *Nucl. Med. Commun.*, **17**, 212–15.

48. Mogensen, P., Munck, O. and Giese, J. (1995) ^{131}I-hippuran renography in normal subjects and patients with essential hypertension. *Scand. J. Clin. Invest.*, **35**, 301–6.

49. Giese, J., Mogensen, P. and Munck, O. (1975) Diagnostic value of renography for detection of unilateral renal or renovascular disease in hypertensive patients. *Scand. Clin. Lab. Invest.*, **35**, 307–10.

50. Nordyke, R.A., Gilbert, F.I. and Simmons, E.C. (1969) Screening for kidney diseases with radioisotopes. *JAMA*, **208**, 493–8.

51. Blaufox, M.D., Middleton, M.L., Bongiovanne, J. and Davis, B.R. (1996) Cost efficacy of the diagnosis and therapy of renovascular hypertension. *J. Nucl. Med.*, **37**, 171–7.

52. Al-Nahhas, A., Marcus, A.J., Bomanji, J. *et al.* (1989) Validity of the mean parenchymal transit time as a screening test for the detection of functional renal artery stenosis in hypertensive patients. *Nucl. Med. Commun.*, **10**, 807–15.

53. Smith, H.W. (1956) Unilateral nephrectomy in hypertensive disease. *J. Urol.* **76**, 685–701.

54. Luke, R.G., Kennedy, A.C., Briggs, J.D. *et al.* (1968) Result of nephrectomy in hypertension associated with unilateral renal disease. *Br. Med. J.*, **3**, 764–8.

55. Datseris, I.E., Sonmezoglu, K., Siraj, Q.H. *et al.* (1995) Predictive value of captopril transit renography in essential hypertension and diabetic nephropathy. *Nucl. Med. Commun.*, **16**, 4–9.

56. Oei, H.Y., Hoogeveen, E.K., Kooij, P.P.M. *et al.* (1994) Sensitivity of captopril renography for detecting renal artery stenosis based on visual evaluation of sequential images performed with ^{99m}Tc-MAG3, in *Radionuclides in Nephrourology* (eds P.H. O'Reilly, A. Taylor and J.V. Nally), Field and Wood, Philadelphia, pp. 43–50.

57. Fommei, E., Ghione, S., Hilson, A.J.W. *et al.* (1993) Captopril radionuclide test in renovascular hypertension: a European multicentre study. *Eur. J. Nucl. Med.*, **20**, 635–44.

58. Nally, J.W., Chen, C., Fine, E. *et al.* (1991) Diagnostic criteria of renovascular hypertension with captopril renography. *Am. J. Hypertension*, **4**, S749–52.

59. Taylor, A. and Nally, J.V. (1995) Clinical applications of renal scintigraphy. *Am. J. Radiol.*, **164**, 31–41.

60. Taylor, A. and Nally, J.V. (1996) Consensus report on ACE inhibitor renography for the detection of renovascular hypertension. *J. Nucl. Med.*, **37**, 1876–82.

61. Maxwell, M.H., Marks, L.S., Varady, P.D. *et al.* (1975) Renal vein renin in essential hypertension. *J. Lab. Clin. Med.*, **86**, 901–9.

62. Datseris, I.E., Bomanji, J.B., Brown, E.A. *et al.* (1994) Captopril renal scintigraphy in patients with hypertension and chronic renal failure. *J. Nucl. Med.*, **35**, 251–4.

63. Blaufox, M.D. (1994) Should the role of captopril renography extend to the evaluation of chronic renal disease? *J. Nucl. Med.*, **35**, 254–6.

64. Britton, K.E., Bomanji, J.B., Datseris, I.E. *et al.* (1997) Captopril renal radionuclide studies in diabetic nephropathy, in Radionuclide Studies in Nephrology, Santa Fe Symposium 1995 (eds A. Taylor, J.V. Nally and M.D. Blaufox) (in press).

65. Farto, A., Soriano, A., Rinon, A. *et al.* (1996) Detection of renovascular hypertension with isotopic techniques; a comparison between basal, post-captopril and post aspirin renography, in *Radiopharmaceuticals in Nephro Urology* (eds G.S. Lemouris and M.M. Melloul), Mediterra Publishers, Athens, pp. 99–103.

66. O'Reilly, P., Aurell, M., Britton, K.E. *et al.* (1996) Consensus in diuresis renography. *J. Nucl. Med.*, **37**, 1872–6.

67. Whitaker, R.M. (1979) An evaluation of 170 diagnostic pressure flow studies of the upper urinary tract. *J. Urol.*, **121**, 602–4.

68. Whitfield, H.N., Britton, K.E., Hendry, W.F. *et al.* (1979) Frusemide intravenous urography in the diagnosis of pelviureteric junction obstruction. *Br. J. Urol.*, **51**, 445–8.

69. Kletter, K. and Nurnberger, N. (1989) Diagnostic potential of diuresis renography: limitations by the severity of hydronephrosis and by impairment of renal function. *Nucl. Med. Commun.*, **10**, 51–61.

70. Britton, K.E., Nawaz, M.K., Whitfield, H.N. *et al.* (1987) Obstructive nephropathy: comparison between parenchymal transit time index and frusemide diuresis. *Br. J. Urol.*, **59**, 127–32.

71. O'Reilly, P.H., Testa, H.J., Lawson, R.S., Farrar, D.J. and Charlton Edwards, E. (1978) Diuresis renography in equivocal urinary tract obstruction. *Br. J. Urol.*, **50**, 76–80.

72. O'Reilly, P.H., Lawson, R.S., Shields, R.A. and Testa, H.J. (1979) Idiopathic hydronephrosis *J. Urol.*, **121**, 153–5.

73. O'Reilly, P.H. (1986) The diuresis renogram 8 years on: an update. *J. Urol.*, **136**, 993–9.

74. Bahar, T.H. (1988) Chronic urinary schistosomiasis: patterns of abnormalities in radionuclide Tc-99m-DTPA diuretic renogram. *Acta Pathol. Microbiol. Immunol. Scand. Suppl.*, 54–58.

75. Bahar, R.H., Kouris, K., Sabha, X. *et al.* (1989) Value of quantitative analysis of radionuclide diuretic renogram in predicting the outcome of surgery in chronic schistosomal obstructive uropathy, in *Dynamic Functional Studies in Nuclear Medicine in Developing Countries*, International Atomic Energy Agency, Vienna, pp. 141–6.

76. Monsour, M., Azmy, A.F. and MacKenzie, J.R. (1987) Renal scarring secondary to vesicoureteric reflux: critical assessment and new grading. *Br. J. Urol.*, **70**, 320–4.

77. Smellie, J.M., Shaw, P.J., Prescod, N.P. and Bantock, H.M. (1988) ^{99m}Tc dimercaptosuccinic acid (DMSA) scan in patients with established radiological renal scarring. *Arch. Dis. Child.*, **63**, 1315–19.

FURTHER READING

Limouris, G.S., Melloul, M.M., Shukla, S.K. and Biersack, H.-J. (eds) (1996) *Radiopharmaceuticals for Nephro Urology, Current status and Future Aspects*, Mediterra Publishers, Athens.

Taylor, A. and Blaufox, M.D. *Radionuclides in Nephrology*, Santa Fe Symposium, Society of Nuclear Medicine, New York (in press).

Vesicoureteric reflux and ureteric disorders

S. R. Payne and H. J. Testa

INTRODUCTION

Vesicoureteral reflux (VUR) may be defined as a backward passage of urine from the bladder into the ureter and possibly the kidney. It is a non-physiological event, which may have pathological consequences for both renal parenchymal function and ureteric motility. The methods of evaluation, and treatment, of VUR are extremely variable due to a generally poor understanding of this condition [1], despite its potentially devastating effects on long-term health.

Under normal circumstances the vesicoureteral junction functions as a one-way valve, allowing antegrade flow of urine from the kidney, however full the bladder is, yet stopping retrograde flow into the ureter when the intravesical pressure has risen. This valve mechanism seems to be consequent upon the ureter passing through the bladder wall with a length-to-width ratio of 4:1. This means that the intramural ureter is compressed over a longish distance when a detrusor contraction occurs, even when that contraction effects only a minor increase in intravesical pressure.

AETIOLOGY AND PRESENTATION

The aetiology of this condition may be a primary abnormality of the vesicoureteral valvular mechanism, or secondary to factors altering the anatomical or functional integrity of that mechanism.

Primary incompetence of the valvular mechanism may be due to a congenital abnormality such as a short submucosal ureteral tunnel or a large laterally placed ureteric orifice; it may also be associated with other congenital abnormalities such as Prune Belly syndrome. The likelihood of spontaneous resolution in reflux is greater in situations of unilateral VUR and when the reflux is of low grade. The precise incidence of primary VUR is difficult to quantify, since reflux may be found in asymptomatic children [2]; it does seem to have some basis in heredity, since it is common in siblings of affected children [3,4] and in the offspring of individuals who have had reflux during their own childhood [5]. The intramural ureter can be expected to lengthen during the childhood years and this process may convert an incompetent mechanism into a non-refluxing one [6].

Secondary reflux may be the consequence of cystitis (in 29–50% of cases), or surgery such as re-implantation or ureteric meatotomy, or due to the placement of a double-J stent as a temporary internal urinary diversion. Structural or functional abnormalities of the lower urinary tract may also result in reflux. Congenital or acquired obstructions to bladder drainage, due to conditions such as urethral valves, prostatic hypertrophy or urethral strictures, or neurological conditions, resulting in a high-pressure detrusor and a high outlet resistance, may cause significant renal damage if the underlying cause for the reflux is not identified. Boys with urethral valves and individuals with spinal dysraphism or spinal injury are groups particularly at risk of developing early renal damage due to asymptomatic high-pressure reflux.

VUR may present clinically in a variety of ways, dependent upon the aetiology. The most common mode of presentation of primary reflux is with urinary tract infection, associated with the dysfunctional voiding symptoms of frequency, urgency, uralgia and occasionally strangury; this symptom set is most commonly seen in girls and tends to present within the first few years of life. Secondary VUR is less likely to present with dysfunctional voiding in young boys with urethral valves, who usually present within the first months of life, although these symptoms may be prominent features of VUR in acquired abnormalities resulting in high intravesical pressures. Urge incontinence and enuresis are particular symptoms that may indicate high-pressure voiding and raise the possibility of VUR. The presence of VUR is often now being suggested by maternal ultrasound scanning during pregnancy. Inference of reflux may be made from transient dilatation of the foetal urinary tract; this behoves investigation of the child at birth to differentiate between dilatation due to reflux, low-pressure dilatation due to

Clinical Nuclear Medicine, 3rd edn. Edited by M.N. Maisey, K.E. Britton and B.D. Collier. Published in 1998 by Chapman & Hall, London. ISBN 0 412 75180 1

dysplastic syndromes, and high-pressure dilatation due to obstruction [7]. Routine, non-selective, ultrasound scanning of all newborn infants has not, however, been shown to be efficient in detecting the presence of reflux in the population at large [8].

PATHOPHYSIOLOGY

Whatever the reason for VUR, the end-result is that bladder emptying is incomplete, with refluxed urine from the urinary tract returning to the bladder after voiding. The degree of reflux, i.e. the volume of urine that refluxes (the grade), has been assumed to determine the likelihood of infection, and therefore, the expected pathophysiological progression of this condition.

Reflux without infection and at normal voiding pressures appears to have little impact on the upper urinary tract. even where the reflux volume is high [9,10]. A number of 'grading' systems have been evolved to quantify the degree of reflux and the morphological changes it has caused in the collecting system. The method illustrated in Table 11.4 utilizes a five-point grading, based upon radiological appearances during micturating cystourethrography, and is perhaps that most widely used [11]. The problem with this, and any other method of classification, is that reflux is a transient phenomenon, and while one study may suggest a certain grade of reflux, this observation may not be seen subsequently without any active anti-reflux treatment having been initiated [12].

In the presence of infection, there is potential for development of acute pyelonephritis with subsequent cortical scarring and permanent loss of

function, if urine refluxes back into the renal collecting system. This acquisition of infection, may occur *in utero*, but is most frequently acquired after birth [13]. Once the scar tissue has become established, and even after the cause of reflux has been treated, there is still a predisposition for further attacks of pyelonephritis, and consequently, further parenchymal scarring [14,15]. This occurs in 22–50% of those who reflux, and can lead to end-stage renal failure in 5–15% of those affected in adult life. The presence of cortical scarring is therefore a pathological process that needs to be prevented [15]; it is the determinant for the long-term outcome from VUR [16], and also determines the follow-up necessary once VUR has been diagnosed [17,18]. However, there does appear to be a direct correlation between the grade of the VUR and the subsequent development and progression of cortical scarring [19], and so information about the degree of reflux is probably an important clinical prognostic tool.

Reflux into the ureter associated with dilatation of the ureter or pelvicalyceal system will result in morphological change in the ureter, dependent upon the degree and duration of ureteric dilatation. A decrease in the muscular component of the ureter due to this dilatation will impair urine bolus transmission from the kidney to the bladder, and in the long-term may further compound problems with parenchymal function. Established structural changes in the ureter will not be improved by anti-reflux treatment, and prevention of dilatation should be a secondary objective of therapy.

DIAGNOSIS OF VESICOURETERAL REFLUX

Various methods for the non-invasive determination of reflux and its sequelae have been widely evaluated and compared. It seems important for these various investigations to:

- be able to differentiate urinary tract infection without reflux from that associated with VUR due to the secondary effects of even minor degrees of reflux on renal scarring [18];
- grade the reflux to determine the likely progression of that scarring dependent upon the severity of the reflux [19]; and
- determine whether the scarring is progressing and is likely to have a deleterious effect on the total renal function.

Table 11.4 Classification of grades of vesicoureteral reflux [11]

Grade I	The micturating cystourethrogram shows reflux into the distal ureters
Grade II	There is evidence of reflux into the collecting system without caliceal dilatation or blunting
Grade III	As above, plus mild dilatation of pelvis and calyces
Grade IV	As above, plus moderate dilatation of pelvis and calyces with some clubbing of calyces
Grade V	As above, plus severe tortuosity of the ureters

Imaging tests used in the investigation of VUR can therefore be divided into those that determine the presence of reflux, and those that demonstrate the sequelae of reflux.

DETECTION OF REFLUX

Radiological techniques

Micturating cystourethrography (MCUG) has been the mainstay of diagnosis of VUR for many years, providing the 'gold standard' by which the grading systems of the severity of reflux have been determined, and against which other investigations must be compared (Figure 11.14). MCUG is an invasive investigation necessitating catheterization, and is associated with a risk of introducing infection into an already compromised urinary tract [9]. This non-physiological technique, which involves passing a catheter into the bladder, filling it rapidly with a hyperosmolar contrast medium and precipitating voiding 'in public,' is associated with a significant variation in the observed result. Use of the intravenous urogram to effect bladder filling has not been found helpful, and because this radiological technique is associated with potentially an increased risk of carcinogenesis in young children, it has generally been displaced from widespread use. The use of expression cystography by filling the bladder with the individual anaesthetized, applying suprapubic pressure, and taking X-ray images to show reflux, is very rarely used for the same reason.

Ultrasound (US)

Ultrasonography, by virtue of its non-invasive nature, has been proposed as an alternative to MCUG for the determination of VUR. However, unless grossly dilated, the ureter is difficult to visualize using this imaging modality, even when colour Doppler imaging or micro-bubble cystographic modifications are used. Because of the transient nature of reflux, US scores poorly against MCUG, and has a low sensitivity and specificity for picking up even high grades of reflux [20]. Inference of the presence of reflux by the sonographic detection of renal scarring is also poor [21]. US is, however, a valuable investigation, particularly in the investigation of secondary VUR, where information about bladder morphology and the efficiency of bladder emptying is essential. Consequently, a urinary tract US is often

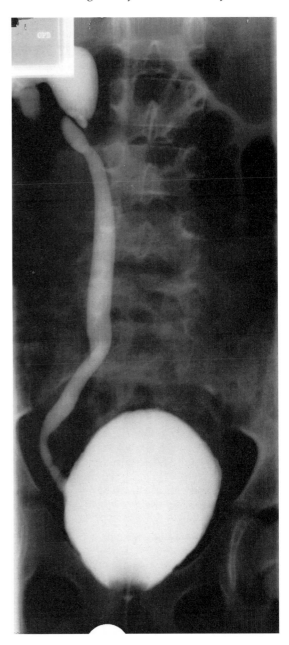

Figure 11.14 An example of grade IV vesicoureteral reflux into the right upper urinary tract. There is both dilatation of the ureter and the pelvi-calyceal system of the kidney.

used to exclude morphological abnormalities that may cause reflux; its sensitivity being improved by combination with other imaging modalities, particularly the use of radionuclides.

Radionuclide techniques

Radionuclide cystography, a radionuclide equivalent to the MCUG, was first described in 1959 by Winter [22]. It was not developed for routine clinical practice until the introduction of the gamma-camera, when dynamic visualization of images of the voiding cycle became possible. Since then, two different techniques of radionuclide cystography have been in use: first, the instillation of radionuclide into the bladder followed by scanning (direct method) [23,24], and second, the observation of radionuclide activity in the ureter following its intravenous administration (indirect method) [25]. More recently, imaging of the direction of flow of the isolated, radionuclide-containing ureteric bolus has been used as an accurate, physiological and operator-independent technique for detecting VUR [26].

Direct radionuclide cystography necessitates the introduction of a bladder catheter, drainage of the residual urine, and the instillation of a non-absorbable radiopharmaceutical, such as ^{99m}Tc-sulphur colloid (20 MBq) in normal saline, until the bladder is full, at which point the patient voids. Continuous dynamic images are acquired during filling, voiding and after voiding, using a gamma-camera computer system; it is important that both kidney areas and the bladder region are in the gamma-camera field-of-view for the whole study. The presence or absence of reflux is visualized directly on a persistence monitor, continuous data being acquired in the computer system for subsequent analysis at the completion of the investigation. Relevant images of the study are then produced for reporting purposes. Since there is no body background, and in particular no renal tract background activity, the method is sensitive even for low-grade reflux [27]. By comparison with MCUG, the radiation dose received by the patient is significantly reduced [28]. This technique is more sensitive than indirect radionuclide cystography in the detection of VUR [29], and in addition, facilitates simultaneous urodynamic measurements of bladder pressures. The limitations of this technique over MCUG are that visualization of the urethra and the bladder neck is not possible, and the risk of precipitating urinary tract infection is similar to the radiological technique.

Indirect radionuclide cystography is carried out as an extension of a renogram. The patient should not void until the bladder feels full. At that time a gamma-camera image of the bladder region is obtained, with further acquisition of continuous dynamic images during voiding in a 'private' environment. A final image is taken once micturition has been completed. Reflux is evident when more activity is seen in the renal area and/or ureters during the elimination phase of the renogram, or during voiding, or following micturition, than on the image acquired before bladder emptying commenced (Figure 11.15). The great advantage of this technique is that it avoids bladder catheterization and allows evaluation of both renal function and urinary elimination under more physiological circumstances. The use of this investigation is, however, limited to cooperative and continent subjects; therefore it is unsuitable for the investigation of children who are not toilet-trained. The technique is as sensitive and specific as MCUG, for the presence of VUR, with sensitivity of 74% and a specificity of 90% [25,30,31].

The investigation of ureteric function, and of *in vivo* ureteric peristalsis in particular, has become possible through the development by Muller-Schauenberg *et al.* of the Nuclear Medicine Space Time Matrix [32]. The technique has been applied to the investigation of ureteric function [33,34], and has been shown to be a reproducible method of imaging ureteric peristalsis [35,36] at a lower

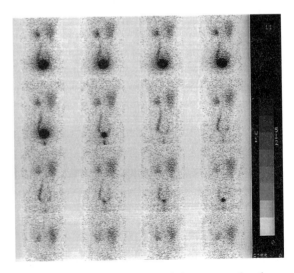

Figure 11.15 Indirect radionuclide cystography showing the left ureter filling with tracer as the bladder empties during voiding.

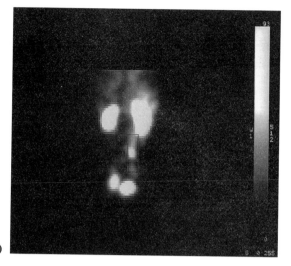

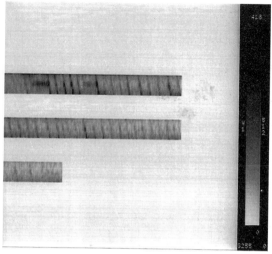

(a)

(b)

Figure 11.16   (a) The region of interest defined over the left ureter to facilitate identification of ureteric spindles by the modified technique [38]. (b) An example of a 'spindle image' of ureteric urine transport. In this display, the x-axis represents time, while the y-axis represents distance from the renal pelvis, located at the top of the display, to the bladder, located at the bottom of the image. The line of negative slope indicates 'normal' antegrade ureteric peristalsis.

radiation dose than the radiological techniques [37].

The technique requires an acquisition interval of 2–2.5 s per frame throughout a renogram, instead of the usual 10-s frames acquired during conventional renography. In this way, the passage of a bolus of urine down the ureter (a spindle that normally takes about 10 s and indicates ureteric peristalsis) is recorded in several frames. To display ureteric peristaltic activity, data acquired from several regions-of-interest (ROIs) of equal size are drawn over the ureter, from top to bottom. A bolus of radioactive urine will first be apparent as a high level of activity in the renal pelvic ROI, and subsequent frames will show the activity passing into the upper, middle and lower ROIs of the ureter as this drains towards the bladder. The ROI for each frame is displayed as a vertical column with sequential frames arranged horizontally, and to the right. This produces a time–distance matrix image of ureteric activity against time.

This method was modified by Rose *et al.* [38]. The frame acquisition rate for the renogram is the same, but the images are filtered temporally and spatially. A single ROI, 3 pixels wide, is created over the whole length of the ureter (Figure 11.16(a)). To produce the display, the ROI from

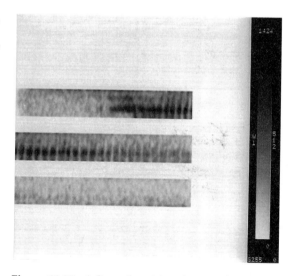

Figure 11.17   A line of positive slope in the 'spindle image' indicates urine flowing retrogradely up the ureter from the bladder towards the renal pelvis. This can intimate vesicoureteral reflux or retrograde peristalsis due to an obstruction in bolus passage.

each frame is aligned in a vertical column and compressed, giving a 1 pixel-wide column. The columns are then positioned in temporal order (Figure 11.16(b)). This method of spindle analysis gives a finer resolution of bolus anatomy than the Muller-Schauenberg technique, with characteristic diagonal lines of negative slope representing antegrade peristalsis in the ureter [39]. The dose of the radiopharmaceutical administered is usually increased (e.g. 100 MBq of ^{99m}Tc-DTPA, 30 MBq of ^{123}I-Hippuran or 75 MBq of ^{99m}Tc-MAG3) to facilitate spindle visualization [40]. These modifications allow detailed investigation of normal [41] and abnormal [26] ureteric function. Reflux can be inferred from the lines of positive slope on the matrix image (Figure 11.17).

EVALUATION OF SEQUELAE

Radiological techniques

The intravenous urogram (IVU) has little place in the determination of renal scarring or the efficiency of upper urinary tract drainage. Even with modification of the examination technique [42], there is still an unacceptable radiation exposure, particularly to children, which means that routine use of the IVU has been all but superseded by the combination of US and radionuclide scanning.

Ultrasound

Ultrasound, in isolation, has proven disappointing in determining the presence or absence of parenchymal scarring in comparison with urography or scintigraphic techniques. The potential for missing upper tract dilatation indicative of high-grade reflux (i.e. grades III–V) is high [20], which promotes the risk of failing to identify those kidneys at risk of scarring; there is also significant inter-observer variation in the diagnosis of parenchymal scarring itself [21].

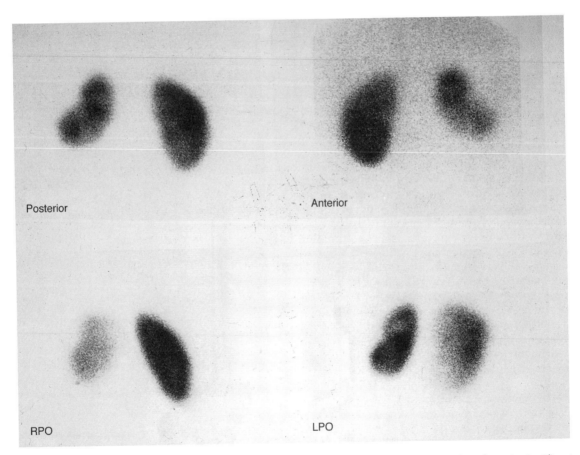

Posterior   Anterior

RPO   LPO

Figure 11.18 The presence of scarring as shown by DMSA scanning. It is noticeable that there is significant decrease in the size of the left kidney and irregularity of its contour and a break in the cortical outline.

Radionuclide techniques

Dimercaptosuccinic acid (DMSA) scanning has been shown to be the most effective method of demonstrating the presence of renal scarring (Figure 11.18). It has a significantly greater sensitivity than IVU [18] and US [21], and is a useful investigation for monitoring disease progression [17]. DMSA scanning is especially helpful in the determination of scarring associated with antenatally diagnosed reflux [14], which gives important prognostic information as far as the child's long-term renal function is concerned [17]. The use of DMSA for accurately determining differential renal function is also helpful for monitoring the progression of scarring. A decrease in unilateral function may indicate increased parenchymal fibrosis and may suggest a need for active intervention.

The possible effects of reflux on upper tract motility and morphology are often forgotten. Impaired excretion of radionuclide from the renal pelvis on sequential renographic scanning may indicate increasing fibrosis of the dynamic components of the pelvicalyceal system and ureter [43]. Renography may be used as an effective non-invasive method of detecting the continued presence of reflux, using indirect radionuclide cystography, of drainage impairment, by interpretation of the excretion curve, of differential function, by analysis of the 2-minute uptake of tracer, and of bolus transmission, by spindle imaging. Although renography cannot be used to determine the presence of scarring, it is a useful technique for the monitoring of renal function and upper tract drainage in vesicoureteral reflux.

REFERENCES

1. Elder, J.S., Snyder, H.M., Peters, C. *et al.* (1992) Variations in practice among urologists and nephrologists treating children with vesicoureteral reflux. *J. Urol.*, **148**, 714–17.
2. Shrestha, G.K., Ikoma, F., Schumacher, S. *et al.* (1994) Asymptomatic vesicoureteral reflux in children. *Int. Urol. Nephrol.*, **26**, 283–91.
3. Noe, H.N. (1992) The long-term results of prospective sibling reflux screening. *J. Urol.*, **148**, 1739–42.
4. Kenda, R.B. and Fettich, J.J. (1992) Vesicoureteric reflux and renal scars in asymptomatic siblings of children with reflux. *Arch. Dis. Child.*, **67**, 506–8.
5. Cooper, A. and Atwell, J. (1993) A long-term follow-up of surgically treated vesicoureteral reflux in girls. *J. Paediatr. Surg.*, **28**, 1034–6.
6. Ransley, P.G. (1982) Vesicoureteric reflux, in *Paediatric Urology*, 2nd edn (eds D.I. Williams and J.H. Johnston), Butterworth, London, pp. 151–65.
7. Whitaker, R.H. and Thomas, D.F.M. (1991) Prenatal diagnosis of urological disorders, in *Recent Advances in Urology/Andrology*, No. 5 (ed. W.F. Hendry), Churchill Livingstone, Edinburgh, pp. 37–51.
8. Scott, J.E., Lee, R.E., Hunter, E.W. *et al.* (1991) Ultrasound screening of newborn urinary tract. *Lancet*, **338**, 1571–3.
9. Hodson, C.J., Maling, T.M.J. and McManamon, P.J. (1975) Reflux nephropathy. *Kidney Int.*, 8, 50–8.
10. Ransley, P.G., Risdon, R.A. and Goldy, M.L. (1984) High pressure vesicoureteral reflux and renal scarring: an experimental study in the pig and minipig. *Contr. Nephrol.*, **39**, 320–43.
11. International Reflux Study Committee (1981) Medical versus surgical treatment of primary vesicoureteral reflux. *Paediatrics*, **67**, 392–400.
12. Fettich, J.J. and Kenda, R.B. (1992) Cyclic direct radionuclide voiding cystography: increasing reliability in detecting vesicoureteral reflux in children. *Paediatr. Radiol.*, **22**, 337–8.
13. Crabbe, D.C., Thomas, D.F., Gordon, A.C. *et al.* (1992) Use of ^{99m}Technetium-dimercaptosuccinic acid to study patterns of renal damage associated with prenatally detected vesicoureteral reflux. *J. Urol.*, **148**, 1229–31.
14. Arima, M., Matsui, T., Ogino, T. *et al.* (1993) Vesicoureteral reflux in infants under one year old. Follow-up study and consideration on development of renal scarring. *Urology*, **41**, 372–7.
15. Weiss, R., Duckett, J. and Spitzer, A. (1992) Results of a randomised clinical trial of medical versus surgical management of infants and children with grades III and IV primary vesicoureteral reflux. *J. Urol.*, **148**, 1667–73.
16. Smellie, J.M. (1992) Commentary: management of children with severe vesicoureteral reflux. *J. Urol.*, **148**, 1676–8.
17. Rushton, H.G., Majd, M., Jantausch, B. *et al.* (1992) Renal scarring following reflux and nonreflux pyelonephritis in children: evaluation with ^{99m}Technetium-dimercaptosuccinic acid scintigraphy. *J. Urol.*, **147**, 1327–32.
18. Arant, B.S. (1992) Medical management of mild and moderate vesicoureteral reflux: follow-up studies of infants and young children. A preliminary report of the Southwest Paediatric Nephrology Study Group. *J. Urol.*, **148**, 1683–7.
19. Elison, B.S., Taylor, D., Van der Wall, H. *et al.* (1992) Comparison of DMSA scintigraphy with intravenous urography for the detection of renal scarring and its correlation with vesicoureteric reflux. *Br. J. Urol.*, **69**, 294–302.
20. Blane, C.E., DiPietro, M.A., Zerin, J.M. *et al.* (1993) Renal sonography is not a reliable screening examination for vesicoureteral reflux. *J. Urol.*, **150**, 752–5.
21. Stokland, E., Hellstrom, M., Hansson, S. *et al.* (1994) Reliability of ultrasonography in identification of reflux nephropathy in children. *Br. Med. J.*, **309**, 235–9.

22. Winter, C.C. (1959) A new test for vesicoureteral reflux: an external technique using radioisotopes. *J. Urol.*, **81**, 105–11.

23. Willi, U.V. and Treves, S.T. (1985) Radionuclide voiding cystography, in *Paediatric Nuclear Medicine* (ed. S.T. Treves), Springer, New York, pp. 105–9.

24. Conway, J.J. (1985) Radionuclide cystography, in *Nuclear Medicine in Clinical Urology and Nephrology* (eds W.N. Tauxe and E.V. Dubovsky), Appleton Century and Crofts, East Norwalk, pp. 305–20.

25. Gordon, I., Peters, A.M. and Morony, S. (1990) Indirect radionuclide cystography: a sensitive technique for the detection of vesicoureteral reflux. *Paediatr. Nephrol.*, **4**, 604–6.

26. Lancashire, M.J.R. (1996) *Ureteric function in pathological states*. Doctorate of Medicine, University of London.

27. Willi, U. and Treves, S.T. (1983) Radionuclide voiding cystography. *Urol. Radiol.*, **5**, 161–73.

28. Rothwell, D.L., Constable, A.R. and Albrecht, M. (1977) Radionuclide cystography in the investigation of vesicoureteric reflux in children. *Lancet*, **i**, 1072–5.

29. De Sadeleer, C., De Boe, V., Keuppens, F. *et al.* (1994) How good is Technetium-99th mercaptoacetyltriglycine indirect cystography? *Eur. J. Nucl. Med.*, **21**, 223–7.

30. Pollet, J.E., Sharp, P.F. and Smith, F.W. (1979) Radionuclide imaging for vesico-renal reflux using intravenous ^{99m} Tc-DTPA. *Paediatr. Radiol.*, **8**, 165–7.

31. Hedman, P.J.K., Kempi, V. and Voss, H. (1978) Measurements of vesicoureteric reflux with intravenous ^{99m}Tc DTPA compared with radiographic cystography. *Radiology*, **126**, 205–8.

32. Muller-Schauenberg, W., Anger, K., Carl, I., Feine, U. and Hippeli, R. (1978) Erste Erfahrungen mit einer neuen nuklearmedizinischen Darstellung der Uretern, in *Proceedings of 16th International Annual Meeting of the Society of Nuclear Medicine 1978* (eds X. Schmidt and X. Berrocal), Schattauer, Madrid, pp. 552–5.

33. Muller-Schaunenberg, W. (1981) Imaging of peristaltic waves and other ureteral kinetics by a highly sensitive space–time-matrix display of one-dimensional motions, in *Information Processing in Medical Imaging, VIIth International Conference, 1981* (ed. M.L. Goris), Stanford University, pp. 264–75.

34. Muller-Schauenberg, W. and Anger, K. (1985) The Nuclear Medicine Space Time Matrix Approach to Ureteral Motility, in *Urodynamics – Upper and Lower Urinary Tract II* (eds W. Lutzeyer and J.H. Hannappel), Springer-Verlag, Berlin, Heidelberg, pp. 154–67.

35. Muller-Suur, R. and Mesko, L. (1987) Analysis of ureteral peristalsis in routine renography using a time–space approach. *Contrib. Nephrol.*, **56**, 232–7.

36. Lewis, C.A., Coptcoat, M.J., Carter, S. *et al.* (1989) Radionuclide imaging of ureteric peristalsis. *Br. J. Urol.*, **63**, 144–8.

37. Muller-Suur, R., Muller-Schauenberg, W., Mesko, L. and Ohlson, L. (1988) Urinary peristalsis investigated by radionuclide and X-ray methods: a comparison. *Scand. J. Urol. Nephrol.*, **22** (Suppl. 110), 285–90.

38. Rose, M.R., Lawson, R.S. and Wujanto, R. (1987) Experience in the use of a fast frame renography to demonstrate ureteric peristalsis and reflux. *Nucl. Med. Commun.*, **8**(4), 244 (abstract).

39. Wemyss-Holden, G., Hosker, G., Rose, M., Payne, S. and Testa, H. (1993) Validation of a non-invasive radioisotope method of imaging ureteric urine transport. *Br. J. Urol.*, **71**, 130–6.

40. Wemyss-Holden, G.D., Hosker, G.L., Rose, M.R., Payne, S.R. and Testa, H.J. (1994) Validation of, and initial evaluation of, a technique for non-invasive measurement of ureteric function, in *Radionuclides in Nephrourology*, Field and Wood Periodicals Inc., pp. 139–53.

41. Wemyss-Holden, G.D., Rose, M.R., Payne, S.R. and Testa, H.J. (1993) Non-invasive investigation of normal individual ureteric activity in man. *Br. J. Urol.*, **71**, 156–60.

42. Smellie, J.M. (1995) The intravenous urogram in the detection and evaluation of renal damage following urinary tract infection. *Pediatr. Nephrol.*, **9**, 213–19.

43. Lupton, E.W., Testa, H.J., O'Reilly, P.H. *et al.* (1979) Diuresis renography and morphology in upper urinary tract obstruction. *Br. J. Urol.*, **51**, 10–14.

Renal transplantation

A. J. W. Hilson

INTRODUCTION

Nuclear medicine has a significant role to play in the management of renal transplant recipients. To understand this role, it is necessary briefly to review the clinical problems.

In the immediate post-operative period, there may be a concern about the vascular supply to the kidney. Over the 24 to 48 hours following surgery, the kidney shows the effect of the (inevitable) ischaemic injury that it has undergone. This process is known as acute tubular necrosis (ATN). It may lead to total anuria by the end of 48 hours. At the same time, the kidney is being exposed to the recipient's immune system, and this inevitably leads to an element of acute rejection. With modern immunosuppression, this is usually mild and occurs more slowly than was the case before the introduction of cyclosporin A as an immunosuppressant. Typically, a mild cell-mediated rejection develops at about 7–10 days (with modern tissue-typing, the full-blown accelerated or hyper-acute rejection of the past, developing in the first 48 hours, is rarely seen). This rejection involves the parenchyma and especially the vasculature (which is, of course, of donor origin). It also involves the donor ureter, which may lose its peristaltic properties.

Over a longer time scale, the management depends on the use of maintenance therapy, including cyclosporin A. This is not straightforward, as a low dosage may lead to rejection, while chronic higher dosage leads to renal damage. This is initially parenchymal but, if maintained or severe, vascular change may result.

Over a period of years, the kidney may also undergo chronic rejection, which is poorly understood, but involves both vasculature and parenchyma.

At any stage – but especially in the immediate post-operative period – there may be surgical complications.

RADIOPHARMACEUTICALS

Experience has shown that there is no significant advantage to either ^{99m}Tc-MAG3 or ^{99m}Tc-DTPA in the investigation of renal transplants, although it is often convenient to use one agent in any given patient until expertise has been gained.

THE IMMEDIATE POST-OPERATIVE PERIOD

If there is no suspicion of surgical complications, and the patient's urine output is good, with the serum creatinine level falling satisfactorily, then it is preferable to leave the baseline study until about 48 hours after surgery, when the effect of ATN is likely to be maximal.

If the patient is passing satisfactory volumes of urine (30 ml/h above any previous urine output), but the serum creatinine is not falling, this most likely represents moderate to severe ATN. Occasionally, patients who have been maintained on regular haemodialysis may develop a 'hypovolaemic circulatory failure' without fluid loss. Treatment consists of fluid replacement, but occasionally a nuclear medicine study may be requested to confirm renal perfusion.

Complete anuria post-operatively is always a cause of alarm. If there is a suspicion of a vascular complication, this represents an emergency, and the kidney must be studied immediately with whatever pharmaceutical is to hand. The study should always be reviewed with either the surgeon concerned or his or her operation note, to be sure what the vascular supply to the kidney was – it is not uncommon for the graft to have two or more arteries, and it may be necessary to look for evidence of a polar or posterior surface infarct.

The image should also be examined for evidence of a photon-deficient area above or around the kidney, representing a collection. If one is seen, a delayed image must be obtained to see whether it fills in with the ^{99m}Tc-DTPA or ^{99m}Tc-MAG3, representing a urine collection. This may happen even if the graft is apparently producing no urine, as the ureter may have become detached from the

Clinical Nuclear Medicine, 3rd edn. Edited by M.N. Maisey, K.E. Britton and B.D. Collier. Published in 1998 by Chapman & Hall, London. ISBN 0 412 75180 1

bladder and there may be a total leak. It is important to remember that all renal transplant recipients have had an incision in the bladder for the reimplantation of the ureter. For this reason, the bladder is always drained with a urethral or supra-pubic catheter. This must never be clamped, as this may produce a leak, especially if the patient is in the polyuric phase of recovery from renal failure.

If the collection does not fill in, but urine is being produced, it may be a haematoma. Ultrasound may be helpful here, as fluid collections such as urine are well shown by ultrasound. If no separate collection is shown ultrasonographically, then a haematoma is more likely, as fresh haematomas in the transplant bed are often not identified on ultrasound, since they consist of solid echogenic clot that cannot be clearly separated from the retroperitoneal muscle on which the graft is lying.

The worst situation that may be seen is that of the dreaded 'black hole' – so named from the early days when images were recorded on Polaroid instant film, and a non-perfused kidney was seen as a black hole surrounded by a rim of inflammatory activity. This is generally considered an indication for instant intervention – the surgeon should be contacted as soon as this is seen on the screen, even before the study is finished, as the only hope is for urgent vascular surgery [1].

THE EARLY POST-OPERATIVE PERIOD

On the baseline study performed at about 48 hours, it is usual to see some evidence of ATN. This is shown on a ^{99m}Tc-DTPA study as a mild to moderate impairment of perfusion, with the presence of a blood pool within the kidney at 2 minutes, but little or no excretion. With ^{99m}Tc-MAG3 the perfusion changes are similar, but the parenchyma shows progressive accumulation of tracer, with varying excretion. Indeed, if no excretion is seen, it may not be possible to exclude obstruction (although this is extremely uncommon in renal transplants). This is one of the very unusual times when a dual pharmaceutical study may be necessary: if a ^{99m}Tc-DTPA study shows gross impairment, a ^{99m}Tc-MAG3 study may be reassuring to show that there is uptake of tracer by tubular cells – which is probably a good prognostic sign. Conversely, if a ^{99m}Tc-MAG3 study shows progressive uptake, a ^{99m}Tc-DTPA study showing that there is

no functional peak, but rather a blood pool, may be taken as proof of ATN.

The impairment of perfusion typical of ATN may be assessed more accurately by use of numerical methods. The most widely used compares the upslope of the curve from a region of interest (ROI) drawn over the transplanted kidney with the upslope of a curve from a ROI over the iliac artery. This gives a 'perfusion index' which reflects renal transplant perfusion (Figure 11.19). In simple ATN there is mild to moderate impairment of perfusion, but this improves steadily with time [2]. It used to be necessary to carry this out on alternate days because of the lack of other methods of investigation and the fear of rejection, but now it is more usual to carry it out once or twice per week in the oliguric period.

Some centres use a measurement of ^{99m}Tc-MAG3 clearance as a measurement of renal blood flow [3]. While there is no doubt that this measurement changes with pathology, this is more complicated, as the clearance reflects not only blood flow, but also extraction fraction, which may change with pathology.

Regardless of the agent used, it is essential to record the presence or absence of excretion, and

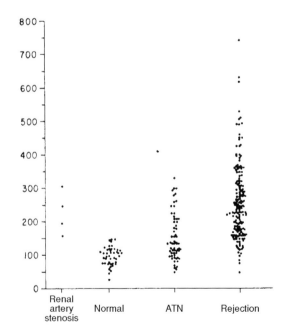

Figure 11.19 Values of perfusion index in 276 studies in patients of known renal transplant status. (After Hilson *et al.*, 1978 [2].)

imaging of the bladder or catheter bag should always be obtained and recorded, even if it contains no activity.

THE LATER POST-OPERATIVE PERIOD

During the first 2–3 weeks following the operation, there is usually slow but definite resolution of the ATN. This is seen as a steady improvement in perfusion (shown as a fall in the perfusion index) accompanied by improving function as measured by a rising glomerular filtration rate (GFR), 2-minute uptake or improved percentage of dose excreted during the study. However, it is not uncommon for an episode of rejection to develop, typically from about 5 or 7 days onwards. Since the introduction of cyclosporin A as anti-rejection therapy this is less dramatic than it used to be in the earlier period when prednisolone and azathioprine were the only agents available (when a rejection episode could 'explode' in a matter of minutes). Now, a more typical time scale is that a rejection will develop slowly over a day or so. This has taken much of the rush and drama out of management.

REJECTION

The features of a full-blown rejection episode are very characteristic, but it is also important to realise that it is relatively uncommon for all the features to be present.

The most important feature is the impairment of perfusion, more easily detected when a measure of perfusion such as a perfusion index is used. Sometimes this may only be a failure of improvement of perfusion in a kidney with ATN. The kidney may also swell, and in a functioning graft there may be deterioration of function. A feature that is often missed is the development of 'pseudo-obstruction'. This is a dilatation of the ureter, due to its rejection, with delay of entry of tracer into the bladder. One key feature is that in true obstruction there is dilatation of the renal calyces, whereas in rejection the calyces are compressed by oedema of the renal pyramids.

With successful treatment of the rejection, the features should all reverse, but the perfusion may take up to 5 days to recover after treatment.

It is important to realise that renal blood flow falls following haemodialysis, so that in the oliguric patient on haemodialysis, the study must be performed at least 6 hours after a dialysis session – in practice this usually means carrying out the nuclear medicine study first thing in the morning before starting dialysis.

During the post-operative oliguric period, it is helpful to study the graft once or twice a week to follow recovery and monitor possible complications.

CYCLOSPORIN A TOXICITY

The third major complication is cyclosporin A toxicity. This drug is used in lower concentrations than initially, and toxicity is less of a problem. At the dose levels now used, it initially produces a parenchymal impairment. If sustained high levels occur, then further vascular changes may follow. Therefore, as might be predicted, the initial feature on a nuclear medicine study is a deterioration in parenchymal function, as measured by uptake or percentage excreted, while perfusion is relatively unaffected [4]. This is the converse of rejection. However, if there is deterioration of both perfusion and parenchymal function it is not possible to distinguish between rejection and cyclosporin A toxicity on nuclear medicine grounds. Nonetheless, to produce vascular changes, cyclosporin A levels will have been high for several days, while for rejection to occur they will have been low.

THE FUNCTIONING GRAFT AND LATER COMPLICATIONS

Once urine output and excretory function have recovered, nuclear medicine studies are indicated if there is subsequent deterioration in function (which may be due to cyclosporin A toxicity or to the development of acute or chronic rejection), or there is a suspicion of a complication.

It is helpful to carry out serial studies at regular intervals after transplantation – it is almost impossible to make helpful comments on a graft that has not been studied for several years, but where the function has suddenly deteriorated.

URETERIC COMPLICATIONS

As mentioned above, ureteric obstruction is uncommon (indeed many surgeons deliberately do not implant the ureter with an anti-reflux incision because they are more worried about obstruction).

Where it is suspected, a 15-minute post-frusemide study may be carried out, but anecdotal experience is that this is unreliable, perhaps because the system is rigid, or because the diuresis is inadequate, and it may be necessary to arrange a formal radiological antegrade pyelogram. However, it is important to recognize the pseudo-obstruction of rejection (see above).

LYMPHOCOELES

The lymphocoele is the most common fluid collection around a transplanted kidney, and may result from damage to the lymphatics in the hilum of the kidney or of the iliac vessels during the operation. Rarely, it may cause obstruction of the ureter. It is seen as a photon-deficient area in relation to the kidney [5].

Very occasionally, a lymphocoele may 'fill in' on delayed images, especially with ^{99m}Tc-DTPA [6]. This probably represents lymphatic fluid forming in the legs (and containing ^{99m}Tc-DTPA which has diffused into the extravascular space) taking some time to pass up into the groin and thence into the lymphocoele.

Further management of the lymphocoele is by aspiration and/or surgery.

RENAL ARTERY STENOSIS

This is an uncommon complication, especially in cadaveric grafts where the arterial anastomosis is performed using a patch of donor aorta. It is slightly more common in live-related grafts, where there is an end-to-end anastomosis. Typically, it presents as either hypertension or a failing graft months to years after surgery. The nuclear medicine study will show deteriorating perfusion, but there are no specific features, and it is important to realise that this condition cannot be separated from rejection or chronic cyclosporin A toxicity. Even the use of captopril does not help, as all these conditions produce a pre-glomerular vascular lesion which may give a positive response to captopril challenge. It is important to remember the condition, and to be prepared to suggest arteriography, which will give the correct diagnosis.

SCARRING

There is accumulating evidence that scarring of the renal transplant is more common than was first thought, especially in patients with abnormal lower urinary tracts. Single photon emission computed tomography (SPECT) studies using DMSA may show this clearly [7].

INFECTION

In the later phases, apparent chronic infection may be a problem, presenting either as a pyrexia of unknown origin (PUO), or as recurrent urinary tract infections. In this setting, gallium-67 scintigraphy is often of value. Particular regions to be studied are the native kidneys and the peritoneum in patients who had been treated with chronic ambulatory peritoneal dialysis (CAPD) before transplantation.

Chronic infection in the native kidneys is a particular problem, especially in patients with polycystic kidneys. Typically, these patients present with infections every 2–3 months. In this setting, it is helpful to perform the gallium study some 4–6 weeks after an acute episode, rather than on admission, when the patient is usually receiving treatment [8].

Patients on CAPD often develop a chronic low-grade chemical peritonitis, which may be seen on the gallium study, but which does not cause a pyrexia. On the other hand, a focal accumulation may represent a localized collection.

It is also important to monitor bowel activity carefully, as small bowel and/or peritoneal uptake may be the only feature of tuberculosis in these patients.

SCINTIGRAPHIC METHODOLOGY AND TECHNIQUE

The scintigraphic study is performed with the patient supine under the gamma-camera, and positioned so that the upper edge of the field of view is at the level of the aortic bifurcation (a marker on the umbilicus gives this level), and the lower edge is below the base of the bladder. In small patients, or when using large cameras, the camera should be zoomed so that the field of view is filled.

The computer is set for a frame rate of 1 per second for 30 or 40s, followed by 1/20s for 20 minutes. A minimum resolution of 64×64 is used, but 128×128 is preferred.

A bolus of 300 MBq of ^{99m}Tc-DTPA or ^{99m}Tc-MAG3 is injected, and the system started. For analysis, ROIs are defined over the graft, the iliac artery distal to the graft, and a background area.

Activity–time curves are generated, and analysed. It is essential to examine images as well as the curves. For further details, the reader is referred elsewhere [2,9].

REFERENCES

1. Fernand, D.C.J. and Young, K.C. (1985) Scintigraphic patterns of acute vascular occlusion following renal transplantation. *Nucl. Med. Commun.*, **7**, 223–31.
2. Hilson, A.J.W., Maisey, M.N., Brown, C.B., Ogg, C.S. and Bewick, M.S. (1978) Dynamic renal transplant imaging with Tc-99m DTPA (Sn) supplemented by a transplant perfusion index in the management of renal transplants. *J. Nucl. Med.*, **19**, 994–1000.
3. Dubovsky, E.V., Russell, C.D. and Erbas, B. (1995) Radionuclide evaluation of renal transplants [review]. *Semin. Nucl. Med.*, **25**, 49–59.
4. Kim, E.E., Pjura, G., Lowry, P.A., Verani, R., Sandler, C.M., Flechner, S. and Kahan, B.D. (1986) Cyclosporin-A nephrotoxicity and acute cellular rejection in renal transplant recipients: correlation between radionuclide and histologic findings. *Radiology*, **159**, 443–6.
5. Bingham, J.B., Hilson, A.J.W. and Maisey, M.N. (1978) The appearances of renal transplant lymphocoeles during dynamic renal scintigraphy. *Br. J. Radiol.*, **51**, 342–6.
6. Fortenbery, E.J., Blue, P.W., Van Nostrand, D. and Anderson, J.H. (1990) Lymphocele: the spectrum of scintigraphic findings in lymphoceles associated with renal transplant. *J. Nucl. Med.*, **31**, 1627–31.
7. Cairns, H.S., Spencer, S., Hilson, A.J.W., Rudge, C.J. and Neild, G.H. (1994) ^{99m}Tc-DMSA imaging with tomography in renal transplant recipients with abnormal lower urinary tracts. *Nephrol. Dial. Transplant.*, **9**, 1157–61.
8. Tsang, V., Lui, S., Hilson, A.J.W., Moorhead, J.F., Fernando, O.N. and Sweny, P. (1989) Gallium-67 scintigraphy in the detection of infected polycystic kidneys in renal transplant recipients. *Nucl. Med. Commun.*, **10**, 167–70.
9. Ayres, J.G., Hilson, A.J.W. and Maisey, M.N. (1980) Complications of renal transplantation: appearances using 99m-Tc-DTPA. *Clin. Nucl. Med.*, **5**, 473–80.

CHAPTER 12

Genital

Testicular perfusion scintigraphy

Q. H. Siraj

INTRODUCTION

The use of perfusion scintigraphy in the evaluation of acute scrotal disease, particularly for reliable and accurate diagnosis of testicular torsion, has been the most widely employed clinical application of radionuclide testicular imaging. Scintigraphic evaluation of testicular perfusion in a patient presenting with an acute hemi-scrotum is one of the few emergency nuclear medicine procedures which has a significant impact on clinical decision making and patient management.

Perfusion scintigraphy with ^{99m}Tc-pertechnetate was pioneered by Nadel *et al.* [1] for investigating the acute scrotum. The procedure primarily aims at differentiating inflammatory hypervascular conditions from the avascular scrotal lesion caused by compromised testicular perfusion due to spermatic cord torsion. Over the years, a substantial number of studies with added refinements and modifications in the original methodology have been reported [2–6]. The clinical effectiveness of testicular perfusion scintigraphy is now well established; it is a widely validated non-invasive technique reputed for its high diagnostic efficiency. In acute or missed testicular torsion, testicular perfusion scintigraphy has a reported sensitivity of 96%, specificity of 89% and an overall accuracy of 96% [7].

ACUTE SCROTUM: CLINICAL PRESENTATION AND PATHOGENESIS

The clinical evaluation of a young patient presenting with an acute onset of unilateral scrotal symptoms poses a diagnostic dilemma. The non-specificity of symptoms and inadequacy of clinical examination in a poorly compliant distressed paediatric patient suffering from pain and extreme local discomfort quite often contributes towards an indeterminate clinical conclusion; clinical diagnosis may be incorrect in up to 50% of the patients [2].

The common causes of an acute scrotum include: bacterial epididymitis and epididymo-orchitis, viral orchitis, testicular torsion, torsion of a testicular appendage, acute hydrocoele and retention cysts (e.g. spermatocoele and epididymal cysts). Uncommon differential diagnoses include: testicular tumour, strangulated inguinal hernia, testicular trauma, scrotal deep vein thrombosis, idiopathic scrotal oedema, inflammation of the scrotal sac, haemorrhage in a testicular tumour or associated with trauma, scrotal fat necrosis; and acute testicular inflammation associated with tuberculosis, Buerger's disease or Henoch–Schönlein purpura.

Epididymitis is the most frequent aetiology of acute scrotum, which is easily treatable by drugs. In contrast, testicular torsion is a true medical emergency requiring immediate surgery to preserve testicular viability and prevent development of ischaemic necrosis. Since clinical distinction between these two entities is usually unreliable, a prompt and accurate diagnosis through evalu-

Clinical Nuclear Medicine, 3rd edn. Edited by M.N. Maisey, K.E. Britton and B.D. Collier. Published in 1998 by Chapman & Hall, London. ISBN 0 412 75180 1

ation of testicular perfusion is pivotal in implementing appropriate therapy and avoiding unnecessary surgery.

TESTICULAR TORSION
CLINICAL FEATURES
Extravaginal testicular torsion
There are two distinct clinical types of testicular torsion, intravaginal and extravaginal. The extravaginal form is uncommon, found almost exclusively in neonates. The condition is caused by the rotation of the testis and its covering fascia, above the level of tunica vaginalis. Neonatal testicular torsion may occur during late intrauterine life or the early post-partum period. Clinical examination of the neonate reveals a firm, smooth and painless scrotal mass with a variable scrotal reaction. The presentation is fairly specific, which makes clinical diagnosis easy and straightforward. Unilateral orchiectomy is the current treatment for extravaginal testicular torsion, since at the time of surgical exploration the testis is invariably necrotic [8]. In this clinical scenario, evaluation of testicular perfusion appears superfluous and the condition will not be discussed further.

Intravaginal testicular torsion
Intravaginal testicular torsion is the most common acute scrotal ailment in the paediatric and young adult age group. Torsion of the spermatic cord, or that of a testicular appendage, develops in one out of 160 males before the age of 25 years, with a peak incidence at puberty between the ages of 12 and 20 years [9]. The patient with testicular torsion usually presents clinically with an acutely painful, swollen and tender scrotum, accompanied by nausea or vomiting. With time, the scrotal skin becomes increasingly congested and oedematous. Frequently there is coexisting inguinal or abdominal pain causing a delay in the diagnosis.

In suspected testicular torsion, timely surgical intervention is crucial in preserving testicular viability, the testicular salvage rates being inversely proportional to the degree and the duration of spermatic cord torsion. The majority of gonads are salvageable until 6 hours, the critical grey zone is the 6- to 12-hour period, and a delay of more than 24 hours produces only anecdotal salvage [10].

It must be emphasized that testicular viability is not synonymous with preserved testicular function. Despite successful surgical restoration of testicular perfusion, a large proportion of the affected testes reportedly suffer histological injury with subsequent decrease in fertility [11].

Appendage torsion
Torsion of testicular or gonadal appendages accounts for roughly 5% of acute scrotal pathology [12]. Unlike testicular torsion, the condition is relatively uncommon in young adults, with the result that a much higher percentage (around 20%) is encountered in the paediatric age population [13]. The majority (about 85%) of cases of appendage torsion have been reported in patients aged 7–14 years [14]. Clinically, the patient usually presents with an abrupt onset of moderate scrotal or groin pain. Usually the pain is less intense than in testicular torsion and the tenderness more focal – at the upper pole of the testis. The clinical features of appendix testis and appendix epididymis torsions are similar as are the scan appearances.

RELEVANT ANATOMY AND EMBRYOLOGY

A basic knowledge of testicular developmental anatomy and its blood supply is helpful in understanding the aetiology of testicular torsion.

Normal developmental anatomy
During normal foetal development, the intra-abdominal testes, situated retroperitoneally near the kidneys, descend through the inguinal rings, into the scrotum. This descent is accomplished by relative shortening of a fibromuscular band, the gubernaculum testis, which attaches the caudal pole of the testis to the scrotal remnant. The descending testis is preceded by the distal end of a tubular extension of the peritoneum, the processus vaginalis, which herniates into the scrotum approximately at birth (Figure 12.1(a)). The abdominal connection closes, leaving the testis enclosed by a serous sac, the tunica vaginalis testis (Figure 12.1(b)). On the posterolateral aspect of the testis, the visceral layer of tunica vaginalis encloses the epididymis between its two layers and helps anchor the testis by reflecting back to line the scrotum as the parietal layer. In addition, the testes are also anchored posterolaterally by the gubernaculum and the broad epididymal mesorchium.

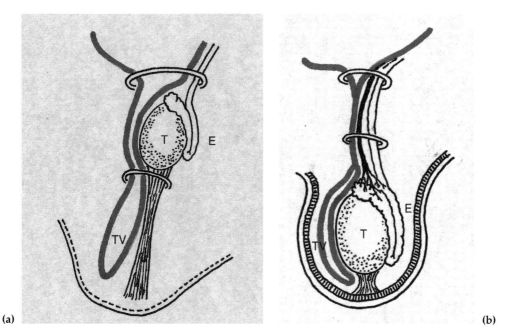

(a)   **(b)**

Figure 12.1 Diagram illustrating: (a) descent of the testes from the abdomen through the inguinal rings into the scrotum, and (b) the formation of tunica vaginalis. T, testis; TV, tunica vaginalis; E, epididymis.

Blood supply

The blood supply of the male genitalia stems from two distinct sources that follow separate routes. The cremasteric, testicular and deferential arteries running along the spermatic cord nourish the testis and are essential to its survival. Spermatic cord torsion may occlude these vessels, causing testicular death. The spermatic cord and epididymis, the testis, and the tunica vaginalis are respectively supplied by the deferential, testicular and cremasteric arteries. The internal pudendal, the superficial and the deep external pudendal arteries supply the scrotum and penis. Testicular torsion does not affect scrotal or penile viability by virtue of their separate blood supply.

Testicular appendages

After birth, vestigial remnants of various structures persist as five testicular appendages including: the appendix testis, a müllerian or paramesonephric duct remnant at the superior pole of the testis; the appendix epididymis, a wolffian or mesonephric duct remnant at the

head of the epididymis; the paradidymis and the superior and inferior vas aberrans, remnants of paragenital tubules. The pedunculated appendages, i.e. the appendix testis and the appendix epididymis are more prone to torsion, representing 98% of the reported cases [15]. Torsion of the appendix testis is about ten times more frequent than that of the appendix epididymis, accounting for 92–95% of the total cases [3,15].

Abnormal developmental anatomy

Occasionally, the visceral layer of the tunica vaginalis encloses the entire testis and the epididymis so that the testis hangs within the scrotum like a bell – the so-called 'bell clapper' deformity (Figure 12.2(a)), which is the major cause of testicular torsion. Patients with this usually bilateral anatomic anomaly have a predisposition to torsion; such testes may rotate and the associated twisting of the spermatic cord (Figure 12.2(b)) compromises testicular and the epididymal perfusion with resultant infarction of the epidi-

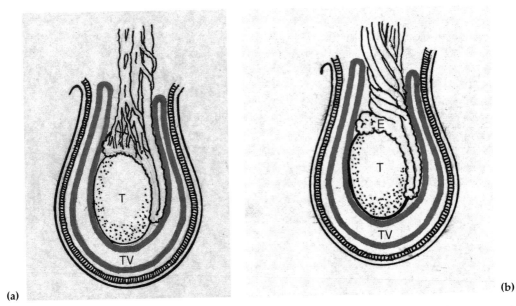

Figure 12.2 'Bell clapper' deformity with complete investation of the testis and epididymis by the tunica vaginalis, leaving the testis anchored in the scrotum solely by the spermatic cord (a); the untethered testis is highly prone to torsion (b). T, testis; TV, tunica vaginalis; E, epididymis.

dymis and loss of testicular viability and/or go-nadal atrophy.

A less common developmental abnormality predisposing to torsion (accounting for about one-third of testicular torsions) is an anomalous mesorchium, which is either elongated, incomplete or has a narrow area of attachment to the testis. Other uncommon anatomic abnormalities that may cause torsion include: partial or total separation of the epididymis and testis, an unusually bulky tunica vaginalis, an abnormally long spermatic cord, and atypical cremasteric muscle fibres that extend more distally than normal – contraction of the muscle, especially during sleep, may cause the cord to shorten and twist.

SCINTIGRAPHIC TECHNIQUE AND INTERPRETATION

The procedure is fairly simple and involves recording early (flow-phase) and delayed (tissue-phase) images of the scrotal region following an intravenous bolus injection of ^{99m}Tc-pertechnetate. The entire study is usually completed in 15 to 20 minutes.

RADIOPHARMACEUTICAL AND EQUIPMENT

Before the start of the study, potassium perchlorate may be administered orally to block the thyroid. Scintigraphy is performed in adults using an intravenous injection dose of 15–20 mCi (555–740 MBq) of ^{99m}Tc-pertechnetate. The dose is reduced proportionally in young patients (200–250 μCi/kg or 7–10 MBq/kg) with a minimum dose of 1.5–2 mCi (55–74 MBq). The radiation dose to the patient is comparable with that of a chest X-ray [16].

Imaging is performed using a standard or large field-of-view gamma-camera with an on-line dedicated computer. For the adult and teenage patients, a general-purpose, low-energy collimator is used whereas a pinhole collimator is needed for paediatric patients.

PROCEDURE

Immediately before the start of the study, the patient is instructed to empty his bladder to reduce bladder activity. The patient is positioned supine on the imaging table, and the penis turned upwards and taped to the pubic region to avoid overlapping of penile and scrotal activity. To obtain a technically satisfactory study, it is important to optimize scrotal visualization by minimizing the distance between the scrotum and the camera head, and reducing the background activity. Scrotal elevation is achieved either by means of a towel placed between the thighs, or through a tape sling under the scrotum stretching from thigh to thigh. In adults, the background radioactivity from the thighs is easily avoided by abducting the thighs. In children, a lead shield interposed between the sling and the scrotum may be used to block background activity. To facilitate interpretation of flow images, the lead shield may be placed under the scrotum after completion of the dynamic phase of the study before the acquisition of the blood pool image, or alternatively a narrow lead shield that allows visualization of the femoral vessels may be used for both phases of the study.

The attending nuclear physician should conduct a brief physical examination of the scrotum and record relevant clinical findings. Examination may reveal *testis redux*, i.e. superior retraction of the testis induced by involuntary contraction of the cremasteric muscle associated with testicular torsion or inflammation. In the presence of *testis redux*, the testis should be gently retracted downwards and taped to the shield. Where the median raphe is displaced by a markedly asymmetric scrotal enlargement, it should be manually realigned and secured in the mid-line position by paper tapes attached to the shield and sideways to the ipsilateral thigh. For the static images, a lead-strip marker placed over the median raphe forms a useful demarcation line between the two halves of the scrotum.

DATA ACQUISITION

The gamma-camera is programmed for dynamic 64×64-matrix word mode acquisition with appropriate computer magnification set to zoom-in the field-of-view extending from below the umbilicus to the proximal one-third of the thighs. Following a bolus injection of ^{99m}Tc-pertechnetate into a suitable antecubital vein, serial images are obtained for 1 minute at a frame rate of 2–5 s. When a pinhole collimator is being used, the dynamic multiframe study is substituted by a 60-s static blood-flow phase image. Immediately after the flow study, a static 500–1000 K-count (word mode, 128×128 matrix or larger) tissue-phase image is obtained with a lead shield placed under the scrotum. Further static images may be obtained with appropriate markers.

INTERPRETATION OF SCINTIGRAPHIC FINDINGS

Normal scan

The early dynamic images show iliac and femoral vessels followed by occasional identification of activity in the regions corresponding to the scrotal and spermatic cord vascular trunks. The late dynamic frames show a very low-grade capillary and venous phase blush of scrotal activity. Tissue-phase images show homogeneous activity in the scrotum, with testicular activity either similar to or slightly less than activity in the adjacent thigh. The testicular, dartos and epididymal activities are indistinguishable.

Testicular torsion

Scrotal image patterns in testicular torsion vary according to the duration of the symptoms. The scan findings can be graded into three stages: early-, mid- and late-phase torsion. Soon after the event, the twisting of the spermatic vascular pedicle occludes the venous return. Even when the degree of twisting is insufficient to occlude the lumen of the testicular artery, compression exerted by the congested veins within the rather rigid sheath of the spermatic cord secondarily blocks the arterial flow. On the flow images, this pooling of blood in the veins and the arterial occlusion may occasionally be seen as the 'nubbin sign,' i.e. increased activity in the vascular pedicle of the cord up to the level of the twist [3]; the pudendal vascular trunk is inconspicuous. The late dynamic and the tissue-phase images show absence of activity in the affected testis.

In undiagnosed or untreated torsion, the ischaemic injury progresses and scintigraphy performed in the mid-phase or early 'missed torsion' stage shows a hyperaemic pudendal vascular trunk with increased activity in the dartos on the af-

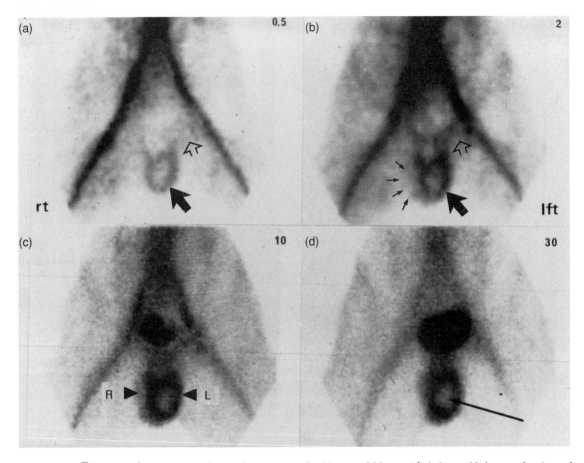

Figure 12.3 ^{99m}Tc-pertechnetate testicular perfusion scan of a 16-year-old boy with 3 days of left scrotal pain and swelling following trauma. The patient was afebrile with a normal urinalysis. Physical examination demonstrated an enlarged tender left testis. Blood flow-phase image (a) and blood pool-tissue phase image at 2 min (b) show pudendal vascular hyperaemia (open arrows) and rim of increased dartos activity (arrows) on the left; the right testis is outlined by small arrows (b). The late tissue-phase images at 10 min (c) and at 30 min (d) show markedly increased peri-testicular uptake (with a higher intensity compared with the activity in femoral vessels), a photopenic left testis (long arrow) and displacement of the right testis. The scan appearances are consistent with mid-phase 'missed torsion' and suggest testicular necrosis. Exploratory surgery revealed haemorrhagic infarction of the left testis due to spermatic cord torsion.

fected side (Figure 12.3(a)). This reactive hyperaemic response in the scrotal tissues is induced by testicular necrosis and is seen as a loop of increased dartos activity surrounding a photopenic testis forming the scrotal bull's-eye or halo sign [17]. If spontaneous detorsion occurs before scintigraphy, the scan may be normal or may show increased activity in the blood-flow and tissue-phase images because of reactive hyperaemia. A similar pattern may be seen in incomplete torsion.

The intensity of the peri-testicular rim of activity is inversely proportional to testicular salvage rates and forms a useful objective parameter for predicting surgical viability. Where the scrotal activity equals or exceeds the activity in the femoral artery in blood pool-tissue phase images (Figure 12.3(b–d)), the chances of successful surgical salvage are poor [5]. Eventually, the testis undergoes atrophy with resolution of the surrounding hyperaemia, and a negative scan pattern ensues.

The large majority of missed torsions will typically demonstrate the rim sign. With time, the intensity of the peri-testicular rim of activity increases, and in the late 'missed torsion' stage a further increase in this activity is evident on the blood-flow and tissue-phase images. Emergency surgery may be deferred as testicular viability in late-phase missed torsion is low at <20% [8,13]. Since immune-mediated anti-spermatogenic effects of an infarcted testis left *in situ* poses a definite threat to the contralateral testis [11], elective surgical exploration is still indicated.

Appendage torsion

The scintigraphic findings in appendage torsion are variable, with the affected side showing either normal, increased or decreased activity. In most of the cases, the scan shows normal activity. In a smaller proportion of patients, focally increased activity is seen near the upper pole of the testis, which may be misinterpreted for an inflammatory condition, in particular with focal inflammation involving only the head of the epididymis. However, the scan finding of focal hyperaemia does not influence the clinical management, which is non-operative, since the usual clinical outcome is appendage atrophy with resolution of symptoms. Occasionally, decreased uptake is seen on the scan, and it is these patients who are likely candidates for exploratory surgery.

Inflammatory disease

In acute bacterial epididymitis, the flow images show unilaterally augmented perfusion through the spermatic cord vessels and a crescentic or C-shaped area of increased activity located laterally in the scrotum, reflecting increased epididymal hyperaemia. In the static images, there is increased uptake corresponding to the inflamed epididymis. The adjacent non-inflamed testis shows normal activity. On occasion, due to a medially displaced epididymis, the curvilinear activity is seen to be located in the medial scrotal region. Infective, traumatic and reactive forms of epididymitis have identical scintigraphic appearance. When there is associated orchitis, the involved testis also shows increased uptake. In viral epididymo-orchitis, there is comparatively a modest increase in activity seen on the flow and static images.

Hydrocoele, haematocoele and spermatocoele

Collection of fluid or blood within the tunica vaginalis are the respective causes of hydrocoeles and haematocoeles. These two conditions are scintigraphically indistinct, with a normal flow-phase and a curvilinear photopenic defect on the tissue-phase images. However, a hydrocoele will transilluminate on physical examination. In spermatocoeles, the vascular studies are normal and static images show a photopenic defect in the region corresponding to the location of the cyst, usually above the testis.

Testicular abscess

Classically, the flow study shows dramatically increased perfusion with enhanced visualization of the spermatic trunk arterial vessels. On the static tissue-phase images, the scrotal abscess is visualized as photopenic or photo-deficient region(s) with surrounding hyperaemia. The scan findings are similar to missed torsion, i.e. increased flow with a scrotal bull's-eye sign.

Testicular tumours

The scan findings are variable. Generally, the flow study shows a diffuse mild increase in scrotal perfusion (less than that seen with epididymo-orchitis or abscess); the tissue-phase image reveals an enlarged testicle with moderately increased uptake, which may either be homogeneously (e.g. seminomas) or heterogeneously distributed (e.g. teratomas). The latter pattern reflects the relative avascular necrotic areas in the tumour. Certain vascular testicular tumours such as seminomas exhibit comparatively more intense activity in the perfusion and the tissue-phase images.

Other acute scrotal conditions

In addition to those listed above, testicular perfusion scintigraphy can also identify inguinal hernia, scrotal trauma, varicocoeles, scrotal involvement by Henoch–Schönlein purpura, etc. In inguinal hernia, the perfusion study is normal and the tissue-phase image shows a photopenic area extending from the involved hemi-scrotum to the level of the inguinal ring. In scrotal trauma, there is diffusely increased perfusion in the flow study and the tissue-phase images show increased uptake with areas of diminished activity due to associated haematoma, haematocoele or hydrocoele formation.

OTHER IMAGING MODALITIES FOR EVALUATING TESTICULAR PERFUSION

Technological advancements in medical imaging have resulted in the application of non-radionuclide imaging modalities for the evaluation of scrotal pathology. It is therefore important to comment briefly on the current clinical role, the advantages and the inherent technical limitations of the individual techniques. The newer diagnostic methods include ultrasonography (US), colour Doppler sonography (CDS) and magnetic resonance imaging (MRI).

Conventional grey-scale US provides high-resolution images of the scrotum and testis. US diagnosis of testicular torsion is based on the presence of equivocal, non-specific and inconsistent morphological changes such as a reduction in testicular echogenicity with an increase in testicular size and the identification of small hydrocoeles. These US abnormalities are similar to those observed in epididymo-orchitis [18]. Further, the method provides no information on testicular perfusion and is therefore of limited value in this clinical context. The sensitivity of US for torsion is poor (47–50%) compared with scintigraphy (94–100%) [19]. In the evaluation of scrotal disease, the US technique has different applications such as differentiating between intra- and extra-testicular conditions (e.g. epididymitis from a testicular abscess). For the evaluation of chronic or painless disorders of the scrotum, scintigraphic imaging is not the primary modality and by merits of its higher specificity, US is the preferred screening test. In selected cases, supplementing scintigraphy with sonography may reduce the incidence of false-positive scans caused by spuriously decreased perfusion (e.g. hernia, hydrocoele and haematocoele), and when the perfusion scintigraphic findings are equivocal, US may help in identifying abnormality or substantiate normalcy [20].

Colour Doppler sonography (CDS) potentially provides the facility to differentiate torsion of the testis from scrotal inflammatory diseases; several studies have reported the use of CDS as a useful imaging modality in children presenting with acute scrotal ailments, particularly for confirming the clinical diagnosis of epididymo-orchitis or testicular torsion [21–23]. However, the detection of testicular blood flow by CDS may be difficult in the paediatric age group due to the small size of the blood vessels [22,23]. The results of a recent CDS study report absence of testicular blood flow in one-third of boys with normal testes [24]. Although CDS is a rapid non-invasive technique that may be helpful in diagnosing testicular torsion, it has a limited clinical role due to its high false-positive rate.

MRI and US are most useful in the evaluation of acute disorders that cause morphological alterations such as acute hydrocoeles, haematomas or testicular trauma [25]. Scrotal inflammatory diseases such as epididymitis or orchitis may be diagnosed by CDS [26], US [27] or perfusion scintigraphy. The Doppler study is more specific and accurate than US with a sensitivity comparable with that of scintigraphy.

In the assessment of testicular perfusion, these newer imaging modalities may in certain circumstances complement testicular perfusion scintigraphy with improvement in diagnostic specificity. However, in the context of spermatic cord torsion, the clinical effectiveness of these techniques remains to be established, and at present, none of these methods can be considered a reliable substitute for testicular perfusion scintigraphy. The scintigraphic patterns of various acute scrotal conditions are well documented and the technique remains the mainstay imaging modality of choice for the diagnosis of testicular torsion.

REFERENCES

1. Nadel, N.S., Gitter, M.H., Hahn, L.C. and Vernon, A.R. (1973) Preoperative diagnosis of testicular torsion. *Urology*, **1**, 478–9.
2. Riley, T.W., Mosbaugh, P.G., Coles, J.L., Newman, D.M., Van Hove, E.D. and Heck, L.L. (1976) Use of radioisotope scan in evaluation of intrascrotal lesions. *J. Urol.*, **116**, 472–4.
3. Holder, L.E., Melloul, M. and Chen, D. (1981) Current status of radionuclide scrotal imaging. *Semin. Nucl. Med.*, **11**, 232–49.
4. Chen, D.C., Holder, L.E. and Melloul, M. (1983) Radionuclide scrotal imaging: further experience with 210 patients. Part I: Anatomy, pathophysiology, and methods. *J. Nucl. Med.*, **24**, 735–42.
5. Chen, D.C., Holder, L.E. and Melloul, M. (1983) Radionuclide scrotal imaging: further experience with 210 new patients. Part 2: Results and discussion. *J. Nucl. Med.*, **24**, 841–53.
6. Mendel, J.B., Taylor, G.A., Treves, S. *et al.* (1985) Testicular torsion in children: Scintigraphic assessment. *Paediatr. Radiol.*, **15**, 110–15.
7. Tanaka, T., Mishkin, F.S. and Datta, N.S. (1981) Radionuclide imaging of scrotal contents, in *Nuclear Medicine Annual* (eds L.M. Freeman and

H.S. Weissman), Raven Press, New York, pp. 195–221.

8. Skoglund, R.W., McRoberts, J.W. and Radge, H. (1970) Torsion of spermatic cord: a review of the literature and an analysis of 70 new cases. *J. Urol.*, **104**, 604–7.

9. Vogt, L.B., Miller, M.D. and McLeod, D.G. (1988) To save a testis. *Emerg. Med.*, **7**, 69–76.

10. Sharer, W.C. (1982) Acute scrotal pathology. *Surg. Clin. N. Am.*, **62**, 955–70.

11. Nagler, H.M. and White, R. (1982) The effect of testicular torsion on the contralateral testis. *J. Urol.*, **128**, 1343–8.

12. Moharib, N.H. and Krahn, H.P. (1970) Acute scrotum in children with emphasis on torsion of spermatic cord. *J. Urol.*, **104**, 601.

13. Williamson, R.C.N. (1976) Torsion of the testis and allied conditions. *Br. J. Surg.*, **63**, 465.

14. Fischman, A.J., Palmer, E.L. and Scott, J.A. (1987) Radionuclide imaging of sequential torsions of the appendix testis. *J. Nucl. Med.*, **28**, 119–21.

15. Skoglund, R.W., McRoberts, J.W. and Radge, H. (1970) Torsion of testicular appendages: presentation of 43 new cases and a collective review. *J. Urol.*, **104**, 598–600.

16. Blacklock, A.R.E., Kwok, H.K.Y., Mason, G.R., Mills, J.A. and Taylor, D.N. (1983) Radionuclide imaging in scrotal swellings. *Br. J. Urol.*, **55**, 749–53.

17. Dunn, E.K., Macchia, R.J. and Soloman, N.A. (1981) Scintigraphic pattern in missed testicular torsion. *Radiology*, **139**, 175–80.

18. Arger, P.H., Mulhern, C.B., Coleman, B.G. *et al.* (1981) Prospective analysis of the value of scrotal ultrasound. *Radiology*, **141**, 763–66.

19. Lutzker, L.G. and Zuckier, L.S. (1990) Testicular scanning and other applications of radionuclide genital tract. [Review]. *Semin. Nucl. Med.*, **20**, 159–88.

20. Mueller, D.L., Amundson, G.M., Rubin, S.Z. and Wesenberg, R.L. (1988) Acute scrotal abnormalities in children: diagnosis by combined sonography and scintigraphy. *Am. J. Roentgenol.*, **150**, 643–6.

21. Middleton, W.D., Siegel, B.A., Melson, G.L., Yates, C.K. and Andriole, G.L. (1990) Acute scrotal disorders: prospective comparison of color Doppler US and testicular scintigraphy. *Radiology*, **177**, 177–81.

22. Burks, D.D., Markey, B.J., Burkhard, T.K., Balsara, Z.N., Haluszka, M.M. and Canning, D.A. (1990) Suspected testicular torsion and ischaemia: evaluation with colour Doppler sonography. *Radiology*, **175**, 815–21.

23. Atkinson, G.O., Partick, L.E., Ball, T.I., Stephenson, C.A., Broecker, B.H. and Woodard, G.R. (1992) Normal and abnormal scrotum in children: evaluation with colour Doppler sonography. *Am. J. Radiol.*, **158**, 613–17.

24. Ingram, S. and Hollman, A.S. (1994) Colour Doppler sonography of the normal paediatric testis. *Clin. Radiol.*, **49**, 266–7.

25. Thurnher, S., Hricak, H., Carroll, P.R., Pobiel, R.S. and Filly, R.A. (1988) Imaging the testis: comparison between MR imaging and US. *Radiology*, **167**, 631–6.

26. Ralls, P.W., Jensen, M.C., Lee, K.P., Mayekawa, D.S., Johnson, M.H. and Halls, J.M. (1990) Color Doppler sonography in acute epididymitis. *J. Clin. Ultrasound.*, **18**, 383–6.

27. Fowler, R.C., Chennells, P.M. and Ewing, R. (1987) Scrotal ultrasonography: a clinical evaluation. *Br. J. Radiol.*, **60**, 649–54.

Impotence

Q. H. Siraj

INTRODUCTION

Impotence, an inability to achieve or maintain an erection suitable for sexual intercourse, is a common male ailment with a reported incidence of 25% at 65 years of age [1]. Erectile dysfunction may be caused by psychogenic, endocrine, neurological, pharmacological or vascular factors. Contrary to the long-held belief, it has now been established that only a small proportion (about one-quarter) of the subjects have purely functional impotence; further, the majority (over 85%) of patients with organic impotence have a vasculogenic aetiology [2].

Current improvements in understanding of erectile dysfunction have spurred the development of new radionuclide tests along with fresh application of old procedures for evaluating vasculogenic impotence. This section aims at: (i) reviewing the various penile radionuclide studies in the light of the present concepts of the neurophysiological, physio-pharmacological and the haemodynamic processes that regulate penile function; (ii) highlighting the unique and specific contribution of radionuclide methods; (iii) clarifying and defining the clinical role of the available scintigraphic techniques for evaluating erectile dysfunction; and (iv) outlining the basic methodology and the underlying theoretical principles of the clinically relevant current scintigraphic tests with emphasis on guidelines for interpretation.

First, the relevant penile anatomy, physiology of erection, aetiology and pathogenesis of vasculogenic erectile dysfunction, and the non-radionuclide penile vascular tests are briefly discussed.

PENILE ANATOMY AND PHYSIOLOGY OF ERECTION

GROSS ANATOMY

The penis is composed of three fibroelastic cylinders: the paired corpora cavernosa lying dorsolaterally, and the corpus spongiosum positioned ventrally in the mid-line. Corpora cavernosa comprise the main body of the penis and are fused with each other in the median plane, but their proximal ends separate to form the crura that attach to the sides of the pubic arch. A strong fibroelastic capsule, the tunica albuginea, surrounds the corpora cavernosa forming a lattice of cavernous spaces in the erectile tissue. The corpus spongiosum is traversed by the urethra and its distal end expands to form the glans penis. All the three corpora are surrounded by a deep (Buck's fascia) and a superficial fascial layer (Colle's fascia).

ARTERIAL SUPPLY

Penile arterial supply arises from the internal iliac artery via the internal pudendal artery, which continues as the penile artery after giving off the superficial perineal branch. The penile artery terminates by dividing into the dorsal and the deep (cavernous) penile arteries. The cavernous arteries arborize into numerous tortuous helicine arteries that open directly into the cavernous spaces via short end-arterioles. They also provide nutrient vessels to the trabeculae and tunica, anastomotic branches that cross the septum, a few branches that end in capillaries within the corpora cavernosa, and small shunt arteries to veins in the corpus spongiosum, which are thought to be responsible for diverting blood away from the cavernosum in the flaccid state.

Each dorsal penile artery courses distally on the dorsum of the penis on either side of the mid-line superficial to the tunica albuginea. Its branches primarily supply the glans penis; the circumflex branches of the dorsal artery may provide blood to the cavernosal bodies through collaterals to the deep arteries on either side.

VENOUS DRAINAGE

The superficial, intermediate and the deep penile venous drainage systems carry the venous efflux from the penis. The superficial system, comprising the single superficial dorsal vein, mainly drains the superficial tissues and empties into the external iliac vein via the external pudendal vein. The

Clinical Nuclear Medicine, 3rd edn. Edited by M.N. Maisey, K.E. Britton and B.D. Collier. Published in 1998 by Chapman & Hall, London. ISBN 0 412 75180 1

intermediate system comprises the deep dorsal vein, the emissary and the circumflex veins. The emissary veins arise from the sub-tunical venous plexuses and pass through the tunica albuginea to emerge from the dorsolateral surface of the corpus cavernosum; compression of these venules during erection between the non-compliant tunica albuginea and the dilated sinusoids is thought to be responsible for venous outflow restriction. The distal portion of the corpus cavernosum empties predominantly through emissary or circumflex veins into the deep dorsal vein of the penis, which also drains the pendulous part of the corpus spongiosum, and empties via the peri-prostatic and peri-vesical plexuses into the internal iliac vein. The deep venous system (cavernous and crural veins) drains the proximal portions of the corpus spongiosum and the corpora cavernosa into the internal pudendal vein.

NERVOUS CONTROL

There are three sets of nerves subserving sexual function: somatic, sympathetic and parasympathetic. Somatic innervation of the penis is through the mixed motor–sensory pudendal nerve, which carries somatic afferent fibres from the penis and efferent nerves to the perineal striated musculature. The autonomic erection centre is located in the intermediolateral grey matter of the spinal cord at S2–4 and T11–L2 levels. The pelvic plexus, formed by the parasympathetic visceral efferent pre-ganglionic fibres from the sacral centre (S2–4) and sympathetic fibres from the thoracolumbar centre (T11–L2), provides autonomic innervation to the pelvic organs and the external genitalia. Some sympathetic fibres coming from the sacral sympathetic chain are included in the pudendal nerve. Cavernous nerves (*nervi erigentes*) from the pelvic plexus represent the final common route for autonomic pathways: its terminal branches innervate the helicine arteries and the trabecular smooth muscles, and are responsible for the vascular events that result in penile erection. The thoracolumbar sympathetic nerves are responsible for ejaculation.

Erection can be psychogenic, elicited by supraspinal stimuli, or reflexogenic caused by local genital and/or visceral stimulation. The former is by sympathetic and parasympathetic pathways and the latter by sacral parasympathetic reflexes.

Normally, the psychic and reflexogenic stimuli act synergistically to produce erection. However, psychogenic factors, endocrine disturbances that influence libido, or the supraspinal centres may interfere with the erectile reflex.

MECHANISM OF ERECTION

Erection is a haemodynamic response to nervous stimuli: non-adrenergic non-cholinergic nerves in the penis are thought to elaborate a relaxant neurotransmitter (nitric oxide), which together with simultaneous withdrawal or counteraction of the smooth muscle contraction produced by noradrenaline, induces a chain of vascular events resulting in erection. During the flaccid state, cavernosal arterial flow bypasses the cavernosal sinusoids. Neurostimulation results in arterial dilatation, an increased penile arterial inflow exceeding the venous outflow, diversion of blood through the helicine arteries into the cavernosal spaces due to constriction of shunt arteries, relaxation of the cavernosal sinusoids, and cavernous venous outflow occlusion due to compression of the outflow venules between the expanding sinusoids and the rigid tunica albuginea.

AETIOLOGY AND PATHOGENESIS OF VASCULOGENIC IMPOTENCE

Erection being a haemodynamic phenomenon, either an inadequacy of the arterial inflow or an excess of venous outflow may result in erectile failure. Arteriogenic impotence is caused by small or large vessel occlusion and venogenic impotence results from venous-occlusive insufficiency. The majority of patients with organic impotence (about 50–70%) have combined arterial and venous dysfunction; arterial insufficiency alone accounts for about 30% of the cases; isolated venous leakage with normal arterial function is even rarer, occurring in approximately 15% of cases [2].

ARTERIOGENIC IMPOTENCE

Erection requires an increased blood supply to the penis, which is not possible if the arterial inflow is greatly impeded. Leriche [3] first documented the relationship between impotence and the limitation of pelvic arterial inflow. Numerous studies have subsequently confirmed the association between impotence and aortoiliac occlusive disease. A link between arterial risk factors (age, smoking, diabetes, hypertension and hyperlipidaemia) and impotence has been well established [4]. Atheromatous disease of the penile arterial tree, post-traumatic alterations, sequelae of local infection and even congenital dysplasia, are aetiologies of vascular alterations that may give rise to clinically isolated erectile impotence. Vascular damage caused by irradiation of the pelvis in malignancies may also result in impotence. Vascular surgical procedures that produce a reduction of blood flow in the internal pudendal artery can result in impotence; internal iliac ligation or transcatheter embolization for uncontrolled pelvic haemorrhage, and renal transplant surgery with end-to-end anastomosis of the internal iliac and the renal arteries, may compromise penile perfusion.

VENOGENIC IMPOTENCE

Penile venous-occlusive insufficiency can prevent cavernous pressure from rising sufficiently for rigid erection. Venous leakage may cause primary erectile dysfunction in young men. Its incidence increases with age. Surgical procedures for treating priapism such as anastomosis of the saphenous vein to corpus cavernosum or the creation of cavernous–spongiosal shunts can result in venous-occlusive insufficiency. Significant post-traumatic venous leakage may occur due to rupture of tunica albuginea or by mechanical disruption of the delicate structures responsible for cavernosal venous-occlusion.

INVESTIGATION OF VASCULOGENIC IMPOTENCE: NON-RADIONUCLIDE TECHNIQUES

EARLY STUDIES

Among the early non-radionuclide screening techniques for the functional evaluation of penile circulatory status, penile pulse–volume recording using strain-gauge plethysmography, penile blood pressure measurement by various methods, and Doppler ultrasound estimation of flaccid penile blood flow are among the better-known tests. Although useful, these techniques had an unacceptably low sensitivity and specificity. The most popular and widely employed tests are briefly discussed.

Nocturnal penile tumescence

Nocturnal penile tumescence (NPT) is a physiological phenomenon with normal healthy males experiencing sleep-related erections, accounting for about one-third of the total sleep time. NPT testing has been a widely popular non-invasive screening technique. However, the accuracy of the NPT test is low: there is a high incidence of false-positive test results in potent men; depression may cause a temporary reduction or inhibition of NPT; and false-negative NPT responses may be seen in subjects with sensory neuropathies, pelvic steal syndrome and corporal leakage impotence.

Penile blood flow measurements

The average velocity of a column of red cells coursing through a vessel can be measured by a Doppler device. Malvar *et al.* [5] first used the Doppler flowmeter to record the flow through the penile arteries in the flaccid penis. In an attempt to quantify flow, a penile blood flow index was later derived, which however showed a poor correlation with angiographic abnormalities. The technique is of limited value in the diagnosis of vasculogenic impotence.

CURRENT STUDIES

Pharmacologically induced penile erections

The achievement of a normal erection following intracavernosal injection of vasoactive drugs is useful in differentiating between vascular and functional impotence: rapid onset of an adequately rigid and durable erection obviates the need for further invasive investigations. Intracavernosal injections of papaverine (with or without an alpha-receptor blocker) or prostaglandin E_1 are commonly used for this purpose. A normal response is consistent with psychogenic or neurogenic aetiology, whereas vasculogenic impotence patients show impaired penile tumescence. One limitation of this test is its inability to differentiate between arteriogenic and venogenic causes, but the main drawback of the technique is an anxiety-related poor erectile response in patients without organic erectile dysfunction due to psychological factors.

Pelvic and internal pudendal angiography

The current technique involves performing pelvic angiography with selective internal pudendal arteriography in conjunction with intracavernosal and/or intra-arterial vasoactive agents. Arteriography confirms the underlying pathology, provides anatomic localization of the site of occlusion, and may help direct any possible surgical intervention. However, the technique is invasive, has a potentially high risk of complications, requires special skills and equipment, is generally difficult to interpret, and provides no physiological information. Further, the extent of the disease demonstrated arteriographically may bear little relation to the symptoms: aortic or bilateral internal iliac occlusion is not invariably accompanied by impotence, and short symptomatic lesions of the pudendal arteries are not demonstrable on arteriography. Therefore, this investigation is not used as a routine diagnostic test, but is indicated in selected cases of pelvic injury, in patients with a suspicion of isolated arterial disease, and in patients being considered for penile revascularization surgery.

Cavernosometry and cavernosography

Dynamic pharmacocavernosometry and cavernosography are employed for the functional evaluation of the corporeal venous-occlusive mechanism. The technique involves intracavernosal injection of a vasoactive drug, followed by infusion of saline into the cavernosa at a controlled variable rate with concomitant recording of intracavernosal pressure. The flow rate required to obtain and sustain an erection adequate for intromission (cavernosal pressure ≥ 90 mmHg) is determined; this maintenance flow rate correlates with the degree of corporeal leakage. Dynamic cavernosography is next performed by infusion of diluted iodinated contrast and may allow visualization of the site(s) of venous leakage.

Doppler flow imaging of pharmacological erection

Pulsed duplex sonography is performed for real-time imaging and measurement of flow through the cavernosal arteries during drug-induced erection. Arterial insufficiency is suggested by a failure of the arteries to dilate and flow velocity to increase; an abnormally increased venous outflow can also be documented. Although the peak velocities show a wide variability and are strongly influenced by technical factors, despite these limitations it is currently widely used for vasculogenic screening.

RADIONUCLIDE INVESTIGATION OF VASCULOGENIC IMPOTENCE: EARLY STUDIES

The potential importance of radionuclide methods for penile vascular evaluation has long been recognized. Radionuclide penile vascular studies were pioneered by Shirai and Nakamura from Japan in the 1970s, who employed non-imaging probes for monitoring penile radioactivity changes following injection of blood pool radiopharmaceuticals [6,7].

In 1982, Fanous and associates performed dynamic flaccid penile blood pool imaging using ^{99m}Tc-pertechnetate and quantified the change in the penile blood volume induced by an intravenous vasodilator, which parameter reportedly correlated well with the penile blood pressure index [8]. Although the data presented by the investigators did not substantiate their claim [9], nonetheless, the technique offered an objective method for the assessment of penile vascular status.

Measurement of the rate of washout of a diffusible tracer such as ^{133}Xe is the standard radionuclide method for assessing organ perfusion. Clearance of ^{133}Xe following subcutaneous injection into the dorsal coronal sulcus of the flaccid penis was first reported by Nseyo et al. [10] and subsequently by other investigators; lower flow rates were seen in patients with penile arterial insufficiency and in patients with mixed arteriogenic–venogenic impotence, with normal results in subjects with isolated venous leakage and non-vasculogenic impotence. The subcutaneous ^{133}Xe washout rate reflects superficial penile perfusion and can potentially identify major arterial disease; however, it is a crude and non-specific technique, which does not provide any information about cavernosal flow.

The design flaws in the earlier studies were partly attributable to the contemporary state of knowledge about the physiology of penile haemodynamics and the pathophysiology of vasculogenic impotence. Nevertheless, the major contribution of the original radionuclide investigations was the application and elaboration of innovative radionuclide methodologies, providing archetypes for later developments.

RADIONUCLIDE INVESTIGATION OF IMPOTENCE: CURRENT METHODS

The current radionuclide techniques used for the diagnosis and quantitation of the arteriogenic and venous elements in vasculogenic erectile dysfunction commonly employ two main strategies:

1. Estimation of penile arterial inflow using blood pool agents.
2. Assessment of the venous outflow by measuring the rate of clearance of an intracavernosally injected diffusible tracer (usually ^{133}Xe).

The studies can be performed both in the flaccid state and in conjunction with drug-induced erections.

CLEARANCE STUDIES

Flaccid ^{133}Xe clearance studies

The clearance rate of ^{133}Xe following an intracavernosal (IC) injection in the flaccid penis reflects basal cavernosal blood flow. Wagner and Uhrenholdt [11] reported lower penile washout rates of IC ^{133}Xe in patients with arteriogenic impotence with no difference in the washout rates between normal subjects and patients with venous leakage. Other investigators have reported slower flaccid penile washout rates of IC ^{133}Xe in venous leakage patients, compared with that in normal controls or non-venous impotence, which factor was attributed to incompetent venous valves with backflow of blood into the penis [12]. However, this hypothesis is not supported by the current medical opinion: venous restriction during erection is not dependent upon the presence or the absence of venous valves.

The discordant findings by different workers, together with the lack of a plausible explanation for the abnormal clearance results in venous impotence patients and an inability to differentiate between arteriogenic and venogenic forms of vasculogenic impotence, has caused an uncertainty about the relevance and clinical value of flaccid IC ^{133}Xe clearance test.

Erection ^{133}Xe clearance studies

Washout of IC ^{133}Xe from the erect penis reflects the egress of blood during tumescence. Erection IC ^{133}Xe clearance studies generally show de-

creased penile washout during erection in normal subjects, whereas an increased clearance rate is documented in patients with venous disease.

Diagnostic role

Flaccid state cavernosal ^{133}Xe clearance rate is predominantly dependent on the arterial inflow. During the induction phase of erection, the arterial inflow and the venous outflow both influence the xenon clearance times; after achievement of full erection at steady-state or maintenance arterial flow rates, the measure mainly reflects venous outflow. Technical factors, such as a variable dilution of the cavernosal blood pool caused by the non-radioactive vasodilator injection [13], together with the volume of the injected xenon with different energy, may be a source of error. These confounding physiological variables and technical factors undermine the significance and reliability of xenon clearance studies for an objective evaluation of the penile venous outflow or venous-occlusive mechanism.

BLOOD POOL TECHNIQUES

Flaccid studies

Siraj et al. [14] developed the Fanous technique by performing dynamic penile scintigraphy (radionuclide phallography) using ^{99m}Tc-red blood cells (^{99m}Tc-RBCs), a superior blood pool agent. Penile arterial inflow function was objectively evaluated by quantifying the haemodynamic response to intravenous vasodilator stress: the change in penile blood volume was quantified using a modification of the Fanous index, which improved the diagnostic accuracy; a quantitative parameter of blood flow was also derived. This non-invasive technique was effective in screening impotent patients for penile arterial insufficiency.

Erection studies

The main limitation of penile vascular studies in the flaccid state was their inability to exclude venous leakage. To evaluate penile vascular function during the process of erection, Siraj et al. [15] performed dynamic erection phallography, which allowed continuous monitoring of the penile circulatory changes during the various stages of drug-induced erections. The technique provided an objective assessment of the normal erectile haemodynamic response and yielded specific data, which was helpful in the differential diagnosis of psychogenic, arteriogenic and venous leakage patients.

Penile blood volume can be estimated by measuring the activity of a venous blood sample taken from the patient [16,17]. This allowed absolute quantification of peak arterial flow rates (ml/min) following papaverine injection by calculating the maximal rate of change in penile activity from the slope of the penile time-activity curve [18], which parameter showed a good correlation with the angiographic extent of penile arterial disease. Another estimate of arterial inflow during early erection, calculated from the ratio of penile blood volume 60s before and 60s after the peak flow, further improved the correlation with angiographic scoring [19]. This latter parameter that measures the relative difference between the flaccid and erection flow rates is basically similar to the flow index described by Siraj *et al.* [15]; in this context there appears no clear-cut benefit of venous sampling.

COMBINATION TESTS

Dual-isotope combination studies using a blood pool agent for estimating arterial inflow and the clearance of intracavernosally injected ^{133}Xe or ^{127}Xe for assessing venous outflow, have been employed for evaluating the penile haemodynamic status during pharmacologically-induced erection. Schwartz and Graham [19] performed a dual-isotope (^{127}Xe/^{99m}Tc-RBCs) study for calculating arterial and venous flow following papaverine-induced erection. Their results, however, showed that measurement of xenon clearance alone was unreliable in predicting the competency of venous-occlusive mechanism. In a combination blood pool (^{99m}Tc-RBCs) and washout (^{133}Xe) study, Miraldi *et al.* [20] estimated the peak arterial and venous flow rates after induction of pharmacological erection; the vascular flow parameters were reported to be helpful in differentiating normal, arteriogenic and venous leakage subjects. However, the relevance of the venous outflow parameter for evaluating the erectile venous-occlusive integrity has been questioned on the basis that xenon was injected in the flaccid state before the papaverine injection [21]. Using a similar dual-isotope (^{133}Xe/^{99m}Tc-RBCs) technique, Kursh *et al.* [22] computed arterial and venous flow rates in the flaccid and erect states and described specific patterns for distinguishing normal subjects

from patients with arterial insufficiency and venous leakage.

Diagnostic role

In theory, the dual-isotope combination studies can potentially be used for simultaneous measurement of penile arterial inflow and venous outflow, and should ideally provide a continuous record of arterial and venous flow rates in the flaccid state and during various phases of erection. The dual-isotope approach is a sophisticated radionuclide research test for studying the penile haemodynamic function; however, the full potential of the technique is yet to be realised. In view of the technical complexity of the test, it is unlikely to become a routine clinical nuclear medicine test for evaluating impotent patients.

EVALUATION OF VASCULOGENIC IMPOTENCE BY FLACCID AND ERECTION PHALLOGRAPHY

An ever-increasing awareness of vasculogenic dysfunction as the major underlying cause of organic impotence has fostered the development of new methods for evaluating the presence, extent and nature of vascular erectile dysfunction. However, most of the currently available penile vascular tests are still in evolution, and their diagnostic efficiency and clinical role is yet to be fully established [21]. Radionuclide penile vascular tests, like their non-radionuclide counterparts, are also in the evolution stages. However, on the basis of the familiarity and long experience with the techniques used for studying a large number of patients with erectile dysfunction, and the practicality and ease of performance of the tests, an effective investigative approach is presented, which is based on contemporary physiological principles and provides maximum diagnostic information for minimum patient discomfort.

FLACCID PHALLOGRAPHY PROTOCOL

Procedure and data analysis

The methodology of flaccid radionuclide phallography is briefly described. The study is performed using *in vivo*-labelled ^{99m}Tc-RBCs; potassium perchlorate (400mg) is administered orally to block the thyroid and improve labelling efficiency. Scintigraphy is performed using a large or standard field-of-view computer-linked gamma-camera equipped with a low-energy, all-purpose collimator. The patient is positioned supine on the imaging couch and a lead mask is placed under the penis to shield background activity from the scrotum and thighs. The camera computer is programmed for dynamic 64×64 matrix (word mode) acquisition with appropriate magnification set to cover the region extending from the umbilicus to the proximal one-third of the thighs. Serial 30-s images are obtained for 55 minutes following a bolus injection of ^{99m}Tc-pertechnetate (dose 10 MBq/kg); intravenous isoxsuprine hydrochloride (dose 10 mg) is administered after 10 minutes.

Computer processing involves generating time-activity curves (TACs) from a background-subtracted penile region-of-interest and computation of quantitative indices of penile volume and flow. The methods of calculating the various numerical indices are detailed elsewhere: the maximum increase in the penile blood volume in response to the vasodilator stress is estimated through the penogram index [8,14,17], and the magnitude of change in penile blood flow quantified through flow indices [14,17,23].

Findings and interpretation

Early flow images may help in assessing the gross morphology of the internal iliac vasculature: there is generally better visualization of the internal iliac blood pool in the non-arteriogenic patients (Figure 12.4(a)) than in patients with advanced atherosclerotic disease of the internal iliac vessels (Figure 12.4(b)).

The penile TACs (phallogram curves) are assessed qualitatively and their general shape and pattern noted. Visual curve assessment reveals fairly characteristic patterns. Normal subjects and most patients with psychogenic impotence show rising curves with secondary pulsations, consistent with phasic increase in penile blood pool due to concomitant penile vascular and trabecular smooth muscle relaxation. There is also an appreciable increase in the steepness of the slope after the vasodilator injection reflecting increased arterial flow (Figure 12.5(a)). Patients with arteriogenic impotence typically show a convex-shaped curve with an insignificant change in the slope after the vasodilator injection, suggesting a poor flow response; there is impairment of normal rhythmic pulsations (Figure 12.5(b)), which may be attributed both to an inadequacy of resting penile arterial inflow and to sinusoidal dysfunction subsequent to penile ultrastructural damage brought about by an altered nutritive environment associated with chronic penile arterial insufficiency [23–25]. The phallogram curves of patients with cavernous-sinusoidal dysfunction show loss of pulsatile activity, whereas patients with isolated venous incompetence due to mechanical venous leakage display preserved pulsatile flow [23–25]. Hence, early subclinical

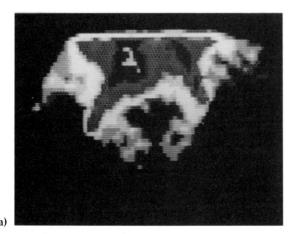
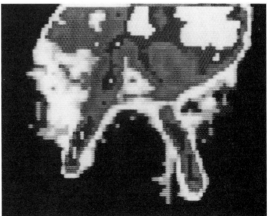

(a)   (b)

Figure 12.4   Early flow images showing: (a) clear visualization of the internal iliac vascular flow in a patient with psychogenic impotence; (b) poor internal iliac blood pool in a patient with advanced atherosclerotic disease of the internal iliac vessels.

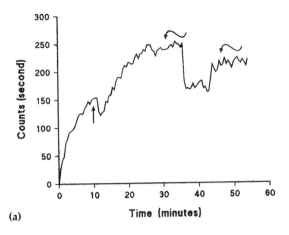

(a)

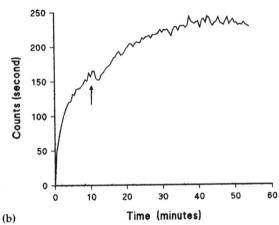

(b)

Figure 12.5 Representative flaccid phallogram curves. (a) A psychogenic impotence patient showing normal pulsatile activity (curved arrows) as well as increased penile activity following vasodilator injection (straight arrow). (b) An arteriogenic impotence patient showing impairment of secondary pulsations and no significant change in curve slope after intravenous vasodilator stress (arrow).

sinusoidal dysfunction can be documented by the absence of normal cavernosal pulsatile flow, which also helps explain the delayed flaccid state cavernosal xenon clearance reported in patients with venogenic impotence [12].

Quantitative haemodynamic parameters allow an objective evaluation of the penile vascular response to the systemic vasodilator injection; the penile volume and flow indices have a high accuracy (>90%) for the diagnosis of arteriogenic impotence [14,23,24].

ERECTION PHALLOGRAPHY PROTOCOL

Procedure and data analysis

The radiopharmaceutical, methodology and analysis of erection and flaccid phallography techniques are essentially similar; the erection test can be performed either following completion of the flaccid study or on a separate occasion. To minimize the effect of anxiety, the study is performed in a quiet and private atmosphere, and 10mg diazepam is injected intramuscularly to relax the patient. The penis is loosely but securely strapped by means of strips of adhesive tape to the lead mask covering the scrotum and upper thighs. A 21-gauge butterfly needle is inserted in the lateral aspect of the mid-shaft of the penis into either cavernosum and the patient positioned under the gamma-camera. Following a bolus injection of ^{99m}Tc-pertechnetate, the computer is activated to acquire a dynamic study comprising of 60 frames, each of 30-s duration; 10 minutes later, 10µg PGE_1 or 60mg papaverine HCl is injected into the corpus cavernosum via the indwelling butterfly needle. The attending nuclear physician should note the time of onset of erection and periodically assess the erectile response during the acquisition period. After completion of the study, the erection is graded by: manual palpation, assessing penile tumescence by recording the penile circumference change, and penile rigidity by measuring the erectile angle.

The data may be analysed in a variety of ways. A background-subtracted, decay-corrected penile TAC is generated. The erectile haemodynamic function may be quantified through parameters of flow and volume: the penogram index calculated from the amplitude of the TAC provides a measure of the peak change in penile blood volume, and a flow index derived from the slope of the TAC estimates the relative change in penile flow following intracavernosal vasodilator injection compared with the resting flow rate [15].

Findings and interpretation

The characteristics of the normal erectile haemodynamic response are evaluated qualitatively through the phallogram curves. In normal subjects and psychogenic impotence patients with good erectile response, the penile TACs characteristically show a sharp increase in the upslope immediately after the injection of the vasoactive drug followed by a plateau (Plate 24(a)). The technique is helpful in differentiating between primarily arteriogenic and venous aetiologies: in patients with mild to moderate arterial insufficiency the penile TAC shows a slowly rising curve with delayed time-to-plateau; when the arterial inflow is severely compromised, there is a gradually rising curve that fails to plateau (Plate 24(b)). The penile TACs of patients with isolated venous leakage typically show an initial rapid rise succeeded by a fall (Plate 24(c)), since the increase in cavernosal blood volume secondary to an increased arterial inflow cannot be maintained due to venous-occlusive insufficiency. In patients with coexisting arterial insufficiency and venous leakage, the penile TAC shows a poor upslope due to concomitantly reduced inflow and increased outflow, and a failure to plateau because of venous-occlusive dysfunction.

There is a good correlation between the flow index (FI) and the erectile angle, a physical measure of penile rigidity [15]. The FI provides an accurate and objective assessment of the rapid penile arterial flow during early tumescence. Erection is achieved by greater than five-fold increase in the penile blood flow over the resting state as judged by the FI values. Patients with arteriogenic impotence have low FI values indicative of poor arterial inflow, whereas venous leakage patients with short-lived erections have higher FI values indicating adequate arterial inflow [15].

An anxiety-related false-positive response may be seen in some psychogenic impotence patients with poor drug-induced erections: the penile TAC pattern may be similar to that seen in arteriogenic impotence with low FI values [15]. However, a normal inflow rate and pattern documented on the flaccid phallogram helps differentiate these cases [24].

CLINICAL DIAGNOSTIC ROLE

In clinical practice, a pharmacological erection test is now routinely performed in all patients reporting with erectile dysfunction; a normal response effectively excludes significant vasculogenic dysfunction. However, a false-positive response is seen in a large number of subjects without organic disease, due to anxiety-related increased sympathetic activity [26], which reduces the arterial inflow and increases the venous outflow [13,15]. Further, the increase in penile blood flow after intracavernous vasodilator injection depends not only on the integrity of the penile arterial supply but also on the cavernosal smooth muscle function. Congenital fibrosis and atrophy of cavernosal smooth muscle [27], and alteration of the fibroelastic properties of the corporal smooth muscle induced by hypercholesterolaemia, ischaemia or hypertension [28], may result in a non-compliant sinusoidal compartment. Poor sinusoidal compliance may impair the erectile haemodynamic response by secondarily diminishing penile arterial inflow along with inadequate restriction of venous outflow.

Techniques that rely solely on evaluating penile haemodynamic parameters following intracavernosal injections may not be able to differentiate poor responders due to anxiety, patients with primary venous–sinusoidal disease, and subjects with cavernosal dysfunction secondary to penile arterial insufficiency. Therefore, functional evaluation of penile arterial inflow during the flaccid state appears a more rational approach since the measured response is not dependent on cavernosal compliance [9,23]. However, the current non-radionuclide penile vascular techniques are limited in their technical ability to provide a sensitive record of the flaccid penile vascular function.

Flaccid radionuclide phallography with intravenous vasodilator stress is a sensitive test for evaluating penile arterial insufficiency, which also provides supplementary information about cavernous sinusoidal function. In patients who show a poor erectile response to intracavernosal injection but with normal arterial function on flaccid radionuclide phallography, cavernous–venous incompetence can be assumed by default [9,23]. This can be further confirmed by erection phallography, which will show an inability to achieve a sustained increase in cavernous blood volume due to venous leakage. Patients showing evidence of cavernous–venous dysfunction on phallography are candidates for further evaluation by cavernosography and cavernosometry.

CONCLUSIONS

Arteriogenic impotence and/or cavernous–venous insufficiency are the major vasculogenic causes of impotence. The clinical management of patients in these categories differs significantly – isolated arteriogenic impotence patients with normal cavernosal smooth muscle function are suitable candidates for intracavernous pharmaco-therapy or revascularization surgery; venous in-competence patients with cavernosographically documented leakage sites are likely candidates for venous ligation surgery; whereas in patients with venous–sinusoidal dysfunction or mixed vascular disease, implantation of a penile prosthesis is a more suitable option. Non-invasive vascular screening techniques must therefore be capable reliably of distinguishing between the various aetiologies of vasculogenic impotence.

Currently, the Doppler ultrasound technique is the prime contender against radionuclide penile vascular studies as a front-line test for screening impotent patients for vasculogenic erectile dys-function. Despite improvements in equipment design, the sonographic technique is limited by inherent technical factors. High ultrasound fre-quencies provide better spatial resolution at the cost of poor depth selectivity, with a proportional increase in the imprecision of the measurement at high blood flow velocities. Also, the physical measurement of flow is highly affected by varia-tions in the transducer angle and inherent diffrac-tion and side-lobe artefacts. Furthermore, Doppler devices measure velocities, not the actual blood flow rates, and the recording is not altogether dy-namic, since measurements are made in a specific segment of a particular vessel at certain points during the development of erection. On the other hand, the radionuclide phallography technique can objectively measure whole-organ blood flow and continuously monitor penile blood volume changes from flaccidity through various phases of erection. Evidence of a sustained increase in the penile blood pool seen during erection helps in differentiating haemodynamically significant ve-nous leakage from minor leaks, which when com-pensated by an increased arterial inflow following pharmacological vasodilation and aided by sexual stimulation, will still allow adequate performance [9].

Radionuclide phallography of the flaccid penis with intravenous pharmacological stress in combi-nation with erection phallography is helpful in differentiating between psychogenic, primary arteriogenic, venous, venous–sinusoidal, and mixed arteriogenic–venogenic aetiologies. The two tests can be performed on a single outpatient visit, minimizing radiation exposure, time and expense.

REFERENCES

1. Kinsey, A.C., Pomeroy, W.B. and Martin, C.E. (1948) Age and sexual outlet, in *Sexual Behaviour in the Human Male*. W.B. Saunders Co., Philadelphia, London.
2. Krysiewicz, S. and Mellinger, B.C. (1989) The role of imaging in the diagnostic evaluation of impotence. *Am. J. Roentgenol.*, **153**, 1133–9.
3. Leriche, R. (1923) Des obliteration artérielles hautes obliteration de la termination de l'aorte comme cause d'une insuffisance circulatoire des membres inferiers. *Bull. Soc. Chir. (Paris)*, **49**, 1404.
4. Virag, R., Bouilly, P. and Frydman, D. (1985) Is im-potence an arterial disorder? *Lancet*, **i**, 181–4.
5. Malvar, T., Baron, T. and Clark, S.S. (1973) Assess-ment of potency with the Doppler flowmeter. *Urology*, **2**, 396–400.
6. Shirai, M. and Nakamura, M. (1970) Differential di-agnosis of organic and functional impotence by the use of ^{131}I-Human Serum Albumin. *Tohoku J. Exp. Med.*, **101**, 317–24.
7. Shirai, M. and Nakamura, M. (1975) Diagnostic dis-crimination between organic and functional impo-tence by radioisotope penogram with ^{99m}TcO$_4$. *Tohoku J. Exp. Med.*, **116**, 9–15.
8. Fanous, H.N., Jevtich, M.J., Chen, D.C.P. and Edson, M. (1982) Radioisotope penogram in the diagnosis of vasculogenic impotence. *Urology*, **20**, 499–502.
9. Siraj, Q.H. and Hilson, A.J. (1993) Penile radio-nuclide studies in impotence: an overview [edito-rial]. *Nucl. Med. Commun.*, **14**, 517–19.
10. Nseyo, U.O., Wilbur, H.J., Kang, S.A., Flesh, L. and Bennett, A.H. (1984) Penile xenon (^{133}Xe) washout: a rapid method of screening for vasculogenic impo-tence. *Urology*, **23**, 31–4.
11. Wagner, G. and Uhrenholdt, A. (1980) Blood flow measurement by the clearance method in the human corpus cavernosum in the flaccid and erect states, in *Vasculogenic Impotence* (eds A.W. Zorgniotti and G. Rossi), Thomas, Springfield, pp. 41–6.
12. Yeh, S.H., Liu, R.S., Lin, S.N., Wu, L.C., Chao, I.B., Chen, M.T., Peng, N.J. and Chang, S.S. (1991) Radionuclide imaging clinical study. Corporeal ^{133}Xe washout for detecting venous leakage in impo-tence. *Nucl. Med. Commun.*, **12**, 203–9.
13. Siraj, Q.H., Hilson, A.J.W., Bomanji, J. and Ahmed, M. (1992) Volume-dependent intracavernous hemo-dilution during pharmacologically induced penile erections. *J. Urol.*, **148**, 1441–3.
14. Siraj, Q.H., Hilson, A.J., Townell, N.H., Morgan, R.J. and Cottrall, M.F. (1986) The role of the radioisotope phallogram in the investigation of vasculogenic impotence. *Nucl. Med. Commun.*, **7**, 173–82.
15. Siraj, Q.H., Bomanji, J., Akhtar, M.A., Rana, M.H., Sadiq, M. and Ahmed, M. (1990) Quantitation of pharmacologically-induced penile erections: the value of radionuclide phallography in the objective

evaluation of erectile haemodynamics. *Nucl. Med. Commun.*, **11**, 445–58.

16. Shirai, M., Nakamura, M., Ishii, N., Mitsukawa, S. and Sawai, Y. (1976) Determination of intrapenial blood volume using ^{99m}Tc-labeled autologous red blood cells. *Tohoku J. Exp. Med.*, **120**, 377–83.

17. Siraj, Q.H. (1984) *Radioisotope Studies of Penile Blood Flow*, MSc Thesis, University of London.

18. Schwartz, A.N., Graham, M.M., Ferency, G.F. and Miura, R.S. (1989) Radioisotope penile plethysmography: a technique for evaluating corpora cavernosal blood flow during early tumescence. *J. Nucl. Med.*, **30**, 466–73.

19. Schwartz, A.N. and Graham, M.M. (1991) Combined technetium radioisotope penile plethysmography and xenon washout: a technique for evaluating corpora cavernosal inflow and outflow during early tumescence. *J. Nucl. Med.*, **32**, 404–10.

20. Miraldi, F., Nelson, A.D., Jones, W.T., Thompson, S. and Kursh, E.D. (1992) A dual-radioisotope technique for the evaluation of penile blood flow during tumescence. *J. Nucl. Med.*, **33**, 41–6.

21. Seftel, A.D. and Goldstein, I. (1992) Vascular testing for impotence [editorial]. *J. Nucl. Med.*, **33**, 46–8.

22. Kursh, E.D., Jones, W.T., Thompson, S., Nelson, D. and Miraldi, F. (1992) A dynamic dual isotope radionuclear method of quantifying penile blood flow. *J. Urol.*, **147**, 1524–9.

23. Siraj, Q.H. and Hilson, A.J. (1994) Diagnostic value of radionuclide phallography with intravenous vasodilator stress in the evaluation of arteriogenic impotence. *Eur. J. Nucl. Med.*, **21**, 651–7.

24. Siraj, Q.H. (1993) *The Study of Penile Vascular Physiology and Pathology using Radiotracer Techniques*, PhD Thesis, University of London.

25. Siraj, Q.H., Hilson, A.J.W., Bomani, J. and Ahmed, M. (1993) A pilot study of flaccid penile blood patterns in normal subjects and patients with erectile dysfunction. *Nucl. Med. Commun.*, **14**, 976–82.

26. Kim, S.C. and Oh, M.M. (1992) Norepinephrine involvement in response to intracorporeal injection of papaverine in psychogenic impotence. *J. Urol.*, **147**, 1530–2.

27. Aboseif, S.R., Baskin, L.S., Yen, T.S.B. and Lue, T.F. (1992) Congenital defect in sinusoidal smooth muscles: a cause of organic impotence. *J. Urol.*, **148**, 58–60.

28. Azadzoi, K.M. and Goldstein, I. (1992) Erectile dysfunction due to atherosclerotic vascular disease – the development of an animal model. *J. Urol.*, **147**, 1675–81.

Infertility

M. P. Iturralde

The Urge to reproduce Runs Deep in the Human Spirit

INTRODUCTION

Infertility, defined as failure of a couple to conceive after one year or more of unprotected intercourse, is a common problem affecting one in seven marriages [1]. For those affected, it can become a major tragedy with significant psychological and physical disturbances.

Aetiologies of infertility include problems of spermatozoa and oocyte availability and tubal occlusion [2]. A significant number of couples will have more than one cause, requiring that the diagnostic investigation be complete and thorough in each case. The single most common gynaecological disorder relating to infertility is the high (30–50%) prevalence of tubal factors. Congenital or acquired anatomical (various malformations, synechia, post-inflammatory occlusion, etc.) or functional (periodical spastic occlusion, decreased peristaltic activity, spasmus of the isthmus, etc.) tubal lesions are reported to be the cause. Male abnormalities are essentially those involving sperm production and transportation.

The number of infertile couples has increased in the past decade, due to growth in the population and an increase in the incidence of sexually transmitted disease. This has caused a greater demand for specialized services for the diagnosis and management of infertility.

In approximately 15% of infertile couples, no reason for infertility can be identified. The term 'unexplained infertility' refers to the failure of a couple to establish a pregnancy when no specific cause can be identified utilizing currently available and acceptable diagnostic techniques. Consequently, the possible presence of a 'tubal factor' justifies the renewed interest in anatomical and functional studies as fundamental in the investigation of the infertile couple, primarily to assess patency, but also to determine the possibility of patent but 'non-functional' oviducts. Evaluation of the male partner is extremely important. However, current imaging techniques are generally of only secondary importance as assessment of the semen is the most valuable diagnostic element in this evaluation.

RELEVANT ANATOMY AND PHYSIOLOGY

THE FALLOPIAN TUBES

Each fallopian tube is about 12 cm long, and opens medially into the uterine cavity and laterally into the peritoneal cavity, near the corresponding ovary. The uterine ostium of the uterine tube is small, while the peritoneal opening or abdominal ostium is located deep within a trumpet-shaped expansion. The infundibulum and its circumference is prolonged by a varying number of fimbriae. The fimbriae are lined by mucosa with longitudinal folds continuous with those in the infundibulum. The infundibulum opens into the ampulla, which is thin-walled, has a tortuous lumen and is more than half the tube's length. The ampulla leads into the isthmus, which is rounded and firm, and forms approximately the tube's medial third. The intramural uterine part is about 3 cm long.

The fallopian tube has an external serosa, an intermediate muscular stratum and an internal mucosa. The serosa is a fold of the peritoneum with subjacent connective tissue. The muscular layer has external longitudinal and internal circular layers of non-striated muscle. A labyrinth of mucosal folds project into the lumen with a smaller number of simpler longitudinal folds. The tubal mucosa has an epithelium and underlying connective tissue containing a rich substrate of blood and lymph vessels and nerves. The simple columnar epithelial lining of the uterine tube is made up of ciliated cells interspersed with intercalated (indifferent) and nonciliated secretory cells that are believed to produce a nutritive secretion.

The ciliated cells of the oviduct have a common structural and functional pattern of internal tubules, with propulsive action as that of most of the respiratory tract, some of the tympanic cavity and auditory tube, efferent ductules of the testis and spermatozoid flagellum (Figure 12.6).

Clinical Nuclear Medicine, 3rd edn. Edited by M.N. Maisey, K.E. Britton and B.D. Collier. Published in 1998 by Chapman & Hall, London. ISBN 0 412 75180 1

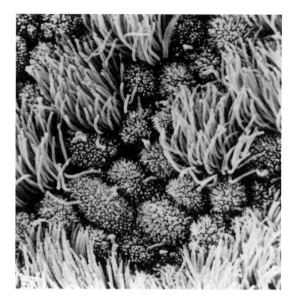

Figure 12.6   Electron microscopy of the ciliated epithelium of the fallopian tubes.

Ciliated cells in the fallopian tubes are most prominent in the epithelial surface of the fimbriated infundibulum where they form dense arrays, while large number of cilia may also be found in the ampulla. In general, ciliated cells are less frequent in the isthmus.

Growth of the ciliated epithelium appears to be under the influence of ovarian hormones, and data from humans and animals (rabbit and monkey) indicate that their growth is promoted by oestrogens. Treatment with progesterone, by contrast, antagonizes the oestrogen-driven cell growth. Ciliated and secretory cells begin to increase in height shortly after menstruation, and by the time of ovulation they are approximately 30 μm high.

A recent report by Paltieli and co-workers [2] described a method for measuring the beat frequency of fallopian tube cilia using laser light-scattering technique as part of the laparoscopic evaluation in infertile women. They determined the normal ciliary beat frequency to be about 5.6 Hz. These measurements revealed changes in the ciliary beat frequency at different stages of ovulation as the fallopian tubes prepare for ovum pickup and transport under the influence of sex hormones. In the fimbria, the highest frequency 6.0 Hz, was measured during the late follicular phase before ovulation. This figure dropped to 4.9 Hz after ovulation. Measurements of ciliary beat frequency also correlated with the percentage of ciliated cells in the fallopian tubes (known as the 'ciliary index'). The ciliary index was determined in 19 women. In 12 of the 13 women whose ciliary beat frequency was normal, the ciliary index was normal as well – above 50%; in five of the six, whose ciliary beat frequency was below normal, the ciliary index was also below normal.

FERTILIZATION

Upon ejaculation into the anterior vagina, the pool of highly concentrated semen bathes the external cervical os and spermatozoa gain access to the mucus-filled cervical canal largely under the influence of their own motility. Contractions of smooth muscle in the vagina and in the cervical walls, as well as active directional beating of some ciliated cells in the cervical canal, may assist this surprisingly rapid process. Migration of spermatozoa through the uterus to the fallopian tubes depends on myometrial contractions while sperm motility, which maintain the spermatozoa in suspension in the uterine fluids, prevent their adhesion within the uterus (Figure 12.7). The existence of upward transportation processes at the time of conception implies that the motility of spermatozoa may not be the only relevant factor for their ascension. Indeed, union of the spermatozoon and the oocyte depends not only on the active role of spermatozoa, but also on actions of the female reproductive tract. The mechanism by which this migration (of spermatozoa or radiolabelled particles) takes place is poorly understood, but it is assumed that it is a combination of muscular peristaltic movements, changes in peritoneal pressure, and ciliary motion. There also appears to be a cyclical hormonal component regulating this process, and it is suggested that migration is facilitated during the period of ovulation [2]. Muscular peristalsis and rate of beat of cilial activity in the fallopian tubes respond to the circulating concentrations of ovarian steroid hormones, although the autonomic nervous system directly regulates the myosalpinx. The rate of cilial beat and muscular contraction seems to be greatest just at or after the time of ovulation, thereby ensuring effective transport of eggs to the site of fertilization. However, progression of eggs to the

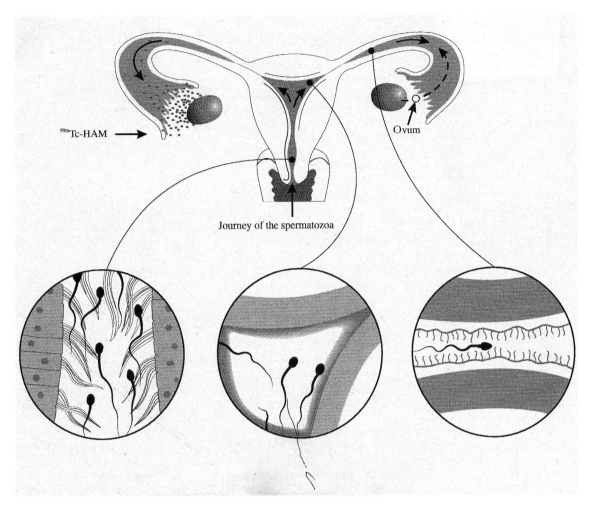

Figure 12.7 The journey of the spermatozoa through the female reproductive tract showing ciliated epithelium of the cervix and tubes facilitating this migratory process. The same mechanism possibly occurs for the migration of radiolabelled microspheres during radionuclide hysterosalpingography (HERS).

ampullary–isthmic junction is not continuous, but consists of intermittent waves of contraction in the ampulla. Just after ovulation – and around the time of fertilization when eggs are descending the ampulla while spermatozoa are ascending the isthmus – the fallopian tube becomes birectional. Male and female gametes are transported in the tube and must meet at a specific site during a specific time-frame for fertilization to take place. Because of the key role of ovarian steroids in regulating these events, anomalous levels of oestrogens and progesterone would certainly upset the normal mechanisms and timing of gamete trans-

port. But most of all, healthy and patent oviducts facilitate conception.

Following fertilization, the principal mechanisms regulating the passage of embryo into the uterus involve activity of myosalpinx and cilia, the reduction of oedema in the mucosa, and the directional flow of fluid in the tubal lumen.

Seen in the context of their structure the fallopian tubes appear to be modest passive uterine appendages. Functionally, they are extremely sensitive organs responding to hormonal, biochemical and neural stimulation that facilitate fertilization, on the few special occasions that the oviducts are required to act, they constitute the most important element in the process of conception.

PHYSIOPATHOLOGY

In the adult female, the peritoneal cavity communicates with the outside via the fallopian tubes, the uterus and the vagina, and there is evidence for the migration of different substances in either direction. For example, malignant cells from ovarian carcinoma can be demonstrated in the posterior fornix of the vagina; retrograde menstruation is also a well-known phenomenon. Peritonitis is said to occur more frequently in females, because infection of the vagina, uterus, or the uterine tube may spread directly to the peritoneum, via the abdominal ostium. Tubal inflammation (salpingitis), which is the most common cause of infertility, is usually secondary, having spread from the vagina or the uterus. For pregnancy to occur, spermatozoa have to move up the uterus as the ova moves down the tube. After insufflation, air and gases pass easily from the vagina into the peritoneal cavity up to the diaphragm. Radio-opaque contrast media are introduced through the uterus and tubes into the peritoneal cavity, and tubal patency is demonstrated during laparoscopy by injection of a dye through the cervix and into the fallopian tubes (chromopertubation).

If transit can take place so easily, it is probable that the same happens with chemical substances used for hygienic, cosmetic or medicinal purposes, many of which may have potential carcinogenic or irritating properties (Table 12.1). Such migration could well explain the aetiological role of chemical substances in certain gynaecological diseases, such as ovarian carcinoma and infertility.

Table 12.1 Chemicals with suspected carcinogenic properties used in the vagina for cosmetic, hygiene and medicinal purposes

Arsenicals	Nitrosamine*
Hydroxiquinolines	Spermicides
Nitrofurantion	Asbestos[†]
Ichthammol	Talc
Sulphonamides	Gentian violet
Metronidazole	

*Possible formation by chemical reduction; [†] As a contaminant.

INVESTIGATIONS

Diagnostic procedures where gases, fluids, dyes and contrast medium are introduced through manual intervention under positive pressure, from the uterine cervix into the peritoneum, are anatomically accurate and safe in the hands of those performing them regularly, but do not fully portray fallopian tube patency or function.

Laparoscopy under general anaesthesia provides visual information about the gross anatomy of the pelvis. Pelvis adhesions, endometriosis, and post-surgical scarring limiting tubal motility, are the most common findings which are not necessarily diagnosed radiographically [1].

Hysterosalpingography (HSG) is an important outpatient radiological procedure for evaluating uterine, tubal and peritoneal causes of infertility. Its advantages include immediate information about proximal and distal occlusion and cornual lesions, and the assessment of intratubal architecture. A major limitation of HSG is its inability to demonstrate peritubal disease with consistency, and to evaluate the status of the tubal fimbria [3,4]. HSG is indicated early in the investigation of the infertile female, particularly in those with a history of previous abdominal surgery, known episodes of pelvic inflammatory disease, post-partum infection, and/or palpable adnexal pathology compatible with hydrosalpinges or endometriosis. It is also indicated in women with previous sterilization who request tubal ligation reversal, or to confirm tubal occlusion after tubal sterilization.

Transcervical hysteroscopy has been utilized to visualize the tubal ostium and the intramural portion of the fallopian tubes. Evidence of proximal tubal occlusion, polyps, adhesions and salpingitis isthmica nodosa may be found.

All the above are invasive procedures, uncomfortable for the patient, at times painful, and restricted under certain conditions. HSG is not free of the risks of hypersensitivity reactions, uterine perforation and tubal rupture, haemorrhage, endometriosis, shock, granuloma formation or pulmonary oil embolism.

Ultrasonography does not use radiation but the tubes are difficult to visualize during ultrasonographic examination of a normal pelvis. The difficulties are probably due to their small diameter, variable position within the pelvis and absence of fluid/tissue interfaces. Blockages at or near the junction of the uterus and oviduct may not give rise to any ultrasonographically detectable alteration.

RADIONUCLIDE HYSTEROSALPINGOGRAPHY

Using a radionuclide imaging method for evaluating fallopian tube function – radionuclide hysterosalpingography (HERS) – Iturralde and Venter studied 53 females to demonstrate the upward migration of non-motile, inert chemical substances. During the course of the study, it became apparent that the value of the images obtained describing the female reproductive system pathways functionally reflected the dynamic state of this system and could be used as an additional diagnostic method of evaluating tubal patency or obstruction in clinical practice [5,6]. Patients in this first study were divided into two groups: group I comprised 24 adult white females, admitted for elective gynaecological operations; group

II comprised 29 young white adult women referred by the infertility clinic for evaluation of their tubal patency.

Patients were placed in the supine gynaecological examination position with the buttocks slightly elevated or in the Trendelenburg position. Commercially available human serum albumin microspheres (HAM) were labelled with technetium-99m. The size of > 95% of HAM ranged between 10 and 40μm with an average diameter 20μm. This roughly approximates the size of a human sperm, which measures 8μm in diameter of the head and is about 40μm long. The cervix and posterior fornix were exposed with a vaginal speculum and 370MBq (10mCi) (for patients of group I) and 70MBq (2mCi) (for patients of group II) of ^{99m}Tc-HAM in a volume of <1ml were deposited in the posterior fornix, or close to the cervical external os. The plastic cover of the needle (37mm) was kept in place so that the exposed tissue was not accidentally traumatized. The radionuclide was quickly discharged and the

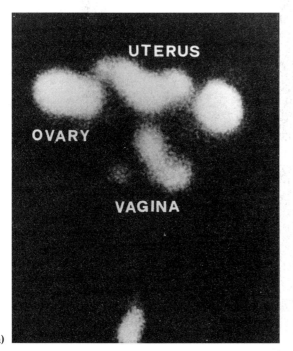

(a)

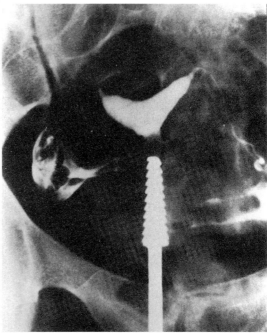

(b)

Figure 12.8   (a) Normal radionuclide hysterosalpingography (HERS) showing the pattern of flow of radiolabelled microspheres from the vagina, through the uterus to the fimbriated peritoneal opening of the patent fallopian tubes, and (b) contrast spillage into the peritoneal cavity during hysterosalpingography.

vaginal speculum carefully withdrawn while trying not to let the radioactive fluid leak out of the vagina. The vulva was then covered with a sanitary towel or tampon and the legs pressed or crossed together. The patient was kept in this position for the next 3 hours.

Images (400–500 K-count) were obtained 1, 2, 3 and 24 hours after deposition of the radioactive tracer by a large field-of-view gamma-camera with a low-energy, all-purpose collimator. The usual was an anterior view over the lower pelvic region. In selected cases, images were also obtained shielding the high activity in the vagina in order to enhance the image of the uterus and tubes, while using a ×2 zoom to enlarge the small field-of-view.

All patients in group II had contrast HSG and laparoscopic chromopertubation (LPC) done after HERS. Spillage of the contrast media into the peritoneal cavity during HSG or appearance of the dye in the fimbria during LPC was evidence of tubal patency. The pressure required to introduce these substances from the uterine cervix to the peritoneal cavity was also considered. Results of the three diagnostic procedures were later compared and evaluated.

CLINICAL RESULTS

The normal pattern of gamma-camera images obtained with this procedure is a central elongated area of high activity over the vagina. Directly on top of this area appeared a narrow stretch of activity corresponding to the endocervix. The uterus was seen as a smaller area of varying size, position and shape (in most cases it was triangular), possibly because of impression of the bladder upon the uterus. The tubes were seen extending laterally or upward in a diverging angle with a distal 'hot' spot of high intensity corresponding to the fimbria and ovaries. In some cases, activity in the region of the tubal isthmus could not be visualized, although there was high activity in their distal segment. In most cases, activity progressed within the first hour simultaneously through both tubes, while in others, activity moved faster in one tube than in the other, showing increased activity on one side. Scans were interpreted as abnormal if there was no activity in one or both tubes and specially if the distal focal area of high activity in the fimbria did not show up to 3 hours after deposition. The course and migra-

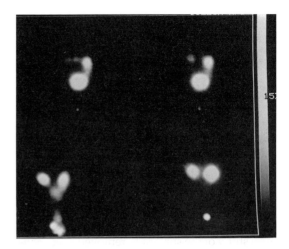

Figure 12.9 Normal HERS at 30 minutes (top left), 60 minutes (top right), and 90 minutes (lower left), with asymmetric migration of radiolabelled microspheres appearing early in the left fimbria, to bilateral tubal patency finally at 3 hours (lower right).

Table 12.2 Radionuclide hysterosalpingography (HERS); summary of results (group I)*

Outcome	No. of patients
Positive migration	16
Negative	
No passage to uterus	2
No passage to adnexae	2
Technically defective	3
Total patients examined	24

* For study details, see text.

Table 12.3 Radionuclide hysterosalpingography (HERS) versus hysterosalpingography (HSG) and laparoscopic chromopertubation (LPC) (group II)*

Outcome	No. of patients
Agreement between HERS, HSG and LPC	21
Disagreement between HERS/HSG and LPC	
HERS (–)[†]; HSG and LPC (+)[†]	5
HERS (+); HSG and LPC (–)	1
Technically defective	2
Total patients examined	29

* For study details, see text; [†] Tubes patent (+); tubes not patent (–).

tion of ^{99m}Tc-HAM by the propulsive action of the tubal ciliary mechanism during HERS was expressed as the transit time from deposition in the vagina until appearance of activity in either fimbria. In healthy females with patent tubes the transit time varies from 1 to 3 hours (Figures 12.8 and 12.9).

In 14 of 21 cases of group I, it was possible to measure high radioactivity levels in the adnexa separately from the uterus. Nine of these showed marked radioactivity in the tubes (most of it localized in the fimbria). In five cases, radioactivity in the tubes was not much higher than the background. In these patients, severe tubal occlusion due to previous infection was confirmed by pathological study of the surgically removed specimens. In the two patients where pieces of the anterior peritoneum, peripheral blood, and lymphatic glands were counted, the radioactivity levels in

the samples was as low as background. This showed that the ^{99m}Tc-HAM had not reached the adnexa through the blood supply owing to local reabsorption or lymphatic drainage from the vaginal mucosa where activity had been deposited.

When HERS was compared with the results of HSG and LPC in patients from group II, it was found that in 21 patients there was complete accordance between the three diagnostic modalities, whether the tubes were patent or occluded (Tables 12.2 and 12.3). In six cases there was no agreement between HERS and HSG and LPC. In five of these, both HSG and LPC showed that the tubes were patent when the contrast media and the dye were introduced under extreme pressure. In these five cases, HERS showed no evidence of migration in one or other tube. In only one case did HERS show patency in one tube, while HSG and LPC did not,

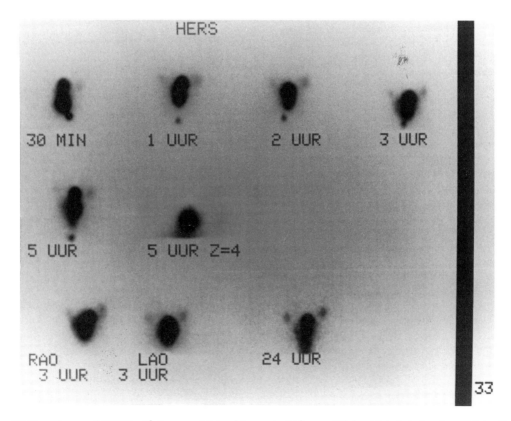

Figure 12.10 Abnormal HERS with images obtained for up to 24 hours. Bilateral tubal obstruction (faint activity is portrayed bilaterally in ampulla of fallopian tubes).

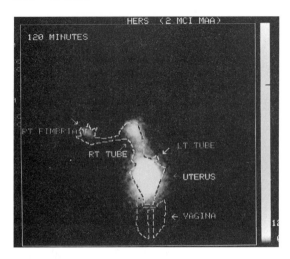

Figure 12.11 Radionuclide hysterosalpingography of a patient who underwent tubal ligation, showing radiolabelled microspheres migration through the right tube to the fimbria beyond the level of ligation.

this was in the case of a woman with a septum in her vagina and a double uterus where manipulations for HSG and LPC were difficult.

In two cases the results were equivocal because at least two of the three diagnostic procedures were technically deficient (Figures 12.10 and 12.11).

The results from the original study with HERS in patients from group I demonstrate the upward migration of a particulate radioactive tracer such as ^{99m}Tc-HAM from the vagina through the uterus and tubes into the peritoneal cavity and ovaries. This correlates with findings on the surgically removed specimens, proving the accuracy of this radionuclide procedure. This supports previous evidence for the migration of inert, non-motile chemical substances from the vagina to the peritoneum and ovaries, and could help explain the role that some of these apparently innocent and frequently used substances play in the aetiology of certain gynaecological diseases.

Although the ^{99m}Tc-HAM molecules differ biochemically and immunologically from human spermatozoa, their diameter roughly approximates the size of human spermatozoa. It is therefore suggested that the radiolabelled tracer molecules are transported by the same mechanisms which were originally designed for support of spermatozoal migration to the ovum during the period of fertilization and that tubal migration of the radionuclide reflects the ascending flow of spermatozoa (see Figure 12.7).

As far as the radionuclide imaging process is concerned, it was encouraging to find a close correlation of this procedure when compared with HSG and LPC. However, most important of all is the fact that HERS functionally reflects the dynamic state of the female reproductive system by showing particulate migration, which is not the case of the other anatomically dependant diagnostic modalities used to evaluate tubal patency. In this initial small series it was found that in five cases, HSG and LPC were reported showing anatomical tubal patency only because both the contrast media and the dye were injected under extreme pressures, opening kinked tubes that under other circumstances would not be patent. HERS proved in these five patients (19% of the series) that there was no migration of ^{99m}Tc-HAM through the fallopian tubes, this being the probable cause for their infertility.

There are some additional circumstances in which HERS seems particularly attractive. The increasing number of sterilizations being performed on relatively young women of low parity, together with the availability of improved microsurgery techniques has led to an increased demand for reversal. Patients who have had surgical reanastomosis for previously ligated or fibrosed tubes are at an unacceptable risk (3.3%) of developing tubo-ovarian abscess or granuloma as a complication of contrast HSG performed during the first few weeks following surgery or being deceived by the diagnosis of tubal patency when in fact the tubes may be patent but non-functional due to deciliation in the blind loop resulting from ligation, while HERS is a simple method used to confirm the success of surgical reanastomosis or of a tubal ligation for sterilization purposes. This is a practical problem with potential legal implications for the surgeon (see Figure 12.11).

From the initial study performed by Venter and Iturralde [5] it was clear that HERS allows the investigation of tubal function with ease of performance, patient comfort, functional relevance and reduced cost. The other advantage of HERS is that the procedure is readily available in most nuclear medicine departments with conventional nuclear imaging equipment.

Comparison between HERS and contrast HSG and LPC may seem inadequate, as the nature of the procedures differs fundamentally, but at present there is no other method in use that can reveal actual tubal function. While contrast HSG has methodological limitations, laparoscopy usually requires general anaesthesia. Furthermore, studies have shown a great discrepancy between HSG and LPC, with correlation between these two techniques in only 50% of infertile women [7,8]. Nonetheless, radionuclide hysterosalpingography continues to be under-utilized at most centres.

If the functional nature of HERS could be shown to predict outcome better than contrast HSG, then gynaecologists may be willing to exchange the superior spatial resolution of contrast HSG for the functional superiority of HERS.

Since the initial description of the procedure, extensive evaluation has taken place to determine the role of HERS in the investigation of tubal dysfunction compared with other diagnostic examinations. Technical refinements were introduced to improve the imaging quality, reduce the radiation dose and increase awareness of the study on part of nuclear medicine and referring physicians.

Iturralde and Venter later reported results obtained on a third group of patients with presumed normal fallopian tubes who were scheduled for tubal ligation for conservative reasons (group III). Patients in this group showed evidence of a hormonal regulatory process of tubal ciliary function as migration of ^{99m}Tc-HAM was faster during the period of ovulation and slower in the luteal phase. During the time patients were using oral contraceptives migration was also slower. Studies in baboons, where the procedure could be repeated in the same animal, confirmed the findings suggested in the human series [9].

McCalley *et al.* [10], in a prospective study of 26 patients referred from an infertility clinic, introduced some procedural modifications including reduction of the administered dose to 37 MBq (1 mCi). The radiotracer was suspended in 1 ml of saline and placed directly onto the cervical mucosa. Anterior pelvic images were acquired between 15 and 30 minutes later by SPECT gamma-camera using pinhole collimation and caudal angulation to improve visualization of the region behind the uterus. Lateral obliques were also obtained when needed. Imaging was terminated as soon as the study was interpreted as being normal or after 4 hours in cases where

obstruction was suspected. Patency of a fallopian tube was inferred if a relatively intense focus of activity was seen in the area of the adjacent adnexa. If no such activity was evident on images one or more hours after radiotracer administration, then that tube was considered obstructed. Direct observations of surgical pathology, peritoneoscopy and contrast HSG were used as comparison studies. Efficiency of HERS for evaluation of fallopian tube patency was over 94%.

In this series two tubes that appeared obstructed on the radionuclide study, but were judged patent by correlative examination, were found at surgery to be immotile with peritubal and periadnexal adhesions which probably rendered them functionally incapable of transport of radiolabelled particles. These results lent further support to the contention that the radionuclide study is a more physiological indicator of tubal function than the radiographical contrast study.

McCalley *et al.* have estimated an ovarian dose of 0.75 mGy/MBq (1.8 rad/mCi) for HERS, assuming that 5% of the administered dose resides on each ovary for the duration of the physical decay of ^{99m}Tc ($t_{\frac{1}{2}} = 6$ h) [10,11]. Stabin [12] (Oak Ridge Radiopharmaceutical Internal Dose Information Center), corrected this dose estimate, suggesting that the actual dose to each ovary is 1.5 mGy/MBq. The gonadal radiation doses received during the radionuclide procedure are comparable with those received during the radiographic contrast examination, not including the dose due to fluoroscopy. Kennedy *et al.* [13] estimate the dose to be much lower because the maximum uptake in the ovaries was found to be 4.6% of the administered activity, giving a maximum dose of 2.35 mGy per ovary. Using ^{99m}Tc-pertechnetate, Yang *et al.* [14] reported a dose of 1.08 mGy (108 mrad) per study. During radiographic fallopian tube recanalization, the average absorbed dose to the ovaries was calculated at 8.5 mGy.

Radionuclide hysterosalpingography (HERS), when compared with the 'gold standard' of laparoscopy and direct observation of tubal motility at surgery, in 77 females referred by the infertility clinic, showed a sensitivity for detection of tubal patency of 93% and a specificity of 94%. For the detection of tubal obstruction, the calculated sensitivity was 94% and the specificity 93%. The overall predictive value of the test for tubal patency was 96% and for tubal obstruction 90%. The overall efficiency (percent of tubes correctly diagnosed for obstruction or patency) of HERS was 97% [15].

Brundin *et al.* [16] reported in a study of 19 infertile women that by using HERS it was possible to verify active passage in cases of tubal spasm during contrast HSG, lack of transport in cases of normal patent oviducts at contrast HSG as well as presence or absence of active transport through hydrosalpinges with or without fimbrial passage to the abdominal cavity as seen at normal contrast HSG. The oviducts were found to be patent with normal contrast HSG but lacked transportation capacity when compared with HERS in 41%. Two patients with normal contrast HSG and normal HERS had conceived in the 18 months following the study. However, none conceived in the group of women showing no radionuclide oviductal transportation capacity in spite of having a normal contrast HSG. This would imply that the capacity of transporting luminal content in those patients with damaged, but apparently patent tubes on HSG, on whom microsurgery is performed to restore luminal passage, could be seriously questioned [16]. Because recent developments in physiological and surgical approach to infertility could be aided by knowledge of fallopian tube function, HERS could constitute an important tool for referring the infertile patient to an optimal choice of therapy for infertility due to a 'tubal factor'.

If ciliary function is normal, the infertile patient should be directed to an *in vitro* fertilization programme. If a woman is found to have pelvic adhesions, but HERS shows normal ciliary function, she may require surgery. However, for women with abnormal tubal ciliary function, HERS tells the gynaecologist that gamete intrafallopian transfer (GIFT) or zygote intrafallopian transfer (ZIFT) will not work. IVF and embryo transfer will be needed instead.

Uszler *et al.* [17] reported on a series of 46 infertile patients, that no patient whose tubes were non-functional on HERS has become pregnant without IVF, and five live, healthy births have resulted in patients showing function of at least one tube. Uszler stated that HERS is the only method to visualize fallopian tubal function, that can aid infertility evaluation [17].

Earlier, McQueen *et al.* [18], following strict criteria for the classification of infertility, prospec-

tively studied 96 infertile women, in which once again HERS was compared with laparoscopy and contrast hysterosalpingography. They introduced a technical modification by taking 'squat' views with the patient sitting upright and the camera under the couch, directed at the perineum. This view facilitated identifying anatomical landmarks [18].

The radionuclide test correlated with laparoscopy in the diagnosis of patency or blockage in 83 cases (86%). In nine patients, where 'blockage' was diagnosed on the radionuclide test but patency found at laparoscopy, a higher prevalence of pelvic abnormality was found, compared with the 78 patients where both tests demonstrated patency ($P < 0.02$). Those results which did not correlate provide evidence that impaired radionuclide migration may occur in diseased, but patent, tubes. Most of these showed some migration of radionuclide into the tube, but not through to the peritoneum, suggesting abnormal tubal function. Peritubal adhesions may be associated with mucosal damage and may affect function. There was a significant increase in radionuclide blockage in laparoscopically patent tubes which are affected by these conditions, suggesting that the radionuclide test may be valuable in their functional assessment. Conversely, some cases, where a diagnosis of patency was made on the radionuclide image but where the tubes appeared blocked at laparoscopy, were found either where the pelvis was completely normal or where there was a hydrosalpinx. It has long been recognized that spasm of a normal tube may occur at the time of chromopertubation, giving a false impression of blockage. This is probably due to the forced injection of relatively large volumes of fluid, which does not occur with the radionuclide test and may explain the finding of radionuclide patency in two patients with apparent blockage of anatomically normal tubes at laparoscopy.

A similar study conducted by Steck *et al.* [19] reported congruent findings between tubal patency on contrast HSG and tubal migration on HERS in 23 out of 28 patients, with an overall correlation of 61%. When bilateral patency was reported on HSG, correlation with HERS results was 18/27 (67%). In three out of eight patients with unilateral patency, the good side was adequately diagnosed by HERS, but scans were reported as bilaterally abnormal in the remaining five patients. As expected, HERS imaging showed no tubal migration of the tracer in all three individuals with anatomical blockage at HSG. For the detection of tubal obstruction, the sensitivity of radionuclide imaging was 86% and the specificity 66% when using the HSG as the standard, and the percentage of tubes correctly classified was 67%. Congruent findings between tubal migration on HERS and patency on laparoscopy were found in 18/31 patients (overall correlation of 58%). When bilateral patency was reported on laparoscopy, the correlation with HERS results was 14/21 (67%). Unilateral patency was revealed on laparoscopy in seven patients, but the normal side was correctly diagnosed by HERS in only one patient (correlation 14%) while scans were reported as bilaterally abnormal in five and equivocal in one patient. Again, HERS did not show tubal migration in all three individuals with anatomical obstruction. For the detection of tubal occlusion, the figures for sensitivity and specificity of HERS were 91 and 60%, respectively, with an overall efficiency of 69% [19].

Barrada *et al.* [20] inserted an insemination catheter into the cervical canal, during the late follicular phase, delivering a smaller dose of radiolabelled particles into the uterine cavity (7.4–11.0 MBq) which allowed for the reduction of the absorbed dose to the ovaries to levels 50% lower than conventional contrast HSG. As with other investigators, this group found once again that none of the patients showing bilateral dysfunction on HERS became pregnant, even if the fallopian tubes had shown patency on contrast HSG and/or chromopertubation on LPC. They further suggested that radionuclide hysterosalpingography be accepted, with the other correlative imaging procedures, on a routine basis as part of the investigation of infertile women [20].

CILIARY FUNCTION AND RADIONUCLIDE STUDIES

Various factors, such as the increasing air pollution and cigarette smoking, are apt to cause a reduction and sometimes total cessation of the beating of the respiratory cilia (ciliostasis), and a consequent reduction in the rate of transport of mucus by the cilia which may lead to the development of bronchial disease, and possibly infertility. This finding, although somehow expected, was important as it appeared that there was now some evidence of a ciliary connection between respira-

tory and fallopian tubes ciliary damage during cigarette smoking [21–23].

If the ciliotoxic effect of cigarette smoke is due to a systemic factor(s), rather than a local action, then it is possible that sperm tails and the oviduct ciliary mechanism might also be damaged.

The association of chronic and recurrent infections of the respiratory tract and male infertility described as the immotile cilia syndrome (ICS) due to reduced tracheobronchial mucociliary clearance, and the production of spermatozoa with straight immotile tails, lends further credibility to the 'ciliary connection' which suggests that the systemic ciliotoxic effects of cigarette smoke may be implicated as the cause of infertility and chronic bronchitis in cigarette-smoking females. After all, sperm tails, flagella and cilia of the respiratory tract, endocervix and oviducts have a common structural and functional pattern of internal tubules with propulsive action.

In women undergoing fertility treatment, the chances of successful fertilization is reduced by some 30% if they smoke. Reproduction in men also appeared to be influenced by smoking. This is probably caused by the same cigarette smoke ciliotoxic constituents, which if systemically transmitted could affect the quality and frequency of the beating of the ciliated epithelium of the

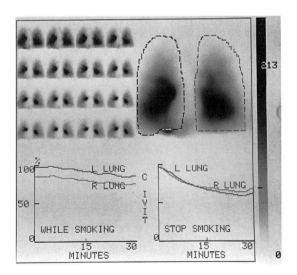

Figure 12.12 Tracheobronchial mucociliary clearance with curves during cigarette smoking and after stopping smoking.

TUBOCILIARY FUNCTION IN SMOKERS
Migration of ^{99m}Tc-HAM from uterus to fimbria

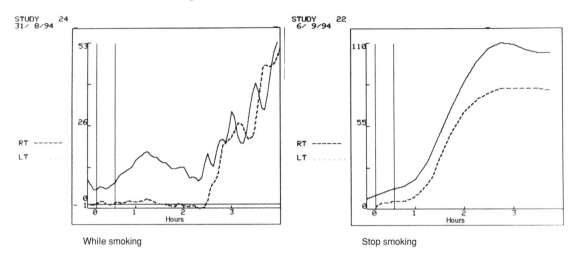

While smoking   Stop smoking

Figure 12.13   Radionuclide hysterosalpingography (HERS) tubociliary clearance of the same infertile woman as in Figure 12.12, showing curves of the arrival of radiolabelled activity in the fimbria for up to 4 hours, during cigarette smoking and after stopping cigarette smoking. This apparently infertile woman eventually conceived after stopping smoking.

fallopian tubes resulting in a critical delay of gamete transport that inhibits conception.

The observation of these clinical and epidemiological factors prompted a further study carried out by Iturralde and Venter [24] to demonstrate – by using nuclear medicine procedures – the validity of this hypothesis.

Two nuclear medicine procedures, based on the same physiological principle, were utilized to portray the tracheobronchial and oviductal ciliary function in a group of infertile cigarette smoking females: the scintigraphic display of tracheobronchial function following radioaerosol inhalation of ^{99m}Tc-colloid particles was the method used for the visualization of the mucociliary function of the lungs, while hysterosalpingo radionuclide scintigraphy (HERS) was the method used to evaluate the active transportation mechanism of the ciliated epithelium of the fallopian tubes.

Of the 28 tubes examined in 14 cigarette-smoking females, eight were found to be obstructed while the rest appeared patent on HSG and LPC. However, when studied by HERS, all the tubes examined showed markedly delayed (>8 h) to totally absent tubociliary migration. In

those patients who decided to stop smoking, ciliary function of the tracheobronchial tree, nasal, and fallopian tubes improved remarkably by 3 months after stopping (Figures 12.12 and 12.13). Three out of the 14 women with unexplained infertility conceived 6 months later and a further four conceived 18 months after stopping smoking with a total success rate of 50%.

None of the infertile women who continued smoking became pregnant in spite of their tubes being patent on HSG and LPC. The fact that this process can be reversed after completely stopping cigarette smoking, and return to fecundity, is encouraging.

Using nuclear medicine procedures such as radioaerosol lung cinescintigraphy and HERS, Iturralde and Venter [24] were able to correlate and demonstrate that epithelial cilia from different organs have a similar behaviour and that the ciliotoxic effect of cigarette smoking in infertile women not only inhibits their tracheobronchial mucociliary escalator function, but also affects oviductal ciliary function possibly causing a critical delay in gamete transport that inhibits conception. Indeed, perhaps illuminating these adverse effects that smoking imparts on reproductive health might persuade individuals to stop.

HERS is the only non-invasive method for visualizing and evaluating *in vivo* the ciliary transportation capacity of the luminal epithelium lining of the inaccessible fallopian tubes.

This simple procedure can play an important role in the evaluation of infertility, especially in patients who suffer from 'unexplained' subfecundity due to a 'tubal' factor.

REFERENCES

1. Winfield, A.C., Fleischer, A.C. and Moore, D.E. (1990) Diagnostic imaging of fertility disorders. *Curr. Probl. Diagn. Radiol.*, 9.
2. Paltieli, Y. (1994) New laser technique can help pinpoint infertility due to fallopian tube pathology. *Med. Chronicle*, 7.
3. Hunt, R.B. and Siegler, A.M. (1993) *Hysterosalpingography: Techniques and Interpretation*, Year Book Medical Publishers, Chicago.
4. Rajah, R., McHugo, J.M. and Obhrai, M. (1992) The role of hysterosalpingography in modern gynaecological practice. *Br. Med. J.*, **65**, 649–51.
5. Venter, P.F. and Iturralde, M.P. (1979) Migration of a particulate radioactive tracer from the vagina to the peritoneal cavity and ovaries. *S. Afr. Med. J.*, **55**, 917–19.
6. Iturralde, M.P. and Venter, P.F. (1981) Hysterosalpingo-radionuclide scintigraphy (HERS). *Semin. Nucl. Med.*, **11**, 301–14.
7. Brosens, I.A. and Gordon, A.G. (1990) *Tubal Infertility*, J.B. Lippincott, Philadelphia.
8. Lindequest, S., Justesen, P., Larsen, C. and Rasmussen, F. (1991) Diagnostic quality and complications of hysterosalpingography. *Radiology*, **179**, 69–74.
9. Iturralde, M.P., van der Merwe, J.V., Goosen, D.J. and Dormehl, I.C. (1983) Dynamic hysterosalpingo radionuclide scintigraphy (HERS), in *Nuclear Medicine and Biology Advances* (ed. C. Raynaud), Pergamon Press, Oxford, pp. 1589–91.
10. McCalley, M.G., Braunstein, P., Stone, S., Henderson, P. and Egbert, R. (1985) Radionuclide hysterosalpingography for evaluation of fallopian tube patency. *J. Nucl. Med.*, **26**, 74.
11. van der Weiden, R.M.F. and van Xijl, J. (1989) Radiation exposure of the ovaries during hysterosalpingography. Is radionuclide hysterosalpingography justified? *Br. J. Obstet. Gynaecol.*, **96**, 471–2.
12. Stabin, M. (1989) Radiation dosimetry in radionuclide hysterosalpingography. Letter to the editor. *J. Nucl. Med.*, **30**, 415–16.
13. Kennedy, S.H., Mojiminiyi, O.A., Soper, M.D.W., Shepstone, B.J. and Barlow, D.H. (1989) Radiation exposure of the ovaries during hysterosalpingography. Is radionuclide hysterosalpingography justified? (Letter to the Editor) *Br. J. Obstet. Gynaecol.*, **69**, 1359.
14. Yang, K.T.A., Chiang, J.-H., Chen, B.-S. *et al.* (1992) Radionuclide hysterosalpingography with 99mTcO$_4$; application and radiation dose to ovaries. *J. Nucl. Med.*, **33**, 282–6.
15. Iturralde, M.P. and Venter, P.F. (1988) Comparison of diagnostic accuracy of laparoscopy, hysterosalpingography and radionuclide hysterosalpingography in the evaluation of female infertility. Proceedings 4th Asia and Oceania Congress of Nuclear Medicine, Taipei, Taiwan.
16. Brundin, J., Dahlborn, M., Ahlber-Ahre, E. and Lundberg, H.J. (1989) Radionuclide hysterosalpingography for measurement of human oviductal function. *Int. J. Gynecol. Obstet.*, **28**, 53–9.
17. Uzler, M., Jacobson, A., Warnich, A. and Nassor, G. (1003) Radionuclide hysterosalpingography – appropriate for the new assisted reproduction techniques. *J. Nucl. Med.*, **164**, P797.
18. McQueen, D., McKillop, J.H., Gray, H.W., Bessent, R.G. and Black, W.P. (1991) Investigation of tubal infertility by radionuclide migration. *Hum. Reprod.*, **6**, 529–32.
19. Steck, T., Wurfel, W., Becker, W. and Albert, P.J. (1991) Serial scintigraphic imaging for visual passive transport processes in the human fallopian tube. *Hum. Reprod.*, **6**, 1186–91.
20. Barrada, M., Buxbaum, P., Schatten, C., Pateisky, N., Seiffert, M., Strohmer, H. and Vytiska, E. (1995) Hystero-salpingo scintigraphy: a routine investigation in sterile women? *Nucl. Med. Commun.*, **16**, 447–51.
21. Panayiotis, M. and Zavos, E.D.S. (1989) Cigarette smoking and human reproduction: effects on female and male fecundity. *Infertility*, **12**, 35–46.
22. Dalhamn, T. (1970) In vivo and in vitro ciliotoxic effects of tobacco smoke. *Arch. Environ. Health*, **21**, 633–4.
23. London Press Service (1993) Smoking can harm fertility. *Specialist Med.*, 44.
24. Iturralde, M.P. and Venter, P.F. (1994) Radionuclide studies of fallopian tubes ciliary function in infertile cigarette-smoking females. *Eur. J. Nucl. Med.*, **21**, 547 (abstract 179).

FURTHER READING

Gurgan, T., Kisnisci, H.A., Yarali, H. *et al.* (1991) Evaluation of the functional status of the fallopian tubes in unexplained infertility with radionuclide hysterosalpingography. *Gynecol. Obstet. Invest.*, **32**, 224–6.

Jaffe, R., Pierson, R.A. and Abramowicz, J.S. (1994) *Imaging in Infertility and Reproduction Endocrinology*. J.B. Lippincott, Philadelphia.

Gynaecological cancer

K. E. Britton and M. Granowska

INTRODUCTION

Cancers of the ovary, cervix and uterus are becoming increasingly common. Ovarian cancer is one of the most malignant tumours, and accounts for 6% of deaths from cancer in women in the Western world [1]. Whereas screening for cervical cancer has had some benefits and uterine cancer demonstrates itself usually with post-menopausal bleeding, ovarian cancer typically remains concealed until late in its course.

Opportunities for screening women for ovarian cancer include abdominal and transvaginal ultrasound and serum markers such as CA125. Both have their problems. In a survey of 500 women with transabdominal ultrasound, 234 abnormal masses were discovered in the pelvis. All these women were operated upon, and 225 of them did not have ovarian cancer [2]. The incidence of ovarian cancer is more than doubled if there is a family history in a close relative, and so patients at risk are being screened with transvaginal ultrasound, with approximately 1 in 60 pick-up rate of ovarian cancer [3]. Combinations of CA125, ultrasound and menopausal status improves the pre-operative diagnostic accuracy for ovarian cancer [4]. The CA125 marker by itself is insufficient to diagnose early ovarian cancer, since a certain tumour mass has to be present to release enough antigen to increase the blood level over its normal variation [5]. For the same reason, it is a relatively insensitive marker of recurrent ovarian cancer. Finkler et al. [6] showed that the sensitivity of clinical examination for the diagnosis of ovarian cancer was 43% compared with 62% for ultrasound and 68% for CA125.

Radiological techniques rely on detecting cancer as a physical entity: features of malignancy on MRI, CT or ultrasound include a thick irregular cyst wall, solid areas in a cyst, irregular septa, papillary-like projections from the cyst wall, or evidence of metastases, or ascites associated with an ovarian mass. Colour Doppler uses the increased flow of an ovarian cancer as the basis of its detection; however, other ovarian masses such as a corpus luteum cyst, which is benign and usually self-limiting, and ovarian infection or abscess, also increase flow to the mass. CT scanning is widely used, but is relatively insensitive and often inconclusive in the pre-operative diagnosis of ovarian cancer [7]. It is also relatively insensitive for recurrent disease [8]. MRI is gaining ground as a means for assessing primary and recurrent ovarian cancer [8–10].

RADIOIMMUNOSCINTIGRAPHY

The intention here is to use a property of the surface of the cancer cell, that differs qualitatively and quantitatively, from that of the benign ovarian tumour and the normal ovary, so that malignancy can be distinguished. Because of the relative vascularity of ovarian cancer ensuring good antibody delivery, radioimmunoscintigraphy (RIS) has generally been successful. There is a wide range of antibodies used to detect this cancer (Table 12.4).

Many monoclonal antibodies have been used for targeting gynaecological cancer. Anti-HCG has been used to detect the choriogonadotrophic hormone [22]. The polymorphic epithelial mucin antigen has many different monoclonal antibodies made against it. It is a normal constituent of the lining of the ducts of the breast or the follicles of the ovary. Such antigens are remote from the bloodstream, so a monoclonal antibody against them will not normally react in vivo. However, the architectural disruption caused by the cancerous process brings large quantities of such cell-bound antigens into contact with the blood where they are detectable using RIS. HMFG1, HMFG2 against the human milk fat globules, surface-lining protein of the milk duct, and ovarian follicles are in this class. SM3, a monoclonal antibody against the stripped mucin core protein has a high specificity for breast and ovarian cancer and a low reactivity with normal tissues and benign tumours. Whereas the malignant-to-benign uptake ratio for an HMFG antibody is about 8:1, that for SM3 is about 17:1, and therefore enables it to be used for distinguishing malignant from benign tumours in addition to detecting the tumour [23]. Some cancer cell proteins are produced in larger

Clinical Nuclear Medicine, 3rd edn. Edited by M.N. Maisey, K.E. Britton and B.D. Collier. Published in 1998 by Chapman & Hall, London. ISBN 0 412 75180 1

Table 12.4   Radioimmunoscintigraphy of ovarian cancer

Cancer-associated antigen	Monoclonal antigen	Ovary	Reference
Polymorphic epithelial	HMFG1 and 2	+	[11,12]
Mucin antigens	SM3	+	[13,14]
Folate binding protein	MoV-18	+	[15,16]
TF antigen	170 H.82	+	[17,18]
TAG72	B72.3	+	[19]
Released antigen	OVTL3	+	[20]
Released antigen	OC125	+	[21]

Table 12.5   Management of ovarian cancer with radioimmunoscintigraphy

Detection of primary	Clinical examination
	Ultrasound
	Trans abdominal
	Trans vaginal
	Doppler colour
Distinction of benign	Ultrasound, XCT, MRI poor
from malignant	Tc-99m SM3
	Tc-99m MoV-18
Extent of surgery	Per-operative probe
Detection of recurrences	Serum markers
	Radioimmunoscintigraphy
Localization of recurrence	Radioimmunoscintigraphy
	Radiological techniques poor
Effect of chemotherapy	Radioimmunoscintigraphy
	Radiological techniques poor
	'Second-look' surgery
Confirmation of suitability	Radioimmunoscintigraphy
for radioimmunotherapy	

amounts in the cancer cell than in normal cells. These include: anti-placental alkaline phosphatase PLAP (H17-E2), which reacts with ovarian cancers and seminomas [12,24]; OC-125, which is also used as a tumour marker; OVTL [25]; and MoV-18 [15].

Synthetic antigens have been created with monoclonal antibodies such as 170-H82, which is called a panadenocarcinoma monoclonal antibody because of its wide range of reactivity [17,18]. The success of imaging using radionuclide-labelled monoclonal antibodies in the detection of recurrent ovarian cancer has been demonstrated in a correlative imaging study by Peltier *et al.* [26]. It may be concluded that RIS is a reasonable way of imaging recurrent ovarian cancer and evaluating the effects of chemotherapy without 'second-look' laparotomy. It is also able to demonstrate that a mass seen on X-ray, CT or ultrasound contains or does not contain viable tumour.

OVARIAN CANCER

There are basically four types of ovarian cancer patient.

1. Patients with an abdominal or pelvis mass that may have been diagnosed by ultrasound screening of well women or women at risk of ovarian cancer or through some other gynaecological presentation, and there is a reasonable clinical suspicion that ovarian cancer is the cause of the mass.

2. Patients with clinically or radiologically obvious ovarian cancer in whom it is required to determine the extent of the disease pre-operatively, as far as possible. The extent of the tumour and the metastatic spread are assessed at surgery, and the per-operative probe may be used as part of this assessment [27].

3. Patients who have been operated on for ovarian cancer with histological confirmation of the di-

agnoses, and who are then referred to a specialist centre for their continued treatment that may include further surgery.

4. Patients with ovarian cancer who have had primary surgical resection, either maximal or suboptimal, and have then received chemotherapy, and in whom a 'second-look' procedure for debulking or evaluation of the effect of chemotherapy may be suggested to determine the presence of residual disease as a guide to further treatment. Such 'second-look' surgery has now been shown not to affect mortality materially, and so non-invasive imaging procedures are being sought to obtain the same information. The evaluation of chemotherapy has become increasingly important as new drugs are introduced. Laparoscopy with peritoneal washings is one approach; RIS is also effective.

Radiological techniques (including MRI), are unable to distinguish post-therapy fibrosis caused by surgery or radiotherapy from viable tumour recurrence, whereas monoclonal antibodies have this potential ability (Table 12.5).

PATIENTS AND METHODS

The patient protocol requires a good explanation of the whole procedure to the patients before they enter the camera room. Such studies are usually carried out under Ethics Committee approval. No thyroid blockade is required, and provided that 1 mg (or less) of whole monoclonal antibody is used, a patient reaction is no more common than for a bone scan or kidney agent. However, it is an absolute rule that patients with a known allergy to foreign protein or severe atopy should be excluded. Skin testing is useless and only sensitizes the patient to the monoclonal antibody. Human anti-mouse antibody (HAMA) responses may occur and may be detectable in the serum. However, these are not directly related to clinical reactions. After about the third imaging injection, there may be an increased rate of clearance of the antibody, but in only a very small percentage of subjects does this interfere with tumour detectability [28]. An ^{111}In-labelled agent will show high uptake in the liver and usually quite marked bowel and marrow activity, whereas the ^{99m}Tc-labelled agent usually shows mainly renal excretion (the compound is usually a dicysteine complex of ^{99m}Tc) with low activity in the liver, marrow and bowel.

Typically, 3 mCi (120 MBq) of ^{111}In or 15 mCi (600 MBq) of ^{99m}Tc-labelled monoclonal antibody (0.5 mg) is injected. (The protocol is set out in Chapter 17, Radioimmunoscintigraphy.)

There are some important rules for imaging and image interpretation. First, specific uptake increases with time, so if a blood pool image is taken at 10 minutes, it will usually show no specific antibody (whole antibody) uptake in any tumour (see Figure 17.5). Images taken at 6 and 24 hours for ^{99m}Tc, or at 24 and 48 hours for ^{111}Indium-labelled monoclonal antibodies, will show increasing uptake with time (Figure 12.14; see also Figures 17.4 and 17.5). This should be contrasted with non-specific uptake, e.g. in a uterine fibroid, which after the initial distribution decreases with time during the first 24 hours (Figure 12.14; see also Figure 17.4). The initial blood pool image at 10 minutes acts as a template with which later images may be compared. This allows the detection of (visually and subsequently by image analysis) very small lesions that may not be detected without the blood pool image as a guide. Thus, a series of images, at least a pair or preferably a triplet, separated in time give the best visual interpretation for RIS.

The count content of the image is important, and a minimum of 800 K count should be obtained per image, using a general-purpose or preferably a high-resolution, low-energy, parallel-hole collimator, and the camera peaked at 140 keV for ^{99m}Tc. In order to provide comparable contrasts for the two images, a repositioning protocol for the patient is advised, whereby an image of markers on prominent bony landmarks is taken before and for each set of images, so that on the second and third visits the patient can be repositioned in the same place. The markers are positioned on the costal margins, xiphisternum, iliac crests and symphysis pubis. In this way the same amount of liver appears on an abdominal image giving the same image contrast, which allows comparisons to be made much more easily. SPECT images are essential for the pelvis, and often helpful for the liver and para-aortic regions in patients with ovarian cancer. Serial squat views are also of benefit in examining the pelvis. Accurate repositioning of the patient between images is a requirement for image analysis protocols using change-detection algorithms, kinetic analysis and probability mapping [29]. The challenge for RIS in patients with ovarian cancer is in distinguishing benign from

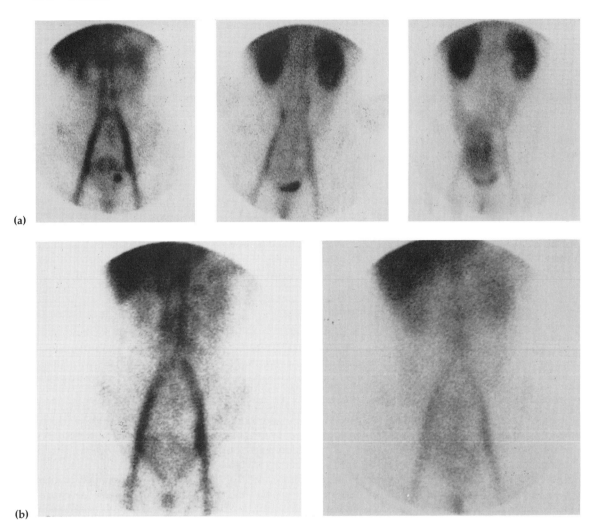

(a)

(b)

Figure 12.14 A 19-year-old woman developed ascites and an ovarian mass due to poorly differentiated serous cystadenocarcinoma FIGO 3c. At operation, it was disseminated in the pelvis and related peritoneal lymph nodes. (a) Radioimmunoscintigraphy with ^{99m}Tc before surgery. Anterior view at 10 minutes (left), 6 hours (centre) and 24 hours (right). The 10 minute image shows initial vascular, uterine, renal and bladder activity. At 6 hours, the non-specific vascular activity has faded. At 24 hours, irregular increased uptake is seen in the centre and right of the pelvis with some lateral extension of uptake on each side of the abdomen. (b) Radiommunoscintigraphy was repeated after surgery and full chemotherapy with intravenous carboplatin and intraperitoneal cisplatin. Anterior views at 10 minutes (left) and 24 hours (right) show no residual abnormal uptake. Second-look surgery showed no microscopic disease. (Reproduced courtesy of the *European Journal of Nuclear Medicine*, 1993).

malignant disease, for which SM3, OC125 and Mov-18 appear the preferred antibodies. It is expected that 75% of women with ultrasound-diagnosed lesions could be demonstrated not to have cancer using ^{99m}Tc-SM3 [30], if RIS were to be interposed between the ultrasound investigation and the laparotomy.

In conclusion, RIS has an important clinical role in the management of patients with suspected or known ovarian cancer, particularly in identifying whether surgery and chemotherapy have been successful (Table 12.5). Its wider application is limited by man-made problems, including over-regulation, which contributes over half the expense of commercializing these techniques and preventing them from becoming readily available.

REFERENCES

1. Williams, C. (1992) Ovarian and cervical cancer. *Br. Med. J.*, **304**, 1501–4.
2. Campbell, S., Bhan, V., Royston, P. *et al.* (1989) Transabdominal ultrasound screening for early ovarian cancer. *Br. Med. J.*, **299**, 1363–7.
3. Bourne, T.H., Whitehead, M.I., Campbell, S. *et al.* (1991) Ultrasound screening for familial ovarian cancer. *Gynecol. Oncol.*, **43**, 92–7.
4. Jacobs, I., Oram, D., Fairbanks, J., Turner, J., Frost, C. and Gurdzinskas, J.G. (1990) A risk of malignancy index incorporating CA 125, ultrasound and menopausal status for the accurate preoperative diagnosis of ovarian cancer. *Br. J. Obstet. Gynaecol.*, **97**, 922–9.
5. Kenemans, P., Yedema, C.A., Bon, G.G. and von Mensdorff-Pouilly, S. (1993) CA 125 in gynaecological pathology – a review. *Eur. J. Obstet. Gynecol. Reprod. Biol.*, **49**, 115–24.
6. Finkler, N.J., Benacerraf, B., Lavin, P.T., Wojciechowski, C. and Knapp, R.C. (1988) Comparison of serum CA 125, clinical impression, and ultrasound in the preoperative evaluation of ovarian masses. *Obstet. Gynecol.*, **72**, 659–64.
7. Petru, E., Schmidt, F., Mikosch, P. *et al.* (1992) Abdominopelvic computed tomography in the preoperative evaluation of suspected ovarian masses. *Int. J. Gynecol. Cancer*, **2**, 252–5.
8. Buist, M.R., Golding, R.P., Burger, C.W. *et al.* (1994) Comparison and evaluation of diagnostic methods in ovarian carcinoma with emphasis on CT and MRI. *Gynecol. Oncol.*, **52**, 191–8.
9. Stevens, S.K., Hricak, H. and Stern, J.L. (1991) Ovarian lesions – detection and characterization with gadolinium-enhanced MR imaging at 1.5 T. *Radiology*, **181**, 481–8.
10. Semelka, R.C., Lawrence, P.H., Shoenut, J.P. *et al.* (1993) Primary ovarian cancer: prospective comparison of contrast-enhanced CT and pre- and post-contrast, fat-suppressed MR imaging, with histologic correlation. *J. Magn. Reson. Imaging*, **3**, 99–106.
11. Taylor-Papadimitrou, J., Paterson, J.A., Arkie, J. *et al.* (1981) Monoclonal antibodies to epithelium specific components of the human milk fat globule membrane, production and reaction with cells in culture. *Int. J. Cancer*, **28**, 17–21.
12. Epenetos, A.A., Britton, K.E., Mather, S.J. *et al.* (1982) Targetting of iodine-123 labelled tumour-associated monoclonal antibodies to ovarian, breast and gastrointestinal tumours. *Lancet*, **ii**, 999–1005.
13. Burchell, J., Taylor-Papadimitrou, J., Boshell, M. *et al.* (1989) A short sequence, within the amino acid repeat of a cancer-associated mucin, contains immunodominant epitopes. *Int. J. Cancer*, **44**, 691–6.
14. Girling, A., Bartkora, J., Burchell, J. *et al.* (1989). A core protein epitope of the polymorphic epithelial mucin detected by monoclonal antibody SM3 is selectively exposed in a range of primary carcinomas. *Int. J. Cancer*, **43**, 1072–6.
15. Crippa, F., Buraggi, G.L., Di Re, E. *et al.* (1991) Radioimmunoscintigraphy of ovarian cancer with the MoV-18 monoclonal antibody. *Eur. J. Cancer*, **27**, 724–9.
16. Crippa, F. (1991) Radioimmunotherapy of ovarian cancer. *Int. J. Biol. Mark.*, **8**, 187–91.
17. McEwan, A.J.B., Maclean, G.D., Hooper, H.R. *et al.* (1992) Mab 170 H.82: an evaluation of a novel panadenocarcionoma monoclonal antibody labelled with ^{99m}Tc and with ^{111}In. *Nucl. Med. Commun.*, **13**, 11–19.
18. Alexander, C., Villena-Heinsen, C.E., Trampert, K. *et al.* (1995) Radioimmunoscintigraphy of ovarian tumours with Technetium-99m labelled monoclonal antibody-170: first clinical experience. *Eur. J. Nucl. Med.*, **22**, 645–51.
19. Jusko, W.J., Kung, L.P. and Schmelter, R.P. (1992) Immunopharmacokinetics of ^{111}In-CYT-103 in ovarian cancer patients, in *Diagnosis of Colorectal and Ovarian Carcinoma* (eds R.T. Maguire and D. Van Nostrand), Marcel Dekker, New York, Chapter 10, pp. 177–90.
20. Massuger, L., Claessens, R., Kenemans, P. *et al.* (1991) Kinetics and biodistribution in relation to tumour detection and 111-In-labelled OV-TL3 F(ab')$_2$ in patients with ovarian cancer. *Nucl. Med. Commun.*, **12**, 593–609.
21. Maughan, T.S., Haylock, B., Hayward, M. *et al.* (1990) OC 125 immunoscintigraphy in ovarian carcinoma: a comparison with alternative methods of assessment. *J. Clin. Oncol.*, **2**, 199–205.
22. Begent, R.H.J., Stanway, G., Jones, B.E. *et al.* (1980) Radioimmunolocalisation of tumours by external scintigraphy after administration of ^{131}I antibody to human gonadotrophin. Preliminary communication. *J. R. Soc. Med.*, **73**, 624–50.
23. Van Dam, P.A., Watson, J.V., Shepherd, J.H. and Lowe, D.G. (1990) Flow cytometric quantification of tumour-associated antigens in solid tumors. *Am. J. Obstet. Gynecol.*, **163**, 698–9.
24. Epenetos, A.A., Snook, D., Hooker, G. *et al.* (1985) Indium-111 labelled monoclonal antibody to placental alkaline phosphatase in the detection of neoplasms of testis, ovary and cervix. *Lancet*, **ii**, 350–3.
25. Tibben, J.B., Massuger, L.F.A.G., Claessens, R.A.M.J. *et al.* (1992) Tumour detection and localization using 99Tcm-labelled OV-TL-3Fab' in patients suspected of ovarian cancer. *Nucl. Med. Commun.*, **13**, 885–93.
26. Peltier, P., Wiharto, K., Dutin, J.-P. *et al.* (1992) Correlative imaging study in the diagnosis of ovarian cancer recurrences. *Eur. Nucl. Med.*, **19**, 1006–10.
27. Ind, T.E.J., Granowska, M. and Britton, K.E. (1994) Peroperative radioimmunodetection of ovarian carcinoma using a hand held gamma detection probe. *Br. J. Cancer*, **70**, 1263–6.

28. Hertel, A., Baum, R.P., Auerbach, B., Herrmann, A. and Hor, G. (1990) Klinische Relevanz Humaner Anti-Maus-Antiokorper (HAMA) in der Immunszintigraphie. *Nucl. Med.*, **29**, 221–7.

29. Granowska, M., Nimmon, C.C., Britton, K.E. *et al.* (1988) Kinetic analysis and probability mapping applied to the detection of ovarian cancer by radio-immunoscintigraphy. *J. Nucl. Med.*, **29**, 599–607.

30. Granowska, M., Britton, K.E., Mather, S.J. *et al.* (1993) Radioimmunoscintigraphy with Technetium-99m monoclonal antibody, SM3, in gynaecological cancer. *Eur. J. Nucl. Med.*, **20**, 483–9.

Prostate cancer

K. E. Britton and V. U. Chengazi

INTRODUCTION

Cancer of the prostate is the most common cancer in men, and third after lung and colorectal carcinoma in order of cancer-related deaths. Its frequency and incidence are both increasing, as they are age-related. Prostate cancer may be discovered accidentally, for example, during digital rectal examination or following symptoms of bladder dysfunction. In 20% of cases, transurethral prostatectomy may reveal malignancy within the excised tissue. The primary cancer may be undetected with the patient presenting as a consequence of bone metastases.

Prostate cancer spreads by the lymphatic route to the obturator lymph nodes, followed by internal and external iliac nodes. The prognosis falls – from 80% 5-year survival to 30% 5-year survival – if a single related node is found to show microscopic involvement. Radioimmunoscintigraphy (RIS) has now shown that nodal extension to the para-aortic glands and into the mediastinum is more frequent than previously expected. The blood-borne spread of prostate cancer, particularly to the bone, is well-recognized, and the bone scan is widely used, either actively for symptoms or passively to monitor therapy at regular intervals. The recognition of the fact that it is the soft tissue metastases rather than the bone metastases that usually kill the patient, and that this may be shown by a rising prostate-specific antigen (PSA) in the patient with a negative bone scan, has increased the need for identification of such metastases. Palliation of bone metastases using strontium-89, and more recently samarium-153 and rhenium-186 phosphonate derivatives, is discussed in Chapter 1.

PROSTATE CANCER IMAGING

Primary prostate cancer may be staged using transrectal ultrasound, pelvic X-ray, transmission computed tomography (CT) and/or magnetic resonance imaging (MRI). All of these techniques are prone to the requirement to identify an abnormal node by its size rather than by its cancerous level. Thus, enlarged (i.e. >1 cm diameter) nodes due to non-specific inflammatory causes may be called malignant, and normal size nodes with micrometastases may be called benign. Resultant sensitivities of the order of 50% for accurate staging of prostate cancer when compared with the findings at radical prostatectomy are current [1,2]. Transrectal ultrasound and needle biopsy are the mainstay of the diagnosis of the primary tumour, but detecting the degree of local spread remains an important clinical problem.

There have been four main approaches to imaging of the prostate and prostatic cancer:

1. The use of a metal, such as zinc-65, which appears in higher concentration in the prostate than in the tissues.
2. The use of substrates for prostate uptake such as ^{75}Se-selenomethionine or ^{18}F-deoxyglucose [3].
3. The use of tumour-associated enzymes and antigens such as prostatic acid phosphatase (PAP), prostate-specific antigen (PSA) and prostate membrane-specific antigen (PMSA).
4. Hormone–receptor-related agents such as fluorinated androgens and androgen analogues.

An alternative approach is to use pelvic lymphoscintigraphy with a transrectal injection of ^{99m}Tc-antimony sulphide colloid or phytate. These can delineate the sites of nodes in the pelvis, but not whether they are involved.

Initial studies with anti-PAP [4] failed when the PAP was raised in the blood, since the antibody bound to the circulated enzyme and was located ultimately in the liver as an immune complex, with resultant poor imaging of the prostate. PSA is widely used as the most important serum marker of prostate cancer. It needs a sufficient size of tumour (or tumour metastases) to release sufficient antigen that is detectable in the blood. Therefore, its use as a screening test for prostate cancer remains controversial, but it is an established marker once prostate cancer has been diagnosed to indicate recurrence or assess the effects of therapy. Imaging with anti-PSA monoclonal antibody has been tried, but again found unsatisfac-

Clinical Nuclear Medicine, 3rd edn. Edited by M.N. Maisey, K.E. Britton and B.D. Collier. Published in 1998 by Chapman & Hall, London. ISBN 0 412 75180 1

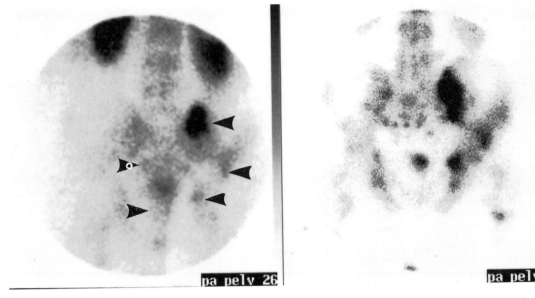

Figure 12.15   Left: prostate radioimmunoscintigraphy with CYT-351 in metastatic disease. Planar views taken at 26 hours post-injection show specific uptake into soft tissue (arrowheads pointing right) and bone (arrowheads pointing left) metastases. Right: the bone scan performed a day later shows only the bone disease.

tory due to the mopping up of the injected antibody with circulating PSA, reducing its sensitivity.

PMSA is found in membranes of benign and malignant prostate cancer with much greater expression in the malignant cell. It is not found in other human organs and in other tumours. The antigen is a 100 kDa glycoprotein, and it is recognized by an antibody, 7E11C5. This antibody is an IgG_1 of murine origin, produced by a hybridoma immunized against an LNCaP cell line. It has been labelled with indium-111 and presented by the Cytogen Corporation as ^{111}In-CYT-356. It is currently completing its Phase 3 clinical trials and receiving FDA approval so that it will become commercially available. The indium conjugate consists of a DTPA–GYK linker – the GYK standing for glycine, tyrosine and lysine – which takes the DTPA group a little away from the antibody so that the addition of indium does not affect its immunoreactivity. Neil and Meis [2] showed that ^{111}In-CYT-356 correctly identified negative nodes in 42 out of 44 patients and correctly identified positively involved nodes in 11 of 21 patients, as compared with CT images, which were positive in only 4/21. Babaian *et al.* [5] showed similar

success in involved pelvic nodes. A particular feature of these studies has been the identification of unsuspected para-aortic, mediastinal and even left neck nodes involved by prostate cancer, in patients with normal bone scans, revealing an extent of disease previously unexpected.

Difficulties in the interpretation of these scans have been helped by undertaking early SPECT during the first hour to provide the blood pool image, since in the age group of these patients, tortuous arteries and veins are more frequent. This aids interpretation of subsequent SPECT images at 1 and 3 days. A revision of pelvic anatomy is required to distinguish obturator and other nodes from the normal internal and external iliac vessels, and to distinguish the bulb of the penis below the prostate and the base of the bladder above. A definite learning curve is required to undertake reliable reporting of these images.

Disadvantages of ^{111}In include a considerable bone marrow uptake, occasional activity in the rectum because of bowel excretion, reduced availability and increased expense, and the need to order the indium. For these reasons, ^{99m}Tc has been used as an alternative label, either using the direct reduction method of Mather and Ellison [6] called

CYT-351, or using a Cytogen linker [7] called CYT-422. With ^{99m}Tc, there is no bowel activity, much less marrow uptake, a higher count-rate suitable for SPECT, and a lower absorbed radiation dose. The study can be arranged and completed within 24 hours. The main disadvantage is increased urinary excretion of ^{99m}Tc-labelled peptides as a result of metabolism of the antibody. Feneley *et al.* [8] found about 13% of the injected dose excreted in the urine within 24 hours with a mean blood clearance half-life of 33 hours. The success of this approach to imaging primary and recurrent prostate cancer was confirmed and the series has been extended by Chengazi *et al.* [9] to 39 patients, with a 92% accuracy. Examples are shown in Plate 25 and Figure 12.15. The problem of rising PSA with a normal bone scan in a patient with known prostate cancer is solved by radioimmunoscintigraphy.

CONCLUSION

Radioimmunoscintigraphy provides cancer-specific imaging of the prostate, with information about local involvement of nodes required for an assessment of radical prostatectomy, its spread to soft tissues and, indeed, to bone. Once the availability of the CYT-356 kit is established, it will take its place in the regular clinical evaluation of prostate cancer.

REFERENCES

1. Gulfo, J.V. (1994) Clinical Utility of Monoclonal Antibodies in Prostate Cancer, in *Prostate Cancer*, Wiley Liss, New York, pp. 77–94.
2. Neil, C.E. and Meis, L.C. (1994) Correlated imaging and monoclonal antibodies in colorectal, ovarian and prostate cancer. *Semin. Nucl. Med.*, **24**, 272–85.
3. Effert, P.J., Bares, R., Handt, S. *et al.* (1996) Metabolic imaging of untreated prostate cancer by positron emission tomography with 18 fluorine labelled deoxyglucose. *J. Urol.*, **155**, 994–8.
4. Vihko, P., Heikkila, J., Konturri, M. *et al.* (1984) Radioimaging of the prostate and metastases of prostate carcinoma with Tc-99m labelled prostate acid phosphatase specific antibodies and their Fab fragments. *Ann. Clin. Res.*, **16**, 51–2.
5. Babaian, R.J., Sayer, J., Podoloff, D.A. *et al.* (1994) Radioimmunoscintigraphy of pelvic lymph nodes with ^{111}Indium labelled monoclonal antibody CYT-356. *J. Urol.*, **152**, 1952–5.
6. Mather, S.J. and Ellison, D. (1990) Reduction-mediated Technetium-99m labelling of monoclonal antibodies. *J. Nucl. Med.*, **31**, 692–7.
7. Stalteri, M.A., Mather, S.J., Chengazi, V.U. *et al.* (1995) Site specific conjugation and labelling of prostate antibody 7E11C5 with Tc-99m. *Nucl. Med. Commun.*, **15**, 241 (abstract).
8. Feneley, M.R., Chengazi, V.U., Kirby, R.S. *et al.* (1996) Prostatic radioimmunoscintigraphy: preliminary results using Technetium-labelled monoclonal antibody CYT-351. *Br. J. Urol.*, **77**, 373–81.
9. Chengazi, V.U., Feneley, M., Nimmon, C.C. *et al.* (1997) Prostate cancer imaging with the monoclonal antibody Tc-99m-CYT-351. *J. Nucl. Med.*, **38**, 675–81.

CHAPTER 13

The abdominal contents

S. S. Tumeh

HEPATOBILIARY SCINTIGRAPHY

INTRODUCTION

The biliary system is the drainage system of the liver into the small bowel. Bile drains from the liver into the hepatic ducts. The left and right hepatic ducts join to form the common hepatic duct, that is joined by the cystic duct to form the common bile duct, which empties into the second portion of the duodenum via the ampulla of Vater. Bile flows down the common hepatic duct into the cystic duct to be stored in the gallbladder. The gallbladder contracts in response to cholecystokinin (CCK), a hormone secreted by the duodenum in response to fatty compounds and proteins reaching it. CCK causes relaxation of the sphincter of Oddi, allowing the flow of bile excreted by the gallbladder into the small bowel.

RADIOPHARMACEUTICALS

The most commonly used radiopharmaceuticals are ^{99m}Tc-labelled iminodiacetic acid (IDA) derivatives. Generically, these compounds are referred to as HIDA, an abbreviation of hepatobiliary-IDA. These compounds are organic anions that function as bichelates. On one side they chelate the radionuclide and on the other the acetanilide analogue of lidocaine; the latter is responsible for the biologic behaviour of these molecules. IDA compounds are excreted by the liver and, although they are thought to follow a similar excretory pathway to that of bilirubin, they do not undergo conjugation or a significant change in their structure. When these compounds are labelled with a radionuclide, they form stable dimers, with two molecules of IDA binding with one molecule of pertechnetate.

The first HIDA compound to be used widely for biliary imaging was lidofenin, or dimethyl IDA. About 80% of this compound is excreted by the liver and 20% by the kidneys, depending on the status of the liver function. One limitation of HIDA is its relatively slow transit through the liver which, while not a problem in patients with normal liver function, is associated with poor visualization of the extrahepatic structures when serum bilirubin levels reach 5 mg/dl or higher. This was overcome by the synthesis of the now more commonly used IDA derivatives, such as PIPIDA and DISIDA. About 10% of these compounds is excreted by the kidneys and 90% by the liver, which along with their faster clearance by the liver, results in higher concentration in the bile ducts, and hence a more consistent visualization of extrahepatic structures. This attribute is particularly important in patients with elevated serum bilirubin levels.

PATIENT PREPARATION

In the patient suspected of having cholecystitis, we require patient fasting for 3–4 hours before the examination. In patients who have been fasting for more than 24 hours, or who are on parenteral nutrition, the gallbladder is stimulated with a fatty meal given orally (or via a nasogastric tube if the patient has one) or by an intravenous infusion of 0.15 μg of cholecystokinin/kg body weight about 1 hour before the examination. This helps to empty

Clinical Nuclear Medicine, 3rd edn. Edited by M.N. Maisey, K.E. Britton and B.D. Collier. Published in 1998 by Chapman & Hall, London. ISBN 0 412 75180 1

the gallbladder from any thick sludge that may have collected as a result of biliary stasis. A large amount of sludge may block the gallbladder and prevent entry of the radiopharmaceutical, thus resulting in a false positive test.

If the test is being performed to evaluate the bile ducts, for bile leak for example, no fasting is required.

IMAGING PROTOCOLS AND NORMAL APPEARANCES

Acute cholecystitis

The patient receives an intravenous injection of 3–6 mCi of ^{99m}Tc methyl-bromo-IDA (Mebrofenin) or di-isopropyl-IDA (Disofenin). With high serum bilirubin levels, up to 10 mCi could be given. We do not obtain a dynamic flow phase because in our, as well as others', experience it adds no useful information. We obtain multiple sequential static images of the upper abdomen in the 30° left anterior oblique projection, which separates the gallbladder (an anterior structure) from the duodenum (a posterior structure) in most cases. The first image is obtained for 1×10^6 counts immediately at the end of the injection, while the remainder of the images are taken for the same amount of time as the first image, namely at 10-min intervals over 60 minutes. If the gallbladder is not visualized by 60 minutes, 0.04 mg morphine/kg body weight is infused intravenously over 3 minutes and, depending on the amount of radioactivity left in the liver, 2–3 mCi of the same radiopharmaceutical may need to be given. Imaging is then continued for another 30 minutes. In some cases, radioactivity in the second portion of the duodenum may overlap the gallbladder fossa and be confused with gallbladder activity. If this issue is not resolved by left and right anterior oblique and right lateral images, the patient is given water by mouth; this washes away radioactivity from the duodenum. The LAO image is repeated 10–15 minutes later. Persistence of radioactivity in the gallbladder fossa indicates that it is located in the gallbladder, while a significant decrease in that radioactivity suggests that it was in the duodenum.

Biliary leak

If a bile leak is suspected, whether secondary to trauma or surgery, 1-min images of the upper abdomen are obtained for 60 minutes. Static planar images are obtained using the same parameters as detailed under acute cholecystitis above. A cine display is created to visualize and localize an early leak before it becomes obscured by radioactivity in the gastrointestinal tract. In cases where the leak has sealed off, forming a biloma, delayed images are necessary to allow radioactivity to accumulate in detectable amounts.

Gallbladder dyskinesia

This condition is suspected in patients who have chronic biliary symptoms. In these cases the patient is prepared by fasting for 3–4 hours. The patient is injected intravenously with 3–6 mCi of the radiopharmaceutical and imaging obtained on a computer at a rate of one frame every 5 minutes. When the gallbladder is well visualized, usually by about 30–40 minutes, an intravenous infusion of 0.15 µg/kg bodyweight of Kinevac, diluted in 20 ml of normal saline, is carried out over 10 minutes. Faster infusion rates are associated with nausea in many patients and vomiting in some, which would interfere with data acquisition. Images are continuously acquired during the Kinevac infusion, and continued for 30 minutes thereafter. In addition to visual inspection of the images, computer analysis of the gallbladder radioactivity is displayed as a function of time. In most cases, the gallbladder is visualized by 30–40 minutes. Gallbladder contraction is evaluated qualitatively by inspecting the images and quantitatively by obtaining an ejection fraction. We consider an ejection fraction of ≥25% as normal.

Normal appearance

Depiction of the normal hepatobiliary tract depends on physiological uptake and excretion by the liver. In normal people, the liver uptake is rapid, clearing most of the radiopharmaceutical from circulation by 5 minutes. Persistence of radioactivity in the circulatory system correlates with hepatocyte dysfunction. Because of the rapid excretion of these compounds by the liver, the test is of very limited value in evaluating liver morphological abnormalities, although occasionally a mass or metastases are detected. This rapid excretion by the liver is associated with early visualization of the extrahepatic bile ducts and small bowel in about 15–30 minutes. If the cystic duct is patent, the gallbladder should be visualized within 1 hour (Figure 13.1). If visualization of the bile ducts and

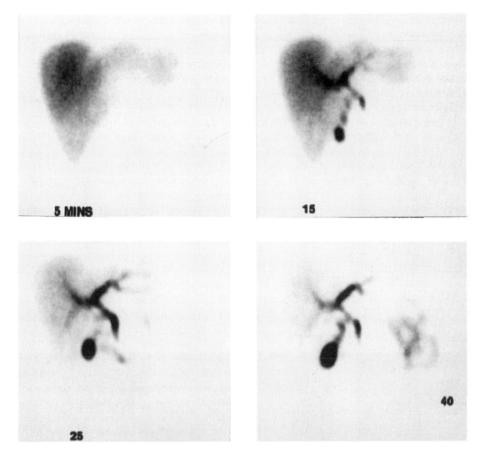

Figure 13.1 Normal hepatobiliary scan. Four images obtained from a hepatobiliary scan at 5, 15, 25 and 40 minutes show normal uptake and excretion by the liver. Notice the visualization of the biliary tree including the common bile duct and the appearance of radioactivity in the gallbladder by 15 minutes and the small bowel by 25 minutes.

gallbladder, but not the small bowel, is achieved by 60 minutes, gallbladder contraction is stimulated by either a fatty meal or CCK to force radioactivity into the duodenum, whose visualization is achieved then in most patients without biliary obstruction.

CLINICAL APPLICATIONS

Congenital anomalies

Biliary atresia and neonatal hepatitis Those uncommon disorders present with neonatal jaundice. Although the work-up of the patient includes a battery of laboratory tests and other imaging modalities, biliary scintigraphy provides the physiological data needed to reach the diagnosis.

In general, neonatal hepatitis is associated with poor uptake and excretion by the liver. Prolonged clearance of the blood pool and very poor visualization, if any at all, of extrahepatic structures are signs of hepatocyte dysfunction. On the other hand, biliary atresia is associated with adequate liver uptake, and relatively fast clearing of blood pool radioactivity, but no excretion from the liver.

Cystic malformations of the biliary tract Caroli's disease is congenital cystic dilatation of the intrahepatic bile ducts. The diagnosis can be made by sonography if those intrahepatic cystic structures are shown to communicate with the bile ducts. If these communications are not depicted, biliary scintigraphy may be helpful in confirming the diagnosis by demonstrating foci of increased uptake within the liver due to the increased volume and stasis in these structures.

Choledochal cyst is cystic dilatation of the common bile duct that may be large enough to present in the neonatal period or infancy due to its size or symptoms of compression of the common bile duct or duodenum. The imaging work-up of the patient starts with sonography, which can differentiate a hydronephrotic kidney from other cystic malformations of the right upper quadrant of the abdomen, such as duplication cyst, mesenteric cyst and choledochal cyst. The differentiation of a choledochal cyst from the other two entities may be difficult, however, unless the communication between the cyst and the common bile duct is clearly demonstrated. Biliary scintigraphy may be very helpful in the ambiguous case. If the cystic structure is filled with radioactivity, usually on delayed images, the diagnosis of choledochal cyst is made (Figure 13.2). If the differentiation of choledochal cyst from the gallbladder is difficult, an infusion of CCK is used, in response to which only the gallbladder contracts.

Acquired disorders

Acute cholecystitis This clinical condition is secondary to cystic duct obstruction, by a stone in most cases. A small minority of patients have acute acalculus cholecystitis, which is an acute inflammatory condition not associated with calculus disease. It usually occurs in patients with predisposing factors such as debilitating diseases, diabetes, burns or recent surgery. The inflammatory reaction and thick inspisated bile may cause cystic duct obstruction. Biliary scintigraphy is the most sensitive and specific imaging modality for the diagnosis of acute cholecystitis approaching 96–100% and 81–100%, respectively [1]. If the

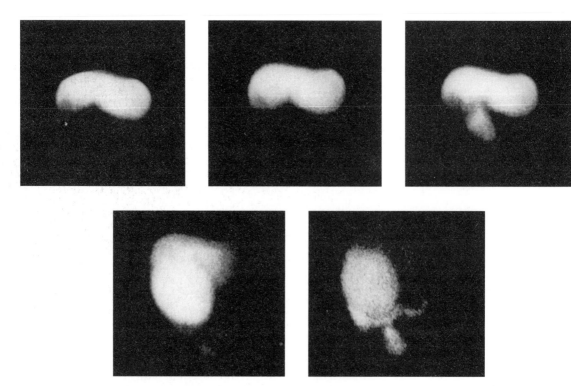

Figure 13.2 Choledochal cyst. Five images from a biliary scan of an infarct with a right upper lobe mass obtained at 5, 15, 30, 45 and 90 minutes. Notice the photopenic defect in the inferior aspect of the right lobe of the liver. On the last two images (bottom row) a large, round structure is seen filled with radioactivity displacing the bowel activity inferiorly. These findings are highly suggestive of a choledochal cyst, which was proven at surgery.

gallbladder, bile ducts and small bowel are visualized by 60 minutes from the time of injection the procedure is stopped and the scintiscan considered normal. If the gallbladder is not visualized by that time, the diagnosis of cholecystitis is made (Figure 13.3). However, to differentiate acute from chronic conditions, delayed images up to 4 hours are obtained. If the gallbladder does not fill with radioactivity by 4 hours, a diagnosis of acute cholecystitis is made. If filling does occur, the diagnosis of chronic cholecystitis prevails. Recently, morphine augmentation has been used to make that differentiation at 90 minutes, obviating the need for delayed images [2–4]. Morphine increases the contraction of the sphincter of Oddi, resulting in increased intraductal pressure, which forces the flow of bile into the gallbladder if the cystic duct is not blocked. Therefore, following morphine augmentation persistent non-filling of the gallbladder is indicative of acute cholecystitis. In contrast, visualization of the gallbladder is suggestive of a non-acute condition (Figure 13.4). One has to ensure, however, that sufficient radioactivity is still present in the liver at the time of morphine augmentation in order to avoid potentially a false-positive result [3]. When compared with conventional delayed imaging, morphine augmentation has a statistically significant higher specificity and positive predictive value for acute cholecystitis, and statistically insignificant lower sensitivity and negative predictive value [4].

Morphine augmentation does not obviate the need for delayed imaging in all cases, however. In cases with severe chronic cholecystitis, or shrunken stone-laden gallbladders, filling of the gallbladder by radioactivity may not be achieved by 30 minutes post-morphine injection, and, therefore, further delayed images may be necessary to avoid a false-positive scan [2,3]. Also in some cases where the cystic duct obstruction is more proximal (closer to the gallbladder) the distal segment of the cystic duct (closer to the common bile duct) may fill with radioactivity. This 'nubbin' of radioactivity, or 'the cystic duct sign' (Figure 13.5) is an uncommon finding in acute cholecystitis [5]. In these cases morphine augmentation may dislodge the calculus back into the gallbladder, resulting in a false-negative scintiscan. These cases are better evaluated with conventional delayed imaging [3,5].

Another cause of false-negative scintiscan is acute acalculus cholecystitis, an uncommon condition that accounts for about 5% of cases of acute

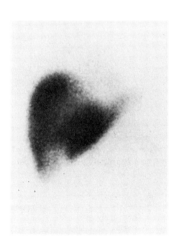 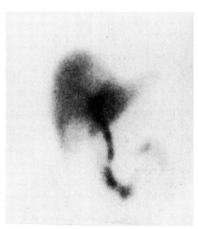 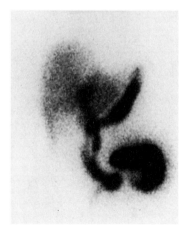

Figure 13.3 Acute cholecystitis. Three images obtained from a hepatobiliary scan at 5, 40 and 60 minutes (left, centre and right, respectively). Notice the prompt uptake by the liver on the initial image and the large photopenic defect on its inferior surface suggestive of large gallbladder fossa or a very dilated gallbladder. In the middle image there is a mild medial bowing of the common bile duct, which in association with the large gallbladder fossa indicates a distended gallbladder. By 60 minutes (far right) there is visualization of the small bowel and reflux into the stomach. Although this last finding is not specific, some investigators believe it indicates a more severe inflammatory process of the gallbladder which involves the duodenum and forces back-flow of bile into the stomach. It usually correlates with bile gastritis.

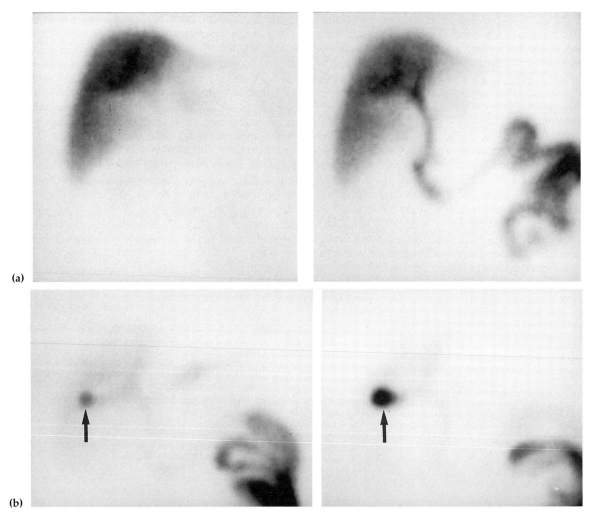

Figure 13.4 Morphine augmentation in differentiating acute from chronic cholecystitis. (a) Two images from a biliary scintiscan obtained at 5 and 60 minutes show prompt uptake and excretion of radioactivity by the liver. There was no filling of the gallbladder by 60 minutes (right image). (b) Two images obtained 15 minutes (left) and 30 minutes (right) following the intravenous infusion of 2.5 mg of morphine show filling of the gallbladder and, hence, ruling out cystic duct obstruction. This case demonstrates the utility of morphine augmentation in differentiating acute cholecystitis (no visualization of the gallbladder after morphine augmentation) from chronic cholecystitis (visualization of the gallbladder following the morphine augmentation).

cholecystitis. In most cases of acute acalculus disease, the inflammatory reaction and associated oedema are severe enough to produce sufficient narrowing of the cystic duct and prevent radioactivity from entering the gallbladder. However, in some cases the narrowing is not severe enough to prevent such entry, especially after morphine augmentation, resulting in a false-negative examination. In some cases, radioactivity in the second

portion of the duodenum may overlap the gallbladder fossa and be confused with gallbladder activity (Figure 13.6), potentially causing a false-negative test. If this issue is not resolved by left and right anterior oblique and right lateral images, the patient is given water by mouth, which washes away radioactivity from the duodenum, and the LAO image is repeated in 10–15 minutes. Persistence of radioactivity in the gallbladder fossa indicates that it is in the gallbladder, while a significant decrease in that radioactivity suggests that it was in the duodenum. Another potential cause of false-negative scintiscan is persistence of radioactivity in the gallbladder fossa, or what has been described as the 'rim sign' (Figures 13.7 and 13.8). The sign, originally described in association with gangrenous cholecystitis, results from an area of progressively increased accumulation of radioactivity in the gallbladder fossa (Figures 13.7 and

13.8). It is thought to represent hyperaemia, manifested by increased flow and early uptake, and localized inflammatory cholestasis, manifested by slower clearance of radioactivity in comparison with the rest of the liver, and hence the paradoxical increased uptake on delayed images that may be confused with gallbladder. This sign is seen mostly in patients with severe acute cholecystitis, only a minority of whom have gangrenous condition.

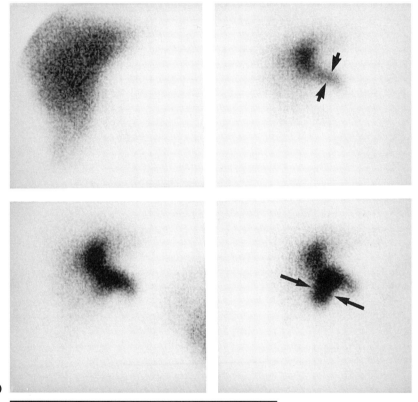

(a)

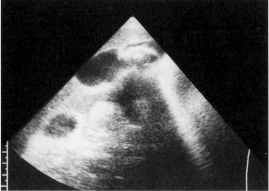

(b)

Figure 13.5 'Nubbin' sign. (a) Four images from a biliary scintiscan demonstrate normal uptake by the liver (upper left). The biliary tree was then visualized. On the last image (lower right) there is radioactivity in a structure that could be confused with a normal gallbladder. However, it represents filling of only the neck region of the gallbladder due to the presence of a large stone. The stone has obstructed the gallbladder and prevented the flow of radioactivity to the region of the fundus. (b) Sonogram of the gallbladder demonstrates a large calculus which has separated the neck of the gallbladder from the fundus.

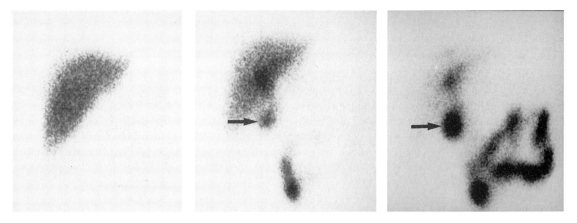

Figure 13.6 False-negative biliary scan due to stasis in the second portion of the duodenum. Three images from a biliary scan obtained at 5, 20 and 40 minutes (left, centre, right) show an area of increased uptake of radioactivity just lateral to the common bile duct. This was interpreted as a gallbladder. In this situation, a small glass of water given orally would have helped to wash the radioactivity from the duodenum, while it would not affect radioactivity in the gallbladder, helping differentiate those two entities. This patient had acute cholecystitis with stones obstructing the cystic duct at surgery.

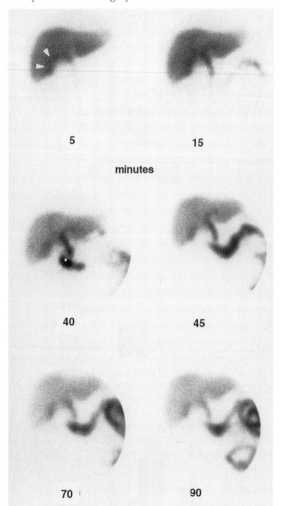

Figure 13.7 Rim sign. Multiple images from a hepatobiliary scan obtained at different times show early appearance of radioactivity in the gallbladder fossa (arrowheads) which became more intense with time, mostly because of the clearance of radioactivity from the rest of the liver. There was no visualization of the gallbladder at 90 minutes, indicating cholecystitis. The rim sign indicates a more severe inflammatory reaction. In this case, the gallbladder was gangrenous.

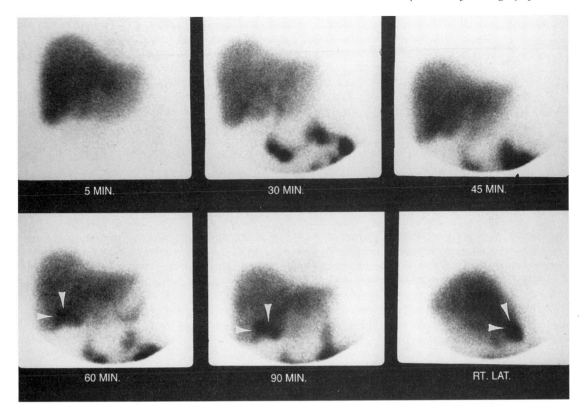

Figure 13.8 Severe rim sign. Hepatobiliary scintiscan demonstrates increased uptake in the gallbladder fossa which becomes more apparent with time due to the clearance of radioactivity from the liver. The intensity of uptake, progressive, increased uptake, and location (particularly on the right lateral image) misled the reader to think that this was the normal filling of the gallbladder. Potentially, this could be reason for a false-negative scan, while it actually indicates a very severe, acute cholecystitis.

False-positive examinations have also been reported, the leading causes being sepsis, prolonged fasting and/or parenteral nutrition. We find stimulation of the gallbladder, whether by CCK or by a fatty meal, to empty it of sludge, before cholescintigraphy, to be helpful in decreasing the false-positive rate.

Chronic cholecystitis This is a chronic inflammatory process of the gallbladder, associated with gallstones. Patients complain of chronic dyspepsia and abdominal discomfort. The combination of the clinical symptoms and the demonstration of gall stones by sonography clinches the diagnosis. On scintigraphy, the gallbladder may show normal (within 1 hour) or very delayed (up to 4 hours) filling with radioactivity. Morphine augmentation helps to fill the gallbladder in 60–90 minutes (Figure 13.4), obviating the need for delayed imaging in most patients.

To evaluate the contractile function of the gallbladder, we perform a biliary scintiscan and, if the gallbladder visualizes normally, it is stimulated with CCK infusion and imaging is continued for at least another 30 minutes. Gallbladder contraction is evaluated qualitatively by inspecting the images and quantitatively by obtaining a time–activity curve from the gallbladder (Figure 13.9) and calculating an ejection fraction. We consider an ejection fraction of ≥25% as normal. In our laboratory, values <25% and reproduction of patient symptoms with the Kinevac infusion correlate well with gallbladder dyskinesia. However, it should be mentioned that different laboratories use different values for gallbladder ejection fraction. Such variation is due to the lack of a 'gold standard' for gallbladder dyskinesia that could be used to verify these values.

Common bile duct obstruction When the extrahepatic bile ducts are occluded acutely, the intraductal pressure rises before the ducts dilate. At that stage, while sonography may still demonstrate normal-calibre ducts, the most common scintigraphic appearance is that of 'liver scan' [6] (Figure 13.10). Uptake by the liver and the clear-

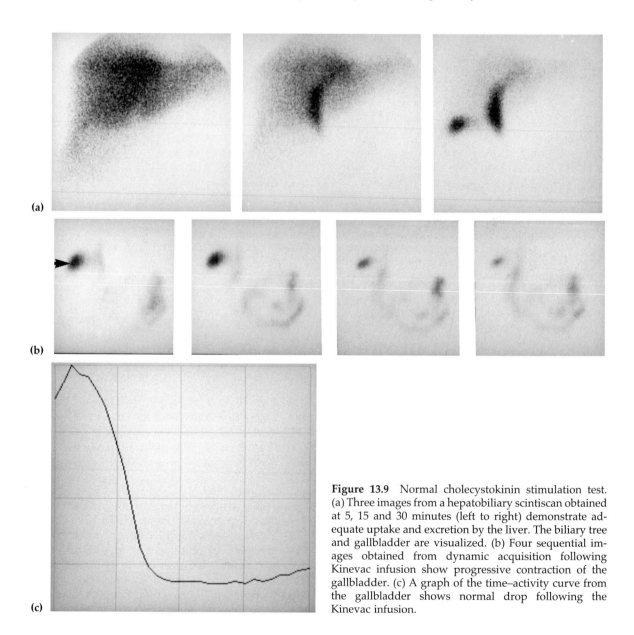

(a)

(b)

(c)

Figure 13.9 Normal cholecystokinin stimulation test. (a) Three images from a hepatobiliary scintiscan obtained at 5, 15 and 30 minutes (left to right) demonstrate adequate uptake and excretion by the liver. The biliary tree and gallbladder are visualized. (b) Four sequential images obtained from dynamic acquisition following Kinevac infusion show progressive contraction of the gallbladder. (c) A graph of the time–activity curve from the gallbladder shows normal drop following the Kinevac infusion.

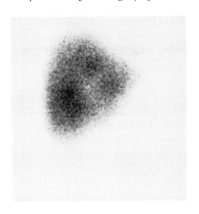

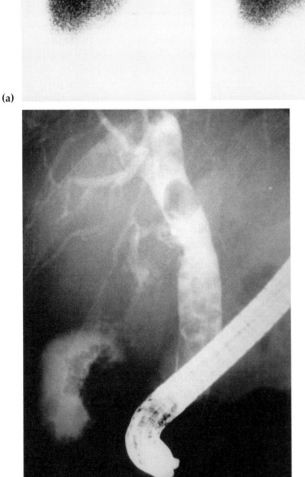

Figure 13.10 Common bile duct obstruction. (a) Three images from a hepatobiliary scan obtained at 5, 45 and 90 minutes (left to right) from the time of injection show normal uptake in the liver given the appearance 'liver scan'. Notice the large photopenic area in the hilum of the liver (arrow) suggesting a dilated common bile duct. This appearance is very suggestive of high-grade common bile duct obstruction. (b) ERCP with injection of contrast medium into the common bile duct shows a markedly dilated common bile duct with numerous filling defects, suggestive of stones. Incidentally, a tumour of the gallbladder is also demonstrated.

ance of radioactivity from the blood are normal, but delayed images fail to demonstrate radioactivity in the bile ducts or small bowel. This lack of liver excretion is thought to be due to the transmission of the elevated intraductal pressure back to the canalicular level, which probably shuts down the excretion by hepatocytes. If the bile ducts are dilated, a photopenic defect may be seen in the region of the porta hepatis (Figure 13.10).

The differential diagnosis of the 'liver scan' pattern includes cholestatic jaundice [7], which is probably a form of 'intrahepatic obstruction'. In cases of partial common bile duct obstruction, visualization of the extrahepatic system varies from normal to delayed. An important differentiation is between high-grade biliary obstruction and diffuse liver disease which, if severe enough, will result in absent excretion of radioactivity from the liver. However, in the latter condition the uptake by the liver is poor and visualization of radioactivity in the circulatory system is prolonged (Figure 13.11).

Bile leak This could be spontaneous or, more commonly, secondary to trauma or surgery. Since the management of blunt abdominal trauma has become conservative in the haemodynamically stable patient, the diagnosis of bile leak could be delayed. The appearance of abnormal perihepatic fluid collections on CT or sonography performed a week or more after trauma to follow up abdominal injury should alert the imager to the possibility of a bile leak, which may have become organized into a biloma. Scintigraphy is very useful in this setting (Figure 13.12).

Iatrogenic injury to the biliary tree is uncommon. Surgical disruption of the bile ducts has been reported to be 0.1–0.2% following open cholecystectomy and 1.6% following laparoscopic cholecystectomy [8]. Patients with such bile leaks usually present with abdominal pain 2–9 days later. Mild leucocytosis (12000–19000/mm^3) and a low-grade fever are commonly seen. Although CT and sonography are very sensitive to demonstrating abnormal fluid collections, they are not specific as to the aetiology of the fluid [8]. The differentiation of haematoma from an abscess, or biloma is usually difficult. We have shown the utility of biliary scintigraphy in this setting [9]. Although the diagnosis is straightforward when

the radioisotope accumulates in the area of a fluid collection that has been demonstrated by CT or sonography, it may be less obvious under certain circumstances, requiring delayed images in multiple projections. Extrahepatic flow of radioactivity in a pattern inconsistent with small bowel, such as direct flow to the right paracolic gutter, is very suggestive of a bile leak (Figure 13.13). The leaking radioactivity may trickle deep to the porta hepatis, since the patient is usually supine during imaging, and then into the sub- and perihepatic spaces. It may be completely obscured by radioactivity in the liver on the early images [9]. Special attention should be paid to the delayed images that would show differential or asymmetric wash out of radioactivity from the 'liver silhouette'. While the liver washes out, the extravasated radioactivity becomes relatively more intense and obvious. Delayed images have another advantage in depicting a biloma. Since bilomas are well-encapsulated bile collections that usually keep their connection with the leak, they have high intraluminal pressure. Filling the high-pressure biloma with radioactivity may be a slow process (Figure 13.12).

Enterobiliary anastomosis The patency of an enteric-biliary anastomosis may be difficult to evaluate. Barium given by mouth may not fill the afferent loop and, therefore, renders it unevaluable. On the other hand, scintigraphy has the advantage of filling the afferent loop anterogradely. Detailed knowledge of the altered

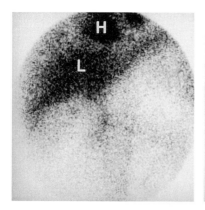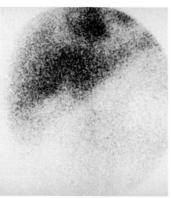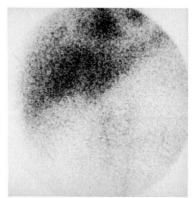

Figure 13.11 Diffuse liver disease. Three images from a hepatobiliary scintiscan obtained at 5, 45 and 90 minutes (left to right) show poor uptake of radioactivity by the liver (L) with persistence of radioactivity in the heart (H) by 90 minutes. This appearance is very suggestive of diffuse liver disease with failure of hepatocytes to extract the radiopharmaceutical from the circulation.

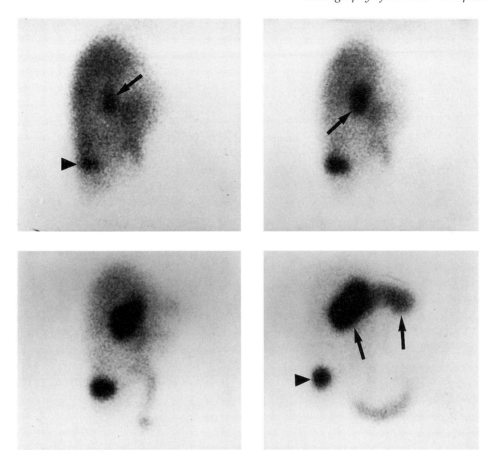

Figure 13.12 Bile leak with biloma. This patient had blunt abdominal trauma 1 week before the scan. The four images from a hepatobiliary scintiscan obtained at 5, 30, 60 and 90 minutes show good uptake and excretion by the liver. There is progressive accumulation of radioactivity in the centre of the liver which becomes dumbbell-shaped on the last image (arrows) (lower right). This patient had laceration of the liver demonstrated by CT at the time of the injury. Follow-up CT examination had shown fluid collection in the region of the laceration and could not differentiate a haematoma from a biloma. The scan was able to demonstrate the biloma. Also, this scan demonstrates the need to obtain the delayed images if a biloma is suspected because it usually fills slowly due to the elevated intraluminal pressure. There is also a focus of progressively increased uptake at the tip of the right lobe of the liver due to bile leak (arrowhead).

anatomy is essential for accurate interpretation of the images, and to avoid significant misinterpretations.

SCINTIGRAPHY OF THE LIVER AND SPLEEN

LIVER SCINTIGRAPHY

The liver has three compartments from the imager's point of view which, by utilizing differ-ent radionuclides, may be imaged. The first compartment is composed of the hepatocytes and biliary system (hepatobiliary system), which could be successfully imaged with the HIDA complexes (see above for detailed discussion). The second compartment is the reticuloendothelial system (RES), the cells of which – also known as Kupffer cells – line the sinusoids of the liver and function as the local macrophages. Some 90% of RES cells are in the liver and spleen and 10% in the bone marrow and lungs. The most commonly

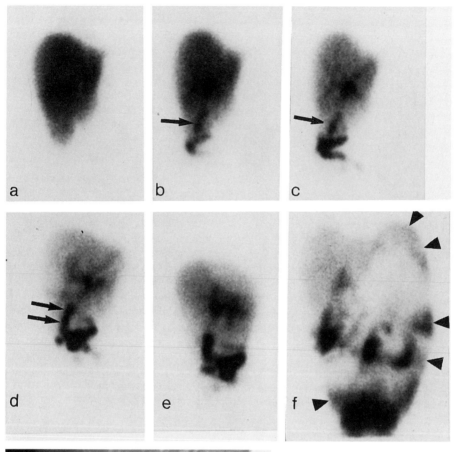

(a)

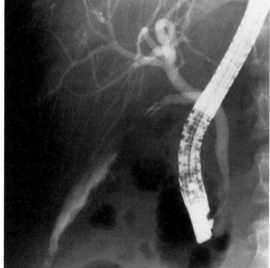

(b)

Figure 13.13 Bile leak following laparoscopic cholecystectomy. This patient has had laparoscopic cholecystectomy 3 weeks before the scan. She returned to the
hospital with abdominal pain and elevated white cell
count. (a) Six images from a hepatobiliary scan demonstrate prompt uptake and excretion of radioactivity by
the liver. At 15 minutes (image b), an abnormal structure
underneath the liver is seen filled with radioactivity (arrow), which became more intense with time. Notice also
the abnormal pattern of flow of radioactivity into the
right lower quadrant instead of the left upper quadrant
where the jejunum is located. This abnormal flow pattern
is suggestive of a bile leak. The last image (f) demonstrates radioactivity in the peritoneal reflections (arrowheads). (b) A radiograph obtained from an ERCP after
injection of contrast medium into the bile ducts shows
extravasation underneath the liver, most likely from the
ducts of Luschka. These small communications suppos-
edly connect the bile canaliculi of the right lobe directly
to the gallbladder and are violated at cholecystectomy.

used radiopharmaceutical to image this compartment is sulphur colloid labelled with 99m-technetium (^{99m}Tc). The third compartment is that of the blood pool; this is usually imaged by labelling red blood cells with ^{99m}Tc. Alternatively, labelled albumin could be used to achieve the same purpose.

The reticuloendothelial compartment

Imaging protocols and normal appearance This system is best imaged with colloid particles labelled with ^{99m}Tc. The injected particles are about the size of ordinary bacteria, ranging between 0.1 and 1 micron. They are rapidly removed from circulation, with a half-life of about 3 minutes, by phagocytosis by the Kupffer cells, where they remain for long periods, ranging between days and months. The radiopharmaceutical uptake depends on the functional status of these macrophages.

After injecting the patient intravenously with 3–5 mCi of ^{99m}Tc sulphur colloid, multiple planar images of the liver and spleen are obtained in different projections.

The shape of the normal liver varies, the right lobe being usually larger than the left. Different measurements of liver size have been used. We use a cephalocaudad span of 18 cm in the anterior axillary line as top normal. The distribution of radioactivity in the liver is homogeneous, except for areas of relatively decreased uptake in the gallbladder fossa, right renal fossa, porta hepatis and the confluence of the hepatic veins and inferior vena cava. If the heart is enlarged it may produce a smooth impression on the cephalad aspect of the left lobe of the liver. A semilunar attenuation defect in the dome of the liver is commonly produced by large breasts. The spleen has a lentiform shape and is located in the left upper quadrant of the abdomen. Its cephalocaudad span varies, but should not exceed 12 cm in adults. The distribution of radioactivity in the spleen is homogeneous, with an area of decreased uptake in the region of the hilum. On routine scintiscans, more radioactivity is seen in the liver than the spleen, with no visible uptake elsewhere at typical film density.

Diffuse liver disease This is a loose term applied to a variety of acute and chronic processes that affect the liver in a diffuse pattern. It includes, but is not limited to, inflammatory processes such as viral and alcoholic hepatitis, heavy-metal or chemotherapy intoxication, infiltrative processes and cirrhosis. Basic to the interpretation of scintigraphy is the concept that any process that involves the liver parenchyma results in some degree of destruction of reticuloendothelial cells. On liver/spleen scintiscan, the liver size could be normal, small or large depending on the severity of the process, the associated inflammatory reaction and whether the dominant feature is that of acute or chronic fibrotic nature. The distribution of radioactivity in the liver is inhomogeneous to a degree that correlates with the severity of the pathological process. In severe cases, the inhomogeneity may be so prominent that it would be impossible to exclude focal lesions, such as metastases. A shift of accumulation of radioactivity to the spleen and subsequently the bone marrow is noted. Splenomegaly is the hallmark of portal venous hypertension. However, the absence of splenomegaly does not exclude it because enough collateral circulation may develop to shelter the spleen from the effects of the elevated pressure. In some cases of acute alcoholic hepatitis superimposed on chronic disease, the Kupffer cells of the liver may be rendered practically nonfunctional, under which condition there will be very little uptake in the liver, if any (Figure 13.14). Unlike patients with terminal liver disease, who might display similar scintigraphic findings, patients with acute alcoholic hepatitis are usually not very sick, despite the severe scintigraphic findings. Furthermore, the markedly diminished or absent uptake by the liver is partially reversible with appropriate treatment (Figure 13.14).

The presence of ascites can be diagnosed on liver/spleen scintigraphy by the presence of a photopenic area around the liver and spleen that separates them from the abdominal wall (Figure 13.15). Diffuse lung uptake may be seen in patients with chronic debilitating disorders particularly cirrhosis.

Benign liver tumours The most common benign hepatic tumours are cavernous haemangioma, adenoma, focal nodular hyperplasia and macroregenerating nodules.

Cavernous haemangioma This is the most common benign tumour of the liver, with an incidence of about 5–7% from autopsy series [10]. Since this tumour is composed predominantly of vascular

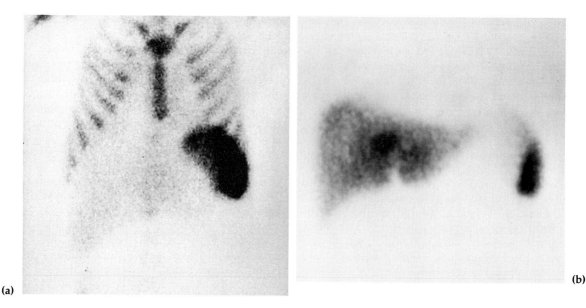

(a)

(b)

Figure 13.14 Alcoholic hepatitis. (a) Anterior image of the chest and abdomen obtained following intravenous administration of radiocolloid demonstrated intense uptake of radioactivity in the spleen and the bone marrow. There was extremely faint visualization of the liver. (b) Repeat examination several months following the treatment of the patient for alcoholism reveals markedly improved uptake of sulphur colloid by the liver. This case demonstrates the dramatic change associated with alcoholic hepatitis and the significant improvement following its treatment.

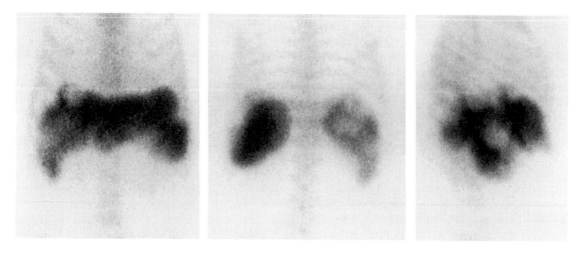

Figure 13.15 Liver cirrhosis with hepatoma anterior (left), posterior (centre), and right lateral (right). Images from a sulphur colloid scan demonstrate small size of the liver, enlargement of the left lobe, shift of colloid uptake to the spleen (posterior image) and bone marrow. Multiple photopenic defects are seen in the liver. Although these are more commonly seen with metastatic disease, the presence of extensive cirrhosis should always alert the reader to the possibility of hepatoma which was proven by biopsy. There is also slight separation of the right lobe of the liver from the rib cage (anterior image on the left). This indicates the presence of ascites.

spaces, it is best examined by radionuclides that label the vascular compartment of the liver rather than colloids. This will be discussed below.

Liver adenoma This uncommon neoplasm occurs almost exclusively in women of child-bearing age. It has been associated with the use of oral contraceptives [11]. It is usually a well-circumscribed lesion with a partial capsule [12,13], typically located in the right lobe of the liver. Although it is usually discovered incidentally by physical examination or imaging, it can be the cause of significant morbidity. It can bleed, infarct, undergo necrosis or even rupture [11,13]. Although typically it produces a photopenic defect on colloid scintigraphy, very rarely it may accumulate radiocolloid. Pathologically, adenomas contain Kupffer cells [12,14]. The lack of uptake of radiocolloid in most adenomas is attributed to the decreased number of Kupffer cells, decreased phagocytic activity by those cells, and the altered blood flow secondary to haemorrhage, necrosis and lack of portal ramifications [12]. Other imaging modalities are as non-specific as radionuclide scintigraphy. Sonography demonstrates areas of decreased as well as increased echogenicity depending on whether haemorrhage is present. CT depicts low-density lesions on non-enhanced scans and a wide range of enhancement following intravenous contrast enhancement. On MRI, the signal characteristics of adenoma are similar to those of hepatocellular carcinoma [15].

Focal nodular hyperplasia (FNH) This solitary liver neoplasm is seen most commonly in young women. Its association with the use of oral contraceptives remains controversial [11]. Most cases are discovered incidentally since complications such as haemorrhage and necrosis are rare. Pathologically, FNH has a thin capsule and contains a central fibrous scar with radiating septae. A variable number of Kupffer cells is seen. This is the reason why these tumours have variable appearance on colloid scintigraphy. While about 30% are photopenic, many others show similar or even more intense uptake than that of the liver. Intense accumulation of radioactivity, which is seen in about 10% of FNH, is a very specific finding. Scintigraphy is more specific for FNH than other imaging modalities. By sonography, FNH may be hypo-, iso- or even hyper-echoic [16]. While the demonstration of a hypoechoic scar is highly sug-

gestive of FNH, it is seen in a small percentage of cases. While unenhanced CT detects most of the cases, contrast enhancement adds to the sensitivity of the test by depicting lesions that are isodense with the liver, a transient hyperdensity being demonstrated by such lesions. The demonstration of a hypodense central scar, while uncommon, is a characteristic finding. On MRI, the presence of a lesion that is isointense on T1- and T2-weighted images with a hyperintense central scar is characteristic of FNH, although it is seen in no more than 10% of cases [17].

Focal fatty infiltration (FFI) Fatty infiltration of the liver is a diffuse process that involves the entire liver in most cases. It is commonly associated with diabetes mellitus, obesity, malnutrition, alcoholism, chemotherapy and other toxic agents. However, this process may have regional or focal distribution, or may involve the liver diffusely while sparing some areas, mimicking a mass lesion on sonography or CT. Since fatty infiltration does not affect the reticuloendothelial cells, colloid uptake remains intact and the colloid scintiscan shows normal uptake in the area of suspected mass lesion [18] (Figure 13.16).

Primary malignant tumours

Hepatocellular carcinoma (HCC) This is the most common primary tumour of the liver. It affects more men than women. There is a strong association between HCC and hepatitis B [19], and hepatitis C [20]. Most cases in North America occur in patients with liver cirrhosis, which renders the diagnosis particularly difficult to make. Since HCC may present as a solitary, multifocal or diffuse infiltrative process, it may be very difficult to differentiate from the fibrosis and regenerating nodules of cirrhosis. These are some of the reasons why HCC presents at an advanced stage with poor prognosis. Although the various radiological modalities are more sensitive than scintigraphy for the detection of small HCC, none has characteristic findings. The presence of surrounding fibrosis and regenerating nodules obscures small HCC on all modalities. Scintigraphy has a very low sensitivity for lesions <2cm in diameter. Deeply seated lesions may be obscured by overlying radioactivity; however, the presence of focal lesions in a cirrhotic liver is very suspicious for this tumour (Figure 13.15). On sonography, HCC

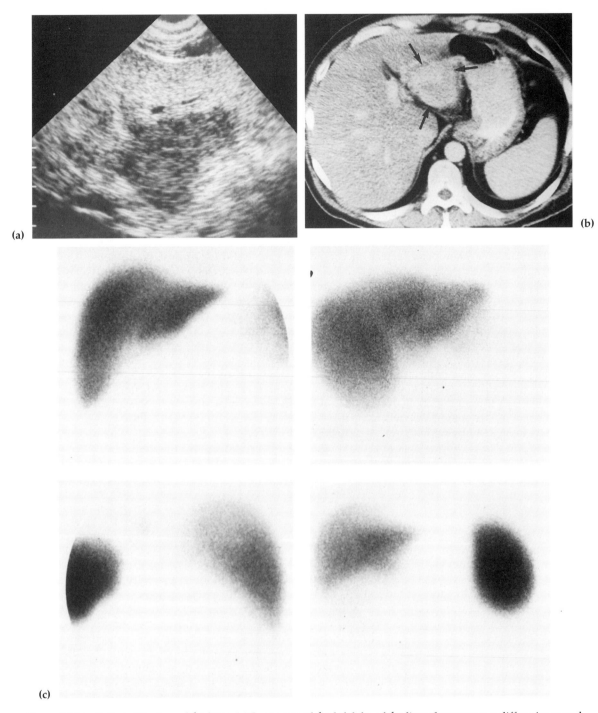

(a)

(b)

(c)

Figure 13.16 Fatty infiltration of the liver. (a) Sonogram of the left lobe of the liver demonstrates diffuse increased echogenicity with an area of decreased echogenicity. This is suggestive of a mass lesion. (b) CT image of the liver obtained following intravenous contrast enhancement shows decreased density in the liver with high density in the posterior aspect of the medial segment of the left lobe (arrows). (c) Multiple images of the liver obtained from a sulphur colloid scan show normal uptake and no focal abnormality. This constellation of findings indicates the presence of diffuse fatty infiltration of the liver with focal sparing of normal parenchyma in the posterior aspect of the left lobe.

may be hypo-, iso- or hyper-echoic. On CT, HCC appears as a discrete hypodense lesion before contrast enhancement, with dense enhancement on dynamic imaging. Despite these non-specific features, CT remains invaluable in determining the inoperability of those tumours by demonstrating tumour invasion of adjacent structures, venous thrombosis, lymphadenopathy or distant metastases.

Cholangiocarcinoma (CCA) This is the second most common primary malignant tumour of the liver. The differentiation of CCA from other vascular lesions of the liver is difficult by all imaging modalities. On sulphur colloid scintigraphy, centrally located CCA appears as a solitary photopenic defect. If other conditions such as sclerosing cholangitis coexisted, the sulphur colloid scan may show a diffusely heterogeneous pattern with no definite focal abnormality, making the diagnosis rather difficult. Sonography demonstrates a non-specific heterogeneously echogenic mass. CT demonstrates a low density mass before contrast enhancement, with variable enhancement pattern after intravenous injection of contrast medium. This variability in contrast enhancement makes characterization by CT inaccurate. The presence of calcifications, smaller satellite lesions and dilatation of the biliary tract favour CCA over other similar lesions, such as HCC. The most sensitive imaging modality for the detection of small CCA remains contrast cholangiography (ERCP or percutaneous).

Secondary malignant tumours Metastases are the most common malignant tumours of the liver in Europe and North America. Since the proper management of the patient varies depending on, among other factors, whether metastatic disease is present, it is important to utilize the imaging modality with the highest sensitivity and specificity. In a prospective study of patients with liver metastases from colon or breast cancer, CT had a higher sensitivity and specificity than sonography and colloid scintigraphy [21]. However, the recent introduction of significant improvement in these technologies, such as helical CT, intraoperative sonography and SPECT, respectively, makes the data outdated.

Colloid scintigraphy suffers from two main weaknesses. First, metastases, like other lesions, produce photopenic defects (Figure 13.17), a non-

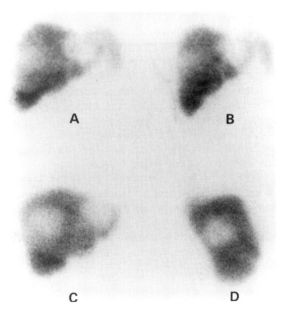

Figure 13.17 Liver metastases from colon cancer. Four images obtained from a sulphur colloid scan show large photopenic defects suggestive of metastatic disease. However, these findings are not specific and may represent cysts, abscesses, or other space-occupying lesions.

specific finding. Furthermore, some metastases spread by perisinusoidal infiltration, such as breast and lung cancers, producing a picture of inhomogeneity without focal defects on colloid scintigraphy, which would be very difficult to differentiate from other diffuse liver diseases. Second, lesions <2 cm in size, especially if they are located deeply in the liver, are likely to be obscured by scatter photons. SPECT, by its ability to separate target radioactivity from those coming from overlying tissue, should improve the sensitivity of scintigraphy, although unfortunately, this has not yet been substantiated [22]. The introduction of labelled tumour-specific monoclonal antibodies and peptides is likely to improve the specificity of scintigraphy, especially when combined with SPECT.

Sonography has similar sensitivity and specificity to colloid scintigraphy for the detection of liver metastases. Unlike scintigraphy, it can accurately differentiate tumours from cysts. Metastases have variable sonographic features, being hypo-, iso- or hyper-echoic. CT remains the imaging modality of choice for the evaluation of intra-abdominal metastatic disease, because of its superior sensitivity and its ability to detect metastatic lesions in other abdominal organs as well as lymph nodes. It depicts metastases as hypodense lesions before contrast enhancement, with variable enhancement patterns, depending on the tumour vascularity and the delay in scanning after the injection of contrast medium. If the images are obtained when the lesions are isodense with the liver, they can be missed.

MRI is a promising modality that seems, by utilizing different techniques and contrast enhancement, reasonably accurate in evaluating metastatic liver disease. However, large prospective studies are needed to compare MRI with CT in order to define its exact role in the management of patients with liver metastases.

The blood pool compartment

Imaging protocol and normal appearance This compartment is best imaged by labelling autologous red blood cells with ^{99m}Tc. We use 20 mCi of the radiotracer and *in vitro* labelling, which produces the highest labelling efficiency of about 98%. We obtain a dynamic flow phase of 3- to 5-second frames for 3 minutes, followed by 1×10^6 count static images at 5, 15, 30 and 60 minutes. Images are obtained in multiple projections depending on the site of the lesion. We reserve SPECT for small and deeply seated lesions that are not depicted by planar images. The heart and major blood vessels are routinely visualized. The liver shows homogeneous distribution of the radiotracer. The spleen shows more intense uptake of radioactivity than the liver. On SPECT, large veins are seen as foci of relatively increased uptake. It is important to demonstrate the continuity of these structures into a central vein in order to differentiate them from cavernous haemangioma.

Cavernous haemangioma of the liver This is the most common benign hepatic tumour, with an incidence of 3–7% from autopsy data [10]. It is of mesodermal origin and is composed of closely adjacent vascular channels, capillary to cavernous, which are lined with a single layer of endothelium. The capillary lesions may be solitary or more commonly part of a systemic disease, Osler-Weber-Rendau disease. In infants, the presence of dermal lesions should alert to the possibil-

ity of liver lesions. Cavernous haemangiomas are usually solitary, small, dark-red, compressible vascular lesions that are composed of large confluent vascular spaces filled with blood and lined with a layer of flat endothelium. Thin fibrous septae are seen which project into the vascular spaces; occasionally these may thrombose. Although they commonly range in size between 1 and 4 cm, they can achieve enormous size (giant cavernous haemangioma). While solitary lesions are seen more commonly, multiple tumours are detected in about 10% of cases.

With the increasing use of abdominal imaging, more cavernous haemangiomas are being incidentally discovered, for they are unlikely to be symptomatic. Since most of these lesions are <5 cm – at which size they tend to have a classical sonographic appearance – sonography is considered satisfactory to make the diagnosis. The classic ultrasound features are a small, well-circumscribed, homogeneously echogenic mass with smooth borders and moderate posterior enhancement. However, as mentioned previously these lesions may become larger, with commensurate change in their internal structure. Haemorrhage, myxomatous changes, thrombosis and calcifications may be seen, which alter the sonographic appearance. The lesion borders become less regular, with variable heterogeneous echogenicity and anechoic areas due to thrombosis, echogenic foci due to calcifications and loss of the posterior enhancement. Several studies have documented this variation of the sonographic appearance as a function of lesion size, and how less reliable sonography is in the evaluation of larger lesions [23–25]. Computed tomography has also been used in the evaluation of cavernous haemangiomata of the liver. Three criteria are needed to make the diagnosis. First, low attenuation on precontrast scan, present in about 90% of cases; second, peripheral enhancement on images obtained during the first 2 minutes after intravenous contrast enhancement, which is seen in about 75–83% of cases; and third, progressively increasing enhancement until it is completely isodense with the surrounding liver on delayed scans up to 60 minutes after contrast administration. This finding is present in about 34–72% of cases. Only 44% of cases will meet all three criteria, making CT unreliable in the majority of cases. Several investigators have examined the MRI characteristics of cavernous haemangiomas versus other tumours

[26,27]. They found that haemangiomas tend to have longer T2 than other tumours. However, as haemangiomas undergo thrombosis and calcification, and tumours undergo necrosis, MRI becomes less reliable in differentiating them. Most investigators agree that there is a 10% overlap.

Radionuclide scintigraphy utilizing labelled red blood cells is the most reliable imaging modality for the evaluation of suspected haemangioma. Two-phase planar imaging, a flow phase and static images, is performed. Haemangiomas are characterized by decreased uptake on the flow phase and increased accumulation on delayed imaging. Hepatomas and metastatic lesions, because of their rich supply from the hepatic artery, show increased flow initially and decreased delayed accumulation on the early images in comparison with the adjacent liver tissue. False-negative planar blood pool scintigraphy has been reported in two conditions. First, since the accu-

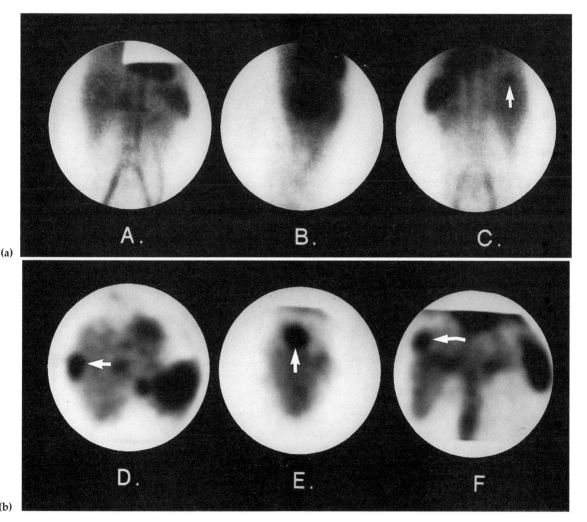

(a)

(b)

Figure 13.18 Cavernous haemangioma of the liver. (a) The scintiscan was done to evaluate a lesion that had been depicted by sonography. Anterior (A), right lateral (B) posterior planar images from a blood pool scan demonstrate a very faint focus of increased uptake in the dome of the liver noted on the posterior image (C). (b) Transaxial (D), sagittal (E) and coronal (F) SPECT images demonstrate a focus of intense uptake of radioactivity in the lateral aspect of the dome of the liver, highly suggestive of cavernous haemangioma (arrows).

mulation of radioactivity is a function of the blood volume in the venous spaces, cavernous haemangiomas may show inhomogeneous or absent uptake if they are partly or completely thrombosed, respectively. Second, depending on size and location, a haemangioma may be missed. Lesions <2 cm, particularly if deeply located in the liver, may go undetected. SPECT imaging, by separating activity in overlying normal tissue, improves contrast resolution (Figure 13.18), and, hence, sensitivity, which we have previously demonstrated [28]. However, SPECT images should be interpreted in conjunction with a morphological examination for two reasons. First, large veins seen in cross-section have a similar intensity as a haemangioma, and may be confused with one, particularly near the liver hilum. Second, since the imager is usually evaluating a lesion that has been diagnosed by sonography or CT, he or she should be sure that the abnormality on the morphological examination corresponds to that depicted by scintigraphy.

SPLEEN SCINTIGRAPHY

Under certain clinical circumstances, splenic imaging is important. Evaluation of the polysplenia/asplenia syndrome, the search for residual splenic tissue after splenectomy and for splenosis are the most common. Although the spleen can be well-visualized by blood pool scintigraphy, damaged red cell scintiscan achieves a higher target-to-background ratio. Usually the red cells are labelled *in vitro* and then heat-damaged before being re-injected. The main advantage of heat-damaging the red blood cells is that they are sequestered from the circulation by splenic tissue, leaving fewer cells in circulation, and, hence, achieve a higher target-to-background ratio.

GASTROINTESTINAL BLEEDING

INTRODUCTION

The diagnosis of bleeding from the gastrointestinal (GI) tract is based on clinical findings. However, the management of the bleed relies on adequate localization and assessment of its magnitude. Chronic upper and lower GI bleeds are best evaluated by endoscopy or contrast radiological examinations. Acute life-threatening haemorrhage requires immediate surgical and/or angiographic attention. In these two groups of patients scintigraphy offers no added benefit to the management of the patient.

However, scintigraphy is very helpful in haemodynamically stable patients with active GI bleeding. Upper GI bleeding is most commonly due to peptic gastroduodenitis, ulcer disease or oesophageal varices. These are best diagnosed, localized and sometimes managed by endoscopy. Brisk rectal bleed is commonly due to tumours, diverticula or haemorrhoids. These are best localized and diagnosed by endoscopy. However, it is not uncommon for endoscopy to fail to localize the site of haemorrhage or diagnose the underlying process because of the presence of a large amount of blood that obscures the bleeding site, and because blood moves forward as well as backward in the GI tract. Despite the major role that arteriography plays in the treatment of GI bleeds, it should not precede scintigraphy in evaluating these patients for two reasons. First, because of the intermittent nature of GI bleed, angiography may miss it unless the contrast medium is injected while the patient is actively bleeding. Second, the smallest bleeding rate that could be detected by arteriography is about 2 ml/min, which makes it a much less sensitive test than scintigraphy. Furthermore, scintigraphy offers two additional advantages. First, since angiography is unlikely to be abnormal in view of a normal scintiscan, a positive scan helps to select patients who are more likely to have positive angiograms. Second, since cinescintigraphy is very accurate in localizing the bleeding site, it can help direct arteriography, and therefore shorten the procedure time and decrease the total amount of contrast medium the patient receives.

IMAGING PROTOCOL AND NORMAL APPEARANCE

Two radiopharmaceuticals can be used to evaluate GI bleeding, ^{99m}Tc-labelled sulphur colloid and red blood cells. No patient preparation is needed for either examination.

^{99m}Tc sulphur colloid

Ten mCi of the radiopharmaceutical are injected intravenously and imaging started immediately. A large field-of-view gamma-camera is used, 1-minute frame-anterior images of the entire abdomen are required for a total of 30 minutes. At that time imaging is discontinued since the radiotracer will have been cleared by the reticuloendothelial system.

The blood pool of the heart, major vessels and major abdominal organs are visualized immediately. With time, the liver and spleen become more visible as they take up radioactivity, while the other organs fade away. By 30 minutes only the liver and spleen, and in some cases the bone marrow, are seen. The other abdominal structures are not visualized.

^{99m}Tc red blood cells (RBCs)

Between 20–25 mCi of the radionuclide are used to label the patient's RBCs. There are several ways of labelling RBCs. The easiest method is the *in vivo* approach, which includes an intravenous injection of 2 mg of stannous ion to reduce the pertechnetate from the −7 valence state to the −5 to make it amenable to labelling; 30 minutes later a separate injection of pertechnetate is made. This method achieves a labelling efficiency of about 80%, resulting in significant soft tissue, urinary and gastric activity. It has been shown that considerable gastric activity occurs in up to 50% of non-bleeding control subjects with this method, necessitating frequent nasogastric suctioning to minimize the likelihood of false-positive results [29, 30]. The second method is *in vitro*, which entails drawing 5–10 ml of the patient's blood, labelling it *in vitro*, using a commercially available kit, and re-infusing the labelled blood. This method, though time consuming, achieves the highest labelling efficiency, of about 95%. The third method is a hybrid of the two preceding methods. Stannous ions are injected intravenously; 30 minutes later blood is drawn into a heparinized syringe containing 20–25 mCi of the radionuclide and is incubated in the syringe for about 10–15 minutes at room temperature, and re-infused into the patient. Although this method saves the price of the labelling kit, it does not achieve the same labelling efficiency as the *in vitro* method. Achieving the highest possible labelling efficiency is sought, since free pertechnetate diffuses rapidly to the extracellular space, raising background activity which may obscure small bleeds. Furthermore, the excretion of free pertechnetate in the stomach may be confused with small upper GI bleeds.

Imaging is performed in a similar fashion to sulphur colloid scintigraphy except that it is carried out for 90 minutes, during which period

about 83% of bleeding occurs [31]. Delayed imaging is obtained if the patient rebleeds, but not routinely. Normally, the heart, major blood vessels and major abdominal organs are visualized immediately and, unlike sulphur colloid scintigraphy, for the duration of the examination. The stomach, small and large bowel are not visualized. If stomach activity is detected, one should suspect free pertechnetate. The urinary bladder is seen in most cases, which is thought to be due to free pertechnetate and labelled small plasma components filtered in urine. In some cases, bladder activity is so prominent that it may obscure small rectal bleeds. The kidneys are not visualized because of their posterior position. Prominent blood pool genital activity is detected in some men; while this is of no clinical significance, it should not be confused with a bleeding site.

GASTROINTESTINAL BLEEDS

Sulphur colloid scintigraphy

Extravasation of radiocolloid into the GI tract is diagnostic of active bleeding [31]. Since the colloid is cleared from circulation by the RE system, hence, lowering background activity rapidly, small bleeds are theoretically easier to detect than with RBC scintigraphy. In the upper abdomen, where the very high background activity in the liver and spleen may obscure small bleeds, the sensitivity is lower. Since the test is only good for as long as adequate radioactivity is present in circulation and radiocolloid is cleared from circulation with a half-life of 2 minutes, this examination is adequate for a short period of time. Since most GI bleeds are intermittent in nature, one can expect a high false-negative rate for this technique. Although this shortcoming could be overcome by repeated injections, the radiation burden to the liver, spleen and bone marrow is too high.

Red cell scintigraphy

This technique has the advantage of being valid for a longer period of time, since red cell labelling is very stable *in vivo*, and there is no active excretion or extraction of the radiopharmaceutical. It has been shown to be more sensitive and specific than colloid scintigraphy [31]. However, several pitfalls may be encountered. First, if the labelling efficiency is not adequate, free pertechnetate may appear in the stomach, mimicking a bleed. Second, excretion of radioactivity in urine may lead to false-positive cases if ureteral activity is confused with that of bowel, and false-negative cases if small rectal bleeds were obscured by prominent urinary bladder activity. Third, the presence of inflammatory lesions, such as gastritis and inflammatory bowel disease may have such a hyperaemic response that they would accumulate radioactivity. However, this radioactivity is usually stable throughout the examination and does not show the movement characteristic of GI bleeds.

The diagnosis of active GI bleeding depends on the demonstration of progressive accumulation of radioactivity with time outside the vascular struc-

tures, kidneys and bladder (Figure 13.19). The depiction of extravasated radioactivity depends on the target-to-background ratio, which depends on the rate of extravasation, or bleeding, and on the presence of a minimal lump sum of extravasated radioactivity. While it is thought generally that radioactivity should extravasate at a rate of no less than 0.5 ml/min to be detectable by current technology, the 'critical volume' of radioactivity needed is very difficult to quantitate, because it depends on the amount of fluid in the bowel that would dilute the extravasated radioactivity and on the peristaltic activity of that bowel segment it is collecting in. Less active bowel segments render smaller amounts of radioactivity more readily

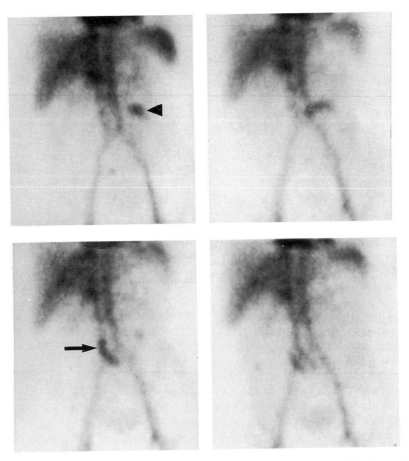

Figure 13.19 Gastrointestinal bleeding scintiscan. Four images from a gastrointestinal bleeding scintiscan obtained following *in vitro* labelling of red blood cells at 10, 20, 30 and 40 minutes reveal an initial focus of abnormal uptake in the left lower quadrant (arrowhead), which than moves across the midline and then crosses cephalad (arrow). The location and pattern of motion is suggestive of a small-bowel bleed which was proven by angiography.

depictable. Extravasated radioactivity usually moves quickly because of bowel peristalsis. In the colon it may move forward, backward or in both directions. The course of movement of extravasated radioactivity usually differentiates small from large intestinal bleeds (Figure 13.19). It is very important, therefore, to monitor the examination continuously to detect the first site of abnormal accumulation of radionuclide and to assess its pattern of motion. While hard-copy images remain the most common method of demonstrating bleeding sites, we [33] and others [34] have shown that cinematic display improves the accuracy of this examination.

MECKEL'S SCINTISCANS

Meckel's diverticulum is a remnant of the embryonic omphalomesenteric duct. It attaches the distal ileum, usually within 15 cm of the ileocaecal valve, to the anterior abdominal wall. This congenital abnormality was found to be present in 2% of cases in one autopsy series. About 50% of the cases of Meckel's diverticula have ectopic gastric mucosa. The complications associated with this abnormality are intestinal obstruction, inflammation and bleeding. Bleeding is due to ulceration of the unprotected mucosa secondary to gastric mucosal secretions. The great majority of bleeding Meckel's diverticula are seen in childhood, and very rarely in adults.

IMAGING PROTOCOL AND NORMAL APPEARANCE

The basic principle of the scintiscan is the uptake of free pertechnetate by the goblet cells in normal gastric mucosa. Ten mCi of $^{99m}TcO_4$ (pertechnetate) are injected intravenously and imaging started immediately. Anterior images of the entire abdomen are obtained for 750 000 counts each every 5 minutes for 30 minutes. The circulatory system, liver and spleen are visualized immediately. The stomach becomes visible 5–10 minutes into the examination. It empties into the small intestines which become visualized between 20 and 30 minutes. Urinary activity accumulates with time [35].

Abnormal appearance

Initial images show rapid diffusion of the radiopharmaceutical to the extracellular space.

Meckel's diverticulum accumulates radioactivity at about the same rate as the stomach, and is located most commonly in the right lower quadrant of the abdomen [36]. Caution should be exercised not to confuse a Meckel's diverticulum with intestinal filling from gastric secretion, which takes place 20–30 minutes after the stomach. Other conditions that may have a positive scintiscan are ileal duplication, inflammatory lesions and active GI bleed from other causes [36]. Ileal duplication is a rare disorder that has ectopic gastric mucosa and, therefore, can accumulate and secrete pertechnetate. Inflammatory bowel disease may be associated with diffusion of pertechnetate due to capillary leak. Also, since pertechnetate is excreted in urine, radioactivity in an ectopic right kidney, extrarenal pelvis, right ureter or a bladder diverticulum may give a false-positive result.

The overall sensitivity of the test is about 85–90% for diverticula that present with bleeding. The scintiscan does not depict diverticula that do not have gastric mucosa, and therefore should not be used in patients who do not present with GI bleeding. Because the scintiscan may not detect very small amounts of gastric mucosa, pharmacological interventions have been tried, without gaining wide acceptance, to enhance the sensitivity and specificity of this examination. Cimetidine, a histamine-2 (H_2) receptor antagonist, blocks the secretion of pertechnetate into the lumen, and therefore enhances the target-to-background ratio improving the detectability of gastric mucosa. Pentagastrin, which stimulates gastric secretion, is less frequently used. Furthermore, neither pharmaceutical has been investigated thoroughly to establish its exact role.

TUMOUR IMAGING

The detection of tumours by radiopharmaceuticals has been the quest of medical investigation for many decades. While initial work utilized simple radionuclides such as ^{131}I and ^{67}Ga, recent work has focused on more complex compounds such as antibodies and peptides. The role of these compounds in early detection, staging, follow-up after treatment and in some cases treatment of different tumours has been investigated. Despite significant progress in radionuclide techniques, morphological examinations, particularly CT, remain the cornerstone in tumour imaging.

RADIOIMMUNOSCINTIGRAPHY (RIS)

Several antibodies have been manufactured for medical use in the past two decades. Knowledge of the target antigen and the antibody is necessary for appropriate clinical use. Most commonly a monoclonal antibody (MAb) is used. It is usually of one immunoglobulin class, is antigen-specific, stable to chemical reaction and relatively easily labelled with radionuclide without any change of its immunoreactivity [37]. Knowledge of the expressivity of the antigen in normal tissue helps understand the biodistribution of the MAb, which along with understanding of its catabolism helps assess radioactive dosimetry to critical organs. Several factors affect the biodistribution of MAb including dose, concomitant metabolic and other disorders, medications, and the presence and levels of human anti-mouse antibodies (HAMA). See Chapter 17.

Although the extent of antigen expression in a tumour determines its expected relative uptake of the radiolabelled MAb, other factors also play a role. Heterogeneity, modulation, tumour specificity, poor tumour vascularity and poor diffusion and whether a whole or fragment of MAb is used influence tumour uptake. The most commonly used radionuclides are ^{99m}Tc, ^{123}I, ^{131}I and ^{111}In. The first two isotopes have short half-lives, and consequently lower radiation doses. Their abundant photon flux and favourable energy peaks make them highly suitable for imaging. They are used to label antibody fragments, which have rapid clearance. The latter two radionuclides, which have longer half-lives, and consequently higher radiation exposure rate, have to be used in small doses. Their small dose and high energy make them less desirable for imaging. However, they are used in preference to whole antibodies (which have a slower clearance rate), and to image tumours with poor vascularity and diffusion, where uptake of the MAb is slow.

Although several labelled immunoglobulins have been investigated for imaging abdominal tumours in the USA, only CYT-103 has been approved by the FDA for routine clinical use. The antibody used in CYT-103 or CR/OV (Oncoscint) is a whole murine IgG$_1$ immunoglobulin known as B72.3. It targets a mucin-like, tumour-associated glycoprotein known as TAG 72.3. This antigen is expressed by a variety of epithelial tumours with little expression by normal tissues. Immunohistological studies have shown that this antigen is expressed by 83% of colorectal and 97% of ovarian carcinomas. This immune complex is safe when introduced by intravenous infusion. In one series [38], 3.5% of patients developed mild side effects, though no patient had any serious reaction. Indeed, 39% of patients developed human antimouse antibody (HAMA), whose titres tended to decrease toward baseline with time.

Imaging protocol and normal appearance

Procedure CR/OV (1 mg) is labelled with 5 mCi of ^{111}In and infused intravenously over 5 minutes. Multiple planar 1000 K images of the torso are obtained on a large field-of-view camera at 48 and 72 hours. Repeat planar and SPECT images are obtained as needed. Visualization of the vascular bed, liver and spleen is routinely achieved. Intense testicular uptake and diffuse faint visualization of the colon are not uncommonly seen.

Colorectal carcinoma This is the third most common non-cutaneous malignancy in the USA. The disease is considered potentially curable if diagnosed and treated early. The 5-year survival correlates inversely with disease stage, being 85% for localized disease, 50% for disease with regional spread, but only 7% for disease with distant metastases. Most of these tumours are adenocarcinomas, their presenting symptoms varying from local to systemic. The spread of these malignancies is by direct invasion of adjacent structures or metastasis to lymph nodes, liver and lungs. Carcinomas of the right colon are more likely to metastasize to the liver, mesenteric and portal lymph nodes, while tumours of the rectum are more prone for local recurrence and pelvic and retroperitoneal lymph node metastases.

Recurrence of colon carcinoma occurs commonly in the liver and lungs, and less commonly in other abdominal foci, while recurrence of rectal carcinoma is very commonly local at the site of the original tumour, or in regional lymph nodes.

Patients are followed-up after treatment clinically, by carcinoembryonic antigen (CEA) levels. While rising CEA titres are a very sensitive indicator of recurrent disease, about 30% of patients with recurrence do not elicit this change. Computed tomography (CT) has been the most widely accepted imaging modality for evaluating patients for presurgical staging and suspected recurrence. While this modality has exquisite spatial resolution, it has limitations. The CT diagnosis of lymph node metastases is strictly based on size criteria; only lymph nodes ≥1.5 cm are considered suspicious for disease involvement, which means that early metastases which have not caused lymph node enlargement will be missed. CT is unable to differentiate a soft tissue mass due to fibrosis from that of a tumour; this is a very common problem with rectal carcinoma. Under these circumstances, RIS with CR/OV would be helpful. In a large multicentre study, Collier *et al.* [38] found in 169 patients with suspected primary or recurrent colorectal carcinoma, who subsequently had surgical verification, that the sensitivity of RIS and CT was 69% and 68%, respectively. The specificity was 77% for both. However, RIS had a statistically significant higher sensitivity in detecting pelvic tumours (74% versus 57%) and extrahepatic abdominal tumours (66% versus 34%) than CT, while CT had a higher sensitivity for hepatic metastases (84% versus 41%). The positive and negative predictive values for RIS were 97% and 19%, respectively. We feel that the best indication for RIS is in a previously treated patient with rising CEA titres and a negative or equivocal CT. In this scenario, a positive RIS is basically diagnostic of recurrent disease. Unfortunately, a negative test is not reliable in excluding recurrence.

Ovarian carcinoma This is the second most common gynaecological malignancy, accounting for the highest mortality rate of all the female genital tract cancers, and the fourth most frequent cause of cancer death in women. The most common histological type is adenocarcinoma. The onset of symptoms is insidious, and many patients have extensive tumour involvement at presentation. This tumour spreads directly to the peritoneum and metastasizes most commonly to abdominal lymph nodes. Extra-abdominal metastases are uncommon, but are seen in late stages. Unfortunately, most patients present at an advanced stage, when the diagnosis is made on the basis of clinical and surgical criteria, while imaging has not contributed significantly to alter the outcome of these patients. However, imaging plays an important role in initial staging and more so in the follow-up

of these patients. The results of initial surgery and the amount of residual disease affect the kind of adjuvant therapy and the prognosis of the patient. Patients are followed-up closely by physical examination, CA-125 serum levels, chest radiography and abdominal and pelvic CT. The physical examination is very crude and CA-125 serum level determination has a high false-negative rate and does not correlate with the extent of disease. Unfortunately, none of the currently available imaging modalities is sensitive or specific for disease <2 cm in size. While, intuitively, RIS may fill the need for an imaging modality that is both sensitive and specific, initial results of CR/OV scintiscanning were disappointing. In two independent series [39,40], the sensitivity and specificity of Oncoscint were 58–68% and 60–65%, respectively. The positive and negative predictive values were 83% and 29%, respectively. This technique may be helpful in some patients with clinical suspicion of recurrent disease and negative or equivocal CT (Figure 13.20). See Chapter 12.

PEPTIDE SCINTIGRAPHY (PS)

Somatostatin is a small peptide hormone of 14 amino acids. It is found in high concentration in the cerebral cortex, hypothalamus, brainstem and the gastrointestinal tract. It inhibits the release of growth hormone, glucagon, insulin and gastrin. It has been also noted to inhibit proliferative activity of human neuroendocrine tumours *in vivo*.

Neuroendocrine tumours of the digestive system are rare. They are comprised of carcinoids of the gastrointestinal tract and islet cell tumours of the pancreas. These tumours show low histological malignant characteristics, but high metastatic potential. They tend to secrete potent hormones that make the patient symptomatic. Also, carcinoids are associated with extensive fibrosis that may produce luminal obstruction or destruction of cardiac valves. They spread by direct invasion or metastasis to the liver and eventually other sites. They are usually small at presentation, but produce significant symptoms due to the hormones they produce. Since they are potentially curable if excised, pressure is put on the imager to find them. None of the conventional imaging modalities including CT, sonography and MRI is sensitive or specific enough for small tumours. Venography with venous sampling requires spe-

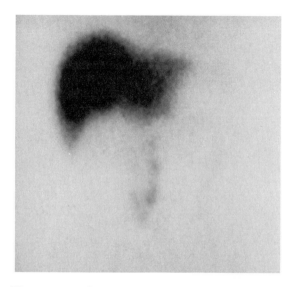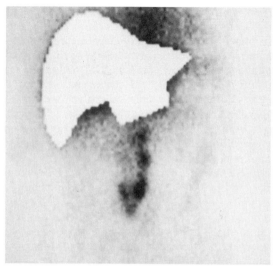

Figure 13.20   Ovarian carcinoma metastatic to retroperitoneal lymph nodes. This patient had resection of an ovarian carcinoma and was considered free of disease after surgery. However, her CA-125 titres showed progressive rise. CT scan of the abdomen and pelvis obtained just before the Oncoscint scan was negative for recurrent disease or metastases. These two images from the Oncoscint scintiscan obtained at 48 hours without (left) and with (right) liver masking to enhance the visualization of the multiple foci of abnormal uptake in the midline. These were proven to represent metastatic retroperitoneal lymphadenopathy.

cial skills, is time-consuming and invasive. Therefore, there is a need for a simple non-invasive imaging technique to localize those tumours.

Imaging protocol and normal appearance

Imaging is by 3–5 mCi ^{111}In-octreotide being infused intravenously and anterior and posterior images of the torso being obtained 24–48 and 72–96 hours later. Radioactivity in the vascular bed is seen on early images. Intense uptake in the kidneys, and less so in the liver, spleen and urinary bladder is normally depicted.

Clinical applications

Preoperative localization of neuroendocrine tumours of the digestive tract has not been successful, mostly due to the small size of these tumours. Morphological imaging modalities including sonography, CT and MRI have low sensitivity and specificity. In comparing the different imaging modalities in a small series of patients, the sensitivity of sonography, CT and PS was 44%, 33% and 55%, respectively [41] (Figure 13.21). All modalities showed similar sensitivities for metastases (Figure 13.22), though PS seems to

be the most promising for the preoperative localization of neuroendocrine tumours in the abdomen.

GASTRIC EMPTYING

The stomach occupies the mid portion of the upper abdomen. Although it is divided anatomically into the fundus, body, antrum and pylorus, functionally it has two compartments. The fundus functions as a reservoir with a remarkable ability to distend to accommodate large meals. The body and antrum function as a unit to break down large chunks of food and to homogenize it. Food fragments are moved through the body of the stomach, by prominent peristaltic waves, into the antrum, which in turn squeezes fragments of food back to the body. This back-and-fro movement grinds the food and mixes it with gastric juice, resulting in a thick semi-liquid mixture, which is passed through the pyloric canal in boluses into the small intestine for further digestion. Under pathophysiological conditions, the stomach may have rapid emptying (dumping syndrome) or slow emptying. Although radionuclide techniques can be used to examine either condition, the latter

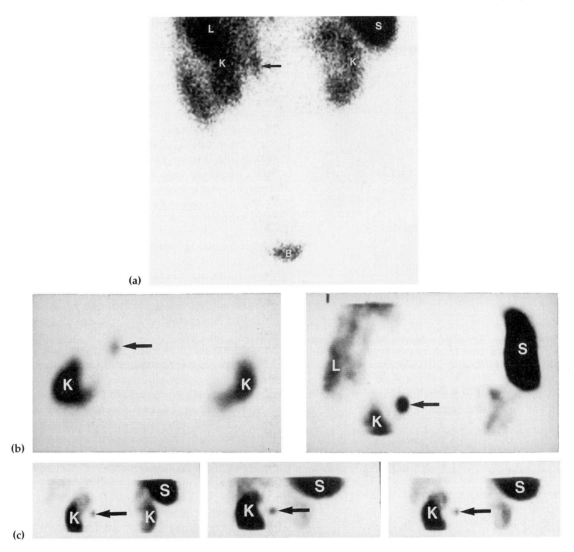

Figure 13.21 Gastrinoma depicted by ^{111}In-octreotide scintiscan. (a) Anterior planar image of the abdomen and pelvis reveals a vague suspicious focus of abnormal uptake medial to the left kidney (arrow). (b) Transaxial (left) and coronal (right) SPECT images from the same scintiscan show the focus of abnormal uptake (arrow) to be medial and slightly anterior to the right kidney. (c) Three-dimensional images from the same SPECT scintiscan in the anterior (left), right anterior oblique (centre), and left anterior oblique (right) show the focus of abnormal uptake to be medial to the hilum of the right kidney. This case illustrates the utility of SPECT in depicting small foci which may be obscured by normal uptake by the kidneys, liver and spleen. In this case, the CT was negative. At surgery, a 4.0-mm gastrinoma was resected from the posterior aspect of the head of the pancreas. B, urinary bladder; K, kidneys; L, liver; S, spleen.

is much more common and has been studied more extensively. Delayed gastric emptying could be due to either anatomical or physiological causes. Anatomically, obstructive lesions can be excluded by contrast X-ray or endoscopic examinations. Delayed gastric emptying secondary to pathophysiological conditions is better evaluated by radionuclide examinations. Gastric stasis could be acute or chronic. Acute gastric paresis, or adynamic ileus, is seen following major trauma or

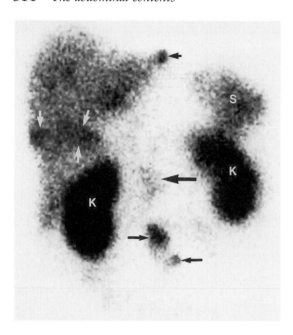

Figure 13.22 Metastatic carcinoid to the liver, retroperitoneal and mesenteric lymph nodes. An anterior image from a ^{111}In-octreotide scintiscan shows a small focus at the tip of the left lobe of the liver (small arrow), multiple foci in the right lobe of the liver (white arrows), an area of faintly increased uptake between the kidneys (large black arrow) representing retroperitoneal lymphadenopathy, and two foci of intense uptake of radioactivity more anterior representing metastatic mesenteric lymphadenopathy. All of these foci of abnormal uptake were corroborated by CT of the abdomen.

surgery, and in association with metabolic disorders, such as acidosis, hyperglycaemia and hypokalaemia, hormones such as glucagon, cholecystokinin, somatostatin, oestrogen and progesterone, and anticholinergic drugs. Gastric paresis in this situation is reversed when the primary disorder is corrected or treated. Radionuclide scintigraphy does not add significantly to the management of gastric paresis under these circumstances. Chronic gastric paresis, which is seen in association with diabetes mellitus, hypothyroidism and collagen vascular disorders, has been more thoroughly studied with radionuclide techniques. It has been shown that scintigraphy provides useful information about the severity of the problem and the efficacy of a treatment regimen.

Imaging protocol and normal appearance

There is no universally accepted standard method to perform the test, probably because of the sensitivity of gastric emptying to many factors and conditions whether psychological, metabolic or otherwise. The contents of the ingested meal affect the rate of gastric emptying, with liquid meals having the fastest rate and solid meals the slowest. Each laboratory should establish its own method taking into account the patient population, available equipment (e.g. single- versus dual-headed cameras), and the type of meal given. In our laboratory we examine gastric emptying of a liquid meal initially and a solid meal later, but simultaneous dual-imaging methods are also used. Immediately following ingestion of the radioactive meal the patient is placed under a single head, large field-of-view gamma-camera. Images are acquired at 5-min intervals for 90 minutes. Because of the position of the stomach with the fundus being posterior in location and the body and antrum anterior, and since we utilize a single-headed camera, we obtain the images in the 45° left anterior oblique (LAO) projection to avoid the problem of attenuation correction and the need for geometric mean. At the end of the examination, a region of interest is drawn around the stomach on a summation image. After correcting for decay, a time–activity curve is obtained. Many quantitative parameters have been used to measure gastric emptying, such as emptying rate, percent emptying at a certain point in time and $t_{1/2}$ of emptying.

Liquid phase One mCi of ^{99m}Tc sulphur colloid in water is given orally to the patient. This radiopharmaceutical dissolves readily in water, in which it becomes homogeneously distributed, and is not absorbable from the GI tract. Liquid meals move quickly through the stomach. A $t_{1/2}$ of emptying of up to 30 minutes is considered normal.

Solid phase One mCi of ^{99m}Tc sulphur colloid is scrambled with egg-white and given to the patient. Sulphur colloid binds to albumen to form a very stable compound. Gastric emptying of such a meal starts after a 'lag phase', the length of which is affected by the factors mentioned earlier. Gastric emptying to the small intestines begins after this lag phase. Emptying of a solid meal usually takes longer than emptying of a liquid meal. We accept a $t_{1/2}$ of emptying up to 90 minutes as normal. Expressing gastric emptying by this parameter assumes an exponential emptying, and some investigators prefer to use percent emptying at different points in time [42].

REFERENCES

1. Weissman, H.S. (1981) The clinical role of Tc 99m iminodiacetic acid cholescintigraphy, in Nuclear Medicine Annual – 1981 (eds L.M. Freeman and H.S. Weissman), Raven Press, New York, pp. 35–90.
2. Keslar, P.J. and Turbiner, E.H. (1987) Hepatobiliary imaging and the use of intravenous morphine. *Clin. Nucl. Med.*, **12**, 592–6.
3. Fink-Bennett, D., Balon, H., Robbins, T. and Tsai, D. (1991) Morphine augmented cholescintigraphy: its efficacy in detecting acute cholecystitis. *J. Nucl. Med.*, **32**, 1231–3.
4. Kim, O.K., Tre, K.K.M., Juweid, M. *et al.* (1993) Cholescintigraphy in the diagnosis of acute cholecystitis: morphine augmentation is superior to delayed imaging. *J. Nucl. Med.*, **34**, 1866.
5. Coleman, R.E., Freitas, J.E., Fink-Bennett, D. and Bree, R.L. (1984) The dilated cystic duct sign – a potential cause of false negative cholescintigraphy. *Clin. Nucl. Med.*, **9**(3), 134–6.
6. Noel, A.W., Velchic, M.G. and Alavi, A. (1985) The 'liver scan' appearance in cholescintigraphy: a sign of complete common bile duct obstruction. *Clin. Nucl. Med.*, **10**, 264–9.
7. Lee, A.W., Ram, M.D., Shih, W.-J. and Murphy, K. (1986) Technetium 99m-BIDA biliary scintigraphy in the evaluation of the jaundiced patient. *J. Nucl. Med.*, **27**, 1407–12.
8. Walker, A.T., Shapiro, A.W., Brooks, D.C., Braver, J.M. and Tumeh, S.S. (1992) Bile duct disruption and biloma after laparoscopic cholecystectomy: imaging evaluation. *Am. J. Roentgenol.*, **258**, 785–9,
9. Walker, A.T., Brooks, D.C., Tumeh, S.S. and Braver, J.M. (1993) Bile duct disruption after laparoscopic cholecystectomy. *Semin. Ultrasonogr. CT and MRI*, **14**(5), 346–55.
10. Ishak, K.G. and Rabin, L. (1975) Benign tumours of the liver. *Med. Clin. North Am.*, **59**, 955.
11. Kerlin, P., Davis, G.L., McGill, D.B. *et al.* (1983) Hepatic adenoma and focal nodular hyperplasia: clinical, pathologic and radiologic features. *Gastroenterology*, **84**, 994–1002.
12. Lubbers, P.R., Ros, P.R., Goodman, Z.D. *et al.* (1987) Accumulation of technetium-99m sulphur colloid by hepatocellular adenoma: scintigraphic pathologic correlation. *Am. J. Roentgenol.*, **148**, 1105–8.
13. Welch, T.J., Sheedy, P.F., Johnson, C.M. *et al.* (1985) Focal nodular hyperplasia and hepatic adenoma: comparison of angiography, CT, US, and scintigraphy. *Radiology*, **156**, 593–5.
14. Goodman, Z.D., Ulrika, V.W., Lubbers, P.R. *et al.* (1987) Kupffer cells in hepatocellular adenoma. *Am. J. Surg. Pathol.*, **11**, 191–6.
15. Rummeny, E., Weissleded, R., Stark, D.D. *et al.*

(1989) Primary liver tumors: diagnosis by MR imaging. *Am. J. Roentgenol.*, **152**, 63–72.
16. Rogers, J.V., Mack, L.A., Freeny, P.C. *et al.* (1981) Hepatic focal nodular hyperplasia: angiography, CT, sonography and scintigraphy. *Am. J. Roentgenol.*, **137**, 983–90.
17. Lee, M.J., Saini, S., Hamm, B. *et al.* (1991) Focal nodular hyperplasia of the liver: MR findings in 35 proved cases. *Am. J. Roentgenol.*, **156**, 317–20.
18. Lipman, J.O., Stomper, P., Kaplan, W.D. and Tumeh, S.S. (1985) Detection of hepatic metastases in diffuse fatty infiltration by CT: the complementary role of scintigraphy. *Clin. Nucl. Med.*, **13**, 602–5.
19. DiBisceglie, A.M., Rustgi, V.K., Hobfnagle, J.H. *et al.* (1988) Hepatocellular carcinoma. *Ann. Int. Med.*, **108**, 390–401.
20. Colombo, M., Kuo, G., Choo, Q.L. *et al.* (1989) Prevalence of antibodies to hepatitis C virus in Italian patients with hepatocellular carcinoma. *Lancet*, **2**, 1004–6.
21. Alderson, P.O., Adams, D.F., McNeil, B.J. *et al.* (1983) Computed tomography, ultrasound, and scintigraphy of the liver in patients with colon or breast carcinoma: a prospective comparison. *Radiology*, **149**, 225–30.
22. Fawcett, H.D. and Sayle, B.A. (1989) SPECT versus planar liver scintigraphy: is SPECT worth it? *J. Nucl. Med.*, **30**, 57–9.
23. Bruneton, J.N., Drouillard, J., Fenart, D. *et al.* (1983) Ultrasonography of hepatic cavernous haemangioma. *Br. J. Radiol.*, **56**, 791.
24. Mirk, P., Rubatelli, L., Bazzocchi, M. *et al.* (1982) Ultrasonographic patterns in hepatic hemangiomas. *Clin. Ultrasound.*, **10**, 373.
25. Gandolfi, L., Solmi, L., Bolondi, L. *et al.* (1983) The value of ultrasonography in the diagnosis of hepatic hemangiomas. *Eur. J. Radiol.*, **3**, 222.
26. Ohtomo, K., Itai, Y., Yoshkawa, K. *et al.* (1988) Hepatocellular carcinoma and cavernous hemangioma: differentiation with MR imaging. Efficacy of T2 value at 0.35 and 1.5 T. *Radiology*, **168**, 621.
27. Stark, D.D., Felder, R.O., Wittenberg, J. *et al.* (1985) Magnetic resonance of cavernous hemangioma of the liver: tissue-specific characterization. *Am. J. Roentgenol.*, **145**, 213.
28. Tumeh, S.S., Benson, C., Nagel, J.S. *et al.* (1987) Cavernous hemangioma of the liver: detection with single photon emission computed tomography. *Radiology*, **164**, 353.
29. Winzelberg, G.G., McKusik, K.A., Strauss, H.W. *et al.* (1979) Evaluation of gastrointestinal bleeding by red blood cells labelled in vivo with technetium-99m. *J. Nucl. Med.*, **20**, 1080–6.
30. Winzelberg, G.G., Froelich, J.W., McKusik, K.A. *et al.* (1981) Radionuclide localization of lower gastrointestinal hemorrhage. *Radiology*, **139**, 465–9.
31. Bunker, S.R., Lull, R.J., Tanasescu, D.E. *et al.* (1984) Scintigraphy of gastrointestinal hemorrhage: superiority of ^{99m}Tc red cells over ^{99m}Tc sulphur colloid. *Am. J. Roentgenol.*, **143**(3), 543–8.
32. Alavi, A. (1982) Detection of gastrointestinal bleeding with 99mTc-sulphur colloid. *Semin. Nucl. Med.*, **12**, 126–38.

33. Tumeh, S.S., Parker, J.A., Royal, H.D. *et al.* (1983) Detection of bleeding from angiodysplasia of the jejunum by blood pool scintigraphy. *Clin. Nucl. Med.*, **8**, 127–8.

34. Maurer, A.H., Rodman, M.S., Vitti, R.A. *et al.* (1992) Gastrointestinal bleeding improved localization with cine scintigraphy. *Radiology*, **185**, 187–92.

35. Sfakianakis, G.N. and Conway, J.J. (1981) Detection of ectopic gastric mucosa. in Meckel's diverticulum and other aberrations by scintigraphy: II. Indications and methods: a 10-year experience. *J. Nucl. Med.*, **22**, 732–8.

36. Sfakianakis, G.N. and Conway, J.J. (1981) Detection of ectopic gastric mucosa. in Meckel's diverticulum and other aberrations by scintigraphy: I. Pathophysiology and 10-year clinical experience. *J. Nucl. Med.*, **22**, 647–54.

37. Hellstrom, K.E., Hellstrom, I. and Brown, J.P. (1982) Human tumour associated antigen identified by monoclonal antibodies. *Springer Semin. Immunopathol.*, **2**, 127.

38. Collier, B.D., Abdel-Nabi, H., Doerr, R.J. *et al.* (1992) Immunoscintigraphy performed with 111-In-labelled CYT-103 in the management of colorectal carcinoma: comparison with CT. *Radiology*, **185**, 179–86.

39. Gallup, D.G. (1992) Multicenter clinical trial of 111In CYT-103 in patients with ovarian Cancer, in *Diagnosis of Colorectal and Ovarian Carcinoma: Applications of Immunoscintigraphic Technology* (eds R.T. Maguire and D. Van Nostrand), Marcel Dekker, Inc., New York, pp. 111–24.

40. Surwit, E.A. (1992) Impact of ^{111}In CYT-103 on the surgical management of patients with ovarian cancer, in *Diagnosis of Colorectal and Ovarian Carcinoma: Applications of Immunoscintigraphic Technology* (eds R.T. Maguire and D. Van Nostrand), Marcel Dekker, Inc., New York, pp. 121–40.

41. Weinel, R.J., Neuhaus, C., Stapp, J. *et al.* (1993) Preoperative localization of gastrointestinal endocrine tumours using somatostatin receptor scintigraphy. *Ann. Surg.*, **218**, 640–5.

42. Zeissman, H.A. (1995) Gastrointestinal Scintigraphy: Esophagus and Stomach, in *National Institutes of Health Series in Nuclear Medicine* (eds R. Neumann, J. Harbert and W. Eckelman), Thieme Medical Publishers, Inc., New York, pp. 585–649.

CHAPTER 14

Blood, bone marrow and lymphoid

Lymphomas

H. M. Abdel-Dayem and
H. A. Macapinlac

INTRODUCTION

Malignant lymphoma usually arises from the hae-matopoietic cells of B- or T-cell origin, and only rarely from the reticular supporting cells of the bone marrow and lymph nodes. It is one of the rapidly increasing malignancies with a more than 50% increase in incidence over the past 15 years. This is due to several predisposing factors such as the acquired immunodeficiency syndrome, either due to HIV infection or following the use of immu-nosuppressive drugs for organ transplantation; other predisposing factors include pesticides, pre-vious radiation exposure and viral infection. The course of the disease differs significantly in adults and children.

ADULT LYMPHOMA

There are two main varieties of lymphoreticular neoplasia in adults: Hodgkin lymphoma (HL) and non-Hodgkin lymphoma (NHL). Each has several subtypes as defined by a variety of histological classifications and clinical staging schemes. For example, the Ann Arbor classification – typically used for staging Hodgkin disease, is based on the sites of lymph node involvement, the presence of bone marrow and extranodal involvement, and

association of systemic symptoms of fever, pruri-tus and weight loss (Table 14.1).

Non-Hodgkin lymphoma may affect any age group, though the most common incidence is in the elderly. Unlike HL, blood-borne spread is usual and extranodal involvement is much more common. Staging of NHLs is less important as 70% has widespread disease at presentation; how-ever, the NHLs can be divided into three groups:

1. Low-grade, with predominantly small lympho-cytes or cells arranged in a follicular pattern.
2. Intermediate-grade, with mixed follicular cell, centrocytes and centroblasts.
3. High-grade, with predominance of centroblasts or immunoblasts with total destruction of nodal architecture.

PAEDIATRIC LYMPHOMA

Non-Hodgkin lymphoma is seen with a slightly greater frequency than HL in the paediatric popu-lation. The disease has a different behaviour in the paediatric than the adult population: for example, childhood NHL spreads in a non-contiguous fash-ion with involvement of extranodal sites in the majority of cases. Table 14.2 highlights the major differences between the adult and childhood NHLs.

Almost 70% of childhood NHL occurs in male patients, but this strong male predilection is not seen in adult NHL. Childhood NHL primarily manifests as extranodal disease, with only 14% of cases showing primarily nodal involvement. Al-most all cases of childhood NHL are considered

Clinical Nuclear Medicine, 3rd edn. Edited by M.N. Maisey, K.E. Britton and B.D. Collier. Published in 1998 by Chapman & Hall, London. ISBN 0 412 75180 1

Table 14.1 Ann Arbor staging of Hodgkin disease

Stage	Description
I	Involvement of a single lymph node region or structure (e.g. spleen Waldeyer's ring; thymus)
II	Involvement of two contiguous lymph node regions on the same side of the diaphragm
III	Involvement of lymph node regions on both sides of the diaphragm
IIIi	Splenic hilar, coeliac, portal lymph nodes
IIIii	Para-aortic, iliac, mesenteric nodes
IV	Involvement of extranodal sites, beyond that designated E A – no symptoms B – symptoms E – a single site of extranodal involvement contiguous to a node-bearing area X – bulky disease, mediastinal disease >1/3 the width of the mediastinum nodal mass >10 cm in diameter

high-grade lymphomas that show a tendency for early and widespread dissemination. Many similarities exist between childhood NHL and childhood leukaemia. Because NHL may involve both the peripheral blood and bone marrow, distinction from leukaemia in some cases may be difficult.

DIAGNOSIS AND STAGING OF LYMPHOMAS

Success in treating lymphomas relies on proper staging and evaluation of treatment response. The approach to the patient begins with a thorough history and clinical examination with special emphasis on systemic symptoms including fever, itching and weight loss. Lymph nodes should be examined for possible enlargement. Imaging techniques contributed to the accuracy of initial staging of the disease, monitoring of treatment response and in the follow-up for early detection of recurrence. The role of each imaging modality varies at different time periods of patient management, the histological type and the stage of the disease, the organ involved, and the age of the patient.

Lymphoangiography and laparotomy had a major role in the late 1960s and 1970s. The advances in chemotherapy at that time required adequate staging. Radiological and nuclear medicine procedures were not advanced to their present status. As developments progressed with time, there had been conflicting reports comparing lymphoangiography with computed tomography (CT) and exploratory laparotomy. The reported results vary. For prediction of para-aortic lymph node involvement, Castellino [1] reported the positive predictive value of lymphoangiography at 89% compared with 65% for CT, with a negative predictive value of 97% for lymphoangiography and 92% for CT. On the other hand, Mauch *et al.* [2] reported positive lymphoangiograms in 106 patients out of 571 (19%); only 41% of these had pelvic and para-aortic lymph node involvement at laparotomy, i.e. 59% were false-positive. In the negative lymphoangiography group, only 3% had para-aortic or pelvic nodal involvement. Another 23% had disease outside the pelvic and para-aortic nodes. In 92% splenic involvement was observed [2].

Despite optimal imaging studies, laparotomy is sometimes essential for appropriate staging in the pelvis and abdomen. In childhood NHL, when the disease extent is uncertain, it is not necessary to proceed to laparotomy for staging, since the patients are assumed to have disseminated disease. In all patients, the initial studies serve as an important baseline from which response after therapy can be evaluated.

Table 14.2 Differences between adult and childhood non-Hodgkin lymphoma (NHL)

Characteristics	Adult NHL	Chidhood NHL
Primary site of occurrence	Nodal	Extranodal
Histological architecture	50% follicular, 50% diffuse	Diffuse
Grade	Low, intermediate, high	High
Histological subtype	Many	Three
Sex predilection	None	Male

RADIOLOGICAL TECHNIQUES

Morphological imaging techniques include plain chest X-ray, barium studies of the gastrointestinal tract, intravenous pyelogram, CT, magnetic resonance imaging (MRI), ultrasonography (US) and lymphoangiography. A chest radiograph is ordered routinely for all lymphoma patients. The presence of a mediastinal mass is helpful when planning radiation ports and is predictive of prognosis. The chest X-ray is important for the assessment of tumour response, and is routinely performed in the follow-up at frequently identified periods.

CT is the primary imaging modality used in the staging and follow-up of lymphoreticular neoplasia. Peritoneal and mediastinal lymph nodes >2 cm in diameter are usually considered to be involved. CT is superior to other radiological modalities in several respects. It is sensitive in the detection of mediastinal, pleural, pericardial and tracheal disease. CT delineates areas of involvement in the lung parenchyma; detects blastic or lytic lesions in the bones, pericardial involvement and both extrapleural and pleural spread; and also identifies axillary and pericardiac adenopathy. CT provides a survey of enlarged lymph nodes that might be overlooked with lymphoangiography, including nodes in the mesentery, porta hepatis, splenic hilum, and coeliac and retrocrural regions. It provides additional benefit of assessment of intra-abdominal organs including the liver, spleen and kidneys. However, lymphomatous deposits in lymph nodes that are not enlarged will not be detected by the CT [3].

MRI is the modality of choice for the evaluation of lymphomatous involvement of the central nervous system. Like CT, MRI readily demonstrates focal brain parenchymal involvement, but MRI is superior to CT in the demonstration of the more common diffuse leptomeningeal tumoral spread and spinal disease. MRI and CT are comparable in the evaluation of the mediastinum; adenopathy, vascular encasement, and pericardial involvement can be easily demonstrated. Unfortunately, neither MRI nor CT allows differentiation of residual lymphoma from fibrosis or lymphomatous thymic involvement from rebound thymic hyperplasia. Because of the poor sensitivity of US and CT in the detection of lymphomatous involvement of the liver and spleen, it was hoped that MRI would be a more sensitive alternative. Unfortunately, MRI has also shown poor sensitivity in the detection of lymphoma in the liver and spleen [4,5]. MRI may play a role in the evaluation of lymphomatous bone marrow involvement. Because lymphomatous marrow deposits are frequently focal or patchy in distribution, routine iliac crest aspiration may yield false-negative results. MRI permits a survey of larger areas for bone marrow involvement, but very small deposits may be overlooked. On the basis of available data, Shields *et al.* [6] have proposed that MRI should be a complementary study to bone marrow biopsy.

Ultrasonography is a relatively inexpensive imaging modality that is well suited for use in the paediatric population, and it may provide a better evaluation of retroperitoneal lymphadenopathy than CT or MRI in those patients with a marked paucity of body fat. US may be helpful in discriminating a lymphomatous mass from non-opacified bowel in cases in which there has been inadequate bowel opacification with CT. In some situations, US may actually be the imaging modality of choice. It is particularly useful in the assessment of genitourinary tract, for testicular imaging, the female pelvis, and for renal involvement, especially in childhood NHL. Because US is less sensitive for the detection of bowel abnormalities, barium studies should be the initial radiological examination in cases in which there is a strong suspicion of gastrointestinal tract abnormalities. However, not uncommonly, US serves as a screening study for patients referred for a possible abdominal mass. In these situations, US may be helpful in the detection of lymphomatous bowel involvement, manifested as the 'pseudokidney' or 'hydronephrotic pseudokidney' or intussusception related to lymphomatous mesenteric node(s) or bowel involvement [7,8].

NUCLEAR MEDICINE TECHNIQUES

Nuclear medicine procedures have an important role in the management of malignant lymphoma. The radionuclide imaging techniques include gallium-67 citrate scans, which have been widely performed for more than two decades. Thallium-201 chloride, ^{99m}Tc-MIBI and ^{111}In-octreotide, are still of limited use and their values have not been fully explored. A number of labelled monoclonal antibodies are on trial. However, the available antibodies have a limited application and are still in the investigational phase. Recent studies with

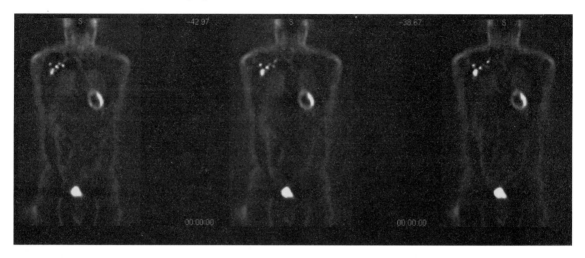

Figure 14.1   A 45-year-old man with biopsy-proven non-Hodgkin lymphoma in a right axillary lymph node referred for evaluation of extent of disease before therapy. Serial coronal emission PET scans acquired 45 minutes after injection of ^{18}F-FDG showing multiple nodes in the right axilla, subpectoral and infraclavicular regions. Note heterogenous activity in myocardium and normal urine activity in the bladder. Minimal activity noted in the liver, spleen, kidney and gut.

positron emission tomography using ^{18}F-FDG or ^{11}C-methionine appear very promising.

Although the mechanism of cellular uptake of all radiopharmaceuticals is different, they all reflect tumour viability. [67]Ga uptake is due to transferrin receptors on the cell membrane, which are more abundant in the intermediate- and high-grade or undifferentiated types, and less in the low-grade or well-differentiated disease [9–17]. Thallium-201 chloride is a potassium analogue, and its cellular uptake is related to ATP-ase activity, sodium–potassium pump and energy consumption. ^{99m}Tc-MIBI uptake is related to a potential difference across the cell membrane, and is taken up by intracellular mitochondria [18]. Preliminary reports have demonstrated the affinity of ^{99m}Tc-MIBI for PGP glycoprotein, which is coded for by the multi-drug resistance gene, indicating a potential utility in identifying tumours resistant to chemotherapy. It has been reported that the uptake of thallium (contrary to gallium), is higher in low-grade, well-differentiated lymphomas, and low in the high-grade, undifferentiated types [19]. This could be due to the presence of necrosis and inflammatory components in the undifferentiated types. The total-body application of both thallium and ^{99m}Tc-MIBI is limited by sites of normal physiological uptake – they are unhelpful in the abdomen and their use in the chest is limited by myocardial activity. For ^{67}Ga, ^{201}Tl and ^{99m}Tc-MIBI, high-dose SPECT imaging improves the sensitivity. However, the dose of thallium is limited only not to more than 4mCi (148MBq) [18].

The future role of PET radiopharmaceuticals, ^{18}F-FDG or ^{11}C-methionine, has yet to be fully explored. Although the studies reported in the literature include a limited number of patients, they all favour PET for initial staging, evaluation of treatment response and for follow-up. A higher degree of FDG uptake has been reported in high-grade tumours, while lower uptakes (and sensitivities) are seen in low-grade lymphomas [20–23]. The current generation of PET scanners have definite advantages with larger fields-of-view (usually 15cm), capable of performing transmission scans in the presence of emission activity allowing shorter and more tolerable whole-body scan times. A particular advantage is the capability of performing quick three-dimensional images of the brain, which typically require 5–10 minutes for acquisition. FDG-PET imaging with state-of-the-art scanners have the advantage of image acquisition at 45–60 minutes post-injection (Figure 14.1). The relatively modest activity in the liver, spleen and gut is also an added advantage. Preliminary reports indicate excellent accuracy of FDG-PET imaging for thoracoabdominal lymphoma, and with successful imaging of all grades of NHL [20]. Furthermore, a limited series indicates that FDG-PET can predict malignancy grade in NHL in contrast to ^{11}C-methionine, which was previously not possible with ^{67}Ga citrate [24].

There are only a few reports on the use of ^{111}In-octreotide imaging for the initial staging and follow-up of patients with malignant lymphoma. Regardless of the degree of differentiation, most lymphomas express somatostatin receptors, and are seen if imaged with ^{111}In-octreotide [25]. For both the initial staging and monitoring the response to chemotherapy, the reports have shown correlation with other imaging modalities. These reports conclude that ^{111}In-octreotide is not reliable for initial staging because of the variable and usually low uptake. It could be useful for the evaluation of residual active tumour tissue after treatment [26]. Our preliminary data (Figure 14.2)

indicate that somatostatin-receptor imaging is a safe procedure, but has been inconsistent in predicting disease involvement, and therefore its routine clinical application is not recommended [27].

At the present time, ^{67}Ga citrate is the most commonly used radiopharmaceutical in malignant lymphoma. The use of high doses (8–15 mCi) and the new state-of-the-art, multi-headed gamma-cameras for planar and SPECT imaging is essential to achieve good results [28]. The uptake of gallium by the tumour reflects its viability since it is not taken up by necrotic or fibrotic tissues. Although in the early stages, it is less sensitive than CT or MRI in diagnosis and does not help in accurate staging. Indeed, a pre-treatment baseline gallium scan is recommended in order to determine if the tumour is gallium-avid in order to decide on its role in the follow-up and treatment assessment.

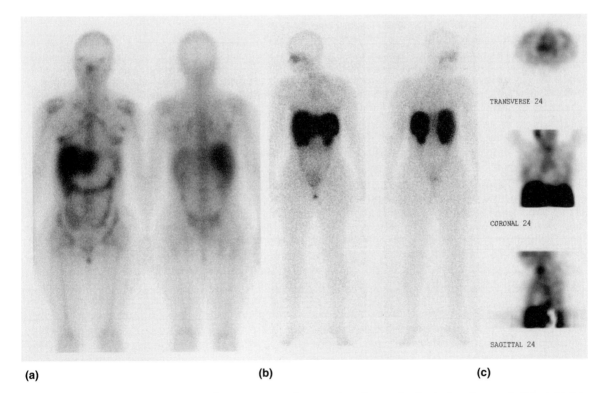

(a)   **(b)**   **(c)**

Figure 14.2 A 28-year-old woman with Hodgkin lymphoma on baseline evaluation before therapy. Left to right: (a) anterior and posterior planar images 48 hours after 10 mCi of ^{67}Ga showing gallium-avid disease in the left axilla, mediastinum, both hila, supraclavicular regions and normal breast activity; (b) 24-hour anterior and posterior planar images after 6 mCi of ^{111}In-pentetreotide, showing faint left supraclavicular and chest uptake. Note intense normal activity in the liver, spleen, and kidneys; and (c) ^{111}In-pentetreotide SPECT images at 24 hours showing bilateral hilar uptake.

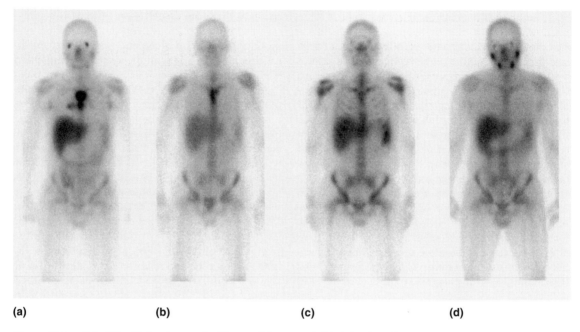

(a)   **(b)**   **(c)**   **(d)**

Figure 14.3   67Ga (10 mCi dose) scan of a 25-year-old man with Hodgkin lymphoma. Anterior planar images (from left to right): (a) baseline pretreatment scan showing gallium-avid disease in both axillae, mediastinum and hila; (b) persistent uptake in the mediastinal mass at mid-chemotherapy cycle; (c) no evidence of gallium-avid tumour at the end of chemotherapy cycle, before radiation treatment; and (d) 1 month after the last radiation treatment. Note the rebound uptake in the salivary glands, which is a common finding after radiation treatment in the chest.

Up to 64% of lymphoma patients with mediastinal disease may show a residual mass after treatment (Figure 14.3); only 18% of these relapse. A follow-up gallium scan helps diagnose the presence of a recurrence (or residual tumour) in a post-therapy mediastinal mass. In this regard, gallium-SPECT is superior to CT or MRI. The post-treatment gallium scan should be performed 3 weeks after the last treatment. Radiotherapy or chemotherapy might affect gallium uptake, and could be the cause of a false-negative scan in the early post-therapy period.

Early detection of recurrence – when the lesion is impalpable and systemic symptoms absent – is important for initiating early treatment before the bulk of the disease becomes larger. Recurrences of lymphoma occur outside the original sites in 25–27% of the cases. A total-body gallium scan has been more helpful than CT or MRI. Early recurrence can be detected on a ^{67}Ga scan, months before the patient becomes symptomatic, and the initial follow-up scan should be performed at 6–12 months after treatment and thereafter once yearly.

An imaging agent that can evaluate treatment response while the patient is on treatment will be of great value for two main reasons. If the patient shows no response after two to three cycles of chemotherapy, treatment can be modified and other chemotherapy agents / regimens substituted. The second advantage is the rapidity of response. There is a statistical difference in survival between those patients who have a complete response without any residual disease after a smaller number of chemotherapy cycles and those who need to be given additional chemotherapy doses to eradicate the disease. Gallium scans performed at mid-cycle or after four cycles of chemotherapy are being used in certain centres for this purpose. Finally, image co-registration could be used in selected cases to allow the functional strengths of SPECT and PET imaging to be combined with the anatomic resolution of CT and MRI [29].

Extranodal involvement, especially of the brain and the heart, is common in immunosuppressed patients. In cardiac lymphoma, the gallium scan is more helpful than other imaging modalities or other radiopharmaceuticals such as ^{201}Tl or ^{99m}Tc-MIBI. We recommend its use for staging purposes once the diagnosis is established and for follow-up in other locations.

The differentiation between toxoplasmosis and intracranial lymphoma is a problem that occasionally cannot be resolved by CT or MRI. The use of thallium brain SPECT or FDG-PET has been helpful in making this differentiation. In our experience, ^{201}Tl is better than ^{99m}Tc-MIBI, because the latter has the disadvantage of choroid plexus uptake, which is a problem since the majority of these lesions are either in or near the basal ganglia. Treated toxoplasmosis might be a cause of false-positive scans due to high thallium or MIBI uptake. We therefore recommend that the ^{201}Tl or ^{99m}Tc-MIBI study should be performed before anti-toxoplasmosis treatment is initiated.

REFERENCES

1. Castellino, R.A. (1990) Diagnostic imaging of abdominal and pelvic lymph nodes in lymphoma. *Radiol. Clin. North Am.*, **28**, 801–31.
2. Mauch, P., Larson, D., Osteen, R. *et al.* (1990) Prognostic factors for positive surgical staging in patients with Hodgkin's disease. *J. Clin. Oncol.*, **8**, 257–65.
3. Nyman, R., Rehn, S., Glimelius, B. *et al.* (1988) Magnetic resonance imaging, chest radiography, computed tomography, and ultrasonography in malignant lymphoma. *Acta Radiol.*, **28**, 253–62.
4. Cohen, M.D., Klatte, E.C., Smith, J.A. *et al.* (1985) Magnetic resonance imaging of lymphomas in children. *Pediatr. Radiol.*, **15**, 179–83.
5. Zimmerman, R.A. (1990) Central nervous system lymphoma. *Radiol. Clin. North Am.*, **28**, 697–721.
6. Shields, A.F., Porter, B.A., Churchley, S. *et al.* (1987) The detection of bone marrow involvement by lymphoma using magnetic resonance imaging. *J. Clin. Oncol.*, **4**, 225–30.
7. Strauss, S., Lisbon, E., Schwartz, E. *et al.* (1986) Renal sonography in American Burkitt lymphoma. *Am. J. Roentgenol.*, **146**, 549–52.
8. Sener, R.N., Alper, H., Demirci, A. and Diren, H.B. (1989) A different sonographic 'pseudokidney' appearance detected with intestinal lymphoma: 'Hydronephrotic pseudokidney'. *J. Clin. Ultrasound*, **17**, 209–12.
9. Tumeh, S.S., Rosenthal, D.S., Kaplan, W.D., English, R.J. and Holman, B.L. (1987) Lymphoma: evaluation with Ga-67 SPECT. *Radiology*, **164**(1), 114–14.
10. Rossleigh, M.A., Murray, P.L., Mackey, D.W., Bargwanna, K.A. and Nayanar, V.V. (1990) Pediatric solid tumors: evaluation of Ga-67 SPECT studies. *J. Nucl. Med.*, **31**, 168–72.
11. Israel, O., Front, D., Epelbaum, R. *et al.* (1990) Residual mass and negative Ga-67 scintigraphy in treated lymphoma. *J. Nucl. Med.*, **31**, 365–8.
12. Front, D., Benen-dashHaim, S., Israel, O. *et al.* (1992) Lymphoma: predictive value of Ga-67 scintigraphy after treatment. *Radiology*, **182**, 359–63.
13. Drossman, S.R., Schiff, R.G., Kronfeld, G.D., McNamara, J. and Leonidas, J.C. (1990) Lymphoma of the mediastinum and neck: evaluation with Ga-67 imaging and CT correlation. *Radiology*, **174**, 171–5.
14. Turner, D.A., Fordham, E.W. and Ali, A. (1978) Gallium-67 imaging in the management of Hodgkin's disease and other malignant lymphomas. *Semin. Nucl. Med.*, **8**, 205–14.
15. Weiner, M., Leventhal, B., Cantor, A. *et al.* (1991) Gallium-67 scans as an adjunct to computed tomography scans for the assessment of a residual mediastinal mass in pediatric patients with Hodgkin's disease. *Cancer*, **68**(11), 2478–80.
16. Neuman, R.D., Kemp, J.D. and Weiner, R.E. (1996) Gallium-67 imaging for detection of malignant disease, in *Diagnostic Nuclear Medicine* (ed. M.P. Sandler, R.E. Coleman, F.J.Th. Wackers *et al.*), 3rd edn, Williams & Wilkins, pp. 1243–60.
17. Front, D. and Israel, O. (1995) The role of gallium scintigraphy in evaluating the results of therapy in lymphoma patients. *Semin. Nucl. Med.*, **25**(1), 60–71.
18. Abdel-Dayem, H.M., Scott, A., Macapinlac, H.A., Elgazzar, A. and Larson, S.M. (1994) Role of Tl-201 chloride and Tc-99m sestaMIBI in tumour imaging. *Nucl. Med. Annual*, 181–234.
19. Waxman, A.D., Eller, D., Ashook, G. *et al.* (1996) Comparison of gallium-67 citrate and thallium-201 scintigraphy in peripheral and intrathoracic lymphoma. *J. Nucl. Med.*, **37**(1), 46–50.
20. Newman, J.S., Francis, I.R., Kaminski, M.S. and Wahl, R.L (1994) Imaging of lymphoma with PET with 2[F-18]-fluoro-2-deoxy-D-glucose: correlation with CT. *Radiology*, **190**, 111–16.
21. Okada, J., Yoshikawa, K., Itami, M. *et al.*(1992) Positron emission tomography using fluorine-18-fluorodeoxyglucose in malignant lymphoma: a comparison with proliferative activity. *J. Nucl. Med.*, **33**, 325–9.
22. Okada, J., Yoshikawa, K., Itami, M. *et al.* (1987) The use of FDG-PET in the detection and management of malignant lymphoma: correlation of uptake with prognosis. *J. Nucl. Med.*, **28**, 288–92.
23. Paul, R. (1987) Comparison of fluorine-18-2-fluorodeoxyglucose and Ga-67 citrate imaging for detection of lymphoma. *J. Nucl. Med.*, **28**, 288–92.
24. Rodriguez, M., Rehn, S., Ahlstrom, S., Sundstrom, C. and Glimelius, B. (1995) Predicting malignancy grade with PET in Non-Hodgkin's Lymphoma. *J. Nucl. Med.*, **36**, 1790–6.
25. Hiruma, K., Koike, T., Nakamura, H., Sumida, T., Maeda, T., Tomioka, H., Yoshida, S. and Fujita, T. (1990) Somatostatin receptors on human lymphocytes and leukaemia cells. *Immunology*, **71**, 480–5.
26. Sarda, L., Duet, M., Zini, J.M., Berolatti, B., Benelhadj, S., Tobelem, G. and Mundler, O. (1995) In-111 Pentetreotide scintigraphy in malignant lymphomas. *Eur. J. Nucl. Med.*, **22**, 1105–9.
27. Goldsmith, S.J., Macapinlac, H.M. and O'Brien, J. (1995) Somatostatin receptor imaging in lymphoma. *Semin. Nucl. Med.*, **25**(3), 262–71.

28. Macapinlac, H.A., Scott, A.M., Larson, S.M., Divgi, C.R., Yeh, D.J. and Goldsmith, S.J. (1994) Gallium-67 citrate imaging in nuclear oncology. *Nucl. Med. Biol.*, **21**(5), 731–8.

29. Scott, A.M., Macapinlac, H.A., Zhang, J.J., Kalagian, H., Graham, M.C., Divgi, C.R, Goldsmith, S.J. and Larson, S.M. (2994) Clinical applications of fusion imaging in oncology. *Nucl. Med. Biol.*, **21**(5), 775–84.

Blood disorders

A. M. Peters and D. M. Swirsky

INTRODUCTION

Nuclear haematology is a broad, wide-ranging discipline based as much on *in vitro* investigations as on imaging, and in many institutions is the responsibility of departments of haematology rather than nuclear medicine. Nuclear haematology plays a crucial role in the diagnosis and clinical management of many haematological disorders; the diseases where the discipline makes an important contribution include polycythaemia, myelofibrosis, aplastic anaemia, idiopathic thrombocytopenic purpura (ITP), haemolytic anaemia and diseases associated with the loose term, 'hypersplenism'. Because nuclear haematology is basically technique-orientated with a wide range and variety of techniques, this chapter is set out according to techniques rather than diseases.

The investigations can be broadly grouped according to the cell type of interest: red cells (including ferrokinetics and investigation of megaloblastic anaemias), platelets and leucocytes. Whereas labelled leucocytes are important in nuclear medicine for imaging inflammation, they offer little clinical value in the investigation of blood disorders.

RADIOLABELLED RED CELLS

Studies based on labelled red cells include *in vitro* measurements of red cell mass (RCM), mean red cell life span (MRCLS), detection and quantification of gastrointestinal (GI) bleeding, and compatibility testing, and *in vivo* measurement of splenic function, quantification of splenic red cell pooling, and detection of sites of red cell destruction [1].

RED CELL LABELLING

Chromium-51

Mean red cell life span and quantification of gastrointestinal blood loss are based on ^{51}Cr red cell labelling. A 14-ml sample of venous blood is taken into a syringe containing 2 ml ACD (NIH formula A). The blood is centrifuged at 1000 g for 5 minutes, following which the plasma supernatant is removed. Care should be taken not to disturb, and inadvertently remove the reticulocyte-rich upper surface of the red cell column, which makes an important contribution to MRCLS. About 100 µCi sodium chromate [^{51}Cr] is added to the red cells and mixed for 5 minutes. The unbound ^{51}Cr (usually <10%) is removed by washing the cells in saline. An anticipated very short MRCLS may be measured using red cells labelled with indium-111 (see below).

Technetium-99m

Short-term investigations, such as splenic red cell pooling and tests of splenic function based on blood clearance measurements, should be performed with a short-lived radionuclide such as ^{99m}Tc. The principle of labelling with ^{99m}Tc is to allow the radionuclide to diffuse into the red cells and then to trap it by reduction with stannous ion. The red cells are first 'tinned' by exposure to stannous fluoride and labelled 15 minutes later by exposure to pertechnetate. It is essential to label the cells *in vitro* and then wash them, although the tinning can be performed *in vivo* by prior intravenous injection of tin. This so-called '*in vivtro*' labelling consists of *in vivo* tinning followed by venesection into a syringe containing anticoagulant and pertechnetate. After gentle agitation, the blood in the syringe is then infused back into the patient or the cells can first be washed *in vitro*.

Indium

Two isotopes of indium are useful in nuclear haematology: ^{113m}In, which is generator-produced but no longer available, and ^{111}In. Blood cells are labelled with indium by exposure to lipophilic metal chelate complexes of indium, such as indium-tropolonate or oxinate, which, following penetration of the cell membrane, bind tightly to intracellular proteins. For labelling platelets and neutrophils, the cell of interest has first to be isolated from other blood cell types because the labelling is indiscriminate. Since red cells greatly outnumber other cell types, the indium complex needs only to be added to whole blood *in vitro* for red cell labelling, followed by washing to remove

Clinical Nuclear Medicine, 3rd edn. Edited by M.N. Maisey, K.E. Britton and B.D. Collier. Published in 1998 by Chapman & Hall, London. ISBN 0 412 75180 1

unbound complex. The labelling efficiency is improved if the complex is added to washed red cells.

Elution of label from red cells is least with ^{51}Cr and greatest with ^{99m}Tc. Indium isotopes label red cells with a stability almost as high as ^{51}Cr [2].

RED CELL VOLUME (RCV)

Measurement of RCV is the most frequently performed nuclear investigation in haematology. A high venous haematocrit in isolation should never be assumed to be due to red cell polycythaemia (erthrocytosis). It may equally be the result of a reduced plasma volume, causing relative or pseudo-polycythaemia. It is important to identify cases of pseudo-polycythaemia as the treatment is venesection rather than myelosuppressive drug therapy. In the occasional patient, usually obese or a smoker, an RCV in the upper normal range and a plasma volume (PV) in the lower normal range combine to give a modestly raised venous haematocrit, so-called 'physiological polycythaemia' [3]. Cases of pseudoanaemia can be identified where the RCV is normal but the PV is expanded, for example in splenomegaly, cirrhosis and glomerulonephritis. Pseudoanaemia is a normal feature of pregnancy and accounts for the reduction in venous haematocrit. When measurement of RCV establishes true polycythaemia, the cause should be sought (Table 14.3).

RCV is preferably measured with ^{51}Cr- or ^{113m}In-labelled red cells, unless splenic red cell pooling is also imaged when ^{99m}Tc is satisfactory. Elution of ^{99m}Tc gives a slight over-estimation of red cell volume [2]. RCV measurement is based on the dilution principle; a blood sample is taken at about 20 minutes after injection of a known amount of labelled cells, when complete mixing within the circulation can be assumed. In clinical practice, it is vital to relate the measured RCV to body habitus. Adipose tissue is avascular relative to muscle. In obese patients the RCV expressed in ml/kg may significantly underestimate the degree of polycythaemia unless the lean body mass is measured or estimated. Without such correction, true polycythaemia may be missed or mis-classified as pseudopolycythaemia. Methods of estimating RCV from body dimensions have recently been reviewed by Pearson *et al.* [4].

Equilibration is prolonged in splenomegaly [5] so the sample should be delayed until 60 minutes

Table 14.3 Causes of increased red cell volume

1. Primary proliferative polycythaemia
2. Idiopathic erythrocytosis
3. Autonomous high erythropoietin production
4. Secondary polycythaemia
   (a) *Hypoxic (with activation of normal erythropoietin mechanism)*
       High altitude
       Hypoxaemic lung disease (including intrinsic lung disease, hypoventilation, sleep apnoea)
       Cyanotic congenital heart disease
       High oxygen affinity haemoglobins
       Smoking
       Methaemoglobinaemia
       Red cell metabolic defect
   (b) *With 'inappropriate' secretion of erythropoietin*
       Renal tumour – hypernephroma, nephroblastoma
       Renal ischaemia (e.g. cysts, hydronephrosis, renal transplant)
       Hepatoma and liver disease
       Fibroids
       Cerebellar haemangioblastoma
       Bronchial carcinoma
       Phaeochromocytoma
   (c) *Miscellaneous*
       Androgen therapy
       Cushing's disease
       Hypertransfusion

post-injection (but see platelets, below). Measurement of RCV should be combined with estimation of plasma volume (PV) (using ^{125}I-labelled albumin), for which at least three samples, usually taken at 10, 20 and 30 minutes after injection, are obtained. As a result of a slow extravascular protein loss, these three samples are used to obtain the appropriate dilution factor for measurement of PV by extrapolation to zero time. On the other hand, the three samples should agree with each other in their estimates of RCV because the limitation here is intravascular mixing which should be complete by 10 minutes unless there is splenomegaly.

MEAN RED CELL LIFE SPAN (MRCLS)

Because of the requirements of intracellular stability and long physical half-life, ^{51}Cr is used for measurement of MRCLS. Blood samples are taken daily after injection of ^{51}Cr-labelled autologous red cells for an appropriate duration judged from the rate of loss of radioactivity from the blood. Because of slow, on-going elution of ^{51}Cr from the cells, the percentage of ^{51}Cr remaining in blood has

Table 14.4 Normal range for ^{51}Cr survival curves with correction for elution

Day	% ^{51}Cr (corrected for decay; not corrected for elution)	Elution correction factors
1	93–98	1.03
2	89–97	1.05
3	86–95	1.06
4	83–93	1.07
5	80–92	1.08
6	78–90	1.10
7	77–88	1.11
8	76–86	1.12
9	74–84	1.13
10	72–83	1.14
11	70–81	1.16
12	68–79	1.17
13	67–78	1.18
14	65–77	1.19
15	64–75	1.20
16	62–74	1.22
17	59–73	1.23
18	58–71	1.25
19	57–69	1.26
20	56–67	1.27
21	55–66	1.29
22	53–65	1.31
23	52–63	1.32
24	51–60	1.34
25	50–59	1.36
30	44–52	1.47
35	39–47	1.53
40	34–42	1.60

to be multiplied by a correction factor, which increases with the passage of time. This varies from 1.03 at 24 hours after injection to 1.6 at 40 days (Table 14.4).

The MRCLS is decreased in haemolytic anaemias. It may also be usefully measured in conjunction with GI blood loss studies. In clinical practice, it is usually measured when the cause of an anaemia is obscure or multifactorial, for example in patients with known GI blood loss who also have a positive direct anti-globulin (Coombs) test, or in patients with an unexplained transfusion requirement. Blood loss in the stools and sites of red cell destruction can be quantified simultaneously by surface counting (see below).

SPLENIC FUNCTION

Splenic function is most conveniently measured from the rate of blood clearance of red cells modified for selective splenic uptake. Modification includes heat treatment (to produce pyrospherocytes), coating with immunoglobulin and – almost never used nowadays – chemical denaturation. ^{111}In-labelled platelets (see below) also provide information on splenic pooling.

Heat-damaged red cells

A few years ago, splenic function was frequently assessed with heat damaged red blood cells (HDRBC) in the belief that the reticuloendothelial system was being tested. The rate of disappearance of HDRBC from the circulation is, however, more a function of splenic blood flow. Normal red cells are highly deformable while pyrospherocytes are not. As a result of their stiffness, therefore, HDRBC pass through the spleen slowly (with a mean time of 10 minutes in contrast to <1 minute for normal cells) and are ultimately trapped irreversibly [6]. Erythrophagocytosis occurs some hours later [7]. The initial fractional rate of disappearance from blood is equal to the ratio of splenic blood flow to total blood volume. The disappearance curve is bi-exponential because, as soon as the cells start to return to the circulation from the spleen, the curve 'bends', concave upwards, on semi-logarithmic display, away from its initial course. The simplest way to quantify the rate of disappearance is the $t_{1/2}$ measured from 3 minutes, or the 'C20', which is the difference in activities between 8 and 28 minutes as a percentage of the activity at 8 minutes [1]. The C20 is preferable as it minimizes the influence of hepatic clearance, which is completed by about 8 minutes. Alternatively, the disappearance curve can be analysed into its two exponentials, from which splenic blood flow, intrasplenic transit time and fractional irreversible splenic retention can be obtained.

The kinetics of HDRBC disappearance from the circulation may be useful to assess whether physiological hypersplenism is present if an anaemia seems out of proportion to spleen size. ^{99m}Tc-labelled HDRBC allow accurate assessment of spleen size, which may be useful, as an alternative to ^{111}In-labelled platelets, for the detection of splenunculi in thrombocytopenic patients following splenectomy.

Immunoglobulin-coated red cells

Antibody-coated red cells are almost of no clinical use but have research potential. Their kinetics depend on the nature and source of the antibody. Ideally the antibody should have affinity only for splenic Fc receptors, in which case there is no liver uptake [8]. The disappearance from blood is then monoexponential with a rate constant equal to splenic clearance (which is splenic blood flow multiplied by splenic extraction efficiency) divided by total blood volume. Extraction efficiency depends on splenic function (specifically the availability of splenic Fc receptors) and the number of immunoglobulin molecules on the red cell surface [9].

GASTROINTESTINAL (GI) BLOOD LOSS

Gastrointestinal blood loss is quantified by measuring ^{51}Cr in a 7-day stool collection after the intravenous injection of ^{51}Cr-labelled red cells. The count rate from daily faecal samples is recorded in an *in vitro* counter and compared with the counts from a sample of blood of accurately measured volume (3–5 ml) taken the previous day, placed in a similar carton and diluted to 100 ml. Correction for intravascular ^{51}Cr elution is not usually made. Since the elution correction factor at 7 days is only 1.11, the maximal possible error is 10%. Measurement of GI blood loss can also be based on whole body counting, analogous to the measurements of ^{59}Fe absorption, GI protein loss [10] and granulocyte migration into bowel lumen in inflammatory bowel disease [11]. It should be emphasized that ^{51}Cr-labelled red cells are used to prove and quantify GI blood loss, but not to localize GI bleeding in a patient known to be bleeding.

COMPATIBILITY TESTING

Compatibility testing takes two forms: a short-term test to confirm that blood for transfusion will survive adequately in the recipient; and a longer-term test to identify a suitable donor for a recipient with multiple antibodies. For the former, a few millilitres of the unit of red cells is removed and labelled with any of the radionuclides mentioned above (usually ^{99m}Tc or ^{113m}In). Following injection into the recipient, there should be a survival or recovery >90%, at 60 minutes after injection if the blood is compatible. In the longer-term test, red cells from the potential donor are labelled with ^{51}Cr and administered to the recipient. In the absence of antibodies the cells will show a normal survival, at least initially. If the recipient develops antibodies to the transfused cells, the survival curve abruptly falls at the first appearance of the antibodies several days after injection of the labelled cells. This is called a 'collapsing' survival curve.

IMAGING THE SPLENIC RED CELL POOL

Abnormal splenic pooling of blood cells may be an important feature of several specific conditions including polycythaemia vera (red cells), thrombocytopenia and more rarely granulocytopenia. The term hypersplenism is often used, but it is a misleading term that fails to distinguish between abnormal pooling and abnormally increased cell destruction in the spleen. Pooling is a term which itself requires defining and distinguishing from the term sequestration. Pooling implies free exchange of cells between the circulating blood and pool, and as such can be measured as the mean transit time of cells through the pool. Sequestration is a process whereby cells are temporarily trapped in a vascular bed and are not freely exchangeable with circulating cells. An example is the pulmonary sequestration of granulocytes that have been activated *in vitro* during labelling. Sequestered cells ultimately re-enter the circulation although they may then be rapidly destroyed elsewhere. Irreversible loss of blood cells from the circulation results from cell destruction or consumption (as in thrombosis) or from migration into the interstitial space. The use of the word sequestration in this context is confusing and should be avoided.

Normally, red cell transit time through the spleen is 30–60 seconds. This is longer than for plasma so the intrasplenic haematocrit is higher than whole-body haematocrit. In contrast, red cells streamline in the hepatic vasculature and consequently the intrahepatic haematocrit is lower than the whole-body haematocrit. In splenomegaly there appears to be an additional red cell pool, with a mean transit time considerably longer than 1 minute. This has been inferred from a biphasic uptake of radioactivity in the spleen following bolus injection of labelled red cells [5]. Owing to the presence of this more slowly exchanging pool, equilibration of red cells is longer in the enlarged spleen compared with the normal; this is the reverse to platelets. The markedly enlarged spleen may pool red cells sufficiently to produce pseudo-anaemia (reduced venous haematocrit in the presence of normal red cell volume), although it more readily causes thrombocytopenia. The normal splenic red cell pool is less than 5% of the red cell mass. It is expanded in polycythaemia vera to between 5 and 20%, and is higher in myelofibrosis, typically reaching 30%. The massive splenomegaly of myelofibrosis may cause significant pseudo-anaemia as a result of splenic red cell pooling. Measurement of the splenic red cell pool may be helpful for predicting the benefits of splenectomy in patients who are severely transfusion-dependent. In pseudo-polycythaemia, the splenic red cell pool is normal. In early primary polycythaemia, an increased splenic pool is an important diagnostic aid in a patient with a spleen of normal size. In some conditions associated with splenomegaly (e.g. hairy cell leukaemia), the splenic red cell volume is increased but not in proportion to the splenomegaly.

DETERMINATION OF SITES OF RED CELL DESTRUCTION

The importance of identifying sites of blood cell destruction is essentially related to the decision to perform splenectomy in diseases like haemolytic anaemias and idiopathic thrombocytopenic purpura in which accelerated cell destruction in the spleen may be pathological. In normal subjects, virtually all of the red cells, granulocytes and platelets are destroyed in the reticuloendothelial system. In particular, the notion that granulocytes are destroyed in the tissues as a result of a continuous on-going migration into the extravascular space in a sub-clinical defence of infection, as widely suggested in haematological textbooks, has not been borne out by imaging studies of granulocyte kinetics (see below).

Because of the relatively long normal life span of red cells, it is usually necessary, even in haemolytic anaemias, to label red cells with ^{51}Cr (half-life 27.8 days). Sequential surface counting with a scintillation probe over the spleen, liver, precordium and lumbar spine gives a semi-quantitative indication of the major sites of cell destruction. Spleen and liver counts can be corrected for their contained blood pool by normalization to, and comparison with, precordial counts. Thus, assuming that the organ counts immediately after injection of the labelled cells arise only from blood, the 'excess' counts represent the difference between spleen or liver counts and precordial counts. In

hereditary spherocytosis, excess counts in the spleen are markedly elevated but not accompanied by an increase in excess hepatic counts. In autoimmune haemolytic anaemia, both are increased, although detection of excess counts over the spleen may be helpful in predicting a favourable response to splenectomy. Equivalent studies with labelled platelets in thrombocytopenia are less reliable in this prediction. In sickle cell disease, the liver typically shows increased destruction, but, because of autosplenectomy, the spleen does not. ^{111}In has been used in severe haemolytic anaemias associated with a very reduced red cell life span [12]. Nevertheless, although its imaging characteristics are superior, it still has a significant rate of elution.

FERROKINETICS AND METABOLIC STUDIES

Ferrokinetic studies, including erythropoietic bone marrow imaging, are useful in the investigation of suspected aplastic and other dyserythropoietic anaemias and diseases associated with myeloid metaplasia, especially myelofibrosis. Iron-59 (^{59}Fe) is administered either orally as the chloride for gastrointestinal absorption studies or intravenously, as citrate for other studies [13]. The interpretation of abnormal findings is summarized in Table 14.5.

IRON ABSORPTION

Iron absorption is measured following an oral dose of ^{59}Fe, given with unlabelled oral ferrous sulphate and ascorbic acid to reduce the radioactive iron to the ferrous form. The unabsorbed iron is then measured by faecal counting. Iron absorption can also be measured by whole-body counting in terms of the percentage difference between counts acquired immediately after ingestion and at 7 and 9 days. The average normal value of iron absorption is about 30%, but the normal range is wide. Values of less than 10% are abnormal. It is increased up to about 90% in iron-deficiency anaemia (not due to malabsorption).

PLASMA IRON CLEARANCE

Plasma iron clearance is measured as the rate constant of clearance of intravenously injected, transferrin-bound, ^{59}Fe citrate. If the patient has a

Table 14.5   Ferrokinetic patterns in various diseases

	Plasma Clearance $t_{1/2}$	Plasma iron turnover	Red cell utilization
Normal	60–140 min	70–140 μmol/l/day	70–80%
Iron deficiency	↓	N	↑
Aplastic anaemia	↑	N	↓
Secondary anaemia	Slightly ↓	N	N
Dyserythropoiesis	Slightly ↓	↑	↓
Myelofibrosis	↓	↑	↓
Haemolytic anaemia	↓	↑	↑

↓ = short/decreased, ↑ = prolonged/increased.

reduced transferrin binding capacity, or if transferrin is already saturated (as in aplastic anaemia) then ^{59}Fe bound to donor plasma should be used, otherwise the iron is taken up rapidly by the liver, to form ferritin. Group AB fresh frozen plasma is a convenient source of donor transferrin. If autologous plasma is used, it should be passed through a resin column before injection in order to remove any free ^{59}Fe. The plasma disappearance of radioactivity is monoexponential, over a wide range of clearance values, with a normal $t_{1/2}$ ranging between 60 and 140 minutes. The clearance rate is decreased, with a $t_{1/2}$ of up to 300 minutes, in aplastic anaemia, and increased in myelofibrosis, polycythaemia vera, iron-deficiency anaemia and haemolytic anaemias, with $t_{\frac{1}{2}}$ values typically 20–40 minutes. Since the disappearance is monoexponential, plasma volume can be measured from the extrapolated zero-time ^{59}Fe plasma concentration.

PLASMA IRON TURNOVER

Plasma iron turnover (PIT), the product of plasma ^{59}Fe clearance and the plasma protein-bound native iron concentration, is an absolute measure of the rate of iron removal from plasma in units of mg/ml/min. It clearly reflects plasma iron clearance values, and adds little useful clinical information to iron clearance.

RED CELL IRON UTILIZATION

Red cell utilization (RCU) is the fraction of an injected dose of ^{59}Fe that is incorporated into circulating red cells, and is therefore a measure of effective erythropoiesis. Blood samples are taken on alternate days for 12–14 days following intravenous iron administration and the whole body red cell volume (RCV) is multiplied by the red cell ^{59}Fe concentration in each sample:

$$RCU = \frac{RCV \times RBC \; ^{59}Fe \; concentration}{^{59}Fe \; dose}$$

The RCV can be obtained routinely from the plasma volume as determined from the plasma iron clearance, and the whole body haematocrit (determined as the peripheral venous haematocrit multiplied by 0.9). It is necessary to assume that RCV remains constant over the period of measurement. This can be partially checked by daily venous haematocrit estimations. The daily RCU values rise to a plateau of 70–80% at about 10 days in normal subjects. It is reduced to <10% in aplastic anaemia and to between 10 and 50% in myelofibrosis. In iron-deficiency anaemia, haemolytic anaemia and true polycythaemia, RCU is increased, usually approaching 100%. Where erythropoiesis is ineffective – for example in myelodysplasia or thalassaemias – the red cell utilization is variably reduced, depending on the severity of the disorder.

^{59}Fe SURFACE COUNTING

An overall picture of ferrokinetics can be constructed from day-to-day surface counting with a scintillation probe positioned over the liver, spleen, sacrum (for bone marrow) and heart (for blood pool) after an intravenous injection of ^{59}Fe. The counts, corrected for physical decay, give information on sites of erythropoiesis (from early counting), which may be extramedullary, and on sites of red cell destruction (from later counting). Surface counting is rarely performed but does have some clinical value for determining the extent of extramedullary erythropoiesis in the spleen before splenectomy. Positron emission tomography (PET) with ^{52}Fe has demonstrated that active bone marrow may have a patchy distribution, underlining the uncertainty of surface counting.

^{52}Fe POSITRON EMISSION TOMOGRAPHY (PET)

The radionuclides of iron, ^{59}Fe and, in centres with facilities for PET, ^{52}Fe, label the erythron and are used to identify sites of erythropoiesis in aplastic anaemia and myelofibrosis. ^{52}Fe is a positron-emitter which, using PET, gives high-resolution

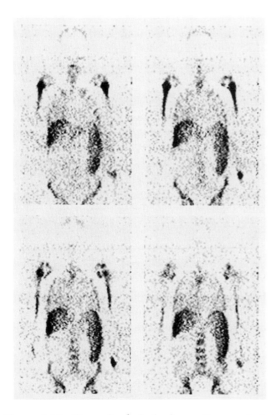

Figure 14.4 Coronal whole body positron emission tomograms in a patient with polycythaemia rubra vera following intravenous injection of Fe-52. Although bone marrow uptake is clearly visible, the presence of myeloid metaplasia confirms transition to myelofibrosis.

images of the distribution of erythropoietic tissue (Figure 14.4). The detection of splenic erythropoiesis, absent in uncomplicated polycythaemia and invariably present in myelofibrosis, is helpful in documenting the transition from polycythaemia to a myelofibrotic state. In doubtful cases of essential thrombocythaemia, detection of splenic erythropoiesis confirms the presence of a myeloproliferative disorder rather than reactive thrombocytosis. PET can also identify unusual sites of erythropoiesis, for example in retrosternal tissue or lymph nodes.

The indications for ^{52}Fe imaging are the same as for ^{59}Fe surface counting. However, the possibilities with ^{52}Fe extend beyond ^{59}Fe surface counting, such as the demonstration of deep internal sites of erythropoiesis. Although PET imaging maximizes the value of ^{52}Fe, the physical half-life of 8 hours is long enough for the isotope to be exported from a cyclotron and imaged with a rectilinear scanner or a gamma-camera fitted with a high-energy collimator suitable for 511 KeV photons.

INVESTIGATION OF MEGALOBLASTIC ANAEMIA

Patients with a macrocytic anaemia and low serum vitamin B_{12}, or incidental finding of a consistently low serum vitamin B_{12}, need to be investigated to determine the cause as dietary deficiency, gastric malabsorption or ileal malabsorption. Increasingly, this is performed using a kit (Dicopac test, Amersham International) that combines the traditional parts 1 and 2 of a Schilling test. The 24-hour urinary excretions of 'free' ^{58}Co-labelled cyanocobalamin and ^{57}Co-labelled cyanocobalamin prebound to human gastric juice, both administered orally, are compared after a saturating dose of 1 mg intramuscular B_{12}. The normal 24-hour urinary excretion of ^{57}Co is >12% and of ^{58}Co, 11%. The ratio of ^{58}Co to ^{57}Co in urine should be >1.3. An increased ratio suggests gastric malabsorption, while reduced excretion of both agents with a urine ratio of <1.3 suggests ileal malabsorption. The two main causes of error or uncertainty are incomplete 24-hour urine collection, and subnormal excretion of both isotopes but with a ^{58}Co/^{57}Co ratio of >1.3. The latter is thought to be due to B_{12} deficiency secondary to ileal malabsorption. The manufacturer recommends that, although ratios of >1.3 are abnormal, only a ratio of >1.7 can be confidently ascribed to low intrinsic factor, but this is probably too stringent. The subject is reviewed by Atrah and Davidson [14], who suggest that a ratio of >1.3 is always suggestive of intrinsic factor deficiency except when the 24-hour urine collection is grossly deficient (<500 ml).

STUDIES BASED ON LABELLED PROTEINS

PLASMA VOLUME

Plasma volume can be measured with several radiolabelled proteins, including ^{59}Fe-transferrin, although it is usually measured with ^{125}I-labelled human serum albumin (HSA). As for red cell volume, the technique is based on the dilution principle. Plasma ^{125}I concentration, measured in samples taken at 10, 20 and 30 minutes after injection, is plotted logarithmically as a function of time in order to establish the fractional rate of loss of albumin from the intravascular compartment. Plasma volume is then calculated from the injected dose and the extrapolated zero-time plasma ^{125}I concentration. The plasma volume should always be measured independently of the red cell volume in patients with a raised haematocrit to identify patients with pseudo-polycythaemia (relative polycythaemia).

GASTROINTESTINAL PROTEIN LOSS

Protein-losing enteropathy can be diagnosed and quantified by measuring the faecal excretion of intravenously injected ^{51}Cr-labelled albumin, analogously to the measurement of gastrointestinal bleeding with ^{51}Cr-labelled red cells. ^{111}In-labelled transferrin can also be used and combined with imaging in order to localize the site of loss. Whole-body counting for quantification of gastrointestinal protein loss is also possible with ^{111}In-transferrin [10]. For localization by imaging without quantification, the best agent may be ^{99m}Tc-labelled human immunoglobulin, which is more stable than ^{99m}Tc-HSA and thereby minimizes pitfalls such as the gastrointestinal secretion of free pertechnetate.

RADIOLABELLED PLATELETS

Studies based on labelled platelets include measurements of platelet production rate, mean platelet life span and splenic platelet pooling. They are generally used in the investigation of thrombocy-topenia. Radionuclides for platelet labelling are the same as those for red cell labelling: ^{51}Cr, ^{111}In, ^{113m}In and ^{99m}Tc. ^{51}Cr offers no advantages over ^{111}In and is now obsolete for this application partly because it has an accelerated rate of elution from platelets coated with immunoglobulin. Furthermore, measurement of platelet life span (normally 9 days) should be accompanied by imaging for the identification of the sites of platelet destruction. ^{111}In is the isotope of choice for platelet kinetic studies [15]. When it was available, ^{113m}In was used for short-term studies, mainly related to splenic function.

PLATELET LABELLING WITH ^{111}In

The volume of blood required is not critical, although for thrombocytopenic patients, up to 100 ml may be necessary; about 25 ml is required for patients with normal counts. The blood should be taken into a syringe already containing acid citrate dextrose (NIH formula A) (1 part/7 parts whole blood). Following separation from whole blood by gentle centrifugation at 200 g, platelet-rich plasma (PRP) is further acidified with ACD (1 volume to 10 volumes). The PRP is then centrifuged at 850 g to pellet the platelets. Platelets undergo irreversible clumping if the PRP is not acidified. The pellet is resuspended in 1 ml platelet-poor plasma (PPP) and indium chelate added, preferably ^{111}In-tropolonate. Adequate labelling is achieved after 5 minutes, following which 5–10 ml of acidified PPP is added. After centrifugation at 850 g, the supernatant is discarded and the platelets resuspended in 5 ml PPP for reinjection.

SPLENIC PLATELET POOLING

Platelet pooling within the spleen is a poorly understood, and little studied – but very prominent – physiological phenomenon, which results in the platelet spending about one-third of its entire life span within the spleen. Increased platelet pooling in the spleen is an important cause of thrombocy-topenia [16], although thrombocytopenia due to abnormal pooling is more often over-diagnosed than under-diagnosed. Platelet pooling in the spleen is much more pronounced than red cell pooling in that the mean intrasplenic transit time is about 10 minutes (very similar to labelled granulocytes), in contrast to <1 minute for red cells. Abnormal platelet pooling in the enlarged spleen results from increased splenic blood flow rather than increased platelet transit time through the spleen [17]. This applies to splenomegaly of almost any cause, although very occasionally an enlarged spleen is associated with a normal-sized splenic platelet pool. Increased pooling in a normal-sized spleen as a result of increased splenic blood flow has been described in some rheumatological disorders [17a].

The size of the splenic platelet pool as a fraction of the total platelet population is most easily measured from the blood disappearance curve following injection of labelled platelets which equilibrate between the splenic platelet pool and the circulating blood. For a normal-sized spleen, this takes about 30 minutes, but is faster in splenomegaly. The enlarged spleen has an increased blood flow, which on theoretical grounds, would be expected to accelerate equilibration. The reason why red cells equilibrate more slowly in the enlarged compared with normal spleen is not entirely clear, but is probably related to the existence of a red cell pool with a slow turnover, which is not present in the normal spleen. As a result of net entry into the splenic platelet pool, the concentration of labelled platelets in blood decreases after injection over a period of about 30 minutes, to a value representing the fraction of the injected dose (the recovery, R) present in blood at equilibrium. So

$$R = \frac{\text{total blood volume} \times \text{concentration/ml wholeblood}}{\text{injected dose}}$$

Since almost all the viable non-circulating, labelled platelets are in the spleen, apart from about 5% sequestered in the liver, the splenic platelet pool (SPP), as a fraction of the total platelet population, is approximately equal to $1 - R$. In the normal subject, R is 0.6–0.7 but may be as low as 0.1 in a patient with massive splenomegaly.

Separating splenic blood flow from platelet transit time in the evaluation of the splenic platelet pool requires dynamic scintigraphy over the spleen and cardiac blood pool, with measurement of the rate constant of equilibration of labelled platelets between the splenic platelet pool and circulating blood (Figure 14.5). Provided that platelets are not significantly removed from the circulation by another organ (either by pooling,

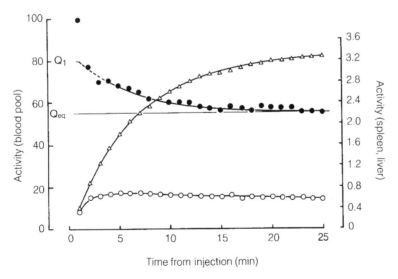

Figure 14.5 Time-activity curves recorded in regions-of-interest over the cardiac blood pool (●), liver (○) and spleen (Δ) in a normal subject following injection of ^{111}In-labelled platelets. Ordinate (left): percentage of maximum (blood pool); ordinate (right): counts per frame per pixel (liver and spleen). The subject was supine with the gamma-camera below. The blood pool curve approaches an asymptote (Q_{eq}) which represents the recovery. Extrapolation of the blood pool curve to 1 minute yields Q_1, which represents the total activity equilibrating between the blood and splenic pools, such that at equilibrium (reached at 20–25 minutes), splenic activity is represented by Q_1-Q_{eq} and blood activity by Q_{eq}. (Reprinted from *Thrombosis and Haemostasis*.)

sequestration or destruction), then the rate constant of equilibration, k_s, is equal to the sum of k_{in} and k_{out} where k_{in} is the ratio of splenic blood flow to total blood volume and k_{out} is the reciprocal of the mean splenic platelet transit time. The ratio k_{in}/k_{out} can be obtained from the quantity, Q_{eq}, of platelets in the spleen at equilibrium (Figure 14.5), since k_{in}/k_{out} is equal to the ratio of respective quantities of labelled platelets in the spleen and blood. Thus

$$\frac{k_{in}}{k_{out}} = \frac{Q_1 - Q_{eq}}{Q_{eq}}$$

where Q_1 is the blood pool signal at 1 minute (Figure 14.5) and $k_{in} + k_{out} = k_s$.

k_{in}, which reflects splenic blood flow, is increased in splenomegaly whereas k_{out}, which reflects mean intrasplenic platelet transit time, tends to remain unchanged [17]. The sum $k_{in} + k_{out}$ is therefore elevated, leading to early equilibration (Figure 14.6).

PLATELET PRODUCTION RATE

Although platelet production rate (PPR) can be measured by cohort labelling, it is almost exclusively measured by random labelling as part of a platelet life span study. Assuming similar platelet production and destruction rates, it then equals the ratio of the total circulating platelet population to the platelet life span, i.e. as a number/litre of blood per day. The total platelet population is not simply represented by the peripheral count but also includes the splenic platelet pool (SPP), measurement of which is therefore necessary for the calculation of PPR from mean platelet life span. Then

$$PPR = \frac{\text{peripheral platelet count}}{MPLS \times (1 - SPP)}$$

This is approximately equal to

$$\frac{\text{peripheral platelet count}}{MPLS \times R}$$

MEAN PLATELET LIFE SPAN (MPLS)

Platelet life span is based on blood samples taken after equilibration of platelets between the circulating blood and splenic platelet pool. If at the time of labelling: (i) the age distribution of platelets in the sample is the same as in the subject's total platelet population; (ii) the affinity for the label is independent of platelet age; (iii) there is no elution or reutilization of label; (iv) there is no significant spread of platelet life spans; and (v) no platelets are destroyed at random, then the graph of platelet-associated radioactivity in post-injection

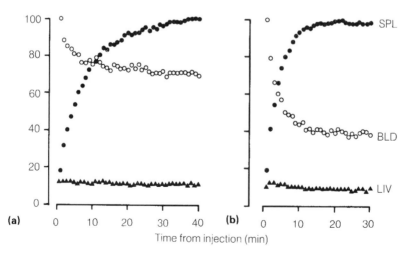

(a)   0   10   20   30   40   (b)   0   10   20   30

Time from injection (min)

Figure 14.6   Time–activity curves recorded in regions-of-interest over the cardiac blood pool (○), liver (▲) and spleen (●) following injection of ^{111}In-labelled platelets in a norml subject (a) and a patient with splenomegaly (b). Ordinate (blood pool): percentage of initial value; ordinate (liver and spleen): percentage of maximal splenic activity (counts per pixel per frame). Note the lower recovery and earlier equilibration between blood and splenic platelet pool in splenomegaly.

blood samples will be a straight line over time, decreasing with a gradient proportional to platelet destruction rate and cutting the time axis at a point equal to the platelet life span. In normal subjects, the platelet disappearance profile is very close to linearity and gives a platelet life span of about 9 days. When mean platelet life span is reduced as a result of disease, the profile becomes curvilinear and cuts the time axis earlier than 9 days. The curvilinearity means that the platelet life spans are non-uniform and implies an element of random destruction. Cutting the time axis earlier than 9 days indicates a reduction in maximum life span (this is the life span of a platelet that avoids random destruction and is finally removed only when it is senescent – so-called deterministic life span). Methods for measuring the MPLS under these circumstances are rather complex and include the gamma function fitting method of Murphy and Francis [18] and the equation based on the studies of Mills [19] and Dornhorst [20], for computing the probability of random destruction [21]. When the MPLS is severely reduced, the mathematics become simple again because the destruction is almost exclusively random and can be described as a simple monoexponential function. Under these circumstances, MPLS is equal to the reciprocal of the rate constant of destruction, which itself is equal to the natural logarithm of 2 divided by the $t_{1/2}$.

The most important role for measurement of MPLS is in idiopathic thrombocytopenic purpura and other causes of obscure thrombocytopenia in which the clinical problem is to distinguish between a production defect and/or a reduced platelet life span. A megakaryocyte-rich bone marrow does not necessarily indicate that thrombocytopenia is due to reduced platelet life span. The third general cause for thrombocytopenia is an increased splenic platelet pool. The spleen has to be considerably enlarged to produce a thrombocytopenia of any real severity.

Isolation of platelets in sufficient numbers for labelling with ^{111}In is difficult when the platelet count is below about 50000/mm³, and is virtually impossible below about 10000/mm³, necessitating the use of homologous platelets. The pathophysiological interpretation of a platelet kinetic study is facilitated if labelled autologous, rather than homologous, platelets are used. For instance, a thrombocytopenic patient who has acquired antiplatelet antibodies may destroy homologous platelets in the liver but autologous platelets in the spleen. Nevertheless, it is occasionally useful to determine where transfused platelets are destroyed in patients whose platelet increments are sustained for only a few hours (or even minutes) after transfusion.

IMAGING SITES OF PLATELET DESTRUCTION

Identification of abnormal platelet destruction in the spleen is based on ^{111}In-labelled platelets. Isotope elution from both platelets and their ultimate sites of deposition is very slow. Identifying sites of platelet destruction is usually combined with measurement of the splenic platelet pool and MPLS. An interesting feature of platelet destruction in the spleen is that, in the absence of

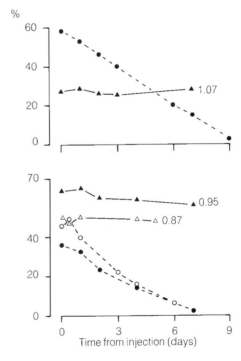

Figure 14.7 Time–activity curves based on peripheral venous blood samples (●) and a region-of-interest over the spleen (▲) following injection of ^{111}In-labelled platelets in a normal subject (upper panel) and two patients with splenomegaly and reduced platelet survival (lower panel). Ordinate: percentage of injected dose. The figures are the $D:P$ ratios, and indicate that in each case the spleen destroys almost the same fraction of the total platelet population as it pools. (Reprinted from *British Journal of Haematology*.)

anti-platelet antibodies, its magnitude is matched by the capacity of the splenic platelet pool. Thus, in the normal subject, about 30% of circulating platelets are pooled in the spleen and about 35% are destroyed there. As pooling increases in splenomegaly, so does the fraction of platelets destroyed in the spleen. This means that the extent of platelet destruction in the spleen increases appropriately as spleen size increases [17] (Figure 14.7).

Several techniques have been used to quantify platelet destruction in the spleen. When ^{51}Cr was used, 'excess' counts were measured in the spleen using a scintillation probe and surface counting, analogously to the excess counts in a ^{51}Cr-labelled red cell study. This is the difference between total counts in the spleen and those due to labelled platelets pooling in the spleen. The latter fraction is obtainable from the circulating activity. Thus, since the pooled platelets and circulating platelets are in equilibrium, the ratio of the count rate recorded over the spleen (as soon as equilibration is achieved before there has been significant destruction) to the count rate in circulating blood can be used to calculate the fraction of the subsequent splenic signal that is due to platelet pooling.

Perhaps the most rational approach to quantification of platelet destruction in the spleen is a comparison of the counts at the time when all the labelled platelets have disappeared from the circulation (which reflects destruction) with the counts at the time of equilibration after the platelets are injected (which reflects pooling). This destruction:pooling ratio is then a measure of destruction which takes into account the tendency for destruction to be increased appropriately in splenomegaly [17]. Re-direction of destruction towards or away from the spleen, as induced by antiplatelet antibodies, will give ratios respectively less than or greater than unity (Figure 14.8). The technique becomes less sensitive for detecting abnormal splenic destruction as the spleen enlarges, since there is less 'room' for an increased destruction:pooling ratio. The reverse of this, i.e. detection of abnormal destruction elsewhere would, however, be enhanced. Increased destruction: pooling ratios are seen in ITP with splenic destruction and patients who have developed antibodies to homologous labelled platelets. Decreased destruction:pooling ratios are seen in patients with abnormalities resulting in hepatic destruc-

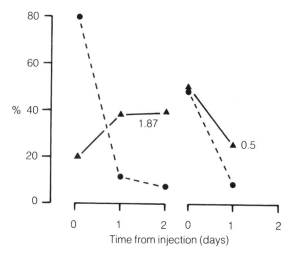

Figure 14.8 Platelet kinetics in severe ITP. Left panel: this patient has markedly reduced ^{111}In-labelled platelet survival (based on peripheral blood sampling, ●) and splenic activity (▲) which increase during the course of ^{111}In-labelled platelet removal from blood. Right panel: this patient also had markedly reduced platelet survival, but in this case the splenic activity falls. Ordinate: percentage of injected dose. The numbers shown are the destruction:pooling ratios.

tion or in patients with thrombocytopenia due to peripheral platelet consumption.

Non-immune causes include: (i) intrinsic platelet defects; (ii) abnormalities of the circulation, such as prosthetic valves or severe atherosclerosis, which lead to premature platelet senility; and (iii) abnormal peripheral consumption as in thrombotic dyscrasias and arterial disease.

INTERPRETATION OF THROMBOCYTOPENIA

Although there are many causes of moderate thrombocytopenia, they can be divided into three categories:

1. Failure of production.
2. Increased pooling in an enlarged spleen.
3. Increased destruction or consumption.

Increased destruction is further subdivided into immune and non-immune causes. In the clinical setting, examination of the bone marrow and testing for anti-platelet antibodies is usually sufficient to identify the cause. The non-immune causes of destruction include: (i) abnormalities of the circulation, such as prosthetic heart valves and severe atherosclerosis, which lead to premature platelet senility, and haemangiomas; and (ii) microangiopathic disorders such as thrombotic thrombocytopenic purpura, haemolytic uraemic syndrome, pre-eclampsia and malignant hypertension. In some congenital disorders, such as Bernard–Soulier syndrome and May–Hegglin anomaly, the cause is unclear. Failure of production may be difficult to identify in early myelodysplastic disorders when morphological changes are not yet fully developed. It is also becoming clearer that in chronic viral hepatitis, especially hepatitis C, there may be thrombocytopenia as a result of reduced production, despite normal megakaryocyte numbers and only moderate splenomegaly. Splenunculi in idiopathic immune thrombocytopenia relapsing after splenectomy are most appropriately detected by imaging with ^{111}In-labelled platelets, which can be used at the same time to quantify platelet kinetics, although more easily with ^{99m}Tc-labelled HDRBC in the severely thrombocytopenic patient.

The splenic platelet pool (SPP), as a fraction of the total circulating platelet population, is slightly less than the difference between the recovery and unity, and is normally about one-third. Because of significant early hepatic uptake, the SPP is more reliably obtained by dynamic camera imaging, as described above, when a correction for hepatic uptake can be made.

Splenomegaly causes thrombocytopenia by a dilutional effect. This thrombocytopenic tendency can be quantified as an equivalent reduction in MPLS. For example, the blood platelet volume is normally about twice the splenic platelet volume. A fourfold increase in splenic platelet volume would, in the absence of a thrombopoietic response, reverse this ratio, give an SPP of two-thirds of the total circulating platelet volume, a recovery of about 30%, and halve the peripheral platelet count. This would be the thrombocytopenic equivalent of a reduction in MPLS to half normal. If thrombopoiesis is sensitive to the total platelet population (the platelet biomass) rather than the peripheral platelet count (P) then the latter can be predicted from the size of the SPP from

$$P = \frac{[1 - SPP] \times P(norm)}{[1 - SPP(norm)]}$$

P(norm) is the platelet count that would result from a reduced MPLS in the absence of splenomegaly. To whatever extent platelet production is regulated by the peripheral platelet count, then increased thrombopoiesis would tend to reverse thrombocytopenia resulting from splenomegaly.

RADIOLABELLED LEUCOCYTES

The main clinical use for labelled leucocytes is the localization of inflammatory foci and abscesses. Leucocytes have a wide range of life spans, though that of an individual leucocyte is generally much longer than the time it spends in the circulation. A neutrophil for instance matures in bone marrow over about 15 days before release into the circulation and may survive for up to 4 days in the tissues if it undergoes extravascular migration. Its intravascular residence time, however, is only about 10 hours. In general, *in vitro* haematological tests based on labelled granulocytes are seldom used clinically. Thus, a reduced granulocyte residence time in the circulation is not recognized as a cause of granulocytopenia, which is usually due to deficient production and occasionally to increased splenic pooling. Increased intravascular granulocyte residence time may be recorded in rare diseases where there is deficient expression of endothelial adhesion molecules and therefore a deficiency in extravascular granulocyte migration [22].

Methods for labelling leucocytes for imaging inflammation are described elsewhere in this book. For haematological studies on granulocyte kinetics, it is essential to label 'pure' granulocytes, which can be separated from a mixed leucocyte population by density gradient centrifugation. Columns may be made from Ficoll-hypaque, Metrizamide or Percoll. Because granulocytes are very sensitive to *in vitro* manipulation, especially isolation from plasma, the columns should be diluted to the appropriate densities using autologous plasma rather than saline. It is not possible to do this with Ficoll since commercial preparations are not dense enough to be diluted with plasma. After removal from the column and washing in plasma, the granulocytes are labelled with ^{111}In using essentially the same approach as for platelets.

Granulocytes activated *in vitro* during labelling undergo prolonged lung transit, probably as a result of cell stiffness, and are removed prematurely from the circulation, mainly by the liver. The distribution of activity between the liver and spleen is comparable with that seen after injection of colloidal materials. Activation is promoted by complete isolation from plasma. In contrast, the normal early distribution of granulocytes is dominated by pooling in the reticuloendothelial system, especially the spleen and bone marrow, and to a lesser extent the liver and lungs [23]. Transit time through the spleen is very similar to that of platelets. Normally, granulocytes are removed from blood by the reticuloendothelial system; blood disappearance is exponential with a $t_{1/2}$ of 7 hours. Extravascular migration into tissues only occurs in inflammation.

Granulocyte activation *in vivo*, which is probably cytokine-mediated, is a feature of several systemic inflammatory diseases including inflammatory bowel disease, systemic vasculitis and graft-versus-host disease, and can be quantified by several techniques, most simply by shape change [24]. Using labelling techniques which do not themselves cause activation, *in vivo* activation is associated with a granulocyte distribution significantly different from that seen following activation *in vitro*. Physiological splenic pooling is retained, liver activity is not increased and pulmonary activity remains elevated in proportion to the circulating activity, a relationship compatible with dynamic equilibrium of cells between the pulmonary vascular pool and whole body pool. Thus, although increased lung accumulation is seen with *in vivo* activation, granulocyte distribution is otherwise physiological with a normal recovery.

With recent improvements in labelling techniques and ability to image activated endothelium [25], granulocyte kinetic studies may be exploited more widely in the investigation of blood disorders associated with abnormalities of granulocytes or endothelium.

BONE MARROW IMAGING

Bone marrow sinusoids are lined by fenestrated endothelium with a high permeability to macromolecules. Blood is supplied to marrow through a portal system via a periosteal network that also supplies bone. Several haematological disorders involving bone marrow, especially granulocytic leukaemia and myelofibrosis, give rise to bone scans with superscan features as a result of increased marrow flow. Normal mean bone perfusion measured with PET shows regional variations around a value of about 10 ml/minute/100 ml. Total bone blood flow is difficult to measure but is about 300 ml/minute.

There are two cellular systems within bone marrow, coexisting throughout red (active) marrow: the reticuloendothelial system (RES) and the haematopoietic system. The distribution of active marrow throughout the skeleton varies with age. Although usually confined to the central skeleton in the adult, experience with bone marrow imaging has shown that occasionally it extends into the shafts of long bones. Active marrow can be imaged using tracers which target either of the systems, although in disease – aplastic anaemia for example – the distribution of the two systems may be divergent.

The indications for bone marrow imaging include: (i) evaluation of a haematological disorder, often as part of a ferrokinetic study; (ii) detection of malignant infiltration either from a haematological malignancy such as lymphoma or myeloma or from metastases, which initially infiltrate marrow; and (iii) to complement another imaging procedure, for example identification of active bone marrow in the interpretation of a white cell scan performed for musculoskeletal infection or suspected marrow infarction showing increased uptake on a bone scan.

Radiolabelled colloids target the RES, including bone marrow. Small-particle size colloids, such as antimony sulphur colloid, have a relative selectivity for marrow. Radionuclides of iron target the haematopoietic component; high-resolution images of sites of erythropoiesis can be obtained by PET using ^{52}Fe, although the high radiation dose limits the amount that can be given. ^{111}In-transferrin is taken up by both components and cannot therefore be used as a surrogate for iron. Indeed, Chipping *et al.* [26] observed a distribution of ^{111}In and ^{52}Fe that was concordant in only two of 15 patients with various haematological conditions. Granulocytes pool in bone marrow with kinetics similar to those in the spleen [27]. Radiolabelled leucocytes therefore give clear images of bone marrow within minutes to hours of injection, becoming more prominent over 24 hours. Because of its wide distribution, granulocyte pooling in the bone marrow is not as obvious as in the spleen. Nevertheless, the size of the marrow pool is comparable with that of the spleen since the mean granulocyte transit times through, and total blood flows of the two organs are broadly similar.

Labelled anti-granulocyte monoclonal antibodies, recently developed for imaging inflammation, give very prominent images of bone marrow because of the large size of the myeloid cell population expressing the appropriate antigens and are currently the imaging agent of choice for the marrow. Indeed, only a tiny fraction of antibody labels the circulating granulocytes, which is not surprising when it is recalled that normally the maturation time in bone marrow is 15 days compared with a granulocyte life span in the circulation of 10 hours. These antibodies, if they become more generally available, have the potential to become much more widely used in the management of patients with cancer [28].

REFERENCES

1. Dacie, J.V. and Lewis, S.M. (1991) *Practical Haematology*, 7th edn, Churchill-Livingstone, Edinburgh.
2. Radia, R., Peters, A.M., Deenmamode, M. *et al.* (1981) Measurement of red cell volume and splenic red cell pool using 133 m-indium. *Br. J. Haematol.*, **49**, 587–91.
3. Marsh, J.C.W., Liu Yin, J.A. and Lewis, S.M. (1987) Blood volume measurements in polycythaemia: when and why? *Clin. Lab. Haematol.*, **9**, 452–6.
4. Pearson, T.C., Guthrie, D.L., Simpson, J. *et al.* (1994) Interpretation of measured red cell mass and plasma volume in adults: expert panel on radionuclides of the International Council for Standardization in Haematology. *Br. J. Haematol.*, **89**, 748–56.
5. Toghill, P. (1964) Red cell pooling in enlarged spleens. *Br. J. Haematol.*, **10**, 347–57
6. Peters, A.M., Ryan, P.F.J., Klonizakis, I. *et al.* (1982) Kinetics of heat damaged autologous red blood cells. Mechanisms of clearance from blood. *Scand. J. Haematol.*, **28**, 5–14.
7. Klausner, M.A., Hirsch, L.J., Leblond, P.F. *et al.* (1975) Contrasting splenic mechanisms in the blood clearance of red blood cells and colloidal particles. *Blood*, **46**, 965–76.
8. Peters, A.M., Walport, M.J., Elkon, K.B. *et al.* (1984) The comparative blood clearance kinetics of modified radiolabelled erythrocytes. *Clin. Sci.*, **66**, 55–62.
9. Elkon, K.B., Ferjencik, P.P., Walport, M.J. *et al.* (1982) Evaluation of heat damaged and IgG-coated red cells for testing reticulo-endothelial function. *J. Immunol. Methods*, **55**, 253–63.
10. Carpani de Kaski, M., Peters, A.M., Bradley, D. and Hodgson, H.J.F. (1996) Detection and quantification of protein-losing enteropathy with indium-111-transferrin. *Eur. J. Nucl. Med.*, **23**, 530–3.
11. Carpani de Kaski, M., Peters, A.M., Knight, D. *et al.* (1992) In-111 whole body retention: a new method for quantification of disease activity in inflammatory bowel disease. *J. Nucl. Med.*, **33**, 756–62.
12. Heyns, A. du P., Lotter, M.G., Kotze, H.F. *et al.* (1985) Kinetics, distribution and sites of destruction of ^{111}In-oxine labelled red cells in haemolytic anaemia. *J. Clin. Pathol.*, **38**, 128–32.
13. Cavill, I. (1986) Plasma clearance studies. *Methods Haematol.*, **14**, 214–44.
14. Atrah, H.I. and Davidson, R.J.L. (1989) A survey and critical evaluation of a dual isotope (Dicopac) vitamin B12 absorption test. *Eur. J. Nucl. Med.*, **15**, 57–60.
15. Heyns, A. du P., Lotter, M.G., Badenhorst, P.N. *et al.* (1980) Kinetics, distribution and sites of destruction of indium-111 labelled platelets. *Br. J. Haematol.*, **44**, 269–80.
16. Harker, L.A. and Finch, C.A. (1969) Thrombokinetics in man. *J. Clin. Invest.*, **48**, 963–74.
17. Peters, A.M., Saverymuttu, S.H., Wonke, B. *et al.* (1984) The interpretation of platelet kinetic studies for the identification of sites of abnormal platelet destruction. *Br. J. Haematol.*, **57**, 637–49.
17a. Walport, M.J., Peters, A.M., Elkon, E.B. *et al.* (1985) The splenic extraction ratio of antibody coated erythrocytes and its response to plasma exchange and pulse methylprednisolone. *Clin. Exp. Immunol.*, **65**, 465–73.
18. Murphy, E.A. and Francis, M.E. (1971) The estimation of blood platelet survival II. The multiple hit model. *Thromb. Diath. Haemorrh*, **25**, 53–80.
19. Mills, J.N. (1946) The life span of the erythrocyte. *J. Physiol.*, **105**, 16P–17P.
20. Dornhorst, A.C. (1961) The interpretation of red cell survival curves. *Blood*, **6**, 1284–92.
21. Schilling, R.F., Ferrant, A., Cavill, I. *et al.* (1988) Recommended method for indium-111 platelet survival studies. *J. Nucl. Med.*, **29**, 564–6.
22. Davies, K.A., Toothill, V.J., Savill, J. *et al.* (1991) A 19-year-old man with leucocyte adhesion deficiency. *In vitro* and *in vivo* studies of leucocyte function. *Clin. Exp. Immunol.*, **84**, 223–31.
23. Peters, A.M., Saverymuttu, S.H., Keshavarzian, A. *et al.* (1985) Splenic pooling of granulocytes. *Clin. Sci.*, **68**, 283–9.
24. Haslett, C., Guthrie, L.A., Kopaniak, M.M. *et al.* (1985) Modulation of the multiple neutrophil functions by preparative methods of trace concentrations of bacterial lipopolysaccharide. *Am. J. Pathol.*, **119**, 101–10.
25. Chapman, P.T., Jamar, F., Keelan, E.T.M. *et al.* (1996) Imaging endothelial activation in inflammation using a radiolabelled monoclonal antibody against E-selectin. *Arthr. Rheum.*, **39**, 1371–5.
26. Chipping, P., Klonizakis, I. and Lewis, S.M. (1980) Indium chloride scanning: a comparison with iron as a tracer for erythropoiesis. *Clin. Lab. Haematol.*, **2**, 255–63.
27. Ussov, Yu., Aktolun, C., Myers, M.J. *et al.* (1995) Granulocyte margination in bone marrow: comparison with margination in the spleen and liver. *Scand. J. Clin. Lab. Invest.*, **55**, 87–96.
28. Reske, S.N. (1994) Marrow scintigraphy, in *Nuclear Medicine in Clinical Diagnosis and Treatment* (eds I.P.C. Murray and P.J. Ell), Churchill Livingstone, Edinburgh, pp. 705–9.

Lymphoscintigraphy

H. M. Abdel-Dayem,
Q. H. Siraj and B. D. Collier

INTRODUCTION

Lymphoscintigraphy, the radionuclide technique of imaging the lymphatic system using interstitially injected particulate radiopharmaceuticals, was introduced more than four decades ago [1–3]. During this period, with technological developments in nuclear medicine equipment and the introduction of improved radiopharmaceuticals, the technique has evolved into an important diagnostic tool for the evaluation of the lymphatic system.

The different modalities currently available for evaluating the lymphatic system include radiocontrast lymphoangiography, computed tomography (CT), ultrasound (US), magnetic resonance imaging (MRI) and radionuclide lymphoscintigraphy. Although radiocontrast lymphoangiography gives the best morphological assessment of the lymphatic system, it is contraindicated in cases of oedema and carries the risk of pulmonary embolism. In addition, the technique is tedious and lengthy as the contrast medium has to be injected directly into a lymph vessel. Computed tomography can conveniently and accurately outline the lymphatic morphology but is limited by its inability to dynamically evaluate the kinetics to lymphatic flow. The structural imaging modalities (CT, US and MRI) can accurately delineate enlarged lymph nodes, but lymphoscintigraphy has the advantage of differentiating between normal lymph nodes, non-malignant hyperplastic nodes and normal-sized neoplastic nodes.

Lymphoscintigraphy is a simple and non-invasive functional test for the evaluation of the lymphatic system. The safety, ease-of-performance and the benign nature of the technique has contributed to its popularity. The present role of lymphoscintigraphy in clinical oncology as well as in the evaluation of benign disease(s), especially for the assessment of lymphatic functional status in patients presenting with lymphoedema are discussed in this chapter.

RELEVANT ANATOMY AND PATHOPHYSIOLOGY

ANATOMY

There are two main components of the lymphatic system: the lymphatic channels and the lymph nodes. Lymph is drained through an extensive network of lymph capillaries, which join to form the thin-walled lymphatic vessels that are beaded in appearance due to the presence of numerous valves and vary from 0.5–1.0 mm in diameter. The lymph vessels usually accompany veins (draining the same areas) and are interrupted by lymph nodes that act as lymph filters. The wall of the lymphatic capillary is made of a single layer of loosely connected endothelial cells that are attached to the surrounding connective tissue by anchoring filaments. The edges of adjacent endothelial cells usually overlap to form a minute valve that is free to flap inwards. These open junctions allow passage of fluid and large molecules; smaller molecules pass directly through the endothelial cell membrane into the lymphatic lumen.

In the extremities, there are two systems of lymphatics: the deep system (underneath the deep fascia and in the muscles) and the superficial system (in the subcutaneous tissues and the skin). The skin is richer in lymphatics than the subcutaneous tissues.

Superficial lymphatics from the upper limb converge either medially along the axillary veins or laterally along the cephalic veins to the axillary and infraclavicular lymph nodes before proceeding to the supraclavicular nodes and the thoracic duct.

In the lower limbs, the lymphatic channels in the superficial compartment converge medially and follow the long saphenous vein to drain into the lower and upper inguinal lymph nodes, then proceed to the external iliac, internal iliac, retroperitoneal and posterior thoracic chain nodes, and finally into the thoracic duct.

The body trunks are divided into four zones by a vertical mid-line anteriorly and posteriorly, and a transverse line across the umbilicus. Lymphatics drain away from the mid-line in these different regions, converge to the corresponding axillary or inguinal lymph nodes, and there is a watershed

Clinical Nuclear Medicine, 3rd edn. Edited by M.N. Maisey, K.E. Britton and B.D. Collier. Published in 1998 by Chapman & Hall, London. ISBN 0 412 75180 1

area 2.5cm (1 inch) on either side of the mid-line anteriorly and posteriorly and on each side of a transverse line running across the umbilicus. Lymphatic drainage from this watershed area, can cross the mid-line to both the ipsilateral or the contralateral axillary or inguinal lymph nodes. A lesion in the peri-umbilical area may drain to both the axillary and the inguinal lymph nodes.

PHYSIOLOGY OF LYMPH FORMATION AND FLOW

The interstitial fluid formation is regulated by pressures acting across the capillaries, i.e. the hydrostatic pressure and the colloid osmotic pressure. The average filtration of the fluid by the capillaries exceeds the reabsorption. This excess amounts to 2–4 litres of interstitial fluid containing 100g of plasma proteins. This fluid (i.e. lymph) is removed by the lymphatic channels, filtered by the lymph nodes, and finally drained back into the intravascular circulation through the thoracic duct. A total of approximately 120ml of lymph flows per hour into the circulation in the normal resting state.

Flow against gravity in the lymphatic channels is achieved in part by the lymphatic pump. Valves exist in all lymph channels; they allow the flow of lymph in only one direction, i.e. towards the thoracic duct. Each segment of the lymph vessel between successive valves functions as a separate automatic pump. When a lymph vessel becomes stretched with fluid, an increased intra-lymphatic pressure initiates contraction of the smooth muscle in the wall of the vessel, thereby opening the lymphatic valves allowing movement of the lymph into the adjacent lymphatic segment. This is followed by relaxation of the walls of the lymphatic channel, which generates a negative pressure, with subsequent closure of the proximal valves and opening of the distal valves. This sequence of contraction and relaxation of the lymphatic channels normally occurs every 2–3 three minutes. These successive contractions of the lymphatic segments help to propel lymph along the lymphatic channels.

Lymphatic capillaries are also capable of pumping lymph. Each time excess fluid causes the tissues to swell, the anchoring filaments attached to the lymphatic capillary pull it open and allow fluid to flow into the capillary through the junctions between the endothelial cells. Then, when the tissue is compressed, the pressure inside the capillary increases and tends to push the fluid forward into the collecting lymphatic.

In addition to the pumping caused by intrinsic contraction of the lymph vessel wall, any external factor that compresses the lymph vessel can also cause lymph propagation. In order of importance, these factors include contraction of the skeletal muscles, movements of body parts, arterial pulsations, negative intrathoracic pressure generated by respiratory movement and compression of the tissues by objects outside the body. Because of these factors, the lymph flow increases 10- to 30-fold above the basal resting value during exercise.

AETIOLOGY AND PATHOGENESIS OF LYMPHOEDEMA

A balance between extravascular diffusion, reabsorption and drainage through the lymphatics is normally maintained, with an imbalance often leading to swelling and oedema. The different factors involved in the aetiology of oedema include: increased capillary pressure, decreased plasma protein concentration, lymphatic obstruction, increased capillary permeability and sodium retention.

Lymphoedema is a progressive condition characterized by an excess of tissue proteins, oedema, chronic inflammation and fibrosis. Early in the course of the disease, reversible oedematous components predominate, but persistent oedema promotes chronic inflammation and irreversible fibrosis. Complications of lymphoedema include lymphocutaneous fistula, elephantiasis, and angiosarcoma. Lymphoedema can be due to congenital conditions like lymphatic aplasia, hypoplasia, or lymphangiectasia; but is more commonly due to secondary factors such as infection, inflammation, trauma, malignancy and iatrogenic causes (e.g. post-surgical or irradiation-induced).

Venous lymphoedema may result from increased lymph production either secondary to venous obstruction or due to increased venous pressure. Increased venous pressure leading to leg oedema can be due to congestive heart failure, an incompetent venous system (as in varicose veins) leading to venous stasis, or increased pressure within the lymphatics and veins such as might be caused by pelvic tumours.

Lymphoedema might be due to increased production of lymph beyond the capacity of reabsorption and drainage by the lymphatics – for example, inflammatory or traumatic lymphoedema.

Obstructive lymphoedema often is due to replacement of the lymph nodes by metastatic tumour. Lymphatic obstruction leading to obstructive lymphoedema also can be due to filariasis, repeated subcutaneous infections, post-operative or post-radiotherapy fibrosis.

RADIOPHARMACEUTICALS

An ideal radiopharmaceutical for lymphoscintigraphy should meet the following requirements:

1. Radiation dose to the injection site should be as low as possible. The absorbed dose depends on the physical and biological characteristics of the compound. The radiopharmaceutical should have a physical half-life of a few hours and should emit only γ-rays. ^{99m}Tc-labelled compounds are therefore the most favourable radiopharmaceuticals.
2. The compound should clear rapidly from the injection site. This allows early visualization of the lymphatics and shortens the study time. Faster clearance also lowers the absorbed dose at the site of injection. The clearance depends on the particle size and the molecular weight of the pharmaceutical. A narrow particle size distribution in the range of 20–50 nm and molecular weight of 70 kDa is appropriate. Homogeneity of particle size and the molecular weight is important for reproducibility of the study.
3. The compound should have high uptake with a relatively long residence in the lymph nodes. This is particularly important if the lymph nodes are to be localized intra-operatively using a probe several hours after injection of the radiopharmaceutical.
4. High labelling efficiency and a high specific activity is desirable. Often, multiple intradermal injections around the margins of a malignant lesion must be performed. The volume of each injection should be from 0.1–0.2 ml and should contain not more than 0.1–0.2 mCi. Free pertechnetate, due to an undesirably low labelling efficiency, would rapidly diffuse into the lymphatics and be excreted by the kidneys into the urinary bladder. This unwanted background activity would obscure the inguinal and iliac lymph nodes.
5. The compound should be commercially available as a simple ready-to-use kit form with a reasonable cost.

Colloidal gold (^{198}Au) was first used in the 1950s [1–4]. It has an ideal particle size of 9–15 nm but with a high photon energy (412 keV) and a long half-life (2.7 days). It is a beta-emitter and the radiation dose at the site of injection unfortunately is several hundred rems, which may cause radiation necrosis.

^{99m}Tc-sulphur colloid with variable particle size in the 100–300 nm range is also not suitable [5–10]. Because of the large particle size, clearance from the site of injection is minimal with resultant suboptimal lymphatic visualization and unreliable imaging of the lymph nodes. A modified sulphur colloid preparation, with smaller particle size, obtained by filtering the radiopharmaceutical, is used today at some clinical sites with satisfactory results.

^{99m}Tc human serum albumin is widely available in kit form for easy preparation [12]. It clears rapidly from the injection site allowing clear visualization of the draining lymphatics and is suitable for lymphatic imaging in patients with lymphoedema. However, there are concerns for its use in localization of sentinel nodes. Some investigations suggest that the agent may not be retained in the lymph nodes long enough for intra-operative localization, which is usually performed 2–3 hours later. This has not been our experience, and we have been able to detect nodes intra-operatively 3 hours post-injection using the probe localization technique.

^{99m}Tc HSA nanocolloid with a particle size of 10–20 nm is one of the newer agents for lymphoscintigraphy. ^{99m}Tc-antimony sulphide colloid with a particle size of 4–12 nm is one of the best radiopharmaceuticals currently available for lymphoscintigraphy. It is stable under normal conditions with a physiological pH. It has high lymphatic uptake and provides a reliable representation of lymph node anatomy [12].

The use of other ^{99m}Tc-labelled compounds such as dextran and hetastarch has been reported [13,14]. These agents all need special expertise for preparation and are not yet available in commercial kits.

INJECTION SITE AND TECHNIQUE

Intradermal injection is most commonly used and is preferred over subcutaneous injection. Lymphatics are richer in the dermis and therefore clearance is faster. The technique is easily learned [15]. A syringe with a 22-gauge needle is often used. The skin should be pinched between the thumb and index finger to provide a site for easy intradermal injection. The injection will form a small swelling in the skin.

For malignant melanoma lesions, injections are given about 1 cm from the edge of the lesion or the surgical incision [16–19]. A total of four to six injections are made approximately 2 cm apart around the periphery of the malignant melanoma lesion. For head and neck skin lesions, injection should be done only at the upper edge of the lesion. Injections below these lesions might obscure sentinel nodes.

For dynamic lymphoscintigraphy of the lower limbs, injections are made intradermally in the web space between the first and second toe on the dorsal aspect of the foot [11]. For the upper limbs, the cutaneous injection is given on the dorsum of the hand between the second and middle fingers or the middle and fourth fingers. For internal mammary lymphoscintigraphy the injection is given in the posterior rectus sheath 2.5 cm (1 inch) below the xiphisternum and 2.5 cm (1 inch) from the mid-line, starting with the side involved with breast cancer [20–22].

CLINICAL APPLICATIONS OF LYMPHOSCINTIGRAPHY

Lymphoscintigraphy has been applied to a wide variety of disease entities including the evaluation of malignant (e.g. melanoma and cancers of the breast, rectum, prostate, etc.), benign (e.g. lymphoedema) and congenital (e.g. Nonne–Milroy disease) diseases.

STAGING OF MALIGNANCY

Accurate staging of malignant diseases, including lymph node involvement, is necessary for treatment planning and prediction of prognosis. Replacement of lymph node follicles by tumour cells leads to decreased lymph flow and appearance of 'filling defects' on either contrast lymphoangiography or lymphoscintigraphy. Starting in the 1950s, lymphoscintigraphy with radioactive colloidal gold was used to visualize the inguinal, iliac, pelvic or peri-aortic lymph nodes [23,24]. Because of the physical and biological disadvantages of colloidal gold and the long waiting period for visualizing the lymph nodes, this procedure had only limited clinical application. Development of more suitable radiopharmaceuticals eventually led to more desirable clinical applications.

Breast cancer

In the mid-1970s, internal mammary lymphoscintigraphy was developed by Ege and other investigators using ^{99m}Tc-antimony colloid [20,21]. The technique consists of bilateral subcostal injections into the posterior rectal sheath of a small volume (0.1–0.2 ml of radiocolloid). When used to evaluate patients with breast cancer, the technique has been shown to be useful both for detecting metastatic involvement of internal mammary lymph nodes and for mapping the pathway of lymphatic flow through the parasternal lymph node chains. Using the criteria of diminished radiocolloid uptake in parasternal internal mammary lymph nodes to identify sites of probably metastatic nodal disease, Ege showed that the prognostic significance of this technique in the staging of breast cancer was comparable to that of axillary dissection with histological evaluation of axillary lymph nodes. In Ege's experience, the percentage of internal mammary lymph node involvement increased with the stage of breast cancer. Furthermore, the mammary lymph nodes were at risk for metastatic involvement regardless of the site of the primary tumour within the breast. As reported by Ege, abnormal parasternal lymphoscintigraphy occurred in 35% of the patients with and 18% of the patients without axillary lymph node metastases from breast cancer. However, the initial enthusiasm for using internal mammary lymphoscintigraphy to stage most women presenting with breast cancer has not led to widespread clinical application.

The technique can also have an impact on radiotherapy planning in patients with breast cancer [25,26]. At times, based on the results of lymphoscintigraphy, radiotherapy portals are extended to include additional parasternal lymph nodes. For example, a woman with cancer involving the medial quadrant of the right breast shown to have cross-over of lymphatic flow from the right to the left internal mammary lymph node chains might have the usual parasternal radiation therapy portal extended to include the left-sided internal mammary lymph nodes that are at risk for metastatic disease.

The technique also can be used to determine the depth of the internal mammary lymph nodes. Such data is needed when planning for electron beam therapy, so as to deliver adequate nodal doses without excessive radiation of the myocardium or the mediastinal structures. However, most of these therapy objectives are currently being met by CT or MRI.

Malignant melanoma

More recently, there has been interest in applying lymphoscintigraphy in the early stages of malignant melanoma of the skin [16–19,27–29]. The success of the treatment depends on accurate staging of the disease. Such staging depends mainly on the extent of local dermal invasion in the subcutaneous tissues and on the presence or absence of lymph node involvement. At many centres, lymph node dissection is routinely practised for stage I and II disease, even in the absence of palpable lymph nodes in the draining areas. Pathological examinations of resected lymph nodes in early-stage patients reveal absence of tumour involvement in as many as 84% of the cases. Thus, many patients undergo unnecessary lymph node dissection. In malignant melanoma, lymphoscintigraphy can be used to visualize the lymphatic pathways leading away from the primary lesion, localize the sentinel node, and determine which group of lymph nodes require surgical dissection. This is of utmost importance in lesions located anteriorly and posteriorly in the trunk close to the mid-line, and around the waist in the watershed

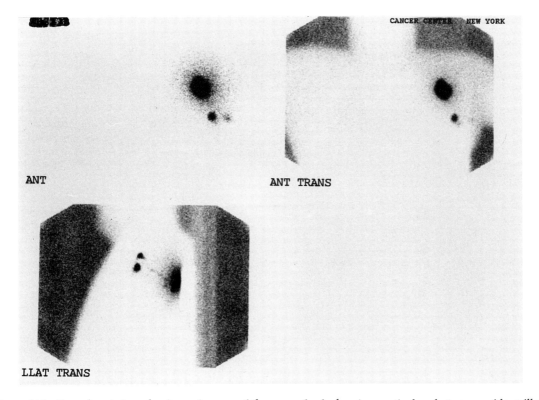

Figure 14.9 Lymphoscintigraphy for melanoma of the upper back showing sentinel node to same side axillary nodes. By permission from Samuel D.J. Yeh, M.D., Sc.D. Attending Physician, Nuclear Medicine Division, Department of Radiology, Memorial Sloan Kettering Cancer Center, New York, New York.

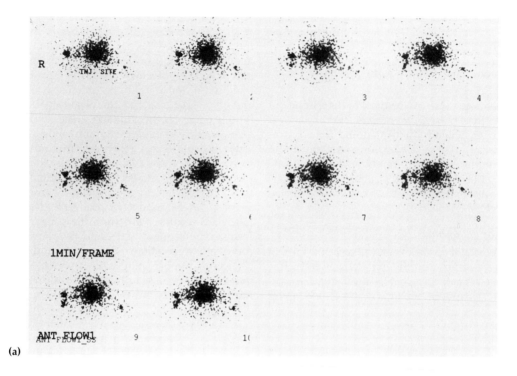

(a)

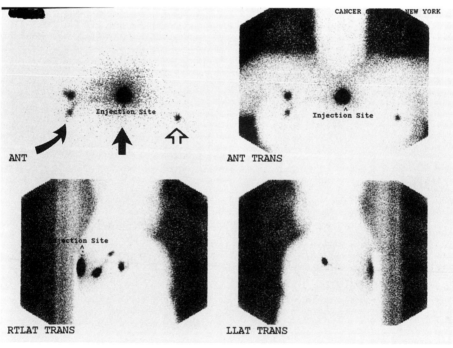

(b)

Figure 14.10 Dynamic (a) and static (b) lymphoscintigraphy for malignant melanoma of the back showing bilateral axillary lymph nodes. Injection site (straight arrow), right axillary nodes (curved arrows), left axillary node (open arrow). By permission from Samuel D.J. Yeh, M.D., Sc.D. Attending Physician, Nuclear Medicine Division, Department of Radiology, Memorial Sloan Kettering Cancer Center, New York, New York.

areas – all these regions have a variable lymphatic drainage.

Sentinel node lymphoscintigraphy

The sentinel node is the closest node draining the lymphatic basin of a malignant lesion and the histological status of the sentinel node is the best indicator of lymph node involvement by metastatic tumour cells. The concept of localizing the sentinel node in malignant melanoma was first introduced by Morton using methylene blue dye [28,29]. However, the dye dilutes rapidly and disappears quickly from the draining lymph nodes. In 1990, Alex and Krag [30] described a lymphoscintigraphic technique for the visualization of the sentinel node in malignant melanoma. This approach was further enhanced by the introduction of commercially available intra-operative probes that can scan and localize the area of maximum activity in the operation field – this corresponds to the sentinel node. Presumably if the sentinel node can be visualized and localized perioperatively, and is found to be free of malignant cells by frozen-section examination, then there is no need for full dissection of the draining regional lymph nodes. However, if the sentinel node is found to be involved with tumour cells, the surgeon should proceed to dissection of the draining regional lymph nodes. Recent results show that lymphoscintigraphy and localization by intra-operative probes is more accurate than localization by methylene blue dye. Figures 14.9–14.11 are examples of sentinel node localization in malignant melanoma.

In addition, the concept of sentinel node lymphoscintigraphy has been extended to breast carcinoma whereby the radionuclide is injected around the breast lesion [31,32,32a]. The sentinel node is then localized by imaging and by intra-operative probes with a view to removal and frozen-section examination.

Localization of the sentinel node by imaging and frozen-section evaluation, in order to avoid unnecessary additional surgery, is only useful in the early stages of malignancy. In the presence of palpable lymph nodes in advanced stages of malignant disease, there is no place for sentinel node localization. Recent reports indicate that when properly used, this technique has changed the surgical management including the extent and location of lymph node dissection, in 33–50% of patients with malignant melanoma. The reproducibility of sentinel node localization by lymphoscintigraphy was reported as high as 85% [31].

EVALUATION OF LYMPHOEDEMA

Lymphoscintigraphy is useful in the evaluation of primary and secondary lymphoedema, lymphangioma of lymphatic leakage, lymphangiectasia, chylous ascites and chylothorax. Lymphoscintigraphy, especially in cases of lymphoedema, is preferable to the radiographic technique of contrast lymphoangiography, which has notable disadvantages including surgical dissection to locate the lymphatic channels, lymphatic infusion pump of the contrast over several hours and contrast reactions (both acute and chronic) [11,33–36].

Dynamic lymphoscintigraphy allows direct visualization of lymphatic flow through the limbs. The technique can be used to differentiate between various types of oedema such as primary, congenital, obstructive or inflammatory, etc. Recent improvements in physiotherapy and surgical management of obstructive lymphoedema have generated increased interest in dynamic lymphoscintigraphy (and other non-invasive techniques) for differentiating between the different types of lymphoedema as well as for treatment evaluation.

Technique

Generally images are acquired every 30–60 seconds. However, data acquisition depends on the radiopharmaceutical used. For example, agents such as ^{99m}Tc-HSA with rapid clearance from the intradermal injection site are good for dynamic studies. Patients should be injected under the gamma-camera and dynamic acquisition should be performed every 30–60 seconds for a total of 45–60 minutes. Gentle massage of, or hot sponges at, the site of injection, will enhance the lymphatic clearance. After dynamic imaging, the patient should be asked to walk around, with delayed images of the draining lymph nodes acquired 3 hours later.

Data analysis

Quantitation significantly improves the sensitivity and specificity of the technique. For cases of lymphoedema, nodal time–activity curves can be generated from regions-of-interest drawn over the draining lymph nodes and are helpful in qualitative and semi-quantitative assessment. Quantitative parameters including the time-of-arrival of activity at the lymph nodes and the percentage of activity cleared from the injection site as well as the fraction of the injected dose taken up by the lymph nodes can be calculated.

Scintigraphic findings

Normal study The activity is seen in the lymphatic channels in the immediate post-injection phase with subsequent and progressive accumulation of activity by the major lymph node groups, and at 10 minutes the activity is seen in the liver. A normal pattern of nodal uptake on qualitative lymphoscintigraphy comprises bilaterally symmetrical and uniform uptake of the radiocolloid in the lymph nodes. An abnormal study appears as heterogeneous nodal uptake, an asymmetric lym-

phatic chain, total absence of the tracer in the chain, or failure to fill the distal lymphatics (Figure 14.12).

Primary lymphoedema Primary lymphoedema is caused by a developmental defect of the lymphatic system. The majority of cases present at puberty and the disease has a higher incidence in females, with the left lower extremity being more frequently involved. In primary lymphoedema, hypoplastic or aplastic channels are suggested by poor visualization, cut-off of lymphatic channels or poor nodal uptake. There might be dermal backflow.

In the less common hyperplastic form of primary lymphoedema, there is pooling of radiocolloid in the dilated channels or an increased number of lymphatic channels are scintigraphically evident.

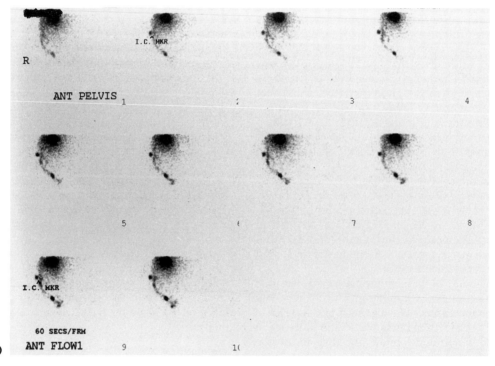

Figure 14.11   Lymphoscintigrams for malignant melanoma of the right buttock: (a) early dynamic phase; (b) static image showing drainage from the injection site (straight arrow) to the right groin (curved arrow), and (c) lymph nodes in the right axilla (open arrow). By permission from Samuel D.J. Yeh, M.D., Sc.D. Attending Physician, Nuclear Medicine Division, Department of Radiology, Memorial Sloan Kettering Cancer Center, New York, New York.

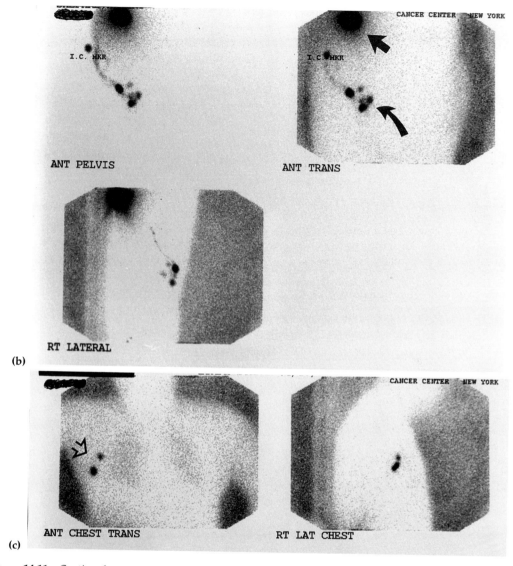

(b)

(c)

Figure 14.11 *Continued*

Nonne–Milroy disease is a form of primary lymphoedema with an autosomal dominant pattern of inheritance. There is extremity lymphoedema with associated findings of chylous ascites, protein-losing enteropathy and chylous pleural effusion. Lymphoscintigraphic findings include lower-extremity oedema that ranges from total obstruction of flow to lymphatic pooling. Pelvic and periaortic nodes of the affected side when visualized are seen to be sparse and small in size.

Secondary lymphoedema Secondary lymphoedema may occur due to obstruction at any level in the lymphatic system. Aetiologies include surgery, specially regional node dissection; trauma, neoplasia/tumour, radiation and infection. Venous obstruction complicates many cases of

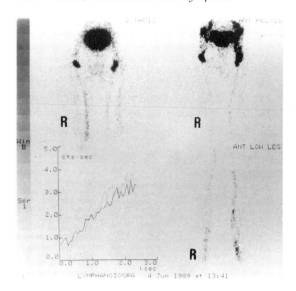

Figure 14.12 Normal dynamic lymphoscintigraphy of the lower extremity showing normal lymphatic channels and normal iliofemoral lymph nodes with bilaterally symmetrical nodal time-activity curves.

secondary lymphoedema. In secondary lymphoedema, a slow transit of radiocolloid, with interrupted delineation of lymphatic channels and dermal backflow with reduced nodal uptake have been described (Figure 14.13).

Dermal backflow results from the radiocolloid uptake in the dermal lymphatics acting as collaterals when deep lymphatics are absent or

obstructed. It is seen as a cut-off of lymphatic channels with accumulation of tracer in the superficial tissues distal to the lymphatic obstruction. This localized accumulation of activity can be differentiated from the activity in the inflamed tissues by the presence of patent lymphatic channels above the accumulation in cases of inflammatory oedema (Figure 14.14). The dermal backflow pattern is not specific for a particular disease, but may be observed with any of the various aetiologies of acquired lymphatic obstruction in the extremities.

Other conditions In cases of lymphangioma, lymphoscintigraphy typically shows accumulation of activity during the vascular phase; the delayed images are usually normal as the radiopharmaceutical is deposited in nodes and has cleared from the vascular compartment.

Lymphoscintigraphy is useful in documenting lymphatic leakage, whether congenital or acquired. Common sites of leakage include the thorax and abdomen. Chylous ascites may be primary (e.g. fistulous, exudative), or acquired (e.g. trauma, neoplastic).

In intestinal lymphangiectasia, lower-extremity lymphoscintigraphy demonstrates normal inguinal lymph nodes, abdominal nodes and liver; however, accumulation of radiopharmaceutical can also be identified in the gastrointestinal tract. Lymphoscintigraphy in cases of pulmonary lymphangiectasia will show tracer accumulation in regions of dilated lymphatics within the lungs.

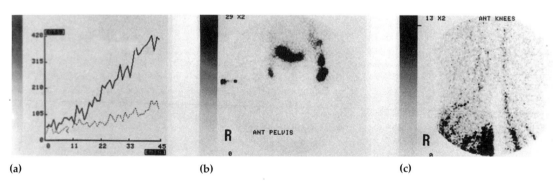

(a)　　　　(b)　　　　(c)

Figure 14.13 Dynamic lymphoscintigraphy in a patient with obstructive lymphoedema of the right leg showing: (a) low-amplitude slowly rising right nodal time-activity curve due to slow transit of the radiocolloid, (b) poor uptake in the right inguinal nodes; and (c) dermal backflow in the right lower extremity. By permission from article 'Tc-99m Human Serum Albumin Lymphoscintigraphy in Lymphoedema of the lower Extremities' by Nawaz MK, Hamad MM, Abdel-Dayem HM, Sadek S, and Eklof BGH. *Clin Nucl Med* 1990;15(11):794–799.

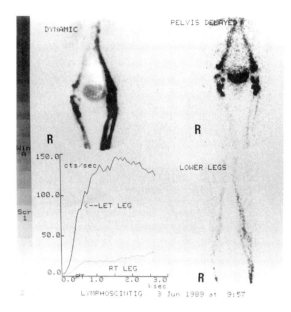

Figure 14.14 Dynamic lymphoscintigraphy in a patient with inflammatory lymphoedema of the left leg. Note the rapidly rising high-amplitude nodal time-activity curve on the left consistent with lymphatic hyperactivity.

Chylothorax can be idiopathic or secondary to neoplasm or trauma. Lymphoscintigraphy has two roles in the evaluation:

1. It can confirm that the fluid in the chest is chyle – by demonstrating the flow of the injected activity into the involved hemi-thorax.
2. It can be used to quantify the amount of chyle accumulating in the chest, which can be a useful parameter for assessing the results of conservative management.

Lymphoscintigraphy can be used to detect chylous ascites but cannot distinguish the aetiology. The radiopharmaceutical is seen to accumulate in the peritoneal cavity and there is non-visualization of the abdominal nodes, liver and spleen.

CONCLUSIONS

Lymphoscintigraphy is a safe and non-traumatic nuclear medicine imaging procedure for the qualitative and quantitative analysis of the lymphatic system. Lymphoscintigraphy has proved to be of value in pre-operative staging of different carcino-mas. The technique has been used extensively for the evaluation of internal mammary, axillary and internal iliac lymph nodes in carcinomas of the breast, rectum and prostate. Lymph node groups that are a risk for metastatic involvement can be identified and localized accurately, thus aiding in the irradiation therapy planning. The technique is also useful in determining the lymphatic flow pattern in cases of melanoma. Lymphoscintigraphy is currently the diagnostic modality of choice for evaluating lymphoedema. Lymphoscintigraphic images allow characterization of lymphatic morphology and quantitation improves the sensitivity of the technique in detecting incipient lymphoedema.

REFERENCES

1. Sherman, A. and Ter-Pogossian, M. (1953) Lymph node concentration of radioactive colloidal gold following interstitial injection. *Cancer*, **6**, 1238.
2. Sage, H.H. and Gozun, B.V. (1958) Lymphatic scintigrams: a method for studying the functional pattern of lymphatics and lymph nodes. *Cancer*, **11**, 200.
3. Hultborn, K.A., Larsson, L.G. and Ragnhult, I. (1955) The lymph drainage from the breast to the axillary and parasternal lymph nodes, studied with the aid of colloidal Au-198. *Acta Radiol.*, **43**, 52.
4. Handley, R.S. (1964) The early spread of breast carcinoma and its bearing on operative therapy. *Br. J. Surg.*, **51**, 206.
5. Warbick, A., Ege, G.N., Henkelman, R.M., Maier, G. and Lyster, D.M. (1977) An evaluation of radiocolloid sizing techniques. *J. Nucl. Med.*, **18**, 827–34
6. Bronskill, M.J. (1983) Radiation dose estimates for interstitial radiocolloid lymphoscintigraphy. *Semin. Nucl. Med.*, **13**(1), 20–5.
7. Bergqvist, L., Strand, S.E., Persson, B.R.R., Hafstrom, L. and Jonsson, P. (1982) Dosimetry in lymphoscintigraphy of Tc-99m antimony sulfide colloid. *J. Nucl. Med.*, **23**, 698–705.
8. Atkins, H.L., Hauser, W. and Richards, P. (1990) Factors affecting distribution of Tc-99m sulfur colloid. *J. Reticuloendothelial Soc.*, **8**(2), 176–84.
9. Kaplan, W.D., Piez, C.W., Gelman, R.S. *et al.* (1984) Quantitative comparison of two radionuclides for lymphoscintigraphy (Abstract). *J. Nucl. Med.*, **25**, P40.
10. Bergqvist, L., Strand, S. and Persson, B. (1983) Particle sizing and biokinetics of interstitial lymphoscintigraphic agents. *Semin. Nucl. Med.*, **13**, 9–19.
11. Nawaz, M.K., Hamad, M.M., Abdel-Dayem, H.M. *et al.* (1990) Tc-99m human serum albumin lymphoscintigraphy in lymphedema of the lower extremities. *Clin. Nucl. Med.*, **15**, 794–9.
12. Kramer, E.L. (1990) Lymphoscintigraphy: radiopharmaceutical selection and methods. *Nucl. Med. Biol.*, **17**(1), 57–63.

13. Sadek, S., Owunwanne, A., Yacoub, T. and Abdel-Dayem, H.M. (1989) Technetium-99m Haemaccel: a new lymphoscintigraphic agent. *Am. J. Physiologic Imaging*, **4**, 46–9.

14. Sadek, S., Owunwanne, A., Abdel-Dayem, H.M. and Yacoub, T. (1989) Preparation and evaluation of Tc-99m hydroxyethyl starch as a potential radiopharmaceutical for lymphoscintigraphy. *Lymphology*, **22**, 157–66.

15. Weissleder, H. and Weissleder, R. (1988) Lymphedema: evaluation of qualitative and quantitative lymphoscintigraphy in 238 patients. *Radiology*, **167**, 729–35.

16. Berman, C., Norman, J., Cruse, C.W., Reintgen, D.S. and Clark, R.A. (1992) Lymphoscintigraphy in malignant melanoma. *Ann. Plast. Surg.*, **28**, 29–32.

17. Norman, J., Cruse, C.W., Espinosa, C. *et al.* (1991) Redefinition cutaneous lymphatic drainage with the use of lymphoscintigraphy for malignant melanoma. *Am. J. Surg.*, **162**, 432–7.

18. Uren, R.F., Hofman-Giles, R.B., Shaw, H.M., Thompson, J.F. and McCarthy, W.H. (1993) Lymphoscintigraphy in high risk melanoma of the trunk: predicting draining node groups, defining lymphatic channels and locating the sentinel node. *J. Nucl. Med.*, **34**, 1435–40.

19. Slingluff, C.L., Stidham, K.R., Ricci, W.M., Stanley, W.E. and Seigler, H.F. (1994) Surgical management of regional lymph nodes in patients with melanoma: experience with 4682 patients. *Ann. Surg.*, **219**, 120–30.

20. Ege, G.N. (1976) Internal mammary lymphoscintigraphy – the rationale, technique, interpretation, and clinical application. *Radiology*, **118**, 101.

21. Ege, G.N. (1983) Lymphoscintigraphy – techniques and applications in the management of breast carcinoma. *Semin. Nucl. Med.*, **13**, 26.

22. Dionne, L., Fried, L. and Blais, R. (1983) Internal mammary lymphoscintigraphy in breast carcinoma – a surgeon's perspective. *Semin. Nucl. Med.*, **13**(3), 41.

23. Kaplan, W.D., Garnick, M.B. and Richie, J.P. (1983) Iliopelvic radionuclide lymphoscintigraphy in patients with testicular cancer. *Radiology*, **147**, 231.

24. Boak, J.L. and Agwunobi, T.C. (1978) A study of technetium-labelled sulphide colloid uptake by regional lymph nodes draining a tumour bearing area. *Br. J. Surg.*, **65**, 374.

25. Dufresne, E.N., Kaplan, W.D., Zimmerman, R.E. and Rose, C.M. (1980) The application of internal mammary lymphoscintigraphy to planning of radiation therapy. *J. Nucl. Med.*, **21**, 697–9.

26. Bronskill, M.J., Harauz, G. and Ege, G.N. (1979) Computerized internal mammary lymphoscintigraphy in radiation treatment planning of patients with breast carcinoma. *Int. J. Radiat. Oncol. Biol. Phys.*, **5**, 573.

27. Sullivan, D.C., Croker, B.P., Jr, Harris, C.C., Deery, P. and Seigler, H.F. (1981) Lymphoscintigraphy in malignant melanoma: Tc-99m-antimony sulfur colloid. *Am. J. Roentgenol.*, **137**, 847–51.

28. Morton, D.L., Wen, D.R., Wong, J.H. *et al.* (1992) Technical details of intraoperative lymphatic mapping for early stage melanoma. *Arch. Surg.*, **127**(4), 392–9.

29. Morton, D.L., Wen, D.R., Foshag, L.J., Essner, R. and Cochran, A. (1993) Intraoperative lymphatic mapping and selective cervical lymphadenectomy for early-stage melanomas of the head and neck. *J. Clin. Oncol.*, **11**, 1751–6.

30. Alex, J.C. and Krag, D.N. (1993) Gamma-probe-guided localization of lymph nodes. *Surg. Oncol.*, **2**, 137–43.

31. Krag, D.N., Weaver, D.L., Alex, J.C. and Fairbank, J.T. (1993) Surgical resection and radiolocalization of the sentinel lymph node in breast cancer using a gamma probe. *Surg. Oncol.*, **2**, 335–40.

32. Alazraki, N. (1995) Lymphoscintigraphy and the intraoperative gamma probe. Editorial. *J. Nucl. Med.*, **36**(10), 1780–3.

32a. Veronesi, U., Paganelli, G., Galimberti, V. *et al.* (1997) Sentinel node biopsy to avoid axillary dissection in breast cancer with clinically negative lymph nodes. *Lancet*, **349**, 1864–7.

33. Ohtake, E., Matsui, K., Kobayashi, Y. and Ono, Y. (1983) Clinical evaluation of dynamic lymphoscintigraphy with Tc-99m human serum albumin. *J. Nucl. Med.*, **24**, P41.

34. McNeill, G.C., Witte, M.H., Witte, C.L. *et al.* (1989) Whole-body lymphoangioscintigraphy: preferred method for initial assessment of the peripheral lymphatic system. *Radiology*, **172**, 495–502.

35. Kaplan, W.D., Slavin, S.A., Markisz, J.A., Laffin, S.M. and Royal, H.D. (1983) Qualitative and quantitative upper extremity radionuclide lymphoscintigraphy (Abstract). *J. Nucl. Med.*, **24**, P40.

36. McConnell, R.W., McConnell, B.G. and Kim, E.E. (1983) Other applications of interstitial lymphoscintigraphy. *Semin. Nucl. Med.*, **13**, 70–4.

CHAPTER 15

Head and neck disease

Cancer of the head and neck

M. N. Maisey and E. B. Chevretton

INTRODUCTION AND BACKGROUND

Cancer of the head and neck is relatively uncommon in Western countries, representing about 5% of all malignant tumours. However, it is extremely common in India and South-East Asia where oral cavity cancer represents 35% of all cancer cases [1,2]. Men are three times more likely than women to develop this form of cancer, with a peak incidence over the age of 50. Risk factors include tobacco and alcohol consumption (these have a synergistic effect), dietary factors, viruses, and exposure to chemicals and fumes. When treating head and neck cancer improved results are achieved when patients are treated in specialized centres with experienced multi-disciplinary teams including head and neck surgeons, radiotherapists and medical oncologists [3]. On account of the site of the tumours, treatment is directed at maintaining both the form and the function of the head and neck structures as well as eradicating the disease. Imaging is important for the management of head and neck cancer [4,5].

ANATOMY AND PATHOPHYSIOLOGY

The majority of head and neck cancers arise from the upper aerodigestive tract (including the lar-

ynx, the pharynx, the oral cavity, the nose and the sinuses), but others arise in structures such as the skull base, the orbit, the thyroid gland and the salivary glands. Although grouped together largely for convenience of management, head and neck cancers behave differently according to the individual site and histopathological type. Over 90% of the tumours are squamous cell in origin, the remainder being adenocarcinomas, lymphomas, mucoepidermoid carcinomas, adenoid cystic carcinoma and other rarer tumours. The prognosis after treatment varies depending on the site of the primary tumour and the stage of the tumour at presentation. The overall 5-year survival rate for all sites and stages is approximately 50%, but there is a wide variation from early cancers of the lip and glottic larynx (5-year survival rate in excess of 85%) to advanced cancers of the hypopharynx and cervical oesophagus (5-year survival of approximately 10%).

Staging is of great importance in the management of head and neck cancer as it acts as a guide to appropriate treatment and prognosis, and also allows comparison of results between different centres. The TNM systems proposed by the UICC and the AJC are widely used (Table 15.1) [3]. The T stage for the oral cavity and oropharynx is based on tumour dimensions, whereas at other sites it is based on local extension. The N and M stages are the same for all primary tumour sites [3]. The most important prognostic variables are the T stage and the presence or absence of regional lymph node involvement. For early disease, radiotherapy is effective and preserves function but for more

Clinical Nuclear Medicine, 3rd edn. Edited by M.N. Maisey, K.E. Britton and B.D. Collier. Published in 1998 by Chapman & Hall, London. ISBN 0 412 75180 1

Table 15.1   TNM staging system

Staging		
T-Size (oral cavity and oropharynx)	Stage I	$- T_1N_0M_0$
T_1 = <2 cm	II	$- T_2N_0M_0$
T_2 = 2–4	III	$- T_3N_0M_0$
T_3 = >4		$T_1,T_2T_3N_1M_0$
T_4 = invasion of local structures	IV	$- T_4,N_0N_1M_0$
N_0 No nodes		Any T,$N_2N_3M_0$
N_1 Ipsilateral node <3 cm		Any T, Any N M_1
N_2a Single ipsilateral node 3–6 cm		
b Multiple ipsilateral nodes <6 cm		
c Bilateral or contralateral node <6 cm		
N_3 Lymph node >6 cm		
M_1 Distant metastases		

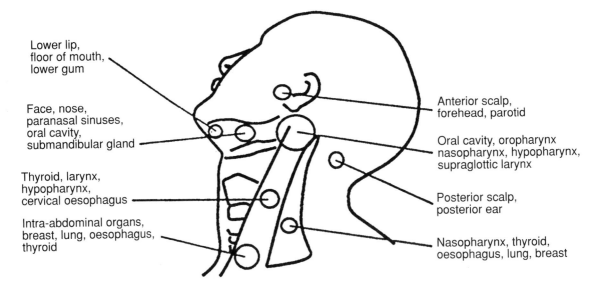

Figure 15.1   Likely sites of metastases from various sites of the head and neck [4].

advanced disease combined surgery (with reconstruction if necessary) and post-operative radiotherapy gives better loco-regional control at many sites in the head and neck. An understanding of the distribution of cervical lymph nodes and the likely sites of local metastatic spread of the primary tumour is of importance in imaging and staging head and neck tumours. Conversely, the precise location of a nodal metastasis may give a clue to the site of primary tumour if it is not clinically evident. The cervical lymph node groups are shown in Figure 15.1 with the likely origins of the metastases. Primary tumours of the head and neck

rarely metastasize to distal sites except in very advanced disease.

RADIONUCLIDES FOR INVESTIGATING HEAD AND NECK CANCER

The ideal radiopharmaceutical for tumour imaging should have a high target-to-background ratio and a low incidence of non-malignant causes of abnormal accumulation. Various tracers have been used including gallium-67, thallium-201, ^{99m}Tc-Sesta-MIBI, ^{99m}Tc pentavalent DMSA and ^{18}F-fluorodeoxyglucose (^{18}F-FDG). With the increasing availability of ^{18}F-FDG a significant number of clinical studies have been published, which have demonstrated that FDG has an important clinical role in the evaluation of head and neck tumours and when available is the radiopharmaceutical of choice [6–12]. The normal physiological sites of FDG uptake in the head and neck include the tonsils, sub-lingual lymphoid tissue, the intrinsic laryngeal muscles during phonation and photopenic areas can normally be identified in the mandible teeth and dental fillings.

CLINICAL MANAGEMENT ISSUES AND THE ROLE OF RADIONUCLIDE IMAGING

Imaging has an important role in the initial management of head and neck tumours because of the need to plan treatment and because local nodal spread is an important prognostic factor. About one-third of patients will suffer from loco-regional recurrence and may benefit from early re-treatment. However, the conventional anatomical imaging procedures are less useful after treatment because of the distortion of the normal anatomy. FDG-PET can therefore have a particularly important role in follow-up of patients and in suspected recurrence.

Staging of head and neck tumours before treatment is usually achieved by a combination of clinical examination (including endoscopy) and anatomical imaging such as CT and MR. These modalities may over-estimate tumour size because of oedema and inflammatory reactions surrounding tumour tissue. FDG-PET scans may provide further clinical information.

Anatomical imaging of regional lymph nodes has also been shown to be extremely unreliable. MR and CT examinations which are dependent on lymph node size and the presence of tumour necrosis have a sensitivity of approximately 80% and a specificity of approximately 70%. FDG-PET scans are as sensitive as MR and CT, but are more specific [13]. In most series there has been 100% sensitivity for the primary tumour and often over 85% sensitivity for regional lymph nodes. Non-malignant causes of increased uptake are relatively uncommon and associated with sites of infection, but clinically have not proved to be a significant problem. Because of the complex anatomy of the head and neck, associated anatomical imaging is frequently essential for the proper interpretation of radionuclide studies and this is an area where co-registration of anatomical imaging and functional imaging has shown to be of value [12]. As with all imaging techniques – both anatomical and functional – the ability to detect micrometastases will always be lower than node dissection and histology.

Some 5% of patients present with nodal disease detected by find needle aspiration cytology (FNAC) without an obvious primary lesion. The reported detection of the primary site of such an occult primary head and neck tumour with CT and MR is 15–20%. The sensitivity of PET FDG may be helpful in identifying the occult primary.

Early detection of recurrent or residual disease is important as this gives an additional chance of cure with further treatment. Both radiation and surgery can lead to changes that mask the detection of disease by anatomical imaging. Detecting recurrent or residual disease is therefore probably the most important role at the present time for nuclear medicine. ^{18}F-FDG-PET has greater accuracy in recurrent disease and surveillance of high-risk patients where the incidence of recurrence may be up to 50% in the first year. As increasing numbers of patients are treated with radiotherapy and chemotherapy, monitoring of response becomes increasingly important, as does the assessment of pre-surgical down-staging of disease. Failed or equivocal biopsy for both primary or recurrent disease is a further problem causing clinical difficulties where FDG-PET can be significantly helpful. Thus, the indications for FDG-PET scans and current clinical indications (in order of importance) in patients with head and neck cancers may be summarized:

- Investigation of suspected recurrence especially when anatomical imaging is equivocal.
- Following a negative biopsy when the clinical suspicion remains high.
- Selectively for surgical planning (especially maxillary sinus).
- Searching for the primary when presenting with nodal metastases.
- Assessment of response to therapy.
- Routine surveillance in groups at high risk for early recurrence.

REFERENCES

1. Tobias, J.S. (1994) Cancer of the head and neck. *Br. Med. J.*, **308**, 961–6.

2. Shah, J.P. and Lydiatt, W. (1995) Treatment of cancer of the head and neck. *Cancer J. Clinicians,* **45**, 352–68.

3. TNM Classification of Malignant Tumours, IUCC (1996) 4th edn, (eds P. Hermanek and L.H. Sobin), Springer-Verlag, Berlin.

4. Noyek, A.M., Witterick, I.J. and Kirsh, J.C. (1991) Radionuclide imaging in otolaryngology-head and neck surgery. *Arch. Otolaryngol. – Head Neck Surg.,* **117**(4), 372–8.

5. van den Brekel, M.W.M., Castelijins, J.A. and Snow, G.B. (1994) The role of modern imaging studies in staging and therapy of head and neck neoplasms. *Semin. Oncol.,* **21**, 340–48.

6. Reisser, C., Haberkorn, U. and Strauss, L.G. (1993) The relevance of positron emission tomography for the diagnosis and treatment of head and neck tumours. *J. Otolaryngol.,* **22**, 231–8.

7. Braams, J.W., Pruim, J., Freling, N.J., Nikkels, P.G., Roodenburg, J.L., Boering, G., Vaalburg, W. and Vermey, A. (1995) Detection of lymph node metastases of squamous-cell cancer of the head and neck with FDG-PET and MRI. *J. Nucl. Med.,* **36**(2), 211–16.

8. Mukherji, S.K., Drane, W.E., Tart, R.P., Landau, S. and Mancuso, A.A. (1994) Comparison of thallium-201 and F-18 FDG SPECT uptake in squamous cell carcinoma of the head and neck. *Am. J. Neuroradiol.,* **15**(10), 1837–42.

9. Laubenbacher, C., Saumweber, D., Wagner-Manslau, C. *et al.* (1995) Comparison of fluorine-18-fluorodeoxyglucose PET, MRI and endoscopy for staging head and neck squamous-cell carcinomas. *J. Nucl. Med.,* **36**(10), 1747–57.

10. Lapela, M., Grenman, R., Kurki, T., Joensuu, H., Leskinen, S., Lindholm, P., Haaparanta, M., Ruotsa-lainen, U. and Minn, H. (1995) Head and neck cancer: detection of recurrence with PET and 2-[F-18] fluoro-2-deoxy-D-glucose. *Radiology,* **197**(1), 205–11.

11. Anzai, Y., Carrol, W.R., Quint, D.J., Bradford, C.R., Minoshima, S., Wolf, G.T. and Wahl, R.L. (1996) Recurrence of head and neck cancer after surgery or irradiation: prospective comparison of 2-deoxy-2-[F-18]fluoro-D-glucose PET and MR imaging diagnoses. *Radiology,* **200**(1), 135–41.

12. Wong, W., Husain, K., Chevretton, E., Hawkes, D., Baddeley, H. and Maisey, M. (1996) Validation and clinical application of computer combined CT and PET-FDG head and neck images. *Am. J. Surg.,* **172**, 628–32.

13. Wong, W., Chevretton, E. *et al.* (1997) A prospective study of PET-FDG imaging for the assessment of head and neck squamous cell carcinoma. *Clin. Otolaryngol.,* **22**, 209–14.

Salivary glands

N. D. Greyson

INTRODUCTION

Salivary gland scanning using ^{99m}Tc pertechnetate provides quantifiable, physiological images of the salivary gland, demonstrating morphology, function and drainage, analogous to that of a renal scan [1–3]. Gallium 67 citrate, or labelled white cells demonstrate active inflammation.

ANATOMY AND PHYSIOLOGY

The salivary glands comprise three paired exocrine glands including small salivary acini within the mucosa of the tongue and oropharynx, which secrete saliva directly into the mouth. Saliva is a complex fluid containing serous and mucoid secretions, salts, polypeptides, glycoproteins, and the digestive enzyme salivary amylase. Salivary lysozymes and immunoglobulins provide antibacterial and anti-fungal properties [4]. The saliva plays an important role in oral hygiene, lubricates food for swallowing, and initiates the digestion of starch. Each individual pair of salivary glands secretes slightly different salivary constituents: the parotid saliva is predominantly serous; the submandibular secretions are mixed serous and mucous; and sublingual gland saliva is predominantly mucous. The structure of the salivary glands is superficially like the kidneys – with acini and ductules representing glomeruli and tubules, and the salivary ducts simulating ureters. These organs are afflicted with similar pathology – obstruction, infection, tumour and dysfunction.

The parotid gland drains through the short Stensen's duct, which opens opposite the second upper molar tooth. Thus, its orifice is susceptible to trauma and bacterial invasion. Parotid glands are more likely to be inflamed, while the submandibular glands with their more viscous secretions, and drainage through the longer Wharton's duct, are more likely to be affected by obstruction or calculi.

Parasympathetic stimulation of salivary secretion is mediated via the facial and glosso-pharyngeal nerves. Olfactory (stimulus of smell), gustatory (sight or thought of food), mechanical (the physical presence of food in the mouth or the act of chewing), and chemical stimuli (especially sour taste) enhance salivation. Sympathetic fibres are inhibitory, causing the all too familiar dryness of mouth and throat at times of stress.

Radioiodinated MIBG, an analogue of noradrenaline, localizes in the neurosecretory tissues. The salivary glands are a normal feature on a MIBG scan [5]. Interruption of sympathetic innervation may decrease salivary secretion. The unilateral absence of salivary uptake of MIBG may indicate neuropathic dysfunction of the gland, such as is seen in Horner's syndrome [6].

NUCLEAR IMAGING

The radiopharmaceutical, ^{99m}Tc pertechnetate ion is analogous to iodide in ionic size and charge. Both iodide and pertechnetate are secreted by the ductal epithelial cells (oncocytes) of the salivary glands, but not by the acinar cells.

The patient is placed in the Water's position (nose and chin against the high resolution collimator). Following an intravenous injection of 555 MBq of ^{99m}Tc pertechnetate, rapid sequential 3- to 5-second images are obtained for 1 minute to show the salivary gland blood flow. Next, serial images are acquired every 2–3 minutes for up to 20 minutes, which show progressive concentration of activity in the glands and gradual washout, with accumulation in the mouth. The intensity of the activity of the normally functioning salivary and thyroid glands are approximately equal (Figure 15.2).

After 20 minutes the patient is given some lemon juice or sour candy. This causes prompt salivation, draining the glands if the salivary ducts are patent (Figures 15.3 and 15.4). Oblique views should be taken before and after salivary stimulation, to help detect subtle changes. Palpation, or ultrasound findings should be correlated with the radionuclide images. Masses may be characterized as being either vascular or non-vascular on the flow phase image, and functioning or non-functioning on sequential images.

The relative blood flow, as well as differential excretory function of each salivary gland can be

Clinical Nuclear Medicine, 3rd edn. Edited by M.N. Maisey, K.E. Britton and B.D. Collier. Published in 1998 by Chapman & Hall, London. ISBN 0 412 75180 1

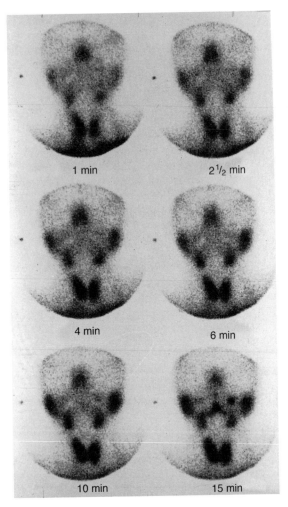

1 min   2½ min

4 min   6 min

10 min   15 min

Figure 15.2 Normal ^{99m}Tc-pertechnetate salivary gland scan. Sequential images show progressive accumulation of activity in the parotid and submandibular glands. The sublingual and minor salivary glands are not seen. Activity is noted in the mouth at 15 minutes. The intensity in all of the salivary glands is approximately equal, and similar to that in the thyroid gland.

assessed either visually or with a computer. Quantification of salivary gland function can be achieved by generating time–activity curves (TACs) from regions-of-interest drawn over the salivary glands. This technique is useful in assessing salivary gland function and diagnosing obstruction of major salivary glands [1,7]. A normal scintiscan essentially excludes significant pathology, but if there is a suspicion of salivary duct obstruction, then contrast sialography is necessary for further evaluation [8] (Table 15.2).

NEOPLASMS AND MASSES

Benign neoplasms of the salivary gland usually present as asymptomatic swellings. Tumours can arise from any of the constituent cell types of the gland. The most common are benign mixed adenomas, derived from a variable mixture of acinar and duct epithelial cells, followed in frequency by the Warthin's tumour. Depending on the proportions of cell types, tumours are cool or cold on the ^{99m}Tc-pertechnetate scan [9].

Malignant neoplasms, usually adenocarcinomas, are generally vascular on the flow and blood pool images, but appear cold or non-functioning on the delayed images. Lymphomas, metastatic tumours, and abscesses also show a similar scan pattern. Simple cysts appear non-vascular and non-functioning on the scan.

WARTHIN'S TUMOUR

Warthin's tumours arise from the salivary duct epithelium. They are almost invariably benign [10,11] and most commonly affect the parotid glands of middle-aged men. Occasionally, they may be multiple, or bilateral. Warthin's tumours also contain lymphatic elements, suggesting that they may be derived from embryologic remnants of the parotid lymph nodes [12]. The ductal components do not make true tubules, but there are multiple cystic clefts within the tumour. These do not communicate with the duct system, and do not drain (Figures 15.5 and 15.6).

Warthin's tumours, and oncocytomas (which are tumours derived exclusively from duct epithelium), accumulate pertechnetate because of the secretory activity of those cells [13]. Thus, they appear as foci of increased uptake within the salivary gland. Following stimulation by lemon, the normal components of the salivary glands drain, but activity trapped in the cystic spaces remains. Thus, the 'post-washout' image is important in detecting the tumour with up to 100% sensitivity. Pre-washout static images have a low sensitivity (detecting only 33% of tumours) because the lesion may be obscured by normal tissue [14,15]. An obstructed salivary gland, shows retention throughout the gland, while a Warthin's tumour will show as a localized focus of retained activity.

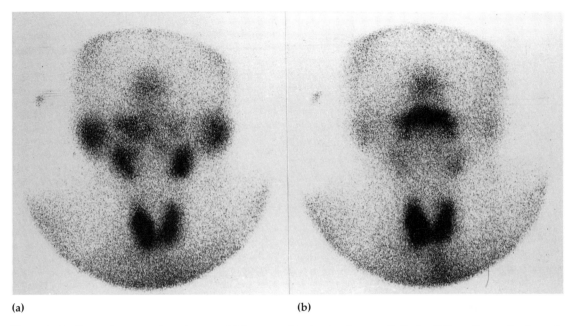

(a)   **(b)**

Figure 15.3 Pre and post-washout images. (a) Image at 20 minutes shows activity in all the salivary glands, and a small amount in the mouth. (b) Following lemon juice, complete washout from the salivary glands is noted.

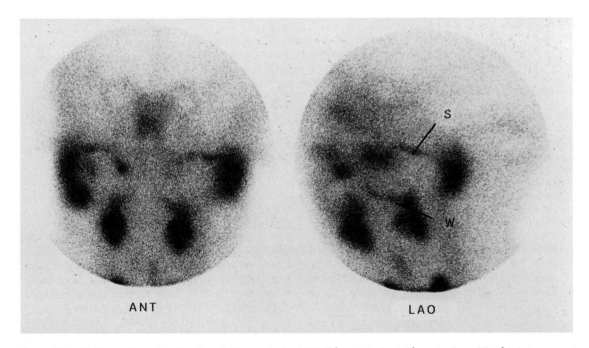

Figure 15.4 Salivary duct visualization. S, Stensen's duct; W, Wharton's duct. There is also a Warthin's tumour at the inferior margin of the right parotid (see Figure 15.5 arrowhead).

Table 15.2 Summary of salivary scan findings*

	^{99m}Tc-pertechnetate			$^{67}Gallium$
	Flow	*Function*	*Washout*	
Benign mixed tumour	→ ↑	↓ usually	→	→
Malignant tumour	↑	↓	→	↑↑
Warthin's tumour	↑	↑	↑	→
Cyst	↓	↓	↓	↓ ↑
Sjogren's syndrome	↓	↓	→	↑
Chronic obstruction/inflammation	↓	↓	↑	→ ↑
Acute inflammation	↑	↑	↑	↑↑
Obstruction	↓	↓	↑	→

* Arrow direction depicts activity compared with normal.

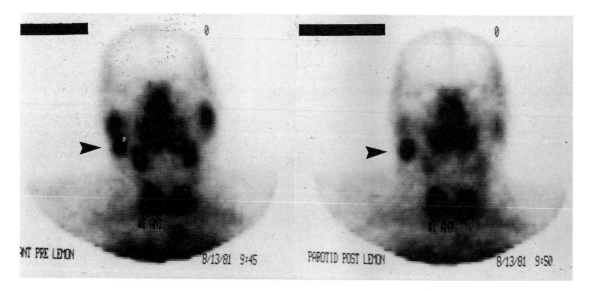

Figure 15.5 Warthin's tumour. Left: a functioning mass is seen at the lower pole of the right parotid gland (arrowhead). Right: after lemon, the normal glands washout, but the activity trapped in the cystic spaces of the tumour do not drain. Post-washout images enhance detection of these lesions.

In parotitis, washout is more uniform throughout the gland [16].

Demonstrating that these tumours are functioning gives the surgeon assurance that they are benign, and that surgery with the associated risk of damage to the facial nerve and fistula formation may be avoided. The absence of uptake of ^{67}Ga in a Warthin's tumour also confirms the benign nature of the pathology.

INFLAMMATION

Salivary glands are vulnerable to a variety of infectious agents, as well as aseptic inflammation. Due to the shortness of Stensen's duct, the parotid glands are more susceptible to bacterial infection, but may also be involved in virus-induced mumps parotitis. Salivary glands may be involved in HIV-related systemic disease, and these patients have frequent complaints of a dry mouth.

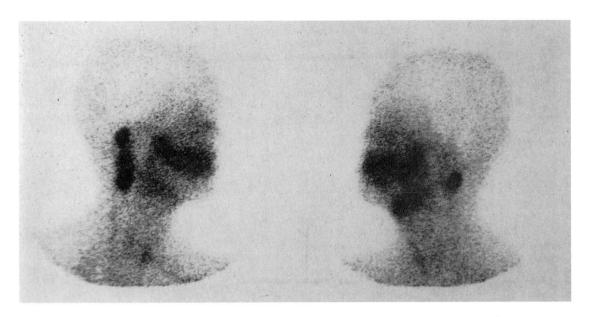

Figure 15.6 Multiple, bilateral Warthin's tumours. Oblique, post-washout images show at least three tumours in the right parotid, and one in the left parotid.

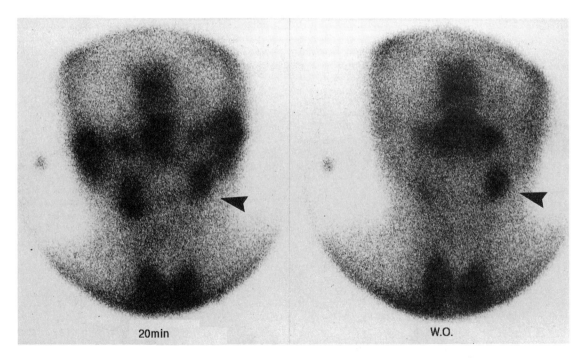

20min

W.O.

Figure 15.7 Sialadenitis. Left submandibular sialadenitis shows good concentration on the 20-minute image. Following lemon, there is retained activity in the gland (arrowhead). Subsequent contrast sialography showed no obstruction, but there was sialectasis. The apparent concentration in the gland and delayed drainage are likely the effects of hyperaemia, stasis in the dilated ductules and damaged acini.

Obstructed submandibular glands may become secondarily infected, but primary acute pyogenic sialadenitis is rare, except in debilitated or immunosupressed individuals. Tuberculosis of the salivary gland occasionally occurs.

Aseptic inflammation with dysfunction is a common occurrence in sarcoidosis, and Sjögren's, or the sicca syndrome, but may also occur with autoimmune diseases such as rheumatoid arthritis, lupus erythematosus and Wegener's granulomatosis.

After intravenous injections of iodinated contrast, or oral Lugol's iodine administration, high concentrations of iodine may be secreted from the salivary glands. This results in an acute painful swelling ('iodide mumps') [17]. The irritating effect of iodinated contrast is also commonly noted after sialography [18,19].

Active inflammation on a pertechnetate scan shows as increased blood flow, and apparent increased concentration, probably due to hyperaemia with increased capillary permeability, permitting extravasation and intracellular distribution of the tracer. Decreased washout is due to intra-glandular obstruction of the ductules, and retention within ectatic ducts and necrotic acinar spaces (Figure 15.7). Occasionally, a fistula tract may be identified.

The appearance of increased vascularity and apparent hyperconcentration in acute inflammation may be confused with a functioning mass. However, the focal appearance of a Warthin's tumour and its usual asymptomatic presentation

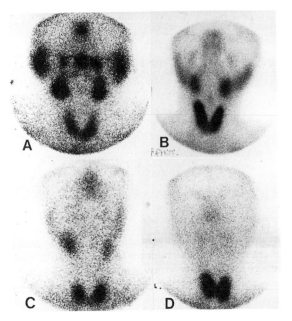

Figure 15.8 Sjögren's syndrome. Various degrees of severity in several patients. (A) Normal salivary function; note comparison with the thyroid gland. (B) Mild Sjögren's involvement affecting the parotid glands. (C) The parotids are more severely involved, and the submandibular function is reduced. (D) Very severe dysfunction of all salivary glands.

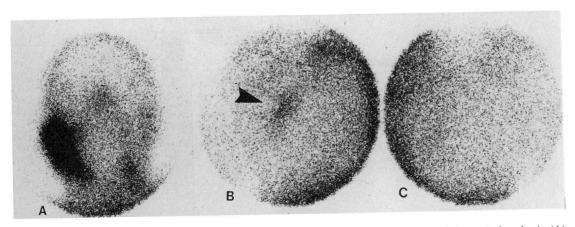

Figure 15.9 Gallium uptake in lymphoma of the right parotid. Note abnormal uptake in left cervical nodes in (A), and a right axillary node (arrowhead) in (B).

helps differentiate it from the more painful sialadenitis, with a diffuse uptake pattern.

SJÖGREN'S SYNDROME

Sjögren's syndrome is a chronic autoimmune inflammatory disease with infiltration by lymphocytes, plasma cells, and ultimately replacement by fibroblasts [20–22].

The pertechnetate salivary gland scan is useful in detecting and monitoring the progress of these patients with complaints of dry mouth. In the early stages, the parotid glands are usually first affected. The activity is less than that of the submandibular glands and the normal thyroid gland. In more severe involvement, the submandibular glands also show decreased function. In the most severe form, scarcely any concentration is seen in any of the salivary glands (Figure 15.8).

In Sjögren's syndrome radionuclide salivary imaging has a very high negative predictive value of 90%. However, a high false-positive rate with a positive predictive value of only 25% has been reported for analogue imaging [23]. Nonetheless, Kohn *et al.* [7] found that quantification is useful in assessing salivary gland images, as their results correlated with salivary gland flow rates.

Quantitative sialography TACs demonstrate the rate of accumulation and washout of tracer from the gland. Flattened TACs are a sensitive indicator of destruction of the salivary gland tissues [24]. When compared with contrast sialography and with histopathology of minor salivary gland biopsy evidence of inflammation, there is excellent correlation [25].

^{67}Ga-CITRATE SALIVARY IMAGING

^{67}Ga has wide usage in the detection of sepsis and some malignant neoplasms, but it does not distinguish between these diseases. Images obtained 48 hours after intravenous administration of 3 mCi (110 MBq) of ^{67}Ga show faint and symmetrical uptake in the normal salivary glands. Focal increased accumulation may represent a primary or secondary malignant neoplasm or infection.

The combination of ^{99m}Tc pertechnetate, and ^{67}Ga citrate imaging is useful in differential diagnosis of various salivary diseases. There is 90% sensitivity in the detection of Warthin's tumours, and 89% specificity for sialadenitis [26]. The differentiation of benign from malignant tumours is less reliable. However, a negative gallium scan

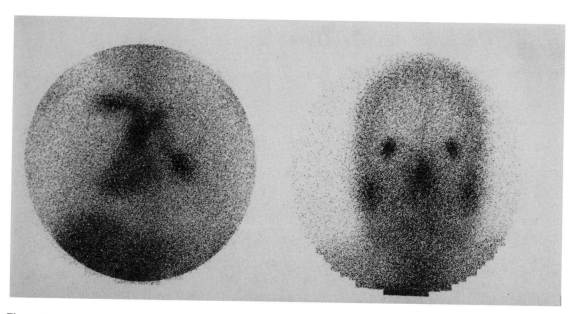

Figure 15.10 Gallium uptake in sarcoidosis. There is a 'lambda' (λ) sign in the view of the mediastinum, due to bilateral perihilar, and right peritracheal node involvement. The face shows a 'panda' sign due to lacrimal and parotid uptake of gallium. This combination is virtually diagnostic of sarcoidosis.

has a 91% negative predictive value in excluding malignant tumours of the salivary gland [27]. Although the sensitivity for detection of neoplasms varies with the histology, positive scans are generally seen only with malignant soft tissue tumours (Figure 15.9). In Sjögren's syndrome, salivary gland gallium uptake correlates with biopsy evidence of inflammatory infiltration, while decreased pertechnetate uptake is a test of dysfunction [28].

Following irradiation to the neck, localized inflammatory reaction results in radiation sialadenitis, and possible fibrosis of the salivary glands. During the first 6 months following radiotherapy, increased vascular permeability, oedema and inflammatory changes in the salivary glands can result in increased gallium uptake. Knowledge of the history of previous irradiation should prevent misinterpretation of this uptake as being due to recurrent tumour [29,30].

A positive gallium scan correlates well with the degree of inflammation, whether due to infectious or aseptic causes. Diffuse increased uptake occurs in aseptic inflammatory diseases such as sarcoidosis or the Mickulicz's syndrome. Salivary symptoms in sarcoidosis may be mild and overlooked in the presence of systemic or pulmonary manifestations. Serial whole-body gallium imaging in sarcoidosis is used to evaluate the distribution of the disease, the effect of therapy, or progression of disease [31]. Pulmonary uptake was present in 83% of the patients with Sjögren's syndrome with normal chest X-rays [28].

Bilateral lacrimal and salivary gallium uptake produces an image reminiscent of the face of a panda (Figure 15.10). The 'panda sign' is the most characteristic extrapulmonary radiogallium finding in sarcoidosis (seen in 41% of 114 patients) [32,33]. HIV patients, despite abnormal chest radiographs and salivary gallium uptake, did not show the panda or lambda findings.

[67]Ga citrate uptake is commonly seen in HIV-infected patients. Some 54% of patients with diffuse infiltrative lymphocytosis syndrome (DILS) complain of dry mouth. Salivary uptake was less common in patients with AIDS [34].

OBSTRUCTION

Drainage of the salivary glands may be obstructed by intraluminal causes, including opaque or non-opaque calculi, food or other foreign bodies, vis-

cous mucous plugs, inspissated pus, or post-inflammatory strictures. Benign or malignant tumours, cysts, surgery or trauma, may cause extra-luminal compression of a salivary duct. Patients typically complain of painful swelling, aggravated by eating, when the salivary flow rates are high.

Acute pyogenic sialadenitis may develop proximal to the obstruction (Figure 15.11). A fistula tract or a communicating abscess cavity is occasionally demonstrated [35]. However, more commonly, chronic inflammatory reaction and progressive atrophy due to back-pressure compromises salivary gland function. In obstruction without dysfunction, the initial images appear normal, but when secretion is stimulated by lemon juice, the activity is retained in the gland, and occasionally the dilated duct will be visualized. When there has been damage to the gland, concentration is markedly reduced. The decision to

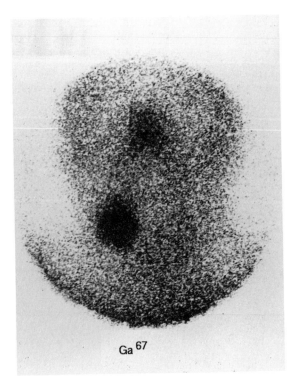

Figure 15.11 Gallium uptake in an acute right submandibular gland pyogenic infection. This condition is usually seen in debilitated, or immunosuppressed patients. This man was undergoing chemotherapy for carcinoma of the lung.

operate and salvage, or to sacrifice an obstructed gland may be based on its residual function as demonstrated by salivary gland scanning with pertechnetate.

CONCLUSIONS

The ability of the salivary glands to secrete and drain may be visually and quantitatively assessed with ^{99m}Tc pertechnetate scanning. Where indicated, salivary gland imaging with ^{67}Ga citrate may help in differentiating between malignant and benign tumours and in the detection and monitoring of inflammatory disease.

REFERENCES

1. Schall, G.L. and Di Chiro, G. (1972) Clinical usefulness of salivary gland scanning. *Semin. Nucl. Med.*, **2**, 270–7.
2. Greyson, N.D. and Noyek, A.M. (1982) Radionuclide salivary scanning. *J. Otolaryngol.*, **11**(10), 1–47.
3. Ohrt, H.J. and Shafer, R.B. (1982) An atlas of salivary gland disorders. *Clin. Nucl. Med.*, **8**, 370–6.
4. Schenkels, L.C., Veerman, E.C. and Nieuw Amerongen, A.V. (1995) Biochemical composition of human saliva in relation to other mucosal fluids. *Crit. Rev. Oral Biol. Med.*, **6**(2), 161–75.
5. Elgazzar, A.H., Gelfand, M.J., Washburn, L.C. *et al.* (1995) I-123 MIBG scintigraphy in adults: a report of clinical experience. *Clin. Nucl. Med.*, **20**(2), 147–52.
6. Sandler, E.D., Hattner, R.S. and Parisi, M.T. (1992) Asymmetry of salivary gland I-123 metaiodobenzylguanidine (MIBG) uptake in a patient with cervical neuroblastoma and Horner's syndrome – possible etiologic mechanisms. *Pediatr. Radiol.*, **22**(3), 225–6.
7. Kohn, W.G., Ship, J.A., Atkinson, J.C. *et al.* (1992) Salivary gland 99m Tc-scintigraphy: a grading scale and correlation with major salivary gland flow rates. *J. Oral Pathol. Med.*, **21**(2), 70–4.
8. Pilbrow, W.J., Brownless, S.M., Cawood, J.I. *et al.* (1990) Salivary gland scintigraphy – a suitable substitute for sialography? *Br. J. Radiol.*, **63**(747), 190–6.
9. Ishikawa, H. and Ishii, Y. (1984) Evaluation of salivary gland tumours with 99m Tc-pertechnetate. *J. Oral Maxillofac. Surg.*, **42**(7), 429–34.
10. Gnepp, D.R., Schroeder, W. and Heffner, D. (1989) Synchronous tumours arising in a single major salivary gland. *Cancer*, **63**(6), 1219–24.
11. Weinstein, G.S., Harvey, R.T.T., Zimmer, W. *et al.* (1994) Technetium-99m pertechnetate salivary gland imaging: its role in the diagnosis of Warthin's tumour. *J. Nucl. Med.*, **35**(1), 179–83.
12. Hwang, B.T., Sugihara, K., Kawashima, K. *et al.* (1987) Scanning electron microscopic study of Warthin's tumour. *J. Oral Pathol.*, **16**(3), 118–23.
13. Higashi, T., Murahashi, H., Ikuta, H. *et al.* (1987) Identification of Warthin's tumour with technetium-99m pertechnetate. *Clin. Nucl. Med.*, **12**(10), 796–800.
14. Sostre, S., Medina, L. and de Arellano, G.R. (1987) The various scintigraphic patterns of Warthin's tumour. *Clin. Nucl. Med.*, **12**(8), 620–6.
15. Blue, P.W. (1988) Failure of washout following gustatory stimulation in Warthin's tumour. *Nucl. Med. Commun.*, **9**(6), 431–3.
16. Liu, R.S., Yeh, S.H., Yen, T.C. *et al.* (1990) Salivary scintigraphy with vitamin C stimulation: an aid in differentiating unilateral parotitis from Warthin's tumour. *Eur. J. Nucl. Med.*, **16**(8), 689–91.
17. Golberg, R.E.A. and Miraldi, F. (1987) Radionuclide imaging of potassium iodide-induced sialadinitis. *Clin. Nucl. Med.*, **12**(5), 370–2.
18. Hardoff, R. and Nachtigal, D. (1989) Unilateral gallium-67 uptake in submandibular salivary gland following sialography. *Clin. Nucl. Med.*, **14**(1), 65.
19. Higashi, T., Mori, Y., Ikuta, H. *et al.* (1988) Salivary gland uptake of gallium-67 citrate after sialography. *Clin. Nucl. Med.*, **13**(2), 110–13.
20. Cleland-Zamudio, S., Demuth, M. and Trune, D.R. (1993) Pathology of labial salivary gland cellular aggregates in Sjögren's syndrome. *Otolaryngol. Head Neck Surg.*, **108**(1), 44–50.
21. Fox, R.I. and Kang, H.I. (1992) Pathogenesis of Sjögren's syndrome. *Rheum. Dis. Clin. North Am.*, **18**(3), 517–38.
22. Huguet, P., Bosch, J.A., Raventos, A. *et al.* (1995) Sjögren's syndrome: histologic and immunohistochemical study. *Ann. Med. Interne*, **146**(4), 233–4.
23. Markusse, H.M., Pillay, M. and Breedveld, F.C. (1993) The diagnostic value of salivary gland scintigraphy in patients suspected of primary Sjögren's syndrome. *Br. J. Rheumatol.*, **32**(3), 231–5.
24. Arrago, J.P., Rain, J.D., Brocheriou, C. *et al.* (1987) Scintigraphy of the salivary glands in Sjögren's syndrome. *J. Clin. Pathol.*, **40**(12), 1463–7.
25. Sugihara, T. and Yoshimura, Y. (1988) Scintigraphic evaluation of the salivary glands in patients with Sjögren's syndrome. *Int. J. Oral Maxillofac. Surg.*, **17**(2), 71–5.
26. Higashi, T., Shindo, J., Everhart, F. *et al.* (1989) Technetium-99m pertechnetate and gallium-67 imaging in salivary gland disease. *Clin. Nucl. Med.*, **14**(7), 504–14.
27. Arbab, A.S., Koizumi, K., Uchiyama, G. *et al.* (1995) The usefulness and limitations of combined ^{99m}Tc pertechnetate and ^{67}Ga citrate imaging of salivary gland disorders. *Clin. Nucl. Med.*, **20**(1), 5–12.
28. Collins, R.D., Jr, Ball, G.V. and Login, J.R. (1984) Gallium-67 scanning in Sjögren's syndrome: concise communication. *J. Nucl. Med.*, **25**(3), 299–302.
29. Beckerman, C. and Hoffer, P.B. (1976) Salivary gland uptake of ^{67}Ga citrate following radiation therapy. *J. Nucl. Med.*, **17**(8), 685–7.
30. Lentle, B.C., Jackson, F.I. and McGowan, D.G. (1976) Localisation of gallium-67 citrate in salivary glands following radiation therapy. *J. Can. Assoc. Radiol.*, **27**(2), 89–91.

31. Lubat, E. and Kramer, E.C. (1985) Gallium-67 citrate accumulation in parotid and submandibular glands in sarcoidosis. *Clin. Nucl. Med.*, **10**, 593.
32. Sulavik, S.B., Spencer, R.P., Weed, D.A. *et al.* (1990) Recognition of distinctive patterns of gallium-67 distribution in sarcoidosis. *J. Nucl. Med.*, **31**(12), 1909–14.
33. Sulavik, S.B., Spencer, R.P. and Castriotta, R.J. (1991) Panda sign – avid and symmetrical radiogallium accumulation in the lacrimal and parotid glands. *Semin. Nucl. Med.*, **21**(4), 339–40.
34. Rosenberg, Z.S., Joffe, S.A. and Itescu, S. (1992) Spectrum of salivary gland disease in HIV-infected patients: characterisation with Ga-67 citrate imaging. *Radiology*, **184**(3), 761–4.
35. Mrhac, L., Zakko, S. and Parikh, Y.H. (1995) Saliva leakage from the parotid gland. *Clin. Nucl. Med.*, **20**(2), 178–9.

Lacrimal apparatus

N. D. Greyson

INTRODUCTION

Tears play a vital role in protecting vision by: moistening and lubricating the sclera, maintaining optical uniformity, providing nutrition for the cornea, and washing away foreign particles. The presence of antibacterial substances, including lysozyme and antibodies in tears protects the eyes from infection.

The quantity of the liquid film over the eye is a balance between production and drainage of tears. Due to the involvement of secretory elements, the volume of tears may be decreased in certain inflammatory conditions such as sarcoidosis. An excessive amount of tears ('epiphora') may be the result of overproduction or impeded drainage. Overproduction occurs in allergic reactions, rhinitis, corneal irritation due to abrasion, irritation by foreign bodies, noxious smells, and emotions. Decreased drainage may be the result of obstruction.

Functional obstruction occurs when the duct system is patent but the drainage mechanism is inefficient, e.g. ectropion, facial palsy, orbicularis oculi muscle paralysis or exophthalmos, etc.

A variety of invasive techniques such as probing, cannulation, irrigation and contrast dacrocystography are available for demonstrating the patency and anatomy of the nasolacrimal duct system. Radionuclide imaging provides a non-invasive, physiological approach to the evaluation of tear duct drainage [1–4].

ANATOMY AND PHYSIOLOGY

The lacrimal apparatus comprises the lacrimal glands, lacrimal ducts, lacrimal canals, lacrimal sacs and the nasolacrimal ducts.

The compound tubuloacinar lacrimal glands located in the superolateral part of the orbital cavity secrete a watery saltish fluid. Tears produced by the lacrimal glands drain through 6 to 12 small ducts into the upper eyelids and spread by capillary action to form a film over the eyes that is kept refreshed by blinking. The lacrimal secretion or tears mix with an oily mucoid secretion derived from the sebaceous glands in the eyelids and mucous glands in the conjunctiva, which helps lubricate and protect the delicate surfaces of the eye and slows down fluid evaporation. Tear secretion averages about 1 ml/day. However, the amount produced is variable and 'reflex' tear flow may occur under parasympathetic stimulation due to corneal or conjunctival irritation in response to a foreign body, irritating odours, allergy and emotions, and excessive drying due to a deficiency of the oily component.

Normally, much of the tears evaporate; excess tears accumulate in the inferior and medial recesses of the eyes. Tiny orifices or puncta in the upper and lower eyelids in the medial canthus of the eye provide entrance for the tears to the superior and inferior canaliculi that merge medially to form the common canaliculus, leading to the lacrimal sac. The lacrimal sac has a thin fibroelastic wall lined by a mucous membrane, and drains into the nasolacrimal duct that lies medial to the maxillary antrum. The nasolacrimal duct opens into the nose, below the inferior turbinate bone. Imperfect valves occur between the sac and ducts, and at the lower end of the nasolacrimal duct (Figure 15.12).

For efficient drainage by capillary action, the punctum must be in contact with the cornea. The canaliculi are surrounded by the orbicularis muscles; blinking causes contraction and stretching of the common canaliculus, resulting in a pump-like action, which enhances tear drainage through a vacuum effect [5].

RADIONUCLIDE DACROCYSTOGRAPHY

TECHNIQUE

The passage of tracer through the lacrimal duct system is visualized using a gamma-camera (fitted with a fine pinhole collimator) for demonstrating the patency of the lacrimal drainage system or localizing the level of obstruction.

For optimal imaging of the fine-calibre lacrimal ductal system (the canaliculi measure 10 mm in

Clinical Nuclear Medicine, 3rd edn. Edited by M.N. Maisey, K.E. Britton and B.D. Collier. Published in 1998 by Chapman & Hall, London. ISBN 0 412 75180 1

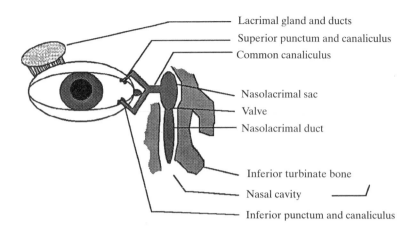

Figure 15.12   Schematic drawing of components of the lacrimal apparatus.

length and 0.5 mm in diameter), the use of a fine pinhole collimator with a 1- to 2-mm orifice is preferable to a standard 3- to 5-mm pinhole collimator (Figure 15.13). Smaller pinhole apertures improve image resolution, but the decrease in sensitivity prolongs the imaging time, which increases the likelihood of image degradation due to patient motion.

The patient is seated in front of the gamma-camera with head stabilized to prevent motion. A tuberculin syringe is filled with 100 μCi (3.7 MBq) 99mTc-pertechnetate in a volume of 10 μl. After removing the needle, a tiny droplet of pertechnetate is gently pushed onto the syringe hub. This droplet is touched to the upper lateral portion of the surface of the eye; it rapidly spreads by capillary action to coat the eyeball. Radiation dose to the lens is 4–14 mrads [6].

Some authors have reported an imaging protocol using 10-s image frames with computer-generated regions of interest. Although useful for research purposes, this rapid imaging sequence is not necessary for general clinical use.

Normally, activity passes through the canaliculi into the nasolacrimal sac within seconds, but transit through the sac and duct into the nasal cavity may take up to 2–5 minutes. The symptomatic eye is studied first, and sequential 60-s images are recorded for 5 minutes following tracer administration (Figure 15.14). Acquisition is continued if the drainage is slow, but imaging beyond 15–20 minutes is unnecessary. Next, the tracer is instilled into the normal eye. Changing the distance between the patient and the aperture of the pinhole

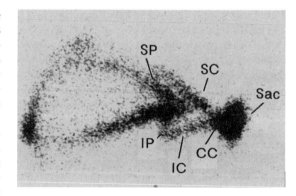

Figure 15.13   High-resolution image of the right eye using a 1-mm tungsten pinhole collimator, 5 minutes following administration of a droplet of 99mTc-pertechnetate onto the surface of the eye. Note the fine detail of the canaliculi. Here, the activity does not extend distal to the nasolacrimal sac, as this patient had an obstruction at that level. IP, inferior punctum; SP, superior punctum; IC, inferior canaliculus; SC, superior canaliculus; CC, common canaliculus; Sac, nasolacrimal sac.

collimator changes the magnification of the field-of-view, and permits either imaging of one eye at a time or simultaneous imaging of both eyes.

INTERPRETATION

The normal pattern is characterized by visualization of the lacrimal sac usually within 1 minute of instillation of activity, and drainage of the nasolacrimal duct into the nasal cavity within 5

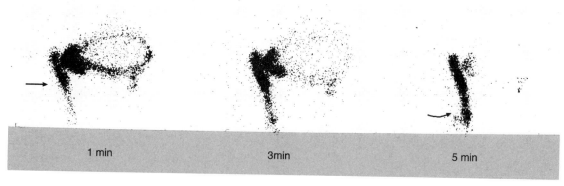

Figure 15.14 Normal radionuclide dacrocystogram. Sequential images of the left eye show prompt and progressive drainage of the tracer through the lacrimal sac (straight arrow) to reach the nasolacrimal duct (curved arrow).

minutes. If there is no patient motion, images acquired with a fine-pinhole collimator will show excellent anatomical resolution, often including the detail of the canaliculi. Artefactual patterns include activity on the eyelashes and tears running down the cheeks. Special attention should be paid to tears on the medial side of the cheek, adjacent to the nose, which could simulate the appearance of the nasolacrimal duct. However, the stream of tears along the nose deviates laterally, while the nasolacrimal duct typically terminates with a medial curvature into the nasal cavity.

Normally, the transit of the tracer is rapid, outlining the drainage pathways within a few minutes. A delay in drainage time or termination of the bolus proximal to the nasal cavity, indicates partial or complete obstruction. Common causes of obstruction include acute and chronic inflammation, mucus plugs, dacroliths, strictures due to trauma, neoplasm, radiation, and congenital failure of nasolacrimal duct canalization [7].

Common sites of obstruction are: the common canaliculus, the junction between the lacrimal sac and the nasolacrimal duct, and the distal end of the nasolacrimal duct (Figures 15.15–15.17). In 85% of the cases, the level of obstruction demonstrated by radionuclide dacrocystography correlates with the contrast results, but in 15% the scintigraphic site of obstruction appears more proximal. This has been attributed to the high sensitivity of the technique [3], but this may be due to back pressure, stasis, debris, mucus, or pus proximal to the obstruction.

If the suspected cause of obstruction is inflammatory oedema due to allergy, a repeat study

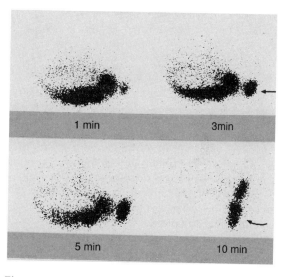

Figure 15.15 Partial obstruction between the lacrimal sac and nasolacrimal duct of the right eye. Note filling of the lacrimal sac (straight arrow) and the delayed visualization of the nasolacrimal duct (curved arrow).

following administration of vasoconstrictor medication may show restoration of normal drainage pattern [8].

If, in a patient presenting clinically with epiphora, the duct system is felt to be patent through probing or irrigation, it may be that the obstruction has been overcome by the pressure of the injection and that a drainage problem does exist [9]. It is also possible to have a 'functional obstruction' with a patent duct system: the patient

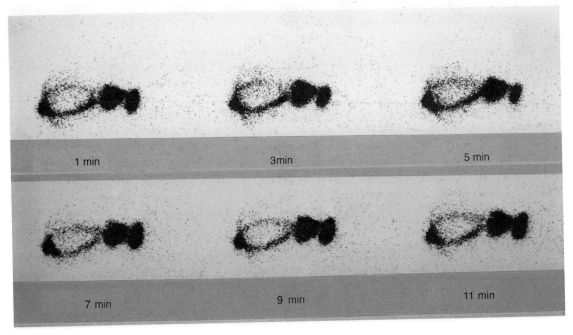

Figure 15.16   Complete obstruction between the lacrimal sac and nasolacrimal duct of the right eye.

may have ectropion or eversion of the eyelid, preventing the punctum from coming into contact with the tears, or a dysfunction of the 'tear-pump' mechanism of the orbicularis oculi muscles. In these circumstances, surgical intervention may be unsuccessful. If the radionuclide test shows normal drainage, no further investigation is needed [10].

CLINICAL VALUE

Non-physiological techniques such as irrigation, probing or contrast dacrocystography may fail to establish the presence of obstruction, if the injection pressure overcomes the resistance of the obstructing lesion. These techniques also do not assess the function of the 'tear-pump' mechanism.

The surgical approach to correcting obstruction of the lacrimal drainage system depends on location of obstruction. Surgical repair by dacrocystorhinostomy produces an anastomotic mucosa-lined connection between the lacrimal sac and the nasal cavity. This is only useful if the obstruction is distal to the sac. For obstructions proximal to the sac, microscopic canalicular anastomoses, balloon dilatation and stents may be used. Following repair, patency of the pathway may be demonstrated non-invasively by radionuclide dacrocystography for assessing the results of surgery.

Radionuclide dacrocystography is an underutilized tool in the assessment of the common complaint of epiphora. It can rapidly and sensitively diagnose the presence of obstruction and accurately demonstrate the site of obstruction of the lacrimal drainage system. The technique is useful in the management of patients following surgical repair or trauma.

LACRIMAL GLAND DISORDERS

The lacrimal gland is subject to involvement by a number of diseases, similar to those affecting the salivary glands. These include acute or chronic inflammation, benign or malignant tumours, and atrophy. In autoimmune inflammatory conditions such as rheumatoid arthritis, or aseptic inflammations such as sarcoidosis, there is lymphocytic infiltration of the lacrimal and salivary glands with an increase in plasma cells, degeneration and necrosis of the glandular epithelium, and ultimately fibroblastic activity that results in atrophy. This is manifested by complaints of dry eyes and dry mouth (Sjögren's syndrome or keratconjunctivitis sicca).

The lacrimal glands and tears are high in lactoferrin, which accounts for the visualization of the lacrimal glands on a gallium-67 scan. On a normal gallium scan of the face, lacrimal activity may be seen in a high proportion of patients. The intensity of uptake is mild and the distribution invariably symmetrical, but the absence of lacrimal activity is not abnormal.

Intense or asymmetric lacrimal gallium-67 uptake may indicate either unilateral or bilateral inflammatory infiltration, or a malignant neoplasm. We have noted unilateral absent gallium uptake in the lacrimal gland in patients with facial nerve injury, following direct trauma to the lacrimal gland, and as a result of previous infection.

In systemic aseptic inflammation, such as in sarcoidosis, lacrimal involvement accompanies the lymphatic, pulmonary or other manifestations in up to 88% of patients [11,12]. Lacrimal uptake with lymphoma is unusual. The combination of hilar adenopathy and lacrimal uptake, with or without salivary involvement, is much more suggestive of sarcoidosis than lymphoma [13] (Figure 15.18). The frequent combination of hot lacrimal

Figure 15.17 Complete obstruction proximal to the lacrimal sac – at the level of the common canaliculus of the right eye. This image pattern persisted for 15 minutes when the test was terminated.

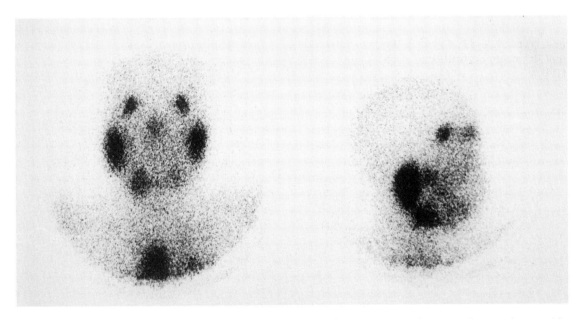

Figure 15.18 ^{67}Gallium citrate images of a 26-year-old female with lacrimal and salivary involvement by sarcoidosis. The patient complained of dry eyes and a dry mouth. Mediastinal lymph node uptake is noted.

and salivary glands in sarcoidosis produces the typical 'panda-face' appearance on a gallium scan [14]. Uveitis is observed in 26% of patients with sarcoidosis. A positive gallium scan is useful in detecting ophthalmic involvement in patients despite the absence of ophthalmic symptoms [15].

Other infiltrative disorders, such as amyloidosis of the lacrimal glands, are a much less common cause of the sicca syndrome, and are usually not associated with increased gallium accumulation.

REFERENCES

1. Rossomondo, R.M., Carlton, W.H., Trueblood, J.H. *et al.* (1972) A new method of evaluating lacrimal drainage. *Arch. Ophthalmol.*, **88**, 523–5.
2. Carlton, W.H., Trueblood, J.I. and Rossomondo, R.M. (1973) Clinical evaluation of microscintigraphy of the lacrimal drainage apparatus. *J. Nucl. Med.*, **14**(2), 89–92.
3. von Denffer, H., Dressler, J. and Pabst, H.W. (1984) Lacrimal dacryoscintigraphy. *Semin. Nucl. Med.*, **14**(1), 8–15.
4. Hurwitz, J.J. and Victor, W.H. (1985) The role of sophisticated radiological testing in the assessment and management of epiphora. *Ophthalmology*, **92**(3), 407–13.
5. White, W.L., Glover, A.T. and Buckner, A.B. (1991) Effect of blinking on tear elimination as evaluated by dacryoscintigraphy. *Ophthalmology*, **98**(3), 367–9.
6. Heyman, S., Katowitz, J.A. and Smoger, B. (1985) Dacryoscintigraphy in children. *Ophthalmic Surgery*, **16**(11), 703–9.
7. Hulsey, J.M. and Smith, R. (1988) Obstructive pattern in dacryoscintigraphy. *Semin. Nucl. Med.*, **18**(1), 65–7.
8. Kim, C.K., Palestro, C.J., Solomon, R.W. *et al.* (1989) Serial dacryoscintigraphy before and after treatment with pseudoephedrine. *Clin. Nucl. Med.*, **14**(10), 734–5.
9. Hanna, I.T., MacEwen, C.J. and Kennedy, N. (1992) Lacrimal scintigraphy in the diagnosis of epiphora. *Nucl. Med. Commun.*, **13**(6), 416–20.
10. Rose, J.D. and Clayton, C.B. (1985) Scintigraphy and contrast radiography for epiphora. *Br. J. Radiol.*, **58**(696), 1183–6.
11. Savolaine, E.R. and Schlembach, P.J. (1990) Gallium scan diagnosis of sarcoidosis in the presence of equivocal radiographic and CT findings: value of lacrimal gland biopsy. *Clin. Nucl. Med.*, **15**(3), 198–9.
12. Israel, H.L., Albertine, K.H., Park, C.H. *et al.* (1991) Whole-body gallium 67 scans. Role in diagnosis of sarcoidosis. *Annu. Rev. Resp. Dis.*, **144**(5), 1182–6.
13. Sulavik, S.B., Spencer, R.P., Weed, D.A. *et al.* (1990) Recognition of distinctive patterns of gallium-67 distribution in sarcoidosis. *J. Nucl. Med.*, **31**(12), 1909–14.
14. Sulavik, S.B., Spencer, R.P. and Castriotta, R.J. (1991) Panda-sign: avid and symmetrical radiogallium accumulation in the lacrimal and parotid glands. *Semin. Nucl. Med.*, **21**(4), 339–40.
15. Karrna, A., Poukkula, A.A. and Ruokonen, A.O. (1987) Assessment of activity of ocular sarcoidosis by gallium scanning. *Br. J. Ophthalmol.*, **71**(5), 361–7.

Technical topics

CHAPTER 16

Radiopharmaceuticals

Introduction

C. R. Lazarus

Recent years have witnessed developments not only in the practice of radiopharmacy, but also in the introduction of new radiopharmaceuticals. New radiopharmaceuticals are giving us the potential to localize and study structures such as antigens with radiolabelled antibodies, receptors with radioligands, enzyme and hormonal systems, localization of infection, inflammation, and early detection of cancers. Progress has also been made in the development of radiolabelled compounds for treatment.

The introduction of new radiopharmaceuticals is now based on more scientific and rational approaches than the earlier, more traditional agents which were often based on the fortuitous finding that a certain radionuclide or molecule localized in a certain body organ. Britton [1], in his review of the development of radiopharmaceuticals makes the point that the way to develop a new radiopharmaceutical is first to ask the clinical question, then examine the physiological basis of how a molecule enters and binds within a cell, and then to look at the molecular basis of these interactions with the possibility of genetic engineering. However, he warns that this development work is being hampered by regulatory authorities who express an unjustified risk-related fear and unreasonable concern in relation to biological products such as antibodies. The continued development of radiopharmaceuticals from biomolecules will undoubtedly continue to attract the attention of the authorities.

RADIOPHARMACEUTICAL USE

Many new radiopharmaceuticals have been very expensive to develop and bring to the market, and this is reflected in their high price. The high price in turn has led to practices in the provision of radiopharmaceuticals which can lead – and have led – to ethical and patient-related problems. Factors to be considered in the introduction of a new radiopharmaceutical are discussed later in this chapter. There is a need to apply more caution in the provision and use of radiopharmaceuticals. To this end, there have been several advances in the practice of radiopharmacy, including dispensing techniques and professional activities such as audit and reporting schemes.

AUTOMATION

Attempts have been made over recent years to introduce some form of automation into the preparation of routine radiopharmaceuticals. The short half-lives of positron-emitting radionuclides, which in turn requires the handling of very large amounts of radioactivity, has already stimulated the application of automatic techniques in PET. This equipment tends to be a single automated device for each radiopharmaceutical prepared, and is not suitable for routine daily

Clinical Nuclear Medicine, 3rd edn. Edited by M.N. Maisey, K.E. Britton and B.D. Collier. Published in 1998 by Chapman & Hall, London. ISBN 0 412 75180 1

preparation of ^{99m}Tc-labelled radiopharmaceuticals. Here, the continuing and increasing demand has led to increased radiation finger-doses from handling larger quantities of radioactivity. Equipment has been developed that will automatically elute a ^{99m}Tc generator, prepare kits and measure the radioactivity. These devices undoubtedly reduce body and finger radiation doses to the operators, but significant problems are associated with their use. For example, the use of fluid-filled tubing can result in the cross-contamination of radiopharmaceuticals with other preparations, while it is also necessary to maintain the whole system in a sterile state – a condition which can be difficult to achieve.

A new device, which involves the use of a robotic arm, capable of eluting a generator, preparing radiopharmaceuticals and subsequently transferring into multi-dose vials or syringes, has been investigated [2]. This approach is different in that no fluid-filled tubing is involved. Sterility is maintained by siting the robotic arm and all associated equipment in a containment isolator, which provides a sterile environment conforming to the guidelines. The robotic arm imitates the manual operation and uses a fresh syringe and needle for each dispensing manipulation. The manufacturer's (Amercare, UK Ltd) intention is that the Amercare Pharmaceutical Automation (APA) system should reduce finger and eye doses to the operator to as low as practically possible, while producing sterile radiopharmaceuticals in a consistent manner and minimizing chances of error. The system allows complete documentation of the process and traceability of all doses. It has been shown [2] that the robotic arm is capable of dispensing over 100 doses per hour with activity and volume errors of <5%. Furthermore, the radiation dose to the operator is virtually eliminated. The APA system is operated from a desktop personal computer (PC), with preparation data being entered through the keyboard into a database. Reports are generated from a printer attached to the PC. There must, of course, be safeguards that any automatic system is capable of achieving its ends. The Good Automated Manufacturing Practice (GAMP) [3] helps suppliers of automated systems to the pharmaceutical industry to ensure that systems are developed with built-in quality and to provide documented evidence that the system meets agreed specifications.

PREPARATION TECHNIQUES AND CONTROL

Radiopharmaceuticals are prepared in hospitals by an aseptic technique, which requires that the handling and transfer of injectables should be within a specified and carefully controlled environment in order to maintain sterility. This has usually been achieved using vertical laminar flow cabinets in traditional pharmaceutical clean rooms. A new innovation has been the introduction of isolators, which are containment devices utilizing barrier technology for the enclosure of a controlled work space. In addition to protecting the product during manipulations, they can be designed to work under a negative pressure, which helps provide protection to the operator from radiation hazards. One advantage of isolators is that they can be used in a background environment of a lower standard than that required for open-fronted laminar flow cabinets.

The increasing awareness of the responsibility to patients by producing radiopharmaceuticals that are safe and efficacious has led radiopharmacies in many countries to review the activities carried out within their unit. In the UK, audit of the radiopharmacy is now an expected part of professional practice. A protocol for auditing radiopharmacies has been developed [4] and the audit document can be used by a radiopharmacy for self-assessment, or it can form the basis for peer review. The radiopharmacy audit looks at various aspects of the operation. A series of questions are asked about the facilities and their compliance with relevant regulations and guidelines is recorded as a 'yes' or 'no' answer. Similar questions are asked regarding documentation, quality assurance, radiation safety, training, health and safety, and professional practice matters. Peer audit provides a very useful means of highlighting deficiencies within a radiopharmacy, and enables programmes to be developed to raise standards to a high level common to all radiopharmacies.

RADIOPHARMACEUTICAL INTERACTIONS

Practitioners of nuclear medicine who have spent many years in the field are now aware that it is possible to alter the behaviour of a radiopharmaceutical in the body. These alterations can be unexpected, and can sometimes be traced to *in vivo* interactions between the radiopharmaceutical and a concomitant medicine, which the patient is taking at the time of the study. It may be useful to have the patient's drug history available to help explain an unusual image. Further difficulties can arise if a patient is self-treating with undeclared 'over the counter' medicines. Conversely, it has now become common practice to deliberately alter the behaviour of a radiopharmaceutical with interventional drugs and procedures to provide more diagnostic information from a nuclear medicine study, e.g. dipyridamole as a stress agent in cardiac studies. A detailed discussion of these interactions is given later.

Radiopharmaceuticals have proven to be extremely safe to administer to patients. However, occasionally there is an untoward reaction to an administered radiopharmaceutical. Reporting schemes in USA, Europe and other areas of the world have been in existence for many years. Estimation of the frequency of these reactions is hampered by a reluctance of many to report them to these schemes. If reporting rates were to be improved, it would also enable an estimation of the probability of the association of the reaction with the radiopharmaceutical in question. The various schemes and reactions are reviewed later in this chapter.

The European Association of Nuclear Medicine uses its 'adverse reaction reporting form' to also report radiopharmaceutical defects. Reporting takes the form of indicating which of a series of given defects applies, and a description of the problem and action taken. The reporting and collation of these defects can subsequently be used to encourage manufacturers and suppliers of radiopharmaceuticals to rectify the defect(s), and raise standards in the process.

PROCESS VALIDATION

An activity which radiopharmacies are increasingly being required to perform is that of equipment and process validation. This requires the radiopharmacist to prove that all procedures, processes (including quality control), equipment, material, activity or system leads to the expected result. When any new procedure or equipment, etc. is introduced into the radiopharmacy, its suitability for its purpose should be demonstrated. A significant amendment to procedures, processes or equipment that may affect quality, should also be validated. Furthermore, these activities should periodically be revalidated to ensure that they continue to achieve their intended purposes.

COSTS

A common complaint with the introduction of new radiopharmaceuticals is their high cost. Manufacturers claim that it is necessary to charge these prices for their new products in order to recoup the costs incurred in product development and bringing it to the market. A substantial portion of the incurred costs is spent on providing the necessary documentation and other data necessary to obtain the national licences required to market the product in various countries. Users of these new products reply that there are several implications to these higher costs. The cost of the new product may be beyond the budget of the department, and so not be available to them. If a decision to adopt the product is taken, it is necessary to pass on the cost to whoever referred the patient. Again, this cost may be prohibitive, and may persuade a referring physician either not to repeat the test or to send his patient elsewhere for a cheaper test.

'SPLITTING' KITS

The increased cost of a new 'cold' kit has led many radiopharmacies and nuclear medicine departments to try to extend the use of the kit by getting more doses from a vial of the product. Such techniques often include reconstituting a product vial with physiological saline, and dividing the resulting solution into portions in fresh vials, which are then stored frozen. When a dose is required, a frozen vial is allowed to come to room temperature, and then radiolabelled. Often, the quantities of radioactivity used for the total of the split vials is far in excess of that recommended by the manufacturer. In the UK, the cold kits are licensed by the licensing authority once the manufacturer has demonstrated that the product is safe, efficient and conforms to their high standards of quality. The manufacturer will define the limits of radioactivity and volume, in the instructions on reconstituting the product in the package insert. Providing that these limits and instructions are carefully followed, the product will comply with the intended specification. Manufacturers have no control over the quality of a product made outside their recommended preparation limits. They also have no responsibility for any problems caused by such a product in a patient. If a radiopharmacy or nuclear medicine department does decide to 'split' kits and reconstitute them outside the manufacturer's recommendations, then the responsibility lies entirely with the department. Many of the new kits appear very sensitive and unstable under certain conditions, and problems can occur even if manufacturer's limits and instructions are followed, e.g. the quality of ^{99m}Tc to be used with exametazime is defined within narrow limits, and failure to observe this can lead to the presence of high levels of pertechnetate in the product; it is now established that dilution of ^{99m}Tc with physiological saline from some plastic ampoules may interfere with the radiolabelling of MAG3. A radiopharmacy, which 'splits' kits, must validate beyond any doubt that this practice produces a product that is safe and efficient to use with patients. Safety requires that no microbiological contamination is introduced during the 'splitting' process and subsequent storage. It must be established that the resulting product is chemically identical to that intended by the manufacturer, and its biodistribution in the body organs has not been altered by, for example, a change in concentration,

or administration of smaller doses of the radiolabelled material. In addition to sterility, other pharmaceutical questions must be answered. Does freezing and thawing affect the chemical nature of the product? Does the product adhere to or interact with the container or rubber closure when present in more dilute solutions in a vial? The act of 'splitting' and reconstituting a cold kit produces in effect, a new product, since it certainly lies outside the manufacturer's specification, and may behave differently in the patient to that expected. A manufacturer has subjected their new product to rigorous testing and quality control before bringing it to the market. It may be necessary for a 'kit-splitter' to subject his or her new product to equally rigorous testing and trial before allowing it to be used in their patients.

REFERENCES

1. Britton, K.E. (1990) The development of new radiopharmaceuticals. *Eur. J. Nucl. Med.*, **16**, 373–85.
2. Solanki, K., Gill, R. and Stoker, M. (1993) A case for automated radiopharmaceutical dispensing. *Nucl. Med. Commun.*, **14**, 914.
3. UK Pharmaceutical Industry Computer Validation Forum (1995) *Good Automated Manufacturing Practice. Supplier Guide for Validation of Automated Systems in Pharmaceutical Manufacture*, London (second draft).
4. Cox, J.A., Hesslewood, S.R. and Palmer, A.M. (1994) A mechanism for professional and organizational audit of radiopharmacy departments. *Nucl. Med. Commun.*, **15**, 890–8.

Interactions

S. R. Hesslewood

INTRODUCTION

The diagnostic or therapeutic efficacy of a radiopharmaceutical is highly dependent on its biodistribution within the body after administration. Unintended alteration of this biodistribution can lead to sub-optimal outcome of a nuclear medicine procedure. It is highly likely that most patients will be taking some form of medication, and the possible effects of these drugs on the biodistribution of radiopharmaceuticals need to be considered. Therefore, an awareness of the potentially important interactions between radiopharmaceuticals and drugs is important for nuclear medicine departments. Such knowledge can be used to prevent occurrence of potentially detrimental effects by modifying the patient's drugs before the procedure, thereby reducing the possibility of alteration in radiopharmaceutical biodistribution. For diagnostic investigations, unintended alteration may lead to an erroneous result or require a repeat investigation, thus causing inconvenience to the patients and increasing their radiation burden. With therapeutic radiopharmaceuticals, an altered biodistribution may result in ineffective treatment and can have marked effects on radiation dosimetry by irradiation of the non-target organs of the body.

There have been many articles and textbooks quoting examples of drug–radiopharmaceutical interactions. The earliest reports were mainly related to the effects of drugs on thyroid uptake of iodine radiopharmaceuticals. Grayson [1] described drugs including radio-opaque contrast media and dietary factors, which could interfere with such studies. In addition, the well-established mechanisms by which these interactions occur were described. However, this is not true for all reports of drugs affecting nuclear medicine procedures. Mechanisms are not clear in many cases and the reports are sometimes anecdotal. The clinical significance of some of the reports is also unclear, and the occurrence of an event in a particular patient does not necessarily mean that it will be universal. Neither is it always possible to extrapolate experimental results into clinical significance. For example, *in vitro* labelling of erythrocytes was found to be adversely affected by dipyridamole [2], whereas clinical studies in which dipyridamole was present in the patient's blood during erythrocyte labelling did not demonstrate the same problem [3]. One of the explanations offered was the large difference in drug concentration in the two circumstances. Many published reports concern radiopharmaceuticals, which are now in limited use and hence of historical interest. It is not intended in this chapter to list every reported instance, and reference should be made to the texts listed in the further reading for comprehensive lists. Mechanisms by which drug–radiopharmaceutical interactions can occur and examples of potential clinical significance in current nuclear medicine practice will be discussed.

CLASSIFICATION OF RADIOPHARMACEUTICAL–DRUG INTERACTIONS

Several methods have been used to categorize these interactions, including classification according to the radiopharmaceutical involved [4], the investigation or treatment being undertaken [5], or the drug involved [6]. Each of these methods has its merits in providing look-up tables for speedy reference. However, with the introduction of new radiopharmaceuticals and therapeutic drugs, such tables are in need of regular updating. A more generalized, all-encompassing scheme based on mechanisms involved has been proposed [7] and offers a convenient basis for discussion. The four different types of mechanism include pharmacological, pharmacokinetic, toxicological and pharmaceutical.

PHARMACOLOGICAL INTERACTIONS

In this situation, the intended or secondary effect of the therapeutic drug alters the biodistribution of the radiopharmaceutical. Many of these interactions are regarded as detrimental to the investigation. However, recognition of interactions has, in

Clinical Nuclear Medicine, 3rd edn. Edited by M.N. Maisey, K.E. Britton and B.D. Collier. Published in 1998 by Chapman & Hall, London. ISBN 0 412 75180 1

some cases, led to the development of deliberate drug interventions within the nuclear medicine department in order to enhance the efficacy of the investigation. In other cases, it has enabled use to be made of the radiopharmaceutical to monitor the effect of the drug – for example, in determination of receptor-binding affinity of a drug or monitoring the toxic effects of chemotherapeutic agents. The use of deliberate drug interventions has been recently reviewed [8]. In current practice, one of the most important interventions is the use of pharmacological stress techniques as opposed to exercise tests in the determination of myocardial perfusion. Vasodilators such as dipyridamole or adenosine now have an important place in such tests, since they can be used in patients unable to exercise and can produce a more satisfactory increase in myocardial blood flow, thus increasing the sensitivity of detection of myocardial ischaemia [9]. These vasodilatory effects can be inhibited by caffeine and theophylline, which compete for the same α_2 receptor on the cell membrane. Caffeine blood levels of 5 mg/l can produce this effect and lead to false-negative results [10]. Abstinence from caffeine for 24 hours is recommended, and has been found to produce caffeine levels of <1 mg/l in 81 of 86 patients [11]. Adenosine and dipyridamole also possess bronchoconstrictor effects, and are therefore contraindicated in asthmatic patients. An alternative agent that has been used in these circumstances is the β-agonist dobutamine, which has primarily β_1 activity, increasing muscle contractility with little effect on heart rate. The haemodynamic effects observed closely resemble those produced by exercise. More recently, arbutamine, which has β-receptor activity together with some α-receptor activity, has been used [12]. This agent has equipotent activity on contractility and heart rate.

Other deliberate interventions that are of current clinical interest are the use of captopril in the assessment of renal function and determination of renal artery stenosis (see Chapter 11) and the use of acetozolamide as a vasodilator in determination of regional cerebral blood flow.

Thyroid studies

One of the most widely recognized drug–radiopharmaceutical interactions is the effect that thioureylene drugs such as carbimazole and propylthiouracil have on the thyroid uptake of iodide. These drugs inhibit the intrathyroidal oxidation of iodide by thyroid peroxidase, thus preventing formation of mono-iodotyrosine, and ultimately thyroid hormones. Carbimazole itself does not have *in vitro* activity and is converted *in vivo* to the active methimazole. As a result, radiopharmaceutical uptake by the gland is reduced. Many patients referred for thyrotoxicosis therapy with ^{131}I sodium iodide will be taking one of these drugs, and in order to prevent suboptimal treatment, they must be stopped before radiopharmaceutical administration. Individual practices vary, but a period of at least 5 days is usually recommended.

Uptake can also be adversely affected by foodstuffs rich in iodine, particularly some types of fish, as well as drugs containing iodine such as amiodarone and radiographic contrast media. The quantity of iodine in these preparations is vastly greater than in radiopharmaceuticals and *in vivo* de-iodination leads to a competitive inhibition of uptake. The duration of inhibition of such uptake can range from days to years (Table 16.1). Variation is in at least partly due to the patient's renal function and hence the rate at which the inhibiting agent is excreted.

Sodium (^{131}I) iodide is also used for detection of metastases following thyroidectomy for thyroid carcinoma. Patients are likely to be taking thyroxine as replacement therapy, and the presence of

Table 16.1 Duration of inhibition of thyroid uptake of radioiodine

Agent	Duration
Lugol's solution, tincture of iodine	2–4 weeks
Drugs containing iodine (e.g. amiodarone)	2–12 weeks
Thyroxine	4–6 weeks
Liothyronine	1–2 weeks
Water-soluble contrast media	2–4 weeks
Oil-based contrast media	4 weeks to years

exogenous thyroxine leads to a feedback inhibition of uptake of iodide. This may decrease the sensitivity of the test, and it is therefore necessary to withdraw thyroxine. Its biological half-life is approximately 7 days, and a withdrawal of at least 4 weeks is generally recommended. In order to prevent hypothyroidism developing in this time period, liothyronine, which has a shorter half-life of 2 days, can be used, and stopped for approximately 2 weeks before radioiodine administration.

Bone studies

The use of technetium-labelled diphosphonates, e.g. medronate and oxidronate, remains one of the most frequently performed diagnostic procedures in nuclear medicine. The radiopharmaceuticals bind to hydroxyapatite crystals of bone and give an indication of the rate of bone turnover. Etidronate has also been used as bone-imaging agent, but the non-radioactive compound is now commonly used therapeutically in patients with Paget's disease and more recently, hypercalcaemia of malignancy. By binding to the hydroxyapatite crystals, it slows down their rate of growth and dissolution and produces palliation of bone pain. The potential for reduced uptake of bone-imaging agents in patients taking these agents therefore exists. Sandler *et al.* [13] demonstrated that a decreased bone uptake of the radiopharmaceutical, accompanied by increased soft tissue uptake, occurred in a patient 1 day after receiving a single treatment with 450 mg etidronate. However, detection of lesions in the skeleton was still possible. A repeat bone scan 4 days later still showed reduced bone uptake, but a final bone scan after 3 weeks showed that the uptake had returned to the normal expected levels. Hommeyer *et al.* [14] also reported greatly reduced skeletal uptake of medronate within 36 hours of a patient having received two doses of 500 mg etidronate. There was marked blood pool activity, but uptake into large metastatic sites was observed. There were no follow-up scans in this patient and therefore no information on the duration of the etidronate effect.

Analogues of etidronate, usually termed biphosphonates as opposed to diphosphonates commonly used for imaging agents, are also used in practice for the treatment of hypercalcaemia of malignancy. These include pamidronate, clodronate and alendronate. It is therefore possible that more patients being referred for bone imaging will have received these drugs. The data sheet of one brand of pamidronate ('Aredia', Ciba) states that, in theory, it could interfere with bone scintigraphy. There have not yet been any reports of such effects, but departments should be aware of the possibility. However, a study on 11 patients with breast cancer treated with a daily dose of 300 mg clodronate for 21 days showed no difference in sensitivity of lesion detection, immediately before and after treatment [15]. There has been one report of a bone scan with oxidronate on a patient who had received a single dose of alendronate (a very potent inhibitor of osteoclast activity) 24 hours earlier [16]. No lesions were detected, but the authors did not comment on whether there was generalized decrease uptake in the skeleton.

Adrenal imaging

Two different types of radiopharmaceutical are used in investigating the embryologically and functionally distinct adrenal cortex and medulla. Adrenal cortex imaging is performed with radiolabelled cholesterol derivatives that are taken up by the adrenal gland. The mechanism is described in Chapter 10, and it is therefore not surprising that drugs affecting cholesterol uptake will also affect radiopharmaceutical uptake, and could lead to misleading results. Table 16.2 lists the most important groups of drugs known or expected to affect radiopharmaceutical uptake. In adrenal cortex imaging, pharmaceutical intervention with dexamethasone is sometimes employed to suppress ACTH release from the pituitary, and thereby enhance visualization of abnormalities.

The main agent for investigating the adrenal medulla is radioiodinated MIBG, an analogue of

Table 16.2 Drugs affecting uptake of adrenal cortex imaging agents (adapted from Swanson, 1990)

Drugs reducing uptake
Glucocorticoids
Spironolactone (long-term)
Beta-blockers
Indomethacin

Drugs increasing uptake
Diuretics
Oral contraceptives
Cholestyramine

guanethidine, which accumulates in tissues rich in catecholamine storage vesicles by means of uptake-1 mechanism. Further details are given in Chapter 10. When labelled with iodine-123, MIBG has been used to image phaeochromocytomas, neuroblastomas and paragangliomas. Many drugs are capable of inhibiting the uptake-1 mechanism, and could thus reduce uptake of radiopharmaceutical by the tumour. In addition, many sympathomimetic drugs, which can have this effect are ingredients of cold-cure and decongestant preparations that may be purchased without prescription, e.g. pseudo-ephedrine and phenylephrine. A comprehensive list of such drugs has been published by Solanki *et al.* [17], and this should be consulted when assessing patients for imaging. The major drug groups involved are listed in Table 16.3. ^{123}I-MIBG can be used to determine the appropriateness of therapeutic treatment with ^{131}I-MIBG, and it is essential that potentially interfering drugs are identified and withdrawn before the study.

Receptor-binding radiopharmaceuticals

There has been an enormous increase in the development and availability of radiopharmaceuticals specifically developed to bind to neuroreceptors. These include agents labelled with positron-emitting radionuclides, normally carbon-11, or single-photon emitters of which iodine-123 is currently the most widely used [18]. Such studies help elucidate the biological and biochemical mechanisms within the brain. As molecular biology and biochemistry becomes increasingly sophisticated, the complexity of receptors and their subgroups with differing affinities has become apparent; a comprehensive listing is outside the scope of this chapter. A detailed consideration of the mechanisms involved and the problems to be encountered has been given by Verhoeff [19]. Many psychoactive drugs exert their pharmacological effect by interaction with receptors, and as such, they will be in direct competition with receptor-binding

Table 16.3 Drugs affecting MIBG uptake (adapted from Solanki *et al.*, 1992)

Tricyclic antidepressants	Phenothiazine derivatives
Amphetamines	Sympathomimetic amines
Labetalol	Guanethidine
Reserpine	Haloperidol

radiopharmaceuticals. Table 16.4 lists the most commonly studied receptor systems with the radiopharmaceuticals and drugs involved. By being able to study receptor density and affinity and how this is affected by disease, a better understanding of neurological and psychiatric illnesses can be gained. Radiopharmaceuticals are prepared at very high specific activities to ensure that in the amounts administered, they do not saturate the very small concentration of receptors or have significant pharmacological activity. In such studies, if meaningful results are to be obtained, it is essential to know the drug status of the patient. In the presence of the drug, radiopharmaceutical uptake may be significantly reduced and thus give misleading information about receptor affinity and density. Before performing the study, it is necessary to ensure that there is a sufficiently long withdrawal period for the drug used. Further complications can arise since there may be receptor supersensitization following drug withdrawal. However, studying patients free of medication and again after stabilization of treatment, is an increasingly important technique in assessing drug potency and efficacy [20].

Cocaine, a widely abused highly addictive drug, has been shown to block the dopamine transporter system and produce changes in dopamine receptor function, glucose metabolism and regional cerebral perfusion. Cerebral perfusion defects were found to be more common in the male than in the female cocaine abusers [21], although no mechanism for this sex difference was proposed. Further studies have shown that buprenorphine, a mixed opioid agonist-antagonist, can produce dose-related improvements in cerebral blood flow in such patients [22].

Drugs interfering with blood labelling procedures

Labelled blood cells are used for a variety of diagnostic investigations. Erythrocytes tagged with technetium-99m are used for blood pool labelling for the assessment of left ventricular function, determination of red-cell mass and detection of gastrointestinal bleeding. Leucocytes or occasionally, purified neutrophils, are labelled with either technetium-99m or indium-111 to detect sites of infection or inflammation. Less commonly, platelets or lymphocytes have also been used. The presence of drugs during the labelling procedure can

Table 16.4 Neuroreceptor imaging radiopharmaceuticals

Receptor system	Radiopharmaceutical	Drugs
Dopamine D2	^{123}I-IBZM ^{123}I-epidipride ^{11}C-raclopride	Neuroleptics e.g. haloperidol
Benzodiazepine	^{123}I-iomazenil ^{11}C-flumazenil	Benzodiazepines e.g. diazepam

adversely affect labelling efficiencies of the cells and hence the quality of diagnostic information obtained.

Technetium-99m labelling of erythrocytes

The labelling technique involves pre-tinning the erythrocytes with stannous ion, followed by exposure to technetium-99m pertechnetate, which is reduced within the cell and remains trapped intracellularly by binding beta chain of haemoglobin [23]. Labelling can be performed either *in vitro*, where a blood sample is removed from the patient, the erythrocytes labelled and then reinjected. Alternatively, *in vivo* labelling can be performed, which avoids the need for blood labelling facilities, but has the disadvantage of the lack of a prospective check for labelling efficiency. Other factors that can influence labelling efficiencies include the clinical condition of the patient and the use of intravenous cannulas containing Teflon [24]. Hambye *et al.* [25] have reviewed drugs that may affect *in vivo* labelling. In their series of patients, heparin and chemotherapeutic agents were found to have significant adverse effects. It has been postulated that heparin might compete with the erythrocytes for the binding of stannous ion, and chemotherapeutic agents may cause alterations in the erythrocyte membrane. Eising and Sciuk [26] obtained satisfactory *in vivo* labelling in patients receiving chemotherapy and overcame the problems of Teflon cannulas by using a fast injection of the stannous agent followed by a saline flush. Other agents which have been reported to produce poor labelling are shown in Table 16.5 although a precise mechanism for the interference has not always been established.

Labelled leucocytes False-negative studies with such cells have been reported with patients taking antibiotics or corticosteroids [4], although it was acknowledged that this did not always occur,

Table 16.5 Drugs affecting *in vivo* labelling of erythrocytes

Heparin	Calcium channel blockers
Hydralazine	Propranolol
Cyclosporin	Quinidine
Cytotoxic drugs	Methyldopa
Digoxin	Iodinated contrast media
Prasozin	

since it is likely that patients presenting for a labelled leucocyte study for determination of a focus of infection will be taking antibiotics and patients being assessed for inflammatory bowel disease will be on steroids. It was proposed that the reason for the negative study may be a reduction in the chemoattractant stimuli for the labelled leucocytes. Other studies [27,28] have suggested that antibiotic treatment does not affect sensitivity and specificity of the investigation.

PHARMACOKINETIC INTERACTIONS

In these situations, the absorption, distribution, metabolism or excretion of the drug alters the biodistribution of the radiopharmaceutical. Reports of this kind of interaction are not common, but one example is the effect of nifedipine on retention of ^{131}I-MIBG in phaeochromocytoma [29]. Increased tumour retention of the radiopharmaceutical was observed in some (but not all) patients who were taking the drug. The altered pharmacokinetics were observed in patients with higher plasma concentrations of nifedipine.

Lithium carbonate has been demonstrated to retard release of ^{131}I-sodium iodide, from 29 of 36 lesions in 15 patients with differentiated thyroid carcinoma [30]. However, it does not appear that attempts have been made to exploit this interaction to increase the radiation dose to the tumour.

Table 16.6 Effect of some cytotoxic drugs on radiopharmaceutical biodistribution

Drug	Effect	Radiopharmaceutical
Cyclophosphamide	Increased renal uptake	Diphosphonates, gallium-67
Doxorubicin	Increased cardiac uptake	Diphosphonates, gallium-67
	Increased kidney uptake	Indium-111 antimyosin
Methotrexate	Increased renal uptake	Gallium-67
	Increased bone marrow	Colloids
	Increased liver uptake	Diphosphonates
Vincristine	Increased renal uptake	Diphosphonates, gallium-67
	Increased bone uptake	Gallium-67
	Decreased liver uptake	Gallium-67

TOXICOLOGICAL INTERACTIONS

Such interactions arise as a result of an exaggerated pharmacological activity of the drug producing altered biodistribution of the radiopharmaceutical. This may be due to damage or dysfunction in a particular organ or tissue, and in certain situations can be regarded as instances of drug-induced disease. Many cytotoxic drugs have been reported to cause alterations in expected biodistribution of radiopharmaceuticals by this mechanism. Some examples are given in Table 16.6. Uptake of bone agent in the liver has been observed in a child receiving a high dose of methotrexate [31]. Intense renal uptake was observed in paediatric patients if bone imaging was performed within 1 week of receiving chemotherapy with cyclophosphamide, vincristine or doxorubicin [32]. Biodistribution of gallium-67 citrate has been demonstrated to be affected by a wide range of cytotoxic drugs, causing reduced tumour, abscess and liver uptake, and increased uptake in other organs such as lung and bone [33]. Whether this represents a toxicological interaction as opposed a pharmacological one is open to question. The drugs may cause a decrease in binding sites for gallium within the serum, and as a result more of the agent is available for deposition in the tissues. Doxorubicin has known cardiotoxic effects, which have been shown to result in increased cardiac uptake of several radiopharmaceuticals including pyrophosphate and indium-111 antimyosin. Indeed, the use of the latter radiopharmaceutical as a sensitive technique for assessing doxorubicin toxicity has been described. Increased uptake of the antimyosin occurs before deterioration of left ventricular ejection fraction [34].

PHARMACEUTICAL INTERACTIONS

This type of interaction involves alteration of some nature of the radiopharmaceutical by a physicochemical property of the drug and resulting in an altered biodistribution. Aluminium ions in the plasma, resulting from ingestion of antacid preparations, can cause such effects with a range of radiopharmaceuticals. Although such aluminium salts are relatively insoluble, plasma levels sufficient to cause problems are achievable. No stomach or bladder activity was detectable after administration of pertechnetate to a patient who ingested 7.2 g of aluminium hydroxide daily, producing an Al^{3+} plasma level of 65 µg/l [35]. After discontinuation of the aluminium, a normal biodistribution was observed when the plasma aluminium level was 15 µg/l. Lung uptake of sulphur colloid was observed in a patient whose plasma contained high levels of aluminium [36]. *In vitro* addition of the radiopharmaceutical to a sample of the patient's plasma produced a precipitate, suggesting that the lung uptake was as a result of flocculation of the sulphur colloid. Experiments in rats have shown that addition of a solution containing 20 µg/ml sulphur colloid to technetium-99m MDP resulted in liver and kidney uptake [37]. Chromatography suggested that changes in the radiochemical nature occurred as a result of this manipulation.

Iron overload can also cause alterations in the biodistribution of technetium bone agents. Byun *et al.* [38] demonstrated high uptake of the radiopharmaceutical at the site of iron dextran in the buttocks, and Choy *et al.* [39] observed decreased bone uptake with increased kidney and soft tissue uptake, when the serum ferritin was elevated. A possible explanation for these observations is that transchelation of technetium from the bone agent to an iron-containing complex occurs.

CONCLUSIONS

Awareness of the possibility of drug–radiopharmaceutical interactions is important in the nuclear medicine department. The chemical quantity of administered radiopharmaceuticals is small when compared with that of normal drugs, and in most situations, no pharmacological action is expected. Ideally, prospective action should be taken to prevent detrimental interactions, thus avoiding a sub-optimal or misleading investigation. However, such an ideal state of affairs does not always exist, and in such instances, it is important for the department to recognize that a drug interaction may be responsible for the observed biodistribution.

Many interactions are well documented but, as has been seen, these do not necessarily occur in all patients, as among other factors blood levels of the drug are important and may significantly affect the biodistribution of the administered radiopharmaceutical. Occasionally, unexpected biodistribution of a radiopharmaceutical occur for which no immediate explanation exists. The question of a drug interaction should be considered, and if appropriate, the possibility of one having occurred should be made more widely known. Publication of the findings should be considered, or a report of the observations should be made to a central reporting system such as that operated by the United States Pharmacopoeia in association with the Society of Nuclear Medicine or the European Association of Nuclear Medicine, in order that information can be widely disseminated and greater knowledge of potential problems obtained. Avoidance of these interactions will enhance both the quality and efficacy of the nuclear medicine service.

REFERENCES

1. Grayson, R.R. (1960) Factors which influence the radioactive iodine thyroidal uptake test. *Am. J. Med.*, **28**, 397–415.
2. Callahan, R.J. and Rabito, C.A. (1990) Radiolabelling of erythrocytes with technetium-99m: role of band-3 protein in the transport of pertechnetate across the cell membrane. *J. Nucl. Med.*, **31**, 2004–10.
3. Hicks, R.J., Eu, P. and Arkles, L.B. (1992) Efficiency of labelling red blood cells with technetium-99m after dipyridamole infusion for thallium stress testing. *Eur. J. Nucl. Med.*, **19**, 1050–3.
4. Hladik, W.B., Ponto, J.A., Lentle, B.C. and Laven, D.L. (1987) Iatrogenic alterations in the biodistribution of radiotracers as a result of drug therapy: reported instances, in *Essentials of Nuclear Medicine Science* (eds W.B. Hladik and G.B. Saha), Williams and Wilkins, Baltimore, pp. 189–219.
5. Hesslewood, S. and Leung, E. (1994) Drug interaction with radiopharmaceuticals. *Eur. J. Nucl. Med.*, **21**, 348–56.
6. Sampson, C.B. and Cox, P.H. (1994) Effect of patient medication and other factors on the biodistribution of radiopharmaceuticals, in *Textbook of Radiopharmacy Theory and Practice* (ed. C.B. Sampson), Gordon and Breach Science Publishers, pp. 215–27.
7. Hladik, W.B., Nigg, K.K. and Rhodes, B.A. (1982) Drug-induced changes in the biologic distribution of radiopharmaceuticals. *Semin. Nucl. Med.*, **12**, 184–210.
8. Leung, S.C.E. and Hesslewood, S.R. (1994) Use of drugs to enhance nuclear medicine studies, in *Textbook of Radiopharmacy Theory and Practice* (ed. C.B. Sampson), Gordon and Breach Science Publishers, pp. 225–41.
9. Pennell, D.J. (1994) Pharmacological cardiac stress: when and how ? *Nucl. Med. Commun.*, **15**, 578–85.
10. Smits, P., Corstens, F.H.M., Aengevaer, W.R.M. *et al.* (1991) False-negative dipyridamole thallium-201 myocardial imaging after caffeine infusion. *J. Nucl. Med.*, **32**, 1538–41.
11. Jacobson, A.F., Cerqueria, M.D., Raisys, V. *et al.* (1994) Serum caffeine levels after 24 hours of caffeine abstention: observations on clinical patients undergoing myocardial perfusion imaging with dipyridamole or adenosine. *Eur. J. Nucl. Med.*, **21**, 23–6.
12. Young, M., Pan, W., Wiesner, J. *et al.* (1994) Characterization of arbutamine: a novel catecholamine stress agent for diagnosis of coronary artery disease. *Drug Dev. Res.*, **32**, 19–28.
13. Sandler, E.D., Parisi, M.T. and Hattner, R.S. (1991) Duration of etidronate effect demonstrated by serial bone scintigraphy. *J. Nucl. Med.*, **32**, 1782–4.
14. Hommeyer, S.H., Varney, D.M. and Eary, J.F. (1992) Skeletal non-visualization in a bone scan secondary to intravenous etidronate therapy. *J. Nucl. Med.*, **33**, 748–50.
15. Pecherstorfer, M., Schilling, T., Janisch, S. *et al.* (1993) Effect of clodronate treatment on bone scintigraphy in metastatic breast cancer. *J. Nucl. Med.*, **34**, 1039–44.
16. Koyano, H., Schimizu, T. and Shishiba, Y. (1995) The biphosphonate dilemma. *J. Nucl. Med.*, **36**, 705.
17. Solanki, K.K., Bomanji, J., Moyes, J. *et al.* (1992) A pharmacological guide to medicines which interfere with the biodistribution of radiolabelled meta-iodobenzylguanidine (MIBG). *Nucl. Med. Commun.*, **13**, 513–21.
18. Mazière, B. and Mazière, M. (1990) Where have we got with neuroreceptor mapping of the human brain? *Eur. J. Nucl. Med.*, **16**, 817–35.
19. Verhoeff, N.P.L.G. (1991) Pharmacological implica-

tions for neuroreceptor imaging. *Eur. J. Nucl. Med.*, **18**, 482–502.

20. Kerwin, R.W. and Pilowsky, L.S. (1995) Traditional receptor theory and its application to neuroreceptor measurements in functional imaging. *Eur. J. Nucl. Med.*, **22**, 699–710.

21. Levin, J.M., Holman, B.L., Mendelson, J.H. *et al.* (1994) Gender differences in cerebral perfusion in cocaine abuse: technetium -99m-HMPAO SPECT study of drug abusing women. *J. Nucl. Med.*, **35**, 1902–9.

22. Levin, J.M., Mendelson, J.H., Holman, B. *et al.* (1995) Improved regional blood flow in chronic cocaine polydrug users treated with buprenorphine. *J. Nucl. Med.*, **36**, 1211–15.

23. Srivastava, S.C. and Chervu, L.R. (1984) Radionuclide labeled red blood cells: current status and future prospects. *Semin. Nucl. Med.*, **14**, 68–82.

24. Millar, A.M., Wathen, C.G. and Muir, A.L. (1983) Failure in labelling of red blood cells with 99mTc: interaction between intravenous cannulae and stannous pyrophosphate. *Eur. J. Nucl. Med.*, **8**, 502–4.

25. Hambye, A.S., Vandermeiren, R., Vervaet, A. *et al.* (1995) Failure to label red blood cells adequately in daily practice using an *in vivo* method: methodological and clinical considerations. *Eur. J. Nucl. Med.*, **22**, 61–67.

26. Eising, E.G. and Sciuk, J. (1995) Failure to label red blood cells adequately in daily practice using an *in vivo* method: methodological and clinical considerations. *Eur. J. Nucl. Med.*, **22**, 587.

27. Chung, C.J., Hicklin, O.A., Payan, J.M. *et al.* (1991) Indium-111 labelled leukocyte scan in detection of synthetic vascular graft infection: the effect of antibiotic treatment. *J. Nucl. Med.*, **32**, 13–15.

28. Datz, F.L. and Thorne, D.A. (1986) Effect of antibiotic therapy on the sensitivity of indium-111 labelled leukocyte scans. *J. Nucl. Med.*, **27**, 1849–53.

29. Blake, G.M., Lewington, V.J., Fleming, J.S. *et al.* (1988) Modification by nifedipine of ^{131}I-meta-iodobenzylguanidine kinetics in malignant phaeochromocytoma. *Eur. J. Nucl. Med.*, **14**, 345–8.

30. Koong, S.S., Movius, E.G., Keenan, A.M. *et al.* (1995) The effects of lithium in radioiodine therapy of metastatic well differentiated thyroid carcinoma. *J. Nucl. Med.*, **36**, 15P.

31. Flynn, B.M. and Treves, S.T. (1987) Diffuse hepatic uptake of technetium-99m methylene diphosphonate in a patient receiving high-dose methotrexate. *J. Nucl. Med.*, **28**, 532–4.

32. Lutrin, C.L., McDougall, I.R. and Goris, M.I. (1978) Intense concentration of Tc-99m pyrophosphate in the kidneys of children treated with chemotherapeutic drugs for malignant disease. *Radiology*, **128**, 165–7.

33. Bekerman, C., Pavel, D.G., Bitran, U. *et al.* (1984) The effects of inadvertent administration of antineoplastic agents prior to Ga-67 injection: concise communication. *J. Nucl. Med.*, **25**, 430–35.

34. Carrió, I., Estorch, M. and López-Pousa, A. (1996) Assessing anthracycline cardiotoxicity in the 1990s. *Eur. J. Nucl. Med.*, **23**, 359–64.

35. Wang, T.S., Fawwaz, R.A., Esser, P.D. *et al.* (1978) Altered body distribution of Tc-99m pertechnetate in iatrogenic hyperaluminaemia. *J. Nucl. Med.*, **19**, 381–3.

36. Bobinet, D.D., Sevrin, R., Zurbriggen, M.T. *et al.* (1974) Lung uptake of 99mTc-sulphur colloid in patient exhibiting presence of Al^{3+} in plasma. *J. Nucl. Med.*, **15**, 1220–2.

37. Zimmer, A.M. and Pavel, D.G. (1978) Experimental investigations of the possible cause of liver appearance during bone scanning. *Radiology*, **126**, 813–16.

38. Byun, H.H., Rodman, S.G. and Chung, K.E. (1976) Soft-tissue concentration of 99mTc-phosphates associated with injections of iron dextran complex. *J. Nucl. Med.*, **17**, 374–5.

39. Choy, D., Murray, I.P.C. and Hoschl, R. (1981) The effect of iron on the biodistribution of bone scanning agents in humans. *Radiology*, **140**, 197–202.

FURTHER READING

Laven, D.L., Clanton, J.A., Hladik, W.B. and Shaw, S.M. *Pharmacological Alterations in the Biorouting/Performance of Radiopharmaceuticals*, Vols 1–4. Gammascan Consultants, Bay Pines, Florida 33504-4098, USA

Swanson, D.P., Chilton, H.M. and Thrall, J.H. (1990) *Pharmaceuticals in Medical Imaging*. Macmillan Publishing Co., New York.

Untoward reactions

D. H. Keeling

INTRODUCTION

Radiopharmaceuticals are used for both diagnostic and therapeutic purposes, though the great majority of administrations are for diagnostic investigations. However, the pattern of use is quite unlike that of normal drug therapy. They are not given in courses over a considerable time period, and are frequently administered only once to an individual patient. Further, they are also given in minute chemical quantities, and no pharmacological effect is intended; indeed, most are designed simply to act as tracers and not to perturb the normal or pathological processes of the body which they are tracing. Thus, it is not surprising that adverse effects attributed to them are very infrequent, particularly when compared with normal therapeutic drugs or even the newer non-ionic radiological contrast agents. Equally, it is to be expected that systems of classification that have been devised for normal therapeutic drugs and their adverse reactions may prove less helpful for radiopharmaceuticals, with many pharmacological subdivisions irrelevant.

CLASSIFICATION OF ADVERSE REACTIONS

The classification of Rawlins and Thompson [1], originally proposed almost 20 years ago, is still being widely used for problems with general drug reactions and interactions. Using a logical framework that has proved to be both theoretically and practically valuable, they divided adverse reactions into two main types, A and B.

TYPE A ADVERSE REACTIONS

Type A (augmented) adverse reactions are the result of an exaggerated but otherwise normal response to a drug; the effect is like that of an overdose but is due to the patient's unusual sensitivity to the drug. These effects are frequently dose-related; the threshold for such effects may be lowered by disease or situations that increase absorption, alter metabolism, or delay excretion. With normal acceptable doses, this will only occur in patients at the extreme of the normal dose–response curve; such reactions are common in clinical practice though rarely serious. Type A reactions would also cover undue sensitivity to the recognized side effects of a drug and drug toxicity. It can be seen that there will have been very few examples of type A reactions resulting from diagnostic radiopharmaceuticals, though the nuclear medicine physicians are quite familiar with the effect of amiodarone on the thyroid. The deterministic (side) effects of therapeutic radiopharmaceutical problems could be considered in this group.

TYPE B ADVERSE REACTIONS

Type B (bizarre) adverse reactions are those which are unexpected and unrelated to any normal pharmacological effects of the drug. In clinical practice, these would include the triggering of acute porphyria and several other bizarre and frequently serious effects, as well as many immunological reactions. There is little or no suggestion of dose–response relationship and although in general clinical practice, type B reactions are relatively rare compared with type A, they are frequently serious. This heterogeneous group is usually due to some qualitative difference either in the drug or in the patient, or possibly both. Problems of drug decomposition would be classified as type B reactions, though the majority of cases in nuclear medicine would simply produce a biodistribution abnormality and as such are not reported. Solubilizers, stabilizers and sedimenting agents have been documented as causes of reaction but with these and the primary radiopharmaceuticals themselves, the most common type B reactions appear to be some form of immunological response. Radiolabelled proteins or peptides as well as macromolecules such as the dextrans are capable of acting as complete antigens, but the great majority of radiopharmaceuticals are small molecules and must act as haptens to take part in allergic or hypersensitivity reactions. Little is known about the details of any such covalent com-

Clinical Nuclear Medicine, 3rd edn. Edited by M.N. Maisey, K.E. Britton and B.D. Collier. Published in 1998 by Chapman & Hall, London. ISBN 0 412 75180 1

plexes formed with macromolecules from the patient. Investigation is made more difficult as an immunological response, indicated by detectable antibody production, does not necessarily mean that there will be a clinically allergic response in the subject. Thus, it is known that countless patients receiving penicillin develop antibodies to the penicilloyl group, but only a small minority show clinical evidence of hypersensitivity. Mouse protein antibodies are commonly found in patients receiving monoclonal antibody radiopharmaceuticals, but their prior detection by skin testing has not correlated well with subsequent clinical hypersensitivity, and it has been suggested that the intradermal skin tests may themselves cause more hypersensitivity than intravenous administration.

IMMUNOLOGICAL REACTIONS

The classification of the immunological mechanisms responsible for allergic reactions described by Coombs and Gell [2] is widely used and describes four types of immunological reactions:

1. **Type I** (immediate or anaphylactic) reaction is mediated largely by antibodies of the IgE group of immunoglobulins (present on the surface of the mast cells and circulating basophils) and triggers a release of pharmacological mediators, in particular histamine, but the number of recognized mediators continues to grow. Clinically, type I reactions are recognisable by urticaria and angioedema, rhinitis, bronchoconstriction and anaphylactic shock.
2. **Type II** (cytotoxic/membrane) reactions are those in which IgG and IgM antibodies react with cell-surface or tissue antigens to produce mostly autoimmune and haematological problems. While important in general medicine as causes of thrombocytopenia and haemolytic anaemias, this form has not been encountered with radiopharmaceuticals.
3. **Type III** (immune complex) reactions are usually due to IgG, IgM and IgA antibodies reacting with antigen in tissues where complement is activated and causes immune complex formation and deposition, that results in local tissue damage. Although often called serum sickness from its original cause and description, it is an important form of reaction seen with radiopharmaceuticals, manifesting itself as

low-grade fever, urticaria and maculopapular skin rashes, and late polyarthralgia.
4. **Type IV** (cell-mediated or delayed hypersensitivity) reaction mediated by sensitized T-lymphocytes has not been noted with radiopharmaceuticals.

NON-IMMUNOLOGICAL REACTIONS

Other mechanisms induce some of these reactions by releasing histamine (and other mediators) directly or by the direct activation of the complement system. These are therefore known as anaphylactoid reaction. Many of the acute reactions to iodinated X-ray contrast materials fall into this category, and it is probably important for radiopharmaceuticals.

The use of iron hydroxide precipitates for lung perfusion scanning with ^{113m}In, which co-precipitates with iron, lead to a number of fatalities in susceptible subjects. The 'fluffy' iron precipitate could be seen under the microscope to consist of a mesh of fine, needle-like crystals, and their impaction in the pulmonary capillaries leads directly to serotonin release and further pulmonary arterial constriction. In the patient already compromised with severe pulmonary hypertension, this could lead to acute heart failure. The clinical picture is due to the release of these active mediators and their tissue localization and therefore mimics the true immunological pattern; the acute management is the same for both. In practice, true immunological or anaphylactoid reactions to radiopharmaceuticals are rarely so clear-cut, but present with a variety of clinical patterns. Many reactions are noted with the first known exposure to the agent but this does not preclude an immunological basis.

CUTANEOUS REACTIONS

These are the most common manifestation found with all drugs [3] and form an important group with radiopharmaceuticals. It is frequently unclear whether there is an immunological basis or not and in any event, the skin shows a limited variety of reaction to a great variety of agents. In nuclear medicine, the two common skin reactions noted are urticaria and macular or maculopapular rashes. These can be seen with many radiopharmaceuticals, but the most common among UK scheme reports is the widely used bone scanning agent, methylene diphosphonate (MDP), causing macular or maculopapular eruptions coming on within 12 to 18 hours after injection of radiopharmaceutical. These are irritative, frequently symmetric and most prominent on the trunk, but are occasionally first noted on the injected limb before spreading more widely. Urticaria and 'hives' are also quite common with pruritic red wheals, again mostly noted on the trunk. (When deep dermal and subcutaneous tissues are involved, the diagnosis is angioedema and this can develop rapidly in a very few minutes as a type I anaphylactic reaction.) Untreated, these cutaneous effects take several days to clear. Most new radiopharmaceuticals, like many other drugs with an acceptably low incidence of adverse reactions, will go through their clinical trials without any pattern of adverse reaction being recognized, and with many patients on other drugs who are already symptomatic from their original medical condition, delays can occur before the true cause–effect relationship is recognized. This situation can be greatly helped if a well-supported reporting scheme is in operation, and a number of examples, some serious, have come to light in this way.

REPORTING SCHEMES

It is well over 30 years ago that clinically significant adverse reactions associated with radiopharmaceuticals were first being recognized with any frequency. It was apparent that these reactions were very uncommon but occasionally serious, and if any progress was to be made on their recognition and management, data collection on a large scale such as national level was required. The Society for Nuclear Medicine in the US set up such a scheme in the early 1970s, Atkins *et al.* [4] reported the first series of results. The UK scheme was set up the same year and Williams [5] published results in 1974. The Medical and Pharmaceutical Committee of the Japan Radioisotope Association has produced a long series of reports, but these are in Japanese and so not easily accessible to many. Other national schemes have been started, though judging from the results, not many have been well supported. Now, under the auspices of the European Association for Nuclear Medicine, a pan-European scheme is operating but again a great variation in national report incidence is noted. Schemes vary in the information

they seek to gather. Some, like the US system, effectively limit their interest to the more serious Rawlins and Thompson type B pharmacological or immunological reactions, and thus avoid mis-/maladministrations, overdose problems and vasovagal phenomena. Reports of overdose and therapeutic radionuclide deterministic effects are also frequently excluded and some disregard all radiation problems.

THE UK RADIOPHARMACEUTICAL ADVERSE REACTION SCHEME

This was deliberately widened beyond purely pharmacological problems and respondents were encouraged to notify details of any 'untoward events'. It was felt that it would be useful to publicise any difficulties that can arise in association with radiopharmaceutical administration, the better to help clinicians quickly recognize and treat specific problems. In the UK, this has led to the reporting of a variety of problems and observations at the time of and subsequent to the administration of radiopharmaceuticals, many of which seemed unlikely or very unlikely to be true cause–effect relationships, but the number of reports has never been high enough to be a problem in its own right!

AETIOLOGICAL ALGORITHMS

There have been several suggested algorithms for cause–effect relationship published and used to help identify more objectively the probability of cause–effect relationship [6]; the latest update of the US scheme [7] uses an algorithm that has given very satisfactory results from a prospective scheme involving 18 large centres over a 5-year period. These centres cooperated to use a relatively complex proforma and made regular returns that included overall workload, to yield incidence data. A similar study is underway in Europe.

The US algorithm is simple and divides reports into four categories: 'unrelated'; 'unlikely'; 'possible'; and 'probable'. The 'unlikely' category includes those cases where the adverse experience follows a reasonable time sequence, but does not follow a known response pattern to the material in question or vice versa. The 'possible' category would include cases where both the time sequence and response pattern seem feasible, but it might

REPORT OF AN ADVERSE REACTION ATTRIBUTED TO A RADIOPHARMACEUTICAL

1 Patient................................... Initials........................... Hosp. No.......................................
  Age...Sex................................. Date of Study...............................
  Nature of Study...
  ....
  Clinical Diagnosis...

2 Radiopharmaceutical: Radionuclide...........................Chemical Form............................
  Brief details of materials, sources, preparation and storage...
  ....
  ....
  ....

  Has a commercial manufacturer been informed?   Yes / No

3 Nature of Reaction: Timing, symptoms and clinical observations...
  ....
  ....
  ....
  ....
  ....

  Has the patient any known allergies? ....

4 Other medications currently or recently taken...
  ....

5 Treatment of the Reaction. Drugs and resuscitative measures. Results................................
  ....
  ....
  ....

6 Can you estimate the frequency of this reaction? ....

7 Any other comments..
  ....
  ....
  ....continue on separate sheet

Signed...Print Name...
Address...
....
Phone No. .... Fax No. ....
Please return completed form to your National Scheme Coordinator. In the U.K.: The Medical Assessor British Nuclear Medicine Society, 1 Wimpole St., LONDON, W1M 8AE   or Fax to: 0181 653 9599

have been due to the patient's clinical state or other factors. In the 'probable' group, the first two criteria are met and alternative causes are not thought likely. The criteria for relegation to the 'unrelated' category are more contentious. Thus, the time sequence may be judged unreasonable, or a pattern of response not recognized – rather begging the question that one knows what sort of adverse reaction to expect. With a new or relatively new radiopharmaceutical, this might not be true. Equally, if a reaction does not reappear when a 'rechallenge' occurs, it is judged 'unrelated' yet the literature and experience suggests this is not necessarily so. The time interval may be crucial.

REPORTING FORMS

There is debate about the format of report forms, with some schemes seeking an initial detailed history and observations, while other are greatly simplified. A general inertia towards reporting reactions of any sort seems to be a human failing, and so the UK proforma was deliberately kept to one side of A4 paper (Figure 16.1), albeit with room for further comment if volunteered. With the modest number of reports being received, it has proved little trouble to contact the person reporting if further detail is required.

The UK scheme was started by the professional bodies actively involved in nuclear medicine to encourage reporting of any untoward event, without asking respondents to make judgements as to the likely cause–effect relationship, and this has continued to be the policy. The recognition of a pattern of adverse reaction can only come with experience of a material and rapid developments in the field of radiopharmaceuticals has meant that some materials have almost fallen out of use before their potential for adverse effects is understood.

Radiopharmacists have wanted to collate information on pharmaceutical defects and biodistribution aberrations, and their scheme has now been integrated with the Adverse Reaction Reports, using the reverse side of the form.

UK REPORTING EXPERIENCE

Full records are available for all reports received since January 1976, previous records being incomplete. Because of the continuing development of new radiopharmaceuticals, particularly the expansion of ^{99m}Tc materials, with new replacing old, results are shown in four 4-year periods covering the years 1980–1983, 1984–1987, 1988–1991 and 1992–1995. Reports for technetium-labelled materials (Table 16.7), which account for ~83% total are separated from the others (Table 16.8) for convenience. The changes for any given radiopharmaceutical or group, between the first and the last period, reflect a variety of factors such as changing needs for a test, and replacing old by new radiopharmaceuticals. It is also very likely that knowledge (and use) of the reporting system has increased over this time. In comparing these figures with any other national or international groups, the policy of the UK system in dismissing only the most unlikely related reports, and the inclusion of vasovagal phenomena in these crude figures must be remembered.

PHOSPHONATES AND DIPHOSPHONATES

These account for nearly one-third of all reports, and effectively involve only the two diphosphonates available in the UK. Table 16.9 shows reports over the 20-year period since 1976. Simple vasovagal hypotensive episodes are separately identified, followed by a 'possible' group with less clear-cut signs and symptoms, plus prominent nausea and vomiting. Importantly, the diphosphonates are the major cause of skin reactions noted in nuclear medicine. The 'allergic' group are mainly angioedema and local effects (other than due to known extravasation), but the skin reactions consist of about two-thirds macular rashes and one-third urticaria. Both 'cardiac arrests' in this group (1 Pyp, 1 MDP) occurred within a few minutes of injection, and may have been severe vasovagal attacks – both were resuscitated successfully. Transient mild headache is not uncommon, but rarely mentioned.

ALBUMIN

Table 16.10 shows the results of 20 years' experience with albumin. Very few reports involve straightforward serum albumin. Colloidal forms

---

Figure 16.1   UK adverse reaction report form.

Table 16.7   UK adverse reaction reports: Tc-99m radiopharmaceuticals

	1980–1983	*1984–1987*	*1988–1991*	*1992–1995*
MDP, HDP and Pyp	13	31	32	61
Albumin – all forms	4	5	9	17
DTPA	1	25	22	13
MAG-3	0	0	7	16
DMSA	0	2	1	16
Sestamibi	0	0	5	6
Tetrofosmin	0	0	0	10
HMPAO	0	0	8	7
Colloids	8	5	3	0
TcO$_4$'	1	3	2	8
Other	0	2	2	1
Totals	27	73	91	155

Table 16.8   UK adverse reaction reports: non-Tc-99m radiopharmaceuticals

	1980–1983	*1984–1987*	*1988–1991*	*1992–1995*
I-123/131 mIBG	0	3	10	11
I-123/131 Hippuran	3	2	0	0
I-123/131 Iodide	0	1	4	4
Ga-67	2	2	0	1
Tl-201	0	1	0	2
Other	6	4	5	12
Total	11	13	19	30

Table 16.9   Tc-Phosphate and diphosphonates: adverse reactions, 1976–1995

	Radiopharmacentical		
	PyP	*MDP*	*HDP*
Vaso-vagal			
Probable	1	28	9
Possible + nausea/vomiting		26	3
Early allergic	0	8	1
Late allergic	0	7	4
Local, including phlebitis	0	6	9
Generalized rashes	0	32	6
Indeterminate	0	3	1
Cardiopulmonary arrest	1	1	0
Total	2 (1.5%)	111 (76%)	33 (22.5%)
[Overall total 146 (28.5%)]			

and microspheres (now no longer available) were associated with a number of serious reactions abroad, but the UK records show only a small number of apparent vasovagal effects though several hypersensitivity-type reactions. Albumin macroaggregates, used for very large numbers of lung perfusion scans, have shown a small number of serious 'allergic' reactions requiring urgent treatment and there are no less than ten cardiopulmonary arrests reported. However, two

Table 16.10 Albumin: all reactions: 1976–1995

	HSA	Colloid	Microspheres	MAA
Vasovagal	2	3	4	11
Pain, nausea, etc.	1	2	0	4
Dyspnoea	0	0	1	5
Fever, rigors	1	0	0	1
Rash	0	0	0	4
Late allergic	1	0	0	0
Indeterminate	0	2	0	2
Cardiopulmonary arrest	0	0	0	10*
Total	5 (9%)	7 (13%)	5 (9%)	37 (69%)
[Overall total 54 (10.5%)]				

*four resuscitated, one coronary artery, one unrelated.

Table 16.11 Renal radiopharmaceuticals: adverse reactions: 1976–1995

	I-Hippuran*	DTPA	MAG-3	DMSA
Vasovagal				
Typical	4	39	6	4
Probable/nausea and vomiting	0	6	7	5
Allergic				
Rash and/or asthma	1	5	9	10
Late allergic	1	0	0	0
Indeterminate	0	9	1	0
Cardiopulmonary arrest within 1 h	0	3 (all aerosol)	1	0
Total	6 (5.5%)	62 (56%)	24 (21.5%)	19 (17%)
[Overall total 111 (21.7%)]				

* ^{123}I or ^{131}I labelled.

of these were probably severe vasovagal attacks, but there were two deaths immediately after injection, and of the three that occurred at about 15 minutes post-injection, one could not be resuscitated. Two patients died within the hour but the cause of death is questionable, and another patient was undergoing coronary artery studies and died following the use of MAA. The lesson is that, although a relatively safe radiopharmaceutical, ^{99m}Tc-MAA can cause serious and potentially fatal problems, and departments doing these studies must be prepared.

RENAL RADIOPHARMACEUTICALS

As seen in Tables 16.7 and 16.8, the past 16 years has seen the fall-off of radioiodinated Hippuran reactions – still a major element in the Japanese experience – with the virtual obsolescence of the ^{131}I and ^{123}I tracers in the UK, but in their place

have been increasing numbers of reports featuring DTPA and more recently MAG3. Table 16.11 gives some indication of the symptomatology and, while a major fraction is vasovagal in nature, this appears to be more pronounced than with the general picture with radiopharmaceuticals. In part, it may be explained by alterations in fluid balance often required for renography, and if performed seated, the prolongation and accentuation of the cerebral ischaemia secondary to severe hypotension. The use of intravenous diuretics is likely to exacerbate this situation.

Also, both DTPA and MAG3 cause a significant number of 'hypersensitivity'-type problems, including typical skin rashes. DTPA aerosol must not be forgotten as a potential cause of serious reactions, and three cardiopulmonary arrests are listed as 'likely' to be related. Reports from abroad list a fatal case of status asthmaticus brought on by the DTPA aerosol.

DMSA is increasingly used at present, particularly in paediatric practice, and a number of skin reactions have been documented.

CARDIAC AGENTS

The myocardial agents sestamibi and tetrofosmin are becoming widely used and a small number of reaction reports have been made. Several document little more than the unexpected metallic taste and attendant anxiety, etc. Two patients independently reported headaches and quite widespread myalgia for 48 hours following sestamibi, and three cutaneous reactions lasting 2–3 days with tetrofosmin are recorded, plus another with more acute onset of facial angioedema. The patient's understandable anxiety about his cardiac problem and the myocardial stressing protocol have produced clinical problems where precise aetiology is uncertain, but the stressing protocol has seemed a more likely cause than the radiopharmaceutical. However, clinicians must be aware of the effect of drugs such as adenosine that are used in pharmacological stress tests, as well as the importance of drug interactions.

NON-TECHNETIUM RADIOPHARMACEUTICALS

Of the non-technetium radiopharmaceuticals, the only one that stands out in Table 16.8 is MIBG, labelled with ^{123}I or [131]I. Most reports are essentially type A reactions and follow a 'misadministration' with either an injudiciously fast injection or the use of an indwelling intravenous catheter or even central line to give a transient high blood level. Some patients report local discomfort even in the absence of any evidence of extravasation, and several experienced transient malaise, flushing and cough.

Minor changes in blood oxygen levels have been noted with both perfusion and ventilation studies, but seem unlikely to be important except in gross respiratory failure. Alteration of inspired oxygen percentage to undertake ventilation scans should be done with great care.

INCIDENCE

The modern range of radiopharmaceuticals have substantially fewer adverse effects than their predecessors, and the most recent US survey [7]

showed a figure of 2.3:100 000. A figure of 3:100 000 was reported in the UK in 1980, but excluded minor effects. It is probable, allowing for under-reporting of the commoner minor problems, that a total figure may be nearer 1:10 000, but even this incidence is much lower than with modern X-ray contrast material, and very much lower than general therapeutic drugs – estimated at nearer 1%. While general drug reaction schemes show a higher incidence in women, the UK adverse reports for radiopharmaceuticals show no male:female imbalance.

TREATMENT OF ADVERSE REACTIONS

ANAPHYLACTIC REACTIONS

Type I (immediate) anaphylactic reactions develop within 1–2 minutes of exposure – usually following intravenous and aerosol administration rather than the oral route – and can reach maximum severity in 5 minutes. The serious clinical state of anaphylactic shock may develop, which can be rapidly fatal and therefore prompt treatment is vital [8]. Hypotension can be severe and angioedema may involve the larynx and glottis compromising the airway, which may be further embarrassed by bronchoconstriction. Facial, particularly periorbital, angioedema and urticaria are frequent. These problems arise from local histamine release and should be treated with adrenaline, the physiological antagonist to histamine. Antihistamines, which are competitive inhibitors and therefore more effective given before histamine release, are too slow but are frequently advocated and will at least have some effect against the ongoing release of histamine. Parenteral steroids, such as hydrocortisone, are slow, but have many effects interfering with immune reactions, and are usually administered in the acute situation. However, adrenaline remains the principal agent for treatment of acute anaphylaxis. Subcutaneous injection in cases with severe peripheral circulatory shut-down is ineffective and Adrenaline Injection BP (1:1000, 0.3–0.7 ml) may be given intramuscularly; deep sublingual injection may be effective when peripheral flow is very poor, and an alternative is direct injection into the airway, either via an endotracheal tube or direct into the trachea by transcutaneous injection. These doses may be repeated in 3–4 minutes, but in extreme emergency, the above dose is diluted to 10 ml or use the equivalent 5 ml of Adrenaline Injection BP (1:10 000), given by slow intravenous infusion. This can precipitate ventricular fibrillation and complete resuscitation facilities should be immediately to hand. These measures for counteracting the pharmacological effects of histamine must be accompanied by attention to correct the clinical problems by establishing an adequate airway with intubation if necessary and supplementary oxygen. Severe hypotension, if present, is treated by replacement of fluid with a colloid plasma expander by rapid intravenous infusion. Further details are given in wall charts published by national advisory bodies, which should be in every nuclear medicine department, and familiarized by all staff.

SKIN REACTIONS

Itching macular or urticarial skin reactions are best treated with a non-sedative H_1 antihistamine such as cetirizine 10 mg orally for 2–3 days; this is more effective in dealing with the pruritus than the rash, but the former is often the patient's principal complaint. The problem will usually, but not invariably return, following a further dose of the causative radiopharmaceutical. This variability seems to be related to the time interval between doses and unknown factors within the subject rather than, for instance, between commercial sources of radiopharmaceutical. As can be seen from Tables 16.9–16.11, skin reactions are common with many radiopharmaceuticals. Apart from diphosphonates, the three renal agents (i.e. DTPA, MAG3 and DMSA), which are in widespread use, can all cause skin reactions, whether administered by injection, or in the case of DTPA, as an aerosol for ventilation studies. Injections of gallium-67 citrate have been noted to cause macular type rashes, both in the UK and abroad, and yet the dose injected is in the nanogram range!

Rare cases of biopsy-proven cutaneous vasculitis have occurred with the diphosphonates, producing a serious clinical problem requiring hospitalization and prolonged steroid treatment.

PYROGENS

Pyrogens are protein and polysaccharide products of the metabolism and breakdown of certain microorganisms which are soluble and heat-stable and not removed by either ultrafiltration or heat sterilization. Although exchange resins are now available that will remove many types of pyrogens from pharmaceuticals, the only safe technique is to avoid their introduction in the first place. Pyrogens have found their way into radiopharmaceuticals in the past, largely due to the unorthodox materials and methods required for some radiopharmaceuticals. Materials checked satisfactory for intravenous use by the standard BP pyrogen test may yet cause severe meningism when given by the intrathecal route. This is many times more sensitive for pyrogens, which have been found in phosphate buffers and on resin columns, and as demonstrated by the classic studies of Cooper and Harbert [9], require the much more sensitive limulus amoebocyte test for their detection.

INTRATHECAL RADIOPHARMACEUTICALS

Apart from potential pyrogen problems, formulation of intrathecal pharmaceuticals imposes special constraints not strictly applicable for small volume intravenous injections. The volume of the fluid space is much less than that of the blood plasma, and there is the additional factor of much slower flow and therefore longer equilibration times. In addition, the sensitivity of neural tissue, both to the injected material and to any local changes, may be vital. For renal investigations with DTPA, the commercially available forms – the free acid, the Na_5 and the mixed $CaNa_3$ salts, work perfectly satisfactorily by intravenous injection, and even extravasation will not produce a noticeable problem. However, the free acid (which on injection becomes the tri-sodium salt H_2Na_3) and the penta-sodium salt (Na_5), are very strong chelators of Ca^{2+} and Mg^{2+} ions. In the plasma, the pool of these ions is sufficient for it to be immaterial, but in the cerebrospinal fluid the effects of chelation and the prolonged drop of Ca^{2+} and Mg^{2+} concentration in the cerebrospinal fluid (CSF) can be and have been disastrous. Verbruggen *et al.* [10,11], noting that not all commercial preparations disclosed the chemical nature of the DTPA clearly – even if the user were to appreciate the significance – reported two (out of 15) cases of severe permanent neurological damage, and elsewhere it is thought there were fatalities. This experience highlights the need for extreme care when altering even the detailed make-up of an established radiopharmaceutical, or using one via a novel route.

STERILITY

There have been no reports of clinical problems from lack of sterility with a radiopharmaceutical for many years. All radiopharmacies in the UK are now required to check sterility of 'in-house' radiopharmaceuticals according to the agreed protocols – though this does not require every single production to be so checked. There are variations in the methodology of testing as the standard BP techniques do not necessarily allow for the problems of inter-departmental handling of radioactive samples, or the effects of radiation on microorganisms. This is more fully discussed in texts of radiopharmacy [12]. While this lack of a clinical problem is most satisfactory, it might be remembered that this type of problem was almost non-existent in the early days of nuclear medicine, when lapses might well have been expected due to the relative crudity of early radiopharmacy conditions and technique. Cost–benefit analysis of today's increased requirements remains a very subjective matter, not limited to this question.

MALADMINISTRATION AND MISADMINISTRATION

Maladministration and misadministration, referring to radiopharmaceuticals, are words usually used in an indiscriminate sense and interchangeably but in an admittedly arbitrary manner. It has been suggested [13] that, to aid discussion of the subject, they might usefully be defined to separate two differing varieties of faulty dosage. The term maladministration could be retained for 'wrong' administrations, largely of an organizational nature. Thus, the wrong patient may be injected, or the right patient may be given the wrong radiopharmaceutical or via the wrong route. Great care is required to avoid this sequence with labelled blood components. These types of maladministration are to be avoided by the careful organization of detailed departmental protocols and close adherence to them [14]. The problem is compounded in bigger departments with larger numbers of patients undergoing a greater diversity of investigations and treatment, and where different members of staff are responsible for different stages of 'ordering', radiopharmaceutical batch and individual dose preparation, labelling and administration.

The use of a central venous catheter line for administration has important pitfalls, though on occasion, the 'bolus effect' is desirable. The delivery of a dose to sensitive chemoreceptors in the great vessels, heart and brain, at a concentration many hundred times equilibrium levels, can result in complications. With MIBG, severe type A reactions have developed – a rare example in nuclear medicine. Transient high concentrations can easily reach the tongue via the blood stream and 'odd tastes' are a common complaint. It is likely that these transient symptoms can trigger vasovagal events in susceptible patients, who should be forewarned and reassured.

Misadministration can then be used in a more limited sense to cover the group of problems that are largely the result of operator error, and would cover problems of technique – possibly compounded by an uncooperative patient – when a radiopharmaceutical dose is 'delivered' (e.g. injected) in a faulty manner. These are therefore likely to be mainly local problems. Undoubtedly the most common example would be with intravenous administration when there is partial or even complete extravasation of the dose. All other local problems with injections could be similarly classified, such as the ante-cubital fossa intravenous injection unintentionally entering the brachial artery, often resulting in a biodistribution abnormality or even minor (though usually temporary) ischaemic changes in the forearm and hand from lung scan particulates.

Other local complications reported have involved pain, induration and swelling together with more obvious haematoma formation, phlebitis and lymphangitis. Venous thrombosis up to the level of the axillary vein with both sensory and motor neurological symptoms of some duration have all been noted, though there is nothing specific to radiopharmaceutical administration – these are recognized complications of any intravascular drug administration. Sepsis seems to be an exceptionally rare problem; there are no records of such events. Transient local pain at the site of a (satisfactory) intravenous injection may also be due to an unwanted local 'pharmacological' action. A high local concentration may produce undesirable signs or symptoms. A common report with MIBG has been transient local pain from the injection site in the ante-cubital fossa along the course of the vein to the shoulder area. Subsequent study has shown no evidence of extravasation or later phlebitis.

MANAGEMENT OF EXTRAVASATED RADIOPHARMACEUTICALS

The management of extravasated radiopharmaceuticals can be a difficult problem, with no clear guidance available based on significant experience. Suggested remedial measures have ranged from simple withdrawal of as much as possible by syringe to heat and massage for the extravasation and introduction of hyaluronidase and steroid to the region. Some have even suggested surgical clearance, as is the accepted practice for industrial injuries with radioactive metal fragments. However, these can be seen on X-ray, physically identified and totally removed. Advice for radiopharmaceuticals [13] suggests this would be inappropriate, as operative intervention is unlikely to remove a significant proportion of the dose without much tissue damage, and may interfere with the lymphatic drainage that would otherwise aid the situation. For all ^{99m}Tc and ^{123}I radiopharmaceuticals, it is suggested that no active measures need be taken other than noting the occurrence and its cause, and endeavouring to avoid the particular problem. It is suggested that particular care should be taken with the parenteral administration of the somewhat longer-lived radionuclides such as ^{201}Tl, ^{67}Ga, ^{75}Se, ^{131}I and ^{131}I-MIBG. If, despite this, extravasation occurs, try to withdraw as much as possible into the syringe, monitor the site to try and assess how much of the dose is still in the tissues, and if significant, consider local measures such as massage, application of heat and local injection of steroid or hyaluronidase. It is important to record the event together with any clearance measurements made and any dosimetry calculations.

For intravenous therapy with radionuclides, it is preferable to set up an intravenous line clear of the ante-cubital fossa and check patency with saline before administering the dose. The line will need flushing subsequently and simple precautions to avoid contamination. If extravasation still occurs, proceed as recommended above but follow-up is advised.

There are records attributing late tissue necrosis to radiation damage from extravasation of diagnostic doses of thallium-201, but they are excessively rare. The opportunity for such an occurrence from an indwelling needle inserted before a cardiac exercise-stress test is obvious, and the situation is likely to have arisen on not a few occasions. Indeed, cases have been documented where the extravasation of ^{201}Tl was recognized at the time but its satisfactory clearance monitored during the next 12–24 hours – not the 'worst case' situation adopted for radiation dosimetry purposes – and no long-term sequelae were noted in these cases.

Small superficial radiation 'burns' were occasionally seen following the intradermal injection of colloidal ^{198}Au (many years ago) for lymph clearance studies when clearance turned out to be grossly delayed.

It is recommended that only experienced staff inject ^{201}Tl, ^{67}Ga, ^{131}I and similar longer-lived radionuclides, and they would be advised to avoid the ante-cubital fossa and its many vital structures and consider a temporary venous catheter, which can be rechecked before use. Radiosynovectomy has attendant dangers from misadministration, because of the high radiation dose resulting from errors of injection, both locally if deposited in an extra-articular loculus, and further afield if entering the lymphatics and cleared, perhaps to liver and kidneys. No reports of problems have been noted, but this needs continued monitoring as it is likely to be difficult to differentiate the effects of further progress of disease such as rheumatoid arthritis from the theoretical possibility of endarteritic changes, in for instance, the cruciate ligaments of the knee.

VASOMOTOR EFFECTS

Acute vasomotor phenomena are a major feature of reports to the UK scheme, though many other systems specifically exclude them, on the basis that they are rarely due to the radiopharmaceutical. This is undoubtedly true, but it is often difficult to judge in individual cases and as discussed above, can be influenced by transient high cerebral concentration effects, although this may also have to be in association with a susceptible subject.

The acute vasovagal reaction involves cardiac slowing via the vagus and a sudden withdrawal of peripheral sympathetic tone, and this fall in cardiac output and drop in peripheral resistance results in a sudden and often very marked fall in blood pressure. Excessive vasodilatation may be influenced by drugs, and anaphylaxis can also produce severe hypotension. For this reason alone, it is often impossible to rule out an immunological reaction in many cases of post-injection 'collapse', since rechallenge is usually impractical as well as unethical.

The vasovagal faint or syncopal attack is a result of cerebral ischaemia due to a complex centrally mediated reflex, often initiated when pain or powerful emotional stimulus is inflicted against a background of intense sympathetic stimulation. Could this be the description by an unsympathetic physiologist, of attendance at some nuclear medicine departments? However, it is often possible to avoid or reduce vasovagal reactions. Many patients have quite legitimate anxiety, but reassurance by the referring clinician, as well as a pleasant confident attitude by the staff in the nuclear medicine department, all help to dispel anxiety. Some patients are particularly prone to this reaction with venepuncture and placing the subject supine will help control the labile hypotension, as can a quick uncomplicated venepuncture. Nevertheless, reactions to intravenous injections are common and the hypotension will produce problems ranging from pallor, often extreme, with initial 'light headedness' often with visual and auditory changes. Sweating or rigors may be noted, and pain in the back or abdomen and frequently in the renal areas is not rare; some patients may complain of nausea and even vomit. Ultimately, consciousness can be lost with convulsive movements and incontinence, but unlike true epilepsy, with which it is sometimes confused, there is a prodromal 'warning' phase before consciousness is lost, but no confusion afterwards. True epilepsy has been precipitated in this situation, albeit in subjects already known to be epileptics. If the patient is held upright or in a sitting position, the cerebral ischaemia will worsen, as will the attendant signs and symptoms. While usually transient, symptoms can recur if the patient resumes an upright position. Patients with postural hypotension either related to an autonomic neuropathy as in some diabetics, or drug-induced in patients taking certain antihypertensive drugs or nitrates, may be particularly susceptible to syncopal attacks, though it is less frequent with modern beta-blockers or diuretics.

BASIC LIFE SUPPORT MEASURES

Clinical emergencies can arise in a number of ways in patients undergoing nuclear medicine investigations; some will be acute complications of their original morbid condition and simply happen to take place in the nuclear medicine department, but a few could be a direct or indirect consequence of their investigations or treatment. Additionally, the physical or emotional stress of that investigation may cause or exacerbate problems, and then there are the effects (or side effects) of radiopharmaceuticals and other drugs administered in the department. For all these reasons, and because it will take time for outside help to arrive, it is vital that members of staff of the nuclear medicine department should be familiar with and ready to put into practice, the basic life support techniques for cardiorespiratory collapse. The chances of a satisfactory full recovery after cardiopulmonary arrest fall off by about 20% every minute, so time is very limited. The institution of adequate basic life support measures reduces this deterioration by half – to 10% per minute – allowing more time for expert help and equipment to arrive and greatly increasing the patient's chances of a good recovery. Every nuclear medicine department should have its own 'crash trolley' with emergency drugs and equipment ready for immediate use and all members of staff should be trained in basic life support.

REFERENCES

1. Rawlins, M.D. and Thompson, J.W. (1991) Mechanisms of adverse drug reactions, in *Textbook of Adverse Drug Reactions*, 4th edn (ed. D.M. Davies), Oxford University Press, Oxford, pp. 18–45.
2. Coombs, R.R.A. and Gell, P.G.H. (1968) Classification of allergic reactions responsible for clinical hypersensitivity and disease, in *Clinical Aspects of Immunology*, 2nd edn (eds R.R.A. Gell and P.G.H. Coombs), Blackwell Scientific Publications, Oxford, p. 575.
3. Wintroub, B.U., Stern, R.S. and Arndt, K.A. (1987) Cutaneous reactions to drugs, in *Dermatology in General Medicine*, 3rd edn (eds T.B. Fitzpatrick, A.Z. Eisen, K. Wolf, I.M. Freedberg and K.F. Austen), McGraw-Hill, New York, pp. 1353–66.
4. Atkins, H.L., Hauser, W., Richards, P. and Klopper, J. (1972) Adverse reactions to radiopharmaceuticals. *J. Nucl. Med.*, **13**, 232–3.
5. Williams, E.S. (1974) Adverse reactions to radiopharmaceuticals: a preliminary survey in the United Kingdom. *Br. J. Radiol.*, **47**, 54–9.

6. Cordova, M.A., Hladik, W.B. and Rhodes, B.A. (1984) Validation and characterisation of adverse reactions to radiopharmaceuticals. *Non-invasive Med. Imaging*, **1**, 17–24.

7. Silberstein, E.B., Ryan, J. *et al.* (1996) Prevalence of adverse reactions in nuclear medicine. *J. Nucl. Med.*, **37**, 185–92.

8. Bockner, B.S. and Lichtenstein, L.M. (1991) Anaphylaxis. *N. Engl. J. Med.*, **324**, 1785–90.

9. Cooper, J.F. and Harbert, J.C. (1975) Endotoxin as a cause of aseptic meningitis after radioactive cisternography. *J. Nucl. Med.*, **16**, 809–13.

10. Verbruggen, A., de Roo, M., Dewit, P., Guelinckx, P. and Dom, R. (1982) Complications after intrathecal administration of Tc-99m DTPA, in *Progress in Radiopharmacology*, (ed. P. Cox), Martinus Nyhoff, The Hague, pp. 223–35.

11. Verbruggen, A.M., de Roo, M.J.K. and Klopper, J.F. (1994) Technetium-99m diethylamine triamine penta-acetic acid for intrathecal administration: are we playing with fire? *Eur. J. Nucl. Med.*, **21**, 261–3.

12. Keeling, D.H. (1994) Adverse reactions and untoward events associated with the use of radiopharmaceuticals, in *Textbook of Radiopharmacy*, 2nd edn (ed. C.B. Sampson), Gordon and Breach, Newark, NJ Academic Publishers, London, pp. 285–98.

13. Keeling, D.H. (1994) Maladministrations and misadministrations. *Nucl. Med. Commun.*, **15**, 63–5.

14. Williams, E.D. and Harding, L.K. (1995) Radiopharmaceutical maladministration: what action is required? *Nucl. Med. Commun.*, **16**, 721–3.

Introduction of new radiopharmaceuticals

S. J. Mather

The process of the development of a new radiopharmaceutical will normally follow the direction outlined in Figure 16.2, and will involve a collaboration between a research group in an academic institution, a commercial radiopharmaceutical company, and the nuclear medicine departments of one or, more likely, several healthcare institutions. The entire process will take about 5–10 years and require a financial investment running into tens of millions of pounds or dollars. The main difference between this process and the development of a new therapeutic, i.e. non-radioactive, drug is one of scale, since the cost of a conventional drug development programme will generally run into hundreds of millions of dollars. However, another interesting difference relates to the first step in the process, i.e. drug discovery. Nearly all therapeutics are developed through drug screening programmes in multinational drug companies, while historically most radiopharmaceuticals have arisen initially from ideas pursued in university or teaching hospital departments.

DISCOVERY

The most recent generation of new radiopharmaceuticals have been developed as tracers of perfusion of major organs such as brain or heart. These have largely arisen from basic studies in radiopharmaceutical chemistry which have explored the properties of interesting classes of technetium complexes. Examples include the development of Ceretec from studies on PnAO by Troutner et al. [1] and Cardiolite from isonitriles by Jones and co-workers [2] and in many cases, the first complexes to be synthesized were those of the ground-state technetium-99.

Currently, most interest is directed towards the development of receptor-binding radiopharmaceuticals. The first step is the identification of an interesting biological target, followed by the choice of a suitable binding ligand, and subsequently the development of radiolabelled compounds. Although this may be regarded as an over-simplification, it could be considered that, in the past, the compound preceded the application, while now the application drives the development of the product. This change in direction has made necessary the acquisition of a new battery of skills and techniques by research groups working in this field.

The discovery of an interesting 'lead' compound may be followed by several cycles of development (as indicated in Figure 16.3) in order to improve the biological or biochemical properties of the compound. Ultimately, on completion of a satisfactory phase of pre-clinical development the compound(s) will undergo some preliminary evaluation in humans.

If the compound still looks promising following this evaluation, it is at this stage that an approach is normally made to the radiopharmaceutical industry to explore the possibilities of commercial development. The relationship between academia and commerce is symbiotic. Industry needs the infusion of fresh ideas from academic research, and the university departments depend to a large degree on industrial funding to support their research programmes.

Before agreeing to support a new development programme, industry will have a number of essential requirements.

An indication for the potential product must be identified and the size of the potential market must be predicted as being sufficient to recoup the development costs.

It must be possible to protect the ownership of the intellectual property by filing for a patent. If either the information is already in the public domain through premature publication, or a prior patent exists, then the project is unlikely to attract industrial support.

Sufficient supporting data must be available to underpin the hypothesis that the radiopharmaceutical is working in the manner proposed. The acquisition of this supporting data will normally require the completion of additional work in a feasibility phase.

Clinical Nuclear Medicine, 3rd edn. Edited by M.N. Maisey, K.E. Britton and B.D. Collier. Published in 1998 by Chapman & Hall, London. ISBN 0 412 75180 1

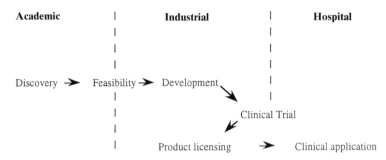

Figure 16.2   Steps in the drug development process.

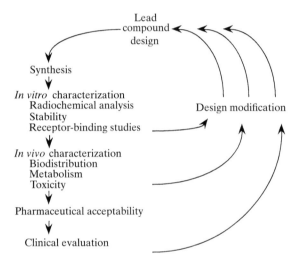

Figure 16.3   Cycles of product development in radiopharmaceutical design.

FEASIBILITY

This phase of the development process may be performed either in the laboratories of the industrial concern, or, with appropriate guidance, in the laboratory of the academic researcher. The primary aims of this phase will be:

- an unequivocal characterization of the identity of the tracer through appropriate analytical techniques;
- a study of its physical characteristics (molecular weight, charge, lipophilicity, etc.) and its interaction with biological systems (protein binding, cellular uptake, biodistribution etc.);
- identification of its mode of action; and
- a measure of the performance of the product in the disease(s) for which it is indicated.

DEVELOPMENT

On successful completion of the feasibility study, the project will be adopted into the development portfolio of the industrial company. Serious sums of money will now start to be consumed by the project and it is essential that the process becomes as streamlined and efficient as possible. Based upon the data obtained thus far, a series of closely related compounds, possibly running into hundreds of molecules, will be synthesized and the relationships between structure and activity identified. An important aspect at this stage is to identify simple but robust assay systems for comparing this large group of compounds. It will not be possible, for example, to perform detailed biodistribution studies on every molecule but, if the critical parameters can be identified, then simple analytical screens such as reverse-phase chromatography (to predict lipophilicity) or automated competitive binding assays (to predict receptor affinity, etc.) can be used rapidly to compare the different analogues. From this process, a small number of optimized compounds will be identified for more complete study. These will undergo much more detailed evaluation including extensive biodistribution studies, initially in suitable animal models and subsequently in humans. The term 'suitable' as a description of animal models is highly appropriate. Many instances exist in which the use of small animal species has failed to accurately predict subsequent biodistribution in humans [3]. At this stage, it is likely that more suitable species, such as primates for brain studies and pigs for heart and kidney investigations, will be employed.

Ultimately, the compound that performs best in this final series of studies and which will go forward through a long series of regulatory hurdles before it receives marketing approval will be selected. At this stage, mention should be made of the question of drug formulation. The ultimate aim of the supplier will be to provide the radiopharmaceutical in the most appropriate and convenient form for its eventual application. This formulation may vary from a simple aqueous salt solution such as, for example, indium-111 chloride, to a freeze-dried kit for labelling with technetium-99m sodium [Tc-99m]. The actual requirements of the formulation will depend upon the complexity of the product concerned, but of paramount importance will be the pharmaceutical and radiochemical quality of the preparation, its stability, robustness and convenience. At this stage in the product development, it is likely that the radiopharmaceutical will exist in a rather primitive formulation. 'Wet chemistry' techniques will normally have been used in the preparation of technetium complexes thus far and the product will go through several mutations during the later stages of its development before the ultimate presentation is finalized.

PRODUCT LICENSING

In nearly all countries of the world, a system of regulations controls the supply of medicinal drugs in order to ensure that they are both efficacious and safe for their proposed application. Until relatively recently, radiopharmaceuticals were, in many countries, exempt from some or all of the rigours of this regulatory process. However, recent changes in legislation in many countries in Europe [4], Asia and Latin America mean that radiopharmaceuticals are now subject to the same systems of regulation as other therapeutic pharmaceuticals.

The detailed requirements for seeking marketing approval are very complex and fall outside the scope of this chapter. Moreover, they vary from one country, or group of countries, to another. The aim in this section, therefore, will be to outline only the types of data required for such applications and the mechanisms by which such approval is obtained from the regulatory authorities. Since 1992, the requirements for obtaining marketing approval within the European Union have been 'harmonized'. Emphasis will be placed on these requirements and, in particular, the mechanisms used in the UK.

A list of the sections in the application for approval of a new radiopharmaceutical can be seen in Table 16.12. Since radiopharmaceuticals are

Table 16.12 Content of EC application for marketing approval [5]

Part I	Summary of the dossier
IA	Adminstrative information
IB	Summary of product characteristics (SPC)
IC	Expert reports
Part II	Chemical and pharmaceutical documentation
IIA	Composition of the medicinal product
IIB	Method of preparation
IIC	Control of starting materials
IID	Control tests on intermediate products
IIE	Control tests on the finished product
IIF	Stability
IIG	Bioavailability/bioequivalence
IIH	Data related to the environmental risk
IIQ	Other information
Part III	Toxicological and pharmacological documentation
IIIA	Toxicity
IIIB	Reproductive function
IIIC	Embryo–foetal and perinatal toxicity
IIID	Mutagenic potential
IIIE	Carcinogenic potential
IIIF	Pharmacodynamics
IIIG	Pharmacokinetics
IIIH	Local toxicity
IIIQ	Other information
Part IV	Clinical documentation
IVA	Clinical pharmacology
IVB	Clinical experience

used only in hospitals, are administered to patients only once or on a small number of separate occasions, and generally have no pharmacological action, the specific requirements for this class of product are somewhat less extensive than for therapeutic drugs, although the same general principles apply.

The first section (Part I) of the application provides summary information on the application and the product itself. Of particular interest are: sections IB, the summary of product characteristics (SPC); and IC, the expert report. The SPC contains information on the chemical nature of the product including the active ingredient and any additives or excipients, and includes details of the formulation, dose, route of administration, indications, contraindications and precautions, etc. The SPC forms the basis of the package insert which must be included in the final presentation and, apart from being an integral part of the licence application, subsequently provides a valuable source of information for the radiopharmacist. Copies of the SPC for approved products will often be supplied by companies on request.

The application also includes three expert reports:

1. One each on the chemical, pharmaceutical and biological section.
2. The toxicological and pharmacological documentation and the clinical section. The expert reports include both a summary of the data presented in the relevant section of the application and a critical evaluation of the methods employed, results obtained and conclusions drawn. As suggested in the title, the authors of these reports are expected to be experts in their particular field; in many cases, they will be employees of the company concerned, but often, especially for the clinical section, well-recognized authorities from outside will be employed.

Part II of the application encompasses the chemical, pharmaceutical and biological data. This section includes a description of the composition of the product, its method of manufacture, and the methods used for analysis and control of the starting materials, intermediates and the final product. Stability data on both the ingredients and the final product are also included.

Part III covers pharmacotoxicological aspects, and it is in this section that perhaps the greatest difference can be seen between radiopharmaceuticals and conventional drugs. For the latter, a detailed study of the pharmacodynamics, pharmacokinetics, acute and chronic toxicity, teratogenicity, mutagenicity and carcinogenicity is required. For radiopharmaceuticals, the specialized nature of the product indicates a special set of requirements. The radiation inevitably associated with these products implies a certain risk, and this is considered separately from the possible toxicity due to the non-radioactive components. A detailed calculation of the radiation dose to individual organs, as well as a whole-body equivalent dose from the quantity of radioactivity to be administered, is presented. While preliminary dosimetric calculations may be performed on the basis of animal biodistribution studies, quantitative imaging investigations in patients will be used to calculate human radiation dosimetry using MIRD formulae.

Toxicity studies will generally be performed using non-radioactive material, either without the addition of the radiolabel, for example in the case of technetium kits or, where the presence of the radionuclide is unavoidable, following decay. The extent of toxicity testing carried out will depend, to a certain degree, on the likely frequency of administration of the radiopharmaceutical. However, in general, despite the very low frequency of administration, toxicity tests involving repeated dosing, in at least two species of small animals will be required. A standard screen for possible mutagenicity on the cold product will be expected, but tests for carcinogenicity and teratogenicity will not normally be required. As indicated above, a pharmacological effect in a radiopharmaceutical will not normally be expected, but a demonstration of the absence of any such effects in the clinical studies performed will be necessary. Pharmacokinetic studies in both animals and humans are presented in order to demonstrate the rate of blood clearance of the radiopharmaceutical, its *in vivo* stability, and the rates and routes of excretion of the product and its metabolites.

Part IV of the application presents the clinical experience gained with this product. These data are normally acquired in three phases. Phase I trials are essentially a preliminary screen for toxicity in man. Only a small number of subjects (about 10) would normally be studied. A detailed search for pharmacodynamic effects would be made, together with a full survey of electrolytes, haematology and enzymes, etc. In phase II, while the surveillance for product safety continues, greater emphasis is placed on efficacy. Approximately 50 patients would be studied. In phase III trials, the efficacy of the new product is judged in comparison to a 'gold standard', which may be an established nuclear medicine technique, an alternative imaging modality or a clinical evaluation. The number of patents studied will depend upon the number of indications for which approval is sought, since a separate assessment of efficacy for each indication is required, but will generally run into several hundreds of subjects.

While much of the data required for this dossier are generated from laboratories and departments within the company, some specialized tests – mutagenicity for example – will be contracted out to specialized agencies. Clearly, clinical trials data can only be acquired in suitably equipped and experienced clinics and hospitals, and industry will normally seek the help of well-established nuclear medicine departments to perform these studies. While this type of work can prove interesting and a useful source of revenue for hospital departments, the amount of work required, in particular the amount of record-keeping, can often be underestimated. This accumulation of data is often particularly onerous, since the findings of much of the pharmacodynamic and toxicological studies are entirely negative. Centres participating in clinical trials must therefore be prepared to pay great attention to detail, follow protocols precisely, and provide complete and comprehensive records on all patients studied, as this information is required by the regulatory authorities when judging the application.

CLINICAL TRIALS

The process of carrying out clinical trials is itself highly regulated [6]. Companies or 'sponsors' must follow what is called 'good clinical practice' (GCP); 'a standard by which clinical trials are designed, implemented and reported so that there is public assurance that the data are credible and that the rights, integrity and confidentiality of subjects are protected'. Among the duties of the sponsor with regard to GCP is the need to appoint expert monitors who constantly survey the progress of the trial to ensure that all appropriate records are rigorously completed and all controls adhered to.

Before the trial can commence, it is necessary to seek the approval of the national regulatory body to ensure that they are satisfied with the proposed study. Various mechanisms exist in many countries for such trials, and the route chosen will depend upon the product under investigation and the investigator involved. All countries require the trial to be initially vetted by the ethics committee or its equivalent at the institution concerned. The main task of this committee is to judge the trial from the point of view of the subject (patient), that the trial is properly conducted, the risks and inconveniences suffered by the subject acceptable and that all legal requirements are adhered to. The ethics committee will also often address the question of liability – who is responsible in the event of a serious adverse effect – the doctor, the hospital or the company concerned.

Many regulatory authorities operate a separate scheme for clinical trials personally sponsored by clinicians. In the UK, this is known as the DDX (Doctors and Dentists exemption) scheme. The responsible clinician must inform the Medicines Control Agency of their intention to perform the trial and provide very brief details of the product, its supplier and the trial protocol. A similar scheme exists in the US known as a physician-sponsored IND (Investigational New Drug) application. The main difference between the various national schemes is the quantity of information the authorities require. The Food and Drug Administration (FDA) in the US, for example, requires detailed information on the chemistry of the product, conditions for its manufacture, methods of control, acute toxicity, pre-clinical biodistribution studies and clinical protocols. This type of scheme can only be used by individual doctors undertaking their own research either on new products developed within their own hospital or on products produced and supplied by commercial companies, which may perhaps be licensed in other countries or for other indications, or be the subject of the company's own trials.

In order to gain approval to conduct their own trials, companies must apply under another scheme. In the US, the appropriate scheme is the company-sponsored IND, similar in principle to the physicians-sponsored IND, but with a greatly increased requirement in terms of data. In the UK, there are two systems: the CTX (clinical trial exemption) and the CTC (clinical trial certificate) schemes. The preferred option is normally the CTX scheme which is a negative vetting system. This requires the submission of a limited dossier of information mostly on pharmaceutical and safety aspects that must be considered by the MCA within 1–2 months. If the regulatory authority has doubts about any aspect of the study, they will reject the application and the company can either correct the deficiencies and make a fresh CTX application or opt for the CTC scheme. This latter requires the submission of a full set of data similar to that in Parts II and III of the product licence application. Apart from the need to supply more information for the CTC scheme, the main disadvantage is that it can take much longer for the application to be assessed, and this may cause an undesirable delay in the commencement of clinical trials.

When all the data required for the marketing approval application have been accumulated, the company will submit this large package to the regulatory authorities responsible for those countries in which it wants to sell the new product. In major markets such as the United States or Japan, a separate application will be sent to the FDA or the Japanese Ministry or Health and Welfare. In Europe, the supplier has the choice of three possible schemes. On rare occasions, they may wish to supply the product in only one country, in which case they will apply to that National Authority. More commonly, they will want to market the product throughout Europe, in which case they have two alternatives: namely the multistate and the concertation procedures.

The multistate (decentralized) procedure involves the submission initially to a single authority known as a rapporteur. This authority will assess the application in the normal way and, on satisfactory completion of all the procedures, will approve the product. The rapporteur then sends his assessment report on to the authorities in those other countries in which the product is to be sold. These authorities can accept the decision of the rapporteur or they can raise objections to the application and these will be referred to the Committee for Proprietary Medical Products (CPMP) who will arbitrate on any disputes.

Under the centralized (concertation) procedure, the rapporteur country refers the application directly to the CPMP for assessment of the data. This procedure was initially developed as an obligatory procedure for high-technology products, but has since been extended to all new products. Once the CPMP has approved the product, its decision is binding on all member states.

The second part of this chapter is concerned with the introduction of a new radiopharmaceutical from the point of view of the radiopharmacist. At some time, all radiopharmacy managers will be asked to supply a new radiopharmaceutical product. Requests will normally fall into three categories:

1. An alternative formulation or supplier for an existing product.
2. A new radiopharmaceutical with the potential to replace an existing one.
3. A completely new radiopharmaceutical, which will not supersede another.

Before undertaking to supply a new product, it is essential to know its legal status. If the radiopharmaceutical has marketing approval, then the indications for which it may be used, together with the recommended dose and preparation method, are an integral part of the package,

and must be adhered to. If a radiopharmaceutical is intended to be used for another indication, then it must be treated in the same way as a non-approved product. If any changes are to be made in the method of preparation or analysis then these must be validated before introducing them into routine use.

If a request is made for an unlicensed product, then thought should initially be given to the possibility of an alternative product or formulation which may be approved, or a product that may be approved in another country. If the product is the subject of company-sponsored clinical trials, then it is possible that the product may be used under the auspices of this trial certificate. If no such opportunity exists, then whatever national regulations control the use of entirely unlicensed materials must be applied. In the UK, separate sets of regulations control both the supply and use of such products. Unlicensed products may only be supplied by manufacturers operating under the control of a manufacturing (specials) licence or under the direct control of a pharmacist.

Under UK regulations, a clinician is permitted to request and administer any pharmaceutical needed for a 'particular' patient under his or her care. This is the so-called 'named-patient' exemption. However, if used as part of a clinical trial, the prescribing clinician must inform the MCA of his or her intentions under the DDX scheme as described above. In addition to these regulations, additional rules controlling the receipt, storage and disposal of radioisotopes apply in most countries. In the UK, such matters are overseen by Her Majesty's Inspectorate of Pollution, who will issue relevant certificates, and inspect stock levels and disposal records. If the radioisotope used in the new product is already being used in the hospital, then no action may be required on this matter, provided existing limits are not exceeded. However, if a new radionuclide is to be used, then the appropriate new certification will be necessary.

The administration of radioactivity to humans is controlled in Europe by the Euratom directives, which require the establishment of a system of prior authorization of the clinicians responsible. In many countries this approval is handled by the same authorities which assess the marketing approval, but in the UK it is handled by the Administration of Radioactive Substances Advisory Committee (ARSAC). Clinicians wishing to administer radioisotopes for the purposes of research, diagnosis or therapy, must apply to ARSAC for permission before they proceed. The committee will assess the training and experience of the applicant, the scientific support services available to them, the research protocol (if applicable), and the radiation dosimetric aspects of the product concerned before granting approval.

The supplier of a new radiopharmaceutical is advised to gather together a dossier of information on the product concerning its clinical use, biodistribution, pharmacokinetics, radiation dosimetry, special precautions, etc. Such information may be available from the requesting clinician, the manufacturer or supplier, or through other recognized sources of drug information such as hospital colleagues or the published literature.

The ability of the radiopharmacy department to produce and supply any new radiopharmaceutical must also be considered. The requirements will clearly depend upon the nature of the radiopharmaceutical, its complexity and availability, and the level of expertise and resources available to the department. While 'ready-to use' products or simple lyophilized technetium 'kits' should present little problem to most radiopharmacy departments, more complex preparations such as labelled blood cells or proteins, or, for example, radiolabelled meals for gastrointestinal transit studies, will require a greater level of expertise. If the preparation of the product is time consuming, an increase in staffing levels may need to be considered. Volatile radionuclides such as radioiodine or radioactive gases and aerosols will require the availability of special containment facilities. Additional equipment such as water baths, centrifuges, or liquid chromatography systems may be required. While commercially available products will provide all the required ingredients, normally in a convenient 'freeze-dried' form, new experimental products usually require 'in-house' formulation. Such a product will require the preparation of suitable starting materials, which will ideally be pre-prepared in a sterile form suitable for aseptic assembly. These materials will need to be produced in a manner that complies with all the regulations controlling the hospital manufacture of medicines, and would normally be the province of the local pharmacy production and quality control departments.

Any new radiopharmaceutical will require the development of a suitable method for radiochemi-cal analysis, which can be applied as part of the preparation procedure. If the radiopharmaceutical is supplied by a commercial manufacturer, then they will normally recommend a fully validated procedure, which should be adopted as the method of choice. 'In-house' preparations will normally be prepared from published papers, which will generally describe a suitable method of analysis; however, any such method should be tried and tested in the radiopharmacy laboratory before the product is introduced into clinical use.

The production of any radiopharmaceutical must be fully documented, and any new product will require the preparation of new standard operating procedures and worksheets which must be written and approved by the individuals responsible for production and quality control in the laboratories concerned. Additional documentation such as labels, special request or consent forms, and information leaflets for staff and patients may also be required.

The implications for the radiation protection of staff involved in the preparation and use of a new radiopharmaceutical should be considered at an early stage, particularly if, for example, large doses of radioactivity are to be used for therapeutic procedures. The adequacy of shielding measures and administration systems should be critically assessed and the radiation dose received by staff should be measured using whole-body and extremity monitoring.

If the administration of the radiopharmaceuticals is to take place at a site distant from the production laboratory, then consideration must be given to the transport arrangements between the two sites. Apart from the need to comply with local regulations governing transport of radioactive materials, the ability of the product to withstand the conditions of transport must be assessed by performing quality control tests before and after transportation.

Before the use of a new radiopharmaceutical becomes routine, consideration must be given to its financial implications. The cost of the radiopharmaceutical will normally be passed on to its user, either internally as part of the departmental budget or to external customers. A detailed pharmacoeconomic analysis is outside the scope of this chapter but interested readers will find detailed advice in the published literature [7,8].

When all these arrangements have been put in

place regarding the supply of a new radio-pharmaceutical, it is recommended that at least one full pre-production test run be performed to test all the systems before commencing supply for clinical use.

ACKNOWLEDGEMENTS

I gratefully acknowledge the helpful assistance of Dr Colin Hewat of Amersham International plc and Dr Suzanne Douglas of Mount Vernon Hospital, Northwood, UK in the preparation of this chapter.

REFERENCES

1. Troutner, D.E., Volkert, W.A., Hoffman, T.J. and Holmes, R.A. (1984) A neutral lipophilic complex of 99m-Tc with a multidentate amine oxime. *Int. J. Appl. Radiat. Isotop.*, **35**, 467–70.
2. Jones, A.G., Abrams, M.J., Davison, A. *et al.* (1984) Biological studies of a new class of technetium complexes: the hexakis(alkylisonitrile)-technetium (I) cations. *Nucl. Med. Biol.*, **11**, 225–34.
3. Kronauge, J.F., Noska, M.A., Davison, A. *et al.* (1992) Interspecies variation in biodistribution of technetium (2-carboxy-2-methyl isocyanopropane) +6. *J. Nucl. Med.*, **33**, 1357–65.
4. Commission of the European Communities (1989) European Council directive [89/343/1989]
5. Commission of the European Communities (1996) *Notice to applicants for marketing authorisatons for medicinal products for human use in the member states of the European Community* [5371196]
6. Commission of the European Communities (1993) *Guidelines on the quality, safety and efficacy of medicinal products for human use.*
7. Clarke, S.E.M., Harding, K., Buxton-Thomas, M. and Shields, R. (1990) The current cost of nuclear medicine. *Nucl. Med. Commun.*, **11**, 527–38.
8. Jolicoeur, L.M., Jones-Grizzle, A. and Boyer, J.G. (1992) Guidelines on performing a pharmaco-economic analysis. *Am. J. Hosp. Pharm.*, **49**, 1741–7.

FURTHER READING

Cartwright, A.C. and Matthews, B.R. (eds) (1991) *Pharmaceutical Product Licensing: Requirements for Europe (1991)*, Ellis Horwood, Chichester.
Mather, S.J. (ed.) (1996) *Recent Developments in Radiopharmaceutical Research and Development*, KIuwer Academic Publishers, Dordrecht, The Netherlands.
Sampson, C.B. (1994) *Textbook of Radiopharmacy, Theory and Practice*, Gordon Breach Publishers.

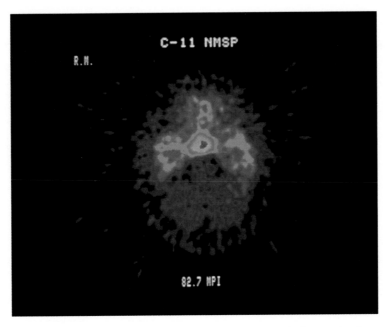

Plate 1 ^{11}C-N-Methlyspiperone concentrates in a pituitary adenoma which contains dopamine receptors.

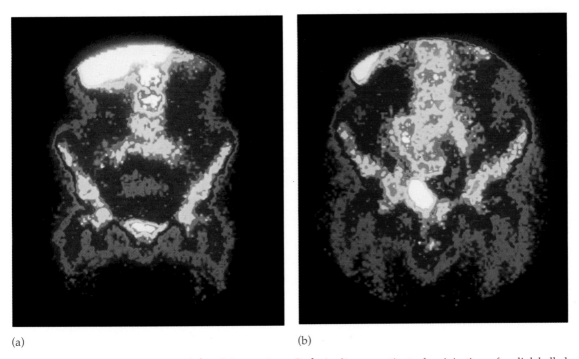

(a)   (b)

Plate 2 Gamma-camera images of the abdomen in a Crohn's disease patient after injection of radiolabelled autologous granulocytes. (a) A negative scan 6 months after surgery; (b) in the same patient, 12 months after surgery, a focal accumulation of radioactivity is seen, suggesting a relapse of the disease in the pre-anastomotic ileum as confirmed by endoscopy.

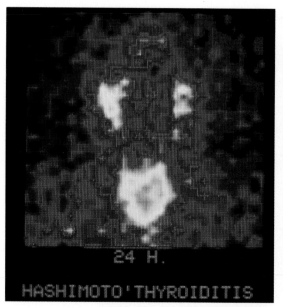

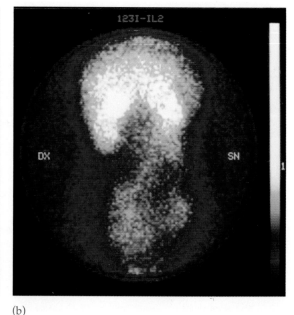

Plate 3 Gamma-camera image of the neck of a patient affected by Hashimoto's thyroiditis 24 hours after administration of radiolabelled autologous lymphocytes. An intense accumulation of radioactivity can be observed in the thyroid, indicating the presence of massive lymphocytic infiltration of the organ.

Plate 4 Gamma-camera images of the neck in a patient with Hashimoto's thyroiditis 1 hour after intravenous injection of ^{99m}Tc-IL-2. High thyroid uptake of the radiotracer is observed, indicating the presence of activated lymphocytes homing into the thyroid.

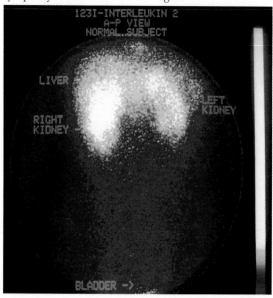

(a)   (b)

Plate 5 ^{123}I-interleukin-2 gamma-camera images of the abdomen of (a) a normal subject and (b) a recently diagnosed coeliac disease patient. Intense and diffuse accumulation of radioactivity can be observed in the jejunum and ileum of the patient, indicating the presence of a severe and diffuse intestinal infiltration by activated T-lymphocytes.

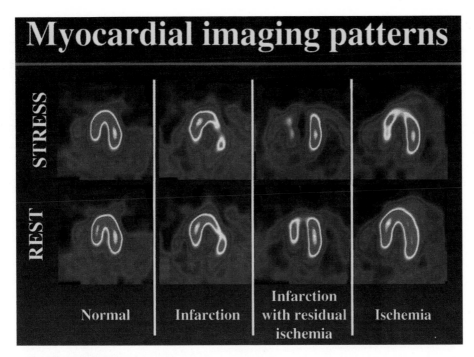

Plate 6 Comparison of stress and rest images in patients with various perfusion patterns : normal, irreversible defects (infarction), partially reversible defects (infarction with residual ischaemia) and reversible defects (ischaemia).

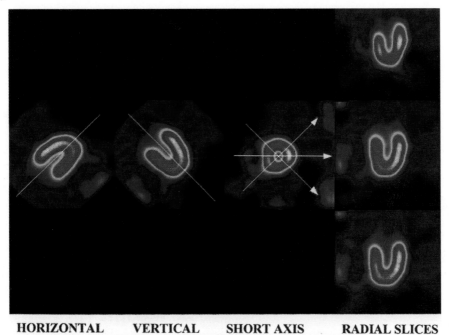

HORIZONTAL   **VERTICAL**   **SHORT AXIS**   **RADIAL SLICES**

Plate 7 Reorientation of cardiac images requires successive steps to first align them in the horizontal plane, then in the sagittal plane. The mid ventricular long axis is then used to cut oblique radial long-axis slices as shown here at three representative angles.

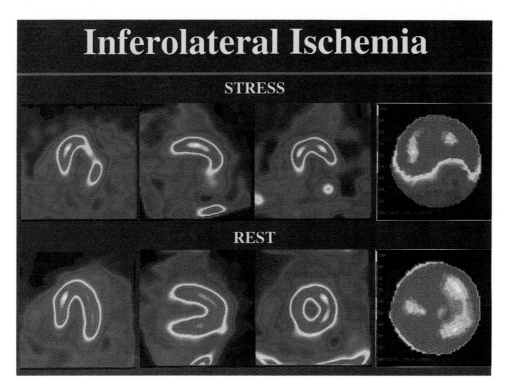

Plate 8 Use of polar map display to visualize the distribution of the myocardial perfusion tracer in a patient with inferolateral ischaemia. The abnormal perfusion at stress (upper panel) is demonstrated by horizontal, vertical and short-axis slices as well as by a polar map display. The resting scan (lower panel) is normal.

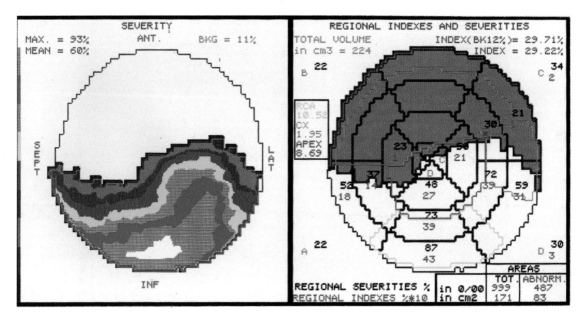

Plate 9 Extent and severity of perfusion defect (same patient as in Plate 8) are demonstrated on this numerical map (right panel) and on this severity map. Maximum severity is expressed in the percentage difference between the mean normal database value for that pixel and the level of background.

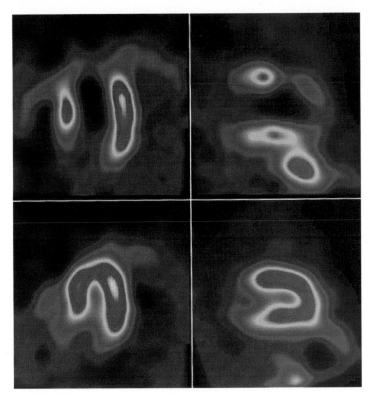

Plate 10 Effect of revascularization in a patient with impending myocardial infarction treated by fibrinolysis and angioplasty. Note the large perfusion defect and cardiac dilatation initially (upper row) and the excellent result with reperfusion (lower row).

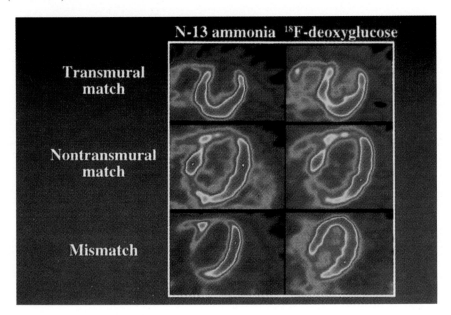

Plate 11 Positron emission tomography (PET) images of myocardial perfusion and metabolism. In myocardial infarction, metabolism is reduced in proportion to blood flow, markedly in transmural infarction, moderately in non-transmural infarction. In hibernating viable myocardium, the uptake of FDG is preserved despite the perfusion abnormality. (Reproduced from Maddahi *et al. J. Nucl. Med.*, **35**, 707–15 (1994), by permission of the Society of Nuclear Medicine.)

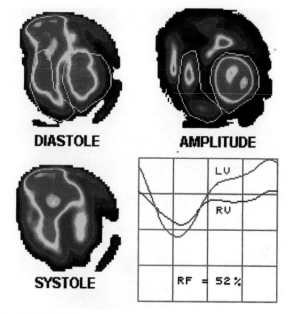

Plate 12 Calculation of the stroke volume ratio (SVR) and the regurgitant fraction (RF) in a patient with aortic regurgitation. Regions-of-interest are traced on the amplitude image but applied on the raw data. The stroke counts of each ventricle are used to calculate the stroke volume ratio (LV stroke counts/RV stroke counts). The formula for regurgitant fraction (RF):

RF = LV stroke counts – RV stroke counts/LV stroke counts ×100

can be modified to correct for the systematic underestimation of the RV stroke volume: (RF = SVR – 1.2/SVR), where 1.2 is the SVR in normals.

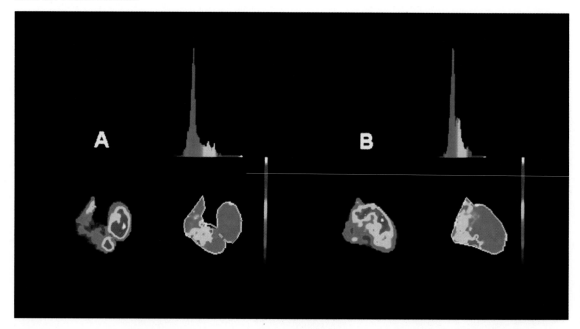

Plate 13 A 32-year-old patient with recurrent ventricular tachycardia resulting from an arrhythmogenic right ventricular cardiomyopathy. Left anterior oblique (A) and right anterior oblique (B) multiharmonic Fourier amplitude and phase images (amplitude bottom left and phase bottom right) demonstrate an inferior wall abnormality in the subtricuspid and free wall regions. The abnormality is best demonstrated on the phase image. (Illustration courtesy of Professor D. Le Guludec, Paris.)

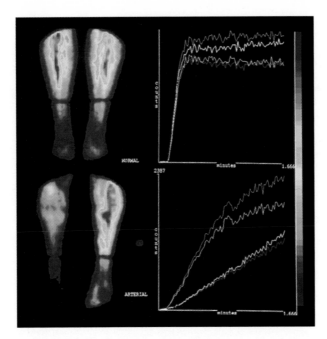

Plate 14 Measurement of limb blood flow: summed images (left) and time-activity curves (right) from a control subject (top row) and a patient with unilateral claudication (bottom row). In the normal control the feet and calves show brisk inflow on both sides In the claudicant the symptomatic leg shows severely impaired inflow (calf, white; foot, red) while the asymptomatic side shows less marked inflow reduction (calf, green; foot, yellow).

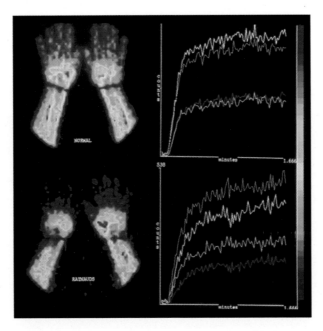

Plate 15 Measurements of forearm and hand blood flow in a control subject (top) and a patient with 'vibration white finger' (VBF; bottom). The summed images (left) show uniform flow into all the digits of the normal subject but patchy loss of flow in the digits of the VBF patient. The control subject shows normal perfusion of both forearms (white and green curves) and both hands (red and yellow curves). Inflow curves in the VBF patient show only minor reduction in forearm flow, worse on the right (white) than left (green) but severe impairment of flow in the hands, again worse on the right (red) than left (yellow).

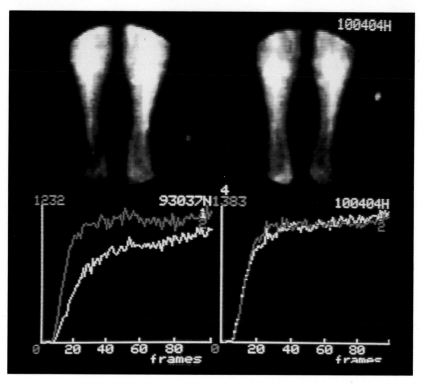

Plate 16 Leg blood flow before (left) and after (right) angioplasty: see also Figure 6.13. Initially, the right leg shows diminished flow on the summed images (top left) and inflow curves (bottom left: red, left leg; white, right leg). After angioplasty (right top and bottom) both legs show equally good inflow.

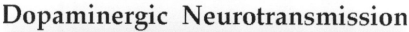

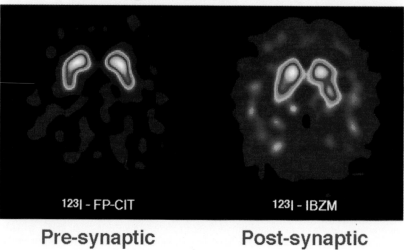

Plate 17 Similar orientation and location transverse slices through the basal ganglia of two normal volunteers to demonstrate the distribution of dopaminergic transporter sites in the pre-synaptic neurone (left) and the post-synaptic dopamine D2 neuroreceptors.

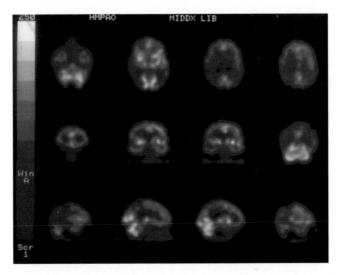

Plate 18 In a case of cortico-basal degeneration (CBD) there are perfusion deficits in the cortex with reduced perfusion ratios to the caudate nuclei.

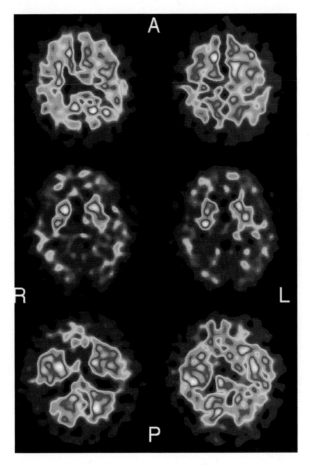

Plate 19 The post-synaptic D2 dopamine receptors show down-regulation in the same individual as in Plate 18. The images show sequential slices from the cerebellum (bottom left) to the dorsolateral fronto-parietal cortex and cyngulate gyri (top right). For description, see text.

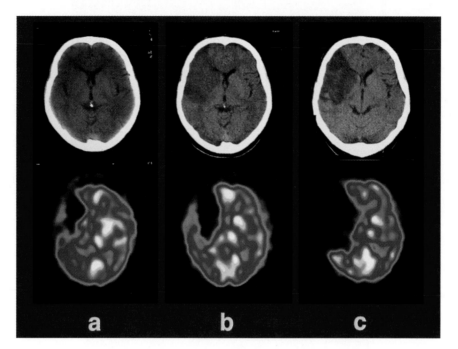

Plate 20 HMPAO-SPECT and CT scans of a patient with a right middle cerebral artery stroke. The scans were acquired at: (a) 3 hours (7 hours for CT); (b) 24 hours; and (c) 11 days after sudden onset of symptoms. There is a slight difference in orientation between SPECT and CT, but for each technique the same slice is shown. The patient received no thrombolytic or reperfusion therapy.

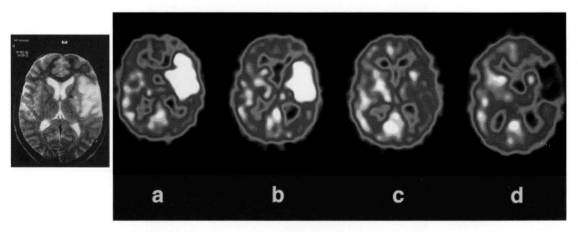

Plate 21 MRI and HMPAO-SPECT scans of a patient with recent left middle cerebral artery (MCA) occlusion. The MRI scan at 7 days shows a large oedematous area of high T2 signal consistent with an infarct involving the left MCA territory. At day 10 (a) there is high uptake of HMPAO in the same region. This uptake gradually decreases from day 13 (b) to day 24 (c) and by day 170 (d) a complete infarct has developed. Reperfusion has been achieved in the subacute stage, several days post ictus, by which stage tissue damage has occurred. The perfusion is non-nutritional and tissue is not salvaged.

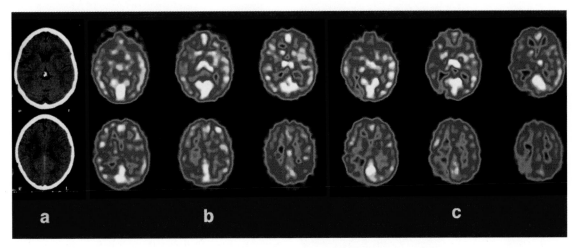

Plate 22   CT and SPECT of a 60-year-old female patient with severe bilateral carotid disease. The CT (a) shows no gross evidence of infarction. The baseline SPECT perfusion image set (b) shows only a slight deficit in the right parietal region. The stimulated scan following acetazolamide (c) shows poor reactivity in the right parietal and occipital regions. This patient was scheduled for carotid artery surgery, but before surgery could be carried out she developed a massive right hemisphere stroke.

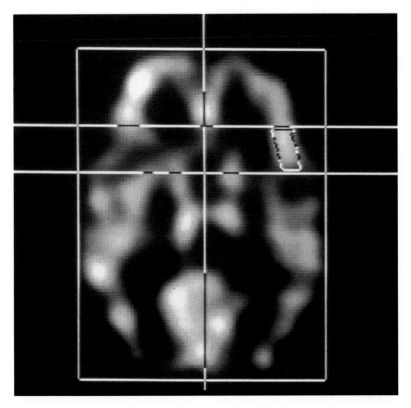

Plate 23   An HMPAO scan of a schizophrenic patient while experiencing verbal auditory hallucinations. There is increased brain perfusion in Broca's area (within the box) during such hallucinations. (Courtesy of Dr P.K. McGuire.)

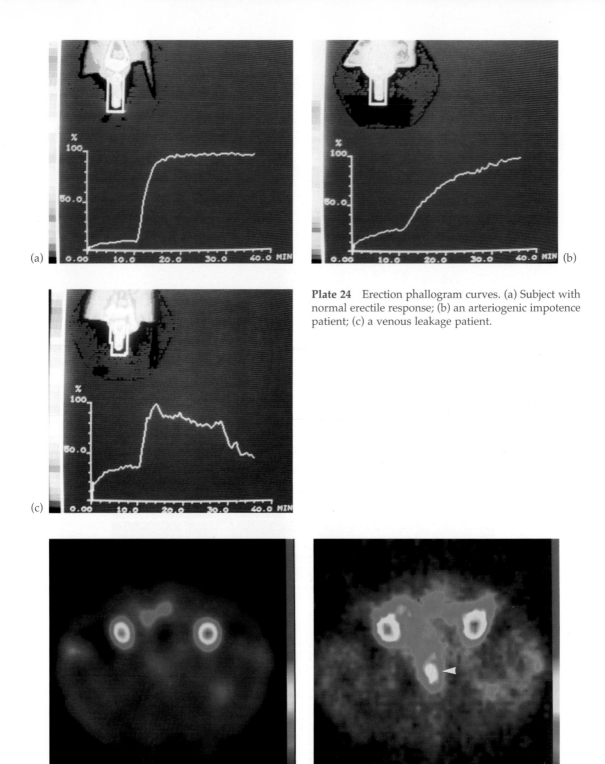

Plate 24 Erection phallogram curves. (a) Subject with normal erectile response; (b) an arteriogenic impotence patient; (c) a venous leakage patient.

Plate 25 Prostate radioimmunoscintigraphy with CYT-351 in recurrent disease. SPECT performed 6 months after radical prostectomy showing the empty prostatic bed in the transverse slice at 6 hours post-injection (left) and the appearance of specific uptake in the recurrence (arrowhead) at 24 hours post-injection (right). The patient had rising PSA levels but a negative bone scan at the time.

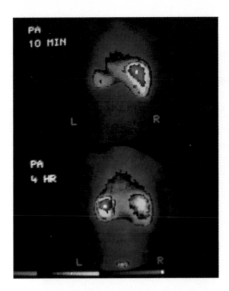

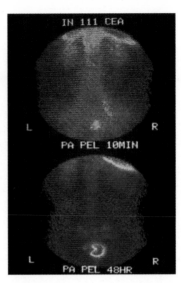

Plate 26 RIS of neuroblastoma using radioiodinated UJ13A in a 4-year-old child. Posterior abdominal images at 10 minute and 4 hour with ^{123}I-labelled UJ13A. At 4 hour the tumour is evident as a focal area of high uptake (red) in contrast to the spleen and liver (green).

Plate 27 RIS with ^{111}In-labelled anti-CEA monoclonal antibody, in a rectal adenocarcinoma. Posterior abdominal views at top, 10 minute, and bottom, 48 hour. Slight vascularity is seen at 10 minute in the pelvis while at 48 hour shows uptake as a reverse 'C' in the pelvis with a small focal area of uptake to its left, probably in lymph nodes. Normal vascular activity is seen at 10 minute, and renal but not urinary activity, high liver, spleen and marrow uptake on both views.

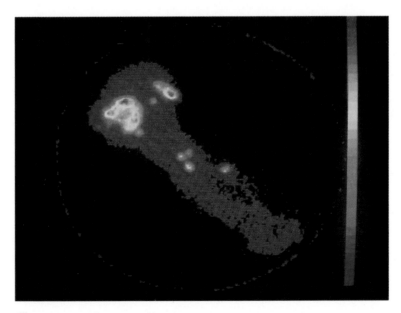

Plate 28 RIS with ^{111}In-labelled anti-CEA monoclonal antibody, in a rectal adenocarcinoma. Image of the surgical specimen taken at 72 hour showing uptake in the tumour in red and yellow (the cut is made opposite to the mesentery to display the bowel lumen; hence, the tumour has been divided) and uptake in lymph nodes. Note none of these lymph nodes contained tumour cells on histology (Dukes' B; see text).

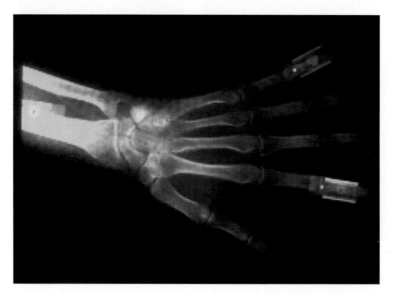

Plate 29 Digitized radiograph of the hand and wrist in grey scale overlaid with a registered image of ^{99m}Tc-MDP distribution displayed as a saturated red scale. Registration was achieved using the markers visible in each modality positioned on the fingers and forearm. The registered scan excludes suspected fracture to the lower pole of the scaphoid. Trauma to the radial carpus is confirmed, but without an intense blood pool activity to suggest fracture.

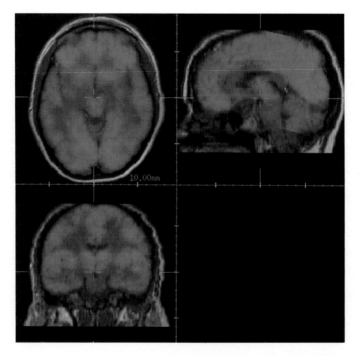

Plate 30 ^{18}F-FDG-PET and MR images of the head registered by identification of corresponding anatomical point landmarks. The PET image is displayed with a saturated green colour scale overlaid on the grey scale of the MR image. Three orthogonal views through the volume are shown.

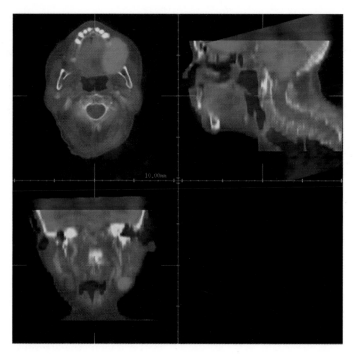

Plate 31 Registered PET and CT images of the head and neck showing accurate anatomical localization of increased uptake of ^{18}F-FDG corresponding to tumour spread. These images were registered by identification of corresponding anatomical point landmarks. Again, the nuclear medicine image is displayed with a saturated green colour scale overlaid on the grey scale of the CT image.

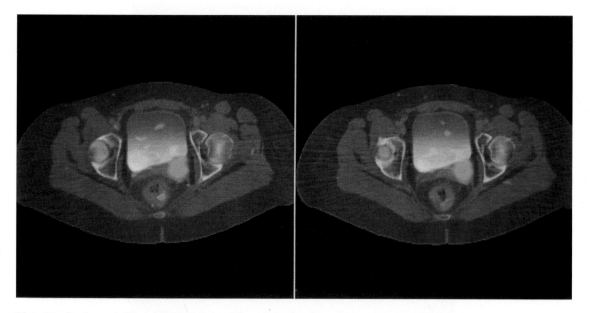

Plate 32 Registered CT and PET images of the pelvis showing clear separation of residual bladder activity from focal [18]FDG activity due to recurrent cervical carcinoma. Findings were confirmed at surgery. Registration was achieved by identification of anatomical point landmarks. Again the FDG-PET image is displayed with a saturated green colour scale.

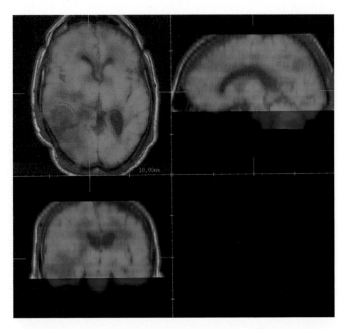

Plate 33 Example of combined image showing the results of a fully automated registration of MRI and PET scans of the head using mutual information as a measure of mis-registration. The algorithm achieved an excellent registration despite the large, space-occupying lesion. The unregistered images formed part of the Vanderbilt study [11]. The images shown on Plate 33 were provided as part of the project 'Evaluation of Retrospective Image Registration', National Institutes of Health, 1 R01 NS33926-02, Principal Investigator, J. Michael Fitzpatrick, Vanderbilt University, Nashville, TN.

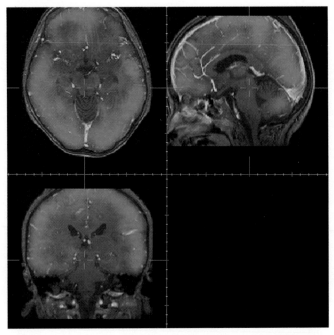

Plate 34 Example of combined image showing the results of a fully automated registration of MRI and SPECT images of the head using the mutual information measure. The study was undertaken to ascertain brainstem activity.

CHAPTER 17

New tracer approaches

Radiopeptides

S. J. Mather

INTRODUCTION

Much of current research in the radiopharmaceutical field is directed towards targeting biological functions in the body, which change as a result of one or more pathological processes. These may be entirely novel targets that may only appear during disease, as is the case, for example, in some tumour-associated antigens, or they may be normal structures, the distribution of which is altered during the diseased state. Among this latter group of potential targets are receptors that may be up-regulated on either normal cells or malignant phenotypes as a result of the disease process.

The complexity of the receptor systems which control homoeostasis is immense and, in all likelihood, there are many thousands of different receptors expressed on cells which could be utilized in this manner. This section is concerned with those receptors for which the normal ligand is a peptide, and which form a major part of the endocrinological and immunological functions of the body. Both peptides and proteins are made up of amino acids. Proteins are larger than peptides, but the dividing line between them is vague. Molecules with a molecular weight below 10 kDa would generally be termed peptides and those above 30 kDa as proteins. The group of large peptides or small proteins which make the transition are often known as polypeptides.

In terms of biodistribution, probably the most important parameter as far as nuclear medicine is concerned, is that an important change takes place at around 50 kDa, above which the proteins become too large to be filtered at the glomerulus. Thus, proteins significantly larger than 50 kDa in mass will have circulation times much greater than those that are significantly smaller. Within the group of larger proteins of interest would be included albumin (c. 60 kDa), transferrin (c. 80 kDa), the IgG immunoglobulins (c. 150 kDa) and many of their fragments, and serum amyloid protein (c. 250 kDa). All have plasma half-lives of the order of many hours, if not several days. Among the smaller peptides, which form the main theme of this section, would be included the cytokines (c. 15–30 kDa), some peptide hormones (c. 1500 Da) and chemotactic peptides (<1000 Da).

PEPTIDE STRUCTURE

All peptides and proteins are composed of amino acids. There are 20 major mammalian amino acids, all of which normally exist in the form of the L-optical isomer. These amino acids, classified in terms of their size and lipophilicity, together with their single-letter and three-letter abbreviations are listed in Table 17.1.

While the amino acids that comprise the primary sequence are fundamental to the properties of the peptide, molecules containing more than just a few amino acids take up secondary configu-

Clinical Nuclear Medicine, 3rd edn. Edited by M.N. Maisey, K.E. Britton and B.D. Collier. Published in 1998 by Chapman & Hall, London. ISBN 0 412 75180 1

Table 17.1   Amino acid characteristics

Amino acid			Mass of residue (Da)	Side-chain structure
Small polar				
Serine	S	Ser	87	CH_2-OH
Glycine	G	Gly	57	H
Aspartic acid	D	Asp	115	CH_2-COOH
Asparagine	N	Asn	114	CH_2-CO-NH_2
Small non-polar				
Cysteine	C	Cys	103	CH_2-SH
Proline	P	Pro	97	CH_2-CH_2-CH_2-(N)
Alanine	A	Ma	71	CH_3
Threonine	T	Thr	101	CHOH-CH_3
Large polar				
Glutamic acid	B	Glu	129	CH_2-CH_2-COOH
Glutamine	Q	Gln	128	CH_2-CH_2-CO-NH_2
Lysine	K	Lys	128	CH_2-CH_2-CH_2-CH_2-NH_2
Arginine	R	Mg	156	CH_2-CH_2-CH_2-NH-C (NH)-NH_2
Large non-polar				
Valine	V	Val	99	CH-$(CH_3)_2$
Leucine	L	Leu	113	CH_2-CH$(CH_3)_2$
Isoleucine	I	Ile	113	CH(CH_3)-CH_2-CH_3
Methionine	M	Met	131	CH_2-CH_2-S-CH_3
Phenylalanine	F	Phe	147	CH_2
Intermediate polarity				
Tyrosine	Y	Tyr	163	
Histidine	H	His	137	
Tryptophan	W	Trp	186	

rations as a result of interactions between the amino acid side-chains within the peptide sequence. These interactions include hydrogen bonding, ionic attractions and hydrophobic interactions. When the peptide sequence contains more than one cysteine residue, the sulphydryl groups may interact to produce a more stable disulphide bridge, resulting in cyclization of the linear sequence. Larger peptides also frequently undergo enzymatic post-translational modification, in particular N-glycosylation at glutamine and O-glycosylation or phosphorylation at serine and threonine residues. The -NH_2 and -COOH termini of the peptide may also be modified by acetylation and amidation respectively.

All of these factors will influence the *in vivo* biodistribution and stability of the peptide, and determine its suitability for use as a radiopharmaceutical. While the biological action of many larger peptides and proteins may be required over an extended period of time, only a brief duration of activity is desired of most of the peptide hormones. Many of these molecules have intense pharmacological activity and are active at extremely dilute concentrations. Following their release from endocrine cells, their duration of activity is limited by the actions of enzymes that are widely distributed in the serum of all mammals. These endo- and exo-peptidases rapidly degrade the structure and biological activities of small peptides following their secretion (or injection) into the blood, and therefore many such hormones in their intact form have half-lives of only a few seconds. For this reason, the usefulness of many naturally occurring peptides as pharmaceuticals (including radiopharmaceuticals) is quite limited. In most cases, some drug development is required to engineer a more stable structure into the natural sequence of the peptide. The most simple approach to this problem is to exchange the natural amino acids, which provide an excellent substrate for the peptidases, with artificial amino acids that block the enzyme digestion. In many cases, the substitution of the D-isomer will slow the rate of cleavage by many orders of magnitude. Alternatively, chemical modification, such as the use of reduced peptide bonds, will fulfil a similar function. Frequently, *in vivo* pharmaceutical development will also use either non-mammalian (e.g. bacterial) or entirely synthetic amino acids.

OCTREOTIDE

In recent years, great interest has been generated within nuclear medicine by the potential of peptides, in particular peptide hormones, to act as radiopharmaceuticals. Much of this interest has been stimulated by the success of one peptide in particular – octreotide – which, when radiolabelled, can be used to image the *in vivo* distribution of somatostatin receptors. Octreotide has almost all the properties that might be considered ideal in a tumour-targeting radiopharmaceutical, including:

- expression of the target receptor is up-regulated in many different tumour types;
- expression of the target receptor on normal tissues is low;
- the affinity of the interaction of the ligand with the receptor is high (approximately 10^{-9} M);
- the molecular weight of the tracer is low (approximately 1500 Da); and
- the tracer is stable *in vivo*.

As a consequence of the combination of these properties, tumours are efficiently imaged within minutes of injection. Remaining circulating peptide clears rapidly from the vasculature and is excreted by the liver or kidneys resulting in high target-to-background ratios [1].

In addition to the properties of octreotide itself, peptides have a number of 'generic' attractions: (i) they can be cheaply and easily synthesized using an automated peptide synthesizer; (ii) because they are entirely synthetic and are not produced in tissue culture they do not suffer from the same potential problems as biotechnological products in terms of viral contamination, mutation, etc., and (iii) since the peptide sequences are essentially 'human', these compounds are not immunogenic, and if required, may safely be administered on many occasions.

The parameters that are likely to determine the targeting properties of a peptide include:

1. its affinity for the target (receptor)
2. the target density
3. the target accessibility
4. non-target expression of receptor
5. the *in vivo* stability of peptide
6. the choice of radiolabel
7. the stability of the radiolabel–peptide complex
8. the physicochemical properties of the radiolabelled peptide (e.g. size, charge, lipophilicity)

In the case of octreotide and its indium-111-labelled analogue, Octreoscan™, many of these parameters are near-optimal. However, it is frequently forgotten that octreotide is not a naturally occurring peptide, but the result of a multi-million dollar R&D programme by a major drug company. Octreotide was originally developed by Sandoz to provide a long-acting drug which can be used to inhibit the secretion of growth hormone by the pituitary [2]. The native hormone, somatostatin, suffers from many of the drawbacks of naturally occurring peptides. Following parenteral administration, it is rapidly cleaved in the blood and has a circulating half-life of only a few minutes [3]. The synthetic analogue octreotide has a very similar structure to somatostatin but, as shown in Figure 17.1, a number of important modifications have been made:

1. The size of the peptide has been reduced from 14 to eight amino acids.

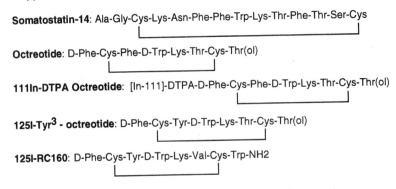

Figure 17.1   Amino acid sequences of somatostatin and some related synthetic analogues.

2. The D-isomer of the N-terminal phenylalanine has been used.
3. An amino-alcohol form of the C-terminal threonine has been used.
4. While the naturally occurring receptor-binding sequence -Phe-Trp-Lys-Thr- has been retained, the L-tryptophan has been replaced by the D-isomer.

The result of these changes is that the peptide is much more stable and has a longer duration of activity *in vivo*. The serum half-life of octreotide following subcutaneous injection is of the order of 2 hours [3].

The number of naturally occurring peptides with properties as advantageous as octreotide is likely to be very few. Some chemical development of the great majority of these peptides is almost certain to be required before an acceptable level of performance as radiopharmaceutical is obtained.

RADIOLABELLING OF PEPTIDES

Many of the methods that are used to radiolabel peptides with gamma-emitting radionuclides were originally developed for much larger proteins such as monoclonal antibodies. While some of these can be directly extrapolated to smaller molecules, some modification of the process is frequently required.

RADIOIODINATION

Electrophilic substitution is normally the method of choice for labelling proteins with iodine. The labelling is mediated by oxidation of the iodide ion to the positively charged iodous ion, which labels the phenolic ring of the tyrosine amino acid side chain in the ortho- and para- positions. Other amino acids such as histidine and tryptophan may also be labelled using this method, but the resultant bonds are much less stable and the compounds would not be stable *in vivo*. Chloramine-T [4] or Iodogen™ [5] remain the most popular oxidants for this purpose and, in general, methods developed for other proteins can be directly applied to most peptides. The majority of medium-to-large size peptides will contain a number of tyrosine residues and, depending on the conditions employed, either one or two atoms of iodine may be substituted into each phenolic ring. Iodination will therefore result in a heterogeneous mixture of labelled compounds. Not all of these will have the same biodistribution and the same receptor-binding capacity. Careful analysis of the reaction products is required to explore the properties of each of the individual components, as well as the mixture, to ensure that compounds with ideal properties are not diluted with those having less-desirable characteristics.

Very small peptides may have the opposite problem, and possess no tyrosine residues at all. Octreotide is a case in point. In these circumstances, it may be possible to replace an amino acid possessing a similar side chain, such as phenylalanine, with a tyrosine. This is the case with octreotide. The Tyr[3] octreotide analogue maintains much of its receptor-binding capacity and provides a compound which can readily be labelled with ^{125}I or [123]I.

Following the radiolabelling procedure, a method of purification is required to remove unwanted contaminants. The most widely applicable technology is called solid-phase extraction (SPE), of which the most widely used form are the SEP-PAK™ cartridges. These preferentially retain lipophilic components such as radiolabelled peptides on the cartridge, while hydrophilic contaminants (such as free iodine) are washed away. The peptide can then be eluted with an organic solvent such as ethanol. It may be necessary to remove this solvent by evaporation before the radiopharmaceutical can be administered to the patient.

RADIOLABELLING WITH ^{111}In

Since the supply of ^{123}I has logistical difficulties, radiometallic isotopes such as ^{111}In may be preferred. Again, the labelling methods of choice are those originally developed for use with monoclonal antibodies, namely the use of bifunctional chelating agents (BFCA). The most widely used chelators are those based on diethylenetriaminepenta-acetic acid (DTPA) [6]. Most BFCAs are conjugated to peptides via free amine groups which are present at the N-terminus of the peptide and also on the side-chains of any lysine residues. In the case of large proteins such as antibodies, there are normally many lysines, and it is unlikely that conjugation will be directed towards an amino acid critical for target binding. In the case of small peptides, however, a limited number of lysines will be present and these may be in parts of the molecule that are critical for biological activity. A typical example again can be seen with octreotide when the single Lys5 resides right in the middle of the receptor-binding sequence. Conjugation of a BFCA at this point will destroy the biological activity of this peptide. To overcome this problem, it may be necessary to temporarily 'block' the lysine ε-amino group in order to direct the conjugation of the BFCA towards the N-terminal amine [7].

Through the use of careful conjugation conditions, it is possible to develop kits of DTPA-peptide conjugates (such as Octreoscan), which can be labelled with ^{111}In to high levels of purity, removing the need for post-labelling purification.

TECHNETIUM-LABELLED PEPTIDES

Since small peptides are delivered very quickly to their targets and show very rapid clearance kinetics, short-lived radionuclides such as technetium-99m are likely to be the radiolabel of choice. The direct methods of labelling developed for monoclonal antibodies will only rarely be applicable to smaller peptides since they normally disrupt sensitive disulphide bridges on which the biological activity of the compound depends. Accordingly, the methods of choice for technetium-labelling of peptides also involve the use of chelating agents. Chelators designed for technetium can be conjugated to peptides in the same way as indium BFCAs [8] (Figure 17.2). Alternatively, chelators can be engineered into the peptide during synthesis [10]. This prevents the need for blocking essential peptide side-chains.

QUALITY CONTROL OF RADIOLABELLED PEPTIDES

Development work with radiolabelled peptides requires two techniques, which are not in widespread use in nuclear medicine laboratories. The first relates to the measurement of radiochemical purity. The method of choice is reverse-phase high-pressure liquid chromatography (HPLC), which separates labelled compounds on the basis of their lipophilicity. This is a very versatile and sensitive technique that can, for example, separate isomers in which radioiodine is attached to different tyrosine residues, and can also separate labelled from unlabelled peptide. However, the equipment is very expensive and could not be justified for routine quality control. Although some simple TLC systems can be developed, the most widely applicable 'low-tech' approach is probably based on the use of SEP-PAK cartridges, widely used for quality control of ^{99m}Tc-MAG3 [11], in which hydrophilic contaminants can be separated from the labelled peptide as described above.

An essential characteristic of radiolabelled peptides is their ability to bind to their specific receptor. Any development programme involving these materials must therefore incorporate an assay to measure the specificity and strength of receptor-binding of the radiopharmaceutical. Since many of these receptors are widely expressed on normal tissues, the best assays involve the use of cell membranes prepared from tissues such as rat brain [12]. Using appropriate methodologies, the affinity of binding of the radiolabelled peptide can be determined and compared with the unlabelled peptide [13].

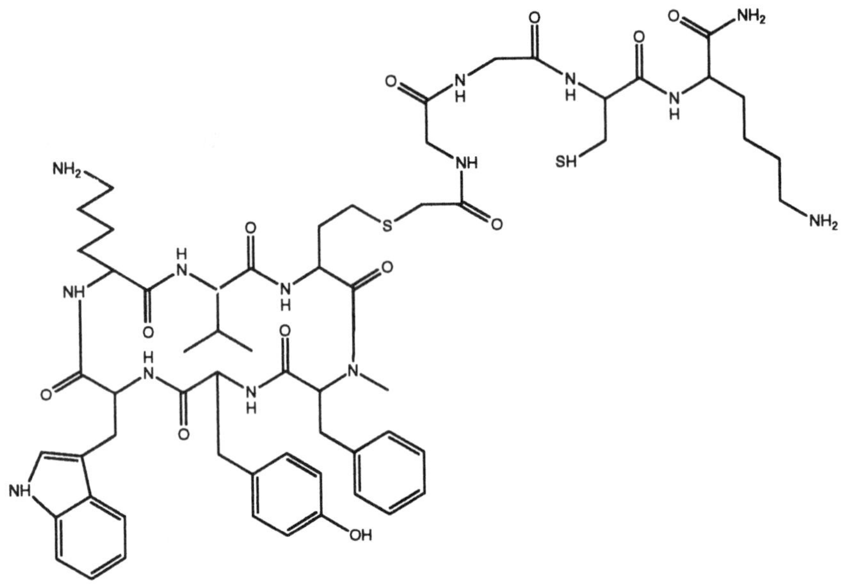

(a)

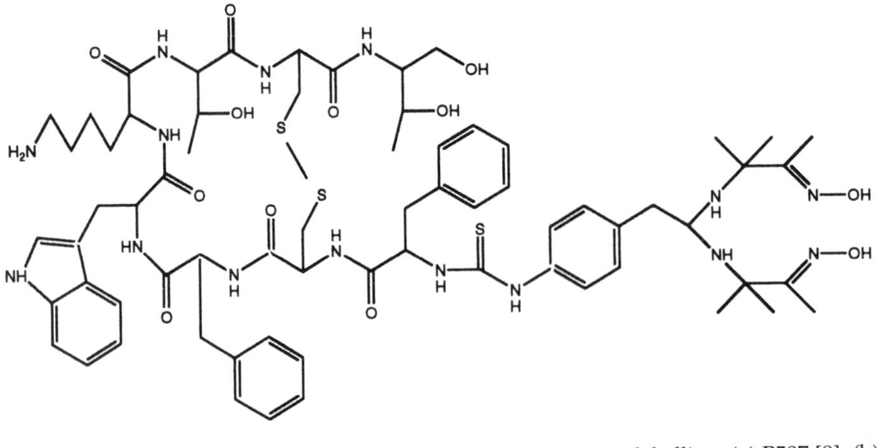

(b)

Figure 17.2 Structures of two somatostatin analogues for technetium-99m labelling: (a) P587 [9]; (b) SDZ 219–387 [8].

BIODISTRIBUTION

Provided that receptor-binding is retained, the success of a labelled peptide will be largely determined by its biodistribution in non-target tissues. As described above, peptides will often clear rapidly from the circulation, giving the potential for high target-to-blood ratios soon after administration. However, metabolism of the peptide in the blood may reduce this rate of clearance, as labelled metabolites may be cleared much less rapidly. Another possible source of increased blood background is protein binding. Depending on the strength of this interaction, the binding of the peptide to circulating plasma proteins can extend the rate of clearance from minutes to several hours.

Apart from the blood, the other tissues of importance are the organs of excretion, namely the liver and kidneys. The route of excretion of a peptide is determined largely by the relative lipophilicity of the compound or its metabolites. Depending upon the balance of polar and nonpolar side-chains in the sequence, the contribution made by the labelling method and the possibility of specific recognition sites within the peptide, the radiopharmaceutical will be routed either towards the hepatobiliary or renal routes of excretion. Since background radioactivity within the hepatobiliary/gastrointestinal tract is much more likely to obscure sites of receptor-mediated uptake of the tracer, peptides which clear through the kidneys are much preferred. Octreotide again provides an excellent example. While ^{123}I-labelled octreotide is cleared largely through the liver, ^{111}In-DTPA-octreotide undergoes mainly renal excretion. In those areas of the body distant from the abdomen, both of the radiopharmaceuticals are equally effective. However, Octreoscan is much more effective for imaging tumours in the liver or gastrointestinal tract.

Since many interesting peptides are naturally occurring hormones, they have great pharmacological activity, and some will be quite toxic when administered to patients in significant amounts. Two approaches can be used to overcome this problem: (i) very small amounts of peptide (<10μg) can be radiolabelled; or (ii) the radiolabelled peptide can be separated from the unlabelled peptide by HPLC before administration. Either solution presents a problem to the developer, since they make the task of producing a simple one-step kit much more difficult.

PEPTIDES OF CURRENT INTEREST

At the present time, the only radiolabelled peptide widely approved for use is Octreoscan. However, a number of other peptides have been explored in greater or lesser detail, though the limited space of this chapter permits only a few to be mentioned. Many other octreotide and alternative somatostatin-receptor binding analogues have been developed for labelling with a variety of radionuclides, but in particular with technetium-99m. Two examples are shown in Figure 17.2. Structure A shows a compound developed by Diatide Inc. [14] in which the ring structure is cyclized through an amide bond rather than a disulphide bridge. The chelation site for technetium is provided by the peptide sequence glycine-glycine-cysteine. In compound B, the PnAO complexing structure has been conjugated to the N-terminus of octreotide [8].

Vasoactive intestinal peptide (VIP) is a 28-amino acid peptide with receptors widely distributed in tumours of the gastrointestinal tract [15]. This peptide presents a challenge to the radiopharmaceutical chemist, since it contains two tyrosine residues and a methionine which is sensitive to oxidation. The peptide is quite toxic and only sub-microgram quantities can safely be administered [16].

The chemotactic peptides based on the formyl-methionine-leucine-proline sequence have been explored as a possible peptide-based method for imaging infection. Again, these peptides suffer from the risk of severe toxicity caused by neutropenia, and this problem has currently limited their study in humans [17]. The chemotactic peptides were one of the first to be studied using the BFCA based on 'HYNIC', a hydrophilic chelator that shows great promise for this type of application [18]. Another group of peptides for which the same chelator has been employed are those based upon the sequence arginine-glycine-aspartic acid (RGD), which bind to the IIb/IIIa receptor of activated platelets [19]. Both synthetic and naturally occurring [20] RGD-based peptides have been explored. In a somewhat different class of larger peptides are the cytokines; both interleukin-1 [21] and interleukin-2 [22] show promise for imaging either infection or auto-immunity respectively.

REFERENCES

1. Krenning, E.P., Kwekkeboom, D.J., Bakker, W.H. *et al.* (1993) Somatostatin receptor scintigraphy with 111-In-D-ThA-D-Phe and 123-I-TyrJ -octreotide: The Rotterdam experience with more than 1000 patients. *Eur. J. Nucl. Med.*, **20**, 716–31.
2. Bauer, W., Briner, U., Doepfner, W.S. *et al.* (1982) SMS 201-995: a very potent and selective octapeptide analogue of somatostatin with pro-longed action. *Life Sci.*, **31**, 1133–41.
3. Pless, I., Bauer, W., Briner, U. *et al.* (1986) Chemistry and pharmacology of SMS 201-995, a long acting analogue of somatostatin. *Scand. J. Gastroenterol.*, **21**(suppl. 119), 54–64.
4. Bakker, W.H., Kremning, E.P., Breeman, W.A. *et al.* (1990) Receptor scintigraphy with a radioiodinated somatostatin analogue: radiolabeling, purification, biologic activity and *in-vivo* application in animals. *J. Nucl. Med.*, **31**, 1501–9.
5. Mather, S.J., Ur, B., Bomanji, I. *et al.* (1993) Radiolabelled Octreotide: what lessons for antibody mediated targeting? *Cell Biophysics*, **21**, 93–108.
6. Hnatowitch, D.J., Childs, R.L., Lanteigne, D. and Najafi, A. (1989) DTPA-coupled antibodies radiolabelled with metallic radionuclides: an improved method. *J. Immunol. Methods*, **65**, 147–57.
7. Bakker, W.H., Albert, R., Bruns, C. *et al.* (1991) 111-In-DTPA-D-PheJ octreotide, a potential radiopharmaceutical for imaging of somatostatin receptor-positive tumors: synthesis, radiolabeling and *in-vitro* validation. *Life Sci.*, **49**, 1583–91.
8. Maina, T., Stolz, B., Albert, R. *et al.* (1994) Synthesis, radiochemistry and biological evaluation of a new somatostatin analogue (SDZ 219-387) labelled with technetium-99m. *Eur. J. Nucl. Med.*, **21**, 437–44.
9. Vallabhajosula, S., Moyer, B.R., Lister-James, I. *et al.* (1996) Pre-clinical evaluation of technetium-99m-labeled somatostatin receptor-binding peptides. *J. Nucl. Med.*, **37**, 1016–22.
10. Mather, S.J., Ellison, D. and Bard, D.S. (1995) Technetium-99m labelled hybrid receptor-binding peptides, in *Technetium and Rhenium in Chemistry and Nuclear Medicine* (eds M. Nicolini, G. Bandoli, U. Mazzi), SG Editorial, Padova. pp. 491–7.
11. Mallinckrodt Medical Inc. (1992) Package insert for Technescan MAG3, R11/92, St Louis, MO, USA.
12. Reubi, J.C., Perrin, M.H., Rivier, I.E. and Vale, W. (1981) High affinity binding sites of a somatostatin-28 analogue in rat brain membranes. *Life Sci.*, **28**, 2191–8.

13. Gammeltoft, S. (1990) Peptide hormone receptors, in *Peptide Hormone Action; a Practical Approach* (eds K. Siddle and J.C. Hutton), IRL Press, Oxford.
14. Lister-James, J., McBride, B., Buttram, S. *et al.* (1995) Technetium-99m chelate-containing receptor-binding peptides, in *Technetium and Rhenium in Chemistry and Nuclear Medicine* (eds M. Nicolini, G. Bandolini and U. Mazzi), SGE Editorial, Padova, pp. 260–74.
15. Virgolini, I., Raderer, H., Kurtaran, A. *et al.* (1994) Vasoactive Intestinal Peptide – Receptor imaging for the localisation of adenocarcinomas and endocrine tumours. *N. Engl. J. Med.*, **331**, 1116–21.
16. Angelberger, P., Virgolini, I., Buchheit, O. *et al.* (1995) Radiopharmaceutical development of 123-I vasoactive intestinal peptide (VIP) for receptor scintigraphy in oncology. *J. Labelled Comp. Radiopharm.*, **37**, 502–3.
17. Fischman, A.J., Rauh, D., Solomon., H. *et al.* (1993) In-vivo bioactivity and biodistribution of chemotactic peptides analogs in non-human primates. *J. Nucl. Med.*, **34**, 2130–4.
18. Abrams, M.J., Juweid, M., Tenkate, C.I. *et al.* (1990) Technetium-99m human polyclonal IgG radiolabelled via the hydrazino nicotinamide derivative for imaging focal sites of infection in rats. *J. Nucl. Med.*, **31**, 2022–8.
19. Shuang, I., Edwards, D.S., Looby, R.J. *et al.* (1996) Labelling a hydrazino nicotinamide-modified cyclic IIb/IIIa receptor antagonist with 99m-Tc using aminocarboxylates as co-ligands. *Bioconjug. Chem.*, **7**, 63–71.
20. Knight, L.C., Maurer, A.I.H. and Romano, I.E. (1996) Comparison of iodine-I 23 disintegrins for imaging thrombi and emboli in a canine model. *J. Nucl. Med.*, **37**, 476–81.
21. Van der Laken, C.J., Boerman, O.C., Oyen, W.J.G. *et al.* (1995) Specific targeting of infectious foci with radioiodinated human recombinant interleukin-1 in an experimental model. *Eur. J. Nucl. Med.*, **22**, 1249–55.
22. Signore, A., Chianelli, M., Ferretti, B. *et al.* (1994) New approach for in-vivo detection of insulitis in type I diabetes: activated lymphocyte targeting with I-123 labelled interleukin-2. *Eur. J. Endocrinol.*, **131**, 431–7.

FURTHER READING

Hider, R.C. and Barlow, D. (eds) (1991) *Polypeptide and Protein Drugs; Production, Characterization and Formulation*, Ellis Horwood, Chichester.
Siddle, K. and Hutton, J.C. (eds) (1990) *Peptide Hormone Action; A Practical Approach*, IRL Press, Oxford.

Radioimmunoscintigraphy

K. E. Britton and M. Granowska

INTRODUCTION

Nuclear medicine techniques are known for their sensitivity to changes of function induced by disease, but not for their specificity in determining the nature of the disease process. To address this problem, nuclear medicine has developed new procedures for tissue characterization additional to functional measurements, by receptor binding techniques and antigen-antibody interactions. The use of radiolabelled antibodies to image and characterize the nature of the disease process *in vivo* is called radioimmunoscintigraphy (RIS).

In principle, the RIS technique is applicable to both benign (as in the identification of myocardial infarction by radiolabelled antimyosin) and malignant pathology.

CANCER RIS

Cancerous tissue differs from the normal tissue in a number of subtle ways that enables it to invade surrounding tissues. This ability appears to be determined mainly by the surface properties of the cancer cell. Differences have been found in the biochemistry, the adhesion properties, the receptor characteristics, the responses to cytokine and autocrine factors, and the antigenic determinants of the cancer cell surface, in comparison with the equivalent population of normal cells.

Thus, the modern approach to cancer detection attempts to exploit these features and to demonstrate the presence of a cancer not by relying on its physical attributes such as size, shape, position, space occupation, density, water content or reflectivity, etc., as for conventional radiology, X-ray computed tomography (CT), magnetic resonance imaging (MRI) or ultrasound (US), but through the essential and specific 'cancerousness' of a cancer. This chapter is concerned with techniques designed to take advantage of the specific antigenic determinants of cancer tissue, in order to demonstrate the tumour, its local recurrence and its metastases. RIS is still some way from achieving the goal of specific cancer detection, but the signposts along the way are becoming clearer.

Four factors are required for RIS:

1. An antibody capable of detecting the cancer.
2. A radiolabel to give the best signal.
3. A radiolabelling method with appropriate quality control to give a labelled antibody suitable for human use while maintaining full immunoreactivity.
4. An imaging system optimized to the radionuclide and the region under study, with single photon emission tomography SPECT and serial image data analysis.

The selective localization of cancer tissue by radiolabelled antibodies carries with it the hope of selective therapy, and explains much of the motivation behind the development of RIS. However, for radioimmunotherapy (RIT) there are two additional requirements: (i) the ratio of uptake of radiolabel by the target cancer compared with that in the most critical non-target organ should be a value of at least 10:1; and (ii) estimates of the absorbed radiation dose delivered to the tumour, to the critical non-target organ such as bone marrow, and to the whole body for which a reasonable maximum would be 2 Gy (200 rad), pose severe limitations on the current techniques.

THE ANTIGEN

The key to RIS is the discovery of an antigen that is specific to the disease process under study. Four decades of saturation analysis techniques using antigen–antibody binding characteristics to measure hormones and other biological substances *in vitro* have shown the feasibility and specificity of this approach when the appropriate antigen or ligand is identified and purified, and an avid and specific antibody is raised against it. The part of an antigen with which an antibody reacts is called an 'epitope' or antigenic determinant.

The first problem for RIS is lack of specificity of the antigen for the disease process. There is no completely cancer-specific antigen, but a range of tumour-associated antigens may be used in the appropriate clinical context for the demonstration of cancer (Table 17.2).

Clinical Nuclear Medicine, 3rd edn. Edited by M.N. Maisey, K.E. Britton and B.D. Collier. Published in 1998 by Chapman & Hall, London. ISBN 0 412 75180 1

The development of the oncogene–anti-oncogene theory of cancer has raised hopes for the demonstration of cancer-specific oncoproteins. The discovery of specific genes involved in the regulation of growth has led to the concept that the uncontrolled growth of cancer cells is due to aberrant expression of these genes – oncogenes, particularly alterations or deletions in 'suppressor' genes that exert control over the cell cycle. Oncogenes may be the final common pathway for genetic damage, and viral or carcinogenic induction of cancer. Such transforming genes have been demonstrated. Since genes are made up of specific DNA sequences, then RNA sequences equivalent to them and thence amino acid sequences equivalent to these can be produced; thus, cancer-related oncoproteins are derived, and give the hope that cancer-specific antigens will be discovered, leading in turn to cancer-specific antibodies. Work in this direction has been undertaken in lung cancer where a monoclonal antibody against the oncoprotein equivalent to the c-myc oncogene was raised and used for RIS [1].

The expression of antigen by the cell is a dynamic process. Clearly it needs to be on the surface accessible to antibody, and the higher its density the greater the amount of antibody binding capacity. The possibility of binding is given by the binding constant K_B of the antigen-antibody reaction; current antibodies have K_B values of 10^{-9} to 10^{-10} l/mol.

Antigen density can be increased by certain circumstances, such as exposure to γ-interferon. Attachment to nuclear antigens would require the internalization of the antibody by endocytosis

Table 17.2   Tumour-associated antigens

1. Epithelial surface antigens
   These are separated from the blood by biological barriers and exposed by the architectural disruption of malignancy.
   Moabs: HMFG1, HMFG2, SM3, PR1A3
2. Oncofetal antigens
   Moabs: anti-CEA, anti-alpha-fetoprotein
3. Tumour-derived antigens
   Moabs: B72.3, Mov 18
4. Viral antigens
   Moab: anti-hepatoma
5. Synthetic antigens
   Moab: 170 H82
6. Receptor antigens
   Moab: anti-EGF receptor

Moab = monoclonal antibody.

or other mechanisms that occur with certain antibodies.

The degree of antigen expression changes with time, and the amount of the antigen on a cell surface can be reduced after exposure to a specific antibody – this process is known as antigen modulation, which can lead to internalization and metabolism of the labelled antibody with either loss of the label or its fixation in the cell. Important for detection, and crucial to radioimmunotherapy, is the requirement that the antigen expression is not too heterogeneous. Ideally, all the cancer cells should express the chosen antigen. However, in practice, this is rare, and more usually some clumps of cells are antigen-positive and others antigen-negative. This does not affect RIS detection, but influences the success of RIT. Some cancers do not express a particular antigen at all. Thus, antibodies against placental alkaline phosphatase (PLAP) are excellent for RIS of ovarian cancer, but only 70% of ovarian adenocarcinomas express this antigen.

Current tumour-associated antigens are chosen in different ways (Table 17.2). The de-differentiation antigens such as carcinoembryonic antigen (CEA), human choriogonadotrophin (HCG) and alpha-fetoprotein (AFP) are widely used. These are expressed in greater numbers on malignant cell surfaces than in normal tissues. They are secreted from such cells and are easily detectable in the blood and body fluids. Surprisingly, the injected antibody is not inactivated by, for example, circulating CEA and immune-complex formation does not appear to be a problem unless serum CEA is over 500 ng/ml. However, these cancer antigens are not specific: CEA expression occurs in lung, bladder, breast and gastric cancers, and also in colorectal cancer. They can be increased in non-malignant disease (e.g. Crohn's disease), and are present in the related normal tissues and colonic mucosa. Virus-related antigens may be used, e.g. anti-hepatitis antibody for liver cancer. Idiotypic antigen may be used for the leukaemias and lymphomas.

An alternative approach is to use normal epithelial tissue antigens lining ducts, which by their situation are not normally exposed to blood. Human milk fat globule (HMFG) is a glycoprotein (one of the polymorphic epithelial mucin, PEM, group) found in the lining epithelium of the lactiferous ducts of the breast, the internal lining of an ovarian follicle and in the crypts of the colon.

The architectural disruption of the malignant process exposes these antigens in increased density directly to the bloodstream and antibodies against these, such as HMFG1, HMFG2 and SM3, are used for RIS. The preferred antigen is membrane-fixed and specific to the cancer. The nearest conventional antigen to this ideal is the high-molecular weight melanoma antigen against which an antibody called 225.28S (Sorin Biomedica) is widely used in Europe for RIS, both for cutaneous and for ocular melanoma. A membrane-stable antigen called TAG72, against which an antibody B72.3 has been made, is commercially available for RIS in colorectal, ovarian and breast cancer. The list is growing rapidly and many malignancies are being studied using RIS.

THE ANTIBODY

Antibodies are bifunctional molecules: one part of the molecule is highly variable in terms of its structure (variable region, idiotype) and is associated with binding to antigen, while the second part varies little between different classes of antibodies (constant region, isotype). Biological functions of antibodies such as complement activation and binding to cell surface receptors are controlled by their constant 'Fc' regions. The basic structure of an IgG antibody molecule contains four polypeptide chains – two heavy and two light chains – held together by a variable number of disulphide bonds (Figure 17.3). It can be cleaved into smaller fragments that retain their ability to

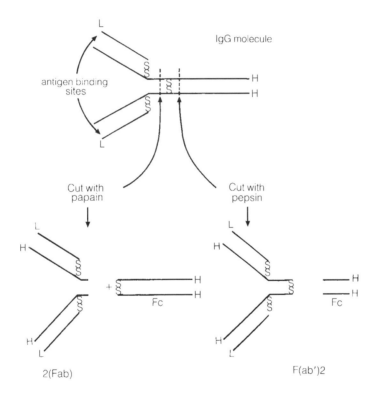

H = heavy chain
L = light chain
S
S = disulphide bonds

Fab = fraction antigen binding – used as imaging reagents
Fc = fraction complement fixing

Figure 17.3 Structure of the IgG molecule.

bind antigen by the two enzymes pepsin and papain. When radiolabelled, these fragments – because of their small size and loss of the biological Fc region – have markedly different pharmacokinetic and imaging properties compared with the whole antibody molecule. The specificity and accuracy of RIS depends on the production of a pure antibody against the selected antigen in a form acceptable for human use. This has been made possible through the development of monoclonal antibody technology.

THE MONOCLONAL ANTIBODY

A monoclonal antibody is the secreted product of a single B-lymphocyte clone. Since each B-lymphocyte and its descendants are genetically destined to make a single antigen-combining site (idiotype), all the antibody molecules produced by a B-cell clone are homogeneous in terms of their structure and antigen-binding specificity. In pathological terms, malignant transformation of a single B-lymphocyte may give rise to a plasma cell tumour known as a myeloma or plasmacytoma, that produces a homogeneous antibody product or myeloma protein. Tumours of this type produce monoclonal gammopathies that can be diagnosed serologically by detecting them as sharp narrow bands on serum electrophoretic scans. In the past, these monoclonal antibodies have been invaluable in elucidating the structure of antibodies (Figure 17.3) but of little use practically. Kohler and Milstein [2] devised a way of making monoclonal antibodies in the laboratory by the technique of somatic cell hybridization. This involved the fusion of B-lymphocytes with a myeloma cell line (adapted for growth *in vitro*) to make hybrid cells known as hybridomas. Essentially, these hybridomas retain the two important functions of their parental cells, namely the ability to produce specific antibodies and to grow indefinitely in tissue culture. To make a hybridoma secrete a single antibody, a non-antibody-secreting myeloma mutant is used.

In a normal antibody response to a foreign antigen, a large number of B-lymphocytes are activated to secrete specific antibodies that bind to antigenic determinants expressed on the surface of the antigen. Added together, these antibodies constitute a polyclonal antibody response to a given antigen, and they will have a range of antibody affinities. The term 'antibody affinity' refers to the summation of the attractive and repulsive forces existing between a single antibody-combining site and its antigenic determinant.

Each time a polyclonal antiserum is made to a given antigen it will contain a different mix of antibody affinities which collectively give a mean value (called avidity) for their binding to the antigen. This means polyclonal antisera are difficult to standardize from one batch to another. Also these antisera will contain only a small proportion (1%) of their total IgG antibody as the antigen-specific antibody, and so further purification steps are required before they can be radiolabelled for RIS. Most of these problems can be avoided by using monoclonal antibodies. A monoclonal antibody differs from a polyclonal. Unlike polyclonal antibodies, monoclonal antibodies bind to antigen with one specificity and one affinity and can be produced in large amounts in the laboratory under standard conditions. All these factors make them ideal standard reagents for a wide range of biological and clinical applications.

BIOLOGICAL FACTORS AFFECTING UPTAKE

At present, only antibodies against tumour-associated antigens have been used for RIS. Apart from specificity, the antibody must have access to the antigen, so that local factors are very important. The arrival of the antibody in the vicinity of the antigenic binding sites on the cells depends on physical factors: the flow to the tumour, the capillary permeability, and the effects of the cellular environment on the diffusion and convection of the antibody. The higher the avidity of the antibody for the antigen, the greater the probability of an interaction and binding on the cell membrane. The tumour blood supply is a major determinant of the kinetics of antibody uptake: the higher the flow, the more rapid the uptake, the earlier the imaging and the more short-lived the radionuclide label may be. Tumour blood supply is not under autonomic control, so attempts are being made to enhance tumour uptake by pharmacological vascular intervention. Tumour capillaries are abnormally leaky, allowing proteins to pass from the circulation to the tumour. This enabled early workers to use radiolabelled albumin or fibrinogen to image tumour, and accounts for the non-specific antibody uptake by tumours. Extracellular fluid-to-cell ratio of tumours is greater than normal tissues, and the charge and composition of this fluid may affect the rate of uptake of antibody onto the tumour cell antigens. Intra-tumour pressure may be greater than its environment and reduce antibody penetration. Locally secreted antigens, such as the CEA from colorectal cancer, may enhance the uptake in the environment of the tumour. Tumour growth leads to deprivation of central blood supply, with necrotic and cystic areas without specific antigen. In general, the larger the tumour, the smaller the fraction of cancer cells to tumour mass, and the greater the degree of non-specific uptake. Thus, the specific uptake of labelled antibody is designed best for demonstrating small tumours. Note also that each cell may have 5000 or more available epitopes to bind the monoclonal antibody. It is this biological magnification factor that helps RIS to compete with physical radiological techniques in tumour detection. Other factors are also important in determining the uptake of antibody by cancer cell antigens. If the amount of antibody administered per study is increased, the amount taken up by both the tumour and its environment is greater, so the tumour-to-mucosa ratio does not change, but this may not be true for doses over 20 mg. The degree of tumour differentiation is important – poorly differentiated tumours taking up much less antibody per gram than the well-differentiated tumours; a four-fold difference in a study of colorectal cancer has been reported [3]. *In vivo* staging of cancer is not possible if normal lymph nodes draining the site of cancer take up a secreted antigen more avidly than the involved nodes, as occurs with CEA. Co-existing disease may compete for the antibody and benign tumours may also take up the antibody. Another considerable influence on detection of small tumours is the degree and distribution of uptake in the blood and tissue background. Kinetic factors play an important part in the differentiation of specific and non-specific antibody uptake and in the choice of radiolabel. Whereas after an initial distribution period, non-specific uptake decreases with time due to a falling blood and tissue fluid concentration and due to local metabolism by reticuloendothelial cells (Figure 17.4), specific uptake of antibody continues to increase with time over the first 24 hours (Figure 17.5), although at a progressively slower rate as its blood concentration in the supplying blood falls.

One of the problems of RIS is the development of human anti-mouse antibodies, HAMA. This occurs in response to most injections of whole mouse monoclonal IgG gamma-globulin, particularly when intradermal skin testing is combined with intravenous injection. This is the main reason why skin testing has been abandoned. There is usually no HAMA response to the first injection of F(ab')$_2$ fragments, but response to a second injection may occur in up to 50%. A strong HAMA response may significantly alter the biodistribution: the presence after the second injection of whole antibody may show a more rapid blood clearance to liver and other reticuloendothelial systems and slightly less tumour uptake.

Occasionally, a systemic reaction occurs (frequency about one per 1000 studies, provided that less than 2 mg antibody is used and patients with known allergy to foreign protein are excluded) and the liver uptake may be rapid. This is illustrated in Figure 17.6: on the left is the normal renal uptake of ^{99m}Tc-labelled F(ab')$_2$ 225.28S anti-melanoma monoclonal antibody with low liver uptake at 20 minutes: on the right, the 20-minute image in a patient with a negative skin test who had an episode of nausea and faintness shortly after injection of the same antibody shows high and rapid liver uptake.

QUALITY CONTROL

Since monoclonal antibodies are a biological product derived from cell culture, stringent quality-control procedures are necessary to prevent undesirable products, particularly genetically active material and virus, from being present in the final product. A reasonable set of guidelines has been set out by a working party on the clinical use of antibodies [4], but the regulations in Europe and USA are much more demanding, including tests for numbers of unlikely mouse viruses at all stages of the production which, apart from the expense, are unnecessary – given proper procedures. The essential requirements are knowledge of:

- the name, source and characteristics of the parent myeloma line;
- the source of the immune parental spleen cell;
- the source of its immunogen and the immunization procedure;

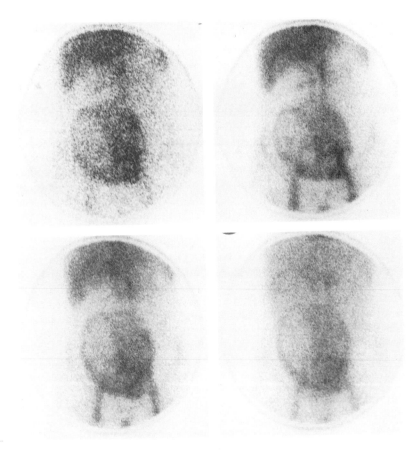

Figure 17.4 Radioimmunoscintigraphy with ^{123}I-labelled HMFG2 in patient with large fibroids in the uterus, anterior abdominal views at top left, 1minute; top right, 10 minutes; bottom left, 4 hours; and bottom right, 22 hours. Note the high early activity fading with time and typical of non-specific uptake (compare with Figure 17.5).

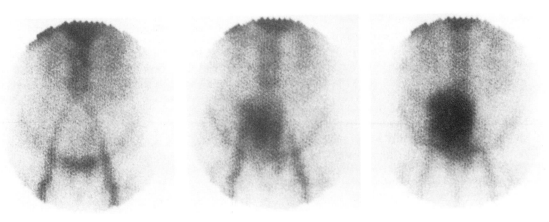

Figure 17.5 Radioimmunoscintigraphy with ^{123}I-labelled HMFG2 in a patient with a large ovarian adenocarcinoma, anterior abdominal views: left, 10 minutes; centre, 4 hours; right, 22 hours. Note the increasing uptake with time typical of specific uptake (compare with Figure 17.4).

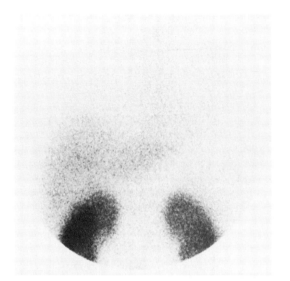

Figure 17.6 Radioimmunoscintigraphy with ^{99m}Tc-labelled F(ab')$_2$ fragment of 225.28S monoclonal antibody against high-molecular weight melanoma antigen. Both images are at 20 minutes. Left: normal distribution with high renal uptake due to filtration, reabsorption, metabolism and deposition of ^{99m}Tc in the proximal tubules. Right: abnormal distribution due to allergic reaction (skin test negative, no previous exposure to antibody). There is very high liver uptake and low renal excretion due to immune complex formation which is too large to be filtered.

- a description of the fusion and cloning processes and the method of cell culture;
- the class and subclass of the monoclonal antibody secreted and the precautions taken to avoid contamination of the cell seed suspension and subcultures; the use and nature of antibiotics in the culture and any preservatives in the purification of the antibody;
- the capacity of the purification procedure to remove DNA and RNA and viruses, the pharmaceutical quality of the final antibody product; and
- its characterization against normal and pathological tissues in terms of its specificity and avidity by immunocytochemistry.

The rationale for its use in RIS should include its demonstrated specificity for the chosen tumour and absence of reactivity with clinical relevant other tissues or tumours. It must be remembered that tissue sections have lost the biological barriers present in living tissues and may give a misleading apparent distribution of a monoclonal antibody in normal tissues. Human tumour xenograft uptake in an experimental animal such as the nude mouse is not required and may give

misleadingly optimistic results since the human tumour antigens have no competition in the mouse, the ratio of tumour mass to mouse is inappropriately large and the tumour stroma is made up by mouse connective tissue. The findings may also be misleadingly pessimistic if antigenic modulation or cytochemical modification has occurred.

HUMAN MONOCLONAL ANTIBODIES

The limitations of monoclonal antibody production have been overcome by genetic engineering. This requires the following:

1. The separation of the immunoglobulin gene sequences and their amplification by the polymerase chain reaction (PCR).
2. The use of an appropriate carrier to grow up ('clone') the product, so that the amplified genes may be expressed.
3. The selection of the 'antibody' for a particular antigen and for high affinity.

In this way the frame or constant part (Fc portion) of the murine monoclonal antibody has been replaced by the equivalent Fc portion of a human monoclonal to give a 'chimaeric antibody'. The next approach was to replace all but the hypervariable region of the murine antibody by the human equivalent. This is called a 'humanized', human reshaped or CDR (complementarity determinant region) grafted antibody. Usually the frame amino acids around the CDR may need to be altered also to improve stability and affinity.

The next advance was to develop phage antibodies. Human B cells, of which there are billions, contain the genes for the heavy and light chains that make up an antibody. Foreign antigen exposure leads to its binding to the B cells causing their differentiation into memory cells and into plasma cells which produce V (variable region) genes which code for the particular antibody, which is released. The V (variable region) genes retained in the memory cells are subject to mutation, one result of which is to increase the binding affinity of the antibodies produced in response to a subsequent encounter with the antigen. It is possible to capture and insert these human V genes into bacteria and infect them with filamentous bacteriophages with the result that antibody components such as the variable region and its frame may be expressed on the 'nose' of the bacteriophage. From immunized or even normal human B cells, all combinations of heavy and light chain V genes can be constructed each expressed on bacteriophages to form a so-called combinatorial library of such potential antibodies. To increase the number of heavy and light (V_H V_H) genes the polymerase chain reaction is used which is a method of amplifying DNA sequences (as in genetic fingerprinting). These genes can be combined to form gene products that are single chain fragments of one heavy and one light chain, called ScFv. These can be grown up and expressed in the bacteriophage system [5–7]. Initially, these phage produced ScFv were of moderate affinity. The selection of the appropriate phage to grow up is done by an 'affinity' column in which the chosen antigen is fixed. Only phages with the appropriate antibody will bind when the mixture of phages is run through the column. The chosen phages are dissociated, grown up in bacteria and rerun through the column containing only a few of the chosen antigens. Only the phage with the highest affinity will then bind. This cloning and selection process gives ScFv of very high affinity which are produced into the culture medium by the phage-

infected bacteria and harvested. In principle, antibodies can be made to any antigen, hapten or ligand without the bother of immunization. Success with an anti-CEA equivalent antibody MFE-23 is reported [7]. This approach circumvents the problems of obtaining human antibodies by immunizing humans which is clearly unethical for a range of toxic substances or malignant cells. The immortalization of human peripheral B lymphocytes, e.g. from a patient who already has a cancer, is a problem which has been overcome in some situations [8,9]. Clearly, the method of genetic engineering with combinatorial libraries is the way forward.

THE RADIOLABEL

What are the properties of an ideal radiolabel for radioimmunoscintigraphy and how do the available radionuclides match up? The key requirement for static imaging of a tumour through the distribution of a radiotracer is a high count-rate delivered from the tissue-of-interest to the imaging system. The major determinant of the suitability of radionuclide for antibody labelling is its half-life. The shorter the $t_{1/2}$, the greater the activity that may be administered and the higher the count-rate obtained, given an upper limit of the absorbed dose of radiation that is permitted for diagnostic nuclear medicine. Ideally, the $t_{1/2}$ should be matched with kinetic information on the rate of antibody uptake by the target. If the uptake of antibody follows the Michaelis–Menten (enzyme–substrate) kinetics, as expected then the uptake rate is initially greatest, with a decrease in the fractional uptake of the amount administered as the blood concentration decreases with time. The temporal requirement concerns the rate of clearance of the injected antibody from the blood and tissues, providing the environment for the target, in relation to its residence time on the target tissue. A typical biological clearance $t_{1/2}$ of clearance of whole-antibody from blood is 43 hours, with a range of 24–64 hours, and an antibody fragment is cleared at approximately twice this rate, a biological half-life of 21.5 hours, with a range of 15–30 hours. For a typical whole-antibody and a typical compact reasonable vascular tumour about 75% of the total uptake of labelled antibody occurs in the first 12 hours, favouring the use of a radionuclide with a physical $t_{1/2}$ of about 12 hours (e.g. ^{123}I, $t_{1/2}$ 13.2 hours). For some antibodies uptake will be more rapid, as Buraggi *et al.* [10] have shown for anti-melanoma antibody, giving an optimal time between 6 and 12 hours, favouring a radiolabel such as ^{99m}Tc with a 6-hour physical $t_{1/2}$. Other malignancies, such as colorectal cancer, and particularly relatively avascular tumours like scirrhous carcinoma of the breast, may show slower uptake requiring a longer-lived radionuclide such as ^{111}In (physical $t_{1/2}$ 67.4 hours).

An appreciation of the need for higher sensitivity in order to detect small tumours requires an understanding of the sources of signal degradation. 'Noise' is a term used generally for anything that degrades the signal and has many sources, but the most important is the signal itself. Since one of the aims of radioimmunoscintigraphy is to visualize recurrences or spread of cancer not detectable by conventional radiology, CT, MRI or US through the properties of a specifically targeted antibody, the optimization of a significant signal from a small target is essential. Most of the noise that prevents this objective is due to the weakness of the signal itself. This primary type of signal degradation severely reduces tumour detectability. Low count-rates give 'noisy' images where the tumour is less separable from the background and the high variability of the background itself may produce 'noise blobs' that may be falsely interpreted as tumour signals.

This may be illustrated by consideration of RIS in a child with neuroblastoma using 40 MBq ^{131}I-labelled UJ13A (an antibody reacting with neuroblastoma) on one occasion (Figure 17.7(a)) and 40 MBq ^{123}I-labelled UJ13A 3 weeks later (Figure 17.7(b)). For the same activity, and the same amount of antibody with ^{131}I as the radiolabel, the tumour is lost in the noisy background of liver, heart and spleen at 21 hours, and can just be visualized at 70 hours. In contrast, with ^{123}I as the radiolabel, the spleen and liver are clearly outlined at 10 minutes, and by 21 hours the space seen superior to the spleen had been replaced by a focal area of high uptake in the tumour. With ^{131}I, the signal-to-noise ratio at 70 hours was 25:1, but the signal was poor, whereas with ^{123}I, at 21 hours the signal-to-noise ratio was 1.5:1, yet the tumour is evident. The tumour is evident at 4 hours on a colour-coded image (Plate 26) when the tumour-to-background ratio was only 1.23:1. This example demonstrates the greater importance of the signal itself, over the calculated signal-to-background ratio. For ^{123}I, the count content per pixel was 25 times that from ^{131}I, for the same administered activity. A good signal enables detection, however high the non-specific background activity [11]. Thus, in principle a pinhead-sized radiolabelled tumour will be visualized, if it gives a good enough signal.

While the avidity, affinity and selectivity of the antibody are crucial to that signal, the choice of a radiolabel itself is very important. Thus, the number of radiolabels allowable per antibody while retaining its immunoreactivity, the efficiency and abundance with which the γ-rays are emitted from the radiolabel, their γ-ray energy, the total number of radioactive molecules that may be injected into the patient and the availability of the radiolabel, all contribute to the choice of ideal radionuclide.

Even ignoring its excessive γ-ray energy, ^{131}I, with its 8-day $t_{1/2}$ and beta-emission that gives 80% of the radiation due to this radionuclide *in vivo*, should no longer be used for modern RIS but limited to RIT.

The immunoreactivity of the antibody must be preserved during the radiolabelling. This usually requires a radiolabel-to-antibody molar ratio of 1:1 or 2:1, since labelling of the antigen-combining site of the antibody must be avoided. Site-specific labelling of the Fc region of the antibody molecule away from the antigen-combining site is being developed to overcome this problem. Methods for labelling must therefore be 'gentle' so as not to denature the molecule by altering its three-dimensional conformation. Genetically engineered mouse antibodies can be 'humanized' to make them less immunogenic, have a specific labelling site introduced, and improvements made to their antigen specificity as well as being produced by a continuous fermentation-like process. All these technological improvements may eventually overcome many of the present problems relating to quality control.

RADIOLABELLING

Radiolabelling with ^{131}I or ^{123}I is usually undertaken using the chloramine T or Iodogen techniques labelling the protein through the tyrosine radical. Radiolabelling with ^{111}In commonly uses the method described by Hnatowich *et al.* [12] in which the bicyclic anhydride of diethylenetri-aminepenta-acetic acid (DTPA) is first coupled to

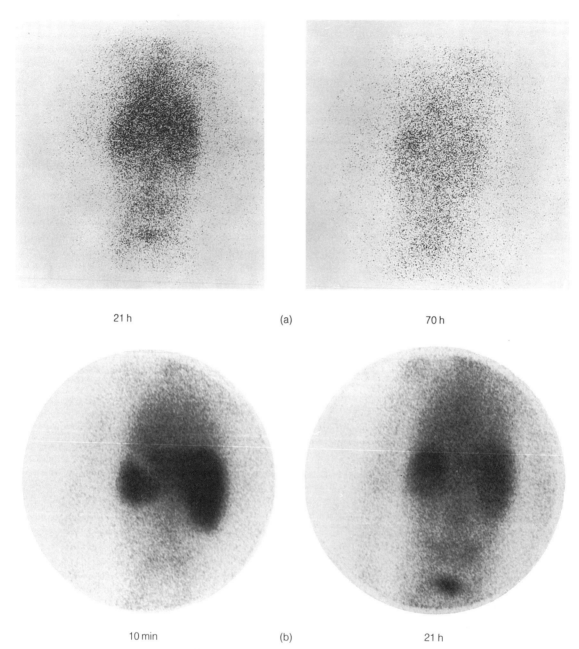

21 h   (a)   70 h

10 min   (b)   21 h

Figure 17.7 Radioimmunoscintigraphy of neuroblastoma using radioiodinated UJ13A in a 4-year-old child. (a) Posterior abdominal images 21 and 70 hours after injection of 40 MBq ^{131}I-labelled UJ13A. General uptake is seen in the liver, spleen and blood pool at 21 hours. Focal low-contrast uptake is seen at 70 hours in the tumour. (b) Posterior abdominal images at 10 minutes and 21 hours after injection of 40 MBq ^{123}I-labelled UJ13A in the same child. At 10 minutes the spleen and liver are identified with an area of reduced uptake superior to the spleen. At 21 hours, a focal area of increased uptake is evident in the tumour superior to the spleen (see also Plate 26).

the antibody with subsequent chelation of ^{111}In with this conjugate.

To achieve good ^{111}In labelling, a balance has to be struck between the amount of DTPA attached to the antibody and the effects of this DTPA coupling on the physicochemical and biological properties of the antibody.

A general finding with all ^{111}In-labelled antibodies given intravenously to patients is the high ^{111}In uptake in the liver. This occurs for a number of reasons: transchelation of ^{111}In onto plasma transferrin (6–10% per day), its binding to liver and sinusoid cells, the localization of antibodies in liver by virtue of its large blood supply, and antibody uptake by Kupffer cells of the reticuloendothelial system. New types of metal chelates and different methods of linking them to antibodies will help reduce this problem in the future.

TECHNETIUM-99m ANTIBODY LABELLING

A few years ago, the *in vivo* stability of ^{99m}Tc-labelled monoclonal antibodies was a major problem, though this has now been successfully overcome by the development of new techniques. The S-S bonds holding the heavy chains are opened using 2-mercaptoethanol (2-ME). The antibody is concentrated by ultrafiltration to approximately 10 mg/ml. To a stirred solution of antibody, sufficient 2-ME is added to provide a 2-ME-to-antibody molar ratio of 1000:1. The mixture is incubated at room temperature for 30 minutes with continuous rotation. The reduced antibody is purified by gel filtration on Sephadex-G50 using phosphate-buffered saline as the mobile phase. The antibody fractions are collated and divided into 0.5-mg aliquots. These are frozen immediately at –20°C and stored ready for use. When imaging is required, the antibody aliquot is thawed and reconstituted [using an Amersham methylene disphosphonate (MDP) kit] with 5 ml 0.9% sterile saline. A 35 µl aliquot of MDP solution is added to the antibody aliquot and mixed. The required amount of ^{99m}Tc-pertechnetate (approximately 700 MBq) is added to the antibody/MDP mixture, which is gently shaken for 10 minutes. The labelling efficiency is assessed by thin-layer chromatography developed in 0.9% saline, and should be over 95%; if below this, the labelled antibody can be further purified by gel filtration on Sephadex-G50. The ^{99m}Tc-labelled antibody is stable *in vivo* with an *in vitro* stability of a few

hours. There is no thyroid uptake of ^{99m}Tc even after 24 hours in patients who have received no thyroid-blocking medication. This technique has been used successfully for five different antibodies in clinical use in this department to date.

CLINICAL PROTOCOLS AND DATA ANALYSIS

A typical protocol is as follows:

1. Before injection of a labelled antibody, the patient must be asked about allergies. A history of severe allergic reactions or sensitivity to foreign protein is a contraindication to RIS. Skin testing is ineffective and sensitizes the patient.
2. The nature of the test is explained to the patient and informed consent is obtained.
3. Potassium iodide, 60 mg twice daily, is given the day before, during and for 3 days after the test for ^{123}I and for 2 weeks in the case of ^{131}I. No such preparation is required when ^{111}In or ^{99m}Tc is the label.
4. The patient is then positioned supine on the scanning couch under the gamma-camera, which is fitted with an appropriate collimator and set up for the particular radionuclide.
5. The labelled antibody (in an appropriate dose) is injected intravenously and, for example, in the context of ovarian or colorectal cancer, anterior and posterior images of the lower and upper abdomen are obtained at 10 minutes, 6 hours and 22 hours for ^{123}I and ^{99m}Tc, and at 10 minutes, 22 hours and 48 or 72 hours for ^{111}In. A minimum of 800 K-counts per view is recommended.

TRANSPARENT FILM DISPLAY

The series of transparent films or workstation displays are evaluated for the distribution of uptake in normal structures: vascular activity, bone marrow, liver, spleen, kidneys, gastrointestinal and urinary activity; for sites of abnormal uptake and how the distribution of uptake varies with time. Thus, the activity in vascular structures, tissue background and at sites of non-specific uptake after an initial increase in distribution seen on the 10-minute images tends to decrease with time (see Figure 17.4), whereas areas of specific uptake may show little or no uptake on the 10-

minute image, but show increasing uptake with time during the first 24 hours (see Figure 17.5). Gastrointestinal, liver and marrow activity for ^{111}In, and urinary activity for ^{123}I and ^{99m}Tc, may increase with time. Focal tumour uptake may be best seen at 6 hours for ^{99m}Tc-labelled F(ab')$_2$ RIS in ocular and cutaneous melanoma [13,14], and at 24 hours for ovarian [15] and colorectal cancer [16], and for ovarian cancer with ^{123}I-labelled HMFG2 [17,18]. In colorectal cancer, 24- or 48-hour images may give the best contrast using ^{111}In-labelled anti-CEA (Plates 27 and 28). The key to identifying the tumour site are the changes occurring in the series of transparent films or workstation displays between the 10-minute and later images.

IMAGE ENHANCEMENT

The following additional techniques are used to improve the contrast between the target and its background:

- Background subtraction using a second radiopharmaceutical [19]
- SPECT [20]
- The use of F(ab')$_2$ fragments [21]
- The use of a second antibody to speed the clearance of the radiopharmaceutical from the blood [22]
- Subtracting an early image from a later image [23]
- The use of a 'chase' in a two-or-three stage system [24,25]
- Kinetic analysis with probability mapping or statistical change detection [18,26]

The Fab' is a monovalent fragment, and the F(ab')$_2$ a bivalent fragment obtained by enzyme digestion of the whole antibody to remove the Fc portion, leaving the active antigen-binding site intact (see Figure 17.3). The advantages of using an F(ab')$_2$ fragment include: the absence of the Fc protein that binds specifically to the reticuloendothelial cells, tending to increase the liver, marrow, lymph node and splenic uptake; a more rapid clearance (about two-fold) from blood; and a more rapid diffusion into the tumour tissue. The disadvantages include: usually lower avidity than the whole antibody; loss by glomerular filtration into the kidney followed by absorption and metabolism in the proximal tubules, depositing the metal ^{111}In and ^{99m}Tc there (but not ^{123}I, which is

released by deiodinases); greater diffusibility into a wider volume of distribution than the whole antibody, contributing to tissue background; and an additional preparative step. However, matched to a short-lived radionuclide such as ^{99m}Tc or ^{123}I, the advantages probably outweigh the disadvantages. For ^{111}In, a reduced liver uptake is balanced by greater renal uptake and the benefits are less evident.

The main requirement for SPECT is a high count-rate from the target, so that the rotation can be completed in a time that is reasonable to expect a patient to remain still. This favours the use of the shorter-lived radionuclides for antibody labelling. It is the registration of sites of suspected abnormality in relation to anatomical landmarks that is the main problem for interpretation. Major vessel activity and incidental bone marrow uptake help, but the presence of activity in the bowel makes for difficulties. Colocation or computer-assisted superimposition of the SPECT and CT images is helpful. The advantage of SPECT is the increased contrast of the target in the plane of the section and particularly the ability to separate objects from in front of and behind the target, e.g. the bladder from a pelvic tumour, which may overlap on a conventional planar image. Another potential advantage is the ability to quantify the amount of activity in a region of the transverse section, for example, for dosimetry purposes. However, this is much more difficult than expected: errors occur due to less than perfect rotation and linearity of response of the camera, Poisson statistical noise, algorithm noise, artefacts due to overlapping tissue activities, the partial volume effect, patient and organ movement, and difficulties in correcting for scatter and for tissue attenuation. Accuracy is thereby considerably reduced and the anatomical relationships of tissues and target may be difficult to visualize and/or interpret. Once created, SPECT sections cannot be repositioned. The SPECT technique is a potentially useful adjunct to, but not a substitute for, planar imaging in RIS. Removal of unwanted objects, such as the bladder activity for prostate imaging, from the SPECT data can be undertaken before to reconstruction by 'image surgery' [27].

In any tumour, part of the uptake is due to nonspecific features such as the blood flow, the tumour blood volume and vascular transit time, the leakiness of the tumour capillaries, the extracellular fluid content, and the lack of lymphatic drainage. Non-specific uptake improves the sensitivity but reduces the specificity of any imaging agent. Thus, if the specificity of a monoclonal antibody against a tumour-associated antigen is to determine the uptake, the tumour or metastasis should be small so that non-specific uptake plays a minimal role.

It is clearly important to distinguish specific tumour uptake from non-specific uptake, and to reduce the effects to tissue and blood background. The concept of subtracting the early post-injection antibody images (showing distribution of activity in the blood and tissue), before significant tumour uptake has occurred, from the delayed images was introduced [23]. This approach overcomes the problem of subtracting the distribution of two radionuclides with differing energies, and allows considerable enhancement of tumour uptake. However, it requires the repositioning and normalization of the two images. The repositioning must be reasonably accurate between the first and second visits of the patient, and then the computer images must be completely superimposed. For each image of the patient, marker images are also obtained. For the latter the patient's bony landmarks (such as xiphisternum, costal margins, anterior superior iliac spines and symphysis pubis) are marked with indelible ink and cobalt-57 radioactive markers are positioned over these. Transparent films of the marker positions on the persistence scope are made at the early visit. At each subsequent visit, the markers are replaced on the patient and the patient is repositioned until the image of the markers on the persistence scope fits that on the previously recorded films placed over the scope. The computer is also programmed so that the recorded images can be moved one pixel at a time, vertically, horizontally or by rotation so that an exact superimposition of the later image over the earlier image may be made in order that detailed analysis of the images may be performed, for example, by proportional subtraction of the early image from the later image [3].

A more sophisticated approach makes use of the kinetic information and also the count-rate distribution. As noted above, the specific tumour uptake increases with time whereas the non-specific blood and tissue activity decreases with time. By analysing pairs of images separated in time, for example, the 10-minute image with the 22-hour image, for temporal changes in the count-rate

distribution between the pairs of images, sites of specific uptake will be identified as positive derivations from a line of correspondence calculated from the count-rate frequency distribution of the two images for the areas where there has been no change between the two images. This technique of kinetic analysis with probability mapping satisfies the basic requirements of detectability of low contrast differences and insensitivity to statistical noise over the range encountered in a typical RIS study. Biopsy-proven 0.5-cm diameter deposits have been correctly identified using this approach [3]. Alternative change-detection algorithms based on statistical comparisons of multiple small regions in each image are being implemented, for example in the determination of axillary node involvement in primary breast cancer [26].

CLINICAL STUDIES

When introducing any new imaging technique the crucial requirement is to define the principal circumstances under which it should be able to contribute to clinical management. Many diagnostic tests are undertaken in relation to a particular clinical problem, and this strict criterion of a successful test is now being met by RIS. A number of generalizations about the technique in the management of malignant disease may be made:

- RIS has no role as a screening test for the presence of cancer in healthy people as it involves the injection of a foreign protein, a radioactive source, and an antibody that is not cancer-specific;
- RIS is gaining a role in the evaluation of patients picked up on a preliminary investigation; e.g. the demonstration of an ultrasound abnormality in the pelvis may be supplemented using RIS to determine whether it contains ovarian cancer; and the demonstration of an eye tumour ophthalmoscopically leads to ultrasound, which if not specific as to the cause, should be followed by RIS, which is 92% specific for ocular melanoma [13].
- RIS is a natural counterpart to the increasing search for tumour markers in serum. However, the ideal antigen for detection in serum has to be released easily from the tumour as is CEA or AFP, and most markers do not show a rise in serum until the tumour has reached a sufficient size to release enough antigen, and/or some

tumour necrosis has occurred. In contrast, for RIS an antigen well fixed to the tumour gives more specific results.

- RIS has a prime role in the re-evaluation of the patient after the management of the primary cancer by surgery, radiotherapy or chemotherapy, or combinations of these. It is of no clinical benefit to image by RIS, the large metastases already evident on ultrasound or CT. It is of particular benefit to show that a mass in the pelvis does not represent post-surgical fibrosis, but is a tumour recurrence; that an enlarged lymph node does not contain metastases; and that a clinically or radiologically normal abdomen does in fact contain tumour, usually in the form of plaques, a few cells thick, which have no 'mass' for radiological detection. This role in demonstrating previously unsuspected metastases has been confirmed in cutaneous melanoma [14], in peritoneal plaques and pelvic recurrence of ovarian cancer [15,18] where ultrasound and CT are unreliable, in colorectal cancer recurrences [16,28,29], in involved nodes that are clinically impalpable, in breast cancer [26], and in recurrences of prostate cancer [30,31].
- RIS is an essential precursor to RIT to demonstrate the *in vivo* uptake of the chosen antibody. Immunohistochemistry showing evidence of specific antibody binding by the patient's tumour cells is important but not sufficient evidence to justify for RIT.

COLORECTAL CANCER

This cancer is used as an example for RIS. The detection of colorectal cancer depends on the history, clinical and digital rectal examination, barium enema and/or endoscopy. Nuclear medicine techniques have no routine role in this phase of the patient's management. Although RIS has a place in staging primary patient colorectal cancer, its main applications are in the detection of para-aortic nodes and liver involvement, in the demonstration of recurrent cancer before serum markers are elevated, in the demonstration of the site of recurrent cancer when serum markers are elevated [28], in the evaluation of the success of chemotherapy and/or radiotherapy, in the demonstration of the distribution of the recurrence for radiotherapy planning and surgery, and in the demonstration of antibody uptake before consideration of RIT.

Radiolabelled monoclonal antibodies may be injected before surgery to enable the use of the per-operative probe. This may aid in the detection of unsuspected disease, in the demonstration that a tumour-bed is free of tumour after operation, in the demonstration that a piece of bowel for anastomosis is free from tumour, and in showing that tissue removed at operation does or does not contain malignancy before its being sent for frozen section [32].

Tumour-associated antigens present in colorectal cancer are of several types. First, the epithelial surface antigens are separated from the blood by being in the inner surfaces of cells and by biological barriers, so do not react with a monoclonal antibody injected intravenously. However, with the architectural disruption that characterizes the malignant process, such antigens become exposed to blood and thus such colorectal tumours may be detected using radiolabelled monoclonal antibodies that react with these antigens. One such example is PR1A3 produced by the Imperial Cancer Research Fund [15,33]. A second well-used group are the oncofetal antigens such as the carcinoembryonic antigen, CEA [3,19,34–37]. Antibodies such as B-72.3 against the tumour-associated antigen TAG 72 are available [38–40]. Antigens may either be fixed to the tumour or released from the tumour. CEA is released from the tumour and therefore is available as a serum marker for cancer. However, a tumour must reach a certain size to release sufficient CEA to overcome uptake by the liver and reticuloendothelial system and the normal biological variations in the blood to make it useful as a serum marker. Both CEA and B-72.3 are released by the tumour into lymphatics and therefore detection of the antigen in lymph nodes does not mean that tumour cells are present [8,41]. Conversely the PR1A3 antigen is fixed to the tumour. It is not found in lymph nodes draining a primary cancer and therefore detection of uptake in lymph nodes represents malignant involvement when PR1A3 is used [16,42]. When the cancer cell dies, the PR1A3 antigen is destroyed with it, whereas the CEA antigen may be still detectable in the environment of dead cancer cells.

It has now been shown that the CEA molecule is very complex. Its three-dimensional structure consists of a large extra-membrane portion with a tail buried in the surface membrane of the cell. The part known as CEA breaks off from this tail and thus is able to diffuse into the lymphatics and the blood vessels. This breaking off process causes a conformational change to conceal the antigen against which the monoclonal antibody PR1A3 is produced. Thus, PR1A3 only binds to the membrane fixed antigen. The sites of the two negative charges that bind to the antigen have been identified in the structure of the monoclonal antibody PR1A3. This information should help in the development of peptides derived from antibodies with even higher binding affinity to the cancer antigen [43].

PATIENT PROTOCOL

The test is explained in detail to the patient. Since these studies are usually performed under ethical committee control, signed informed consent must be obtained from the patient. It is essential to ask the patient whether there is history of an allergy to foreign proteins, and such patients should not be studied. Skin testing which was used previously is inappropriate and leads to immunization of the patient so that human anti-mouse antibodies (HAMA), are produced, which may interfere with the imaging procedure if a series of injections are given for imaging purposes or therapy. The injection consists of 600 MBq of ^{99m}Tc monoclonal antibody or 120 MBq of ^{111}In monoclonal antibody of the chosen type. The amount of protein injected is normally <1 mg, and this reduces the chance of side effects or sensitization. Before the injection, the vital signs are observed and the patient is then set on the imaging couch with the camera over the pelvis.

^{111}In-radiolabelled antibody

For ^{111}In-labelled antibody, the camera is set up with a medium-energy (up to 300 keV) general-purpose, parallel-hole collimator with windows of 15% around the 171 keV and 20% around the 247 keV photo peaks of ^{111}In. The camera is set so that the data are transferred automatically to the mini-computer for subsequent image analysis and presentation. The vial containing the ^{111}In anti-CEA is transferred to a weighed syringe and needle and the amount assayed in an ionizing chamber to make sure that the correct activity is to be injected. After injection, the syringe and needle are re-weighed and the residual activity is reassessed so that the activity and the weight of the antibody injected are recorded. This enables the tumour uptake to be measured in the surgical specimen as a percentage of the injected

dose per gram. The injection is given intravenously into an antecubital vein slowly over 10 seconds. Vital signs are recorded before and after the injection.

A series of images are made over the anterior and posterior lower abdomen, pelvis, upper abdomen and chest, starting about 10 minutes after the injection. Other images are taken at 24 and 72 hours (see Plates 27 and 28) with SPECT at about 24 hours. The camera undergoes a 360° rotation with 64 projections and takes about 32 minutes. It is essential the patient remains still during this period. Each planar image should contain at least 800 K-counts. To aid re-positioning, a similar image to each of the planar images maybe undertaken with radioactive markers over prominent bony landmarks [3,44]. The planar and SPECT images are analysed without clinical and radiological information and decisions are made as to whether a site of abnormal antibody uptake is seen.

Pre-targeted imaging of colorectal cancer undertaken using an ^{111}In bivalent hapten and a bispecific antibody conjugate has given satisfactory results [45].

^{99m}Tc-radiolabelled monoclonal antibody

For ^{99m}Tc, the gamma-camera is set up with a low-energy, general-purpose or preferably a high-resolution, parallel-hole collimator. The photopeak is set at 140 keV with a 15% window and for data transfer on line to the mini-computer. The patient protocol is as above. A 600-MBq ^{99m}Tc-labelled dose of intact monoclonal antibody (either anti-CEA or PR1A3) is injected intravenously over 10 seconds. Images are taken of the upper and lower abdomen and pelvis, upper abdomen and chest anteriorly and posteriorly, at 10 minutes, 5–6 hours and 18–24 hours (Figure 17.8). Each planar image contains a minimum of 800 K-counts. Thyroid blockade is not required. The ^{99m}Tc Fab' fragment of anti-CEA has also been shown to be effective [45].

PRIMARY COLORECTAL CANCER

The identification of primary colorectal cancer is straightforward using ^{99m}Tc anti-CEA or ^{99m}Tc-PR1A3. The 10-minute image shows normal vascular, marrow, renal, urinary and liver uptake. The 5-hour and 22-hour images show the focal area of increased uptake at the site of the cancer. Because of the release of CEA it may be possible to

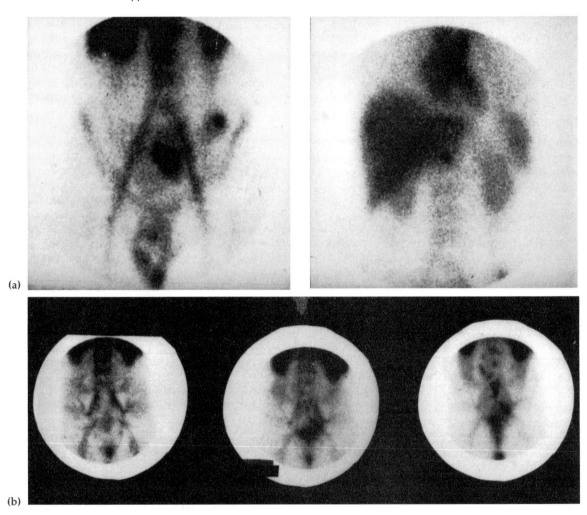

(a)

(b)

Figure 17.8   Colorectal cancer: radioimmunoscintigraphy with ^{99m}Tc-PR1A3. (a) Left: anterior view of the pelvis at 24 hours. Focally increased uptake in the centre of the pelvis due to primary sigmoid adenocarcinoma. In the left iliac fossa, a second unsuspected adenocarcinoma is seen. Right: liver metastasis in the same patient seen as a small focal area of increased uptake in the left lobe, not identified on ultrasound but confirmed at surgery. (b) Posterior view of the pelvis in a patient with recurrent rectal carcinoma. Left, 10 minutes; centre, 5 hours; right, 22 hours. Increasing irregular uptake is seen in the pelvis confirming CT findings, but further focal para-aortic uptake is seen which was unsuspected and made the patient inoperable.

image the normal lymph nodes (Plate 28), and areas affected by inflammatory bowel disease. Through the series of images these areas of bowel show fixed uptake, whereas some secretion into normal bowel contents will show movement between the 5-hour and the 24-hour images. It is not unusual to see some diffuse uptake in the ascending colon, particularly if the patient has undergone bowel preparation before colonoscopy or surgery, where the slightly inflamed bowel becomes somewhat leaky to protein such as the gamma-globulin injected. Besides identifying the primary colorectal cancer, on occasion a second site of focal uptake may be seen; this may represent a second cancer, for example if the distal primary cancer has caused a stricture of the large bowel so that a colonoscope cannot pass (Figure 17.8(a)). The injection of the ^{99m}Tc-labelled monoclonal antibody 24 hours before surgery is useful, and allows the imaging to be combined with the use of the pre-operative probe during surgery.

If rectal cancer is suspected, it is essential to obtain a series of squat views at the three time points, since this may be the best indicator of the fact that a low-lying rectal cancer is posterior to the bladder. The planar anterior and posterior views may not define it due to superimposition with the bladder or genitalia, which usually appear vascular. Some genitalia activity persists with time, and is thought to be due to binding of the Fc portion of the whole antibody to the gonadal tissue. SPECT of the pelvis is always undertaken; this gives a good definition of the position of the bladder in relation to any abnormality in the pelvis, for, with excision of a rectal cancer, the bladder lies more posteriorly than usual. The uterus may be seen as a vascular area on the early image but fades with time.

LIVER METASTASES

Liver metastases from colorectal cancer are mainly supplied by the hepatic artery, rather than the portal vein. Since the hepatic artery supply is less than the portal vein supply per unit volume of the liver, a liver metastasis will usually show as a defect in uptake on the 10-minute image against the normal liver uptake, background and vascularity.

Four patterns of liver metastases are seen on radioimmunoscintigraphy.

1. The first pattern is that of a defect in uptake seen on the 10-minute image, that persists on the 5-hour and 24-hour images. This is usually large and may represent a space-occupying lesion due to a cause other than a liver metastasis.
2. A more typical pattern is a defect on the 10-minute image that appears slightly smaller on the 5-hour image and even smaller on the 24-hour image, often with a halo of increased uptake around its periphery. This is typical of a moderate-sized liver metastasis.
3. A small metastasis in the liver may show as a defect on the 10-minute image but appear undetectable on the 5-hour and 24-hour images since its uptake is balanced by the uptake in the normal liver. Without the 10-minute image,

this sort of liver metastasis, which is not uncommon, would not be detectable.
4. The last pattern is a normal 10-minute image and a normal 5-hour image, with a focal area of increased uptake seen on the 24-hour image (Figure 17.8(a)). This is usually found in a very small metastasis (an accuracy of 92% can be achieved using ^{99m}Tc-PR1A3) [16].

Liver SPECT may help to confirm the presence of a metastasis when interpreted in conjunction with the planar images. A very small focal metastasis with increased uptake may be detected on SPECT when the planar scan is normal. It should be confirmed on all the orthogonal, coronal, transverse and sagittal sections before being called a metastasis. SPECT is not so helpful in large metastases where a defect may be difficult to distinguish from the normal variation of the liver lobes.

Focal areas of increased uptake in the peri-aortic region should be interpreted with caution when anti-CEA is used, but indicates positive involvement when an antibody against a fixed antigen such as PR1A3 is used (Figure 17.8(b)). Rarely, lung metastases are identified but these usually occur only when the liver has been widely invaded. They are however, not uncommon once liver metastases have been treated. Left supraclavicular node metastases may be seen.

RECURRENT COLORECTAL CANCER

This is the main application of RIS, since recurrences may be plaque-like, a few cells thick, over a wide area, and not detectable by CT, MRI or ultrasound. They may be detectable on RIS, before any change in serum markers or symptoms. Dukes' C primary colorectal cancer has up to 50% chance of recurrence at 1 year. Imaging of such patients at a year after primary surgery – at a time when they may have no symptoms and a normal CEA – has shown evidence of recurrence in approximately 30% of cases. The RIS imaging technique is by its nature more sensitive than serum markers, since a tumour has to be a certain size to shed sufficient antigen to raise the serum markers in the blood whereas with a good signal such as ^{99m}Tc, focal recurrences having the pattern of increasing uptake with time can be seen. Indeed, RIS may be the only modality capable of detecting such recurrences. As surgeons become confident with this technique, so surgery (with the help of the probe) or radiotherapy, may be undertaken on the basis of positive RIS alone. When serum markers are elevated, RIS can identify the site(s) of recurrence in the pelvis, abdomen or liver, even when other radiological modalities are negative. CT and MRI can demonstrate an abnormal mass in the pelvis or abdomen in a patient who has had surgery for primary colorectal cancer. However, these techniques are often unable to identify whether such a mass represents post-surgical, post-radiotherapy fibrosis, recurrent viable tumour, or indeed an inflammatory mass. The monoclonal antibody uptake will be absent if the mass is due to fibrosis; uptake will be early, and fade with time if the mass is due to an inflammatory process; and it will show no uptake on the early image with progressively increasing uptake with time, if the mass is due to a viable recurrent tumour. The greater extent of a recurrence in the abdomen may be seen by RIS due to the plaque-like spread of the tumour over the abdomen, whereas only the more mass-like part of the tumour recurrence may be appreciated on CT. Para-aortic lymph node involvement may be well visualized.

REFERENCES

1. Chan, S. and Sikora, K. (1987) The potential of oncogene products as tumour markers. *Cancer Surveys*, **6**, 185–207.
2. Kohler, G. and Milstein, C. (1975) Continuous cultures of fused cells secreting antibody of proven defined specificity. *Nature*, **256**, 495–7.
3. Granowska, M., Jass, J.R., Britton, K.E. and Northover, J.M.A. (1989) A prospective study of the use of ^{111}In-labelled monoclonal antibody against carcinoembryonic antigen in colorectal cancer and of some biological factors affecting its uptake. *Int. J. Colorect. Dis.*, **4**, 97–108.
4. Begent, R.H.J. (1986) Working party on clinical use of antibodies. Br. J. Cancer, **54**, 557–68.
5. McCafferty, J., Griffiths, A.D., Winter, G. and Chiswell, D.J. (1990) Phage antibodies: filamentous phage displaying antibody variable domains. *Nature*, **348**, 552–4.
6. Clackson, T., Hoogenboom, H.R., Griffiths, A.D. and Winter, G. (1991) Making antibody fragments using phage display libraries. *Nature*, **352**, 624–8.
7. Chester, K.A., Begent, R.H., Robson, L. *et al.* (1994) Phage libraries for generation of clinically useful antibodies. *Lancet*, **343**, 455–6.
8. Hanna, M.G., Haspel, M.V., McCabe, R. *et al.* (1991) Development and application of human monoclonal antibodies. *Antibody Immunoconj. Radiopharm.*, **4**, 67–75.
9. Moffat, F.L., Vergas-Cuba, R.D., Serafini, A.N. *et al.* (1995) Preoperative scintigraphy and operative probe scintimetry of colorectal carcinoma using Technetium-99m-88BV59. *J. Nucl. Med.*, **36**, 738–45.
10. Buraggi, G.L., Turrin, A., Cascinelli, N. *et al.* (1985) in *Immunoscintigraphy* (eds L. Donato and K.E. Britton), Gordon and Breach, London, pp. 215–53.
11. Britton, K.E. and Granowska, M. (1987) Radioimmunoscintigraphy in tumour identification. *Cancer Surveys*, **6**, 247–67.
12. Hnatowich, D.J., Childs, R.L., Lanteigne, D. and Najafi, A. (1983) The preparation of DTPA-coupled antibodies radiolabelled with metallic radionuclides: an improved method. *J. Immunol. Methods*, **65**, 147–57.
13. Bomanji, J., Hungerford, J.L., Granowska, M. and Britton, K.E. (1987) Radioimmunoscintigraphy of ocular melanoma with 99-Tc-m labelled cutaneous melanoma antibody fragments. *Br. J. Ophthalmol.*, **71**, 651–8.
14. Siccardi, A.G., Buraggi, G.L., Callegaro, L. *et al.* (1986) Multicentre study of immunoscintigraphy with radiolabelled monoclonal antibodies in patients with melanoma. *Cancer Res.*, **46**, 4817–22.
15. Granowska, M., Britton, K.E., Mather, S.J. *et al.* (1993) Radioimmunoscintigraphy with technetium-99m labelled monoclonal antibody, SM3, in gynaecological cancer. *Eur. J. Nucl. Med.*, **20**, 483–9.
16. Granowska, M., Britton, K.E., Mather, S.J. *et al.* (1993b) Radioimmunoscintigraphy with Technetium-99m labelled monoclonal antibody, IA3, in colorectal cancer. *Eur. J. Nucl. Med.*, **20**, 690–8.
17. Granowska, M., Shepherd, J., Britton, K.E. *et al.* (1984) Ovarian cancer: diagnosis using 123-I monoclonal antibody in comparison with surgical findings. *Nucl. Med. Commun.*, **5**, 485–99.
18. Granowska, M., Britton, K.E. and Shepherd, J.H. (1986) A prospective study of 123-I-labelled monoclonal antibody imaging in ovarian cancer. *J. Clin. Oncol.*, **4**, 730–6.
19. Goldenberg, D.M., Kim, E.E., Deland, F.H. *et al.* (1980) Radio-immunodetection of cancer with radioactive antibodies to carcinoembryonic antigen. *Cancer Res.*, **40**, 2984–92.
20. Berche, C., Mach, J.-P., Lumbroso, J.D. *et al.* (1982) Tomoscintigraphy for detecting gastrointestinal and medullary thyroid cancers: first clinical results using radiolabelled monoclonal antibodies against carcinoembryonic antigen. *Br. Med. J.*, **285**, 1447–51.
21. Wahl, R.L., Parker, C.W. and Philpott, G. (1983) Improved radioimaging and tumour localisation with monoclonal (Fab')$_2$. *J. Nucl. Med.*, **24**, 316–25.
22. Begent, R.H.J., Keep, P.A., Green, A.J. *et al.* (1983) Liposomally entrapped second antibody improves tumour imaging with radiolabelled (first) anti-tumour antibody. *Lancet*, **ii**, 739–41.
23. Granowska, M., Britton, K.E. and Shepherd, J. (1983) The detection of ovarian cancer using 123-I monoclonal antibody. *Radiobiol. Radiother. (Berlin)*, **25**, 153–60.
24. Paganelli, G., Malcovati, M. and Fazio, F. (1991) Monoclonal antibody pretargeting techniques for

tumour localization: the avidin biotin system. *Nucl. Med. Commun.*, **12**, 211–34.

25. Paganelli, G., Belloni, C., Magnani, P. *et al.* (1992) Two step targetting in ovarian cancer patients using biotinylated monoclonal antibodies and radioactive streptavidin. *Eur. J. Nucl. Med.*, **19**, 322–9.

26. Granowska, M., Biassoni, L., Carrol, M.J. *et al.* (1996) Breast cancer Tc-99m SM3 radioimmunoscintigraphy. *Acta Oncol.*, **35**, 19–321.

27. Chengazi, V.U., Nimmon, C.C. and Britton, K.E. (1996) Forward projection analysis and image surgery: an approach to quantitative tomography, in *Tomography in Nuclear Medicine, Present Status and Future Prospects*, International Atomic Energy Agency, Vienna, pp. 31–44.

28. Chatal, J.F., Saccavini, J.C., Furnoleau, P. *et al.* (1984) Immunoscintigraphy of colon carcinoma. *J. Nucl. Med.*, **25**, 307–14.

29. Corman, M.L., Galandiuk, S., Block, G.E. *et al.* (1994) Immunoscintigraphy with 111-In-salumomoab pendetide in patients with colorectal adenocarcinoma: performance and impact on clinical management. *Dis. Colon Rectum*, **37**, 129–37.

30. Babaian, R.J., Sayer, J., Podoloff, D.A. *et al.* (1994) Radioimmunoscintigraphy of pelvis lymph nodes with [111]Indium-labelled monoclonal antibody CYT-356. *J. Urol.* **152**, 1952–5.

31. Feneley, M.R., Chengazi, V.U., Kirby, R.S. *et al.* (1996) Prostate radioimmunoscintigraphy: preliminary results using technetium-labelled monoclonal antibody CYT-351. *Br. J. Urol.*, **77**, 373–81.

32. Howell, R., Hawley, P.R., Granowska, M., Morris, G. and Britton, K.E. (1995) Peroperative radioimmunodetection, PROD, of colorectal cancer using Tc-99m PR1A3 monoclonal antibody. *Tumori*, **81** (Suppl.), 107–8.

33. Richman, P.I. and Bodmer, W.F. (1987) Monoclonal antibodies to human colorectal epithelium: markers for differentiation and tumour characterisation. *Br. J. Cancer*, **39**, 317–28.

34. Bischof Delaloye, A., Delaloye, B., Buchegger, F. *et al.* (1989) Clinical value of immunoscintigraphy in colorectal carcinoma patients: a prospective study. *J. Nucl. Med.*, **30**, 1646–56

35. Goldenberg, D.M. and Larson, S.M. (1992) Radioimmunodetection in cancer identification. *J. Nucl. Med.*, **33**, 803–14.

36. Baum, R.P., Hertel, A., Lorenz, M. *et al.* (1989) Tc-99m anti-CEA monoclonal antibody for tumour immunoscintigraphy: first clinical results. *Nucl. Med. Commun.*, **10**, 345–8.

37. Lind, P., Lechner, P., Arian-Schad, K. *et al.* (1991) Anti-carcinoembryonic antigen immunoscintigraphy (Technetium-99m monoclonal antibody BW 431/26) and serum CEA levels in patients with suspected primary and recurrent colorectal carcinoma. *J. Nucl. Med.*, **32**, 1319–25.

38. Doerr, R.J., Abdel-Nabi, H., Krag, D. and Mitchell, E. (1991) Radiolabelled antibody imaging in the management of colorectal cancer. *Arch. Surg.*, **214**, 118–24.

39. Maguire, R.J. and Van Nostrand, D.V. (1992) *Diagnosis of Colorectal and Ovarian Cancer*, Marcel Dekker, New York.

40. Collier, B.D., Abdel Nabi, G., Doerr, R.J. *et al.* (1992) Immunoscintigraphy performed with In-111-labelled CYT 103 in the management of colorectal cancer: comparisons with CT. *Radiology*, **185**, 179–86.

41. Beatty, J.D., Duda, R.B., Williams, L.E. *et al.* (1986) Preoperative imaging of colorectal carcinoma with ^{111}In-labelled anticarcino-embryonic antigen monoclonal antibody. *Cancer Res.*, **46**, 6494–502.

42. Granowska, M., Mather, S.J. and Britton, K.E. (1991) Diagnostic evaluation of 111-In and 99mTc radiolabelled monoclonal antibodies in ovarian and colorectal cancer: correlations with surgery. *Nucl. Med. Biol.*, **18**, 413–24.

43. Durbin, H., Young, S., Stewart, L.M. *et al.* (1994) An epitope on carcinoembryonic antigen defined by the clinically relevant antibody PR1A3. *Proc. Natl Acad. Sci. USA*, **91**, 4314–17.

44. Britton, K.E., Granowska, M. and Mather, S.J. (1991) Radiolabelled monoclonal antibodies in oncology, I. Technical aspects. *Nucl. Med. Commun.*, **12**, 65–76.

45. Chetanneau, A., Barbet, J., Peltier, P. *et al.* (1994) Pretargetted imaging of colorectal cancer recurrences using an ^{111}In-labelled bivalent hapten and a bispecific antibody conjugate. *Nucl. Med. Commun.*, **15**, 972–80.

45. Sirisriro, R., Podoloff, D.A., Patt, Y.Z. *et al.* (1996) [99]Tc[m]-IMMU4 imaging in recurrent colorectal cancer: efficacy and impact on surgical management. *Nucl. Med. Commun.*, **17**, 568–76.

Radio-oligonucleotides

D. J. Hnatowich

INTRODUCTION

As their name suggests, oligonucleotides (i.e. oligonucleic acids), both ribonucleic acids (RNA) and deoxyribonucleic acids (DNA), are polymers of nucleotides (i.e. nucleic acids). Each nucleotide consists of a nitrogenous base chemically attached to a five-carbon sugar (ribose). To form the polymer, the sugars are linked through a phosphate group. In the case of DNA, the phosphate-sugar backbone supports a sequence of adenine, guanine, cytosine and thymine bases. Figure 17.9 (left) shows the molecular structure of a single-stranded (ss) native DNA, showing a series of bases, the sugar bridge and the phosphate (phosphodiester) backbone. The structure of RNA is identical except for the presence of a hydroxyl group at the 2' position of the sugar, and the replacement of the DNA base thymine, with uracil. These nucleic acids comprise the genetic material of all living matter with the sequence of bases providing the information needed for protein synthesis.

The property of oligonucleotides that best explains the interest these reagents now generate is their ability to hybridize specifically with their complementary sequence. According to Watson–Crick base-pairing rules, thymine and uracil will bind only to adenine, and cytosine will bind only to guanine [1]. This property of hybridization of ss-oligonucleotides can be used to advantage in drug and radiopharmaceutical development. A brief review is presented here of the radiolabelled oligonucleotides that appear potentially useful for imaging and radiotherapy applications in the future.

RADIOLABELLING

The use of radiolabelled oligonucleotides in nuclear medicine requires methods for labelling with radionuclides suitable for imaging and/or therapy. Methods of radiolabelling single- and double-stranded oligonucleotides with beta-emitting radionuclides such as ^{32}P and ^{35}S, have been in use for years. Of more interest to the nuclear medicine community are methods for labelling with γ-emitters for imaging purposes. A method of radiolabelling with the γ-ray-emitting radioisotopes of iodine (iodine-125 and iodine-131) was reported in 1971 [2]. However, radiolabelling of oligonucleotides by chelation would be advantageous for a variety of reasons having to do with convenience and with the superior imaging properties of some of the chelatable metallic radionuclides. Accordingly, Dewanjee and his colleagues [3] and Hnatowich et al. [4] have labelled oligonucleotides using 'bifunctional' chelators (i.e. moieties capable of both conjugating to the carrier and retaining the radionuclide by chelation), which for many years have been successfully applied to radiolabel proteins and peptides. So far, only the ss-oligonucleotides, and only those derivatized on one end with a primary amine, have been radiolabelled in this way.

RADIOLABELLING WITH INDIUM-111

Radiolabelling of oligonucleotides with ^{111}In was first reported by Dewanjee et al. [3]. A 15-base ss-DNA was synthesized to include a primary amine on one end, attached by a six-carbon spacer. An isothiocyanate derivative of DTPA was synthesized according to published procedures, and was coupled to the amine on the DNA. A similar study was performed more recently in this laboratory using the commercially available cyclic anhydride of DTPA in place of the isothiocyanate derivative [4].

RADIOLABELLING WITH TECHNETIUM-99m

Technetium-99m is considered the ideal radionuclide for gamma-camera imaging. It may therefore be assumed that this radioisotope will also be the label of choice for most oligonucleotide imaging applications.

The mercaptoacetyltriglycine (MAG3) chelator of ^{99m}Tc was originally developed as an alternative to radiolabelled hippuran for renal function studies [5]. This N_3S ligand is protected against

Clinical Nuclear Medicine, 3rd edn. Edited by M.N. Maisey, K.E. Britton and B.D. Collier. Published in 1998 by Chapman & Hall, London. ISBN 0 412 75180 1

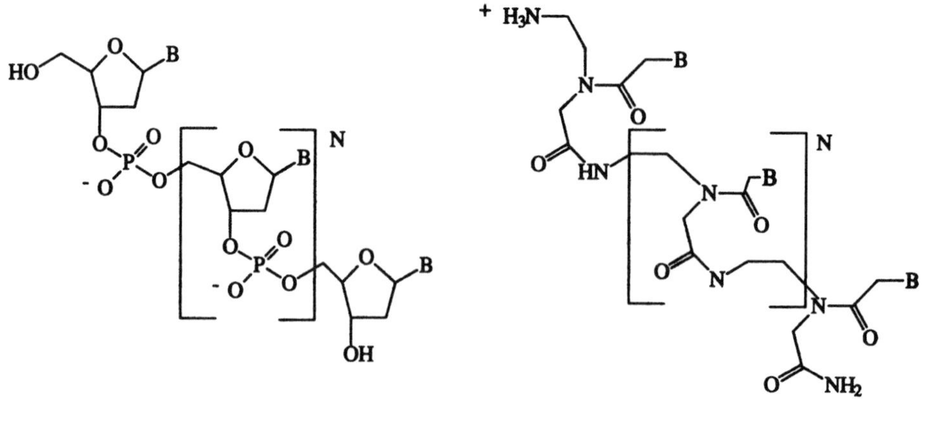

Figure 17.9   The chemical structure of deoxyribonucleic acid (DNA) and peptide nucleic acid (PNA).

disulphide-bond formation by a benzoyl group, which is removed by heating at 100°C for 10 minutes during labelling. The MAG3 chelator has also been used to radiolabel antibodies with ^{99m}Tc [6] and radiorhenium [7]. However, past use of the chelator for protein labelling has been limited, since the benzoyl leaving group requires extreme alkaline pH or boiling temperatures for sulphur deprotection. Accordingly, the chelator is usually radiolabelled before conjugation (preconjugation labelling) to carriers such as proteins or polypeptides which cannot withstand harsh conditions. Preconjugation labelling can be a complex procedure with multiple intermediate purification steps.

Recently, investigators from this laboratory developed an alternative synthesis of MAG3, the important features of which are: (i) the synthesis can be performed in two simple steps; (ii) the end-product is an NHS-ester that facilitates conjugation of the chelator to amines; and (iii) the sulphur atom is protected by an acetyl group in place of the benzoyl group [8]. One result of this [8] and two additional studies from this laboratory [9,10] is that acetyl protection greatly simplifies the synthesis and use of MAG3. The acetyl protection of NHS-MAG3 and MAG3-conjugated amines is stable, apparently indefinitely, to storage even at room temperature, yet the acetyl group will dissociate under standard radiolabelling conditions.

Once radiolabelled, incubated ^{99m}Tc on MAG3-conjugated antibodies was stable in serum [9]. The acetyl-protected NHS-MAG3 bifunctional chelator has been used successfully to radiolabel DNA [9] and peptide nucleic acids (PNA) [10].

POTENTIAL APPLICATIONS

ANTISENSE APPLICATIONS

Of the potential nuclear medicine applications for radiolabelled oligonucleotides, perhaps the most obvious at present is antisense targeting. In nuclear medicine, antisense targeting may be defined as intracellular localization through hybridization of a radiolabelled oligonucleotide with a base sequence opposite (i.e. 'antisense') to a sequence (i.e. 'sense') on the messenger RNA coding for a protein relatively unique to the target [11]. Antisense targeting strategies were first suggested in the mid-1970s [12,13]. The obvious advantage of antisense strategies is the potential for extreme specificity as, in principle, only those cells expressing a particular gene should be targeted. Furthermore, with the explosion of information regarding the human genome in health and disease, the number of potential gene targets is, even now, quite large [14].

The potential of chemotherapy based on antisense strategies has not been lost on the drug industry, who have become the main force in the development of this technology [15]. Preclinical and, in at least five cases at the time of writing, clinical trials are currently under way against viral infection with human immunodeficiency virus, human papilloma virus and herpes simplex virus, to name but a few, and against oncogenes such as c-*ras* and c-*myc* [16,17].

A large number of reports have appeared describing inhibition in animal and, especially in tissue culture studies, by antisense oligonucleotides [18]. In most cases, inhibition was attributed to antisense mechanisms, often on the basis of control studies showing less inhibition with sense or random-sequence oligonucleotides.

That antisense oligonucleotides can interfere with protein expression at the cellular level is no longer in doubt. The pressing question of the moment is whether these effects are due to antisense mechanisms. Unfortunately, very few previous investigations have confirmed transcriptional or translational arrest by measuring intracellular levels of the target mRNA or protein. In the absence of these measurements, the possibility cannot be excluded that the observed effects may be due to some sequence-specific activation of transcription factors or activation of RNA-degrading enzymes such as RNase H. Chemotherapy, of course, may be as effective regardless of whether the mechanism involves true transcriptional or translational arrest, or indeed, whether the effect is even sequence-specific. The mechanism of action is likely to be much more important for imaging and radiotherapy applications, where effective retention of the radiolabel at the target site may depend on mRNA hybridization. Furthermore, just as most therapy strategies are directed at translation arrest [19], because of the potentially much larger number of mRNA targets within a cell, imaging applications are also likely to be more successful when the goal is also translational arrest.

As is readily apparent by even the most cursory examination of antisense mechanisms, a number of barriers to effective targeting need to be overcome [20]. First, the oligonucleotide must survive in circulation long enough to accumulate in the target tissue. Nature has provided us with extracellular and intracellular nucleases designed to degrade foreign oligonucleotides, in particular ss-oligonucleotides, as a defence against viral and other infections. As a consequence, the native phosphodiester DNAs are rapidly degraded such

that their survival time in circulation may be measured in minutes [20]. Fortunately, many chemical modifications to the DNA structure are possible, some of which can greatly stabilize the oligonucleotide against nuclease attack [21]. The most actively pursued modification among these 'first-generation' oligonucleotides is the phosphorothioate DNAs in which one of the non-bonding oxygen atoms, usually in each phosphate group, within the backbone of the phosphodiester is replaced with a sulphur atom [21]. The phosphorothioate DNAs have been shown to be stable [22]; however, they have an unfortunate tendency to bind to tissue proteins, presumably due to an increased lipophilicity resulting from the replacement of oxygen with sulphur [23]. In the chemotherapeutic uses of oligonucleotides, it may be possible to overcome the effects of protein-binding by administering sufficient DNA to saturate these binding sites. This strategy may not be feasible or practical for imaging or radiotherapy applications. We have recently shown that the images obtained with a [99mTc]-labelled 22-base DNA oligonucleotide in normal mice are dominated by interfering radioactivity levels in blood, liver and other organs [24].

Fortunately, 'second-generation' oligonucleotides are under development. Particularly promising at present may be peptide nucleic acids (PNAs), in which the phosphate and sugar backbone of DNA have been replaced with a polyamide linkage [25] (Figure 17.9, right). Since they are not oligonucleotides, PNAs may be more correctly referred to as oligomers. PNAs bind with high affinity to their complement and are reported to be stable. We have recently confirmed the favourable properties of PNA for *in vivo* use [10]. Mice were implanted with beads in both thighs, but only in the target thigh were the beads bound with ss-PNA. Figure 17.10 shows an image obtained 4 hours after administration of [99mTc]-labelled complementary ss-PNA, and shows radioactivity in the bladder, kidneys and the target thigh. This demonstration of *in vivo* hybridization suggests that second-generation oligomers such as PNA may be useful for antisense applications.

A second, and probably more intractable difficulty to antisense applications, is cell-membrane transport. Clearly, the antisense oligonucleotide must gain access to the cytoplasm and possibly even the nucleus. As with any drug, the rate and extent of cellular transport will depend on

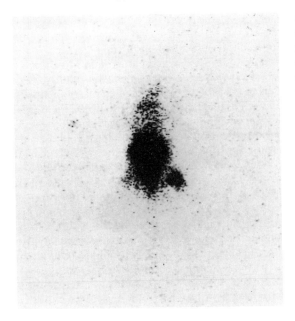

Figure 17.10 Whole-body anterior image of a mouse obtained 4 hours after administration of labelled PNA. Underivatized beads implanted in the right thigh, beads with complementary PNA implanted in the left thigh (on the right in the image) of the animal.

physiochemical properties of oligonucleotides such as their charge, lipophilicity and size [26]. The results of tissue culture studies provide little cause for optimism by showing that generally only a few percent of DNA oligonucleotides are incorporated in cells even under the most favourable circumstances [26]. In case of the phosphodiester and phosphorothioate DNA oligonucleotides, the mechanism of incorporation is thought to be receptor-mediated endocytosis [27]. Thus, depending upon the cell type, the transported oligonucleotides may become en-trapped within endosomal or lysosomal vesicles, and be unable to access their mRNA targets. Just as chemical modification can enhance nuclease stability, changes in chemical structure of oligonucleotides have been used to improve cell-membrane transport, in particular by decreasing the high negative charge of these oligonucleotides [28,29].

A third potential difficulty is also illustrated by the results of tissue culture studies. Not only is the degree of uptake of oligonucleotides into cells se-verely limited, but the rate of incorporation can

also be slow [26]. The rate at which antisense oligonucleotides accumulate in the target cells may be a relatively minor concern in the case of chemotherapy. However, slow incorporation kin-etics will limit the choice of radionuclides for imaging. For example, ^{99m}Tc may possibly be too short-lived for antisense imaging, unless the rate of cellular transport can be improved.

To conclude this brief examination of antisense strategies for nuclear medicine imaging: (i) several barriers must be overcome before antisense imaging and radiotherapy is likely to be success-ful; (ii) new oligomers must be developed which are stable in serum and in cells but without an affinity for proteins – these must incorporate rap-idly into the target cells, in sufficient quantities, and in a form in which they are available to bind to their mRNA targets; and (iii) the oligomers must bind selectively to mRNA in the target cells such that the radioactivity is retained therein for long enough to achieve the clearances elsewhere that are necessary for adequate target/non-target ratios.

While these restrictions may appear daunting, it is encouraging that some success has already been reported in the antisense imaging of tumours. Recently, Dewanjee and co-workers [3] have studied a ^{111}In-labelled 15-base phosphodiester and phosphorothioate ss-DNA oligonucleotide with a sequence antisense to that of c-*myc*, an oncogene thought to be expressed in a variety of malignant diseases. Under the conditions of the investigation, the uptake of label in the culture cells was higher for antisense (70–80%) versus sense (3–4%) DNA oligonucleotides, and the up-take reached a plateau in only 45–60 minutes [3]. The presence of mRNA-antisense DNA was con-firmed by HPLC analysis of cytoplasmic extracts. Further, the whole-body images of tumour-bearing mice showed a slightly better tumour im-age with the phosphorothioate antisense than with the sense probe – a result that could be pre-dicted by the almost ten-fold greater accumulation of radiolabel in tumour reported with the antisense (phosphodiester or phosphorothioate) versus sense DNA probe.

PRETARGETING APPLICATIONS

Because of the difficulties described above in the potential uses of radiolabelled oligonucleotides for antisense targeting, other *in vivo* applications (none of which requires cell-membrane transport) may be more attractive, at least for the present. Several of these are described in this and the subsequent section.

Pretargeting has been variously defined but in each of its strategies the radiolabel is administered on a carrier (usually of low molecular weight for rapid clearance) having a high binding affinity for a targeting molecule previously administered in a first-step and provided with sufficient time to localize in the target and to clear (often with help) from circulation and normal tissues [30]. The importance of high binding affinities to the success of pretargeting localization has been demonstrated by mathematical modelling [31]. In part, because of the very high affinity of biotin for (strept)avidin, these two molecules have assumed a dominant role in recent pretargeting studies in animals and in patients [32,33]. However, difficulties in the *in vivo* use of biotin and (strept)avidin have become apparent. Unless properly constructed, radiolabelled biotins may be subject to plasma biotinidase degradation [34]. Furthermore, when conjugated to antibodies, both streptavidin and avidin generate anti-(strept)avidin antibodies in patients [35]. Finally, and possibly most seriously, is the potential effect of endogenous biotin. We have demonstrated using FACS analysis that one streptavidin-conjugated antibody localized in a nude mouse xenograft becomes saturated with biotin in 2–3 days such that its biotin-binding expression disappears [36]. Circulating biotin levels in mice may be reduced by the intraperitoneal administration of streptavidin, and this can prevent the saturation of streptavidin in the tumour. However, massive doses of streptavidin are required and circulating biotin levels are reduced only temporarily [36]. The influence of endogenous biotin may explain the marginal results obtained using this two-step approach in at least one preliminary clinical trial [37].

These, and other problems, could be eliminated if biotin and (strept)avidin were replaced with another molecular pair with suitable properties for pretargeting. It may be calculated that the binding affinities of ss-oligonucleotides for their complement can approach that of biotin for (strept)avidin ($K_d = 10–15\,M$) [38]. The feasibility of pretargeting by DNA–DNA hybridization has been demonstrated *in vitro* by Bos *et al.* [39] who reported a 15-base ss-DNA covalently conjugated to an anti-tumour antibody and used *in vitro* as the first step in a two-step pretargeting strategy in which the second step employed a radioiodine-labelled complementary ss-DNA.

Because of the superior properties of PNA, we have investigated one pretargeting strategy in mice using PNA in place of DNA [40]. A protein (streptavidin) was conjugated with a 15-base ss-PNA while its complementary ss-PNA was radiolabelled with ^{99m}Tc. The study was performed in two mouse models: an infection model in normal mice in which *E. coli* were injected into one thigh; and a nude mouse tumour model in which the LS174T tumour was implanted in one thigh. The protein-conjugated PNA was administered intravenously and allowed 5 hours to localize through the increased vascular permeability of the lesions. The radiolabelled PNA was then administered intraperitoneally and 4 hours later the animals were imaged and sacrificed. Significantly higher accumulation of label was observed in most tissues at sacrifice in these study animals compared with control animals receiving only the labelled PNA. In particular, in the infection model, the infected-to-normal thigh radioactivity ratio was 3.5 for the study animals, in comparison with 1.7 for control animals ($P = 0.0001$). In the tumour model, these values were 1.7 versus 1.2 ($P = 0.003$). Obviously, *in vivo* hybridization was responsible for this increased radioactivity accumulation. Figure 17.11 presents representative whole-body anterior images of infected mice obtained at 4 hours after intraperitoneal administration of ^{99m}Tc-PNA. The control mouse on the left shows whole-body radioactivity and faint accumulation in the left thigh. The study mouse on the right shows similar whole-body activity and increased activity in the infected thigh. Figure 17.12 shows representative images of tumour-bearing mice obtained at 4 hours after intraperitoneal administration of ^{99m}Tc-PNA. The control mouse on the left shows whole-body radioactivity and faint accumulation in the left thigh. The study mouse on the right shows similar whole-body activity and increased activity in the thigh with the tumour.

MISCELLANEOUS APPLICATIONS

In addition to pretargeting, other applications of radiolabelled oligonucleotides that do not require cell-membrane transport are also possible. We have recently reported on a novel method of

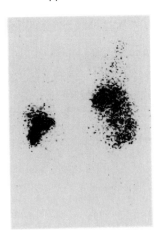

Figure 17.11 Whole-body anterior images of infected mice obtained at 4 hours after administration of ^{99m}Tc-PNA. The control mouse on the left shows whole-body radioactivity and faint accumulation in the left thigh. The study mouse on the right shows similar whole-body activity and increased activity in the infected thigh.

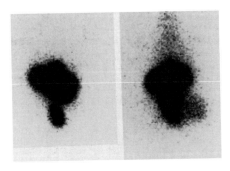

Figure 17.12 Whole-body anterior images of the mouse with tumour obtained at 4 hours after administration of ^{99m}Tc-PNA. The control mouse on the left shows whole-body radioactivity and faint accumulation in the left thigh. The study mouse on the right shows similar whole-body activity and increased activity in the thigh with tumour.

radiolabelling proteins by DNA–DNA hybridization [41]. A ss-DNA was covalently conjugated to an antibody and labelled by hybridization following the addition of the complementary ss-DNA labelled with ^{99m}Tc or ^{111}In. This approach has several advantages in principle: first, only a single modification of the antibody would be necessary to facilitate labelling with a variety of radionuclides, provided that these could be attached to the complementary oligonucleotide. Second, oligonucleotides can withstand pH and temperature conditions which would denature most proteins. Accordingly, if harsh labelling conditions are required, it may often be convenient (if not essential) to attach the radiolabel to DNA first, and then add this to the conjugated protein rather than labelling the protein directly. Third, as we were able to show, the *in vitro* and *in vivo* properties of the oligonucleotides can favourably affect the properties of a radiolabel attached to an antibody in this manner [41].

Hybridization of oligomers may also be used to amplify radioactivity deposited in lesions such as tumours [42]. For example, if a multivalent DNA or PNA can be constructed to consist of several single-stranded oligomers joined in some fashion, then when used in pretargeting applications as the second-step, the number of 'targets' to a third-step will, in principle, have been amplified by one less than the valence of the construct.

As a final example, combinatorial chemistry approaches to drug discovery have been applied to ss-oligonucleotides, with the result that unique and useful structures have been identified. Thus, RNA and DNA 'aptamers' have been developed, which bind at high affinity to diverse molecules such as low-molecular weight dyes [43], antibiotics [44] and thrombin [45]. These studies suggest that aptamers may be developed with high affinities for tumour-associated antigens, for receptor-binding proteins and other potential *in vivo* targets. In principle, when radiolabelled and administered, an aptamer may effectively carry its label to the target.

SUMMARY AND CONCLUSIONS

Radiolabelled oligonucleotides have yet to be administered to patients for nuclear medicine imaging or radiotherapy applications. So far, in the *in vivo* use of oligonucleotides, the emphasis has been on chemotherapy in connection with antisense targeting. However, the very property of ss-oligonucleotides (i.e. their ability to hybridize avidly and specifically to their complement), which fuels the enthusiasm for their use in chemotherapy, may be used to advantage in radiopharmaceutical development. In addition to antisense targeting, other potential applications involve pretargeting, aptamer localization, protein labelling and *in situ* amplification.

Many of the above applications of radiolabelled oligonucleotides must have been obvious for some time. That they have not yet been developed may be attributed in large part to the need for better methods of labelling with ^{99m}Tc and other radioisotopes and the need for more stable oligomers displaying useful pharmacokinetic properties. Both these needs have recently been met. Aminederivatized oligomers may now be radiolabelled with ^{99m}Tc for imaging studies through the use MAG3 [8]. Furthermore, PNAs appear to possess properties suitable for *in vivo* use [10,40]. With the availability of useful labelling methods and oligomer carriers, it is likely that in the next few years we will see a significant increase in the number of research reports describing the use of radiolabelled oligomers in nuclear medicine.

ACKNOWLEDGEMENTS

The author wishes to thank his UMMC colleagues for generously providing the animal images used in this report. This work was supported in part by CA59785 from the United States National Cancer Institute.

REFERENCES

1. Watson, J.D., Gilman, M., Witkowski, J. and Zoller, M. (1992) *Recombinant DNA*, 2nd edn, Scientific American Books, W.H. Freedman & Co., New York.
2. Commerford, S.L. (1971) Iodination of nucleic acids in vitro. *Biochemistry*, **10**, 1993–9.
3. Dewanjee, M.K., Ghafouripour, A.K., Kapakvanjwala, M., Dewanjee, S., Serafini, A.N., Lopez, D.M. and Sfakinakis, G.N. (1994) Noninvasive imaging of c-myc oncogene messenger RNA with indium-111-antisense probes in a mammary tumor-bearing mouse model. *J. Nucl. Med.*, **35**, 1054–63.
4. Hnatowich, D.J., Winnard, P., Jr, Virzi, F. *et al.* (1995) Labeling deoxyribonucleic acid oligonucleotides with 99mTc. *J. Nucl. Med.*, **36**, 2306–14.
5. Fritzberg, A.R., Kasina, S., Eshima, D. and Johnson, D.L. (19986) Synthesis and biological evaluation of technetium-99m MAG3 as a hippuran replacement. *J. Nucl. Med.*, **27**, 111–16.
6. Fritzberg, A.R., Berninger, R.W., Hadley, S.W. *et al.* (1988) Approaches to radiolabeling of antibodies for diagnosis and therapy of cancer. *Pharmaceutical Res.*, **5**, 325–34.
7. Goldrosen, M.H., Biddle, W.C., Pancook, S. *et al.* (1990) Biodistribution, pharmacokinetics, and imaging studies with ^{186}Re-labeled NR-LU-10 whole antibody in LS174T colonic tumor-bearing mice. *Cancer Res.*, **50**, 7973–8.
8. Winnard, P. Jr, Rusckowski, M., Mardirossian, G. and Hnatowich, D.J. (1997) A simplified synthesis of MAG3-coupled oligonucleotides for technetium-99m labeling. *Nucl. Med. Biol.* (in press).
9. Lei, K., Rusckowski, M., Chang, F., Qu, T., Mardirossian, G. and Hnatowich, D.J. (1996) Technetium-99m antibodies labeled with MAG3 and SHNH-an in vitro and animal *in vivo* comparison. *Nucl. Med. Biol.*, **23**, 917–22.
10. Mardirossian, G., Rusckowski, M., Chang, F., Qu, T., Lei, K., Egholm, M. and Hnatowich, D.J. (1997) In vivo hybridization of technetium-99m labeled peptide nucleic acid (PNA). *J. Nucl. Med.*, **38**, 907–13.
11. Milligan, J.F., Matteucci, M.D. and Martin, J.C. (1993) Current concepts in antisense drug design. *J. Med. Chem.*, **36**, 1923–37.
12. Ts'o, P.O.P., Miller, P.S. and Geene, J.J. (1983) Nucleic acid analogs with targeted delivery as chemotherapeutic agents, in *Development of Target-Oriented Anticancer Drugs* (eds Y.C. Cheng, B. Goz and M. Minkoff), Raven Press, New York, p. 183.
13. Zamecnik, P.C. (1991) Introduction: oligonucleotide base hybridization as a modulator of genetic message readout, in *Prospects for Antisense Nucleic Acid Therapy of Cancer and AIDS*, (ed. E. Wickstrom), Wiley-Liss, p. 1.
14. Anonymous (1994) Human genetic disorders. *J. Natl Inst. Health Res.*, **6**, 115–34.
15. Chrissey, L. (1991) An indexed bibliography of antisense literature, 1978–1990. *Antisense Res. Dev.*, **1**, 65–113.
16. Cohen, J.S. (1991) Antisense oligodeoxynucleotides as antiviral agents. *Antivir. Res.*, **16**, 121–33.
17. Tidd, D.M.A. (1990) Potential role for antisense oligonucleotide analogues in the development of oncogene targeted cancer therapy. *Anticancer Res.*, **10**, 1169–82.
18. Wagner, R.W. (1994) Gene inhibition using antisense oligonucleotides. *Nature*, **372**, 333–5.
19. Mirabelli, C.K. and Crooke, S.T. (1993) Antisense oligonucleotides in the context of modern molecular drug discovery and development, in *Antisense Research and Applications* (eds S.T. Crooke and B. Lebleu), CRC Press, Boca Raton, pp. 7–35.
20. Cook, P.D. (1993) Medicinal chemistry strategies for antisense research, in *Antisense Research and Applications* (eds S.T. Crooke and B. Lebleu), CRC Press, Boca Raton, pp. 149–87.
21. Uhlmann, E. and Peyman, A. (1990) Antisense oligonucleotides: a new therapeutic principle. *Chem. Rev.*, **90**, 543–84.
22. Wickstrom, E. (1986) Oligodeoxynucleotide stability in subcellular extracts and culture media. *J. Biochem. Biophys. Methods*, **13**, 97–102.
23. Kumar, S., Tewary, H.K. and Iversen, P.I. (1995) Characterization of binding sites, extent of binding, and drug interactions of oligonucleotides with albumin. *Antisense Res. Dev.*, **5**, 131–9.
24. Hnatowich, D.J., Mardirossian, G., Fogarasi, M., Sano, T., Smith, C.L., Cantor, C.R., Rusckowski, M.

and Winnard, P., Jr (1996) Comparative properties of a technetium-99m-labeled single-stranded natural DNA and a phosphorothioate derivative *in vitro* and *in vivo*. *J. Pharmacol. Exp. Ther.*, **276**, 326–34.

25. Egholm, M., Buchardt, O., Nielsen, P.E. and Berg, R.H. (1992) Peptide nucleic acids (PNA): oligonucleotide analogues with an achiral peptide backbone. *J. Am. Chem. Soc.*, **114**, 1895–7.

26. Crooke, R.M. (1993) Cellular uptake, distribution and metabolism of phosphorothioate, phosphodiester, and methylphosphonate oligonucleotides, in *Antisense Research and Applications* (eds S.T. Crooke and B. Lebleu), CRC Press, Boca Raton, pp. 427–49.

27. Goodarzi, G., Watabe, M. and Watabe, K. (1991) Binding of oligonucleotides to cell membranes at acid pH. *Biochem. Biophys. Res. Commun.*, **181**, 1343–51.

28. Pardridge, W.M. and Boado, R.J. (19991) Enhanced cellular uptake of biotinylated antisense oligonucleotide or peptide mediated by avidin, a cationic protein. *FEBS Lett.*, **288**, 3–32.

29. Quattrone, A., Di Pasquale, G. and Capaccioli, S. (1995) Enhancing antisense oligonucleotide intracellular levels by means of cationic lipids as vectors. *Biochemica*, **1**, 25–9.

30. Goodwin, D.A., Meares, C.F., McTigure, M. *et al.* (1986) Rapid localization of hapten in sites containing previously administered antibody for immunoscintigraphy with short half-life tracers. *J. Nucl. Med.*, **27**, 959 (Abstract).

31. Yuan, F., Baxter, L.T. and Jain, R.K. (1991) Pharmacokinetic analysis of two-step approaches using bifunctional and enzyme-conjugated antibodies. *Cancer Res.*, **51**, 3119–30.

32. Hnatowich, D.J., Virzi, F. and Rusckowski, M. (1987) Investigations of avidin and biotin for imaging applications. *J. Nucl. Med.*, **28**, 1294–302.

33. Hnatowich, D.J. (1994) The in vivo uses of streptavidin and biotin – a short progress report. *Nucl. Med. Commun.*, **15**, 575–7.

34. Rosebrough, S.F. (1993) Plasma stability and pharmacokinetics of radiolabeled desferoxamine-biotin derivatives. *J. Pharmacol. Exp. Ther.*, **265**, 408–15.

35. Paganelli, G., Malcovati, M. and Fazio, F. (1991) Monoclonal antibody pretargetting techniques for tumour localization: the avidin-biotin system. *Nucl. Med. Commun.*, **12**, 211–34.

36. Rusckowski, M., Fogarasi, M., Fritz, B. *et al.* (1997) Effect of endogenous biotin on the applications of streptavidin and biotin in mice. *Nucl. Med. Biol.*, **24**, 263–8.

37. Kalofonos, H.P., Rusckowski, M., Siebecker, D.A. *et al.* (1990) Imaging of tumor in patients with indium-111-labeled biotin and streptavidin conjugated antibodies: preliminary communication. *J. Nucl. Med.*, **31**, 1791–6.

38. Egholm, M., Kim, S.K., Norden, B. and Nielsen, P.E. (1993) PNA hybridizes to complementary oligonucleotides obeying the Watson-Crick hydrogen-bonding rules. *Nature*, **365**, 566–8.

39. Bos, E.S., Kuijpers, H.A., Meesters-Winters, M. *et al.* (1994) *In vitro* evaluation of DNA-DNA hybridization as a two-step approach in radioimmunotherapy of cancer. *Cancer Res.*, **54**, 3478–86..

40. Rusckowski, M., Qu, T., Chang, F. and Hnatowich, D.J. (1997) Pretargeting using peptide nucleic acid (PNA). *Cancer* (in press).

41. Hnatowich, D.J., Mardirossian, G., Rusckowski, M. and Winnard, P., Jr (1996) Protein labelling via deoxyribonucleic acid hybridization. *Nucl. Med. Commun.*, **17**, 66–75.

42. Hnatowich, D.J., Winnard, P., Jr, Virzi, F. *et al.* (1994) Amplification of radioactivity using complementary DNA. *Proceedings, Fifth Conference on Radioimmunodetection and Radioimmunotherapy of Cancer*, Princeton, NJ.

43. Elington, A.D. and Szostak, J.W. (1990) *In vitro* selection of RNA molecules that bind specific ligands. *Nature*, **346**, 818–22.

44. Davis, J., Von Ahsen, U. and Schroeder, R. (1993) Antibiotics and the RNA world, in *The RNA World* (eds R.F. Gesteland and J.F. Atkins), Cold Spring Harbor Laboratory Press, Plainview, NY, pp. 185–204.

45. Griffin, L.C., Toole, J.L. and Leung, L.L.K. (1990) The discovery and characterization of a novel nucleotide-based thrombin inhibitor. *Gene*, **137**, 25–32.

CHAPTER 18

Diagnostic accuracy and cost-benefit issues

M. N. Maisey

New investigations have frequently been introduced with little or no evaluation of either their diagnostic performance or the influence they have on patient management. This deficiency has become particularly important over the past two decades as major new diagnostic technologies, including nuclear medicine, magnetic resonance imaging (MRI), computed tomography (CT) and ultrasound, have been introduced into clinical medicine, and there has been an increasing pressure to contain costs. The Council on Science and Society report in 1983 noted the haphazard manner in which expensive technologies were introduced, and also that an assessment was considered with very little concern for patient reactions or to the social and psychological consequences. The overriding reason for an evaluation is to confirm a positive effect on patient management but there are other reasons for increasing effort in this area, which include constraints on the available resources within the health services and a pressure for evidence-based practice. Clinicians have the right to know whether the diagnostic services that are offered make a real contribution to patient care, and which assessments should be well founded.

This chapter sets out some of the methodologies involved in diagnostic technology performance evaluation, and aims to draw attention to common inadequacies in published studies.

INTRODUCTION

The general methodology for evaluation is common to most diagnostic applications, although the emphasis will depend on the purpose for which the diagnostic method is being used. Diagnostic imaging techniques can be divided into four categories:

1. **Screening of asymptomatic patients for disease:** the prevalence of disease in the referred population will usually be low (e.g. breast or osteoporosis screening); the goal is to detect all patients who have early disease, and usually, to accept the need to investigate a proportion of patients without the disease on the cost of not missing any individuals with disease.
2. **The detection and diagnosis of disease in symptomatic patients:** this is the conventional area of diagnostic imaging techniques in hospital. The patients are symptomatic, the prevalence of disease in the investigated population is intermediate and the goal is to detect and characterize disease.
3. **Staging of disease:** the presence of disease will usually have been established by alternative methods; the goal is to identify further sites or the extent of the disease, e.g. staging procedures for the treatment of lung cancer and perfusion imaging to establish the extent and severity of coronary artery disease (CAD). This will determine optimal management, risk stratification and prognosis.
4. **Monitoring change:** imaging techniques are being increasingly used to assess the progress of disease and the response to treatment.
5. **Targeting disease:** the use of imaging to target lesions for image-guided biopsy or image-guided therapy (e.g. surgery or radiotherapy).

Clinical Nuclear Medicine, 3rd edn. Edited by M.N. Maisey, K.E. Britton and B.D. Collier. Published in 1998 by Chapman & Hall, London. ISBN 0 412 75180 1

THE GOALS OF DIAGNOSTIC TESTS

The preceding section classified the applications of imaging procedures; in order for them to be effective, there must be a gain to the individual and to society when they are used. The demonstration of pathology in a patient is not sufficient as a goal in itself. New information should ultimately benefit the patient in one of the following ways: (i) save lives by diagnosis and consequent treatment; (ii) restore health; (iii) alleviate suffering (physical and/or psychological) by early detection and treatment; (iv) prevent occurrence of symptomatic disease by early detection and treatment; and (v) predict the course of disease (prognosis).

THE COSTS AND BENEFITS OF EVALUATION

Although it appears self-evident that a soundly based evaluation of diagnostic methods in clinical medicine would be beneficial, an argument has to be made for evaluation techniques and it needs to be demonstrated that they are cost-effective.

The benefits of evaluation include: better use of limited resource in patient care within the health service; withdrawal of tests which are not shown to be of value and could even do harm; prevention of early diffusion of unproven tests into widespread clinical practice; and the earlier adoption of good practice.

The direct costs of evaluation may be high because the methods are often difficult and time-consuming to undertake. Further costs may include delay in the introduction of a truly effective test. Similar evaluation costs apply to drug trials and these have undoubtedly been broadly beneficial.

Timing of evaluations is often critical; early evaluation studies are often like 'trying to hit a moving target' because technology changes so rapidly that the results may be regarded as irrelevant. On the other hand, early evaluation may prevent the widespread application of a test or purchase of equipment and dissemination of a method that is ultimately shown to be useless or at best non-contributory. Early evaluation by a well-designed study may detect an unsuspected morbidity associated with the diagnostic technique, which would have taken much longer to uncover if careful evaluation had not been undertaken. Equally, a too-early evaluation can lead to the premature rejection of a potentially valuable technique; and evaluation that is too late may be unable to prevent the use of a technology, which cannot be shown to be useful but is 'believed in' by clinicians and therefore difficult to dislodge. Usually, the advantage of late evaluation is that the technology is stable and therefore the results of evaluation more credible.

HOW SHOULD NEW TECHNOLOGY BE INTRODUCED?

There are three ways that new technologies are introduced:

1. **Random diffusion:** new technology is frequently introduced on a random basis depending on a variety of factors such as source of finance, clinical pressures, institutional prestige, commercial interests, and other outside influences.
2. **Evaluation of every new technique:** with the rapid change of technology and the number of established diagnostic methods, this would not be a cost-effective exercise, and is clearly impractical and not realistically achievable.
3. **Selective evaluation:** both new and old tests can be selectively examined especially if they are expensive, widely used and applied to disease with a high prevalence. Subsequent resource decisions can then be made on well-established quantifiable data. The choice of what should be evaluated should also be influenced by therapeutic impact and downstream costs.

METHODOLOGY AND TECHNIQUES FOR EVALUATING DIAGNOSTIC PERFORMANCE

The performance of diagnostic tests can be measured at several well-defined hierarchical levels, which have been categorized by Feinberg *et al.* [1], and form the basis of a classification, which assists in the understanding of the evaluation process. The levels are:

- technical capacity;
- diagnostic accuracy;
- diagnostic impact;

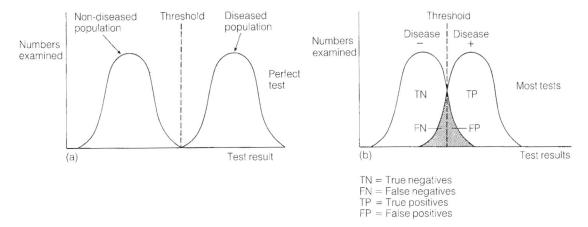

Figure 18.1   The two graphs show how a threshold may be used to separate normal from diseased populations (a); however, this is almost unknown in medicine – the overlap in (b) is the more usual finding.

- therapeutic impact;
- patient outcome; and
- optimal usage.

Diagnostic tests, if they have been evaluated at all, have only been evaluated at the first and second levels, very rarely at the third level, and almost never at the fourth, fifth or sixth levels.

TECHNICAL CAPACITY

Evaluation of test performance at this level is essentially a pilot study concerned with questions of safety: Are there major hazards? Is there morbidity associated with the test? What is the patient acceptability? Does the test perform reliably (i.e. is it repeatable and/or consistent) and does it measure what it claims to measure? What is the reproducibility and the precision of the test?

These studies should include an assessment of the engineering reliability of the equipment and the frequency of non-diagnostic tests, test failures and/or patient failures.

DIAGNOSTIC ACCURACY

At this level of evaluation, the purpose is to assess how good the test is at discriminating between patients with the disease from those without the disease. It is very rare for a test in clinical medicine to distinguish completely between a diseased and a non-diseased population; as a consequence of this overlap, a criterion has to be developed for the optimal separation of the two populations with acceptance of the inevitable false-negative (FN) and false-positive (FP) diagnoses. Figure 18.1 illustrates this general principle. However, Figure 18.2 is more realistic, because it would be unusual for 50% of the population studied to be diseased and 50% normal. In this case, there are fewer diseased than normal people, i.e. the prevalence of disease in the population is less than 50%.

In nuclear medicine, the diagnostic criterion that is used to separate diseased from non-diseased populations may be quantitative (e.g. thyroid uptake or ejection fraction), but often qualitative and reported as positive or negative with varying degrees of confidence or probability, e.g. bone and lung scans. Figure 18.3 shows how by changing the criterion or threshold for diagnosing disease alters the numbers of false-negatives and false-positives.

For any single value of the diagnostic criterion used to separate diseased from non-diseased populations, we can consider the outcome as a 2×2 matrix as shown on p. 648:

DISEASE

		Present	Absent	Total
DIAGNOSTIC TEST	Positive	TP	FP	TP + FP
	Negative	FN	TN	FN + TN
	Total	TP + FN	FP + FN	TP + FN + FP + TN

Different ways of measuring accuracy of a diagnostic test have been developed, which have both advantages and disadvantages.

Accuracy

The accuracy of a test is defined as the ratio of true-positive results (TP) plus true-negative results (TN) to the total number of patients studied.

$$\text{Accuracy} = \frac{TP + TN}{TP + FP + TN + FP} \times 100\%$$

This is a global measure of accuracy that does not distinguish between positives and negatives, and is therefore often misleading as a measure of test performance. This problem can be seen graphically from Figure 18.3 in which the accuracy of the test is the shaded areas divided by the total area under both curves.

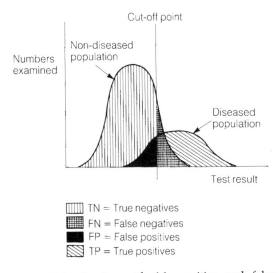

TN = True negatives
FN = False negatives
FP = False positives
TP = True positives

Figure 18.2 Overlap with false-positive and false-negative results when the prevalence in the population studied is less than 50%.

The prevalence of the disease in the population studied affects the accuracy of the test:

Example 1: Prevalence 50%

Disease

Test		+	−
	+	450	200
	−	50	300

$$\text{Accuracy} = \frac{450 + 300}{1000} = 75\%$$

Example 2: Prevalence 2%

Disease

Test		+	−
	+	18	392
	−	2	588

$$\text{Accuracy} = \frac{18 + 588}{1000} \times 100\% = 60.6\%$$

This effect of prevalence is illustrated in Figure 18.4 where the disease prevalence is lower but the threshold remains unchanged.

Sensitivity and specificity

The information from the matrix can be translated into measurements referred to as the sensitivity and the specificity of the test. **Sensitivity** is defined as the ratio of true-positive to true-positive plus false-negative, or

$$\text{Sensitivity} = \frac{TP}{TP + FN} \times 100\%$$

This can be expressed as 'the proportion of people with the disease that will be detected by the test' (diagnosed by the test set at a particular threshold or criterion).

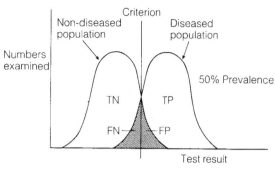

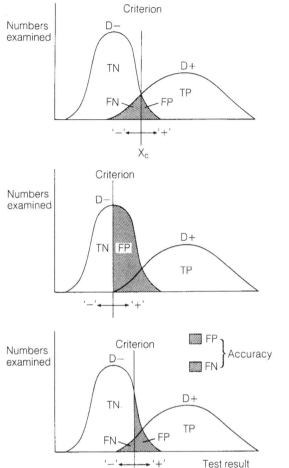

Figure 18.3 Three graphs showing how when the population prevalence and the test remains constant, the sensitivities and specificities can alter by adjusting the diagnostic criterion.

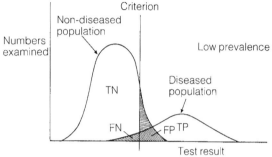

Figure 18.4 Two graphs showing the effect of changing the disease prevalence in the population on the test performance when the diagnostic criterion remains constant.

Specificity is the ratio of true-negative, to true-negative plus false-positive, or

$$\text{Specificity} = \frac{\text{TN}}{\text{TN} + \text{FP}} \times 100\%$$

This can be expressed as 'the proportion of people without the disease that will be confirmed to be free of the disease'. The closer to 100% each of these measurements approaches the better the test is performing.

It can be seen from Figure 18.3 that as the criterion or threshold is changed, the number of true-positive and false-positive cases, and hence the

sensitivity and specificity of the test, varies. When the sensitivity and specificity of the test have been measured using a broad enough spectrum of patients with and without the disease, and with a wide range of disease presentations and severity, the prevalence of disease in the test population **does not** influence the sensitivity and specificity of the test. This can be shown by recalculating the figures in the previous section for sensitivity and specificity.

Example 1: Prevalence 50%

$$\text{Sensitivity} = \frac{450}{450 + 50} = 90\%$$

$$\text{Specificity} = \frac{300}{300 + 200} = 60\%$$

Example 2: Prevalence 2%

$$\text{Sensitivity} = \frac{18}{18 + 2} = 90\%$$

$$\text{Specificity} = \frac{588}{588 + 392} = 60\%$$

This effect can be seen graphically in Figure 18.4 where these ratios remain constant in spite of much lower disease in the population. Although sensitivity and specificity are good objective measures of the performance of a test, they do not provide any information as to the likelihood of an individual patient whose test is positive or negative being normal or having the disease, and this is the information needed by a clinician for decision making. The measures which provide this information are called the positive and negative predictive accuracies (PPA and NPA) or positive and negative predictive values (PPV and NPV) and are heavily dependent on prevalence of the disease.

Positive and negative predictive accuracies

The positive predictive accuracy is the ratio of true-positive, to true-positive plus false-positive results:

$$PPA = \frac{TP}{TP + FP} \times 100\%$$

or the likelihood of a patient with a positive test actually having the disease.
   The negative predictive accuracy is the ratio of true-negative, to true-negative plus false-negative:

$$NPA = \frac{TN}{TN + FN} \times 100\%$$

or the likelihood of a patient with a negative test being free of the disease. These post-test probabilities are dependent on the prevalence of the disease in the population (pre-test probability of disease), which can be seen by working the same example.

Example 1:   Prevalence 50%
Predictive value of positive test = (PPA)

$$= \frac{450}{450 + 200} \times 100\% = 69\%$$

Predictive value of negative test = (NPA)

$$= \frac{300}{300 + 50} \times 100\% = 86\%$$

Example 2:   Prevalence 2%
Predictive value of negative test = (NPA)

$$= \frac{18}{18 + 392} \times 100\% = 4.4\%$$

Predictive value of negative test = (NPA)

$$= \frac{588}{588 + 2} \times 100\% = 99.7\%$$

The measures so far discussed are sometimes expressed as probabilities:

   Sensitivity (true-positive ratio) = P(T+|D+),

where

   P = the probability of an event occurring
   T+ = positive result to a test
   | = given
   D+ = disease present

i.e. the probability of disease being present given a positive test result.

Similarly:

   Specificity (true-negative ratio) = P(T−|D−),

where

   P = the probability of an event occurring
   T− = the negative result to a test
   | = given
   D− = disease absent

and

   False-positive ratio = P(T+ |D+)
   False-negative ratio = P(T− |D+)
Predictive value of a positive test = P(D+ |T+)
Predictive value of a negative test = P(D− |T−)
   Prevalence = P(D+)

Bayes' theorem

Bayes' theorem provides a general basis for decision theory, from which a mathematical formula can be derived to show how sensitivity and specificity combine with probability of disease to give a predictive value of a positive or negative test, i.e. how positive predictive value of a positive or negative test (i.e. how positive predictive value or negative predictive value) can be calculated from sensitivity, specificity and prevalence.
   For example:

$$P(D+|T+) = \frac{P(T+|D+) \times P(D+)}{P(T+)}$$

or

$$= \frac{P(T+|D+) \times P(D+)}{P(T+|D+) \times P(D+) + P(T+|D-) \times P(D-)}$$

where

> P = probability
> B = B occurring
> D+ = disease present
> D− = disease absent
> T+ = positive test result
> | = given

Or

$$PPV = \frac{\text{Sensitivity} \times \text{Prevalence}}{\text{Sensitivity} \times \text{Prevalence} + (1 - \text{Specificity}) \times (1 - \text{Prevalence})}$$

and

$$NVP = \frac{\text{Specificity} \times (1 - \text{Prevalence})}{(1 - \text{Sensitivity}) \times \text{Prevalence} + \text{Specificity} \times (1 - \text{Prevalence})}$$

The measures of accuracy, which have been discussed, only apply to disease being present or absent. When the possibility of various different diseases is introduced (i.e. an ordered differential diagnosis), the problem becomes more complex; for example, a chest X-ray may be abnormal because of tuberculosis, cancer or infection.

When two tests (X and Y) are used then the two sensitivities can be combined as shown below:

Test	Sensitivity (%)	Specificity (%)
Ultrasound (X)	80	60
CT Scan (Y)	90	90
Call positive X *and/or* Y positive*	98	54
Call positive if X *and* Y positive^	72	96

* Positive X+ and/or Y+
Sensitivity = sens X + ((100 − sens X) × sens Y) / 100 = 98
Specificity = spec X × spec Y / 100 = 54

^ Positive X+ and Y+
Sensitivity = sens X × sens Y / 100
Specificity = spec X + ((100 − spec A) × spec Y) / 100

Thus, it means that insisting that two tests are positive, before making a diagnosis, will result in a very high specificity (i.e. few false-positives) but a low sensitivity (i.e. frequent missed cases).

Test selection

The choice of which test to use, as well as the threshold for calling a test positive, will depend on the use to which the test is being put.

High SENSITIVITY picks up most of the patients who have the disease (few false-negatives).

Good for: • excluding disease
• screening especially if there is high morbidity associated with missing the disease.

High SPECIFICITY picks up most of the individuals without the disease (few false-positives).

Good for: • confirming the presence of disease;
• cases when the risk associated with treating unnecessarily is high.

If two or more tests are very sensitive, and the primary purpose of the test is to exclude disease, the gain in sensitivity obtained by using two or more tests may be offset by the decrease in specificity.

RECEIVER-OPERATING CHARACTERISTIC (ROC) CURVE

Another measure of the performance of a diagnostic test is the receiver-operating characteristic curve (ROC curve), which measures the sensitivities and specificities over a range of criteria. These curves demonstrate graphically how the sensitivities and the specificities change when the diagnostic criterion is altered, i.e. the threshold for reporting a test as positive is raised or lowered. If the test has a quantitative measure, the diagnostic criterion for abnormality may be set at different levels, e.g. lymph nodes on CT may be called pathological only if they are 5 mm or 10 mm or 20 mm, etc. Although most imaging techniques are reported qualitatively, it is still possible to express the likelihood of their being abnormal semi-quantitatively with different levels of confidence. For example, a chest X-ray may be absolutely normal, or there may be something suspicious, or something almost certainly abnormal, or a gross abnormality. Different levels of likelihood of disease being present are divided into five categories:

0 – definitely normal
1 – probably normal
2 – possibly abnormal
3 – probably abnormal
4 – definitely abnormal

The evaluation of a test will use these different levels of likelihood and are included in the reporting of the films. From these data, the ROC curves can be constructed and each test, X-ray or imaging method will have its own characteristically shaped curve, which will express the performance of the test quantitatively.

To produce such a curve for an imaging test, a series of scans (using a minimum of 100) are obtained from a representative population with an intermediate prevalence of disease and a wide range of severity of disease. The scans will be read by one individual or a group and put into one of the categories above (i.e. graded 0–4). The positivity of the test is then created five times, i.e. the test is called positive:

1. only when the definitely abnormals are called positive, i.e. very strict threshold;
2. only when definitely abnormal and probably abnormal, are called positive;
3. when definitely abnormal, probably abnormal and possibly abnormal, are called positive (i.e. a lax threshold);
4. even when cases categorized as probably normal are included, and called positive; and
5. when cases categorized as definitely normal are also included, i.e. all cases are called abnormal, in which case, no diseased patient will go undetected (100% sensitivity) but all the patients free of disease will be called diseased (0% specificity).

These results are then plotted in the ROC space, the vertical axis being the true-positive ratio (the sensitivity correct detection of disease or 'hits') and the horizontal axis being the false-positive ratio (1– Specificity) or the 'false alarms' shown in Figure 18.5.

Typical characteristic curves

These curves can be used to compare the overall performance of tests (Figure 18.6). Curve A would result from randomly assigning results to one of the categories referred to above and using the outcome to report whether the test was normal or abnormal, and clearly would have no diagnostic value.

Curve B describes the shape of a perfect curve when there are no false-positive and no false-negative results, and as we have already seen, for practical purposes, never occurs clinically. Most tests will have shapes approximating to C and D, where C is a better test than D for detecting a particular condition, because at every threshold or criterion, there are more true-positives and less false-positives than for curve D. It can be seen from this that if the result of the scan has to be unequivocally abnormal before it is reported to the clinician as abnormal, then the sensitivity of detection of disease will be low, but the specificity will be high. On the other hand, if we report as positive anything which is possibly abnormal, probably abnormal or definitely abnormal, then the sensitivity for detection of the disease will be much higher but with decreased specificity, i.e.

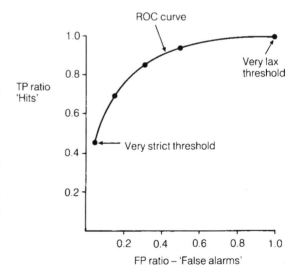

Figure 18.5 An ROC curve from an imaging procedure with five levels of diagnostic probability.

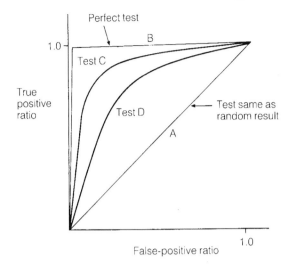

Figure 18.6 Four theoretical ROC curves showing test performance from perfect (B) to random (A). Curves C and D are typical for many imaging procedures.

the diagnostic and therapeutic impact, and the outcome.

DIAGNOSTIC IMPACT

The diagnostic impact of an imaging procedure is a measure of performance that is used to measure the extent by which a test is able to influence the subsequent pattern of diagnostic testing. Does it replace other diagnostic tests? Does it significantly alter the need for or choice of other tests afterwards? The following may occur:

1. The new test may be more accurate and render previously used tests redundant.
2. The new test may be more accurate but cost or morbidity does not justify the improved accuracy.
3. The test may be equivalent to one or more other tests, in which case other factors such as morbidity and cost will determine any change.
4. The new test may be less accurate than the old test, but may have other characteristics such as a significantly decreased morbidity or cost, which justify its introduction.

The general tendency is for more tests to be performed on patients for any particular disease

there will be more false-positives, and will increase the number of patients who are actually free of disease but whom we are diagnosing as having the disease.

The performance of the tests can be assessed by simply inspecting the curves' shapes; however, quantitative values can also be derived from them. The most commonly used method is to integrate the area below the curve and express this as a proportion – the nearer to 1.0, the better the test.

The shape of the ROC curves may be more complex than indicated previously and may crossover as indicated in Figure 18.7. This illustrates how two tests may be similar in accuracy, because the area under the curves are identical but the characteristics are different. In this instance, neither of the tests is necessarily better overall, but performance will depend on the use to which it is put. If false-positive results are to be avoided, e.g. when the consequences of a positive diagnosis would be dangerous treatment, test A would be a better test, provided a strict threshold is used; whereas test B may be a better screening test (provided a lax threshold is used) because the sensitivity is higher in this area of the curve.

Showing that a test has a good sensitivity and specificity and performs well using ROC curve measurement does not prove that it is clinically useful. This can be assessed only by measuring

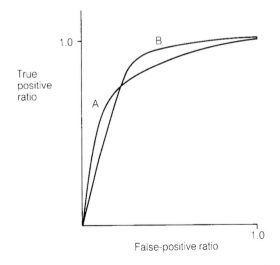

Figure 18.7 An example of an ROC curve when the total accuracy may be similar but performance differs in different areas of the curve.

rather than replacing redundant tests because of the lack of good evaluation procedures and a clear understanding of the diagnostic process. New investigations, unless they have a significantly decreased morbidity, are too often used as 'add-on tests'. It is usually not possible to consider a technology in its entirety because it may have one characteristic in one clinical situation and another for another clinical situation, e.g. MRI can replace CT for posterior fossa disease but has less advantage in supratentorial disease. The concept of 'incremental value of a test' has become important; this will vary in different clinical scenarios, and can be applied so that any test in a diagnostic sequence can be assessed quantitatively for its incremental value in different clinical situations using a statistic such as the 'likelihood ratio' which will demonstrate when the test is more usefully applied. Diamond [2] has described the incremental value methodology and has shown the additive value of tests for the evaluation of CAD.

Kauls and Beller [3] have reviewed the incremental value of a test and identified the importance of incremental value for: (i) assessing the worth of a test in detecting disease; (ii) the worth of a test in risk stratification; and (iii) the worth of a test in predicting the outcome. These authors have also highlighted some of the problems associated with experimental determination of the incremental value.

It is not sufficient to show incremental value of a test but the quantitative value of the incremental value has to be measured against the cost of that test to decide whether it is an appropriate use, the cost in this context being the total costs (the financial costs as well as the clinical costs of complications, etc.).

The really important stages of the Fineberg test evaluation sequence only come in the fourth and fifth levels of the hierarchy, i.e. the impact a test has on patient management and on the clinical outcome. These are at the same time, the most important, and the most difficult and expensive evaluations to undertake, and consequently, rigorous assessments of these levels are almost absent from the literature.

THE THERAPEUTIC IMPACT

The performance of diagnostic procedures can be measured by assessing the effect they have on the therapy and subsequent management of the patient, i.e. number of decisions about patient management that are altered on the basis of their results. The resource expenditures and patient risks associated with these downstream costs are: (i) costs of a false-positive plus inappropriately instituted subsequent treatment; (ii) missed therapeutic opportunities from a false-negative; and (iii) complications associated with delay in making a diagnosis.

THE PATIENT OUTCOME

This is clearly the most important criterion in the evaluation of the impact of diagnostic methods in clinical care. The question that needs to be asked is whether the diagnostic procedure contributes to the improved health of the individual patient. If it does not materially affect the patient in such a way as to lower mortality, alleviate suffering, restore health, prevent symptomatic disease or predict prognosis, then in the final analysis, however accurate, the test is worthless and may even be harmful – for example, by increasing the anxiety among a large section of the population regarded as candidates for the test. Equally, this is the most difficult and the least often attempted measure of the performance of diagnostic procedures. Indicators or measures, which can be used to measure this outcome include: the total lives saved; the life-years saved; the quality-adjusted life-years saved; the disability days avoided; and the age-adjusted disability days saved.

DETERMINING SUCCESS CRITERIA FOR MEASURING THE BENEFIT OF DIAGNOSTIC PROCEDURES

As highlighted above, the benefit of a diagnostic procedure should be measured, not only by the impact of the procedure on the individual patient but also on the integrated healthcare system. Available techniques for achieving this tend to focus on either the resulting clinical or the economic benefits, often to the exclusion of the other. This divergence reflects the agendas of clinicians or planners respectively, rather than those of patients. Therefore, it is appropriate to gain an appreciation of the interests of these three key stakeholder groups in determining the criteria for measuring the 'Cost of Success'.

Planners

The agenda of the planners, who may be the government and/or insurance companies, is a combination of quality and cost-effectiveness. With an ever-increasing awareness of the importance of healthcare outcomes, diagnostic procedures will increasingly need to conform to Hillman's [4] definition of cost-effectiveness: 'If the benefits are sufficiently great to justify the costs, and if equal or greater benefits cannot be obtained through less costly means'.

New evaluation methodologies will need to contain a financial component spanning not just the specific procedure and the disease management process, but also incorporating the capital impact, both initial and long term. In addition, from the healthcare planners point of view, evaluation must be capable of making an assessment of the potential payback the use of a diagnostic procedure may provide in terms, not only of immediate advantages, but also wider benefits that may accumulate throughout the healthcare system.

Clinicians

The focus of the clinician is likely to be increasingly directed towards identifying the most appropriate medical action, which is likely to fall into one of three broad categories:

1. Discharge – confirmation that no further treatment is necessary.
2. Treatment – evidence confirming that treatment is necessary and defining the appropriate treatment.
3. Further testing – insufficient evidence to proceed to either of the other two options.

Patients

Patients, as individuals and collective consumers of health care, are likely to become increasingly focused on receiving the most appropriate treatment pathway, which returns them to their optimal state of well-being with respect to medical history and lifestyle. Furthermore, the appropriate treatment pathway will be one which is associated with minimal risk, pain, radiation, complications and anxiety.

In contrast to the planners, patients as individuals and/or groups will not be as concerned with the associated costs of the treatment pathway, since they may perceive healthcare as their right, irrespective of who is ultimately paying the bill. Their main priority will be to secure the best possible healthcare for themselves and/or their group.

The 'Cost of Success'

The true value of diagnostic testing can only really be appreciated within a 'global healthcare system' context. This may be represented by the catchment area of a hospital, or a more regional perspective, but more critically, take into account benefits that may accrue elsewhere within the system and with time. The true value of a test for the prevention of later illness or the identification of a more appropriate treatment path may take many years to become apparent. Thus, evaluation techniques for diagnostic procedures must be capable of incorporating the 'Cost of Success' of an intervention, i.e. the role of a diagnostic test in achieving the optimal overall cost for each successful outcome.

METHODS FOR MEASURING THE CLINICAL BENEFIT FROM THE PERFORMANCE OF A DIAGNOSTIC TEST

It has usually been regarded as sufficient to measure the accuracy of a diagnostic test, and from this infer a consequential benefit as a result of an accurate test. This is not necessarily the case, and complementary methods are available, which should be increasingly used in an attempt to measure the diagnostic and the therapeutic impact, and the patient outcome. The currently available methods are shown in Table 18.1.

Case reports and case control studies

Case reports and case control studies are the form of clinical study with which we are most familiar in the literature. Case reports may be the first presentation of a new test, but are usually so biased as to have little scientific basis for the assessment of the effectiveness of a test. Case control studies with well-matched controls, if they avoid the well-established problems, can be valuable and can show efficacy (i.e. demonstrate benefit in a single dedicated research centre) but may not be effective in more widespread usage.

Early studies with case series of patients with chest pain and indeterminate ECGs indicate a

Table 18.1   Methods for testing clinical value

1. Case reports and case control studies
2. Consensus evaluation
3. Meta-analysis
4. Databases
5. Computer modelling and simulation
6. Prospective measurement of clinical impact
7. Randomized prospective clinical trials
8. Epidemiology

potential significant cost-effectiveness of ^{99m}Tc-MIBI perfusion scanning in the accident and emergency department where the gains are achieved by reduction of ITU usage and length of stay [5,6].

Consensus guidelines

This method has been increasingly used over the past decade. It usually incorporates some literature review or meta-analysis of the literature with the personal views of experts. Consensus studies may be valuable if the experts are well chosen and the consensus discussion objective, but will still often suffer from some bias in favour of a technology. Consensus studies are relatively quick and inexpensive, and may lead to useful practical results, particularly by developing practice guidelines for the more appropriate application of tests.

Consensus studies are particularly useful when there are big variations in the usage of diagnostic or therapeutic interventions. For example, there is evidence of large variations in use of methods in cardiology: the likelihood of using angiography and coronary artery bypass grafting (CABG) for coronary artery disease (CAD) varies by a factor of three within the USA, and by as much as seven times between the USA and countries such as the UK. In a study by Bernstein *et al.* [7], appropriateness ratings were established for performing angiography in different clinical situations. From 3382 angiograms, a 320 sample was audited (nuclear cardiology procedures had only been used in 2% of those). They rated 49% appropriate, 30% equivocal, and 21% inappropriate and compared them with North American experience. The key finding was that inappropriate usage was not related to usage rate, i.e. it might be expected that in a country where the rate of angiograms per case was low there would be higher appropriate usage; however, the assumption was not corroborated by

this study. The authors concluded that guidelines developed from consensus agreements about appropriateness would increase effectiveness. Recently, Berman *et al.* [8] have developed guidelines for the use of nuclear cardiology procedures in nine clinical situations: the diagnosis of CAD, post-myocardial infarction assessment, poor ventricular function, unstable angina, post-catheterization, before non-cardiac surgery, post-percutaneous transluminal coronary angioplasty (PTCA), post-CABG and long-term medical management. The American College of Cardiology Task Force [9] have also developed similar guidelines for 10 clinical situations using a I, II, III classification of appropriateness, where I is usually appropriate and useful, II is acceptable and useful but less established, and III is generally not appropriate.

Databases

Some databases may be valuable for evaluating outcome in relation to diagnostic methodologies used. However, the incompleteness and doubtful accuracy of many databases limits this method. One example of the use of a database is the study by Topol *et al.* [10], who used an insurance claims database to analyse angioplasty practice. These authors showed that only 29% of the study cohort had any objective measurement of ischaemia (including exercise testing) before angioplasty. They concluded that the relative lack of an objective definition of myocardial ischaemia and the marked variability of the use of procedures suggests a need for further implementation of established 'guidelines'.

Modelling

Modelling is a methodology whereby the effect of diagnostic procedures on clinical care and the costs involved can be evaluated. The model will use assumptions, such as for example, the prevalence of disease in patients who undergo perfusion imaging, and the sensitivity and specificity of the test as well as the costs both of the test itself and the consequences of the results. The model based on these assumptions can then be used to predict the possible benefits of using the test and it can be used to test different usage scenarios or at different stages in diagnostic stratagem. By varying the base assumptions of the model the sensitivity of the predictions can be tested and the key issues that control the benefits of the test can be assessed.

Some of the advantages of the modelling approach to cost-benefit evaluation are:

1. It allows an initial assessment that focuses on areas requiring more research, i.e. where the potential for health gain and improved cost-effectiveness of useful resources is greatest.
2. It provides a method to assess how cost-effectiveness is effected by sensitivity and specificity, and provides information about costs and outcomes.
3. It allows the potential merits of using a diagnostic test in place of others and at different time points in the work-up or management.

In a paper by Lau and Adams [11], the authors use decision analysis methodology in a model system to assess the likely benefit in outcome using various different assumptions to assess whether it is worthwhile doing perfusion stress imaging (or other tests) post-infarction. They showed that there would be little to be gained unless the sensitivity of the test was >90% with a moderate (50%) prevalence of CAD causing silent ischaemia. They are also showed how it can highlight the research that needs to be done. In this case further information about the frequency and extent of silent ischaemia post myocardial infarction.

Cohen and co-workers [12] used a decision analytic model to evaluate the potential cost-effectiveness of stenting for single-vessel disease and showed limited cost-effectiveness for some groups.

Management impact studies

One of the first successful management impact studies was by Wittenberg *et al.* [13], who looked at the impact of CT on abdominal masses. In this type of study, the management plan is determined on the basis of the tests that have been performed and the plan written down. The test under evaluation (e.g. it could be thallium reperfusion and re-injection for hibernating myocardium) is then performed and a final management plan agreed incorporating the new results. This sequence will document whatever impact on patient management has been achieved by the test. Subsequently, patient outcome can be reviewed and an agreed judgement can be made as to the benefits or otherwise effected by the change of management which

occurred. The approach was adopted by Nallamutha *et al.* [14] who looked at the impact of thallium SPECT on management (including angiography) and outcome (death or other hard cardiac events). Of 2700 patients, 2027 had a normal scan (defined as group I) and 673 had abnormal scans (defined as group II); only 3% of the normal scans and 36% of the abnormal scans proceeded to angiography; 2% of the normal group that proceeded to angiography had revascularization procedures subsequently compared with 30% of the abnormal thallium group proceeding to angiography having revascularization. Patients in group I who had angiography but no revascularization, had no cardiac events, but there were 15 cardiac events in group II. This study, although weak in some respects, attempted to look at the potential impact of SPECT thallium imaging on management. Wassertheil-Smoller and colleagues [15] looked at the impact of perfusion scanning on the decision to perform angiography: 98 (61%) of the planned catheter studies were cancelled after scan results were available, and 38 (14%) were referred for angiography which had not been planned previously, i.e. there was a significant management impact in 136 of 439 patients, which resulted in a reduction of total cost as well as better patient care. The weakness of this methodology is partly the lack of a control population – in the absence of such a control arm, it is difficult to compare outcome, and therefore the ultimate effect of the investigation on anything except the management plan.

The clinician will also be aware that further information, in this case from nuclear cardiology, will subsequently be provided, which may influence him and affect any management plan that he or she devises. It may be difficult to blind the clinician to the nuclear cardiology result when he or she is making their first management plan and the studies tend to be complex with difficult logistics.

Randomized control trials

As with therapeutic evaluations, randomized control trials are considered to be the most rigorous way of assessing the clinical benefit of diagnostic procedures such as nuclear cardiology as well as their cost-effectiveness. They are however, complex to undertake and expensive to perform; and consequently, there are few in the literature and they are not generally well understood or as well developed as therapeutic trials.

Many of the issues that apply to randomized drug trials also apply to randomized studies of diagnostic methods. For example, it is not ethical to do a randomized study if the outcome is believed to be known, unless it can be demonstrated that resources would not be sufficient for all patients to have the test. For example, this is the case in PET imaging, so that in spite of the knowledge that it is probably the best test of hibernating myocardium, limited facilities would still make it ethical to undertake a study of this type. If the study is randomized, patient consent is essential and may be difficult to obtain if patients believe they are missing an investigation that could help in their management. There are many possible designs for randomized control studies depending on individual circumstances, probably the most reliable design is one that randomizes between the standard diagnostic stratagem plus the new investigation. In some circumstances, it may be possible to randomize between one test and another, e.g. thallium scanning randomized against echo studies. These studies can measure the affect on management decisions as well as eventually comparisons of outcome.

Utilization of resources in healthcare

The assessment of diagnostic, therapeutic impact and clinical outcome is important but only one side of the coin in any system, which has a finite resource with which to provide healthcare to their population, i.e. in systems where there is healthcare rationing whether explicit or implicit.

For the resources to be used effectively, not only do there need to be discussions about relative priorities (e.g. hip replacements versus bypass grafts) but also the available resources need to be used 'appropriately'. The overall effectiveness will depend on the appropriateness by which resources are used. Any procedure will be 'appropriate' if the expected health benefits exceed the expected negative benefits by a sufficiently wide margin. This is the basis for the cost-effectiveness studies in medicine, which are now becoming used more extensively. It should now be rare for a clinical study to be undertaken in isolation from a cost-benefit evaluation. There are various definitions of cost-effectiveness, probably the best is that of Hillman et al. [4]: 'A medical procedure is cost-

effective, if its benefits are sufficiently great to justify its costs, and if equal or greater benefits cannot be gained through less costly means'. Cost–benefit or cost-effective studies tend to be overarching terms used to cover all types of studies incorporating a measure of cost; however, they are specific methodologies that are used by health economists. Cost–benefit methods are used to assist decision making when choices between options have to be made, these decisions may be being made by purchasers, providers or clinicians in an effort to maximise the gain in health from any budget. Most of the methods depend on ways of drawing up a balance sheet between the advantages (benefits) and disadvantages (costs), and are hence called 'Cost–benefit analyses'.

The health service costs may include:

1. The costs of diagnosis and treatment and resources used.
   (a) type and quantity of tests and treatments.
   (b) resources needed to provide the tests.
   (c) the costs of providing the resources.
2. Patient carers / costs
   (a) direct costs, e.g. travel, baby sitters, etc.
   (b) indirect costs, e.g. time away from normal activities.
   (c) health costs, e.g. radiation, complications, pain, anxiety, etc.

The downstream costs also need to be considered. These are the costs which are incurred as a direct consequence of the result of diagnostic tests. Downstream costs are particularly important in relationship to false-negative and false-positive results, because costs are incurred that have no benefit and may have less benefits. Opportunity costs may also be important; these are alternative uses of the resources, e.g. the gamma-camera that could have been used for other purposes, had the tests not been performed.

The four methods for incorporating costs and benefits are:

1. **Cost minimalization:** this method is used when outcomes are likely to be the same (it is important to be sure than this is in fact true), an example might be comparing ^{201}Tl and ^{99m}Tc-MIBI scanning for the diagnosis of CAD, where the diagnostic accuracy is similar, and this was the basis of a recent study [16].
2. **Cost-effectiveness studies:** these are used

when clinical outcomes are likely to be different, but can be expressed in the same units, e.g. cases of CAD detected or reduction in cardiac events. The results are usually expressed as the cost per unit of outcome and are usually restricted to a single disease, e.g. ischaemic heart disease.

3. **Cost utility studies:** these methods are used when there is a need to compare different treatments and different diseases (or programmes) where the units of outcome will vary, e.g. reduction in cardiac events by angioplasty compared with renal transplant programme. The usual measures used to express results of these comparisons is one of the 'well-being measures' such as the quality-adjusted life-years saved (QALYS), which is a measure of quantity and quality of life gained, for a given cost.

4. **Cost-benefit studies:** these methods specifically attempt to put a monetary value on the benefits (outcomes), e.g. the 'value' of a year of life gained. The methodology is difficult and fraught with problems. In so far as these methods are relatively new techniques in clinical medicine, it is important that evaluations are as rigorous as possible, and standardization is important in order to compare results between studies. Drummond *et al.* [17] have identified the main advantages for attempting to standardize:
   (a) Maintenance of methodological standards.
   (b) Comparison of different interventions (for priority ratings QUALYS, etc.)
   (c) Interpretation from setting to setting, within and between countries.

Generally, there is agreement about some but not all aspects of standardization. The areas of agreement include:

1. The terminology – cost utility, etc.
2. Superiority of marginal testing rather than using average costs.
3. Importance of considering alternatives.
4. Importance of analytical viewpoint and the need to consider the societal view point.
5. Discounting (in principle), not the rate.
6. Sensitivity analysis.

Drummond *et al.* [17] have also proposed a useful checklist for assessing health economy evaluation publications:

1. Was a well-defined question posed in answerable form?
2. Was a comprehensive description of competing alternatives given, i.e. can you tell who did what to whom, where, and how often?
3. Was there evidence that the programme's effectiveness had been established? Was this done through a randomized, controlled clinical trial? If not, how strong was the evidence of effectiveness?
4. Were all important and relevant costs and consequences for each alternative identified?
5. Were costs and consequences measured accurately in appropriate physical units (e.g. hours of nursing time, number of physicians visits, days lost from work or years-of-life gained) before valuation?
6. Were costs and consequences valued credibly?
7. Were costs and consequences adjusted for differential timing?
8. Was an incremental analysis of the costs and consequences of alternatives performed? Were the additional (incremental) costs generated by the use of one alternative over another compared with the additional effects, benefits, or utilities generated?
9. Was a sensitivity analysis performed?
10. Did the presentation and discussion of the results of the study include all of the issues that are of concern to users?

Black and Welch [18] have drawn attention to some extremely important issues relating to cost–benefit, an outcome that may result from improvements in diagnostic techniques. They have shown the misleading effect that an increase in the accuracy of diagnosis (e.g. for coronary artery stenosis) will cause an apparent increase in the prevalence and incidence of the disease, and the apparent improved effectiveness of therapeutic interventions that may result because of the effect of 'lead time' and 'length biases' which wrongly indicate that the early diagnosis seems to confer longer survival. It is critical to compare like with like in the case mix studies.

Costing

The direct cost of a technology under evaluation is often easy to identify, particularly for a new technique being provided under special funding arrangements. However, just as care must be taken in projecting effectiveness from studies of efficacy conducted in 'laboratory' conditions, the use of cost data derived from studies of technologies used in a 'research mode', may not reflect the actual cost of provision in the 'service mode'. The size and direction of this cost-difference may be unpredictable. For example, investigations carried out under a research protocol may take longer because more information is required than is strictly necessary for immediate diagnosis, and patient processing may take longer. On the other hand, use of technology in a research unit may use hidden resources such as special technical and maintenance expertise, the cost of which cannot readily be separated from other overhead costs.

In using any costing information, the appropriate form of presentation varies with the question being addressed. If it is proposed that a new technology should be introduced to completely replace an existing service, then comparison can be made on the basis of total costs. It is more often the case that a new method is a partial replacement for several existing techniques, none of which will completely disappear. Here, a careful assessment of the marginal (or incremental) cost is necessary. The full cost of the new service is still relevant, but the estimates of resource savings from avoidance of other tests will be much reduced, reflecting only the direct operating costs which can be avoided, while maintaining capital equipment and trained staff.

ERRORS ASSOCIATED WITH MEASURING DIAGNOSTIC PERFORMANCES

These sources of error and bias are well-known methodological problems but despite this there are consistent errors in reported evaluation procedures.

INTER- AND INTRA-OBSERVER VARIATIONS

As a part of every test performance evaluation, information about the variations in reporting the images or making the measurements between different interpreters (inter-observer variation) and for the same observer on different occasions (intra-observer variation), must be incorporated as these errors can lead to inconsistent test performances.

INADEQUATE RANGE OF PATIENTS

When a new test is evaluated, it is frequently applied to patients with well-advanced and well-documented disease. When this is the case, and the use of the test is subsequently extended to patients with milder disease and/or a broader range of disease severity, the results of the initial evaluation will no longer apply.

NON-MATCHED CONTROLS

Controls must always be used in a good scientific evaluation. Frequently however, inappropriate controls are chosen. For example, a test may be performed for elderly patients with heart disease and the controls are young fit individuals. In most instances, they should at least be age- and sex-matched.

Exclusion of uninterpretable results or uncooperative patients

Frequently, these are excluded before the calculations are made. This is wrong, and will give quite inaccurate and often optimistic measures of the performance of the test. Such patients should always be included, and it is only possible to exclude them if the exclusion is done before the test is undertaken.

READING THE IMAGES BLIND OR OPEN

For the best non-subjective results the reading should be blind, i.e. the reporting physician should not be aware of the clinical history of the patient. Ideally, they should be read blind initially, and open on a subsequent occasion, together with the other available clinical information. Many studies do not comment on this point and do not specify which was used.

PREVALENCE OF THE DISEASE IN THE POPULATION

As mentioned previously, in a well-conducted study with a broad range of patients and disease stages, sensitivities and specificities will not change with prevalence. However, if positive predictive accuracies are calculated, these are acutely dependent on the prevalence in the population, which must be stated.

THE 'GOLD' OR REFERENCE STANDARD IS INADEQUATE

It is often impossible to obtain a final diagnosis on the basis of well-established 'gold standards' such as histology, and the diagnosis may be assessed with another non-invasive test. When this is so, it is essential to know the test performance parameters of the 'gold standard'.

INADEQUATE SAMPLE SIZE

Too frequently, sensitivities, specificities and even ROC curves are calculated from inadequate numbers. There are well-defined rules based on the prevalence of the disease and the likely accuracy of the test, which enable investigators to estimate the sample sizes needed for accurate sensitivity and specificity measurements. In addition, the confidence range of these sensitivities must be calculated. The size of the samples should be such that the SE is less than half of (100% – % estimated sensitivity) [19], but will also depend on the measured parameter of performance of competing tests.

CONCORDANCE WITH HISTOLOGY

Histology is often regarded as the 'gold standard'. However, if only those patients who have final histology available were used for assessing the test performance, this might introduce a major source of bias, because of the referral patterns.

CLINICAL FOLLOW-UP (FINAL OUTCOME)

Clinical follow-up is often used as the gold standard, which may be entirely appropriate where histology is not available. The follow-up must be long enough to detect disease that may have been present and missed by the diagnostic test, but more importantly, the results of the test must not have been incorporated into this final diagnosis. This is a frequent source of error.

STATISTICAL CALCULATIONS

These are often inappropriate, the most common error being the use of parametric statistics when the numbers are too small and the information inadequate to know that the data are normally distributed. In these instances, non-parametric statistics are usually more appropriate.

LOGISTIC PROBLEMS

The logistic problems of performing evaluation tests are not to be underestimated.

ETHICAL FACTORS

Ethical approval is necessary for most studies, particularly randomized control trials. The patients must give their consent, preferably in writing. This fact should be incorporated in reports of the study design.

RANDOM ORDER

When two tests are compared, the order in which this is done should be randomized.

PUBLICATION BIAS

There is a natural bias towards enhancing the value of a test because of the tendency to report positive findings and not write up negative ones.

GLOSSARY OF TERMS

Cost–benefit analysis Places a monetary value on the benefits and non-monetary costs and compares them with the monetary costs, to produce a net present value. Also net social benefit.

Cost-effective Additional benefits worth the additional costs.

Cost-effectiveness analysis Outcome measure is chosen and expressed as a ratio to the cost.

Diagnostic efficiency Capacity of a test to meet its immediate objectives, i.e. correct diagnosis.

Downstream costs Costs consequent on the result of the test, e.g. treatment costs.

Efficacy The usefulness of a procedure under ideal or pilot conditions.

Effectiveness The usefulness when widely applied.

Incremental cost The additional cost of changing the level of activity or the type of activity. Often referred to as marginal cost, to distinguish it from the total cost of the whole activity.

Offset studies (tests) Those which decrease inappropriate treatment.

Opportunity costs The value of a resource in its best alternative use.

Predictive tests Risk / assessment, e.g. tests to assess risk of myocardial infarction.

ROC curve Receiver-operating characteristic curve.

Specificity A measure of the ability of a test to correctly exclude disease in non-diseased patients.

Sensitivity A measure of the ability of a test to detect disease when it is present.

REFERENCES

1. Fineberg, H.V., Bauman, R. and Sosman, M. (1977) Computerised cranial tomography: effect on diagnostic and therapeutic plans. *JAMA.*, **238**, 224–7.
2. Diamond, G.A. (1989) Future imperfect: the limitations of clinical prediction models and the limits of clinical prediction. *J. Am. Coll. Cardiol.*, **14**(3), A12–22.
3. Kauls, X. and Beller, G.A. (1992) Evaluation of the Incremental value of a diagnostic test: a worthwhile exercise in this era of cost consciousness? Editorial. *J. Nucl. Med.*, **33**(10), 1732–4.
4. Hillman, B.J., Kahon, P.J., Neu, R. *et al.* (1989) Clinical trials to evaluate cost effectiveness. *Invest. Radiol.*, **24**, 167–71.
5. Varetto, T., Cantalupi, D., Altieri, A. *et al.* (1993) Emergency room Technetium 99m sesta MIBI imaging to rule out acute myocardial ischaemic events in patients with non-diagnostic electrocardiograms. *J. Am. Coll. Cardiol.*, **22**, 1804–8.
6. Hilton, T.C., Thompson, R.C., Williams, H.J. *et al.* (1994) Technetium 99m sesta MIBI myocardial perfusion imaging in the emergency room evaluation of chest pain. *J. Am. Coll. Cardiol.*, **23**, 1016–22.
7. Bernstein, S.J., Kosecoff, J., Gray, D. *et al.* (1993) The appropriateness of the use of cardiovascular procedures: British versus US perspectives. *Int. J. Technol. Assessment in Healthcare*, **9**, 3–10.
8. Berman, D.S., Kiath, J., Freidman, J.D. *et al.* (1995) Clinical applications of exercise nuclear cardiology studies in the era of healthcare reform. *Am. J. Cardiol.*, **75**, D3–13.
9. ACC/AHA Task Force Report. (1995) Guidelines for clinical use of cardiac radionuclide imaging. *J. Am. Coll. Cardiol.*, **25**, 521–47.
10. Topol, E.J., Ellis, S.G., Cosgrove, D.M. *et al.* (1993) Analysis of coronary angioplasty practice in the United States with an insurance claimer's database. *Circulation*, **87**, 1497–9.
11. Lau, J. and Adams, M.E. (1993) Non-invasive testing of asymptomatic patients for the detection of silent ischaemia after an infarction, a decision analysis. *Int. J. Technol. Assessment in Healthcare*, **9**(1), 112–23.
12. Cohen, D.J., Breall, J.A., Ho, K.K.L. *et al.* (1994) Evaluating the potential cost-effectiveness of stenting as a treatment for symptomatic single vessel coronary disease. Use of a decision analytic model. *Circulation*, **89**, 1859–76.
13. Wittenberg, J., Fineberg, H.V., Ferrucc, J.T. *et al.* (1980) Clinical efficacy of computed body tomography. *Am. J. Roentgenol.*, **134**, 1111–20.
14. Nallamuthu, N., Pancholy, S.B., Lee, K.R. *et al.* (1995) Impact on exercise single photon emission computed tomographic thallium imaging of patient management and outcome. *J. Nucl. Cardiol.*, **2**, 334–8.
15. Wassertheil-Smoller, S., Steingart, R.M., Wexler, J.P. *et al.* (1987) Nuclear scans: a clinical decision making tool that reduces the need for cardiac catheterization. *J. Chron. Dis.*, **40**, 385–97.
16. Nightingale, B. (1995) Cost effectiveness of thallium 201 versus technetium 99m sesta MIBI in the detection of coronary artery disease. *J. Nucl. Med. Technol.*, **23**, 36–41.
17. Drummond, M., Brandt, A., Luce, B. *et al.* (1993) Standardising methodologies for economic evaluation in healthcare, practice, problems and potential. *Int. J. Technol. Assessment in Healthcare*, **9**(1), 26–36.
18. Black, W.C. and Welch, H.G. (1993) Advances in diagnostic imaging and overestimations of disease prevalence and the benefits of therapy. *Adv. Diagnostic Imaging*, **328**(17), 1237–43.
19. Freedman, L.S. (1987) Evaluating and comparing imaging: a review and classification of study designs. *Br. J. Radiol.*, **60**, 1071–81.

FURTHER READING

Backhouse, M. (1995) Understanding Cost Utility and Cost Benefit. *Economics, Medicines and Health*, 16–18.

Gambhir, S.S., Hoh, C.K., Phelps, M.E., Madar, I. and Maddahi, J. (1996) Decision tree sensitivity analysis for cost-effectiveness of FDG-PET in the staging and management of non-small-cell lung carcinoma. *J. Nucl. Med.*, **37**, 1428–36.

Maisey, M.N. (1996) Evaluating the benefits of nuclear cardiology. *Q. J. Nucl. Med.*, **40**, 47–54.

Maisey, M.N. *et al.* (1996) Determining the cost of success. Dialogues *in Nuclear Cardiology*, No. 4., Kluwer Academic Press, the Netherlands..

Patten, D.D. (1993) Cost-effectiveness in nuclear medicine. *Semin. Nucl. Med.*, **23**(1), 9–30.

Robinson, R. (1993) Economic evaluation and healthcare; what does it mean? *Br. Med. J.*, **307**, 670–3.

CHAPTER 19

Technology and instrumentation

SPECT issues

P. H. Jarritt

INTRODUCTION

Single-photon emission computed tomography (SPECT) refers to the acquisition and reconstruction of cross-sectional images of *in vivo* radionuclide distributions. Specifically, this relates to the detection of emitted photons as single isolated events, as opposed to positron emission tomography (PET), where detection is based upon the 'simultaneous' detection of the two opposed annihilation photons from radionuclides that decay by positron emission. The annihilation photons can be detected as single decays, and most SPECT systems are capable of imaging positron-emitting radionuclides, in both planar and tomographic modes, although with significantly reduced sensitivity when compared with PET systems.

SPECT systems are mainly based upon the Anger gamma-camera [1]. These general-purpose nuclear medicine systems are capable of a wide range of routine acquisition modes. Dedicated instruments are also available that are capable of tomographic acquisition alone, which have been designed to provide greatly enhanced sensitivity and often improved resolution when compared with the planar gamma-camera systems. This chapter will not consider PET systems, although a number of Anger gamma-camera systems are being developed with coincidence-detection capability, and thus tomography systems capable of both SPECT and PET imaging modes will be available commercially. Systems not based on conventional Anger gamma-camera technology will also not be considered in detail, but the principles outlined can effectively be applied to systems utilizing single-photon detection.

The potential user of SPECT technology is faced with a large range of choices. These start with the appropriate choice of detector configuration, and continue through the relevant range and frequency of detector performance checks to data acquisition and reconstruction protocols. The following sections highlight the main areas that users should consider in the implementation of this methodology. SPECT technology is currently undergoing a significant change in the commercial implementation of attenuation and scatter correction. These developments will lead to considerable improvements in the quantitative capabilities of SPECT, and it is hoped in clinical effectiveness. A brief review of these developments is included along with a consideration of factors that contribute to errors in the reconstructed images.

EQUIPMENT AND TECHNIQUES

EQUIPMENT CHOICES

Modern gamma-camera systems reflect the priorities of the clinical service. Systems optimized for whole-body scanning, for SPECT, or for dynamic imaging using single detectors can be purchased.

Clinical Nuclear Medicine, 3rd edn. Edited by M.N. Maisey, K.E. Britton and B.D. Collier. Published in 1998 by Chapman & Hall, London. ISBN 0 412 75180 1

Organ-optimized systems are also available, especially for myocardial and brain perfusion imaging. Clearly, selection will be dependent on the requirements of the clinical service, but choice of the detector configuration can have significant effects on the range of studies and the ease with which these can be performed.

All imaging processes are ultimately limited by spatial resolution and detection sensitivity. In SPECT, these are related directly to the area of scintillation detector available to the imaging process, i.e. the number and area of the detectors, and the characteristics of the collimators used for data acquisition. Unfortunately, resolution and sensitivity are not independent variables. For a fixed detection geometry, improvements in spatial resolution will result in a reduction in system sensitivity, requiring increased patient doses and/or scanning times. Administered doses and scanning times are effectively limited by regulations and practicalities. Optimization of detector configuration and collimation is thus of primary importance in SPECT imaging. At first sight, it might appear that the sensitivity of the detection system is directly proportional to the number of detectors; however, in any practical definition, sensitivity must consider the total time required to complete a patient examination. The user must therefore consider the ease with which detectors can be positioned for SPECT imaging, the proportion of the total acquisition time that is spent on rotating the detector(s), the need for 180° versus 360°

data sampling, and finally, the requirements for measurement of patient attenuation maps using external radioactive sources. Though not exhaustive, the most obvious detector configurations are shown in Figure 19.1. Possible configurations for the incorporation of attenuation coefficient measurements are also shown.

PATIENT POSITIONING

The position of the patient relative to the detector is dependent on the collimator geometry chosen. For systems using parallel-hole collimation, the overriding requirement of the SPECT process is that the detector(s) must maintain an orbit as close to the patient as possible. This does not affect the sensitivity of the detection process, but is critical in maintaining resolution within the reconstructed data. Any component of the detector configuration that prohibits a close approach to the patient for a particular organ study should be investigated. This may include the design of the couch or head-rest, the distance between the field-of-view and the physical edge of the detector, or simply the overall detector size.

A number of different methods are employed to ease patient positioning. While some systems offer fully automated body-contouring facilities, most rely on some form of learning process whereby the operator trains the acquisition controller before starting the acquisition. Two points should be noted. First, due to safety considerations the

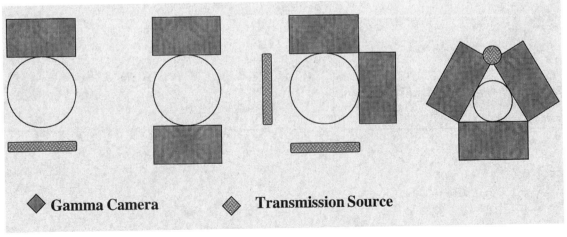

Gamma Camera   **Transmission Source**

Figure 19.1 Gamma-camera detector configurations for single-photon emission tomography, including transmission source locations.

automatic systems operate at a distance of 15–20 mm from the body surface. For studies such as brain perfusion imaging, this distance is too large. With experience, an improvement in image quality can be obtained by using a manually set circular orbit. Second, the time taken in setting up the detector orbit should also be considered carefully. The patient should remain motionless throughout the imaging process, and lengthy set-up times will contribute to patient discomfort and increase the likelihood of patient movement artefacts. It should be noted that there are some detector configurations where the operator must maintain a minimum distance between the patient and the detector. This specifically relates to the need to ensure that the radioactive distribution, particularly between the organ under investigation and the detector, remains within the field-of-view throughout the imaging process (Figure 19.2).

These requirements may have to be modified for non-parallel geometries such as Fan-Beam configurations (Figure 19.2b). Here, the detectors do not use body-contouring orbits, but maintain a circular orbit around the patient. For maximum sensitivity the patient is positioned as close to the focal line of the collimator while ensuring that the organ-of-interest remains within the field-of-view in all projections.

DATA SAMPLING ANGLE

The tomographic process requires that data be sampled from all angles around the object. For SPECT, this usually requires measurements from a 360° arc, since measurements from opposed directions do not give the same data due to attenuation and scattering of photons emitted within the body. Opposed projection views are normally combined to compensate in some degree for these effects. However, where the organ-of-interest resides towards one edge of the patient – as with myocardial perfusion imaging – data can adequately be sampled using an 180° arc from the right anterior oblique projection to a left posterior oblique projection. While this technique has been applied to a number of other organs, its routine use is only recommended for studies of the heart. In this context, several studies have concluded that the contrast and resolution of the images are improved for 180° acquisitions, although at the expense of spatial distortion in the reconstructed image (Figure 19.3) [2]. Methods of image interpretation, whether visual or semi-quantitative, include these distortions within the expected normal image.

The acceptance of these effects from 180° acquisitions supports the use of particular configurations for tomographic heart imaging. Two

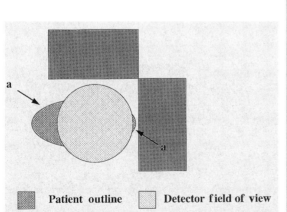

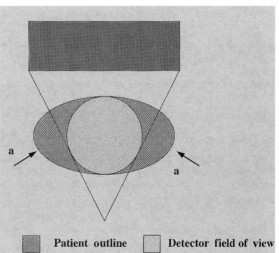

(a)   **(b)**

Figure 19.2 (a) Parallel Hole collimation; (b) Fan-Beam collimation. The patient should remain in the field-of-view at all times. Artefacts may be caused by incomplete sampling due to a limited field-of-view. Areas outside the field-of-view are indicated (a).

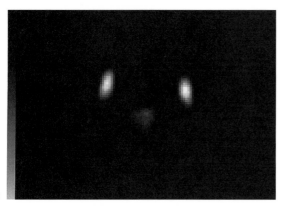

(a)

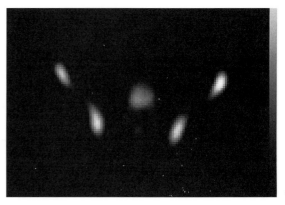

(b)

Figure 19.3 SPECT reconstruction from (a) 180° and (b) 360° showing distortion of the reconstructed data due to incomplete sampling.

Table 19.1 Relative sensitivities of different detector configurations for 180° and 360° rotations

	Sensitivity relative to a single detector	
Configuration	*180°*	*360°*
Single detector	1.0	1.0
Two detectors opposed	1.0	2.0
Two detector right angle	2.0	2.0
Three detectors	1.5	3.0
Four detectors	2.0	4.0

detectors at right-angles or a four-detector square array are optimum. A right-angle configuration further permits the introduction of two radioactive sources for simultaneous measurement of attenuation coefficients. These can all be achieved from a 90° rotation of the gantry, minimizing the time lost in detector motion. Table 19.1 indicates the relative sensitivities of detector configurations for 180° and 360° acquisitions. Systems with variable geometry are available, and allow imaging with two detectors positioned as an opposed pair or at right-angles allowing optimization of study protocols for a range of studies including whole-body planar imaging. It is clearly possible that other, non-orthogonal geometries are possible for such variable geometry systems.

ATTENUATION CORRECTION

The processes of attenuation and scattering of photons within the body are fundamental to the interaction of radiation with matter. Attenuation of photons results in their removal from the imaging process. This attenuation is solely dependent on the physical structure of the body within which the radioactivity is distributed and can therefore be corrected given the availability of a map of the linear attenuation coefficients within the body. This is equivalent to a transmission X-ray CT study of the region-of-interest. CT measurements have been used to correct SPECT data [3]; however, alignment of the two datasets is required. To avoid this added complexity, facilities to perform a low-resolution CT study are being added to the gamma-camera systems, such that both emission and transmission data can be acquired without moving the patient, thus ensuring alignment of the two datasets. Attenuation correction of SPECT studies has typically been performed by assuming a uniform, effective, attenuation coefficient, which is applied post-reconstruction after the delineation of a body outline, usually derived from the edge of the reconstructed image as defined from the scatter distribution in the image. This technique has proved adequate for most clinical studies except where there are significant changes in attenuation coefficients. These include studies in the region of the thorax, the base of the brain and of the legs where both limbs are imaged together having a low attenuation space between two high attenuators. For a reconstruction that does not allow for such changes in attenuation, the result is a significant distortion in the reconstructed images. Quantitative data cannot be obtained without an adequate attenuation correction [4].

Systems currently under commercial development are based on research conducted by a number of groups. Collimated flood sources opposed to a detector with parallel-hole collimation has been proposed [4–6]. This method has not been commercially exploited, primarily due to difficulties in radiation shielding and a higher than necessary radiation burden to the patient. A scanning line source was proposed by Tan *et al.* [7]. Such implementation leads to an insignificant additional dose to the patient. The use of well-shielded solid sources installed within the gantry of the detector ensures no measurable increase in radiation exposure to staff. This technique has been extended on commercial systems to use multiple scanning line sources opposite detectors with parallel-hole collimation (Figure 19.1). For systems which use Fan-Beam collimators, or geometries that do not require a scanning line, a line or a point source can be placed at the focal line or point of the collimator respectively [8]. These systems require no mechanical movement of the source, but often result in limited fields-of-view due to the converging collimator geometry and thus require extreme care during data acquisition and modifications to the reconstruction process to compensate for incomplete data sampling (Figure 19.2).

SCATTER CORRECTION

Scattered photons are those photons that have undergone a Compton scattering event within the patient. These photons lose energy and change direction, yet are detected within the pulse-height analyser window chosen due to the finite energy resolution of NaI. Typically, some 30–50% of the total counts in a SPECT study with ^{99m}Tc are due to scattered photons. Due to the unknown origin of these photons they will be wrongly positioned in the reconstruction process, resulting in a loss of contrast and quantitative accuracy in the transaxial images.

The inclusion of scattered photons in SPECT data renders the attenuation correction methods described above inappropriate, since they assume that no scattered photons are present. It is therefore necessary to apply a scatter correction to the data before attenuation correction. The distribution of scattered photons in the images is dependent on both the attenuation map and the radionuclide distribution. There are two broad classes of correction methods: (i) energy spectrum manipulations; and (ii) pre-reconstruction operations on the projection data and post-processing of the transaxial images.

Energy spectrum manipulations

Since scattered photons lose energy in Compton interactions, an analysis of the pulse-height spectrum during an acquisition may permit the elimination or reduction of scattered photons. In practice, an estimate of the proportion of scattered photons within the photopeak window is required and a correction applied. A reduction of scattered photons can be achieved by using an asymmetric photopeak window. This is a simple and universally available method, although it does require a uniform energy response from the detector to ensure that non-uniformity artefacts are not generated.

Methods of estimating the scatter fraction within the photopeak window include methods based on acquiring data in multiple energy windows. Jaszczak *et al.* [9] introduced a method based on two discrete windows with variations of this method being introduced by King *et al.* [10] and Pretorius *et al.* [11]. Simple spectral modelling based on three energy windows has been proposed by Ichihara *et al.* [12]. Many of these methods have been implemented on commercial systems, although they are not universally available. Considerable effort is being applied for incorporating methods based on a more comprehensive analysis of the pulse-height spectrum. These techniques use many discrete windows, often numbering between 16 and 32 [13,14]. The majority of acquisition interfaces are currently incapable of performing such acquisitions, although the need for accurate scatter correction will promote major changes in this area of SPECT data acquisition hardware.

Pre- or post-reconstruction corrections

These methods provide approximate corrections for scatter within the projection data, and rely upon an analysis of the response of the imaging system to sources at different depths within scatter material. The majority of techniques use data based upon an effective depth for the organ under investigation and then filter the data post-reconstruction, using restoration filters such as

Metz or Weiner [15]. Alternatively, the projection data are convolved with a function to give an estimate of the scatter component, which can then be subtracted from the projection data before reconstruction [16,17].

These methods require pre-calibration of the reconstruction process to generate system- and often organ-specific filters that can be applied to all data without multiple image acquisition. Thus, corrections can be applied retrospectively to any SPECT data and are potentially universally available.

All methods of scatter correction are approximate, although those based on spectral modelling look very promising in delivering a robust method of scatter correction. The clinical evaluation of the impact of attenuation and scatter correction in myocardial perfusion imaging has yet to be completed. It is true to say that, in a small number of patients, the effect of these corrections can be dramatic; however, with an already highly developed technique, significant improvements in clinical outcomes will be hard to quantify, especially as 'gold standards' are often not available for the validation of nuclear medicine studies.

SYSTEM CALIBRATION

The requirements for system calibration can be readily understood in the light of the requirements for SPECT imaging. The tomographic process is based upon a number of fundamental assumptions about the acquisition and reconstruction process. Developments in system calibration and quality control protocols are directed at ensuring that these assumptions are justified. The assumptions can be summarized as follows.

- That the detector, including the digital interface, has a position-independent response to incident radiation. This does not simply imply a uniform response to a uniform source, but a spatially independent energy and spatial resolution and count-rate response. High spatial linearity is required to maintain data alignment.
- That the acquisition angle corresponds to the reconstruction back projection angle. This requires the calibration of a reconstruction parameter which relates the mechanical centre of rotation of the gantry to its projection onto the

planar images and the back projection process – this is often referred to as the centre of rotation calibration.
- That each of the above remain true with rotation and, where the gantry is mobile, the translation of the detection system.

ENERGY RESPONSE

The energy response of gamma-camera systems has improved markedly over the past 10 years. Improvements have been achieved not only in the uniformity of response of the detector to incident radiation, but also to the absolute energy resolution. Energy resolution has improved from approximately 13% at 140 keV to below 9%, and is arguably the most important factor in image quality improvements. An improved energy resolution permits greater rejection of scattered photons, resulting in improved image contrast. An important component of these improvements is the incorporation of an energy correction calibration, resulting in one or more energy correction maps. This calibration may or may not be left to the user. Many systems do require the user to perform this calibration at intervals dependent on the stability of the detector. It may also be integrated with a photomultiplier tuning file to compensate for variations in response due to changes in photomultiplier high-voltage supply and gains. It is essential that the user establishes a calibration schedule based upon the stability of the detector. This should ideally be established during the initial warranty period. Daily quality assurance measures should permit the assessment of the adequacy of the existing correction files.

The energy calibration provides a correction for variations in energy response of the system due primarily to the physical construction of the detector with a discrete photomultiplier array. The correction is applied on a region-by-region basis with energy signals being modified to provide the same response to a monoenergetic source at all positions on the camera face. Since the selection of photons into the imaging process is by pulse-height analysis, this correction has the largest impact of any correction on the uniformity of response of the gamma-camera and hence to providing a spatially independent response.

SPATIAL LINEARITY

Many systems implement a linearity correction map in conjunction with the energy correction map. This map addresses the problem of mispositioning of pulses due to errors within the x and y coordinate position calculations, which in turn are based upon variations in light collection and conversion efficiency within the detector. If the corrections were not applied, images of radioactive line sources would exhibit distortions of 3–4 mm over a 40-cm field-of-view. While this may be acceptable for planar imaging, it is not suitable for tomographic imaging.

This calibration is exclusively in the domain of the manufacturer and may or may not be performed at the site of installation. Its importance must be understood in relation to the requirements for data alignment at acquisition and reconstruction. It can be shown that errors in the alignment of projection data in excess of 1–1.5 mm result in significant degradation of image contrast and resolution. Correctly calibrated detectors are capable of providing a linearity of spatial response within ±0.4 mm over 40 cm. This performance specification enables the requirements for data alignment to be met. Systems that do not meet this specification should be used with care for SPECT imaging.

UNIFORMITY OF SENSITIVITY

Following the application of energy and linearity correction maps, there remain small variations in response of a detector to a uniform source of radioactivity. Typically, these variations are below ±4% and ±3% for integral and differential uniformity respectively, measured to NEMA standards [18]. An analysis of the effects of non-uniformities in response by Gullberg *et al.* [19] led to the recommendation that these should exhibit a standard deviation of less than 1% of the mean. Manufacturers have thus implemented facilities for the use of a uniformity correction based on the response of the detector to uniform irradiation. Typically, this is implemented as a post-acquisition correction often incorporated into the SPECT reconstruction process.

It is necessary to insert a word of caution at this point. The recommendations for uniformity correction were established when detector perform-ance was significantly worse than at present. A more detailed analysis of the factors that effect detector uniformity indicates that if any improvement is to be achieved by the application of a uniformity correction to a modern gamma-camera, then it must be performed under the same conditions as will be encountered in the imaging process. This means that the calibration must be obtained using the same isotope, collimator, count-rate, pulse-height–window setting and scatter component. One could thus argue for a range of corrections, however, the required 'scatter component' is patient-specific and cannot be determined or easily simulated. The routine acquisition of system flood corrections with other than ^{57}Co (solid) and ^{99m}Tc (liquid mixed) sources are prohibited on cost grounds, and the practicalities of disposal of long-lived radionuclides. Acquisitions at count-rates comparable with patient studies may prove impractical due to extended imaging times or impossible within the decay of the radionuclide.

While it is not possible to make a definitive statement, it is necessary to say that, for a modern gamma-camera system, a uniformity correction should be used with care as the process may degrade an image if incorrectly applied.

CENTRE OF ROTATION (COR)

The tomographic reconstruction process has to make an assumption as to which pixel in each of the planar projection profiles is coincident with the point in space about which the detector system rotates. This is a relationship between a mechanical centre of rotation (CoR) and an electronically generated image set. This relationship is influenced by mechanical components such as the gantry rotation mechanism, the directional characteristics of the collimator and the electronic gain and offset adjustments of the image formation process including any analogue-to-digital interfaces. This relationship may be a very simple one expressed as a single value for a detector performing a circular rotation to a very much more complex one where a calibration is required for each projection angle. A particular word of caution is required for multiple detector systems where calibrations are often required for each detector. There is no agreement as to how this information should be encoded within the projection dataset and many of these datasets cannot be reconstructed on other proprietary data processing systems. For instance, datasets with multiple, per projection or per detector calibrations cannot be reconstructed on systems which only allow for a single CoR calibration.

Manufacturers provide protocols for the CoR calibration with recommendations on frequency of performance. In general, this is a very stable calibration and is only significantly affected when the detector head is recalibrated, or when there are electronic failures that affect the position signals from the detectors.

PERFORMANCE EVALUATION

SPECT performance evaluation should be separated from routine detector calibration. Performance evaluation can be used in two ways.

1. To assess the characteristics of a detector system in tomographic mode, which could include spatial resolution, sensitivity, uniformity, reconstructed signal-to-noise ratios, etc.
2. To determine whether the system is performing optimally or whether corrective action is required.

Space does not permit a detailed discussion of the standards for SPECT system characterization. The concepts are derived from the characterization of planar performance and have recently been published by Graham *et al.* [20]. However, it is necessary to highlight a number of useful diagnostic tests which the user may apply to evaluate SPECT functionality.

EVALUATION AT INSTALLATION

The SPECT process assumes that data have been acquired from a unique plane within the patient, i.e. at all angles projection data must be co-planar. This is usually achieved by designing the detection plane to be vertical, parallel to the rotation plane, and perpendicular to the face of the detector. The gantry is installed with the mechanical rotation plane vertical, and SPECT acquisitions performed with the detector adjusted to the horizontal position. The weakest component in this process is the collimator construction. The detection planes are defined by the directions of the holes whether parallel or focused in design. It is

necessary for the user to verify the orthogonal properties of the detection process and the integrity of collimator construction.

These requirements can be easily assessed by performing a series of tomographic measurements with a radioactive point source. A point source can be constructed from an haematocrit glass capillary tube, dipped into a very high specific activity solution of ^{99m}Tc. Capillary action will provide a 3–4 mm column of activity, which can be sealed into the tube with a clay-like material. Tomographic studies should be performed with the point source positioned in air (not resting on an attenuating support such as the patient couch) and offset from the CoR by 15–20 cm. It should however, remain within the field-of-view throughout the tomographic study. The radius of rotation of the detector should be within the range used for clinical studies (i.e. 15–20 cm).

Following the acquisition, the x and y coordinates of the point source in the projection data should be calculated and plotted as shown in Figure 19.4. For an orthogonal system, the y coordinate value (measurement in the direction of the patient axis) should be constant. For multiple detector systems the value should be identical for each detector to ensure correct alignment of data from each head. Errors in this parameter should not exceed 3 mm for a single detector system. For multiple detector systems, this may need to be reduced to 1–2 mm. If a plot of y coordinate against projection angle produces a sinusoidal response, this is evidence of a non-orthogonal detector alignment. A plot of the x coordinate against projection angle should produce a sinusoidal curve, the amplitude of which is proportional to the offset of the point source from the CoR. Subtraction of a 'best fit' sine curve from the data should provide a straight line with a y intercept, which is the CoR calibration value. The residual errors in the values should not exceed ±1–1.5 mm. It is not possible to identify the causes of error in this measurement without further investigation. They may be due to collimator deficiencies, errors in detector motion, linearity correction failures, or even measurement errors. The measurement should be repeated at a number of positions along the patient axis to verify that a single CoR is applicable to all transaxial images. Variations in CoR should not exceed 1–1.5 mm. Variations in CoR with position along the patient axis almost certainly indicate collimator deficiencies requiring

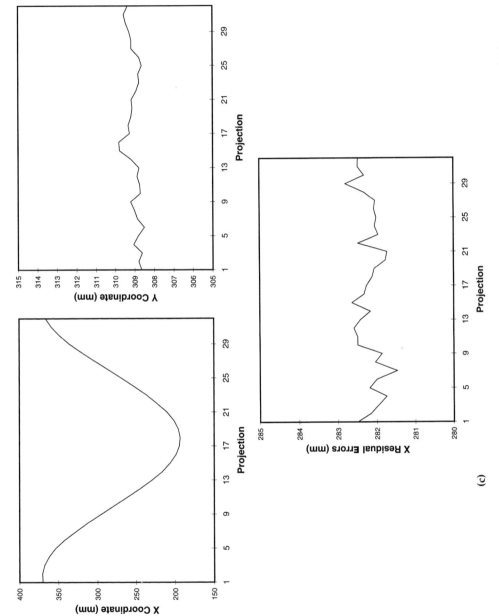

Figure 19.4 Centre of rotation calibration plots. (a) x coordinate; (b) y coordinate; and (c) x coordinate residual errors.

the collimator to be replaced. This measurement can also be used on a regular basis as part of routine quality control protocol.

The final assumption of the tomographic process, that the response of the system remains constant with rotational position, can easily be tested by performing a tomographic study with a source secured to the face of the detector. More than 10K-count should be acquired at each angle. On completion of the study, the total counts in the region of the source should be plotted as a function of rotational position. Following correction for any decay of the source, the observed count-rate should not vary by more than ±1%. There are many factors which can affect this measurement, including environmental electromagnetic field effects, as well as the influence of heat distribution and the Earth's electromagnetic field on the detector. The significance of changes in this measurement should be understood in the light of comments above concerning calibrations for uniformity of response.

ROUTINE EVALUATION PROTOCOL

It is essential that the user implements a daily quality assurance programme to ensure the correct functioning of the SPECT system. The programme should be practical and sensitive to changes in performance that affect SPECT images, and provide action thresholds at which clinical SPECT studies should not be performed until the faults have been corrected [21].

Experience has shown that modern gantry systems are extremely stable and that failures are normally unpredictable. Routine measurements will not help prevent these problems. The most common problems are those related to detector calibration and detector alignment, whether under the control of the operator or robotic systems. Detector alignment can be checked on a patient-by-patient basis using a spirit level once the validity of the adjustment has been determined as described earlier. Issues of detector calibration can be checked either in planar or tomographic mode. A routine measurement of SPECT performance would be ideal, but no practical method has been developed for implementation on a daily basis. The most practical method is to perform a daily planar uniformity measurement. The requirement is to identify changes in response from day to day which may indicate the need for recalibration.

This can be implemented as an intrinsic uniformity measurement using a shielded point source, minimizing radiation exposure to staff as well as cost. This is analogous to a constancy check for a dose calibrator. Trend graphs of integral and differential uniformity as well as detector sensitivity (if a long-lived source is used) can identify sudden as well as progressive failures [22]. This latter aspect permits remedial action to be taken before action thresholds are triggered, thus enabling corrective maintenance to be planned without disruption to clinical services.

This is not a comprehensive system evaluation, and it is essential that planar projection datasets are reviewed to identify failures of the acquisition process.

IMAGE FORMATION

The quality of SPECT data is dependent on many factors. These include the use of the correct detector orbit, the choice of collimator, pixel size, number of projections, pulse-height analyser settings, count density, as well as reconstruction choices such as noise suppression filters, attenuation correction algorithm, reconstructed voxel size and image reorientation angles. In practice, the optimal choices are dependent on each specific patient investigation, clinical problem and detector configuration. It is thus only possible to provide guidelines as to how the correct choices should be made.

ACQUISITION REQUIREMENTS

Patient positioning

As discussed above, it is essential that the detector is correctly positioned in relation to the patient. Resolution sacrificed by the acceptance of poor positioning cannot be recovered during the reconstruction process.

Collimator choice

Where the user is faced with a choice between using a collimator with higher sensitivity but poorer resolution versus one with higher resolution but lower sensitivity, for most routine clinical studies the higher-resolution collimator should be used. The reduced sensitivity may not need to be compensated for with a longer study time, since studies have shown that overall image quality can be maintained even at lower count densities [23].

Spatial sampling

The correct spatial sampling is governed by the collimator choice and the highest spatial resolution thus obtained at the depth of the organ-of-interest. Spatial resolution is defined by the full width at half maximum (FWHM) of a profile drawn across a line source at the relevant camera-to-object distance. For organs such as the brain, this is the resolution at the surface of the head. As a guide, the pixel size should be between the FWHM/2 and the FWHM/3. Finer sampling will provide no greater detail within the reconstructed image; a larger pixel size will result in decreased resolution.

Number of projection angles

The number of projection angles required is theoretically defined by the spatial sampling chosen. The circumferential arc between adjacent projections, measured at the organ-of-interest, should be approximately equal to the pixel size chosen.

$$\text{Number of projections} = 2\pi r / d$$

where r is the distance of the outer edge of the organ from the CoR and d is the pixel size.

For a brain perfusion study where d is set at 4 mm and the radius of the brain is approximately 10 cm, the number of required projections is approximately 176. This is often impractical and fewer projections are used. Degradation of image resolution can be demonstrated in this example below 120 projections.

Energy window settings

For all gamma-camera studies a pulse-height or energy window must be selected. Photons with measured energies within this window are used in the formation of the images. The selection of a pulse-height window is usually expressed as a percentage of the photopeak energy of the radionuclide being imaged, e.g. 20% at 140 keV for ^{99m}Tc. This would provide limits of 126–154 keV. The pulse-height window chosen can have a significant effect upon image contrast. As the width of the pulse-height window is increased, more photons which have undergone a scatter event within the patient will be included. This has the effect of reducing image contrast. The choice of pulse-height window must be related to the energy resolution of the system [24]. As the energy resolution of gamma-cameras is improved, smaller energy windows should be set, typically a 15–17.5% window at 140 keV for a gamma-camera energy resolution of 9–10%. An alternative is to adopt a non-symmetric window where the lower energy window is raised while the upper bound is not reduced [25]. This will permit the rejection of scattered photons but maximize the collection of unscattered photons. Figure 19.5 and Table 19.2 illustrate a number of typical settings and their effect on the upper and lower bounds of the energy window.

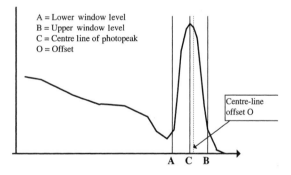

A = Lower window level
B = Upper window level
C = Centre line of photopeak
O = Offset

Centre-line offset O

A   C   B

Figure 19.5 Pulse-height spectrum showing energy window selection settings. (see also Table 19.2)

Table 19.2 Example pulse-height analyser settings for ^{99m}Tc showing the effect of width and offset selection on upper and lower window settings. (See also Figure 19.5)

Energy window width and offset (O)	Lower level (keV) (A)	Upper level (keV) (B)	Centreline (keV) (C)
10% offset 0%	133	147	140
15% offset 0%	129.5	150.5	140
17.5% offset 0%	127.8	152.3	140
20% offset 0%	126	154	140
20% offset 3%	130.2	158.2	144.2

These guidelines apply to radionuclides that decay with the emission of single-energy photons. Where multiple emissions occur, the optimum setting of energy windows is a more complex matter [25]. The measured pulse-height spectrum contains information about both scattered and unscattered photons. Significant progress is being made in the use of spectral analysis techniques to remove the scattered photons from the image formation process.

Count density

The required count density for any particular clinical study is difficult to define. Little evidence exists as to relevant count densities below which clinical diagnosis is compromised. Various guidelines have been produced by special interest groups for particular organ studies and the reader is urged to consult these documents.

PROCESSING METHODS

The most widely used method of image reconstruction in SPECT studies is that of filtered back projection. Under ideal conditions, this is the exact analytical solution to the reconstruction of transaxial sections. However, the non-ideal sampling of the *in vivo* distribution, attenuation, scatter and statistical noise, mean that the process is approximate, although it has proven adequate for most clinical studies. It is known to produce significant errors in studies of the thorax and other areas with large variations in attenuation coefficients. Where an independent measurement of the attenuation map is available, the reconstruction must be performed with an iterative technique. The process involves forming multiple successive estimates of the *in vivo* distribution, which is continued until the estimate produces projection images consistent with the original data. It is possible to incorporate many parameters within this process, including attenuation, scatter and system resolution function. The additional computational resources required for iterative reconstruction can be extremely large. Typically, reconstruction times are 50–1000 times longer than for the equivalent filtered back projection reconstruction.

Noise suppression filters

The filtered back projection method – and often also the iterative technique – require the user to define a noise suppression filter. There are an infi-

nite number of such filters presenting the user with an often confusing problem. There are essentially two classes of filter: first, those that act as low pass filters, suppressing noise above a certain threshold; and second, those that are capable of providing resolution enhancement as well as noise suppression. For each filter definition, the user is required to select one (Hanning filter) or two (Butterworth filter) parameters, which define the amount of smoothing and enhancement to be performed. To ensure uniform noise characterisitics within the three-dimensional reconstructed dataset, the filters should either be applied in two-dimensions to the planar projection images before reconstruction, or preferably in three-dimensionsal post-reconstruction of the transaxial image dataset.

Which filter is optimal is a difficult question to answer. The experiences of others is often a good starting position to adopt; however, the choice of filter is essentially application-dependent. The selection will incorporate considerations of the size of the object under investigation, whether the problem is one of 'cold spot' or 'hot spot' detection and the count statistics in the projection images. Not all filters are implemented on all computer processing systems and the choice may therefore be restricted. In general, the choice should be to use as high frequency a filter as possible within the constraints of the noise present. For studies which are not count-limited, a higher frequency filter can be used. Where studies are to be compared with a 'normal' dataset, the same filtering should be used as was used to establish the 'normal' dataset. While different filters may be used for visual interpretation quantitative studies will require the filter characteristics to be fixed across all studies.

Restoration filters are based on the resolution characteristics of the detection system. These characteristics are dependent on the object-to-camera distance, and thus an approximate filter must be chosen for a particular imaging applications, i.e. a different filter will be used for surface objects such as the skeleton and extended structures such as the liver.

The definition of the 'best' filter could be obtained by undertaking a receiver–operating characteristic (ROC) curve for each particular protocol. This is an extremely time-consuming and often impossible task, and will lead to the use of filters that are specific to each person reporting the images. Experience indicates that most reporters will initially choose a filter which is relatively smooth and progress to a less smooth image as they become more familiar with the noise characteristics of the images. The final filter is often found to be a near-optimal choice.

QUANTIFICATION

The absolute quantification of radionuclide concentrations *in vivo* is dependent on a number of fundamental physical phenomena related to the imaging process. These include a finite system resolution, photon scatter and attenuation and statistical noise. It is also dependent on the reconstruction algorithm used in the SPECT process. It is clear that not all SPECT systems produce the same output for the same input data. These differences are the result of many factors, but essentially point to a lack of validation and verification of software using standard test facilities. These factors continue to impede progress to an absolute measurement from a SPECT study.

The absolute quantification of SPECT data will not necessarily lead directly to improved diagnostic accuracy, as there will still be a need to understand the results of 'normal' anatomy and physiology. This has led to the development of relative quantification techniques based on statistical comparisons with 'normal' datasets where these are generated from a well-characterized group of patients or volunteers.

Relative quantification

The use of relative quantification as an aid to the differentiation of disease processes is dependent on the adoption of standard protocols. This includes all aspects of the imaging process, including radiopharmaceutical, patient preparation, collimation, pixel size, number of projections, reconstruction process and filter, data manipulation and interrogation. This ultimately means that the processes are system- and protocol-specific, and that 'normal' datafiles need to be generated for each system. The system-specific nature of these 'normal' datafiles cannot be over-emphasized. It is essential that any modifications to an existing protocol are carefully validated before routine implementation. What might appear to be an innocuous change to a noise suppression filter may render the 'normal' datafile inappropriate, and would require the 'normal' datafile to be produced with the revised filter and revalidated. This is often a sig-

nificant problem and poses a severe limitation to the development of nuclear medicine, since the replacement of a detector system may render all previous 'normal' datafiles obsolete. Given that a stable routine protocol can be established, the principal persistent problem with this technique is the identification of the correct method for normalization of the 'patient study' to the 'normal' datafile – a selection that is affected by a disease process may lead to the masking of abnormalities.

Despite these limitations, a number of applications have been developed. These include the bull's-eye technique for myocardial imaging [27] and multiple regions-of-interest analysis of cerebral perfusion [28]. Incorporated within the normal file are limitations imposed by the imaging process, including the effects of finite resolution, scatter and attenuation.

Absolute quantification

Where adequate contrast exists within the SPECT data, the absolute quantification of linear size and volume can be performed with considerable accuracy. The limits to this process are the reconstructed resolution and the count statistics. The finite resolution of the imaging process is reflected in the partial volume effect [29] where objects less than twice the FWHM of the reconstructed resolution will appear larger that the actual size. Limited counting statistics will lead to errors in the detection of the edges of count distributions within the images.

The measurement of absolute activity concentrations is dependent not only on partial volume and statistical effects, but also on an adequate correction for photon attenuation and scatter. As already discussed, these corrections will be dependent on the implementation of iterative reconstruction methods enabling the whole imaging process to be modelled. Considerable development is taking place in this area and careful studies show that accuracies in excess of 95% may be obtained in many applications [4].

IMAGE INTERPRETATION AND ARTEFACTS

The interpretation of SPECT images, whether using visual, qualitative or quantitative methods requires a careful assessment of the adequacy of the acquired data. An essential discipline in the reporting of SPECT data is to establish a clinical quality control process whereby the data are evaluated for patient or organ motion during the study. The data should also be evaluated for other technical failures during the process, such as misaligned detectors in multiple detector systems, incorrect CoR calibrations, or the failure to maintain the patient within the field-of-view throughout the acquisition process. Another factor that can affect the reconstructed data is the inclusion within the field-of-view of high concentrations of radioactivity due to an extravasated injection or external contamination on the patient. This can completely invalidate the reconstructed data, especially if the radioactive source lies in the plane of the organ-of-interest. The SPECT process assumes that the distribution does not change during acquisition. This should be verified before reconstruction by displaying the projection data as a cine loop. Various acquisition protocols can be adopted to minimize this effect if it is known that it is likely to occur as, for example, with studies of the pelvis where the urinary bladder may significantly accumulate excreted radioactivity during the study. The most effective method to eliminate this effect is to perform multiple, rapid 360° samples of the data which can be combined before reconstruction.

Problems in interpretation can also be encountered due to anatomical variations and these are often organ-specific. Such effects include breast and diaphragmatic attenuation in myocardial perfusion studies, which can again be evaluated by viewing the projection data as a cine loop to evaluate the anatomical components of the study.

It is true to say that there are very few occasions where rigorous post-acquisition corrections are available for problems encountered during the acquisition process. Studies where technical problems are suspected should be interpreted with care.

Image re-orientation

Provided that an adequate dataset has been acquired, interpretation is dependent on the generation of relevant section images. This often requires a re-orientation of the reconstructed transverse section dataset to produce what are referred to as oblique sections. This may be required to correct for inaccuracies in patient positioning, or more likely to produce a standard projection orientation to correct for anatomical variations. For many SPECT systems this is a manual process requiring the operator to select the modified reconstruction planes. Errors of a few degrees in the choice of these axes may lead to apparent abnormalities in the images and methods should be in place to evaluate this re-orientation process. Where automatic algorithms are available, these should be reviewed on a case-by-case basis, especially as the algorithms will fail as the distribution deviates further and further from the expected distribution. The introduction of automatic re-orientation algorithms will lead to more reproducible SPECT analysis protocols producing a much less operator-dependent process.

CONCLUDING REMARKS

The optimization of SPECT is a continual process. It is extremely difficult to identify one factor which, above all others, will result in high-quality imaging. Care is required at each stage to maximize the information content in the final images. There are clear limits within the process. Injected dose and an imaging time giving a low probability of patient motion set an envelope within which the requirements of adequate statistics and spatial sampling must be set. The user has particular control over the proximity of the detector to the patient during the imaging process. This is probably the most important factor in the SPECT process. Where gamma-camera systems offer automatic orbit contouring, it may even be appropriate to bypass this feature to improve the detector proximity to the patient, especially when imaging the brain.

The current emphasis on the implementation of rigorous attenuation and scatter correction, especially in myocardial perfusion imaging and studies in the thorax, represents a potential major advance in SPECT imaging. Absolute quantification of radiopharmaceutical distributions will renew interest in the investigation of physiological function *in vivo* and lead to the development of dynamic SPECT technology.

REFERENCES

1. Anger, H.O. (1985) Scintillation Camera. *Rev. Scient. Inst.*, **29**, 27–33.
2. Eisner, R.L., Nowak, D.J., Pettigrew, R. and Fajman, W. (1986) Fundamentals of 180 degree acquisition and reconstruction in SPECT imaging. *J. Nucl. Med.*, **27**, 1717–28.

3. Fleming, J.S. (1989) A technique using CT images in attenuation correction and quantification in SPECT. *Nucl. Med. Commun.*, **10**, 83–97.

4. Bailey, D.L., Hutton, B.F. and Walker, B.J. (1987) Improved SPECT using simultaneous emission and transmission tomography. *J. Nucl. Med.*, **28**, 844–51.

5. Malko, J.A., Van-Heertum, R.L., Gullberg, G.T. and Kowalsky, W.P. (1986) SPECT liver imaging using an iterative attenuation correction algorithm and an external flood source. *J. Nucl. Med.*, **27**, 701–5.

6. Tsui, B.M., Gullberg, G.T., Edgerton, E.R., Ballard, J.G., Perry, J.R., McCartney, W.H. and Berg, J. (1989) Correction of non-uniform attenuation in cardiac SPECT imaging. *J. Nucl. Med.*, **30**, 497–507.

7. Tan, P., Bailey, D.L., Meikle, S.R., Eberl, S., Fulton, R.L. and Hutton, B.F. (1993) A scanning line source for simultaneous emission and transmission measurements in SPECT. *J. Nucl. Med.*, **34**, 1752–60.

8. Jaszczak, R.J., Gilland, D.R., Hanson, M.W., Jang, S., Greer, K.L. and Coleman, R.E. (1993) Fast transmission CT for determining attenuation maps using a collimated line source, rotatable air-copper-lead attenuators and fan beam collimation. *J. Nucl. Med.*, **34**, 1577–86.

9. Jaszczak, R.J., Greer, K.L., Floyd, C.E., Harris, C.C. and Coleman, R.E. (1983) Improved SPECT quantification using compensation for scattered photons. *J. Nucl. Med.*, **25**, 893–900.

10. King, M.A., Hademenos, G. and Glick, S.J. (1992) A dual photopeak window method for scatter correction. *J. Nucl. Med.*, **33**, 605–12.

11. Pretorius, P.H., van Rensberg, A.J., van Aswegen, A., Lötter, M.G., Serfontein, D.E. and Herbst, C.P. (1993) The channel ratio method of scatter correction for radionuclide image quantitation. *J. Nucl. Med.*, **34**, 330–5.

12. Ichihara, T., Ogawa, K., Motomura, N., Kubo, A. and Hasimoto, S. (1993) Compton scatter compensation using triple energy window method for single and dual isotope SPECT. *J. Nucl. Med.*, **34**, 2216–21.

13. Gagnon, D., Todd-Pokropek, A., Arsneault, A. and Dupras, G. (1989) Introduction to holospectral imaging in nuclear medicine for scatter subtraction. *IEEE Trans. Med. Imag.*, **TMI-8**, 245–50.

14. DeVito, R.P., Hamill, J.J., Trefert, J.D. and Stoub, E.W. (1989) Energy weighted acquisition of scintigraphic images using finite spatial filters. *J. Nucl. Med.*, **30**, 2029–35.

15. King, M.A., Schwinger, R.B., Doherty, P.W. and Penny, B.C. (1984) Two-dimensional filtering of SPECT images using Metz and Weiner filters. *J. Nucl. Med.*, **25**, 1234–40.

16. Axelsson, B., Msaki, P. and Israelsson, A. (1984) Subtraction of Compton scattered photons in single photon emission computerized tomography. *J. Nucl. Med.*, **25**, 490–4.

17. Masaki, P., Axelsson, B., Dahl, C.M. and Larsson, S.A. (1987) Generalized scatter correction method in SPECT using point source scatter distribution functions. *J. Nucl. Med.*, **28**, 1861–9.

18. NEMA Standards Publication NU 1-1994. Published by National Electrical Manufacturers Association 2101 L Street, NW, Washington, DC 20037.

19. Gullberg, G.T. (1987) An analytical approach to quantify uniformity artefacts for circular and non-circular detector motion in single photon emission computed tomography imaging. *Med. Phys.*, **14**, 105–14.

20. Graham, L.S., Fahey, F.H., Madsen, M.T., van Aswegen, A. and Yester, M.V. (1995) Quantitation of SPECT performance: Report of Task Group 4 Nuclear Medicine Committee. *Med. Phys.*, **22**, 401–9.

21. Young, K.C., Kouris, K., Awdeh, M. and Abdel-Dayem, H.M. (1990) Reproducibility and action levels for gamma camera uniformity. *Nucl. Med. Commun.*, **11**, 95–101.

22. Knight, A.C. and Williams, E.D. (1992) An evaluation of cusum analysis and control charts applied to quantitative gamma-camera uniformity parameters for automated quality control. *Eur. J. Nucl. Med.*, **19**, 125–30.

23. Muehllehner, G. (1985) Effect of resolution improvement on required count density in ECT imaging: a computer simulation. *Phys. Med. Biol.*, **30**, 163–73.

24. Kojima, A., Matsumoto, M., Takahashi, M. and Uehara, S. (1993) Effect of energy resolution on scatter fraction in scintigraphic imaging: Monte Carlo study. *Med. Phys.*, **20**, 1107–13.

25. Koral, K.F., Clinthorpe, N.H. and Roger, W.L. (1986) Improving emission-computed tomography quantification by Compton-scatter rejection throughout offset windows. *Nucl. Instr. Meth. Phys. Res.*, **A242**, 610–14.

26. Li, J., Tsui, B.M., Welch, A., Frey, E.C. and Gullberg, G.T. (1995) Energy window optimization in simultaneous technetium-99m TCT and thallium-201 SPECT data acquisition. *IEEE Trans. Nucl. Sci.*, **42**, 1207–13.

27. Garcia, E.V., DePuey, E.G. and De Pasquale, E.E. (1987) Quantitative planar and tomographic thallium-201 myocardial perfusion imaging. *Cardiovasc. Intervent. Radiol.*, **10**, 374–83.

28. Claus, J.J., van Harskamp, F., Bretler, M.M.B., Krenning, E.P., van der Cammen, T.J.M., Hofman, A. and Hasan, D. (1994) Assessment of cerebral perfusion with single-photon emission tomography in normal subjects and in patients with Alzheimer's disease: effects of region of interest selection. *Eur. J. Nucl. Med.*, **21**, 1044–51.

29. Hoffman, E.J. and Phelps, M.E. (1986) Positron emission tomography: principles and quantitation in *Positron Emission Tomography and Autoradiography: Principles and Applications for the Brain and Heart* (eds M. Phelps, J. Mazziotta and H. Schelbert), Raven Press, New York, pp. 273–6.

FURTHER READING

King, M.A., Tsui, B.M.W. and Tin-Su, Pan (1995) Attenuation compensation for cardiac single photon emission computed tomographic imaging: Part 1. Impact of attenuation and methods of estimating attenuation maps. *J. Nucl. Cardiol.*, **2**, 513–24.

Murray, I.P.C. and Ell, P.J. (eds) *Nuclear Medicine*

in *Clinical Diagnosis and Treatment*, Churchill
Livingstone, Edinburgh, ISBN 0 443 04710 3.

Rosenthal, M.S., Cullom, J., Hawkins, W., Moore, S.C.,
Tsui, B.M.W. and Yester, M. (1995) Quantitative
SPECT Imaging, a review and recommendations by
the Focus Committee of the Society of Nuclear Medi-
cine Computer and Instrumentation Council. *J. Nucl.
Med.*, **36**, 1489–513.

Image registration

D. J. Hawkes

INTRODUCTION

Image registration has emerged as an important application of computational methodology in medical imaging, and particularly so in nuclear medicine. The process allows information derived from one imaging source to be related to information from another. In other application areas such as surveillance, defence and remote sensing this combination of information is often termed 'data fusion'. Image registration methodologies are also being applied to areas of medicine using technologies of virtual reality, augmented reality and telepresence in, for example, image-guided surgery and other interventions.

The purpose of this chapter is to provide a review of the different methods available to solve the registration problem, to outline briefly the range of applications to which this methodology has been applied and, most importantly, what attempts have been made to validate the various approaches for different applications. Practical suggestions gleaned from the author's experiences on 'how to do it' will be described and, finally, as the general area of data fusion is developing rapidly, pointers to future developments will be provided.

Image registration or matching methodology has three broad areas of application in medical imaging.

1. Combination of information on one subject from multiple imaging sources acquired at different times. The images are usually three-dimensional (3D). While common information in these sources is used to establish a single coordinate system, it is the complementary information that leads to a more detailed understanding of the subject's anatomy, physiology and any pathology. The 3D image registration processes is usually restricted to rigid body motion. Rigid body motion, as the name implies, assumes that the subject does not change shape or size between images. The transformation between a coordinate system of the two 3D images can then be described by just six parameters; namely, translations in the three or four orthogonal axes and rotations about these three axes. This also implies that the scale of the image is correct, i.e. the voxel dimensions are known, and that the axes of the 3D image are truly orthogonal to each other, i.e. that the gantry tilt of the X-ray CT scanner for example is accurately known.

2. Labelling of the anatomy in the images by matching to an anatomical model or atlas derived from another individual. In this case, deformation of either the atlas or the image is needed to compensate for the expected range of individual anatomical variation. Detailed labelled 3D digital atlases are becoming available but these are usually derived from one individual. An exception is the atlas produced by the Montreal group [1] which is averaged over many individuals. More details are given later in the chapter. The major problem in defining a deformation between an atlas and an individual scan is that in principle any image can be deformed into any other, as graphically demonstrated in the application of warping techniques in the film industry. Effective constraints need to be applied for the match to have any physical or anatomical meaning. Statistical methods that assess the range of variation expected between individuals are becoming available and are also outlined later in this chapter.

3. Establishing the pose of the 3D representation of the patient for surgical or other therapeutic interventions. The pose can be determined by matching two-dimensional (2D) images acquired as part of the procedure. Examples include X-ray projections, video images or slices from ultrasound, CT or interventional MR. Applications include radiotherapy, image-guided neurosurgery, minimally invasive or 'key-hole' surgery, orthopaedic surgery and interventional radiology. Nuclear medicine images are only rarely acquired during

Clinical Nuclear Medicine, 3rd edn. Edited by M.N. Maisey, K.E. Britton and B.D. Collier. Published in 1998 by Chapman & Hall, London. ISBN 0 412 75180 1

interventional work, primarily because of the requirements for precise spatial information in image-guided interventions and the relatively long acquisition times, although special-purpose probes have been proposed [2]. Nuclear medicine imaging information can, however, provide useful information in constructing the 3D representations used in image guidance.

METHODS
TWO-DIMENSIONAL RIGID BODY

Although most images are still stored and viewed as 2D projections or slices, 2D image registration is of limited value. The human body is a 3D structure and it is rare that image acquisition protocols are sufficiently constrained so that registration in 2D is sufficient to establish correspondence. One exception has been work investigating injury to the wrist. In this method, the hand is constrained to be in the same position for both the radiograph and a 2D image of ^{99m}Tc-MDP distribution. If image scaling is known, there are three degrees of freedom of registration – two translations and one rotation. These are determined from the location of three landmarks attached to the hand. Overlay of the X-ray image on the isotope image provides accurate anatomical localization of any region of abnormal uptake. This has proved to be particularly useful in the assessment of suspected scaphoid fractures [3]. Plate 29 shows an example image of a patient with a suspected scaphoid fracture. Image registration has located the region of increased uptake over the site of the fracture on the radiograph.

THREE-DIMENSIONAL RIGID BODY REGISTRATION

This is the simplest registration paradigm and is by far the most widely used, in particular for images of the head. The skull effectively constrains movements and changes in shape of the brain, and the rigid body transformation is a reasonable approximation to within the resolution of imaging devices used. In the remainder of the body the 3D rigid body transformation is generally a poor approximation except in regions that can be considered locally rigid, such as parts of the pelvis and spine, or when other precautions are taken such as in gating acquisitions to heart rate or breathing for images within the thorax.

TRANSFORMATION

The coordinate transformation can be expressed by a 3×3 rotation matrix and a translation vector or by a single 4×4 matrix in homogeneous coordinates, **U**. The value of each point y in a destination image is computed from the coordinate **x** in the source image by:

$$\mathbf{x}^T = \mathbf{U}^{-1}\mathbf{y}^T$$

As a transformation is very unlikely to map one set of voxels directly over the other set for all locations in the image, this process will require interpolation. The simplest but least accurate is nearest neighbour, the value of the voxel nearest to the coordinates given by $\mathbf{x}^T$ are computed. Usually, however, tri-linear interpolation between the eight nearest neighbours is used but this too can lead to errors in intensity values of a few per cent near sharp boundaries. Higher-order quadratic or cubic interpolation schemes may also be used, at the expense of processing time. The most accurate is *sinc* interpolation, which preserves potentially all information during the transformation process [4,5], but is expensive in computer time. Usually, nearest neighbour or tri-linear interpolation is used in multi-modal work while sinc interpolation is used for applications where the highest accuracy is required, for example in the assessment of very small changes over time using multiple images from the same modality.

In certain circumstances, for example image-guided surgery, it may be sufficient simply to compute the transformations of single points and display their location. Viewing tools could be devised that display orthogonal sections through corresponding points in the two image volumes in their original orientation. However, in general, the complete 3D volume is transformed.

The choice of which image to transform can be important. If a magnetic resonance (MR) image is transformed to PET coordinates then there will be a considerable loss of spatial resolution unless the PET image is sub-sampled. If the PET image is transformed to MR coordinates, then there will be an increase in the volume of the combined data set, and care must be taken to preserve any quantitative intensity information in the original PET image. If the image intensity represents isotope activity per voxel of the original image, and this information is to be preserved, then intensity re-scaling in proportion to the transformed image voxel size is necessary.

METHODS OF 3D RIGID BODY IMAGE REGISTRATION

INTERACTIVE REGISTRATION

The most intuitive method is to re-align interactively the images as they are displayed on the workstation. As registration is a 3D process, care must be taken to establish good registration over the whole volume and not just on a single slice. Therefore, displays that sample the whole volume are used – for example three orthogonal cuts through the volume. Pietzryck *et al.* [6] have reported a technique which first extracts the location of edges of high-intensity gradient. These edges tend to correspond to the boundaries of anatomical structures. This edge image is sparse and therefore can be transformed rapidly, allowing interactive relocation of the edges over the other image.

We have implemented a similar scheme of interactive registration, but by exploiting improved computing power, we can re-compute the complete orthogonal slice image intensity data at each trial. We have found the technique useful for establishing reasonable starting estimates for other more automated methods, but many observers find interactive re-orientation in 3D a difficult task.

EXTERNAL FIDUCIAL MARKERS

A large number of methods have been reported which make use of the location of markers attached to the patient and visible in each modality. Markers can be attached to the skin [7] or using stereotactic frames or similar head-holders or clamps [8,9]. All these approaches have significant problems in that the skin surface can distort or move between scans, and markers can easily be displaced between scans, in particular when there is a significant inter-scan period. Relocatable markers positioned on indelible ink markers on the skin are unlikely to be sufficiently accurate. Markers attached to a frame, which is in turn fixed to a bite block moulded to the patient's upper teeth, have been used successfully in radiotherapy

[10]. Markers screwed into the bone of the skull or attached rigidly to the stereotactic frame used in stereotactic biopsy, tumour resection, electrode placement, other surgery or radiotherapy provide the most accurate registration. Such systems provide the most reliable 'gold standard' against which other methods can be tested, but have a disadvantage of invasiveness leading to discomfort, unless the patient is anaesthetized. These systems also pose a potential risk of infection. The Vanderbilt study [11] of image registration accuracy was based on markers drilled into the skull. The registration process relies on determination of point coordinates in the 3D images. This is best achieved, not by using a very small marker, but by using markers that are much larger than the voxel sizes of the coarsest sampled image, and computing the centre of gravity of the intensity distribution over all the voxels of the image of the marker. Great care has to be taken to remove the effect of any background image intensity. The distribution of material that gives image contrast must be the same for each modality.

Interactive location of three non-co-linear pairs of corresponding points in the two image volumes is sufficient to compute a rigid body registration transformation. In practice, there is always some error associated with identifying corresponding points. If this error is largely random, then identifying a larger number of corresponding points will improve our estimate of the transformation.

The transformation from corresponding point locations can be calculated directly using the Procustes method [12], which was applied to medical images by Arun *et al.* [13]. The centroid of point distribution is computed for each of the corresponding point lists. Rotation about the centroid to minimize the sum of the squared displacements between coordinates in one modality and transformed points in the other is calculated using single-value decomposition. The displacements of the centroids yields the translation vector. When computing the total transformation it is important to remember that rotation and translation transformations do not commute. Computing moments about the centroids yields a single homogeneous scaling factor. This is usually done purely as a check of voxel coordinates delivered by the scanner, which in turn should be checked as part of routine quality assurance.

INTERACTIVELY IDENTIFIED ANATOMICAL LANDMARKS

External fiducials are usually either too invasive or of insufficient accuracy. They also require a decision to have been made before scanning that the images need to be registered. This is not always convenient nor possible in many clinical scenarios. Internal corresponding landmarks were used effectively to register MR and PET images of the head [7], while Hill *et al.* [14] have successfully registered MR and CT images of the head. In both applications between 12 and 16 corresponding pairs of points were identified. With the MR and PET application, inter- and intra-observer reproducibility for identifying point landmarks was about 4 mm. This gives a typical registration accuracy, for 12 points located on the surface of a sphere, of 2 mm at the centroid, rising to 2.8 mm on the surface of the sphere – assuming negligible systematic errors. For MR and CT image registration, point location reproducibility is typically 1–2 mm, which would yield a typical registration accuracy, in the absence of systematic errors of 0.5–1 mm at the centroid and 0.7–1.4 mm on the surface of the sphere.

For a fixed distribution of points these errors reduce as the square root of the number of points selected. The error on the rotation vector is dependent on the point distribution. The points should be distributed so that their centroid corresponds to the region where registration is most critical but, to reduce rotation errors, the points should be distributed as far from this centroid as possible, provided that this does not place the points in regions where significant errors are introduced by image distortion. Research into automated methods for finding point landmarks is underway but as yet no robust methods applicable to multi-modal image registration have been described.

Interactively identified corresponding point landmarks have been used successively to register PET and MR images of the head in studies of brain function (Plate 30); the maxillofacial region to locate regions of high ^{18}F-FDG uptake in the head and neck (Plate 31) [15]; and for registering CT and PET images of the pelvis in assessing tumour spread in cervical carcinoma (Plate 32). Outside the brain, the uptake of ^{18}F-FDG is low and the PET image contains very little anatomical information. To assist in the registration process in studies of the pelvis we routinely inject 350 MBq of ^{18}F fluoride, which provides a bone image with sufficient contrast to identify landmarks. Anatomical landmark-based registration has also been used to register gated MR and ^{99m}Tc-sestamibi images of the heart [16] to relate contractility and perfusion. Fleming has described registration of SPECT and CT images of the liver to improve attenuation correction and quantitation [17].

SURFACE MATCHING

Interactive methods are time consuming and can be prone to user error, particularly in inexperienced hands. This has led to significant efforts in the past few years to develop fully automated methods for image registration.

In their so-called 'head and hat' algorithm Pelizzari *et al.* [18] produced the first system that worked reasonably reliably on real clinical image data. Their method was devised – again for neurological applications – in particular for the registration of MR, PET and CT scans. Corresponding surfaces such as the skin surface or the brain surface are defined – usually by interactive delineation or by defining intensity thresholds corresponding to the surface. One surface is deemed to be the 'head', and the other the 'hat'. Rays are cast from each point from the hat to the centroid of the head points and the distance along each ray to the 'head' surface is computed. Registration then proceeds by minimizing the sum of squares of these distances in an iterative process, akin to fitting a 'hat' to a 'head'. Powell optimization is used in this process. The technique has been used widely and effectively and validation results in the Vanderbilt study [11] (see below) were encouraging. The method has been extended to SPECT and MR studies of the heart by Faber *et al.* [19].

Jiang *et al.* [20] described a closely related method but used a modified distance transformation to compute the separation in the two surfaces. They also modified the distance transform as the registration process proceeded to improve robustness, accuracy and speed. The algorithm is incorporated in the Mayo Clinic's Analyze package [21] which is widely available and in common use.

Both methods are reliant on the accuracy of surface delineation. This delineation is subject to error due to limitations in image contrast and image artefact and lack of correspondence of the surface seen in the two modalities. For example, the location of the outer surface of the brain in PET is very dependent on the intensity threshold chosen. The outer surface of the brain in MR imaging does not correspond exactly to the inner surface of the skull in CT. In addition, many anatomical structures show high degrees of symmetry about certain axes – for example the upper surface of the brain has an axis of near symmetry to craniocaudal rotation. In particular, for small scanned volumes this can lead to erroneous minima of the distance function far from true registration. Hill *et al.* [22] have shown how modifications of the distance function – in the light of anatomical knowledge of the likely distance between adjacent surfaces, might be used to improve the robustness and accuracy of image registration, but this method is difficult to apply in practice. Finally, surface registration uses only a very small proportion of the available data in the registration process. Other potentially useful information is discarded.

Malandain *et al.* [23] have described registration algorithms based on the geometric properties of surfaces, particularly the location of ridges or crest lines. Once the surface is delineated and the crest lines extracted, the registration process is fast. Encouraging results have been shown for the whole-head, high-resolution CT and MR images [23], but results in the Vanderbilt evaluation study were disappointing [11].

Other hybrid feature based methods based on points, lines, planes and/or surfaces have been reported but they tend to be rather *ad hoc* being geared to particular applications and have not found widespread acceptance.

Where complete anatomical features are visible in each modality, alignment of the principal axes, using the moments of the object, has been reported [24]. Unfortunately, medical images are usually heavily truncated, to focus on the region of clinical interest, and the principal axes difficult to compute. The method is highly dependent upon accurate boundary delineation.

VOXEL SIMILARITY MEASURES

Image registration by correlation of image intensities has been proposed as a method of image registration [25]. Unfortunately, for multimodal work, there is little if any linear relationships between image intensities. Correlation methods have, however, proved to be very useful when attempting registration of two (or more) volumes acquired on the same patient, at different times, using the same image modality. This is particularly relevant in MR imaging when assessing tumour growth over a long period or in assessing neurological function or activation [4,5].

Woods *et al.* [26,27] proposed a method in which the standard deviation of intensity ratios between two modalities is minimized. Originally, they developed a method for registering multiple PET studies from the same individual [27]. They subsequently showed that, by recomputing the ratio over a number of narrow bands of image intensities from one of the modalities, they could register PET and MR images of the brain after segmenting the brain from the skull, scalp and other extracranial features [27].

The UMDS group have explored this and other so-called voxel similarity methods [28]. First, they generated plots of image intensity of one modality versus another at registration and a series of mis-registrations. An example of such plots or 'feature spaces' for registration and a range of mis-registrations for MR and PET images of the head is shown in Figure 19.6. There is a striking 'signature' at registration that changes and disperses as the two images are mis-registered. In the plot at registration in this example the regions corresponding to scalp, skull, grey matter and white matter can be clearly identified. These plots show that, in general, there is not a simple linear relationship between the image intensity in one modality and the intensity in the other. However, in certain regions of the feature space plot, linear relationships do exist. Van den Elsen *et al.* [29] exploited this finding to automate registration of MR and CT images of the head. In regions containing bone, there is an inverse relationship between CT and MR image intensities. Other measures include moments and in particular the third order moment of the histogram of the feature space [28].

Of significant current interest is the use of measures based on information theory. The joint entropy of image intensities has been proposed as a suitable measure for registration [30,31]. Collignon *et al.* [32] and Wells *et al.* [33] independently proposed the measure of mutual information.

Joint entropy provides a measure of the information in the combined images. At registration, there should be a minimum of this function. For example, the combined image might contain two eyes and two ears while at mis-registration there might be four eyes and four ears. Unfortunately, this measure is not particularly robust as the algorithm will favour situations that minimize the total information. For example, this will occur purely by overlaying background regions of air outside the patient. The solution is to maximize the difference between the information in the overlapping volumes of the individual images and the information in the combined image. Such a measure is provided by mutual information. Formally, given a pair of images to register and a transformation mapping one set of voxels onto the other, we can find, for corresponding voxels in the volume of overlap of the two images, the intensities $x \in X$ in one image and intensities $y \in Y$ in the other, where X and Y are the sets of all intensity values present in the region of overlap of the two images. Additionally, we can calculate the probability of occurrence of individual intensities $p\{x\}$ and $p\{y\}$ and corresponding intensity pairs $p\{x,y\}$. The mutual information, $I(X;Y)$ is derived from the difference between the sum of the individual entropies $H(X)$ and $H(Y)$ and the joint entropy $H(X,Y)$ of the sets of intensities X and Y. $I(X;Y)$ is given by:

$$I(X;Y) = H(X) + H(Y) - H(X,Y)$$

The individual entropies $H(X)$ and $H(Y)$ are derived from the probabilities of each intensity $p\{x\}$ and $p\{y\}$:

$$H(X) = -\sum_{x \in X} p\{x\} \log p\{x\}$$
$$H(Y) = -\sum_{y \in Y} p\{y\} \log p\{y\}$$

The combined entropy $H(X,Y)$ is given by the probability of occurrence of pairs of intensities $p(x,y)$:

$$H(X,Y) = -\sum_{x \in X} \sum_{y \in Y} p\{x,y\} \log p\{x,y\}$$

The probabilities $p\{x\}$ and $p\{y\}$ are estimated for the histogram of image intensities in the overlapping volume of the two images, and the joint probability $p\{x,y\}$ by the 2D distribution of image intensities from the combined image. The latter is sometimes termed the intensity feature space. Using these probabilities, $I(X;Y)$ can be re-written as:

$$I(X;Y) = \sum_{x \in X} \sum_{y \in Y} p\{x,y\} \log\left(p\{x,y\}/p\{x\}p\{y\}\right)$$

The process of registration is to find the transformation of the coordinate system of one of the images that maximizes $I(X;Y)$.

Mutual information is a measure of the information that is common to two (or more) data sources. It is a measure of how much one data source 'explains' the other, yet it makes no assumption of the functional form of the relationship between two data sources.

This measure has proved to be very successful in a wide range of medical imaging applications.

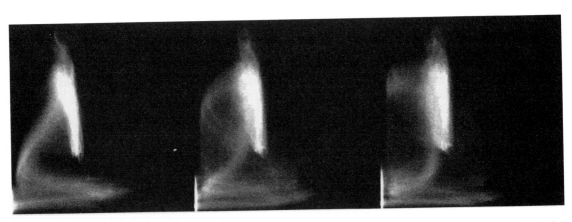

Figure 19.6 Two-dimensional histograms (or joint probability distributions) of voxel intensity at registration (right) and lateral mis-registration by 4 mm (middle) and 10 mm (left). The y-axes represent ^{18}F-FDG-PET image intensity and the x-axes represent MR image intensity. The grey value represents the number (or probability) of voxels in the combined volume having that particular pair of image intensities.

Robust algorithms are now available for registering MR and CT images of the head [34] and MR and PET images of the head [35] without resource to any prior delineation or segmentation of structures. The algorithm is now being extended to other parts of the body [36] and to encompass scaling and skew errors in the image data [37] and deforming structures.

A comparison of a range of voxel similarity methods showed that the mutual information measure performs consistently very well when registering MR and PET images of the head as well as in other applications. The variance of intensity ratios methods also performed well for the MR and PET application [35].

A recent accuracy study conducted by the Vanderbilt group [11] showed that algorithms based on mutual information implemented by two groups [32,34,35] provided reliable registration of MR and PET images of the head which were accurate to between 2.1 and 3.6 mm (median error) as measured at 10 regions selected over the volume of the head. The results were compared with registrations obtained using marker pins embedded in the skull. The estimated accuracy of the 'gold standard' registration was 1.7 mm. The registration using the automated algorithms were undertaken blind by removing the markers from the images distributed for the study. Plate 33 shows an example set of images showing the results of a fully automated registration of MR and PET images of the head using mutual information as a measure of misregistration. The MR voxel sizes were $1.3 \times 1.3 \times 4.0 \text{ mm}^3$ and the PET voxel sizes were $2.6 \times 2.6 \times 8.0 \text{ mm}^3$.

Automated registration using mutual information has also been applied to ^{99m}Tc-HMPAO SPECT images and MR images. Plate 34 shows a registered pair of images taken in a study of brainstem activity.

INTRA-MODALITY REGISTRATION

Accurate registration of images of the same subject taken at different times with the same imaging protocol can permit assessment of subtle changes such as response to therapy over long periods or response to stimulus over very short periods, as in neuroactivation studies. To maximize sensitivity to change, estimation of the transformation parameters and the transformation itself must be

very accurate. The sum of the absolute difference, sum of squared differences or the number of sign changes in difference images have been used to determine registration but are prone to errors in intensity scaling. The most commonly used measures are cross-correlation and voxel intensity ratios [26]. Mutual information can be used and should be equivalent to cross-correlation as a registration measure. Registration to sub-voxel accuracy is possible, assuming that the rigid-body assumption is valid. For accurate assessment of change, the transformation process must be as accurate as possible. Hajnal *et al.* [5] and Hill *et al.* [4] have both shown that, for MR images, interpolation using a sinc function should be used. As images are limited in spatial extent, an appropriate apodizing function should be used in conjunction with the sinc function. While less of a problem for over-sampled nuclear medicine images, which have relatively poorer resolution and signal-to-noise ratio, interpolation errors can still dominate unless care is taken.

LIMITS TO IMAGE INTEGRITY

SCALE AND SKEW

Registration confined to calculation of the six parameters of rigid-body registration (three rotations and three translations) assumes that the voxel data set provided by each scanner is accurately sampled on an orthogonal grid and that the sampling interval, or voxel dimensions are accurately known. Accurate calibration of the imaging system with appropriate phantoms should permit measurement of voxel dimensions and any deviation from an orthogonal coordinate system. These phantom measurements must be performed accurately as current registration algorithms are capable of registration accuracies of 1–2 mm which is less than 1% of the field-of-view. In other words, scaling errors >1% can easily dominate errors in registration. Routine quality assurance procedures should be performed to maintain calibration. These should be performed on a regular basis, and in particular after every service or maintenance work done on the scanners.

Care must be taken to ensure that voxel dimensions are known for the imaging protocols used in registration studies. Significant skew of image axes is unlikely to occur in well-maintained scanners, except in CT where gantry tilt can be adjusted. Scans acquired with a gantry tilt will produce volumes with skewed axes. The angle of tilt is usually accurately recorded and readily available in the non-image information contained within the scan record. Phantom measurements should be used to ensure integrity of these values.

Rigid-body image registration can be extended to include computation of scale and skew parameters. This will increase the six degrees of freedom of the rigid-body match to the 12 degrees of freedom of the so-called 'affine transformation'. This can lead to longer computational times for automated algorithms and potentially can effect robustness as the higher dimensionality of the search space may be more prone to local minima.

Studholme *et al.* [37] have implemented a full 12 degrees of freedom registration algorithm based on the mutual information measure. Testing on MR and CT image registration has enabled them to detect errors in axial scaling when using spiral mode CT acquisitions. In many commercial scanners, bed movement measurement in spiral acquisitions has a relatively poor tolerance (typically ±3%) resulting in potential errors at the periphery of a 200 mm acquisition of ±6 mm which is clearly detectable. A 12 degree of freedom affine search will allow measurement of these discrepancies but cannot, of course, distinguish which scanner is in error. Determining scaling factors for PET or SPECT images in this way may be a risky strategy due to the blurry nature of boundaries visualized using these modalities.

The Leuven group [38] have shown how registration of images to a computational model of a phantom can be used to assess scaling errors accurately.

IMAGE DISTORTION

MR images in particular, are prone to geometric distortion. This distortion can be due to inherent inhomogeneities in the magnetic field and magnetic field gradients, or can be induced by magnetic susceptibility inhomogeneities in the patient's anatomy. Scanner-related effects can be measured and corrected, but patient-induced effects are harder to quantify. In-plane, 2D correction schemes are available, but full 3D correction is still rarely performed [39]. Errors are highly dependent on MR scan sequence, field strength and patient anatomy, but can easily be in the range 2–

5 mm at air–tissue boundaries, for example within the air sinuses of the skull.

In principle, the registration process could be used to compensate for these errors by performing multiple registrations on small fractions of the total field-of-view. A coarse-to-fine resolution strategy could be implemented with appropriate interpolation between the multiple registration solutions. It is not clear however, that there will be sufficient information in either modality to provide this correction robustly.

PATIENT MOVEMENT

A related problem is image artefact or distortion due to patient movement. In conventional CT and 2D MR acquisitions, movement between slices will lead to a distortion of the image volume. For spiral CT, 3D MR and PET or SPECT acquisitions, movement will lead to streak artefacts, ghosting effects and blurring as well as distortion. As with scanner-related scaling and skew errors, distortion of >1% may well dominate registration errors. It is difficult to ensure that patient movement during a scan is less than 1–2 mm.

NON-RIGID METHODS OF REGISTRATION

Registration assuming the validity of the rigid-body registration paradigm breaks down when there is distortion or movement of internal structures between image acquisitions or, as described above, when one or both of the imaging modalities gives rise to geometric distortion. The relatively sparse data and poor spatial resolution in nuclear medicine images makes it rather difficult to warp nuclear medicine images to corresponding anatomical images with any degree of confidence. For structures that change shape with patient pose, precautions must be taken to ensure that the patient is scanned in identical positions (such as in the application in imaging the hand and wrist described above) or regions that have moved are specifically excluded from the matching process (such as the legs when combining MR or CT images with PET images of the pelvis). Little *et al.* [40] have recently proposed a method of allowing rigid structures (such as bone) to move within a deforming substrate (such as soft tissue).

Deformation techniques are also used when a template or atlas of the anatomical structure is to be brought into correspondence with an image, often to assist in identification or delineation of specific anatomical structures. One way of achieving this is by registering the atlas to the specific anatomy of the patient. The registration process must include the deformation between the atlas and the patient's anatomy. Likewise, when combining images from multiple individuals in, for example, building averaged images of the human brain [1], a deformation into a single 'space' is required. This space or coordinate system may correspond to a particular individual's brain, an average brain or some other idealized space such as that of the Tailarach atlas [41]. Once anatomical correspondence is achieved then statistics of image intensities in the population can be studied in order to determine significance of differences in, for example, studies of neuroactivation [42]. Precisely which is the best coordinate system to use is an area of current research. A system that minimizes residual variance in landmark location by defining a series of principal warps has been proposed by Bookstein [43].

Collins *et al.* [1] have proposed a multi-scale matching scheme for deforming one MR image volume of the brain onto another. They use correlation of image intensity across the whole image to find the approximate rigid-body transformation. They then successfully divide the image into octants, to form an oct-tree. Each node of the oct-tree is successfully individually registered, layer by layer, and the final deformation is found by interpolation of the final 'leaves' of the oct-tree. The system behaves well, but errors of correspondence still occur due to topological differences, at fine scale, between individual brains. Thirion *et al.* [44] have proposed a fast deformation algorithm that produces visibly acceptable results, though more work is required to establish precisely which constraints should be used in image deformation.

The widely used Statistical Parametric Modelling (SPM) of Friston *et al.* [45] performs a realignment and statistical measure of significance of differences between groups of brains imaged using PET or SPECT. When performing this analysis it is more appropriate to register the PET or SPECT images to their corresponding MR image volumes and then compute the deformation of a standard brain (or atlas) to the MR image as the latter has much finer anatomical detail.

VALIDATION

In medical imaging, any re-computation, information processing or information extraction must be validated. Validation must take place at three levels: algorithmic validation; application validation; and clinical evaluation. Algorithmic validation is the confirmation that the description of the output as a function of input does indeed match the mathematical or algorithmic definition. In terms of image registration this means, for example, that a rigid-body transformation of one image space to another defined by the transformation that minimizes the squared difference between a number of corresponding point landmarks does produce the defined transformation over the whole image volume. Application validation refers to the accuracy of registration of corresponding regions of two images in a particular application. Clinical evaluation refers to the resulting clinical utility, effectiveness and benefit of the registration process.

Algorithmic validation is relatively straightforward and uncontroversial, at least for rigid-body transformation. Clinical validation is complex and beyond the scope of this chapter. Application validation on the other hand is of vital importance, yet only recently have we seen reasonably effective methodology proposed and tested. A first and necessary stage is the construction and imaging of appropriate phantoms [46], but this will not tell us how the system behaves in the presence of real clinical data with all the compounding effects of image noise, patient-induced artefact, limited field-of-view, etc. Images from one modality can be simulated from images acquired using another modality; for example, the Montreal group have generated a synthetic FDG-PET scan from a segmented MR scan by assigning appropriate ratios of radioactivity to segmented grey and white matter and simulating PET acquisition and reconstruction [47]. This simulated PET scan is, by definition, registered to the original MR scan and can be used to assess registration accuracy. Unfortunately, the simulated PET scan, while visually similar to real PET scans, will never have all the attributes (including artefacts) of real PET scans. Total reliance on such data is therefore difficult.

External fiducial markers attached to the skin surface in patient scans are not recommended.

They can easily move by 4mm or more between scans, which is significantly worse than the potential registration accuracy achievable with existing techniques.

Hemler *et al.* [48] have described a method of insertion of fluid-filled rods into the brains of fresh cadavers before imaging with MR or CT. This careful work was of great benefit to the assessment of registration accuracy of MR and CT image volumes of the head. Unfortunately, its very nature makes it inappropriate for nuclear medicine imaging that uses short-lived isotopes.

To date, the Vanderbilt study has provided the best data sets for assessing the registration accuracy of MR, PET and CT data sets of the head [11]. As part of the standard protocol for image-guided surgery, seven patients had MR, CT and PET scans with specially designed markers screwed into the skull. Each marker contained a void of larger dimensions than the voxel size of the lowest resolution modality (PET). The void was filled with a fluid giving contrast in each modality. The markers were used to compute an accurate rigid-body registration transformation. This provided a 'gold standard' against which a range of registration methods were assessed. Each site participating in the study received the data sets in which all traces of the markers had been removed using an electronic 'air brushing' technique. Their estimates of the registration transformation were returned to Vanderbilt for assessment ensuring a 'blind' study. For the methods that performed well, median errors were 0.7–2.9mm for MR/CT registration and 2.0–4.5mm for MR/PET registration. This compares well with the estimated accuracy of the 'gold standard' registration of 0.4mm for MR/CT registration and 1.7mm for MR/PET registration. Outside the head, accurate application validation has yet to be reported.

VISUAL ASSESSMENT

In the absence of a well-defined 'gold standard', visual assessment remains the only pragmatic way of assessing registration accuracy and is the only method currently available for assessing quality of a particular registration in clinical practice. A study by Wong *et al.* [49] with five observers of 54 trial registrations of MR and FDG-PET volumes of the head showed that all observers could detect transaxial translations of ≥2mm and axial translations of ≥3mm. Axial rotations of ≥2°

were always detected, as were craniocaudal or lateral rotations of ≥4°. Sensitivity of visual assessment will depend on viewing protocols, image quality (especially image resolution) and the presence of pathology. The study by Wong *et al.* [49] was on radiographically normal images, with MR and PET voxel sizes of $1.3 \times 1.3 \times 4.0 \, mm^3$ and $2.6 \times 2.6 \times 8.0 \, mm^3$, respectively. Detection of image registration errors is dependent on the visual perception of misaligned high-contrast boundaries. The study only considered mis-registrations along the six axes of rigid body motion. Visual assessment of mis-registration along combinations of these axes may well be less sensitive due to natural symmetries in anatomical structures.

CONCLUSION

Fully automated image registration using multi-resolution maximization of mutual information [32–35] is now available to register MR-PET images and MR-SPECT images of the head. The technique has been extensively validated by both visual assessment and as part of the Vanderbilt study [11].

Robustness and accuracy are dependent on the volume of head imaged by both modalities and the starting estimate. Generally, for complete volumes, starting estimates that encompass the full range of initial positions encountered in clinical practice can be registered. For smaller volumes of image overlap, better starting estimates may be required. The algorithm appears to be robust for large space-occupying lesions and other pathologies. It has also proved robust in a wide range of different MR acquisition parameters and ranges of image contrast. Obviously, the method applies only to nuclear medicine images where the whole brain has reasonable isotope uptake, as is found in ^{18}F-FDG, H_2 ^{15}O PET or ^{99m}Tc-HMPAO SPECT images. It is unlikely to be robust when registering very sparse images resulting, for example, from ligand studies.

Image registration is dependent upon accurate image scaling, while registration accuracy will be limited by geometric distortion in MR and errors in gantry skew angle and bed-movement in CT. A high level of quality assurance of image acquisition devices is paramount if accurate registration is to be achieved. Automated registration methods may, in the future, be used to assess the integrity of scanner calibration.

Outside the head, registration using anatomical landmarks or skin markers has proved effective for applications in oncology, and in imaging of the heart, lung and liver. Automated methods are being introduced, but deformation and movement of anatomical structures poses a major problem. Compensating for tissue deformation and motion remains a significant challenge requiring further research.

REFERENCES

1. Collins, D.L., Peters, T.M. and Evans, A.C. (1994) An automated 3D non-linear image deformation procedure for determination of gross morphometric variability in human brain, in *Visualisation in Biomedical Computing* 1994 (ed. R.A. Robb), International Society for Optical Engineering, Washington, DC, pp. 180–90.
2. Saffer, J.R., Barrett, H.H., Barber, H.B. and Woolfenden, J.M. (1991) Surgical probe design for a coincidence imaging system without a collimator, in *Information Processing in Medical Imaging* (eds A.C.F. Colchester and D.J. Hawkes), Springer, 1991, pp. 8–22.
3. Hawkes, D.J., Robinson, L., Crossman, J.E. *et al.* (1991) Registration and display of the combined bone scan and radiograph in the diagnosis and management of wrist injuries. *Eur. J. Nucl. Med.*, **18**, 752–6.
4. Hill, D.L.G., Hawkes, D.J., Studholme, C., Summers, P.E. and Taylor, M.G. (1994) Accurate registration and transformation of temporal image sequences. *Proc. Soc. Magnetic Resonance*, **2**, 830 (abstract).
5. Hajnal, J.V., Saeed, N., Oatridge, A., Williams, E.J., Young, I.R. and Bydder, G.M. (1995) Detection of subtle brain changes using subvoxel registration and subtraction of serial MR images. *J. Comput. Assist. Tomogr.*, **19**, 677–91.
6. Pietrzyk, U., Herholz, K. and Heiss, W. (1990) Three dimensional alignment of functional and morphological tomograms. *J. Comput. Assist. Tomogr.*, **14**, 51–9.
7. Evans, A.C., Beil, C., Marrett, S., Thompson, C.J. and Hakim, A. (1988) Anatomical-functional correlation using an adjustable MRI-based region of interest atlas with positron emission tomography. *J. Cereb. Blood Flow Metab.*, **8**, 513–29.
8. Bergstrom, M. (1981) Head fixation device for reproducible position alignment in transmission CT and PET. *J. Comput. Assist. Tomogr.*, **5**, 136–41.
9. Schad, L.R., Boesecke, R., Schlegel, W. *et al.* (1987) Three dimensional image correlation of CT, MR and PET studies in radiotherapy planning of brain tumours. *J. Comput. Assist. Tomogr.*, **11**, 948–54.
10. Thomas, D.G.T., Gill, S.S., Wilson, C.B., Darling, J.L. and Parkins, C.S. (1990) Use of a relocatable stereotactic frame to integrate positron emission tomography and computed tomography images: application in human malignant brain tumours. *Stereotact. Funct. Neurosurg.*, **54/55**, 388–92.

11. West, J., Fitzpatrick, J.M., Wang, M.Y. *et al.* (1996) Comparison and evaluation of retrospective intermodality image registration techniques, in *SPIE Medical Imaging 1996*, International Society for Optical Engineering, pp. 332–47.
12. Schoenemann, P.H. (1966) A generalised solution to the orthogonal Procrustes problem. *Psychometrica*, **31**, 1–10.
13. Arun, K.S., Huang, T.S. and Blostein, S.D. (1987) Least squares fitting of two 3D point sets. *IEEE Transactions on Pattern Analysis and Machine Intelligence*, PAMI-**9**, 698–700.
14. Hill, D.L.G., Hawkes, D.J., Crossman, J.E. *et al.* (1991) Registration of MR and CT images for skull base surgery using point-like anatomical features. *Br. J. Radiol.*, **64**, 1030–5.
15. Wong, W.L., Hussain, K., Chevretton, E. *et al.* (1997) Validation and clinical application of computer-combined computed tomography and positron emission tomography with 2-[18F]fluoro-2-deoxy-D-glucose head and neck images. *Am. J. Surg.*, **172**, 628–32.
16. Hawkes, D.J., Hill, D.L.G. and Bracey, E.C.M.L. (1992) Multi-modal data fusion to combine anatomical and physiological information in the head and heart, in *Cardiovascular Nuclear Medicine and MRI: Quantitation and Clinical Applications* (eds J.H.C. Reiber and E.E. van der Wall), Kluwer Academic Publishers, Dordrecht, Boston, London, pp. 113–30.
17. Fleming, J.S. (1989) A technique for using CT images in attenuation correction and quantification in SPECT. *Nucl. Med. Commun.*, **10**, 83–97.
18. Pelizzari, C.A., Chen, G.T.Y., Spelbring, D.R., Weichselbaum, R.R. and Chen, C. (1989) Accurate three dimensional registration of CT, PET and/or MR images of the brain. *J. Comput. Assist. Tomogr.*, **13**, 20–6.
19. Faber, T.L., McColl, R.W., Opperman, R.M., Corbett, J.R. and Peshock, R.M. (1991) Spatial and temporal registration of cardiac SPECT and MR images: methods and evaluation. *Radiology*, **179**, 857–61.
20. Jiang, H., Robb, R.A. and Holton, K.S. (1992) New approach to 3-D registration of multimodality medical images by surface matching. *International Society for Optical Engineering (SPIE)*, **1808**, 196–213.
21. Robb, R.A. and Barillot, C. (1989) Interactive display and analysis of 3D medical images. *IEEE Transactions on Medical Imaging*, **8**, 217–26.
22. Hill, D.L.G. and Hawkes, D.J. (1994) Medical image registration using knowledge of adjacency of anatomical structures. *Image and Vision Computing*, **12**, 173–8.
23. Malandain, G., Fernandez, M.A. and Rocchisani, J.M. (1994) Rigid registration of 3-D objects by motion analysis. *Proceedings, 12th International Conference on Pattern Recognition*, pp. 579–81.
24. Gamboa-Aldeco, A., Fellingham, L.L. and Chen, G.T.Y. (1986) Correlation of 3D surfaces from multiple modalities in medical imaging. *Proceedings, International Society for Optical Engineering (SPIE)*, vol. **626**, pp. 467–73.

25. Maguire, G.Q., Noz, M.E., Lee, E.M. and Schimpf, J.H. (1986) Correlation methods for tomographic images using two and three dimensional techniques, in *Information Processing in Medical Imaging* (ed. S. Bacharach), Martinus Nijhoff, Dordrecht, Netherlands, pp. 266–79.

26. Woods, R.P., Cherry, S.R. and Mazziotta, J.C. (1992) Rapid automated algorithm for aligning and reslicing PET images. *J. Comput. Assist. Tomogr.*, **16**, 620–33.

27. Woods, R.P., Mazziotta, J.C. and Cherry, S.R. (1993) MRI PET registration with automated algorithm. *J. Comput. Assist. Tomogr.*, **17**, 536–46.

28. Hill, D.L.G., Studholme, C. and Hawkes, D.J. (1994) Voxel similarity measures for automated image registration, in *Visualisation in Biomedical Computing* 1994 (ed. R.A. Robb), International Society for Optical Engineering, vol. **2359**, pp. 205–16.

29. Van den Elsen, P.A., Pol, E.J.D., Sumanaweera, T.S., Hemler, P.F., Napel, S. and Adler, J.R. (1994) Grey value correlation techniques used for automatic matching of CT and MR volume images of the head, in *Visualisation in Biomedical Computing* 1994 (ed. R.A. Robb), International Society for Optical Engineering, vol. **2359**, pp. 227–37.

30. Studholme, C., Hill, D.L.G, and Hawkes, D.J. (1995) Multiresolution voxel similarity measures for MR-PET registration, in *Information Processing in Medical Imaging (IPMI '95)* (eds Y. Bizais, C. Barillot and R. Di Paola), Kluwer, Dordrecht, pp. 287–98.

31. Collignon, A., Vandermeulen, D., Suetens, P. and Marchal, G. (1995) 3D multi-modality medical image registration using feature space clustering, in *Computer Vision, Virtual Reality and Robotics in Medicine* (ed. N. Ayache), Springer, Berlin, pp. 195–204.

32. Collignon, A., Maes, F., Delaere, D., Vandermeulen, D., Suetens, P. and Marchal, G. (1995) Automated multimodality image registration using information theory, in *Information Processing in Medical Imaging* (eds Y. Bizais, C. Barillot and R. Di Paola), Kluwer, Dordrecht, pp. 287–98.

33. Wells, W.M., Viola, P., Atsumi, H., Nakajima, S. and Kikinis, R. (1996) Multi-modal volume registration by maximization of mutual information. *Medical Image Analysis*, **1**, 35–51.

34. Studholme, C., Hill, D.L.G. and Hawkes, D.J. (1996) Automated 3D registration of MR and CT images of the head. *Medical Image Analysis*, **1**, 163–75.

35. Studholme, C., Hill, D.L.G. and Hawkes, D.J. (1997) Automated 3D registration of MR and PET brain images by multi-resolution optimisation of voxel similarity measures. *Med. Phys.*, **24**, 25–36.

36. Studholme, C., Hill, D.L.G. and Hawkes, D.J. (1996) Incorporating connected region labelling into automated image registration using mutual information, in *Mathematical Methods in Biomedical Image Analysis* (ed. A. Amini), San Francisco, California, pp. 23–31.

37. Studholme, C., Little, J.A., Penny, G.P., Hill, D.L.G. and Hawkes, D.J. (1996) Automated multimodality registration using the full affine transformation: application to MR and CT guided skull base surgery, in *Visualisation in Biomedical Computing* (eds K.H. Hoehne and R. Kikinis), Springer, Berlin, pp. 601–6.

38. Maes, F., Collignon, A., Vandermeulen, D., Marchal, G. and Seutens, P. (1996) Multi-modality image registration by maximization of mutual information, in *Mathematical Methods in Biomedical Image Analysis* (ed. A. Amini), San Francisco, California, pp. 14–22.

39. Chang, H. and Fitzpatrick, J.M. (1992) A technique for accurate magnetic resonance imaging in the presence of field inhomogeneities. *IEEE Transactions in Medical Imaging*, **11**, 319–29.

40. Little, J.A., Hill, D.L.G. and Hawkes, D.J. (1996) Deformation incorporating rigid structures, in *Mathematical Methods in Biomedical Image Analysis* (ed. A. Amini), San Francisco, California, pp. 104–13.

41. Tailarach, J. and Tournoux, P. (1988) *Co-Planar Stereotactic Atlas of the Human Brain*, Georg Thieme Verlag, Stuttgart.

42. Christenson, C.A., Rabbitt, R.D., Miller, M.I. *et al.* (1995) Topological properties of smooth anatomic maps, in *Information Processing in Medical Imaging* (eds Y. Bizais, C. Barillot, and R. Di Paola), Kluwer, Dordrecht, pp. 101–12.

43. Bookstein, F.L. (1991) Thin-plate splines and the atlas problem for biomedical images, in *Information Processing in Medical Imaging* (eds A.C.F. Colchester and D.J. Hawkes), Springer-Verlag, Heidelberg, pp. 326–42.

44. Thirion, J.P. (1995) Fast intensity-based non-rigid matching, in *Medical Robotics and Computer Assisted Surgery* (eds A.M. DiGiccia, R.H. Taylor, R. Kikinis and S. Lavallee), Wiley, pp. 47–54.

45. Friston, K.J., Frith, C.D., Liddle, P.F. and Frackowiak, R.S.J. (1997) Comparing functional (PET) images: the assessment of significant change. *J. Cereb. Blood Flow Metab.*, **11**, 690–9.

46. Turkington, T.G., Hoffman, J.M., Jaszczak, R.J. *et al.* (1995) Accuracy of surface fit registration for PET and MR brain images using full and incomplete brain surfaces. *J. Comput. Assist. Tomogr.*, **19**, 117–24.

47. Neelin, P., Crossman, J.E., Hawkes, D.J., Ma, Y. and Evans, A.C. (1993) Validation of an MRI/PET landmark registration method using 3-D simulated PET images and point simulations. *Computerised Medical Imaging*, **17**(4–5), 351–6.

48. Hemler, P.F., Van den Elsen, P.A., Sumanaweera, T., Napel, S., Drace, J. and Adler, J.R. (1995) A quantitative comparison of residual errors for three different multimodality registration techniques, in *Information Processing in Medical Imaging* (Proceedings of IPMI '95) (eds Y. Bizais, C. Barillot and R. Di Paola), Kluwer, Dordrecht, pp. 251–62.

49. Wong, J., Studholme, C., Hawkes, D.J. and Maisey, M.N. (1997) Evaluation of the limits of visual detection of image misregistration in a brain FDG PET-MRI study. *Eur. J. Nucl. Med.*, **24**, 642–50.

CHAPTER 20

Radiation

Radiation risks and patient issues

A. B. Brill, L. K. Harding and W. H. Thomson

INTRODUCTION

The centennial year of Roentgen's discovery of X-rays (1995), and Becquerel's discovery of radioactivity (1996), are important historical markers for radiation medicine. We have just lived through the 50th anniversary of the Hiroshima and Nagasaki A-bomb explosions, and the 10th anniversary of the Chernobyl accident. On the positive side, much credit is given to the remarkable medical diagnostic and therapeutic advances using ionizing and non-ionizing radiations. At the same time, attention should also be devoted to questions regarding the safety of ionizing radiations. This chapter reviews the question of risk and dose limits. It then considers nuclear medicine in the context of legislation regarding radiation safety.

SOURCE OF RISK ESTIMATES

Knowledge of quantitative risks of radiation depends largely on human data relying mostly upon studies of health effects in the follow-up of the Japanese A-bomb survivors. Risk coefficients are derived from the slope of the dose–response curve, extrapolated to the lowest dose levels. Although the data are derived from high-dose, high-dose-rate exposures to a mixed field of γ-rays and

neutrons, the risk coefficients are assumed to apply both to low-dose and low-dose-rate exposures to X- and γ-rays for population, and to occupational radiation exposure guidelines. In 1957, E.B. Lewis (1996 Nobel laureate for work on *Drosophila* genetics), postulated a linear relation between radiation dose and leukaemia incidence in the A-bomb survivors [1]. The risk factor he computed was based upon leukaemia mortality after high doses and high dose-rates, extrapolated to low doses where there was no evidence of an increase. Non-linear dose–response curves can also fit the data, and current estimates of leukaemia risk use a linear–quadratic model, consistent with a reduced effect at low dose-rates. For some cancers such as skin cancer, quadratic (threshold and non-threshold) models are accepted. The Nagasaki leukaemia data show a dip in the very low dose region, where few people were exposed, and some have cited this as evidence of a hormetic effect, but this is not generally accepted.

PROBLEMS OF LOW DOSE-RATES

For many years, the scientific community has known that deleterious effects at low doses, if present, are too low to be observable in epidemiological studies, and it is widely agreed that discrimination of 'nil' versus 'low' effect can only be established when mechanisms of carcinogenesis and body defence mechanisms are better understood. Indeed, some stimulating effects do occur at low doses in animal studies, and more research is needed to understand these observations. Unless new knowledge changes current regulatory para-

Clinical Nuclear Medicine, 3rd edn. Edited by M.N. Maisey, K.E. Britton and B.D. Collier. Published in 1998 by Chapman & Hall, London. ISBN 0 412 75180 1

digms, the linear no-threshold (L-NT) model, is likely to continue to be relied upon. Based on this model, many people have stated that there is no safe dose of radiation, but this notion has been misunderstood and has led to a high level of public anxiety. As a result, we spend very much larger sums of money to counter much lower risks from radiation than from real societal hazards, thereby diminishing funds available for real needs.

One problem that arises from the low-dose extrapolations was highlighted in a recent note in *Science* [2]. In it the author speculated regarding the number of cancers that could be attributed to the increased radiation dose received, if everyone in the world for 1 year wore shoes that made them 1 inch (2.5 cm) taller. Using current risk factors, the minuscule increase in cosmic ray dose was projected to result in some 1500 extra cancer deaths from this change in life style. Accepting the same notions, news reports have attributed 125 000 deaths to the Chernobyl accident, based on the multiplicative propagation of small theoretical risks by very large numbers of purportedly exposed individuals to their lifetime cancer risk.

When attempting to gain approval for siting radiation waste disposal areas one encounters similar risk magnifications. Despite the fact that there is no other kind of waste which is disposed of in a more prudent fashion than radioactive waste, inordinate difficulty has been encountered in obtaining siting approval. In the USA, when a new site is approved, a billion or more real dollars will have been expended to prevent one theoretical radiation death from the time span projected for the containment facility. The logic is so different from that of other accepted societal investments, that one presumes this reflects the consequences of the mathematical distortion noted above, plus a feeling that the risks are worse than they are being stated. In any case, distrust of authority and the 'NIMBY' (not in my backyard) problems are serious; we badly need major improvements in communicating a better understanding of radiation risks balanced against other risks and the competing societal needs. This is true not only for radiation-related matters, but also important for solving many other difficult problems.

In response to the distortion of low levels risk, the Health Physics Society in the United States, issued the following position statement: 'In accordance with current knowledge of radiation health risks, the Health Physics Society recommends against quantitative estimation of health risk below an individual dose of 5 rem (50 mSv) in one year or a lifetime dose of 10 rem (100 mSv) in addition to background radiation. Risk estimation in this dose range should be strictly qualitative accentuating a range of hypothetical health outcomes with an emphasis on the likely possibility of zero adverse health effects. The current philosophy of radiation protection is based on the assumption that any radiation dose, no matter how small, may result in human health effects such as cancer, and hereditary genetic damage. There is substantial and convincing scientific evidence for health risks at high dose. Below 10 rem (100 mSv) (which includes occupational and environmental exposures), health effect risks are either non-existent or too small to be observed.

Current radiation protection standards and practices are based on the premise that any radiation dose, no matter how small, can result in detrimental health effects, such as cancer and genetic damage (L-NT model). There is however, substantial scientific evidence that this model is an oversimplification of the dose–response relationship, and results in an overestimation of health risks in the low-dose range. 'Biological mechanisms including cellular repair of radiation injury, which are not accounted for by the L-NT model, reduce the likelihood of cancers and genetic effects' – this statement by Mossman *et al.* [3] has received a lot of critical comment, but the position statement is indicative of a growing frustration with the way in which low-level risks are being exaggerated, leading to public anxiety and regulatory over-reaction.

RECENT RECOMMENDATIONS

Radiation risk estimates undergo continuous review by international bodies including the International Commission on Radiation Protection (ICRP), the United Nations Scientific Committee on the Effects of Atomic Radiation (UNSCEAR), and various national committees. Between the years 1980 and 1990, the US National Academy of Sciences (NAS) Biological Effects of Ionizing Radiation (BEIR) Committee reports, UNSCEAR and ICRP reported a greater than two-fold increase in the risk coefficients. There a number of problems with the recent risk estimates based on the Japanese A-bomb data. There are errors in the Hiroshima neutron dosimetry, which when corrected, will reduce the risk estimates. Furthermore, the 1990 NAS report included chronic lymphocytic leukaemia in the analyses, which erroneously increased the risk coefficients. Most of the cancers in the A-bomb survivors are gastrointestinal (GI) malignancies, which are attributed to the A-bomb (neglecting consideration of the even higher doses received from annual gastrointestinal fluoroscopies). In the 1996 NCRP Annual Meeting, a review of sources of uncertainty presented by its former Director, W. Sinclair, indicated that NCRP is discussing a two-fold reduction in the risk factors based on current information.

RADIATION RISK AND MEDICAL PRACTICE

From the perspective of the medical practitioner, the balance between the benefits of improved early diagnosis far outweigh the theoretical risks of clinical procedures. Patients do not focus concern on radiation risk, as they know they have a benefit to derive. Subjects who volunteer for research procedures do so for altruistic reasons, probably also believing that medical advances may someday benefit them or their families, as well as the larger community. In the case of societal decisions where the benefit is more diffuse, and public approval is required, the situation is more complex, and the costs assigned to the mitigation of minuscule risks need to be kept in reasonable bounds based on the current state of knowledge of radiation risks. Regulations regarding medical uses of radiation are generally left up to the patient and the physician to decide based on national legislation, the patient's condition, and the best available means of diagnosis or therapy. The ICRP and other international radiation protection bodies are considering lowering the occupational limits from 50 mSv per annum to 20, and subsequently to 10, on the basis of their belief that such changes would not adversely affect current practices and would provide additional safety margins. Since the allowable levels of radiation that can be administered to normal volunteers has in many countries been tied to the occupational dose limit, a five-fold lowering of the permissible dose to normal volunteers would greatly limit the ability of practitioners to obtain needed data on normal subjects, in order to establish normal values for PET and SPECT imaging procedures. Since there are no data to suggest adverse effects at the 50 mSv level, it seems reasonable to detach medical guidelines from changing occupational levels, and keep the medical research procedure guideline at 50 mSv.

EFFECTIVE DOSE

The way in which we calculate dose and express risk from radiopharmaceuticals is based on dose calculations made using the methodology promulgated by the Medical Internal Radiation Dose (MIRD) Committee of the Society of Nuclear Medicine. The tools for doing so are embedded in the newest releases of MIRDOSE III, developed and distributed by the Oak Ridge Radiopharmaceutical Dose Center [4]. This provides the tools needed to calculate absorbed organ generic doses for male and female patients in different age groups. These are average organ dose values, usually derived from studies in normal subjects. The magnitude of the absorbed dose from nuclear medicine procedures depends on the amount administered, the type of emissions and the kinetics of the material in the body. Internal emitters are non-homogeneously distributed, and thus absorbed dose varies widely between different organs. Until recently, the total-body dose was used to compare the dose from different procedures. Non-homogenous distribution however, makes it difficult to use total-body dose as a risk surrogate, when one wants to compare for example, the risk from macroaggregates that lodge in the lungs with the uptake of radiolabelled colloid by the reticuloendothelial system.

An estimation of the risk from partial-body radiation procedures requires knowledge of the dose distribution to the different organs, and the risk of each. In the absence of an accepted method for assigning a well-defined risk that would predict acute and chronic, long-term health consequences, the ICRP generated what they called Effective Dose (ED), the computation of which is based on weighting factors (W_R) for different radiations and a set of weighting factors (W_T) defined for the relative radiosensitivity of irradiated tissues. The current values for the weighting factors are given in Table 20.1. The values of the W_T were intended to take into account the then most recent estimates of the cancer mortality risks (from the Japanese A-bomb survivors), and the risks of severe hereditary effects (in all generations) for irradiated tissues mapped to a 'standard' Western population. They also attempted to include the

Table 20.1 Weighting factors for effective dose calculation

Radiations	W_R	Tissue	W_T
Photons, all energies	1	Gonads	0.20
Electrons, all energies	1	Red marrow	0.12
Neutrons, energy <10 keV	5	Colon	0.12
10 keV to 100 keV	10	Lung	0.12
>100 keV to 2 MeV	20	Stomach	0.12
>2 MeV to 20 MeV	10	Bladder	0.05
>20 MeV	5	Breast	0.05
Protons, other than recoil protons, E > 2 MeV	5	Liver	0.05
Alpha particles, fission fragments and heavy			
nuclei	20	Oesophagus	0.05
		Thyroid	0.05
		Skin	0.01
		Bone surface	0.01
		Remainder	0.05*

*The remainder is composed of the following tissues or organs: adrenals, brain, small intestine, kidney, muscle, pancreas, spleen, thymus, and uterus.

risk of non-fatal cancer and length of life lost, assuming that such effects occur. The inclusion of these risk indicators increases the apparent risk per Sv of diagnostic and occupational exposures, recognizing that it is meaningless for predictions from therapy studies to which they were never intended.

The ED concept has been widely accepted, and has been useful in summing information that is otherwise difficult to integrate and interpret. However, the choice of the values for weighting factors is subject to debate, and the current values (already changed from the initial values used in the ICRP-defined Effective Dose Equivalent) will no doubt undergo a series of further redefinitions as radiobiological knowledge improves.

Although the ED concept has problems, it is nonetheless useful. One of the applications of the method is to rank and thereby compare risk from different types of procedures, e.g. radiographic and nuclear procedures. To calculate ED from radiographic procedures, one needs to know which organs are in the field-of-view, and the dose they receive. After adjustment for the fraction of the different organs in the field of view (e.g. one breast rather than both, or 10% of the body red-marrow space), one applies the weighting factors and sums the products to obtain the ED for the particular procedure [5]. Given knowledge of the parameters of the particular X-ray system, one can be reasonably accurate (reproducible) in computing the ED, whereas there is more uncertainty in the ED from nuclear medicine procedures. Figure 20.1 presents

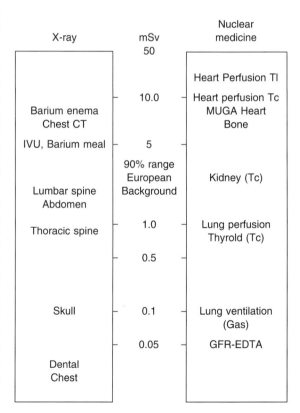

Figure 20.1 Radiation doses from common X-ray and nuclear medicine procedures.

a comparison of EDs for selected radiographic and nuclear medicine procedures.

The MIRD Committee presents its results as the ensemble of organ dose measurements, and has not published ED values for any of the tracers they have analysed to date. They have argued that computed estimates of organ dose are as accurate as the measurements made and the integrity of the computational method [6]. Given that the data are handled correctly, they are not subject to change, whereas ED is also dependent on the changing assignment of values for the weighting factors. The ED however, is useful in presenting a single number when interpreting the risk of procedures to patients. A NRCP report brings together much useful data concerning the different radiation protection issues encountered in nuclear medicine, and provides detailed data on many of the topics only touched upon in this introduction [7]. It also brings up to date references to the long series of related reports that are of interest concerning radiation protection in nuclear medicine.

LEGISLATIVE BACKGROUND

INTRODUCTION TO LEGISLATION

Throughout the world, legislation in nuclear medicine is determined by reference to recommendations of international bodies, notably the International Commission on Radiological Protection (ICRP) and the International Atomic Energy Agency (IAEA).

Within Europe, there are Euratom or other EC Directives, and national legislation is written to comply with these. With the publication of ICRP60 [5], the framework of legislation is currently under review, and revised European and national documents will be available in the next few years.

For the UK, the regulations comprise a series of fairly short documents, described as Statutory Instruments (SI). Associated with these SI are Codes of Practice, which demonstrate how to comply with the law, although the option is open for anyone to establish that they complied with the law in a way differently from that set out in the Code of Practice. There are also Guidance Notes, and these provide advice on good practice, and describe implementation of the law. In practice, it is these latter documents that are used in the day-to-day practice of nuclear medicine.

In other countries, different arrangements will apply, but the principles used are similar. Medical practitioners need to be aware of some of the issues but will be guided by physicists and others in complying fully with the regulations in their individual country. This section brings together the essential requirements for medical practitioners regarding radiation protection in nuclear medicine departments.

THE IONIZING RADIATIONS REGULATIONS 1985 (IRR85) [8]

These implement the Euratom Directives 80/836 [9] with amendments contained in 84/467 [10], which comprise the basic safety standards. Essentially, the IRR85 require employers to protect their employees and other people who work with ionizing radiation. All such work must be notified to the Health and Safety Executive and the radiation doses kept as low as reasonably practicable – ALARP (this term is used synonymously with as low as reasonably achievable – ALARA). Table 20.2 sets out the existing dose limits and those which are recommended in ICRP60. If the dose rate in a room is likely to exceed three-tenths of the 50 mSv limit then the area must be controlled (Table 20.3). There are some exemptions, which are described in Table 20.3. If the dose rates or the dose to a person is likely to exceed one-tenth of the limit, then the area must be supervised. Access to both of these areas must be restricted, and entry into a controlled area must either require workers to be classified or regulated through a written System of Work. The latter defines exactly who can enter the room and in what circumstances. Classified workers have to have regular medical examinations and radiation dose monitoring. Generally

Table 20.2 Yearly dose limits (mSv)

	Current	*ICRP60 [5]*
Employees		
Body dose	50	20
Organ dose (includes skin)	500	500
Lens of eye	150	150
Pregnant woman (declared pregnancy)*	10	1
General public		
Body dose	5	1

*Declared term of pregnancy is from the time a woman tells her employer that she is pregnant.

Table 20.3 UK controlled areas (external irradiation)

General rule: 3/10 of dose limits (see Table 20.2)

1. Instantaneous dose rate – above 7.5 μSv/h (assumes an 8-h working day for 48 weeks a year)
2. Exemptions* – above 7.5 μSv/h, but not a controlled area
   (a) In a person
       Up to 150 MBq·MeV[†] (1000 MBq ^{99m}Tc, 400 MBq ^{131}I)
   (b) Not in a person (i.e. in a bottle or syringe)
       Up to 50 MBq·MeV[†] (400 MBq ^{99m}Tc, 150 MBq ^{131}I)

*There are other exemptions not generally used in nuclear medicine.
[†]MBq·MeV is the product of the activity and total gamma energy per disintegration.

Table 20.4 Notification of overexposure overadministration factor

Diagnostic administrations	
Effective dose equivalent intended:	
>5 mSv	3×
0.5–<5 mSv	10×
<0.5 mSv	20×
Therapeutic administrations	
Beta or gamma emitters [12]	1.2×

in nuclear medicine, workers do not need to be classified, but enter controlled areas under a written System of Work. In addition, patients undergoing investigation or treatment are of course allowed to enter. Indeed, the written Systems of Work and how the department intends to implement the legislation must all be incorporated into a local document (the Local Rules). Radiation Protection Supervisors are appointed within departments to ensure that practices comply with these Local Rules. Also, if there are controlled or supervised areas, as there always are in nuclear medicine departments, the hospital has to appoint a Radiation Protection Adviser (RPA) whose responsibility is to help in writing the Local Rules, and give instruction and training to employees or others so as to satisfy the legislative requirements. RPAs have to be approved by the Health and Safety Executive. In nuclear medicine departments, the radiopharmacy, the radioisotope dispensary (where individual patient doses are dispensed), the injection and imaging rooms and the patient waiting rooms, are all likely to be controlled areas. Monitoring of radiation dose by film badges or other dosemeters is essential for classified persons, and should be undertaken on other staff as appropriate, to ensure that they comply with the dose limits. Such monitoring devices must be assessed by a dosimetry service approved by the Health and Safety Executive. Should there be a suspicion of over-exposure in individuals, they should be examined by a doctor appointed with the agreement of the Health and Safety Executive.

The design of departments, labelling of radioactive sources, and general provisions to ensure that radiation doses are minimized are described in the Guidance Notes to the IRR85 [11]. Monitoring for contamination of controlled and supervised areas, and keeping appropriate records is a requirement placed on employers, as is investigation of a possible over-exposure or loss of a radioactive source. In the event of a patient being over-exposed due to an equipment fault, which results in an exposure greater than that shown in Table 20.4, the Health and Safety Executive must be informed.

THE IONIZING RADIATION (PROTECTION OF THE PATIENT UNDERGOING MEDICAL EXAMINATION OR TREATMENT) REGULATIONS 1988 (IRR88) [13]

These regulations, colloquially known as POPUMET, are derived from 84/466/Euratom [14], which aims to protect the patient with regard to ionizing radiation. At present, the regulations do not include research, but it is likely that future versions of the directive will do so. They define two important groups of people, those clinically directing the exposure, i.e. those who decide that a study should take place, and those physically directing the exposure – in nuclear medicine it is the person who injects the radiopharmaceuticals. When venous access is difficult, particularly in the case of children, it may be necessary for a suitably experienced person to insert a cannula and the person physically directing to inject the radiopharmaceutical through the cannula.

Those clinically directing have overall responsibility for conduct of examinations, and have to ensure that all procedures are in accordance with accepted practice. Department arrangements must ensure that such people are named for each exposure. Those physically directing are also required to act in accordance with the accepted practice and exercise a strategy for dose reduction, which will keep radiation doses as low as reasonably practicable. The phrase 'in accordance with accepted practice' seems innocent, but giving the wrong amount of activity, or giving it to the wrong patient, or not acting in accordance with guidelines produced by professional bodies, could be construed as contravening this regulation. Both the clinically and physically directing staff members need to be trained, and the training syllabus is set out in the schedule to the SI. Practical experience is also required. Training courses are approved by national bodies and approval is generally valid for 5 years. In some instances, these form part of professional training (e.g. radiographers). At present, there is no requirement for refresher courses, although these are likely to be introduced in the revised European Directive.

It is important to note that the referring consultant does not need to hold a certificate of training for POPUMET. Such consultants are considered to have sought a medical opinion from the imaging department.

The employer is required to keep a schedule of any equipment that controls the extent of exposure of the patient (dose calibrators), and also records of employees who are trained under these regulations. For nuclear medicine and for therapy departments, the employer also has to provide the advice of a physicist. The future revision of the patient directive is also likely to encompass research, and to be applicable either to over or under-exposure of the patient. A report of the POPUMET inspectorate has been published and indicates areas where problems have arisen [15], but also notes that there have been no prosecutions under this legislation.

THE MEDICINES ACT

The various parts of the Medicines Act implement European legislation (65/65, 75/319, and 89/343 EEC) [16–18] and are concerned with the preparation of radiopharmaceuticals and who may administer them to human beings. For the latter, the degree of experience and training required varies, and in many countries, once licensing has been achieved, there is little restriction on administered activity. In the UK, this is not the case, and administered activities are tightly regulated. There are some indications (in IAEA documents), that there may be a move to follow the UK model, with restrictions on the administered activities permitted.

The Medicines Act – preparation of radiopharmaceuticals

Legislation 89/343 EC [18] requires that all radiopharmaceuticals be registered by the 1st January, 1993, with the Committee on Proprietary Medicinal Products (CPMP). More recently, a European Medicines Evaluation Agency (EMEA) has been set up under 93/39 EEC [19], and this describes decentralized and centralized procedures for registering radiopharmaceuticals. It is anticipated that the decentralized route will be mainly used with application to individual member states and other states will be given a period in which to object to marketing authorization, subject to binding arbitration by CPMP. The centralized procedure also requires consultation with member states, and this latter process will be mandatory for biotechnology products such as antibodies. Within the UK, preparation of radiopharmaceuticals in hospitals and clinics is also controlled under the Medicines Act [20]. Departments are required to obtain a Manufacturer's Licence (Specials), granted by the Medicines Control Agency of the Department of Health, unless the process is performed under the supervision of a pharmacist, in which case an exemption from licensing can be claimed. Whichever situation applies, the requirements for procedures and standard of facilities is the same.

In considering these requirements for radiopharmaceutical production it is important to remember that radiopharmaceuticals vary from normal pharmaceuticals in several respects. First, they are usually used only once and the chemical amount is so small that chemical toxicity is not an issue; the main hazards are that of radiation and of hypersensitivity (as pharmacological activity is not usually intended). Second, mutagenicity and teratogenicity are not related to the chemical product, but to the potential effects of irradiation. Sterility testing on every batch of radiopharmaceuticals is not possible before their issue because of the short half-life of many of the radionuclides used (notably ^{99m}Tc). However, there are particular problems with testing antibodies where the source of the protein used must be clear-cut, and proper tests should have been undertaken for contaminating viruses. With positron-emitting radionuclides the problems of short half-life are generally greater and the role of the radiochemist in preparation is particularly important. Such radiopharmaceuticals are, however, unlicensed, and because of the problems of testing very short half-life products, the quality assurance of the process is essential.

The Medicines (Administration of Radioactive Substances) Act 1978 (SI 1006) (MARS) [20]

These regulations set out the important guiding rules about administration of radioactive medicinal products to patients and implements 76/579/Euratom [21]. In the UK, such administration may only be performed by doctors or dentists who hold a certificate issued by Health Ministers advised by the Administration of Radioactive Substances Advisory Committee (ARSAC). Such certificates are specific as to the site where administration occurs. Certificate holders need to be those who are responsible for the test procedure rather than being the referring doctor. In order to obtain a certificate, such doctors or dentists will need to indicate their training and experience, and the extent of this will vary depending on the nature of the work to be undertaken. Requirements are therefore more stringent for therapy procedures than diagnostic ones. Applicants also have to establish that they have the equipment, facilities and supporting staff necessary for the application, and generally this would require a radiopharmacist and a physicist with appropriate experience.

Separate certificates are issued for diagnosis, treatment or research, and in addition to established trials of a radioactive medicinal product (RMP), research includes any situation that involves additional radiation exposure of the subject. Research studies also require separate submission to a local Research/Ethics Committee. There is a maximum usual activity (MUA) for diagnostic procedures, but these activities may be exceeded for individual patients – for example, in a particularly obese patient or in a patient with severe bone pain. Regular administration of activities above the MUA would require application for a variation of the certificate. For treatment, the administered activity is considered a matter of clinical judgement, but in all cases this activity must be recorded in the patients clinical records.

Should the activity administered to the patient be incorrect, measures for enhancing excretion must be considered [22]. Such maladministrations of radiopharmaceuticals are fortunately rare; while there is no formal requirement to notify these instances it is recommended that Table 20.4 is used as a guideline for those cases to be reported to the Secretary of State's Inspector for POPUMET [23].

General advice on maladministration and misadministration (where the radiopharmaceutical is correct but there is a problem in administration such as extravasation) has been given by Keeling and Maltby [24]. See Chapter 16.

The ARSAC committee has also produced in its Guidance Notes [25] advice about administered activities for children, thyroid-blocking agents, breast-feeding, avoiding pregnancy after radiopharmaceutical administration, and choosing subjects for research. Notably from the latter is a recommendation that healthy volunteers should, wherever possible, be over the age of 50. In addition, there should be a record of subjects used for research investigations. Employers have to be satisfied that their employees hold valid certificates, that staff with delegated authority can check these certificates and that authority to administer RMP in the absence of the certificate holder is properly documented.

STAFF ISSUES

NUCLEAR MEDICINE STAFF

Body doses to workers in nuclear medicine departments are low. Roberts and Temperton [26] published dose records from film badges for 1809 nuclear medicine staff and these showed mean recorded doses of <0.3 mSv with a maximum figure of 4.9 mSv. It is unlikely that classified workers will be needed in most nuclear medicine departments or radiopharmacies since exceeding three-tenths the annual dose limits is unlikely. Monitoring records in most departments show <0.2 mSv received by workers each month, but in large radiopharmacies the figures quoted by Roberts and Temperton may be exceeded. Hilditch *et al.* [27] found figures of <6 mSv in a radiopharmacy that handled 30 TBq ^{99m}Tc a year. However, Jansen *et al.* [28] found the maximum figure of 10.2 mSv, and interestingly this was to nursing staff from a diagnostic X-ray department in one hospital who rotated on a 3-monthly basis. The authors comment that these nurses were less experienced in working in nuclear medicine departments. A group that needs further consideration is pregnant technicians and this issue is discussed elsewhere in the book.

It is important to understand that, in nuclear medicine, the major part of the body dose to technicians comes from patients, and not from handling radiopharmaceuticals in dispensing and injecting. Harding [29] has provided data for individual patient studies, which clearly demonstrate this point. While clinical care of the patient is paramount, the implication of these data is that whenever possible, all explanation to the patient should take place before injection, and that apart from setting up the imaging procedure, the technologist should maintain a reasonable distance (at least 1 m) from the patient in order to minimize the radiation dose.

Patients with an activity greater than that equivalent to 300 MBq·MeV are described as high-activity patients (= 800 MBq for ^{131}I). Such patients have to be nursed in separate wards and may not leave without being accompanied by a member of staff, and with the approval of the radiation protection supervisor or medical officer. They have to have a radioactive sign on their bed, to use designated toilets, their own crockery, and the ward needs regular monitoring because of possible contamination by the patient. With some radionuclides (especially ^{131}I) this is a particular problem because of radioactive sweat [30]. Detailed precautions for looking after such patients have to be discussed with the radiation protection supervisor.

With beta-emitting radionuclides the levels at which patients become high-activity patients are generally beyond those usually encountered (3000 MBq ^{90}Y, 9000 MBq ^{32}P). The only significant hazard to others is Bremsstrahlung radiation externally, or for example contamination from urine.

Finger doses

Finger doses are the area in nuclear medicine where workers are most likely to approach 3/10 of the dose limit. Data are available [29] for the radiation doses to the finger pulp of those working in a radiopharmacy, in a radionuclide dispensary and in the injection area. These data show a reduction of up to four-fold from using syringe shields, and the latter are of most benefit in the injection area.

This is because measuring radiation doses in the radiopharmacy and radionuclide dispensary generally requires unshielded syringes. If one person injects about 40 GBq of ^{99m}Tc over the period of 1 month, then the finger pulp dose would be 12 mSv; syringe shields reduce this to 3 mSv. The data of Hilditch *et al.* [27] for a large regional radiopharmacy, by careful selection and training of staff, have shown a reduction of radiation dose at the base of the finger from 0.29 mSv/10 GBq to 0.10 mSv/10 GBq. Figures up to 50 mSv per year were recorded. As lightweight syringe shields are now available they should be used routinely, and of course gloves worn so that any contamination can be easily removed. These high radiation doses to fingers without using syringe shields have also been reported by Shuernbrand *et al.* [31] and Jansen *et al.* [28], though data for these two studies are not strictly comparable as the first used ring dosemeters while the second recorded the dose at the base in the middle finger. Doses at the base of the finger are approximately one-quarter of those measured at the finger pulp. The latest recommendations of ICRP made clear that finger doses must be averaged over 1 cm^2 and therefore finger pulp measurements are more appropriate [32].

OTHER HOSPITAL STAFF

Porters

There are few data available on nuclear medicine departments portering staff although Harding and Thomson [32] have estimated that in an old hospital with a long corridor where the porter may have to walk 0.4 km to take the patient back to the ward, the radiation dose from diagnostic studies would only be 0.1 mSv per month.

Ward nursing staff

There are no direct measurements of radiation doses to ward nursing staff from diagnostic procedures, but Harding *et al.* [33] have made estimates based on a nurse staffing formula which assesses the dependency of patients. They showed that a nurse on duty for 8 hours looking after patients who had just left the imaging department would generally receive <20 μSv from the patient. The exception would be those patients who needed a high level of care, where a figure of 100 μSv was not exceeded. Clearly, dependence of patients in different wards varies greatly, and the important points to come from this paper were that nursing procedures that involve the greatest radiation dose were incontinence or catheter care, treatment of pressure areas, and the nurse feeding the patient. In specialized wards, the extent to which these three activities are carried out is therefore the main consideration in deciding if doses to nurses are likely to warrant further consideration.

The precautions necessary for patients in wards after they have undergone nuclear medicine procedures varies from country to country. High-activity patients very properly need special precautions. In other cases, including virtually all patients having diagnostic investigations, local rules should indicate what precautions are needed. Although the patient may represent a supervised area, there is no need for this to be demarcated physically, but nursing staff need to be aware if a given patient is in this category. In our department we would send a letter to the ward when the patient leaves nuclear medicine, although others use a yellow wrist band as a means of identification. The only problem which arises commonly is that of incontinent patients. Proper nursing procedures for dealing with soiled linen or infected urine specimens provide sufficient safety precautions for radioactive contamination. However, there is a UK requirement to label urine which contains only low levels of activity [8] and to keep the urine for more than 24 hours; this is 5 MBq in the case of ^{99m}Tc, and 0.05 MBq for ^{131}I. Such requirements relate to the storage of radioactive sources rather than the urine constituting a serious hazard. Labels should be issued for such urine collections when the patient leaves the nuclear medicine department [29]. The label also warns the pathology laboratory when urine samples need chemical or microbiological analysis.

Laboratory staff

Harding and Thomson [32] have calculated the radiation dose to laboratory staff from radioactive urine and blood. The study was undertaken in a district hospital with a busy nuclear medicine department and calculated on the basis of the processes used in their laboratory. They estimated the dose to clinical chemistry staff at 0.02 mSv from urine and 0.002 mSv from blood. While ^{99m}Tc radiopharmaceuticals could interfere with radioimmunoassay, it is clear that there is not likely to be a problem from direct gamma radiation.

PATIENTS

In order to minimize radiation doses to patients, it is important to decide which is the appropriate examination to undertake, and this depends on the information provided by the referring clinician. A nuclear medicine physician should consider the value of the test and the optimum way in which to undertake it, bearing in mind the other imaging alternatives that may result in less radiation or no radiation. With some examinations there is a choice of radiopharmaceutical, and such a choice will depend on the physical and biological properties of the radiopharmaceutical, together with the imaging equipment available, and availability of the radiopharmaceutical, its shelf life and cost.

The activity to be administered will depend on a number of factors. First, it may vary with the equipment – for example, probe versus gamma-camera, or if the camera is multi-headed. Second, it would depend on the rate of data acquisition, as the arterial phase of an examination or a gated blood pool study will require more activity. Administered activity may occasionally depend on the clinical condition of the patient (e.g. renal or hepatic failure) and in those with marked obesity or severe bone pain from metastases an increased activity is important so that the patient does not have to be still for long periods. Such decisions about administered activity must be made by the nuclear medicine consultant (the person clinically directing the exposure in UK legislation).

A reduced administered activity is appropriate for children, and this may be based on body weight or surface area. The latter has been recommended by the Paediatric Task Group of the European Association of Nuclear Medicine [34]. However, phosphate bone-imaging agents and gallium tend to concentrate in growing bones so that a simple calculation of activity based on weight or surface area is not appropriate. On the other hand, the brain is relatively large in the child and an increased activity for blood–brain barrier or cerebral perfusion agents may be necessary. A further problem arises with very small children and generally, it is undesirable to reduce the administered activity below one-tenth of the adult dose [25].

With children or adults it is important to ensure that the administered activity is sufficient for the diagnostic purpose [22]. Irradiation of a patient without obtaining the necessary clinical information must be avoided, and studies which are prolonged because of low administered activity often result in patient movement with loss of resolution.

THE GENERAL PUBLIC

Irradiation of the general public from patients leaving hospital following nuclear medicine investigations or therapy has been subject to restrictions which, for the most part, have been derived by judgement rather than direct measurements. Such judgements were usually based on dose rates from patients, but of course the difficult factor to take into account was the occupancy factor, that is the distance between the patient and the member of the general public, and the time during which they were at that distance. Figure 20.2 shows the current restrictions on nuclear medicine outpatients as set out in the UK Guidance Notes in relation to the MBq·MeV limits and the corresponding activities with ^{99m}Tc and [131]I. In some of these areas there are now data that will allow a more balanced view of the risks to be taken. An important consid-

eration will be the new dose limits as set out in Figure 20.2 and the recommendation of ICRP60 [5] that those 'knowingly and willingly helping in the comfort and support of the patient' may be treated as medical exposure. It seems possible that they will be subject to a figure of 5 mSv rather than a 1 mSv dose limit. Relatives therefore may be exposed to this higher figure, although the situation regarding children who are relatives is unclear. The particular problem arises as to whether the child can give consent, but by analogy with other clinical situations, e.g. bone marrow transplant, it seems possible that older children may be able to give consent.

Waiting rooms

A number of authors have measured the radiation dose in nuclear medicine department waiting rooms by attaching dosemeters to the wall. However, these measurements do not take into account occupancy of the waiting room, and therefore an early attempt to measure doses to individuals was made by Harding *et al.* [35]. The estimates were based on dose rates from patients and observation of who was sitting in which seat in the waiting room for every 5 minutes of a working day. The work-load is over 3000 patients a year and the waiting room is a small one used solely for the

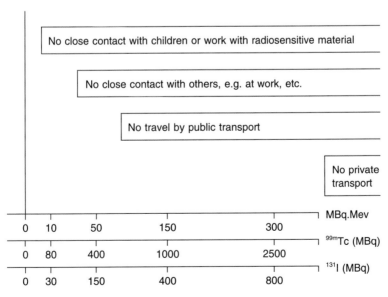

Figure 20.2 Current restrictions on nuclear medicine outpatients as set out in the UK Guidance Note in relation to the MBq·MeV limits and the corresponding activities with ^{99m}Tc and [131]I.

nuclear medicine patients and their relatives. The radiation doses are therefore likely to be higher than those in the average nuclear medicine department, but showed a median dose of only 2 μSv to a relative with a maximum of 33 μSv. The respective times spent by relatives in the waiting room were 85 minutes median and maximum 325 minutes. Subsequent data from a European Group [36] using digital dosemeters have shown a median dose of 13 μSv for one waiting room, and 12 μSv for two waiting rooms, which are not significantly different. This showed that there was no benefit in having a second waiting room for injected patients.

Transport home

The question of radiation dose to fellow travellers from patients administered ^{131}I for thyrotoxicosis has recently been addressed by Barrington *et al.* [37] in a multi-centre trial. As had been predicted by O'Doherty *et al.* [30], such radiation doses in private cars or taxis were small. Barrington's data suggested that there was no need to restrict travel in private cars and that on public transport journeys could last up to 7 hours.

Gunasekera *et al.* [38] have also measured the dose to fellow passengers on bus or train seats, and estimated the radiation dose to the adjacent person would be 230 μSv for a 60-minute journey for an administered activity of 400 MBq.

Home

The radiation dose at home, particularly to relatives of patients having ^{131}I for thyrotoxicosis, has been examined in a number of studies, and reviewed by Thomson and Harding [39]. Buchan and Brindle [40] made the first measurements to family members using thermoluminescent dosemeter sachets worn in a locket around the neck of the relative. Thomson *et al.* [41] carried out direct measurements of radiation doses to relatives using digital dosemeters carried by the relatives at all times, except during the night when the dosemeter was placed under their pillow. Measurements were made over 6 days and the average excretion curve for ^{131}I used to correct the measurements to total excretion. Thomson *et al.* [41] found values of 0.2 and 0.5 mSv for the median and maximum day-time figures respectively in patients administered 200 MBq of [131]I. For night-time figures, the geometric mean of anterior and posterior thermoluminescent dosemeters gave a

median of 1 mSv and a maximum of 2 mSv normalized to 200 MBq of radioiodine administered. The sum of the median day and night values for the spouse was therefore 1.2 mSv for 200 MBq administered, and this was essentially comparable with the data of Buchan and Brindle [40]. These data are for patients sharing a double bed, and to ensure a radiation dose of <5 mSv to the partner they would have to sleep apart for 4 days for 600 MBq administered and for 8 days for 800 MBq. To comply with a dose limit of 1 mSv would require 8 days sleeping apart with only 200 MBq iodine administered. The corresponding figures for 400, 600 and 800 MBq are 16, 24 and 30 days, respectively. Clearly these latter figures are excessive and unrealistic.

The workplace

Not surprisingly, no measurements of radiation dose to the general public in the workplace have been made. O'Doherty *et al.* [30] calculated the time necessary for ^{131}I patients to stay off work in order to ensure doses to other workers of <5 mSv, and also for <1 mSv. They assume that the patient was 1 metre away from their colleague for an 8-hour day, but a more realistic assumption might be that their fellow worker is at 2 metres. In the latter case, there is no need for any restrictions for ^{131}I except for 2 days at 800 MBq. For diagnostic tests, the patient may return to work for the day following the test because of the short half-life of such radionuclides.

RADIOACTIVE SUBSTANCES ACT

Controls must be in place regarding the amount of radioactivity on site at any time and also on the routes of radioactive waste disposal. Within the UK, the Radioactive Substances Act 1993 [42] governs these aspects.

One of the other principal issues relates to the disposal of radioactive waste and the radiological impact of this on members of the public. The major source of radioactive waste in hospitals is usually patient excreta which goes into the sewerage system. The total water outflow from the hospital site usually provides a sufficiently large dilution factor for most radionuclides with the possible exception of [131]I. For patient excreta, a simplified method of excretion calculation is considered adequate based on a percentage of administered activity for each radionuclide. Organic liquid waste is usually accounted for on a separate basis and has separate limits. Modern water-miscible organic scintillants used in beta-counting can be obtained, and with the additional permission of the water authority may be disposed via the sewerage system. Although this may save on incineration costs, this must be balanced against the fact that individual samples may need to be handled and emptied instead of the batch being sent for incineration. The biological hazard associated with patient samples is also relevant.

One of the main problems is that related to solid waste. This arises as a consequence of residues of stock vials, and from the aspects of dispensing and injecting, e.g. syringes, needles, gloves, tissues, etc. Such waste is normally stored for a period to decay and then sent for incineration. The activity limits for incineration are usually small and also the time for which radioactive waste can be stored is carefully controlled. Limits set initially should account for the maximum likely situations. It is important therefore before any new work is started, particularly if this involves a new or infrequently used radionuclides, that the limits for both storage and waste disposal should be checked. Re-application and authorization are expensive, but must be obtained before the work commences.

It is important therefore that the activity of solid waste is kept to a minimum, for example by disposing of longer-lived stock residues via the sewerage system wherever possible.

Other issues relate to generator systems and sealed sources. Where possible, the use of ^{90}Mo-^{99m}Tc generators on an exchange basis simplifies the disposal problem. Other sealed sources such as flood sources and markers may also be disposed of via an exchange system when new sources are purchased. The alternative is usually a landfill site, but this can be both a costly and involved procedure.

TRANSPORT REGULATIONS

Within the UK, there are regulations governing the aspect of transport of radioactive materials by road (Radioactive Substances Regulations 1985) [43] based on the IAEA recommendations [44]. For the purposes of nuclear medicine there are essentially two types of container, the excepted package and the 'type A'.

Excepted packages are those where there is

minimal external radiation dose and a limited activity. The surface dose rate must not exceed $5\,\mu Sv$ per hour and the package must be at least 10 cm on each side. Although ^{99m}Tc is easily shielded and could fall within this category, each package has an activity limit of 800 MBq for ^{99m}Tc.

The next level of container is designated as a type A, and must go through a rigorous series of test procedures. It is important to note that type A package will be approved for a particular type of vial or contents only. There are limits to the external surface radiation dose that a type A package can have, as shown in Table 20.5. A consignment note is also required on each package that is transported. This will contain details of the contents of the package, the radiation rates, the transport index and also the details of the shipper. The transport index relates to the radiation dose rate at 1 metre from the package and a transport index of 1 corresponds to a dose rate of $10\,\mu Sv$ per hour at 1 metre. This gives a useful indicator to the driver of the external radiation dose rate of the packages that he is carrying. Packages should always be placed in the rear boot or container of the vehicle to maximize the distance from the driver. Packages can also be used to self-shield those with the higher transport index.

Excepted packages do not require the vehicle to be placarded. However, type A containers require vehicle signs to be placed on the rear and both sides of the vehicle. A metal fireproof plate also needs to be carried within the vehicle cab. This contains details of who should be contacted in the event of any accident.

There are also separate requirements for drivers to have received training on the carriage of radioactive materials [45]. Relevant radiation protection advice and usually a short course involving practical instruction of about 2 hours' duration is adequate. During the transport of radioactive ma-

Table 20.5 Type A containers: specifications

Classification and package labels	Maximum dose rate at 1 m* ($\mu Sv/h$)	Maximum surface dose rate* ($\mu Sv/h$)
WHITE I	1	5
YELLOW II	10	500
YELLOW III	100	2000

*Maximum activity limits also apply, but are usually in excess of likely activities encountered in nuclear medicine.

terials, it is permissible for the vehicle driver to have a short break if essential, but at all times the vehicle must remain locked when the driver is not within the vehicle.

An essential element of the transport of radioactive materials is that there should be a quality assurance programme governing all aspects of the transport. Procedures should be in place that can demonstrate compliance with the appropriate regulations including design, testing, storage and transit of the packages, and driver compliance with the regulations.

PATIENT EXPLANATIONS

Patients are generally anxious about attending a nuclear medicine department. In order to allay this anxiety, information sent to them before their attendance is invaluable. Furthermore, the patient who is less anxious is more likely to comply with the instructions they are given and thus make the study easier for them and for the technical staff.

Professional staff tend to write information leaflets for patients as though they were scientific papers, whereas the style should be that of the local daily newspapers. The key points in writing such leaflets have been clearly set out by Clarke *et al.* [46]. Writing simple English takes a little practice, but most computers now have a parsing program that will test how easy it is for the information to be read. The two most important points are to keep sentences short, preferably 10–12 words and wherever possible to avoid words of more than two syllables. Important messages should be first and negative or subordinate clauses should be avoided. The use of personal pronouns such as 'you' or 'your child' make the document more friendly to read and it has become usual to use a question and answer format. In some departments to make the leaflets more attractive and interesting icons are used [47,48]. Finally, the minimum type size should be 10 characters per inch, bearing in mind that many patients are elderly, and the document should be presented as attractively as possible. Many of these features can be combined into a leaflet for general nuclear medicine investigations.

In addition, most departments send out a letter specific to the type of study, which indicates the time and date of the appointment, how long the procedure will take, and any special instructions

for the type of study. Sometimes, patients are required to take a lot of fluid, and with occasional exceptions it is useful to indicate that the patient does not have to starve. Such information should include instructions or perhaps a diagram as to where the department is on the hospital site together with details of for example disabled access and car parks. Once the patient reaches the department it is important that they are greeted pleasantly and wherever possible by name. After their identity has been checked, it is very important to repeat the essential points of the procedure, and for this reason both the receptionist and technical staff should be familiar with the procedure for each type of study. At this point it is also important to check whether women might be pregnant or breast-feeding. In addition to asking them as appropriate, it is good practice to have notices in the department – and particularly in the waiting room – asking mothers to indicate if they are breast-feeding, and for patients and staff to indicate if they think they may be pregnant.

Surveys of patient satisfaction [49] often show that the thing which most concerns patients is the injection. The need for an injection should be described in the patient leaflet, and also forms part of the explanation when they reach the department, but many patients still seem surprised about the injection. It is important that this is undertaken efficiently, and in children the use of local anaesthetic cream is recommended. During imaging the technologist should try and stay 1 metre away from the patient for the majority of the study in the interests of minimizing staff radiation doses. It is, however, important to keep in verbal contact with the patient during this period, to ensure that they are comfortable, and to provide encouragement that the study is going well. Should any problems occur and repeat views have to be taken then this should be explained to the patient.

Finally, it is generally the practice to tell patients that the results will be sent to their referring doctor; coupled with this is a need to ensure that all studies are reported promptly.

ETHICAL ISSUES
DIAGNOSTIC INVESTIGATIONS AND THERAPY

It is usually considered that implied consent is sufficient for diagnostic investigations. If the examination is explained to the patient and the patient holds out their arm for the injection then they have implied consent. Many people now feel that, for therapy, written consent should be obtained. For iodine therapy for thyrotoxicosis we would also ask female patients to sign a form to say they understand that they must not become pregnant for 4 months. The same applies to therapy for cancer, although the period may need to be longer. Such written consent does not abdicate the nuclear medicine staff from explaining the procedure thoroughly, but its value is that it provides proof that an explanation was made.

RESEARCH

Considerations about using nuclear medicine investigations for research are different. A detailed consideration of the issues is given in the ARSAC Notes for Guidance [25] and this defines research as where any additional radiation exposure is given, over and above that which the subject would normally receive as part of their routine management. Therefore, even an additional bone scan for research purposes is included. All research should be referred to a local research/ethical committee, in the best interests both of the investigator and the patient. In determining whether the additional radiation burden is justifiable, it is important to consider the effective dose equivalent of the investigation and the number of times that it might be repeated. Clearly, quite different levels of risk are associated with studies where the EDE is <1 mSv, up to 10 mSv, or up to 50 mSv. Only exceptionally should research investigations be considered where the EDE is >50 mSv. ARSAC has also made some pertinent points about the age of the subjects. Those under 18 should not be used for volunteer studies and indeed, research in children should be confined to issues appropriate to their age group. There is a further recommendation that wherever possible volunteers should be over the age of 50. It is especially important not to involve women who may be pregnant as volunteers. A difficulty which arises in some hospitals is that patients with certain diseases tend to have multiple research investigations. It is very important to keep records of those who participate in research studies and also to ask the patient about previous volunteer studies, in order to prevent this happening. Radiation workers should generally not be involved in

any volunteer studies which involve additional radiation.

CONSENT BY RELATIVES

Because patients are radioactive when they leave the hospital they will inevitably cause extra irradiation to their relatives. For diagnostic studies, the amount of this is small and no precautions are necessary. The only exception is young children where it is normal practice to advise patients not to cuddle or sit next to children for long periods after they have had investigations with technetium radiopharmaceuticals. These precautions are only necessary for 24 hours and therefore it is easy to conform with them. With patients having therapy the situation becomes more complex. ICRP60 [5] has a very important phrase concerning those 'knowingly and willingly helping in the support and comfort of a patient'. This allows relatives or friends to give consent to radiation above that of the dose limit to the general public. Considerations of this concept are at an early stage [50]. However, it is clear that friends and relatives must be aware of the risks they are taking and these should be explained simply to them, or to the patient to convey to the relative, who must also consent to receiving this additional radiation. NCRP [51] have pointed out that an ill relative creates anxiety and stress in the family which may be detrimental, but may draw the family together both emotionally and physically. They may therefore wish to spend extra time with the patient, and attempts to restrict this will be met with resistance and failure to comply. This is entirely consistent with taking social and economic factors into account in keeping radiation doses as low as reasonably practicable. It is also important to remember that the chances of having more than one patient in the family receiving radionuclide therapy are very small. However, in some circumstances it may be necessary to keep the patient in hospital, or where possible to arrange a different form of therapy.

A particular area of contention regards the children of those receiving radionuclide therapy. The whole question of consent by children is shifting from the argument that below a certain age the parent must consent on their behalf, to a situation that if the child understands the procedure and risks, then he or she can consent. Clearly, with very young children this is not appropriate and it is in the very young child that the hazards of irradiation are proportionally larger, as set out in ICRP60 [5]. These issues are still unresolved, and sometimes it may be necessary to arrange for the children to be looked after by a relative for a few days so that the radiation dose is minimized.

REFERENCES

1. Lewis, E.B. (1957) Leukaemia and ionizing radiation. *Science*, **125**, 965–72.
2. Goldman, M. (1996) Cancer risk of low level exposures. *Science*, **271**, 1821–2.
3. Mossman, K.L., Goldman, M., Masse, F.X. *et al.* (1996) Radiation risk in perspective. *Health Physics Society Newsletter*, **24**, 3.
4. Stabin, M. (1996) MIRDOSE: Personal Computer Software for Internal Dose Assessment in Nuclear Medicine. *J. Nucl. Med.*, **37**, 538–46.
5. ICRP 60 (1991) *Recommendations of the International Commission on Radiological Protection*, publication 60. Pergamon Press, Oxford.
6. Poston, J.W. (1993) for the MIRD Committee. Application of the Effective Dose Equivalent to Nuclear Medicine Patients. *J. Nucl. Med.*, **34**, 714–16.
7. National Commission on Radiological Protection (1996) *Sources and Magnitude of Occupational and Public Exposures from Nuclear Medicine Procedures – Report 124.* NCRP, Bethesda.
8. *Ionising Radiations Regulations* (1985) HMSO, London.
9. Euratom Directive 80/836 (1980) Amending directives laying down basic safety standards for health protection of general public and workers against the dangers of ionising radiation. *Off. J. Eur. Comm.*, **L246**, 17.9,1.
10. Euratom Directive 84/467 Directive 80/836 Euratom as regards basic safety standards for health protection of general public and workers against the dangers of ionising radiation. *Off. J. Eur. Comm.*, **L265**, 5.10,4.
11. National Radiological Protection Board (1988) *Guidance Notes for the Protection of Persons Against Ionising Radiations Arising from Medical and Dental Use.* NRPB, Oxford.
12. HSE (1992) *Fitness of equipment used for medical exposure to ionising radiation.* Guidance Note PM77. HMSO, London.
13. Ionising Radiation Regulations (1988) *Protection of the Patient Undergoing Medical Examination or Treatment.* Department of Health, London.
14. Euratom Directive 84/466 Laying down basic measures for radiation protection of persons undergoing medical examination or treatment. *Off. J. Eur. Comm.*, **L265**, 5.10,1.
15. Wilson, E. and Ebdon-Jackson, S. (1994) Secretary of State's POPUMET Inspectorate: the first six years. *Health Trends*, **26**, 67–9.
16. EC 65/65 (1965) An approximation of provisions laid down by law regulation or administrative action relating to proprietary medical products. *Off. J. Eur. Comm.*, **22**, 9.2,369.
17. EC 75/319 (1975) Approximation of provisions laid down by law regulation or administrative action relating to proprietary medicinal products. *Off. J. Eur. Comm.*, **L147**, 9.6,13.
18. EC 89/343 (1989) Extending the scope of directives 65/65/EEC and 75/319/EEC and laying down additional provisions for radiopharmaceuticals. *Off. J. Eur. Comm.*, **L142**, 16.5,1.
19. EEC Council Directive 93/39 (1993) Amending Directives 65/65/EEC 75/318/EEC and 75/319/EEC in respect of medicinal products.
20. Medicines (Administration of Radioactive Substances Act 1978): SI1006. DHSS, London.
21. Euratom 76/579 (Re MARS). Laying down revised basic safety standards. *Off. J. Eur. Comm.*, **L187**, 12.7, 1–44.
22. ICRP68 (1993) *Summary of the current ICRP principles for the protection of the patient in nuclear medicine.* ICRP 68, Pergamon Press, Oxford.
23. Williams, E.D. and Harding, L.K. (1995) Radiopharmaceutical maladministration: what action is required? *Nucl. Med. Commun.*, **16**, 721–3.
24. Keeling, D.H. and Maltby, P. (1994) Editorial. Maladministrations and misadministrations. *Nucl. Med. Commun.*, **15**, 63–5.
25. ARSAC (1993) *Notes for Guidance on the Administration of Radioactive Substances to Persons for the purposes of diagnosis, treatment or research.* Department of Health, London.
26. Roberts, P.J. and Temperton, D.H. (1991) Occupational exposure in UK hospitals. *Rad. Prot. Dosim.*, **36**, 229–32.
27. Hilditch, T.E., Elliott, A.T. and Amstee, D.E. (1990) Fifteen years of radiological protection experience in a regional radiopharmacy. *Health Physics*, **59**, 109–16.
28. Jansen, S.E., Van Aswegen, A., Lotter, M.E. *et al.* (1994) Staff radiation doses during 8 years in a nuclear medicine radiopharmacy. *Nucl. Med. Commun.*, **15**, 114–18.
29. Harding, L.K. (1987) Radiation safety in the nuclear medicine department: impact of UK Ionising Radiation Regulations. *Br. J. Radiol.*, **60**, 915–8.
30. O'Doherty, M.J., Kettle, A.J., Eustance, C.M.P. *et al.* (1993) Radiation dose from adult patients receiving ^{131}I therapy for thyrotoxicosis. *Nucl. Med. Commun.*, **14**, 160–8.
31. Schurnbrand, P., Schicha, H., Thal, H. and Emrich, D. (1982) External radiation exposure of personnel working with ^{99m}Tc technetium. *Eur. J. Nucl. Med.*, **7**, 237–9.
32. Harding, L.K. and Thomson, W.H. (1993) Where do we stand with ICRP 60? *Eur. J. Nucl. Med.*, **20**, 787–91.
33. Harding, L.K., Tan, C.P., Conroy, J. *et al.* (1986) The radiation doses to ward nurses from patients having nuclear medicine investigations. *Nuklearmedizin*, Suppl. **22**, 46–8.
34. Paediatric Task Group of the European Association of Nuclear Medicine (1990) A radiopharmaceutical schedule for imaging in paediatrics. *Eur. J. Nucl. Med.*, **17**, 127–9.

35. Harding, L.K., Harding, N.J., Warren, H. *et al.* (1990) Radiation dose to accompanying nurses, relatives and other patients in a nuclear medicine department waiting room. *Nucl. Med. Commun.*, **11**, 17–22.
36. Harding, L.K., Bossuyt, A., Pellet, S. *et al.* (1994) Radiation doses to those accompanying nuclear medicine department patients: a waiting room survey. *Eur. J. Nucl. Med.*, **21**, 1223–6.
37. Barrington, S.F., Kettle, A.G., Thomson, W.H. *et al.* (1996) RCP Guidelines on radiation protection following radio-iodine therapy for thyrotoxicosis: are they appropriate? *Nucl. Med. Commun.*, **17**, 275.
38. Gunesakera, R., Thomson, W.H. and Harding, L.K. (1996) Use of public transport by I-131 therapy patients. *Nucl. Med. Commun.*, **17**, 275.
39. Thomson, W.H. and Harding, L.K. (1995) Radiation protection issues associated with nuclear medicine outpatients. *Nucl. Med. Commun.*, **16**, 879–92.
40. Buchan, R.C.T. and Brindle, J.M. (1971) Radioiodine therapy to outpatients – the radiation hazard. *Br. J. Radiol.*, **44**, 973–5.
41. Thomson, W.H., Mills, A.P., Smith, N.B., Mostafa, A.B., Notghi, A. and Harding, L.K. (1993) Day and night radiation doses to patients' relatives: Implications of ICRP 60. *Nucl. Med. Commun.*, **14**, 275.
42. *Radioactive Substances Act 1993*, HMSO, London.
43. *Radioactive Substances (Carriage by Road) (Great Brit-ain) (Amendment) Regulations 1985* (SI 1985 No 1729), HMSO, London.
44. IAEA Safety Series No. 6 *Regulations for the Safe Transport of Radioactive Material* (1985 as amended 1990): IAEA, Vienna.
45. *Road Traffic (Training of Drivers of Vehicles Carrying Dangerous Goods) Regulations 1992* (SI 1992 No. 744), HMSO, London.
46. Clarke, S.E.M., McKillop, J.H., Prescott, M.C. and Williams, E.D. (1992) Information for patients and staff concerning nuclear medicine. *Nucl. Med. Commun.*, **13**, 271–81.
47. EANM Task Group Explaining Risks (1993) Patient letters. *Eur. J. Nucl. Med.*, **20**, A15–22.
48. EANM Task Group Explaining Risks (1994) Patient letters. *Eur. J. Nucl. Med.*, **21**, BP13–18.
49. Harding, L.K., Griffiths, J., Harding, V.M., Tulley, N.J., Notghi, A. and Thomson, W.H. (1994) Closing the audit loop: a patient satisfaction survey. *Nucl. Med. Commun.*, **15**, 275–8.
50. Harding, L.K. and Thomson, W.H. (1995) 'Knowingly and willingly in the support and comfort of a patient'. *Nucl. Med. Commun.*, **60**, 877–8.
51. National Commission on Radiological Protection Commentary No. 11 (1995). Dose limits for individuals who receive exposure from radionuclide therapy patients; NRCP, London.

Pregnancy and breast-feeding

P. J. Mountford and A. J. Coakley

INTRODUCTION

The administration of a radiopharmaceutical to a pregnant woman will result in exposure of the foetus to radiation emitted from adjacent maternal organs and from radioactivity transferred across the placenta. Administration to a breast-feeding mother will result in the secretion of radioactivity in her milk, and her infant will be exposed to the radiation emitted by the ingested radioactivity. In view of the increased awareness of the general public about the risks associated with ionizing radiation and the growing tendency to question clinical management, nuclear medicine services should adopt a range of measures. These include:

1. Procedures should be implemented to prevent inadvertent (i.e. uncontrolled) exposure of a pregnant or breast feeding patient.
2. All staff should be familiar with the precautions necessary to minimize the dose to the foetus or infant.
3. Senior members of staff must be aware of the risks associated with carrying out nuclear medicine procedures on pregnant and non-pregnant women.
4. A member of staff must always be available to explain these risks to the patient, and where appropriate, the referring clinician.

A pregnant member of staff will be exposed to the radiation emitted from a range of different types of sources and to the potential risks associated with dealing with radioactive contamination. Therefore, nuclear medicine departments may need to modify working practices for pregnant staff by minimizing the possibility of high foetal exposures.

PREGNANCY ISSUES IN ADULTS OF REPRODUCTIVE AGE

THE MENSTRUAL CYCLE

It is now accepted that there is no risk from diagnostic nuclear medicine procedures during the first 10 days of the menstrual cycle, and no special limitations need apply during the remainder of the cycle [1,2]. A woman should be treated as though she was pregnant if her period is overdue or clearly missed. The National Radiological Protection Board (NRPB) considers that exposures of 'tens of mGy' approximately doubles the total natural cancer risk in the unborn child. It recommends that procedures resulting in such foetal doses should be avoided even in early pregnancy; one way of eliminating this risk is by restricting these procedures to the early part of the menstrual cycle [2]. Although this recommendation is tantamount to reinstating the old '10-day rule', it will be seen from the dosimetry section below that only ^{67}Ga-citrate, ^{75}Se-selenonorcholesterol and ^{131}I-iodine scans produce a foetal dose of >10 mGy. At the time of writing, the exact magnitude of this critical dose remains unspecified, but if it is taken to mean a foetal dose of at least 20 mGy, then for diagnostic nuclear medicine the recommendation only applies to ^{131}I-iodine scans for thyroid cancer.

AVOIDANCE OF CONCEPTION

The findings of Gardner *et al.* [3] led to the hypothesis that preconception exposure of men resulted in sperm mutations which increased the risk of leukaemia in their offspring. However, this association is now considered a chance finding [4], and hence there is no need to issue any restriction to male patients to avoid conception following a diagnostic procedure.

In the UK, periods have been recommended for which a female patient should not become pregnant following administration of a long-lived radiopharmaceutical (Table 20.6) [5]. It should be noted that first, no restriction is recommended for radionuclides with a physical half-life of less than

Clinical Nuclear Medicine, 3rd edn. Edited by M.N. Maisey, K.E. Britton and B.D. Collier. Published in 1998 by Chapman & Hall, London. ISBN 0 412 75180 1

Table 20.6   Recommended periods for female patients to avoid conception [5]

Radiopharmaceutical	Activity (MBq)	Period (months)
Diagnostic procedures		
All $t_{1/2}$ < 7 days		0
^{59}Fe (iron metabolism studies)	0.4	6
^{75}Se-selenonorcholesterol	8	12
^{131}I-MIBG	20	1
^{131}I-iodide (thyroid metastases imaging)	400	4
Therapeutic procedures		
^{131}I-iodide (thyrotoxicosis)	800	4
^{131}I-iodide (thyroid cancer)	5000	4
^{131}I-MIBG	5000	3
^{32}P-phosphate	200	3
^{89}Sr-chloride	150	24
^{90}Y-colloid	400	0

7 days, and second, the periods of time are recommended to apply to all activities up to the values given.

LONG-TERM RISKS FROM ^{131}I ADMINISTRATION

Follow-up studies of children, adolescents and adults treated with ^{131}I for hyperthyroidism or cancer have shown no significant differences in the fertility rate, incidence of complications in subsequent pregnancies, or abnormalities in their progeny including stillbirth, prematurity, birth weight, congenital malformation and death during the first year of life [6–10]. Theoretically, irradiation of the ovaries from ^{131}I treatment of thyroid cancer should not increase foetal anomalies and does not warrant permanent sterilization [11]. These empirical data are supported by the fact that ^{131}I treatment of hyperthyroidism produces a lower ovarian dose than a diagnostic X-ray barium enema procedure [12,13].

GENERAL PROCEDURE FOR A PREGNANT OR BREAST-FEEDING PATIENT

AVOIDANCE OF UNCONTROLLED EXPOSURE

The greatest hazard will occur when a radiopharmaceutical is administered to a patient without the nuclear medicine service realizing that she is pregnant or that she is breast-feeding (see p. 713). The following procedures should be adopted to avoid an uncontrolled exposure of a foetus or of a breast-fed infant:

1. Include a section on the request form that asks whether the patient is breast-feeding or pregnant and the date of her last menstrual period.
2. Display signs prominently in the waiting area and in the injection room asking such patients to identify themselves to nuclear medicine staff. These signs may need to ask this question in more than one language, and they should also have an appropriate pictorial representation of the question in case of reading difficulties.
3. Question female patients of a childbearing age directly and discretely just before administration of the radiopharmaceutical.

APPLICATION OF THE ALARP PRINCIPLE

Before a radiopharmaceutical is administered to a pregnant or breast-feeding patient, the principle of ensuring the radiation dose to the foetus or infant will be as low as reasonably practicable (ALARP) should be applied by considering the following questions:

1. Is the requested procedure essential?
2. Is there an alternative procedure not involving the administration of radioactivity?
3. Can the procedure be delayed until the baby has been born or until after the mother has decided to give up breast-feeding?

4. Is there an alternative radiopharmaceutical producing a lower dose to the foetus or infant (see Tables 20.7 and 20.8)? Apart from obvious examples such as using ^{123}I-compounds rather than ^{125}I or ^{131}I, implementation of this precaution for a pregnant patient is hampered by the lack of knowledge of the placental transfer of radiopharmaceuticals.

5. Can a diagnostic result be obtained with less than the usual administered activity?

6. What is the possibility of a further nuclear medicine procedure or any other radiological investigation that will result in a radiation dose to the foetus or infant? When deciding whether to proceed with the nuclear medicine investigation, it is the total radiation dose which will be incurred by the foetus during the entire pregnancy or by the infant while breast-feeding is maintained that must be considered. If a breast-feeding mother is to have any more procedures requiring the *in vivo* administration of radioactivity, then the total effective dose to the infant from all such procedures must not exceed 1 mSv, even if the second procedure is carried out up to 1 year after the first.

PREGNANT PATIENTS

CRITICAL LEVELS OF FOETAL DOSE

In the UK, it is recommended that a procedure resulting in an absorbed dose to the foetus of more than 0.5 mGy requires particular justification [5]. This dose gives a level of risk comparable with that due to variations in natural background radiation found in the UK [14]. The National Radiological Protection Board (NRPB) advises that although a foetal dose of 'tens of mGy' approximately doubles the total natural cancer risk in the unborn child, it is unlikely to be a reason for termination of a pregnancy [2].

FOETAL AND UTERINE DOSIMETRY

According to the MIRD system, the absorbed dose to a foetus is given by the summation over all source organs of the product of the cumulated activity in each source organ and the absorbed dose in the foetus per unit cumulated activity in the source organ (the S-factor) [15]. Foetal radiopharmaceutical dosimetry is limited by the absence of cumulated activity data for the pregnant woman and by the little data available to describe human placental transfer and the foetal biokinetic behaviour of radiopharmaceuticals. Although these latter data are available for animals, human data are limited to fallout radionuclides, radiopharmaceuticals used for placental localization before the advent of obstetric ultrasound, pregnant patients treated inadvertently with ^{131}I, and a few case reports involving diagnostic radiopharmaceuticals. In general, these studies lack foetal clearance measurements. However S-factors for the pregnant female at different stages of pregnancy are contained in the latest MIRD dosimetry software (MIRDOSE 3) [15].

Some of these limitations can be ignored during the early stages of pregnancy, when it can be assumed that the abdominal organs have not yet been displaced or changed in shape. Under these circumstances, the foetal dose is considered equivalent to the dose to the uterus. A comprehensive set of uterine absorbed doses (per unit activity administered) for various different radiopharmaceuticals has been published by the International Commission on Radiological Protection (ICRP) [12]. The uterine absorbed doses corresponding to typical administered activities for radiopharmaceuticals in common use are listed in Table 20.7; it can be seen that for ^{99m}Tc-labelled radiopharmaceuticals, the absorbed doses range from 0.2–4 mGy.

FOETAL RISKS FOLLOWING *IN UTERO* IRRADIATION

The possible deterministic effects to the foetus following *in utero* irradiation include lethality, gross malformations and mental retardation [1,2]. The threshold doses for lethality and gross malformations are well in excess of the foetal doses from radionuclide tests. For a gestational age of 8–15 weeks, there is a possible no-threshold response for the induction of severe mental retardation, but the predicted intelligence quota (IQ) loss of 0.03 IQ points/mGy would not be detectable. Outside this gestational age, mental retardation has either not been observed or it has a threshold dose far greater than foetal doses incurred from diagnostic nuclear medicine procedures.

The possible stochastic effects to the foetus following *in utero* irradiation are heritable disease and cancer. The NRPB gives (assuming a linear hypothesis) a risk for heritable disease and for excess fatal cancer up to the age of 15 years of

Table 20.7   Uterine absorbed doses for radiopharmaceuticals in common use [12]

Radiopharmaceutical	Administered activity (MBq)	Uterine absorbed dose (mGy)
^{51}Cr-EDTA	3	0.008
^{67}Ga-citrate	150	12
^{75}Se-selenonorcholestrol	8	14
^{81m}Kr (gas)	6000	0.0008
^{99m}Tc-IDA derivatives	150	2.0
^{99m}Tc-DTPA	300	2.4
^{99m}Tc-DTPA (aerosol)	80	0.5
^{99m}Tc-DMSA	80	0.4
^{99m}Tc-erythrocytes	800	3.8
^{99m}Tc-diphosphonates	600	3.7
^{99m}Tc-gluconate/glucoheptonate	500	3.9
^{99m}Tc-HMPAO	500	3.3
^{99m}Tc-MAA	100	0.2
^{99m}Tc-MAG3	100	1.2
^{99m}Tc-MIBI	400	3.1
^{99m}Tc-pertechnetate	80	0.7
^{99m}Tc-sulphur colloid	80	0.2
^{111}In-leucocytes	20	2.4
^{123}I-iodide	20	0.3
^{123}I-MIBG	400	4.4
^{123}I-hippuran	20	0.3
^{125}I-HSA	0.2	0.04
^{131}I-iodide	400	22
^{131}I-MIBG	20	1.6
^{201}Tl-chloride	80	4.0

2.4×10^{-2}/Gy (1 in 40000 per mGy) and 3.0×10^{-2}/Gy (1 in 33000 per mGy) respectively [2]. If excess non-fatal cancers are also included, then the latter risk coefficient approximately doubles. In the early stages when pregnancy may not yet have been confirmed, the NRPB considers that although the risk of cancer cannot be assumed to be zero, it should be much lower than in the later stages [2].

RISKS FROM ^{131}I ADMINISTRATION

In addition to the theoretical risk data discussed above, there is some empirical data to describe the risk following inadvertent administration of ^{131}I to pregnant patients for the treatment of hyperthyroidism [16]. No increased risk of spontaneous abortion or foetal abnormalities was observed in children born to mothers treated during the first trimester of pregnancy. For administration during the later stages of pregnancy, there was an increased risk of hypothyroidism in the infant with the possibility of mental deficiency if the hypothyroidism was not detected. These empirical risk data can also be applied to ^{131}I imaging of thyroid cancer because the administered activi-

ties are similar to those used for treatment of hyperthyroidism.

ADVICE TO THE PATIENT

The type of advice that can be given to the patient (and the referring clinician) can be demonstrated by the following example of a ventilation–perfusion scan which is probably the most frequently requested nuclear medicine procedure carried out in pregnant women for suspected pulmonary embolism.

For an administration of 80 MBq ^{99m}Tc-DTPA aerosol and 100 MBq ^{99m}Tc-MAA, the total uterine absorbed dose will be 0.7 mGy [12]. The corresponding risk of heritable disease and fatal cancer is about 1 in 60000 and 1 in 48000 respectively [2]. (It should be noted that firstly using ^{81m}Kr gas for the ventilation scan will reduce these risks to about 1 in 170000 and 1 in 140000, respectively, and secondly some nuclear medicine services may find it diagnostically acceptable to use a lower activity of ^{99m}Tc-MAA.) These risks can be compared with the risk of a baby being born with a congenital malformation (1 in 56 in England and Wales during 1989) [17], and with the natural cumulative risk of fatal childhood cancer (1 in 1300 in England and Wales) [2].

It is also essential to advise the patient of the risks associated with not carrying out the procedure. Occasionally, this explanation should be left to the referring clinician, since the actual risks may depend on the patient's particular clinical condition and circumstances. The above example represents a potentially fatal condition, and hence the risks can be given simply as the number of deaths from pulmonary embolism during pregnancy (16 in the UK during the period 1985–1987) [18].

A more straightforward description of the risk is to compare the foetal dose with the national average dose received from natural background radiation and with that received in a part of the country where the background is higher than the national average. For example, if the above procedure was carried out in the UK, the mother can be advised that her baby will receive an additional dose that is less than one-half of the average dose from natural background radiation during the entire course of pregnancy, and is the average additional dose received above this background value after spending 7 weeks in Cornwall [14].

The patient should also be advised on any precautionary measures that she can take to reduce the foetal dose. For instance, if the radioactivity is excreted in urine, then the bladder will act as a significant source of exposure to the foetus. In which case, the patient should be encouraged to drink plenty and to empty her bladder as often as possible to hasten excretion and reduce the bladder component of the foetal dose.

SUMMARY

The radiation risks to pregnant patients from most routine diagnostic nuclear medicine procedures are small. Particular care is needed with the administration of radioiodine in the treatment of thyroid disorders. Routine radiation protection precautions should minimize the risks that exist. The major problem is an occasional failure to identify a pregnant patient.

PREGNANT STAFF

A large proportion of staff working in a nuclear medicine department are women of childbearing age. If local rules, working practices and procedures assume that female members of staff are pregnant, then there is no need for the employees to adopt special precautions in pre-conception or in the early stages of pregnancy. However, once a member of staff is known to be pregnant, it is good practice to reassure her by minimizing the possibility of high exposures. Pregnant nuclear medicine staff members can usually continue to work throughout their pregnancy, but some adjustment to their pattern of work and monitoring arrangements should be considered to reduce the total foetal exposure, and in particular, any possibility of exposure to known sources of high activity should be eliminated.

In departments with large numbers of staff, drastically reducing or even avoiding any exposure to ionizing radiation by an individual member of staff may be possible, but smaller departments may not be able to function on this basis. In any case, it is recommended that wherever practicable, pregnant members of staff should avoid: radiopharmaceutical dispensing; preparing and handling therapy doses; eluting, preparing and using ^{99m}Tc and ^{81m}Kr generators; dealing with radioactive spills; and imaging very sick patients.

ICRP recommends that the dose limit for members of the public be reduced to 1 mSv (averaged over 5 years), and that the foetus of a pregnant employee should be treated as a member of the public [1]. To achieve this level of protection, a dose limit of 2 mSv to the surface of the mother's abdomen has been recommended [1], which has been translated into a limit of eight imaging studies per day during the declared term of pregnancy [19]. However, a phantom study has shown that under occupational exposure conditions of nuclear medicine staff to ^{99m}Tc and ^{131}I patients, a dose limit of 1 mSv to the foetus would require a limit of 1.3 mSv to the maternal abdominal surface which corresponds to a lower limit of six ^{99m}Tc studies per day or one ^{131}I study per day for the duration of pregnancy [20]. This value of the abdominal dose limit also necessitates that the member of staff would have to wear a more sensitive personal dosimeter than a film badge.

BREAST-FEEDING PATIENTS

If the radiation exposure to a breast-fed infant is too high, then the effective dose should be reduced to an acceptable level by the mother either interrupting or ceasing feeding. An appropriate recommendation can only be issued to the mother if there is prior knowledge of the effective dose to the infant and the effective half-life of the radioactivity in milk. Until a few years ago, there was a dearth of data on the secretion of radioactivity in milk following administration of radiopharmaceuticals; in addition, different methods were being used for data analysis and the decision to resume breast-feeding was subject to assumptions and criteria for which there was no consensus.

Considerable data have recently become available, and a comprehensive set of recommendations have been derived by applying a uniform analytical method [21–24]. These recommendations have been designed to ensure that the effective dose to the infant does not exceed the 1 mSv limit recommended by the International Commission on Radiological Protection (ICRP) for exposure of the public in a year [1].

ADVICE TO THE PATIENT

Before arriving at the nuclear medicine department for her appointment, the mother should be issued with the following advice:

1. To express some breast milk and store it in a refrigerator.
2. To breast-feed her infant immediately before attending the department.
3. To interrupt feeding according to the recommendations given in Table 20.8.
4. To feed her infant with the stored milk during the period of interruption.

If the mother follows the above advice, then the effective dose to her infant will be no more than 1 mSv, and in many cases, much less than this value.

The mother can be reassured by comparing the

Table 20.8 Recommendations for interrupting breast feeding [21–24]

Category	Recommendation	Radiopharmaceutical
I.	Interruption not essential*	^{51}Cr-EDTA, ^{99m}Tc-DISIDA, ^{99m}Tc-DTPA, ^{99m}Tc-DMSA, ^{99m}Tc-diphosphonates, ^{99m}Tc-glucoheptonate, ^{99m}Tc-gluconate, ^{99m}Tc-MAG3 (100 MBq), ^{99m}Tc-HMPAO, ^{99m}Tc-MIBI, ^{99m}Tc-sulphur colloid, ^{111}In-leucocytes (20 MBq), ^{201}Tl-chloride (80 MBq).
II.	Interruption for a definite period†	^{99m}Tc-MAA (13 h: 100 MBq). ^{99m}Tc-pertechnetate (47 h: 800 MBq; 25 h: 80 MBq)
III.	Interruption with measurement‡	^{99m}Tc-erythrocytes, ^{99m}Tc-MAA + technegas, ^{99m}Tc-microspheres, ^{99m}Tc-pyrophosphate, ^{99m}Tc-macroaggregated ferrous hydroxide, ^{99m}Tc-plasmin, ^{99m}Tc-EDTA, ^{99m}Tc-polyphosphate, ^{113m}In-chelate complex, ^{123}I-iodide§, ^{123}I-MIBG§, ^{123}I-hippuran§ ^{125}I-hippuran, ^{131}I-hippuran.
IV.	Cessation	Chromic ^{32}P-phosphate, Sodium ^{32}P-phosphate, ^{67}Ga-citrate, ^{75}Se-methionine, ^{125}I-HSA, ^{131}I-HSA ^{125}I-fibrinogen, ^{131}I-iodide, ^{131}I-MAA.

*An interruption is not essential for each of these radiopharmaceuticals if the administered activity is less than the value given in the succeeding parentheses. If no value is given, then it is much greater than the typical administered activity. In practice, a mother can be reassured by advising a short interruption time (e.g. 4 hours).
†The period of interruption and the corresponding maximum administered activity are given in the succeeding parentheses.
‡This recommendation should also be applied to any of the radiopharmaceuticals listed in category I if their administered activity exceeds the value tabulated in category I above.
§The level of ^{124}I and ^{125}I contamination must also be measured.

magnitude of this effective dose with that received from common diagnostic X-ray procedures (e.g. the thoracic spine), or from natural background radiation. For instance, an effective dose of 1 mSv is less than one half of the average background dose received in the UK, and is the average additional dose received above this national average after spending 10 weeks in Cornwall [14].

Further reassurance if required can be supplied by giving the actual risks associated with 1 mSv. ICRP gives a risk of severe hereditary effects and of fatal cancer of $1.3 \times 10^{-2}/Sv$ and $5 \times 10^{-2}/Sv$ respectively, corresponding to an increase in hereditary effects and fatal cancer of 1 in 77 000 and 1 in 20 000 respectively for an effective dose of 1 mSv [1]. These risks can be compared with an estimated natural frequency of 1–3 in 100 for genetic diseases manifesting at birth, and a cumulative risk of 1 in 1300 for fatal childhood cancer up to the age of 15 years [25].

RECOMMENDATIONS

Categories

The recommended advice for each radiopharmaceutical is selected from one of the following four categories describing a different type of interruption to feeding (Table 20.8) [22–24]:

I. **Interruption not essential**: because the activity in the milk is low enough for the effective dose to the infant to be equal to or less than 1 mSv, breast-feeding need not be interrupted. In practice, a mother can be reassured by applying the ALARP principle and advising a short interruption (e.g. 4 hours), at the end of which time period, milk should be expressed and discarded. This recommendation applies only up to a given maximum administered activity (see Table 20.8).

II. **Interruption for a definite period**: starting from the time at which the radiopharmaceutical was administered to the mother, breast-feeding should be interrupted for a specific period (see Table 20.8). During this interruption period, breast milk should be expressed and discarded at normal feeding times. As long as it is practical for the mother to resume feeding after this period, then the main criteria for including a radiopharmaceutical in this category is the quantity of available data.

III. **Interruption with measurement**: estimations of the effective dose to an infant and inter-

ruption period from published data indicate that it is practical to advise the mother that she will be able to resume feeding, but the available data are too limited for a definite period to be recommended. Instead, the concentration of radioactivity expressed in samples of the mother's milk should be measured, and feeding resumed after a period (derived by the method described below) when the effective dose to the infant has reduced to 1 mSv. This recommendation should also be applied to any of the radiopharmaceuticals listed in category 'I' if the administered activity exceeds the maximum limits given in Table 20.8.

IV. **Cessation**: the mother should discontinue feeding altogether because the period of interruption estimated from the available data is much too long to allow resumption of feeding.

Colostrum

In the early stages of lactation when the patient may still be producing colostrum, the rate of secretion of radioactivity in milk appears to follow a different pattern [26]. However, the relevant data available are sparse and the rate is likely to vary between patients. Therefore, except for category 'IV' radiopharmaceuticals, the patient should be advised to follow category 'III' recommendations for *all* other radiopharmaceuticals, if she is likely to be producing colostrum.

Quality control

The recommendations given above and in Table 20.8 apply to a radiopharmaceutical administered in the radiochemical form stated. It is assumed that no other radiochemical species is administered, which will result in a significant effective dose to the infant. There are three instances where this condition could have a practical implication:

1. Free pertechnetate and free iodide are concentrated in milk to a higher level than in plasma [27–29], and therefore it is essential to ensure that a negligible quantity of the unbound form of the radionuclide is administered with any radioiodinated or any ^{99m}Tc-labelled compound.
2. Binding of radioactivity to breast milk protein either before or after administration leads to high concentrations of radioactivity in breast milk. Such high levels will be unavoidable in the case of ^{67}Ga-citrate (where the ^{67}Ga binds to lactoferrin), and for ^{75}Se-methionine (also a

milk protein). However, for ^{111}In-leucocytes (where the ^{111}In also binds to lactoferrin), high protein-bound activity can be avoided by minimizing the quantity of non-cell-bound ^{111}In in the labelled leucocytes injection/preparation.

3. ^{123}I-labelled radiopharmaceuticals may also contain [124]I and ^{125}I as an impurity, depending on the production method. Therefore the levels of these potential contaminants must be determined on an individual basis before a recommendation for resuming breast-feeding can be issued.

ANALYTICAL METHOD TO DERIVE AN INDIVIDUAL RECOMMENDATION

The following analytical method can be used [21–24] if it is necessary to make individual measurements of activity concentration in expressed milk samples (i.e. category 'III' above) in order to advise when a mother can resume feeding.

Ingested activity

Published data show that generally after radiopharmaceutical administration, the activity concentration decreases exponentially with time from a peak value. The effective decay constant can be calculated by a least-squares fit of an exponential curve to the measured activity concentrations. If the peak activity concentration occurs in the first sample, then the total activity ingested, I, by the infant for all feeds can be calculated from:

$$I = \sum_{j=1}^{m} c_j \cdot V / \left(1 - \exp\{-\lambda_j \cdot \tau\}\right) \quad (20.1)$$

where m is the number of exponential components for each of which c_j is the concentration of activity ingested in the first feed, and λ_j is the effective decay constant. The volume of milk per feed (V) and the time between feeds (τ) are assumed constant, and values can be allocated to these two terms as appropriate to the individual case. If the peak occurs after the first sample, then the fraction ingested in each feed taken before the peak is given by $a \cdot V$, where a is the activity concentration in that feed, and the total ingested activity can be determined by adding each of these contributions to the value given by Eqn (20.1) applied to all feeds taken after the peak value. Analyses of breast milk data on which the above recommendations (Table 20.8) are based have assumed that the infant has

ingested 850 ml per day in six feeds (i.e. 4 hours between each feed of 142 ml) [30].

For most radiopharmaceuticals, the activity concentration in milk decays monoexponentially, and if the decay constant λ is known, then by making just one measurement of the concentration c of radioactivity in milk, the total activity which would be ingested if feeding was resumed at the next occasion can be estimated simply [5] from the equation:

$$I = c \cdot K \quad (20.2)$$

where K is a constant calculated from:

$$K = V \cdot \exp\{-\lambda \cdot \tau\} / \left[1 - \exp\{-\lambda_j \cdot \tau\}\right] \quad (20.3)$$

using values of V and τ appropriate to the individual case as before. It can be seen that K represents a single effective ingested volume which accounts for the intermittency of breast-feeding and for the decay of the radioactivity concentration in milk between feeds.

Dose to the infant

The effective dose D to the infant is given by:

$$D = I \cdot e \quad (20.4)$$

Because of the absence of data describing the variation of e, the effective dose to the infant per unit activity ingested, the ICRP values of the effective dose to an adult per unit activity ingested [31] were increased by the ratio of the standard adult body weight (70 kg) to the infant's body weight (taken to be 4 kg) for the data analyses on which the above recommendations are based.

Interruption period

For a monoexponential decrease in activity concentration with time after administration, the period P (hours) after the time of administration for feeding to be interrupted in order to reduce the infant's effective dose to x mSv can be calculated from:

$$P = t_{1/2}\left(\ln\{D/x\} / \ln\{2\}\right) + t_c \quad (20.5)$$

where $t_{1/2}$ is the effective half-life of the radioactivity in milk, and t_c is the time after administration either at which the milk concentration c_j was expressed if D was derived from Eqn (20.1), or of the subsequent feed if D was derived from Eqns (20.2) and (20.3).

CLOSE CONTACT DOSES

A young infant held in close contact with a parent who has undergone a nuclear medicine procedure will be exposed to the radiation emitted from the radioactivity retained by the parental organs, regardless of whether the parent is breast-feeding or not. However, dosimetry studies have concluded that an infant will receive a close contact dose of <1 mSv from a parent who has undergone a diagnostic nuclear medicine procedure as long as the administered activity does not exceed the typical maximum value [23,32,33]. The only exception is ^{111}In-labelled leucocytes where the maximum close contact period [34] observed between a parent and a fretful infant will result in a dose of 1 mSv if the administered activity exceeds 8 MBq [35].

Close contact will have to be restricted if the parent has undergone an ^{131}I therapeutic procedure. The duration of this restriction should be based on satisfying a statutory requirement or an official recommendation, which could take the form of a dose limit to the infant or a level of activity retained by the parent. The restriction can be derived on an individual basis by estimating the potential dose to the infant. This dose can be obtained by multiplying the dose rate measured on or close to the surface of the patient by an effective exposure time (e.g. 27.4 hours for ^{131}I administered to a euthyroid patient) which accounts for the intermittency of close contact and for dose rate decay [32,33], and which corresponds to the maximum close contact period mentioned above [34]. Alternatively, published values of dose rates at different distances from patients administered ^{131}I for thyrotoxicosis [36,37] and thyroid cancer can be used [38,39].

SUMMARY

There is no reason for denying a breast-feeding woman the benefits of a diagnostic nuclear medicine procedure or causing an unnecessary interruption to her feeding because of ignorance of the passage of radioactivity into her milk and the effective dose to her infant. Apart from ^{67}Ga-citrate and ^{131}I-labelled compounds, mothers should be able to resume feeding within 2 days of administration of the most commonly used radiopharmaceuticals. Indeed, for many of the agents in routine use, particularly those labelled with ^{99m}Tc, there is no need to interrupt feeding at all – although a short period is still recommended for reassurance. The reason why individual measurements have still to be recommended for some of these commonly used radiopharmaceuticals is because of a lack of relevant data describing the concentration of radioactivity secreted into milk and the chemical species of this radioactivity. Nuclear medicine practitioners are urged to acquire these data at every opportunity in order to allow definite periods of interruption to be allocated with confidence.

REFERENCES

1. International Commission on Radiological Protection. (1991) *1990 Recommendations of the International Commission on Radiological Protection*, ICRP Publication 60, Pergamon Press, Oxford.
2. National Radiological Protection Board. (1993) *Board Statement on Diagnostic Medical Exposures to Ionising Radiation During Pregnancy*. Documents of the NRPB, Vol. 4, No. 4, HMSO, London.
3. Gardner, M.J., Snee, M.P., Hall, A.J. *et al.* (1990) Result of a case control study of leukaemia and lymphoma in young people near Sellafield nuclear plant in West Cumbria. *Br. Med. J.*, **300**, 423–9.
4. Doll, R., Evans, H.J. and Darby, S.C. (1994) Paternal exposure not to blame. *Nature*, **367**, 678–80.
5. Administration of Radioactive Substances Advisory Committee. (1993) *Notes for Guidance on the Administration of Radioactive Substances to Persons for Purposes of Diagnosis, Treatment or Research*, Department of Health, London.
6. Safa, A.M., Schumaker, O.P. and Rodriguez-Antunez, A. (1975) Long-term follow-up in children and adolescents treated with radioactive iodine (131I) for hyperthyroidism. *N. Engl. J. Med.*, **292**, 167–71.
7. Sarker, S.D., Beierwaltes, W.H., Gill, S.P. *et al.* (1976) Subsequent fertility and birth histories of children and adolescents treated with ^{131}I for thyroid cancer. *J. Nucl. Med.*, **17**, 460–4.
8. Casara, D., Rubello, D., Saladini, G. *et al.* (1993) Pregnancy after high therapeutic doses of iodine-131 in differentiated cancer: potential risks and recommendations. *Eur. J. Nucl. Med.*, **20**, 192–4.
9. Dottorini, M.E., Lomuscio, G., Mazzucchelli, L. *et al.* (1995) Assessment of female fertility and carcinogenesis after iodine-131 therapy for differentiated thyroid cancer. *J. Nucl. Med.*, **36**, 21–7.
10. Schlumberger, M., De Vathaire, F., Ceccarelli, C. *et al.* (1996) Exposure to radioactive iodine-131 for scintigraphy or therapy does not preclude pregnancy in thyroid cancer patients. *J. Nucl. Med.*, **37**, 606–12.
11. Sobels, F.H. (1969) Estimation of the genetic risk resulting from the treatment of women with 131I iodine. *Strahlentherapie*, **138**, 172–7.
12. International Commission on Radiological Protection. (1994) *Radiation Dose to Patients from Radio-*

pharmaceuticals (including Addendum 1), 2nd edn, ICRP Publication 53, Pergamon Press, Oxford.

13. Shrimpton, P.C., Wall, B.F., Jones, D.G. *et al.* (1986) *A National Survey of Doses to Patients Undergoing a Selection of Routine X-ray Examinations in English Hospitals.* NRPB-R200, HMSO, London.

14. Hughes, J.S. and O'Riordan, M.C. (1993) *Radiation Exposure of the UK Population – 1993 Review*, NRPB-R263, HMSO, London.

15. Stabin, M.G. (1996) MIRDOSE: personal computer software for internal dose assessment in nuclear medicine. *J. Nucl. Med.*, **37**, 538–46.

16. Stoffer, S.S. and Hamburger, J.I. (1976) Inadvertent 131I therapy for hyperthyroidism in the first trimester of pregnancy. *J. Nucl. Med.*, **17**, 146–9.

17. Department of Health (1992) *On the state of the public health. The annual report of the Chief Medical Officer of the Department of Health for the year 1991*, HMSO, London.

18. Department of Health (1992) *Report on confidential enquiries into maternal deaths in the United Kingdom 1985–87*, HMSO, London.

19. Clarke, E.A., Thomson, W.H., Notghi, A. *et al.* (1992) Radiation doses from nuclear medicine patients to an imaging technologist: relation to ICRP recommendations for pregnant workers. *Nucl. Med. Commun.*, **13**, 795–8.

20. Mountford, P.J. and Steele, H.R. (1995) Foetal dose estimates and the ICRP abdominal dose limit for occupational exposure of pregnant staff to technetium-99m and iodine-131 patients. *Eur. J. Nucl. Med.*, **22**, 1173–9.

21. Ahlgren, L., Ivarsson, S., Johansson, L. *et al.* (1985) Excretion of radionuclides in human breast milk after the administration of radiopharmaceuticals. *J. Nucl. Med.*, **26**, 1085–90.

22. Mountford, P.J. and Coakley, A.J. (1989) A review of the secretion of radioactivity in human breast milk: data, quantitative analysis and recommendations. *Nucl. Med. Commun.*, **10**, 15–27.

23. Rubow, S., Klopper, J., Wasserman, H. *et al.* (1994) The excretion of radiopharmaceuticals in human breast milk: additional data and dosimetry. *Eur. J. Nucl. Med.*, **21**, 144–53.

24. Mountford, P.J., Lazarus, C.R. and Edwards, S. (1996) Radiopharmaceuticals, in *Drugs and Human Lactation*, 2nd edn (ed. P.N. Bennett), Elsevier Science, Amsterdam, pp. 609–77.

25. National Radiological Protection Board (1993) *Occupational, Public and Medical Exposure*, Documents of the NRPB, Vol. 4 No. 2, HMSO, London.

26. Heaton, B. (1979) The build up of technetium in breast milk following the administration of $^{99m}TcO_4$ labelled macroaggregated albumin. *Br. J. Radiol.*, **52**, 149–50.

27. Mountford, P.J., Heap, R.B., Hamon, M. *et al.* (1987) Suppression of technetium-99m and iodine-123 secretion in milk of lactating goats. *J. Nucl. Med.*, **28**, 1187–91.

28. Ennis, M.E., Johnson, J.E., Ward, G.M. *et al.* (1989) Technetium metabolism by lactating goats. *Health Phys.*, **57**, 321–30.

29. Honour, A.J., Myant, N.B. and Rowlands, E.N. (1952) Secretion of radioiodine in digestive juices and milk in man. *Clin. Sci.*, **11**, 447–62.

30. International Commission on Radiological Protection (1977) *Report of the Task Group on Reference Man*, ICRP Publication 23, Pergamon Press, Oxford.

31. International Commission on Radiological Protection (1991) *Annual Limits on Intake of Radionuclides by Workers Based on the 1990 Recommendations*, ICRP Publication 61, Pergamon Press, Oxford.

32. Mountford, P.J. (1987) Estimation of close contact doses to young infants from surface dose rates on radioactive adults. *Nucl. Med. Commun.*, **8**, 857–63.

33. Mountford, P.J., O'Doherty, M.J., Forge, N.I. *et al.* (1991) Radiation dose rates from adult patients undergoing nuclear medicine investigations. *Nucl. Medicine Commun.*, **12**, 767–77.

34. Rose, M.R., Prescott, M.C. and Herman, K.J. (1990) Excretion of iodine-123-hippuran, technetium-99m-red blood cells, and technetium-99m-macroaggregated albumin into breast milk. *J. Nucl. Med.*, **31**, 978–84.

35. Mountford, P.J. and Coakley, A.J. (1989) Body surface dosimetry following re-injection of ^{111}In leucocytes. *Nucl. Med. Commun.*, **10**, 497–501.

36. Culver, C.M. and Dworkin, H.J. (1991) Radiation safety considerations for post-iodine-131 hyperthyroid therapy. *J. Nucl. Med.*, **32**, 169–73.

37. O'Doherty, M.J., Kettle, A.G., Eustance, C.P. *et al.* (1993) Radiation dose rates from adult patients receiving ^{131}I therapy for thyrotoxicosis. *Nucl. Med. Commun.*, **14**, 160–8.

38. Culver, C.M. and Dworkin, H.J. (1991) Radiation safety considerations for post-iodine-131 thyroid cancer therapy. *J. Nucl. Med.*, **33**, 1402–5.

39. Barrington, S.F., Kettle, A.G., O'Doherty, M.J. *et al.* (1996) Radiation dose rates from patients receiving iodine-131 therapy for carcinoma of the thyroid. *Eur. J. Nucl. Med.*, **23**, 123–30.

CHAPTER 21

Quantitation

H. D. Royal and B. J. McNeil

INTRODUCTION

Clinicians who are either enthralled by numbers or who are somewhat in awe of them frequently fail to be sufficiently critical of tests with numerical outputs. They assume that such tests have a value or accuracy higher than do tests which have only subjective or qualitative outputs. While this situation is sometimes the case, it is clearly not always the case. In this chapter on quantitative nuclear medicine, we shall focus first on objective measurements of regional physiology and secondly on measurements of the efficacy of diagnotic tests. In both sections we shall try to emphasize basic principles, the likely effects of errors in analysis and the extent to which mathematical approximations provide accurate answers to clinical problems. Since this chapter provides only an introduction to these quantitative techniques, the interested reader is encouraged to consult other more detailed sources which are listed in the references.

QUANTITATIVE TRACER STUDIES

Although nuclear medicine has its origins in utilizing basic radiotracer principles to study non-invasively a variety of physiology processes, the clinical specialty has consisted primarily of subjectively evaluated static images in which changes in structure are often as important as changes in function. Two forces are now at work to mould clinical nuclear medicine into a more quantitative, more physiological, more dynamic specialty. Firstly, for the first time in nuclear medicine's short history, sophisticated digital data acquisition and analysis capabilities are becoming widely available in clinical units. The impetus for rapid dissemination of digital capabilities has come from nuclear cardiology and from high-technology developments which have made sophisticated data analysis systems available at a reasonable cost. Secondly, improvements in spatial resolution of other non-invasive modalities (computed tomography and ultrasound) are redirecting nuclear medicine to exploit its unique capability for studying regional pathophysiology. In this climate, quantitative physiological studies will surely flourish; therefore the need for radiologists and nuclear medicine physicians to become aware of the fundamentals of quantitative tracer studies is more acute than ever.

The examples of quantitative clinical studies which will be presented in subsequent sections have been chosen for a variety of reasons. The cerebrospinal fluid shunt flow study has limited application; however, its simplicity as a quantitative model is attractive for didactic purposes. An understanding of physical, biological and effective half-lives is essential in any quantitative study; therefore these have been discussed. Measurement of glomerular filtration rate provides an example of a quantitative *non-imaging* physiological test. Regional blood flow has many potential clinical applications although it has until now been primarily a research tool. Cardiac output and transit time determination undoubtedly will be routinely obtained as nuclear cardiology becomes more refined. Finally, more sophisticated methods of data analysis such as deconvolution are likely to be widely applied in the future.

Although the details of each section of this half of the chapter differ, the reader should recognize the similarity of approach in each section. When faced with the task of determining a quantitative solution to a problem, the following approach should be taken. First, define the assumptions upon which the solution to the problem is based. Secondly, assess how accurately each assumption is met in reality. Thirdly, test the technique in a broad spectrum of patients to determine what limitations might exist.

CEREBROSPINAL FLUID (CSF) SHUNT FLOW

Measurement of CSF flow through ventriculo-peritoneal or ventriculovenous shunts in patients with non-communicating hydrocephalus is useful in differentiating disease progression from shunt failure [1,2]. To perform this study, 500 µCi of pertechnetate in a small volume (<0.1 ml) are rapidly injected into the reservoir of the one-way valve of the shunt appliance. Sequential digital images are then acquired at a rate of 12 frames min^{-1} for 5 min using a pinhole or parallel-hole collimator and a gamma camera interfaced to a minicomputer. An activity-time curve is generated using an operator-defined region of interest over the reservoir (see Figure 21.1).

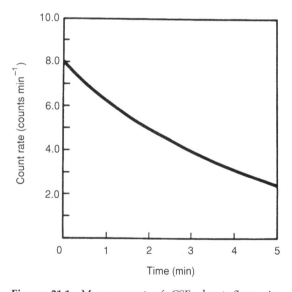

Figure 21.1 Measurement of CSF shunt flow. An activity–time curve obtained from a region of interest over a shunt reservoir is shown. The ordinate is the count rate recorded by the scintillation camera and the abscissa is time. Both scales are linear, and a mono-exponential curve is seen. This curve becomes a straight line when plotted on a semi-logarithmic graph (see Figure 21.3).

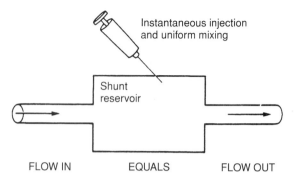

Figure 21.2   Assumptions underlying CSF flow calculation. This diagram shows schematically a shunt reservoir with an entrance (Flow in) from the ventricles and an exit (Flow out), first into the shunt tubing and ultimately into the peritoneum. The injection site for the radiotracer is also illustrated. Calculation of CSF shunt flow assumes that there is instantaneous injection and uniform mixing of the tracer and also that flow into and out of the reservoir are equal. The latter implies that the volume of the reservoir is constant.

Shunt flow (ml min^{-1}) can be measured with this system if the effective volume of the reservoir is known and if two assumptions are made (see Figure 21.2). First, there is instantaneous, uniform mixing of the tracer within the reservoir. Secondly, the volume of the reservoir is constant, and, therefore, flow into and out of the reservoir are equal. Under these conditions, the change in the tracer activity of the reservoir during any small time interval is equal to the flow times the tracer activity of the reservoir divided by the effective volume of the reservoir, all times the time interval. That is:

$$\Delta Q(t) = -F \frac{Q(t)}{V} \Delta t \qquad (21.1)$$

where

$Q(t)$ = tracer activity of the reservoir (mCi)
$\Delta Q(t)$ = the change in the tracer activity in the reservoir at time t (mCi)
F = CSF shunt flow (ml min^{-1})
V = effective volume of the reservoir (ml)
Δt = a small time interval (min).

The minus sign indicates that tracer is lost from the reservoir system.

Since the change in activity of tracer in the reservoir is equal to the change in concentration times the volume, equation (21.1) can be rewritten in terms of concentration

$$\Delta Q(t) = -\Delta C(t)V = -FC(t)\Delta t \qquad (21.2)$$

where

$C(t)$ = tracer concentration of the reservoir ($\mathrm{mCi\,ml^{-1}}$)

$\Delta C(t)$ = the change in tracer concentration of the reservoir at time t ($\mathrm{mCi\,ml^{-1}}$)

If Δt approaches 0, equation (21.2) can be rearranged and written in differential form as

$$\frac{dC(t)}{C(t)} = -\frac{F}{V}dt \qquad (21.3)$$

Integration results in

$$\int_0^t \frac{dC(t)}{C(t)} = -\int_0^t \frac{F}{V}dt \qquad (21.4)$$

The solution to equation (21.4) can be found in standard tables of solutions to integrals and is

$$\ln C(t)\Big|_0^t = -\frac{F}{V}t\Big|_0 \qquad (21.5)$$

Substituting the limits of the integral into equation (21.5) and simplifying, yields

$$\ln C(t) = -\frac{F}{V}t + \ln C(0) \qquad (21.6)$$

Since equation (21.6) has the form of a linear equation, a graph of the logarithm of the concentration against time produces a straight line with a slope of F/V and an intercept of $C(0)$ (see Figure 21.3). The slope of the straight line can be calculated using a least squares fit; therefore, since the effective reservoir volume, V, can be determined experimentally, CSF shunt flow, F, can be calculated from

$$F = -\text{slope} \times V \qquad (21.7)$$

Equation (21.6) is sometimes expressed in exponential form

$$C(t) = C(0)e^{(-F/V)t} \qquad (21.8)$$

Even in this simple example of quantitative analysis, the critical reader will appreciate that the assumptions upon which the analysis was based are not strictly met. For example, flow through the reservoir is more likely to be pulsatile than constant; there may not be instantaneous uniform mixing; and the injection of even a small volume of tracer will cause a transient increase in flow. Moreover, in the more elaborate shunt appliances,

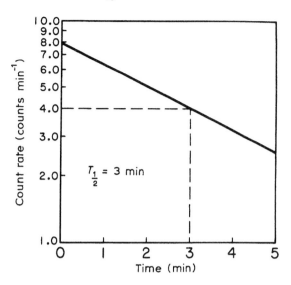

Figure 21.3 Calculation of CSF flow from data presented in Figure 21.1. The ordinate is the activity recorded on a logarithmic scale and the abscissa is time (min). If the volume of the reservoir is known, the slope of the resulting straight line can be used to calculate CSF flow. CSF shunt flow (F) equals the slope times the effective volume (V) of the reservoir. For a Holter valve with an effective volume of 0.18 ml, the flow is 0.042 ml min^{-1}; this is within the range of normal.

CSF shunt flow determination

$$F = (\text{Slope})\,(V)$$

$$\text{Slope} = \frac{0.693}{T_{1/2}} = \frac{0.693}{3\,\text{min}} = 0.231\,\text{min}^{-1}$$

$$V = 0.18\,\text{ml}$$

$$F = (0.231\,\text{min}^{-1})(0.18\,\text{ml})$$

$$= 0.042\,\text{ml\,min}^{-1}$$

eddy currents and turbulence may make the *effective* reservoir volume differ from the *physical* reservoir volume. Despite these differences between the model and the actual situation, this technique has been found to be clinically useful [1,2].

HALF-LIVES

Quantitative analysis of CSF shunt flow described in the previous section is an example of *first-order kinetics* where the rate of change of a substance is directly proportional to the quantity of substance present. That is

$$\frac{dQ(t)}{dt} = kQ(t) \qquad (21.9)$$

where

$Q(t)$ = the quantity of substance present at time t (mCi)

$\dfrac{dQ(t)}{dt}$ = instantaneous rate of change of $Q(t)$ (mCi s^{-1})

k = proportionality constant (s^{-1})

Many physical processes demonstrate the first-order kinetics described by equation (21.9). For example, the rate of radionuclide decay is directly proportional to the number of atoms present, that is

$$\frac{dN(t)}{dt} = -kN(t) \qquad (21.10)$$

where

$N(t)$ = number of atoms present at time t (atoms)

$\dfrac{dN(t)}{dt}$ = the decay rate (atoms s^{-1})

k = decay constant (s^{-1})

Integration and simplification, analogues to equations (21.3–6) and (21.8) results in

$$N(t) = N(0)e^{-kt} \qquad (21.11)$$

where $N(0)$ = initial number of atoms. Since the physical half-life of a radionuclide is well known, equation (21.11) is more useful when k is expressed in terms of physical half-life ($T_{1/2_p}$). By definition

$$\frac{N(0)}{N\left(T_{1/2_p}\right)} = \frac{1}{0.5} = 2 = \frac{N(0)}{N(0)e^{-k\left(T_{1/2}\right)}}$$

$$= \frac{1}{e^{-k\left(T_{1/2}\right)}} \qquad (21.12)$$

Thus, k is defined in terms of $T_{1/2_p}$ by taking the natural logarithm of equation (21.12) and rearranging

$$k = \frac{-\ln 2}{T_{1/2_p}} = \frac{-0.693}{T_{1/2_p}} \qquad (21.13)$$

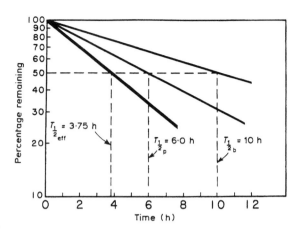

Figure 21.4 Effective ($T_{1/2_{eff}}$), physical ($T_{1/2_p}$) and biological half-lives ($T_{1/2_b}$). In this graph, the percentages of radionuclide remaining if only physical decay or biological clearance was considered are plotted as the light lines. The heavy black line indicates the actual percentage remaining assuming that both physical decay and biological clearance occur. Typically the physical half-life is known and the effective half-life is measured. Biological half-life is then calculated. As shown in the sample calculations, any of the half-lives can be calculated if the other two are known.

Half-life determination

$$T_{1/2_{eff}} = \frac{T_{1/2_p} \times T_{1/2_b}}{T_{1/2_p} + T_{1/2_b}} = \frac{(10h)(96h)}{10h + 6h} = 3.75h$$

$$T_{1/2_b} = \frac{T_{1/2_p} \times T_{1/2_{eff}}}{T_{1/2_p} - T_{1/2_{eff}}} = \frac{(6.0h)(3.75h)}{6.0h - 3.75h} = 10h$$

$$T_{1/2_p} = \frac{T_{1/2_b} \times T_{1/2_{eff}}}{T_{1/2_b} - T_{1/2_{eff}}} = \frac{(10h)(3.75h)}{10h - 3.75h} = 6h$$

In biological systems, the disappearance of a tracer is often the result of both its physical decay and its biological clearance (see Figure 21.4). If the biological clearance follows first-order kinetics, the effective or observed clearance of the tracer will be equal to the sum of the amount cleared biologically and that lost by physical decay

$$\frac{dQ(t)}{dt} = \frac{-\ln 2}{T_{1/2_p}} Q(t) + \frac{-\ln 2}{T_{1/2_b}} Q(t) \qquad (21.14)$$

where

$Q(t)$ = quantity at time t (mCi)

$\dfrac{dQ(t)}{dt}$ = *total* rate of loss of activity (mCi s^{-1})

$T_{1/2_p}$ = physical half-life (s)
$T_{1/2_b}$ = biological half-life (s)

Collected terms yields

$$\frac{dQ(t)}{dt} = -\left(\frac{\ln 2}{T_{1/2_p}} + \frac{\ln 2}{T_{1/2_b}} \right) Q(t) \qquad (21.15)$$

By definition, the effective clearance rate is equal to the sum of the biological and physical clearance rates

$$\frac{\ln 2}{T_{1/2_{eff}}} = \frac{\ln 2}{T_{1/2_b}} + \frac{\ln 2}{T_{1/2_p}} \qquad (21.16)$$

where

$$T_{1/2_{eff}} = \text{effective half-life (s)}$$

Simplifying equation (21.16) yields

$$T_{1/2_{eff}} = \frac{T_{1/2_b} \times T_{1/2_p}}{T_{1/2_b} + T_{1/2_p}} \qquad (21.17)$$

Since the physical half-life is usually known and the effective half-life is usually measured, equation (21.17) can be written in terms of the unknown biological half-life

$$T_{1/2_b} = \frac{T_{1/2_p} \times t_{1/2_{eff}}}{T_{1/2_p} + T_{1/2_{eff}}} \qquad (21.18)$$

GLOMERULAR FILTRATION RATE

Although the clinical usefulness of measuring glomerula filtration rate (GFR) is widely accepted, the existence of multiple methodologies to measure GFR (for example, 24-h endogenous creatinine clearance, inulin clearance, radiotracer clearance) indicates that each one has limitations. One commonly used radiotracer method is based on Sapirstein's mode [3] to measure GFR after a single intravenous injection of non-radioactive creatinine. The simplified method discussed here requires three hourly venous blood samples beginning 2 h after a single intravenous injection of a suitable radiopharmaceutical. Although controversy exists regarding the radiopharmaceutical of choice for this study, the ideal radiotracer would have the following four characteristics: (a) no loss of the tracer due to in-vivo metabolism; (b) no protein binding of the tracer preventing free filtration by the glomerulus; (c) small molecular size;

(d) no secretion or absorption of the radiotracer by the renal tubular cell.

Sapirstein's model of GFR measurement is based on five assumptions. First, the tracer mixed instantly and uniformly in the intravascular space. Secondly, the tracer mixed uniformly in the extravascular space. Thirdly, the volumes of the intra- and extravascular spaces are constant. Fourthly, the rate of loss from the intravascular compartment due to GFR is equal to the glomerular filtration rate times the concentration in the intravascular space. Finally, the tracer diffusion rate between the intravascular and extravascular space varies directly with the difference in tracer concentration in these areas. These assumptions are schematically illustrated in Figure 21.5.

The assumption that the rate of tracer loss due to GFR is equal to the intravascular tracer concentration times the GFR can be stated mathematically

$$\left(\frac{dQ_1(t)}{dt} \right)_{GFR} = GFR C_1(t) \qquad (21.19)$$

where

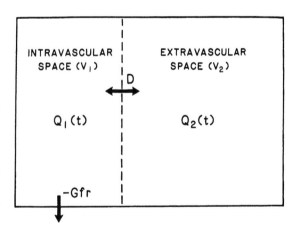

Figure 21.5 Sapirstein's model for measurement of glomerular filtration rate. This model assumes instantaneous intravascular injection with uniform mixing within the intravascular (V_1) and extravascular (V_2) space. The rate of transfer of the tracer between spaces equals the difference between the concentrations in two spaces times the diffusion constant (D) (equation (21.20)). The rate of tracer loss due to glomerular filtration equals the intravascular concentration of tracer times the glomerular filtration rate (GFR) (equation (21.19)).

$\left(\dfrac{dQ_1(t)}{dt}\right)_{GFR}$ = the rate of tracer loss from the intravascular space due to GFR at time t (mCi min^{-1})

GFR = glomerular filtration rate (ml min^{-1})

$C_1(t)$ = intravascular tracer concentration at time t (mCi min^{-1})

Likewise, the assumption that the rate of tracer loss due to diffusion is equal to the diffusion constant time the intravascular and extravascular tracer concentration differences can be stated mathematically

$$\left(\frac{dQ_1(t)}{dt}\right)_{Diff} = -D\left(C_1(t) - C_2(t)\right) \quad (21.20)$$

where $\left(\dfrac{dQ_1(t)}{dt}\right)_{Diff}$ = rate of loss of tracer from the intravascular compartment due to diffusion at time t (mCi min^{-1})

D = Diffusion constant (ml min^{-1})

$C_2(t)$ = extravascular tracer concentration at time t (mCi ml^{-1})

Furthermore, the left sides of equations (21.19) and (21.20) can be expressed in terms of changes in concentration since the change in quantity of a substance is equal to the change in concentration times the volume of distribution

$$\left(\frac{dQ_1(t)}{dt}\right)_{GFR} = V_1\left(\frac{dC_1(t)}{dt}\right)_{GFR} \quad (21.21)$$

where V_1 = the intravascular volume (ml)

$\left(\dfrac{dC_1(t)}{dt}\right)_{GFR}$ = rate of change in concentration due to GFR (mCi ml^{-1}s^{-1})

An analogous relationship exists for changes due to diffusion,

$$\left(\frac{dQ_1(t)}{dt}\right)_{Diff}$$

Therefore, equations (21.19) and (21.20) can now be rewritten solely in terms of concentration

$$\left(\frac{dC_1(t)}{dt}\right)_{GFR} = \frac{-GFR}{V_1}C_1(t) \quad (21.22)$$

and $\quad\left(\dfrac{dC_1(t)}{dt}\right)_{Diff} = \dfrac{-D}{V_1}\left(C_1(t) - C_2(t)\right) \quad (21.23)$

Since the total rate of change in concentration of tracer equals the sum of the rate of change due to GFR and to diffusion, the following equation emerges

$$\left(\frac{dC_1(t)}{dt}\right)_{Total} = \left(\frac{dC_1(t)}{dt}\right)_{GFR} + \left(\frac{dC_1(t)}{dt}\right)_{Diff}$$
$$= \frac{-GFR}{V_1}C_1(t) - \frac{D}{V}\left(C_1(t) - C_2(t)\right)$$

$$(21.24)$$

The equation is not practical to work with since it contains the term $C_2(t)$ which represents the concentration of the tracer in the extravascular space. Since this value cannot be measured clinically, some mathematical manipulations of equation (21.24) are needed to eliminate this term. The interested reader is referred to references 3, 4 and 5 for a full derivation which bridges the gap between equation (21.24) and the following equation which states that the concentration in the intravascular compartment is equal to the sum of two monoexponentials

$$C_1(t) = A_1 e^{\alpha_1 t} + A_2 e^{\alpha_2 t} \quad (21.25)$$

where

A_1 = effective initial concentration for diffusion (mCi ml^{-1})

α_1 = effective transfer rate for diffusion (min^{-1})

A_2 = effective initial concentration for GFR (mCi ml^{-1})

α_2 = effective transfer rate for GFR (min^{-1})

The logarithm of equation (21.25) shown below, is used to calculate GFR since it is the simplest form of the equation

$$\ln C_1(t) = \ln A_1 + \alpha_1 t + \ln A_2 = \alpha_2 t \quad (21.26)$$

As shown in Figure 21.6 equation (21.26) is in the form of the sum of two linear equations. The initial rapid decrease in the intravascular tracer concentration is due to the rapid diffusion of the tracer from the intravascular space to the extravascular space. Once the extravascular tracer

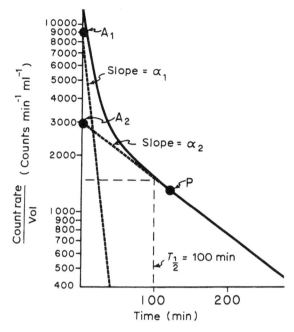

Figure 21.6 Calculation of GFR. GFR is calculated by determining the slope (α_2) and γ intercept (A_2) of the slow component of the blood clearance curve following a single injection of an appropriate radiopharmaceutical. After point P (usually 2 h after injection) the effects of the fast component on the blood clearance curve are negligible; therefore the slope of the slow component can be determined using a semi-logarithmic plot of the concentration–time curve. Extrapolation of this curve identifies A_2 as the γ intercept. The amount of activity injection (I) is determined by measuring the counts g^{-1} of a diluted standard multiplied by the actual number of grams of the injectate and the dilution factor.

GFR determination

$$\text{GFR} = \left(\frac{1}{A_2}\right)(\alpha_2)$$

$$\alpha_2 = \frac{0.693}{T_{1/2}} = \frac{0.693}{100\,\text{min}} = 0.00693\,\text{min}^{-1}$$

$$I = 45\,000\,000\,\text{counts}\,\text{min}^{-1}$$

$$A_2 = 3000\,\text{counts}\,\text{min}^{-1}\,\text{ml}^{-1}$$

$$\text{GFR} = \frac{45\,000\,000\,\text{counts}\,\text{min}^{-1}}{3000\,\text{cts}\,\text{min}^{-1}\,\text{ml}^{-1}}\left(0.00693\,\text{min}^{-1}\right)$$

$$= 104\,\text{ml}\,\text{min}^{-1}$$

concentration approximately equals the intravascular concentration (point P), loss of tracer from the intravascular compartment is due solely to glomerular filtration. Analogous to the calculation of F/V in the GSF shunt flow study

$$\alpha_2 = \frac{\text{GFR}}{V_{\text{eff}}} \qquad (21.27)$$

where

α_2 = slope of the slow component shown in Figure (21.5) (min^{-1})
V_{eff} = effective volume of distribution (ml)

α_2 can be calculated using a least squares fit through the data points after point P. The effective volume of distribution can be calculated from the extrapolated y-intercept, A_2, the effective initial concentration, since the effective volume of distribution equals the injected dose divided by the effective initial concentration, that is

$$V_{\text{eff}} = \frac{I}{A_2} \qquad (21.28)$$

where

V_{eff} = effective volume of distribution (ml)
I = dose injected (mCi)
A_2 = effective initial concentration (mCi ml^{-1})

Substituting equation (21.28) into equation (21.27) and rearranging yields

$$\text{GFR} = \frac{I}{A_2}\alpha_2 \qquad (21.29)$$

Routine clinical use of this technique is promising; however, two obstacles must be overcome. Firstly, the accuracy of this method in patients with moderate to severe renal failure who had expanded extravascular spaces needs further validation. Secondly, an easily prepared chemically stable radiopharmaceutical which meets the previously described criteria for an optimal GFR agent for all pathological states is needed.

REGIONAL BLOOD FLOW

The measurement of regional blood flow is based on principles similar to the ones used for calculation of CSF shunt flow. The main difference between the two techniques is the type of tracer used – diffusible in the case of blood flow measurement and non-diffusible in the case of shunt flow meas-

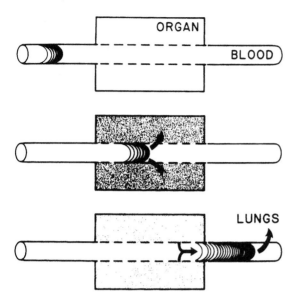

Figure 21.7 Assumptions underlying regional blood flow measurement. (a) Instantaneous injection of the diffusible radioactive tracer into the arterial blood supply of the organ of interest. (b) Rapid diffusion of the tracer into the organ during the first passage of the bolus of radioactivity. (c) Washout of the tracer from the organ into the veins. Note that recirculation of the tracer is prevented by elimination through the lungs.

urements (Figure 21.7). Regional blood flow is measured after the intra-arterial injection of a poorly soluble gas such as ^{133}Xe, which does not recirculate because of rapid elimination by the lungs [6]. The injection is frequently given as part of a contrast angiogram; to avoid the effects of contrast on blood flow, a delay of 30–40 min between the injection of contrast agent and Xe is common.

Measurement of regional blood flow using this technique is based on four assumptions. Firstly, instantaneous injection of the tracer into the organ; secondly, instantaneous equilibrium between blood and tissue; thirdly, no recirculation of tracer; and fourthly, an accurate measurement of organ concentration by external monitoring.

Under these conditions, the regional rate of tracer loss at time t, is equal to the regional blood flow times the regional concentration of the tracer in the venous blood, that is

$$\frac{dQ(t)}{dt} = -FC_v(t) \qquad (21.30)$$

where

$Q(t)$ = regional amount of tracer (mCi)

$\dfrac{dQ(t)}{dt}$ = the regional rate of loss of the tracer (mCi s^{-1})

F = regional blood flow (ml s^{-1})

$C_v(t)$ = concentration of tracer within the venous blood (mCi ml^{-1})

Since external monitoring measures organ concentration (assumption 4), not venous concentration, equation (21.30) must be expressed in terms of organ concentrations. Venous blood–organ concentrations are related in the following manner

$$\lambda = \frac{C_o(t)}{C_v(t)} \qquad (21.31)$$

where λ = blood/organ partition coefficient

$C_o(t)$ = organ tracer concentration (mCi mg^{-1})

In addition, the organ tracer concentration equals the quantity of tracer, $Q(t)$, in the organ divided by the organ weight, W; therefore equation (21.30) can be rewritten

$$\frac{dQ(t)}{dt} = -F\frac{Q(t)}{W\lambda} \qquad (21.32)$$

This can be re-expressed in a form analogous to equation (21.6)

$$\ln Q(t) = \frac{-F}{W\lambda}t + \ln Q(0) \qquad (21.33)$$

where $Q(0)$ = initial organ activity (mCi)

A plot of the logarithm of activity against time yields a single straight line with a slope of $-F/W\lambda$. Thus

$$\frac{F}{W} = -\lambda \times \text{slope} \qquad (21.34)$$

Equation (21.34) applies to regional organ flow for organs with homogeneous blood flow. Generally, however, organs are more complex and consist of several types of tissues, each with their own characteristic blood flow. In the brain [7], for example, a plot of activity against time does *not* yield a single straight line. Rather, a biexponential curve results (Figure 21.8). This occurs because of differences in blood flow between grey and white matter. Grey matter has a high blood flow

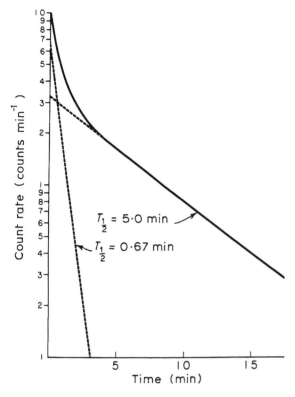

Figure 21.8 Typical brain washout curve after an internal carotid injection of ^{133}Xe. The count rate–time curve representing washout of activity from the brain following an intra-arterial injection of radioactive xenon is plotted on a semi-logarithmic graph. Two components representing blood flow to the white and grey matter are

apparent. The relative blood flow can be determined from the slopes of the two components of the washout curve if the blood/tissue partition coefficients are known. These blood/tissue partition coefficients can be determined experimentally and tables containing their values are available. Blood flow is customarily determined per 100 g of tissue.

Regional blood flow determining (slope method)
$F/W = (-\lambda)$ (Slope)
Grey matter

$$\lambda = 0.77 \frac{\text{ml}}{\text{g grey matter}}$$

$$\text{Slope} = \frac{-0.693}{T_{1/2}} = \frac{0.693}{0.67\,\text{min}} = 1.03\,\text{min}^{-1}$$

$$F/W = 0.77 \frac{\text{ml}}{\text{g grey matter}} \left(1.03\,\text{min}^{-1}\right)$$

$$\left(100\,\text{g grey matter}\right)$$

$$= 79.3\,\text{ml}\,\text{min}^{-1}$$

White matter

$$\lambda = 1.44 \frac{\text{ml}}{\text{g white matter}}$$

$$\text{Slope} = \frac{-0.693}{T_{1/2}} = \frac{0.693}{5.0\,\text{min}} = 0.139\,\text{min}^{-1}$$

$$F/W = 1.44 \frac{\text{ml}}{\text{g white matter}} \left(0.139\,\text{min}^{-1}\right)$$

$$= \left(100\,\text{g grey matter}\right)$$

$$= 20.0\,\text{ml}\,\text{min}^{-1}$$

(78.0–80.5 ml min^{-1} per 100 g tissue) which causes a rapid washout of the tracer. White matter has a lower blood flow (18.7–21.1 ml min^{-1} per 100 g) and hence a slower washout. These two components can be separated mathematically either by simple curve stripping or by a more complicated procedure using a non-linear least squares fit [8].

An alternative mathematical approach to the measurement of regional systemic blood flow using washout has been proposed by Zierler [9]. It is based on the principle that over all time, the change in the amount of tracer, d$Q(t)$, must equal the efferent flow times the efferent concentration, that is

$$\int_0^\infty dQ(t) = -\int_0^\infty FC_v(t)\,dt \qquad (21.35)$$

Equation (21.35) is identical to equation (21.30), except that integration has been performed. Substituting $(1/(\lambda Q)/Q(t)$ for $C_v(t)$ (see equation (21.31)) and rearranging terms, yields

$$\int_0^\infty dQ = \frac{-F}{\lambda W} \int_0^\infty Q(t)\,dt \qquad (21.36)$$

Solving the integration of the left-hand side of equation (21.36) yields

$$Q(0) = \frac{F}{\lambda W} \int_0^\infty Q(t)\,dt \qquad (21.37)$$

Rearrangement yields equation (21.38) which expresses relative flow (F/W) in terms of the measured variables, $Q(0)$ and $\int_0^\infty Q(t)\,dt$

$$\frac{F}{W} = \frac{Q(0)}{\int_0^\infty Q(t)\,dt} = \frac{\lambda H}{A} \qquad (21.38)$$

where

H = height ($Q(0)$) of the washout curve
A = area ($\int Q(t)\mathrm{d}t$) under the washout curve from
    t equals 0 to ∞

The tissue blood coefficient (λ) can be determined experimentally.

The height of the washout curve is proportional to $Q(0)$ and the area under the washout curve is proportional to $\int_0^\infty Q(t)\mathrm{d}t$. Since the same detector geometry is used to measure both, relative flow (F/W) is equal to the blood tissue coefficient (λ) times the height of the washout curve divided by its area. In Figure 21.9 a component of the washout curve from Figure 21.8 ($T_{1/2} = 5.0$ min) has been replotted on a linear graph. The height over

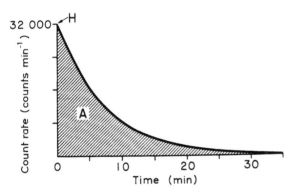

Figure 21.9 Regional blood flow determination (height/area method). The slow component from the biexponential curve obtained in Figure 21.8 is plotted here on linear paper. Note that the same relative flow which was obtained using the slope method in Figure 21.8 is obtained using the height over area method. Regional blood flow determination (height/area method)

$$F/W = (\lambda)\frac{H}{A}$$

$$\lambda = 1.44\frac{\text{ml}}{\text{g white matter}}$$

$$H = 32\,000\,\text{counts min}^{-1}$$

$$A = 229\,200\,\text{counts}$$

$$F/W = \left(1.44\frac{\text{ml}}{\text{g white matter}}\right)$$

$$\left(\frac{32\,000\,\text{counts min}^{-1}}{229\,000\,\text{counts}}\right)(100\,\text{g white matter})$$

$$= 20.0\,\text{ml min}^{-1}$$

area method yields the same relative flow as was obtained using the slope method.

CARDIAC OUTPUT

During the past several years, cardiovascular nuclear medicine has grown dramatically. An important index of cardiac function, cardiac output, can be obtained non-invasively in conjunction with a first-pass radionuclide angiocardiogram performed alone or performed prior to grated equilibrium cardiovascular studies. In fact, if cardiac output, ejection fraction, mean transit time (see the next section) and total blood volume are known, all of the cardiac indices listed in Table 21.1 can be determined non-invasively.

Two problems need to be solved, however, before the simultaneous radionuclide measurement of cardiac output and ejection fraction is widespread. Firstly, a ^{99m}Tc-labelled radiopharmaceutical which can be used for both of these measurements is needed. In-vitro labelled red cells prepared with the Brookhaven kit currently come closest to meeting this need. Secondly, externally monitored activity-time curves must accurately reflect intravascular concentration-time curves. Problems related to detector geometry and deadtime at high count rates with an Anger camera need to be resolved.

Cardiac output determinations are based on the principle of conservation of mass [10,11,12,13]. If a non-diffusible, non-metabolizable tracer is used, the amount of tracer entering the heart must equal the amount of tracer leaving the heart. The amount of tracer entering the heart is equal to the total amount of the tracer injected. The amount of tracer leaving the heart region of interest in any small time interval is equal to the concentration of the tracer at that time times the cardiac output

Table 21.1

Measured
  Cardiac Output
  Ejection Fraction
  Mean Pulmonary Transit Time
  Total Blood Volume
Derived
  End Diastolic Volume
  End Systolic Volume
  Pulmonary Blood Volume

times the time interval. The *total* amount leaving the heart is equal to the sum of all the amounts that left during all of the small time intervals. Mathematically

$$Q = \Sigma FkC(t)\Delta T \qquad (21.39)$$

where

Q = the total amount of tracer injected (mCi)
F = cardiac output (ml min^{-1})
k = proportionality constant to convert counts min^{-1} to mCi ml^{-1}

$$\left(\frac{mCi}{ml} \Big/ \frac{counts}{min} \right)$$

$C(t)$ = externally monitored count rate of the tracer leaving heart region of interest at time t (counts min^{-1})
Δt = small time interval (min)

As Δt approaches 0, equation (21.39) can be integrated

$$Q = Fk \int_0^\infty C(t) dt \qquad (21.40)$$

Estimation of cardiac output requires knowledge of the proportionality constant k. This is difficult to measure since it changes with each patient and with each detector. However, if equilibrium measurements are made using the same detector geometry used to measure concentration changes, then the following relationship exists.

$$Q = kC_{eq}V \qquad (21.41)$$

where

C_{eq} = count rate at equilibrium in the heart region of interest (counts min^{-1})
V = total blood volume (ml).

Substituting equation (21.41) into (21.40), simplifying and rearranging leads to the elimination of k in the final expression. Thus

$$F = \frac{C_{eq}V}{\int_0^\infty C(t) dt} \qquad (21.42)$$

The total blood volume can be determined by simple dilution principles if the red cells have been labelled *in vitro* with high efficiency.

The use of equation (21.42) in measured cardiac output is described in Figure 21.10. In this example 15 mCi of Tc-labelled red cells were injected (Q). A blood sample obtained at equilibrium con-

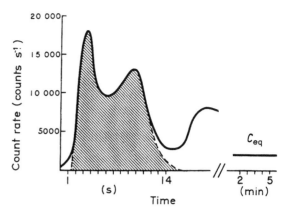

Figure 21.10 Cardiac output determination. The count rate–time curve from a region of interest of the heart is plotted. The crosshatched area under the curve is a graphic representation of the area under the curve when the upslope and downslope have been extrapolated to zero. The total blood volume (V) is calculated from simple dilution principles. Since the injected dose (Q) contains several thousand times the amount of activity as the equilibrium sample (E), an aliquot of the injected dose is usually carefully diluted one thousand-fold to assure a linear response of the well counter. Once total blood volume is known, cardiac output can be determined by measuring the count rate at equilibrium (C_{eq}) and the area under the count rate–time curve. In order to eliminate the effects of background and recirculation the count rate–time curve must be extrapolated to zero.

Cardiac output determination

$$F = \frac{(C_{eq})(V)}{\int_0^\infty C(t) dt}$$

$$V = \frac{Q}{E} = \frac{15\,mCi}{3\,\mu Ci\,ml^{-1}} = 5000\,ml$$

$$C_{eq} = (2000\,counts\,s^{-1})(60\,s\,min^{-1})$$
$$= 120\,000\,counts\,min^{-1}$$

$$\int_0^\infty C(t) dt = 130\,000\,counts$$

$$F = \frac{(120\,000\,counts\,min^{-1})(5000\,ml)}{(130\,000\,counts)}$$

$$= 4615\,ml\,min^{-1}$$

tained $3\,\mu Ci\,ml^{-1}$; therefore, the total blood volume (V) was 5000 cm^3. To calculate cardiac output the equilibrium concentration, C_{eq}, and the area under the activity-time curve are needed. The curve has two peaks representing the passage of the bolus through the right and left side of the heart (see Figure 21.10). When corrections for background and recirculation were made by extrapolating to zero, the area was found to be 130 000 counts-s. The count rate at equilibrium, C_{eq}, was determined several minutes after the injection of the tracer using the same region of interest and without moving the patient. In performing this technique, it is important to note that the gamma camera must have a linear response over a several-fold range in count rates (that is, 2000–18 000 counts s^{-1}) if accurate results are to be obtained. Excessive deadtime will result in underestimation of the denominator of equation (21.42) and therefore will overestimate cardiac output.

TRANSIT TIMES

The current popularity of first-pass radionuclide angiocardiography has stimulated interest in transit times because they can be used to estimate pulmonary blood volume. The calculation of transit times can be understood if the flow of a non-diffusible radioactive marker travelling with a velocity, v, through a pipe of length, L, and an area, A, is considered (Figure 21.11) [14]. If the quantity of nuclide appearing at the exit is monitored as a function of time, no activity is registered at the exit while the marker is in the pipe; once the tracer leaves the pipe, counts are registered. The time to transverse the system from entrance to exit is the transit time (Figure 21.11c).

Because flow, F, can be related to velocity by

$$F = vA \qquad (21.43)$$

where

F = flow of the tracer (ml s^{-1})
v = velocity of flow (cm s^{-1})
A = cross-sectional area of the pipe (cm^2)

and because

$$v = L/t \qquad (21.44)$$

where

L = length of the pipe (cm)
t = transit time (s)

$$F = \frac{LA}{t} = \frac{V}{t} \qquad (21.45)$$

where

V = volume (ml)

and, on rearranging,

$$t = \frac{V}{F} \qquad (21.46)$$

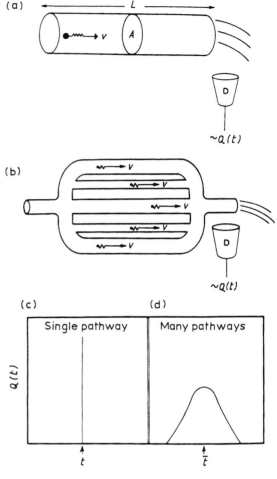

Figure 21.11 Transit time. Transit of tracer through a single pathway (a) yields a single transit time, t (c). Transit of tracer through many pathways (b) yields a mean transit time, t (d). (Reprinted with permission from *Diagnostic Nuclear Medicine* edited by Alexander Gottschalk and E. J. Potchen, MD, Williams and Wilkins Company, Baltimore.)

The transit time, t, then equals the volume of the pipe divided by its flow. This generality applies to all intravascular (non-diffusible) indicators.

For real systems the situation is more complex because several paths through the conduit are possible (Figure 21.11b). In such cases, a distribution of counts against time is expected at the exit (Figure 21.11d); those tracer molecules appearing at earlier times will have traversed a shorter total path length than those appearing at later times. Thus, there is no single transit time but rather many transit times with a mean transit time, $\bar{t}$. located at the centre of gravity of the activity-time plot. Mean transit time is equal to the integral of the activity at time t times the time divided by the integral of the activity-time curve

$$\bar{t} = \frac{\int_0^\infty Q(t)t\,dt}{\int_0^\infty Q(t)\,dt} \qquad (21.47)$$

where

$\bar{t}$ = mean transit time
$Q(t)$ = activity at time t (mCi)
t = time from the initial input of activity (s)

Equation (21.47) is called the first moment of the activity-time curve.

An example of the calculation of mean pulmonary transit time is shown in Figure 21.12. A time activity plot from a region of interest over the lungs is obtained. The upslope and downslope of the pulmonary curve must be extrapolated to zero activity to eliminate the effects of background and recirculation and, thus, obtain a finite value from the integral of the curve. Typically, the extrapolation of the upstroke is linear, whereas the extrapolation of the downslope is mono-exponential. Once this extrapolation has been performed, mean transit time can be calculated using equation 21.47.

Furthermore, as implied in equation (21.46), pulmonary blood volume can be calculated if pulmonary flood flow and mean transit time are known. Mathematically, pulmonary blood volume equals pulmonary blood flow times mean pulmonary transit time. In patients without shunts, pulmonary blood flow equals cardiac output; therefore

$$V_P = Ft_P \qquad (21.48)$$

where

V_P = pulmonary blood volume (ml)
F = cardiac output (ml s^{-1})
$\bar{t}_P$ = mean pulmonary transit time (min)

Since cardiac output and mean pulmonary transit time can be calculated using first-pass radionuclide angiocardiography, an estimate of pulmonary blood volume, which may be useful in evaluation of left ventricular failure, can also be obtained.

An alternative approach to the measurement of

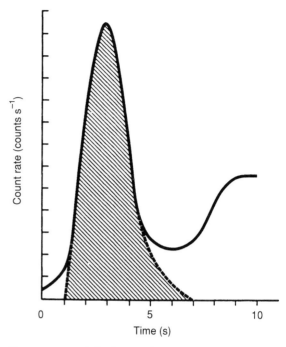

Figure 21.12 Calculation of mean pulmonary transit time. A count rate–time curve is obtained over the lungs after a bolus injection of radiotracer. The activity–time curve is extrapolated to zero to eliminate the effects of background and recirculation (dashed curve). The cross-hatched area graphically represents the integral of the extrapolated count rate-time curve. The integrals in equation (21.47) are calculated from this extrapolated curve and are used to determine mean pulmonary transit time.

Mean pulmonary transit time determination

$$\text{MPTT} = \frac{\int_0^\infty Q(t)t\,dt}{\int_0^\infty Q(t)\,dt}$$

$$\int_0^\infty Q(t)t\,dt = 180\,000 \text{ counts s}^{-1}$$

$$\int_0^\infty Q(t)\,dt = 30\,000 \text{ counts}$$

$$t = \frac{180\,000 \text{ counts s}^{-1}}{30\,000 \text{ counts}} = 6\,\text{s}$$

mean transit time has been proposed, analogous to that described in the measurement of regional blood flow [9]. It states that

$$\bar{t} = \frac{A}{\lambda\sigma H} \qquad (21.49)$$

where

A = area under the washout curve
H = initial height of washout curve
λ = the blood/tissue partition coefficient
σ = tissue density, which for most tissues is
  approximately 1. Therefore, equation (21.49)
  can be simplified to

$$\bar{t} = \frac{A}{\lambda H} \qquad (21.50)$$

The concept of transit time has been confused because two other indices which can easily be calculated have been popularized. In addition to mean transit time, peak-to-peak transit time and mean pool transit time are routinely calculated by one major manufacturer's software for first-pass radionuclide angiocardiograms. Although these two indices are *proportional* to mean pulmonary transit time, the proportionality constant is unknown; therefore, the desired measurement of pulmonary blood volume cannot be made.

Measurement of peak-to-peak transit time is illustrated in Figure 21.13. For this purpose, activity–time curves from right and left ventricular regions of interest are superimposed. The peak-to-peak transit time is equal to the difference in the times that peak activity is in the right and left ventricles.

Calculation of the mean pool transit time is slightly more complex than calculation of peak-to-peak transit time. This index measures the differ-

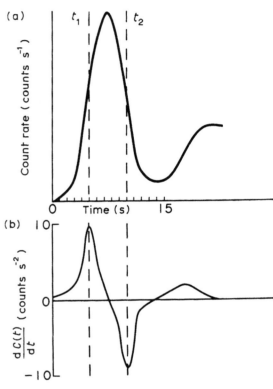

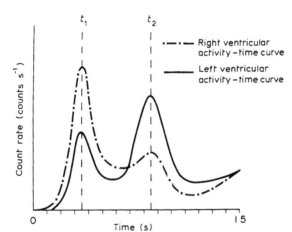

Figure 21.13 Peak-to-peak transit time (T). The dashed curve represents activity–time curve from a region of interest over the right heart. The solid curve represents an activity-time curve from a region of interest over the left heart. The peak to peak transit time is calculated by subtracting the time that peak activity occurs in the right ventricle (t_1) from the time that peak activity occurs in the left ventricle (t_2). These times are determined from right (– · – ·) and left (—) ventricular activity-time curves following a bolus injection of a radiotracer.

Peak to peak transit time determination

$$T = t_2 - t_1 = 8.5\,\text{s} - 3.5\,\text{s} = 5.0\,\text{s}$$

Figure 21.14 Mean pulmonary pool transit time. Curve (a) represents an activity–time curve from a region of interest over the lungs. Curve (b) represents the first derivative of curve (a). Mean pulmonary transit time equals the difference between the time when the maximum activity enters (t_1) and leaves the lung. Since the first derivative (curve b) corresponds to the instantaneous slope of the pulmonary activity–time curve (curve a), the times of maximum upslope and down-slope can be easily calculated from the peaks and valleys of the first derivative.

Mean pulmonary pool transit time determination

$$T = t_2 - t_1$$
$$T = 10\,\text{s} - 5\,\text{s} = 5\,\text{s}$$

ence between the time when the maximum activity enters and the time when it leaves the region. The upper curve in Figure 21.14 is the pulmonary activity–time curve; the lower curve is the first derivative of the upper curve. The pool transit time is equal to the difference between the time of maximum upslope and maximum down-slope. Since the first derivative (the lower curve) corresponds to the instantaneous slope of the upper curve, the times of maximum upslope and maximum downslope of the upper curve can easily be calculated from the peaks and valleys of the lower curve.

CONVOLUTION AND DECONVOLUTION

Although convolution and deconvolution analysis has been widely applied in many quantitative fields, these techniques have only recently been utilized in the analysis of cardiac [15] and renal radiotracer studies [16,17]. In all dynamic studies,

observed organ activity–time curves depend not only on the organ function (the organ response) but also on the manner in which the tracer arrives in the organ (the input function). Deconvolution analysis eliminates the effects of the input function and, therefore, allows more accurate investigation of organ response.

To understand this analysis, let us first look at the interaction of a hypothetical input function and organ response function (see Figure 21.15). Assume that the input to the organ is instantaneous and that the area under the input function is equal to 1.0. This theoretical input function is called a delta or spike function. Let us further assume that the organ of interest instantaneously extracts 50 per cent of the injected tracer, that the minimum time it takes for the tracer to pass through the organ is 10s, and that the elimination of the tracer from the organ is linear. With an instantaneous input, the output function is equal to the organ response. Generally, instantaneous

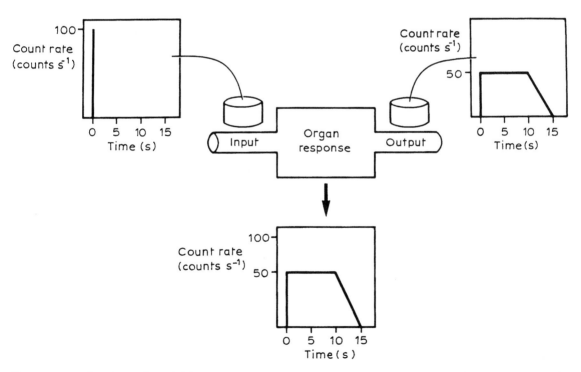

Figure 21.15 The relationship of the input function, organ response and output function. If the input function (the bolus injection) illustrated in the upper left and the output fraction (the activity–time curve for the organ of interest), illustrated in the upper right, are externally monitored, the organ response (below) can be calculated. In the example shown here, the output function is identical to the organ response since the input function is instantaneous (spike or delta function).

input functions do not exist; therefore, in practice, the output function never equals the organ response.

A continuous input function can be approximated by multiple instantaneous input functions. In Figure 21.16a, five instantaneous input functions, 10s apart, have been used to approximate a continuous input function (dashed curve). The organ response from each of these five instantaneous inputs is shown in Figure 21.16b. Under these conditions the output function equals the *sum* of the organ responses to multiple instantaneous inputs.

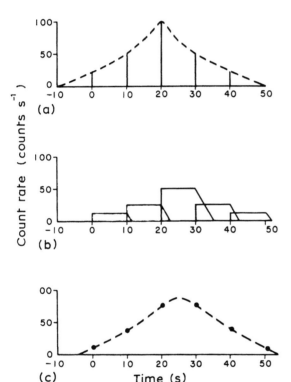

(a)

(b)

(c)

Time (s)

Figure 21.16 Effects of a continuous input function on the output function. (a) The count rate–time curve of a continuous input function is illustrated. A continuous input function can be treated mathematically as an infinite series of instantaneous input functions. For simplicity only five of the instantaneous input functions used to approximate the continuous input function are shown. (b) The instantaneous organ response to the five instantaneous input is illustrated. (c) The externally monitored output function equals the sum of the organ responses illustrated in (b). The shape of output function can be more profoundly affected by the input function than by the organ response.

The sum of the organ responses in Figure 21.16b at six different times is indicated in Figure 21.16c. This process of summing the organ response and input product is called *convolution*. A dashed line connecting the points in Figure 21.16c reveals that the shape of the output function can be affected much more by the input function than by the organ response.

Mathematically, a continuous input function can be treated as an infinite number of instantaneous inputs; therefore any input function can be convoluted with any organ response to yield an output function. Likewise any output function can be deconvoluted so that the organ response is identified if the input function is known. The actual mathematics of the convolution and deconvolution processes are beyond the scope of this text. The formal mathematical statement of the convolution process is as follows

$$C(t) = \int_0^{\infty} I(T)H(t-T)\,dT \qquad (21.51)$$

where $C(t)$ = output function
   $I(T)$ = input function
   $H(T)$ = system (organ) response

These calculations are performed relatively easily on computers by using fast Fourier transforms which change the complex process of convolution/deconvolution to multiplication and division, respectively.

An obvious but sometimes overlooked limitation of deconvolution analysis is that this technique is valid only if the input and output functions are accurately known. If the externally monitored activity–time curves from regions of interest are inaccurate due to poor statistics or due to contamination by activity from surrounding structures, then the deconvolution will be meaningless. Since bolus injections are generally used, determination of the input function can be particularly difficult. Monitoring activity from a region of interest over the heart would give the best counting statistics but would not accurately reflect the input function of an organ which is some distance from the heart. By the time the bolus reached the organ it would have spread out. The time delay from the heart to the organ would also be unknown. Because of these problems, the input function is measured as close to the organ of interest as possible. For renal studies, a region of interest over the abdominal aorta is used to determine the input function. This approach introduces uncertainties because the counting statistics are poor, background activity is high and small changes in position will cause great changes in the detected activity. Since the deconvolution analysis is very sensitive to aberrations in the input function, some

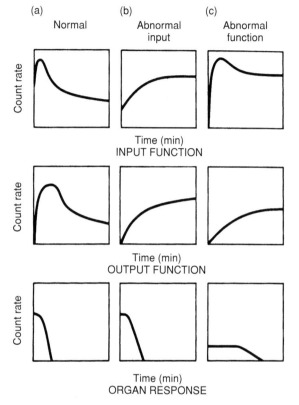

Figure 21.17 Usefulness of deconvolution analysis of renograms. The count rate–time curves for the input function, the output function and the organ response are illustrated for a normal renogram, an abnormal renogram due to an abnormal input function, and an abnormal renogram on all graphs. Column (a), normal input function, normal output function (renogram), normal organ response. Column (b), abnormal input function due to the subcutaneous injection of the radiopharmaceutical. Abnormal output function (renogram) due to the abnormal input function. Normal organ response after deconvolution. Column (c), abnormal input function revealing delayed blood clearance due to poor renal function. Abnormal output function (renogram) due to abnormal organ response and the resulting abnormal input function. Organ response is clearly abnormal after deconvolution indicating the abnormal output function was not due soley to an abnormal input function.

processing of the raw data to remove some of these aberrations is often needed before the deconvolution can be performed [18].

Examples of the clinical usefulness of deconvolution analysis of renograms is shown in Figure 21.17. A normal input function, renogram and deconvoluted renogram are shown in (a), an abnormal input function (due to a subcutaneous injection), the resulting abnormal renogram and the deconvoluted renogram are shown in (b), and an abnormal input function (due to poor renal function), and abnormal renogram and the deconvoluted renogram are shown in (c). Since the height of the deconvoluted renogram is proportional to renal function, and since the transit time increases with decreased renal function, the deconvoluted renogram can be used to differentiate between normal and abnormal renal function independent of the input function. Note that not only does an abnormal input function cause an abnormal renogram (b) but also that abnormal renal function causes an abnormal input function (c) because of slower blood clearance.

REFERENCES

1. Rudd, T.G., Shurtleff, D.B., Loeser, J.D. and Nelp, W.B. (1973) Radionuclide assessment of cerebrospinal fluid shunt flow in children. *J. nucl. Med.*, **14**, 683–6.
2. Harbert, J., Haddard, D. and McCullough, D. (1974) Quantitation of cerebrospinal fluid shunt flow. *Radiology*, **112**, 379–87.
3. Sapirstein, L.A., Vidt, D.G., Mandel, M.J. and Hanusek, G. (1955) Volumes of distribution and clearances of intravenously injected creatinine in the dog. *Am. J. Physiol.*, **181**, 330–6.
4. Bianchi, C. (1972) *Radionuclides in Renal Evaluation*, Vol. 2, Basel and University Park Press, Baltimore, pp. 21–53.
5. Morgan, W.D., Birks, J.L. and Singer, A. (1977) An efficient technique for the simultaneous estimation of GFR and ERPF, involving a single injection and two blood samples. *Int. J. Nucl. Med. Biol.*, **4**, 79–83.
6. Kety, S.S. (1951) The theory and applications of the exchange of inert gas at the lungs and tissues. *Pharmac. Rev.*, **3**, 1–47.
7. Hoedt-Rasmussen, K., Aveisdotter, E. and Lasser, N. (1966) Regional cerebral blood flow in man determined by intra-arterial injection of inert gas. *Circ. Res.*, **18**, 237–47.
8. Dell, R.B., Sciacca, R., Lieberman, K., Case, D. and Cannon, P.J. (1973) A weighted least-squares technique for the analysis of kinetic data and its application in the study of renal 133 Xenon washout in dogs and man. *Circ. Res.*, **32**, 71–84.

9. Zierler, K.L. (1965) Equations for measuring blood flow by external monitoring of radioisotopes. *Circ. Res.*, **16**, 309–21.

10. Donato, L., Guintini, C., Lewis, M.L., Durand, J., Rochester, D.F., Harvey, R.M. and Cournand, A. (1962a) Quantitative radiocardiography – I theoretical considerations. *Circulation*, **26**, 174–82.

11. Donato, L., Rochester, D.F., Lewis, M.D., Durand, J., Parker, J.O. and Harvey, R.M. (1962b) Quantitative Radiocardiography – II technical analysis of curves. *Circulation*, **26**, 183–8.

12. Lewis, M.L., Guintini, G., Donato, L., Harvey, R.M. and Cournand, A. (1962) Quantitative radiocardiography – III results and validation of theory and method. *Circulation*, **26**, 189–99.

13. Kuikka, J., Timisjarvi, J. and Tuominen, M. (1979) Quantitative radiocardiographic evaluation of cardiac dynamics in man at rest and during exercise. *Scand. J. Clin. Lab. Invest.*, **39**, 423–34.

14. McNeil, B.J., Holman, B.L. and Adelstein, S.J. (1976). In *Theoretical Basis for Blood Flow Measurement in Diagnostic Nuclear Medicine* (eds A. Gottschalk and J. Potchen), Williams and Wilkins, Baltimore, ch. 13.

15. Alderson, P.O., Douglass, K.H., Mendenhall, K.G., Guadini, V.A., Watson, D.C., Links, J.M. and Wagner, H.N. (1979) Deconvolution analysis in radionuclide quantitation of left and right cardiac shunts. *J. Nucl. Med.*, **20**, 502.

16. Kenny, R.W., Ackery, D.M., Fleming, J.S., Goddard, B.A. and Grant, R.W. (1975) Deconvolution analysis of the scintillation camera renogram. *Br. J. Radiol.*, **48**, 481–6.

17. Diffey, B.L., Hall, F.M. and Corfield, J.R. (1976) The ^{99m}Tc-DTPA dynamic renal scan with deconvolution analysis. *J. Nucl. Med.*, **17**, 352–5.

18. Fleming, J.S. and Kenny, R.W. (1977) A comparison of techniques for filtering noise in the renogram. *Phys. Med. Biol.*, **22**, 359–64.

Index

Numbers in **bold** refer to figures, numbers in *italics* refer to tables